Pain and Chemical Dependency

Pain and Chemical Dependency

EDITED BY

HOWARD S. SMITH
STEVEN D. PASSIK

OXFORD
UNIVERSITY PRESS

2008

OXFORD
UNIVERSITY PRESS

Oxford University Press, Inc., publishes works that further
Oxford University's objective of excellence
in research, scholarship, and education.

Oxford   New York
Auckland   Cape Town   Dar es Salaam   Hong Kong   Karachi
Kuala Lumpur   Madrid   Melbourne   Mexico City   Nairobi
New Delhi   Shanghai   Taipei   Toronto

With offices in
Argentina   Austria   Brazil   Chile   Czech Republic   France   Greece
Guatemala   Hungary   Italy   Japan   Poland   Portugal   Singapore
South Korea   Switzerland   Thailand   Turkey   Ukraine   Vietnam

Copyright © 2008 by Oxford University Press, Inc.

Published by Oxford University Press, Inc.
198 Madison Avenue, New York, New York 10016

www.oup.com

Oxford is a registered trademark of Oxford University Press

All rights reserved. No part of this publication may be reproduced,
stored in a retrieval system, or transmitted, in any form or by any means,
electronic, mechanical, photocopying, recording, or otherwise,
without the prior permission of Oxford University Press.

Library of Congress Cataloging-in-Publication Data
Pain and chemical dependency / edited by Howard S. Smith, Steven D. Passik.
    p. ; cm.
Includes bibliographical references.
ISBN 978-0-19-530055-0
1. Opioid abuse—Treatment.   2. Opioids—Therapeutic use—Complications.
3. Chronic pain—Chemotherapy—Complications.   4. Opioids—Side effects.
I. Smith, Howard S., 1956–   II. Passik, Steven D.
[DNLM: 1. Substance-Related Disorders—therapy.   2. Analgesics—adverse effects.
3. Analgesics—therapeutic use.   4. Chronic Disease.   5. Pain—therapy.
6. Substance-Related Disorders—etiology.   WM 270 P144 2007]
RC568.O45P35 2007
615'.7822—dc22
                    2007009232

9 8 7 6 5 4 3 2 1

Printed in the United States of America
on acid-free paper

I dedicate this book in loving memory to my mother, Arlene Smith, and to my wife, Joan, and children, Alyssa, Joshua, Benjamin, and Eric, as well as my father, Nathan, and stepmother, Priscilla.

—HSS

I dedicate this book to my mentors in studies of the pain management and addiction interface: to Dr. Russell K. Portenoy, to Dr. Kathleen Foley, to Dr. William Breitbart, and to the memory of Dr. Raymond Houde. All four were incredible mentors in learning about pain, all encouraged me to find the interface of pain research and addiction research, and all recognized the need for academic work that bridged the two fields. Without their attention, nurturance, and support, my contributions to this work would never have been possible and the doors to this interesting field would have remained closed.

—SDP

Foreword

A principal role for health-care providers is the relief of pain and suffering. This is a noble aim, but even today, the treatment of pain is surrounded in controversy. Many issues within the discipline of pain medicine can arouse debate; few arouse such passions as the prescribing of opioid or narcotic drugs. To the phenomenon of fear in the use of such medications the term *opiophobia* is applied. It is present throughout the world.

Many techniques are employed for the relief of pain, and one of the most common is treatment with narcotic medications. The first of these, opium (or morphine), has been in use for many thousands of years. In the early part of last century opium was given the designation Laudanum—a praiseworthy drug that was regarded highly and readily used by the citizens of the time. By the end of the century, medicine's awareness of the phenomenon of drug addiction attracted much scrutiny and led to widespread attitude changes to these medications. Within public and professional minds, they became objects of concern or even denigration. In more recent times, very satisfactory formulations have become available that can be administered safely and effectively to a wide variety of pain patients.

Recent government policies restricting access to such chemicals has exacerbated opiophobia and has had a detrimental effect on notions of suitability of their use for the relief of pain. In the majority of countries, both industrialized and preindustrial, significant undertreatment of pain is one outcome of this fear. The worldwide scourge of "drug addiction" has complicated the matter further, and many governments have developed restrictive legislation in their endeavors to contain or prevent its occurrence. People are often well-versed in the potential harm of nonprescription drug use, and knowingly choose to engage in high-risk behaviors despite the harm these chemicals may cause. It is generally recognized that these substances have been obtained illegally for personal use. However, nonprescribed drug use often results in harm to the users, to one's significant others, and to the broader society. Governments, properly, have attempted to reduce the availability of illicit drugs, but the tightening of regulations inevitably brings in its wake heightened difficulties in accessing narcotics for the treatment of pain patients, and thus has exacerbated the undertreatment of pain.

One outcome for physicians of this developing perception that narcotic medications are "bad" or "evil" further reinforces reluctance to prescribe opioid medications even within clinical situations that make such prescriptions appropriate. Patients, too, though faced with significant pain, worry unduly and perceive that opioid treatment may lead to addiction and thus may be reluctant to use opioids. Patients may well need considerable encouragement to consider opioid use.

More recently, this undertreatment of pain has been recognized in a number of clinical settings and in particular in New York City. Research has shown that a significant number of people on methadone programs have reported that their reason for turning to methadone (by stating the untruth that they were heroin users) or nonprescribed medication, including heroin use, was motivated by their desire to relieve chronic nonmalignant pain untouched, or inadequately managed, by treatment from more regular treatment methods.

Recognition of this trend led to the convening of a series of international conferences on pain and chemical dependency, mostly in New York City. In turn, this has prompted a wider understanding of the problem and highlighted the usefulness of a new category of health practitioner able to treat both pain and chemical dependency. Furthermore, there is now an understanding within many health organizations that it is not possible to effectively and safely treat pain with narcotic medications without an understanding of addiction medicine. It is clearly important for persons who have pain to be treated properly, including those persons labeled "drug addicts." People in this latter group have as much right to pain relief as other citizens, but very frequently they are denied such assistance. They may, however, require close support and monitoring to ensure appropriate and safe medication use.

As a consequence of this new understanding of patient reliance on less orthodox chronic pain self-care strategies, an appreciation that conceptualizing opioid use would benefit from a better understanding of the role of opioid medications and their function in modern society has evolved. Clearly, on the one hand, these drugs bring comfort and quality of life to millions of people around the world who have pain, whether acute or chronic, malignant or nonmalignant, whereas on the other, these medications are also capable of being misused, with resultant harm to people and the societies in which they live. One challenge for health professionals who care for people who suffer chronic pain is to manage this tension and the balance between the two conflicting value systems. There is now concern amongst health professionals to find ways to ensure worldwide access to pain-relieving medication at affordable prices, a major issue for most countries and particularly preindustrial societies. This problematic issue is in urgent need of study if satisfactory solutions are to be found.

The editors and authors of this book have compiled a treatise summarizing many aspects in the management of pain and with a clearer understanding of chemical dependency. Editors and contributors to this publication are to be congratulated. This text maps the twin issues of pain and drug dependency in the attainment of compassionate pain relief. The book is perhaps best read as complementary to the more numerous general publications on pain management techniques. However, the book offers authoritative collective and distinctive voice on a developing perspective within the field of pain management.

Publication of this book should do much to encourage safe prescribing of narcotic medications, and begin to address the problem of undertreatment of pain. In addition, it will do a great deal to encourage practitioners from many professional spheres to join the emerging discipline of pain management, with rational debate about the use of opiate medications.

Ian Buttfield
Chairman, International Association of Pain
and Chemical Dependency

Preface

Comments by Steven D. Passik

The fields of pain management and chemical dependency have always needed unification. Emblematic of the progress being made to bring about a bridge between experts in the field is the creation of this volume. With the formation of the International Association for Pain and Chemical Dependency and their seventh scientific meeting, the timing seemed right to bring together current knowledge for scientists, clinicians, and educators.

When Portenoy and Foley first urged the pain field to take a new look at opioids in noncancer pain, they were not simply advocating for an "opening of the flood gates" with regard to prescribing and clinical practice. Instead, they put forth the observation that if tertiary care–based cancer patients can enjoy favorable outcomes on opioids with regard to meaningful analgesia, improvements in psychosocial function, manageable side effects, and the absence of addiction, then it stood to reason that a subset of the vast and heterogeneous population of people with noncancer pain could also potentially derive such benefits. Important in their writings, and often missed during the time period in the United States when clinical practice jumped forward with regard to opioid prescribing, was their call for a medical, scientific, and health-care based discussion of this issue, as opposed to the more traditionally legal and ethical debates that had dominated to that point.

The need then, as it is now, was to replace rhetoric and opinion with science, knowledge, and reason. But in an aging society with a growing problem of chronic pain, an abysmal track record of undertreatment, and, as Bonica called it, "therapeutic nihilism," the clinical practice took off faster than clinical trials data could accrue. Rhetoric was used in place of science and in their zeal to do good, the pain management community seemed to forget that all pain management goes on against a backdrop of our substance abusing society (which goes, as we know, far beyond opioids, to nicotine, cannabis, alcohol, and other licit and illicit drugs). The result was a perfect storm of rhetoric, increased prescribing, the availability of new opioids and other agents, and the failure to teach about addiction. In the end, we now have the concomitant and growing problem of prescription drug abuse.

The need for bridging pain and chemical dependency includes the empirical, clinical, and didactic domains. To move the science forward, we need dialogue. The endocrinologic effects of opioids, for example, only recently appreciated in the pain management field, were known to researchers in chemical dependency decades ago. For the good of our patients and their communities, all prescribers of controlled substances need to be, as Doug Gourlay puts it, "talented amateurs" in addiction medicine. Educationally, physicians, nurses, psychologists, and others frequently report that their training included little formal teaching about pain. Teaching about addiction lags behind even further. And training on the pain addiction interface is almost nonexistent. It is our hope that this volume can serve as a jump-off point to scientists, clinicians, and educators.

Comments by Howard S. Smith

Furthermore, it is hoped that this text may foster "cross-pollination" of ideas between pain medicine specialists and addiction medicine specialists.

The areas in the brain classically associated with reward from the administration of opioids (working as agonists at the mu opioid receptor; or other drugs/activities of abuse) include the following: anterior bed nuclei/medial forebrain bundle, ventral tegmental area, nucleus accumbens (NAc), olfactory tubercle, ventral pallidum, and medial prefrontal cortex, as well as associated communications (e.g., amygdala, hippocampus). The predominant sites in the brain where opioids are thought to produce analgesia are predominantly in the periventricular-periaqueductal gray regions and include the following: periaqueductal gray (PAG) area of the brain stem, some intralaminar and midline thalamic nuclei, and some lateral reticular nuclei (Pert, 1974). Finally, the two major brain sites associated with physical dependence from microinjection of opioids into the brain are predominantly in the periventricular gray substance and include (1) a region around the PAG and (2) an area close to the mesencephalic isthmus, which encompasses part of the locus ceruleus (Bozarth & Wise, 1984).

Although these areas appear distinct, there also exists significant overlap between pain, pain relievers (e.g., opioids), and addiction in both the clinical and basic science arenas. In humans, central nervous system pathways/circuitry involved in pain and addiction may share a number of common areas. Regions such as the nucleus accumbens, the amygdala, the anterior cingulate cortex, and the hypothalamus are all involved in both pain processing and opioid addiction (Becerra et al., 2001; Sell et al., 1999). Natural rewards (e.g., food/water, sex) as well as "unnatural rewards" (drugs of abuse [e.g., opioids], alcohol, and compulsive activities [e.g., gambling]) lead to increases in extracellular dopamine release from mesocorticolimbic neurons with resultant activation of the "reward circuitry."

Pain appears to reduce addiction liability. Geha et al. (2007) identified brain regions involved in the spontaneous pain of postherpetic neuralgia (PHN), which maps to sensory (thalamus, SI, SII, insula), affective (anterior cingulated cortex, insula), as well as hedonic (ventral striatum, amygdala, ventral tegmentum, and orbital frontal cortex) regions. The short-term responses to topical lidocaine patch therapy were seen predominantly in sensory and affective regions, whereas longer term responses revealed a shift in the brain pain-related circuitry, away from sensory-representational cortical areas, to hedonic-reward subcortical areas, potentially suggesting the evolution of a more "subconscious" condition that may impact motivational drives (Geha et al., 2007).

Pain is an aversive stimulus, and analgesia seems to act as a rewarding stimulus (Franklin, 1989; Seymour et al., 2005). Furthermore, it appears that the reward circuitry may be modulated (albeit perhaps in a different fashion) by noxious stimuli (Becerra et al., 2001), supporting the notion of a shared neural system for processing of aversive and rewarding stimuli (Becerra et al., 2001). This "shared" system has been referred to as the reward-aversion circuitry (RAC; Borsook et al., 2007).

Mediators and signaling of pain and chemical dependency may overlap as well. Zachariou and colleagues (2006) proposed that ΔFosB in the NAc is an essential modulator of the behavioral effects of opioids and that this may contribute to addiction. Zachariou et al. (2006) suggest that enhanced opioid reward may be at least partially explained by opioids leading to overexpression of ΔFosB in the nucleus accumbens and dorsal striatum, which may then mediate features of diminished opioid analgesia and enhanced opioid rewards partly via repression of dynorphin expression. Dynorphin expression (likely via activation of the bradykinin 2 receptor) may contribute to the maintenance of neuropathic pain (Lai et al., 2006).

This textbook explores both the commonalities and differences between pain and chemical dependency issues in basic and clinical science realms. Part I introduces and lays the history and groundwork of pain and chemical dependency. A historical account of the use of opioids for chronic pain is presented. Part II covers a vast spectrum of both basic science and clinical issues relating to chemical dependency and addiction. Some sections of Part II touch on the predisposition or vulnerability for addiction. Although genetics is a strong factor in vulnerability to addiction, the mechanisms that predispose people to becoming addicted remain uncertain; however, even small structural proteins involved in signaling processes could play a role.

It is conceivable that mutations of various cytoskeletal proteins may regulate synaptic transmission and affect neuromodulatory signal transduction in the reward circuitry. Spinophilin (Allen et al., 2006; Satoh et al., 1998) and neurabin (neural tissue-specific F-actin-binding protein; Nakanishi et al., 1997), which bind to protein phosphatase 1 (PP1; a serine/threonine phosphatase that may dephosphorylate and inactivate glutamate receptors), are structurally distinct cytoskeletal proteins closely associated with the postsynaptic density (PSD) proteins (PSDs appear to modify N-methyl-d-aspartate receptor [NMDAR] complex trafficking at synaptic sites; Muly et al., 2004a, 2004b). Without proper function and interaction of PP1 and scaffolding proteins, PP1 may lose modulatory capabilities over glutamatergic responses (Morishita et al., 2001; Yan et al., 1999), with potential effects on dopaminergic and serotonergic signaling (Greengard et al., 1999; Svenningsson et al., 2004). Allen et al. (2006) have established a requirement for synaptic scaffolding (with distinct roles for spinophilin and neurabin) in dopamine-mediated plasticity. Enhancement in the rewarding effects of cocaine seen in spinophilin knockout (KO) mice may be related to preferential expression of long-term potentiation (LTP) over long-term depression (LTD) at corticostriatal synapses (Allen et al., 2006). Corticostriatal LTP has been implicated in reward-related learning (Gerdeman, 2003; Reynolds et al., 2001) and has been proposed to contribute to drug addiction (Berke & Hyman, 2000; Kauer, 2004; Wolf et al., 2004). Spinophilin (via interaction with G-coupled receptor protein [Gq]) may modulate NMDAR complex functioning and therefore could affect nociceptive processing as well.

Impulsiveness is explored in Part II as a potential trait that may predispose people to substance abuse. People afflicted with a type of dementia that causes inappropriate and impulsive social behavior had 74% fewer von Economo neurons (VENs) in their anterior cingulate cortex compared to normal controls (Seeley et al., 2006), and it has been proposed that a similar loss of VENs in particular brain regions may render people more vulnerable to substance abuse (Smith, in press). Drug abusers tend to be impulsive, however. Are they impulsive secondary to drug effects, or are they drug abusers because they are impulsive? Dalley and colleagues (2007) identified spontaneously impulsive rats and found that they had about half as many dopamine D2/3 receptors in the nucleus accumbens as their patient peers (controls) even before exposure to cocaine. Trait impulsivity in rats was predictive of subsequent high rates of intravenous cocaine self-administration (impulsive rats consumed nearly twice as much cocaine as controls; Dalley et al., 2007). It appears, then, that impulsivity may be a key contributor to drug abuse vulnerability and not a consequence of chronic drug exposure.

In Part III, the clinical issues involved in the management of chronic pain are dealt with. Part IV covers multiple approaches to management of the chemically dependent patient. In Part V, a wide variety of special clinical issues, tools, and situations related to the management of pain in patients with chemical dependency are covered. Part VI delves into a number of practical challenges that clinicians may face when treating persistent pain in patients exhibiting aberrant drug-taking behaviors. Finally, Part VII discusses the interface between pain and chemical dependency, addressing the effects of pain on the vulnerability for addiction.

A fundamental appreciation of the complexities and interrelationships of pain, its treatment, and addiction may help clinicians to become more comfortable in these clinical arenas and lead to optimal patient outcomes.

Acknowledgments

The editors would like to acknowledge the enormous efforts of Pya Seidner. Her work helped bring this project to fruition.

The editors would like to thank Dr. Kenneth Kirsh for all his help. His contributions to the project were significant.

References

Allen PB, Zachariou V, Svenningsson P, et al. Distinct roles for spinophilin and neurabin in dopamine-mediated plasticity. *Neuroscience.* 2006; 140: 897–911.

Becerra L, Breiter HC, Wise R, et al. Reward circuitry activation by noxious thermal stimuli. *Neuron.* 2001; 32: 927–46.

Berke JD, Hyman SE. Addiction, dopamine, and the molecular mechanisms of memory. *Neuron.* 2000; 25: 9144–9151.

Borsook D, Becerra L, Carlezon Jr. WA, et al. Reward-aversion circuitry in analgesia and pain: Implication for psychiatric disorders. *Eur J of Pain.* 2007; 11: 7–20.

Bozarth MA, Wise RA. Anatomically distinct opiate receptor fields mediate reward and physical dependence. *Science.* 1984; 224: 516–7.

Dalley JW, Fryer TD, Brichard L, et al. Nucleus accumbens D2/3 receptors predict trait impulsivity and cocaine reinforcement. *Science.* 2007; 315: 1267–70.

Franklin KB. Analgesia and the neural substrate of reward. *Neurosci Biobehavior Rev.* 1989; 13: 149–54.

Geha PY, Baliki MN, Chialvo DR, et al. Brain activity for spontaneous pain of postherpetic neuralgia and its modulation by lidocaine patch therapy. *Pain.* 2007; 128: 88–100.

Gerdeman GL, Partridge JG, Lupica CR, et al. It could be habit forming: drugs of abuse and striatal synaptic plasticity. *Trends Neurosci.* 2003; 26: 184–192.

Greengard P, Allen PB, Nairm AC. Beyond the dopamine receptor: the DARPP-32/protein phosphatase-1 cascade. *Neuron.* 1999; 23: 435–447.

Kauer JA. Learning mechanisms in addiction: synaptic plasticity in the ventral tegmental areas as a result of exposure to drugs of abuse. *Annu Rev Physiol.* 2004; 66: 447–475.

Lai J, Luo MC, Chen Q, et al. Dynorphin A activates bradykinin receptors to maintain neuropathic pain. *Nat Neurosci.* 2006; 9: 1534–40.

Morishita W, Connor JH, Xia H, et al. Regulation of synaptic strength by protein phosphatase 1. *Neuron.* 2001; 32: 1133–1148.

Muly EC, Allen P, Mazioom M, et al. Subcellular distribution of neurabin immunolabeling in primate prefrontal cortex: comparison with spinophilin. *Cereb Cortex.* 2004a; 14: 1398–1407.

Muly EC, Smith Y, Allen P, et al. Subcellular distribution of spinophilin immunolabeling in primate prefrontal cortex: localization to an within dendritic spines. *J Comp Neurol.* 2004b; 469: 185–197.

Nakanishi H, Obaishi H, Satch A, et al. Neurabin: a novel neural tissue-specific actin filament-binding protein involved in neurite formation. *J Cell Biol.* 1997; 139: 951–961.

Pert A, Yaksh T. Sites of morphine induced analgesia in the primate brain: relation to pain pathways. *Brain Res.* 1974; 80: 135–40.

Reynolds JN, Hyland BI, Wickens JR. A cellular mechanism of reward-related learning. *Nature.* 2001; 413: 67–70.

Satoh A, Nakanishi H, Obaishi H, et al. Neurabin-II/spinophilin. An actin filament-binding protein with one pdz domain localized at cadherin-based cell-cell adhesion sites. *J Biol Chem.* 1998; 273: 3470–3475.

Seeley WW, Carlin DA, Allman JM, et al. Early frontotemporal dementia targets neurons unique to apes and humans. *Ann Neurol.* 2006; 60: 660–7.

Sell LA, Morris J, Bearn J, et al. Activation of reward circuitry in human opiate addicts. *Eur J Neurosoci.* 1999; 11: 1042–8.

Seymour B, O'Doherty JP, Koltzenburg M, et al. Opponent appetitive-aversive neural processes underlie predictive learning of pain relief. *Nat Neurosci.* 2005; 8: 1234–40.

Smith HS. VENF-challenged. *Journal of Cancer Pain and Symptom Palliation.* In press.

Svenningsson P, Nishi A, Fisone G, et al. DARPP-32: an integrator of neurotransmission. *Annu Rev Pharmacol Toxicol.* 2004; 44: 269–296.

Wolf ME, Sun X, Mangiavacchi S, et al. Psychomotor stimulants and neuronal plasticity. *Neuropharmacology.* 2004; 47: 61–79.

Yan Z, Hsieh-Wilson L, Feng J, et al. Protein phosphatase 1 modulation of neostriatal AMPA channels: regulation by DARPP-32 and spinophilin. *Nat Neurosci.* 1999; 2: 13–17.

Zachariou V, Bolanos CA, Selley DE, et al. An essential role for DeltaFosB in the nucleus accumbens in morphine action. *Nat Neurosci.* 2006; 9: 205–11.

Contents

Contributors *xvii*

Part I. Introduction

1. History of Opioids and Opiophobia *3*
   Kenneth L. Kirsh, Anya Kerith Vice, and Steven D. Passik

2. The Language of Pain and Addiction *9*
   Seddon R. Savage

3. Opioids for Chronic Pain: Historical Notes *15*
   Russell K. Portenoy

4. The Growth of Prescription Opioid Abuse *19*
   Sandra D. Comer and Judy B. Ashworth

5. Pain Management and the Medical Profession: What Is Our Responsibility? *25*
   Richard Payne

Part II. Addiction and Related Issues

6. The Basic Science of Addiction *33*
   Roberto I. Melendez and Peter W. Kalivas

7. Neuroimaging in Addiction *39*
   Tim M. Williams, Shrikant Srivastava, Anne R. Lingford-Hughes, and David J. Nutt

8. Reward and Addiction *49*
   Susan E. Best and Bryon Adinoff

9. Neurobehavioral Mechanisms of Compulsive Drug Seeking *59*
   Louk J. M. J. Vanderschuren

10. Neurochemical Approaches to Addiction Treatment *71*
    William R. Millington and Gökhan Göktalay

11. Neurobiology of Opioids in Dependency *81*
    Linda I. Perrotti

12. The Regulation of Cellular Mechanisms in Antinociception and Dependency *89*
    Jeffery N. Talbot and John R. Traynor

13. "Impulsology": A New Paradigm for Addiction *97*
    Kara Lee Shirley, Lisa J. Norelli, and Howard S. Smith

14. Natural and Synthetic Ibogamines: A Novel Approach to Treating Opioid Dependency *105*
    Stanley D. Glick and Isabelle M. Maisonneuve

15. Opioid Tolerance *109*
    Jianren Mao and Lucy Chen

16. Methadone Pharmacology in Pain and Addiction *113*
    Howard S. Smith, Mary Jeanne Kreek, Carrie L. Johnson, and Kenneth L. Kirsh

17. Cannabinoids in Pain and Addiction *123*
    Billy R. Martin, Aron H. Lichtman, and Sandra P. Welch

18. Alcohol Use Disorders and Their Treatment *131*
    Barbara Flannery and David Newlin

19. Benzodiazepines: Misuse, Abuse, and Dependence *137*
    Danielle M. Ciraulo and Domenic A. Ciraulo

20. Treating Cocaine Dependence *145*
    Tracy A. Steen and Charles A. Dackis

21. Smoking, Pain, and Addiction 153
    Lara K. Dhingra and Jamie S. Ostroff

Part III. The Problem of Clinical Pain

22. The Pathophysiology of Chronic Pain 161
    Daniel Brookoff

23. Opioid Pharmacology for Pain 175
    Charles E. Inturrisi

24. Opioids for Pain 183
    Howard S. Smith, Todd W. Vanderah, and Gary McCleane

25. Adjuvants for Pain 203
    Craig K. Chang and Marco Pappagallo

26. Behavioral Medicine Approaches to Pain Management 211
    Akiko Okifuji

27. Physical Medicine Approaches to Assessing and Treating Pain 217
    Steven Stanos and Lynn R. Rader

28. Interventional Pain Medicine 233
    Michel Y. Dubois and Roshni Patel

Part IV. Current Approaches to Management of the Chemically Dependent Patient

29. Pharmacologic Approaches to Opioid Dependence and Withdrawal 247
    Eric D. Collins

30. Behavioral Medicine Treatment in the Management of the Chemically Dependent Patient 253
    Joshua Wootton

31. Traditional Chinese Medicine for Pain and Addiction 259
    Gira Patel and David Euler

32. Support Groups and Twelve-Step Programs in the Treatment of the Chronic Pain Patient 271
    Douglas M. Ziedonis, Jeffrey A. Berman, M. Dale Lehn, and Stephen Colameco

Part V. Clinical Management of Pain in Chemical Dependency

33. Treatment of Acute Pain in the Opioid-Dependent Patient in the Perioperative Setting 285
    Raymond S. Sinatra and Sukanya Mitra

34. Management of Persistent Pain in the Opioid-Treated Patient 291
    Thomas Simopoulos

35. Chemical Coping: The Clinical Middle Ground 299
    Steven D. Passik and Kenneth L. Kirsh

36. Buprenorphine in Pain and Addiction 303
    Howard A. Heit and Douglas L. Gourlay

Management in Distinct Settings

37. Pain and Chemical Dependency in the Emergency Department 309
    Knox H. Todd

38. Management of Pain in Chemical Dependency in the Primary Care Clinic 317
    Bill H. McCarberg

Management in Special Populations

39. The Palliative Care Patient 321
    Lida Nabati and Janet Abraham

40. Managing Pain and Substance Abuse in the Patient With HIV/AIDS 329
    William Breitbart and Lara K. Dhingra

41. Sickle Cell: A Disease of Molecules and a Disease of Race 339
    Lauren Shaiova, Craig Blinderman, Daniel Brookoff, and Marc Goloff

Special Management Considerations

42. Urine Drug Testing in Pain and Addiction Medicine 353
    Douglas L. Gourlay and Howard A. Heit

43. The Opioid Contract 359
    Felix A. Chen, Scott M. Fishman, and Paul G. Kreis

44. Opioids and the Treatment of Chronic Pain 367
    Daniel S. Bennett, Pamela Squire, and Daniel Brookoff

45. Federal and State Policies at the Interface of Pain and Addiction 377
    Martha A. Maurer, Aaron M. Gilson, and David E. Joranson

46. Documentation and Potential Documentation Tools in Long-Term Opioid Therapy 385
    Kenneth L. Kirsh and Howard S. Smith

Part VI. Aberrant Drug-Taking Considerations

47. Screening for the Risk of Substance Abuse in Pain Management 395
    Lynn R. Webster

48. Aberrant Drug-Taking: Empirical Studies and Clinical Application   *405*
Kenneth L. Kirsh and Steven D. Passik

49. Abuse Liability Assessment of Prescription Opioids in Chronic Nonmalignant Pain Patients   *411*
James P. Zacny

50. Aberrant Behavior and Drug Abuse Treatment in Pain Patients   *419*
Peggy Compton

Part VII. Pain and Chemical Dependency: The Interface

51. Pain Management and the So-Called "Risk" of Addiction: A Neurobiological Perspective   *427*
Eliot L. Gardner

Index   *437*

Contributors

Janet Abrahm, MD
Associate Professor, Harvard Medical School; Co-director, Pain and Palliative Care Program, Dana-Farber Cancer Institute

Bryon Adinoff, MD
Professor, University of Texas Southwestern Medical Center at Dallas, and VA North Texas Health Care System

Judy B. Ashworth, MD
Director, Center of Excellence for Abuse Liability, Grunenthal USA, Inc.; Visiting Lecturer, Department of Psychiatry, College of Physicians and Surgeons of Columbia University, New York State Psychiatric Institute

Daniel S. Bennett, MD, DABPM
Integrative Treatment Centers, Denver

Jeffrey A. Berman, MD, MS
Department of Psychiatry, Robert Wood Johnson Medical School

Susan E. Best, MD, PhD
Associate Professor, University of Texas Southwestern Medical Center at Dallas, and VA North Texas Health Care System

Craig Blinderman, MD, MA
Palliative Care Service, Massachusetts General Hospital; Instructor, Harvard Medical School

William Breitbart, MD
Department of Psychiatry and Behavioral Sciences, Pain and Palliative Care Service, Department of Neurology, Memorial Sloan-Kettering Cancer Center

Daniel Brookoff, MD, PhD
Medical Director, Center for Medical Pain Management, Presbyterian–St. Luke's Medical Center, Denver, CO

Craig K. Chang, MD
Teaching Faculty, Virginia Commonwealth University School of Medicine, Inova Campus

Felix A. Chen, MD, PhD
Department of Anesthesia and Pain Medicine, Division of Pain Medicine, University of California, Davis

Lucy Chen, MD
Massachusetts General Hospital Pain Center, Harvard Medical School

Danielle M. Ciraulo, BA, MA, LMHC
Instructor, Division of Psychiatry, Boston University School of Medicine

Domenic A. Ciraulo, MD
Professor and Chairman, Division of Psychiatry, Boston University School of Medicine

Stephen Colameco, MD, MEd
Assistant Clinical Professor, Department of Family Medicine, Thomas Jefferson University School of Medicine

Eric D. Collins, MD
Assistant Professor of Clinical Psychiatry, Department of Psychiatry, Columbia University

Sandra D. Comer, PhD
Associate Professor of Clinical Neuroscience, Department of Psychiatry, College of Physicians and Surgeons of Columbia University, New York State Psychiatric Institute

Peggy Compton, RN, PhD, FAAN,
Associate Professor of Nursing, Acute Care Division, School of Nursing, University of California, Los Angeles

Charles A. Dackis, MD
University of Pennsylvania School of Medicine

Lara K. Dhingra, PhD
Department of Psychiatry and Behavioral Sciences, Memorial Sloan-Kettering Cancer Center

Michel Y. Dubois, MD
Professor of Anesthesiology, Director of Education and Research, New York University Medical Center

David Euler, LicAc
Co-Director, Structural Acupuncture Course, Harvard Medical School Department of Continuing Education

Scott M. Fishman, MD
Department of Anesthesia and Pain Medicine, Division of Pain Medicine, University of California, Davis

Barbara Flannery, PhD
RTI International, Transdisciplinary Behavioral Science Program

Eliot L. Gardner, PhD
Chief of the Neuropsychopharmacology Section, Intramural Research Program, National Institute on Drug Abuse, National Institutes of Health

Aaron M. Gilson, MS, MSSW, PhD
Director of U.S. Program, Pain and Policy Studies Group, Paul P. Carbone Comprehensive Cancer Center, University of Wisconsin-Madison

Stanley D. Glick, PhD, MD
Center for Neuropharmacology and Neuroscience, Albany Medical College

Gökhan Göktalay, MD, PhD
Department of Pharmacology and Clinical Pharmacology, Uludag University School of Medicine

Marc Goloff, PhD, ABPP
Director of Psychology in Primary Care, VA New York Harbor Healthcare System, New York Campus

Douglas L. Gourlay, MD, MSc, FRCPC, FASAM
Wasser Pain Management, Mount Sinai Hospital, Toronto, Ontario

Howard A. Heit, MD, FACP, FASAM
Assistant Clinical Professor, Georgetown School of Medicine

Charles E. Inturrisi, PhD
Weill Medical College of Cornell University; The Pain and Palliative Care Service, Memorial Sloan-Kettering Cancer Center

Carrie L. Johnson, PharmD
Assistant Professor, University of Kentucky College of Pharmacy

David E. Joranson, MSSW
Distinguished Scientist, Pain and Policy Studies Group, Paul P. Carbone Comprehensive Cancer Center, University of Wisconsin-Madison

Peter W. Kalivas, PhD
Department of Neurosciences, Medical University of South Carolina

Kenneth L. Kirsh, PhD
Assistant Professor, University of Kentucky College of Pharmacy, Department of Pharmacy Practice and Science

Mary Jeanne Kreek, MD
Professor, Laboratory of the Biology of Addictive Diseases, Rockefeller University

Paul G. Kreis, MD
Department of Anesthesia and Pain Medicine, Division of Pain Medicine, University of California, Davis

M. Dale Lehn
Co-founder Chronic Pain Anonymous

Aron H. Lichtman, PhD
Department of Pharmacology and Toxicology, Virginia Commonwealth University

Anne R. Lingford-Hughes, MA, PhD, BM BCh, MRCPsych
Reader in Biological Psychiatry and Addiction, University of Bristol

Isabelle M. Maisonneuve, PhD
Center for Neuropharmacology and Neuroscience, Albany Medical College

Jianren Mao, MD, PhD
Massachusetts General Hospital Pain Center, Harvard Medical School

Billy R. Martin, PhD
Department of Pharmacology and Toxicology, Virginia Commonwealth University

Martha A. Maurer, MSSW, MPH
Assistant Researcher, Pain and Policy Studies Group, Paul P. Carbone Comprehensive Cancer Center, University of Wisconsin-Madison

Bill H. McCarberg, MD
Founder, Chronic Pain Management Program, Kaiser Permanente San Diego; Assistant Clinical Professor (voluntary), University of California, San Diego

Gary McCleane, MD
Rampark Pain Centre

Roberto I. Melendez, PhD
Department of Neurosciences, Medical University of South Carolina

William R. Millington, PhD
Department of Pharmaceutical Sciences, Albany College of Pharmacy

Sukanya Mitra, MD
Research Associate in Anesthesiology, Yale University School of Medicine

Lida Nabati, MD
Associate Professor of Medicine, Harvard Medical School; Director, Pain and Palliative Care Program, Dana-Farber Cancer Institute

David Newlin, PhD
RTI International, Transdisciplinary Behavioral Science Program

Lisa J. Norelli, MD, MPH, MRCPsych
Department of Psychiatry, Albany Medical College

David J. Nutt, MB BChir, DM, FRCP, FRCPsych, FMedSci
Professor of Psychopharmacology, University of Bristol

Akiko Okifuji, PhD
Pain Research and Management Center, University of Utah

Jamie S. Ostroff, PhD
Department of Psychiatry and Behavioral Sciences, Memorial Sloan-Kettering Cancer Center

Marco Pappagallo, MD
Director, Pain Medicine Research and Development, Professor, Department of Anesthesia, Mount Sinai School of Medicine

Steven D. Passik, PhD
Psychiatry and Behavioral Services, Memorial Sloan Kettering Cancer Center

Gira Patel, LicAc
Arnold Pain Management Center, Beth Israel Deaconess Medical Center, Boston; Clinical Research, Osher Institute, Harvard Medical School

Roshni Patel, MD
Fellow in Pain Medicine, New York University Medical Center

Richard Payne, MD
Director, Institute on Care at the End of Life, Duke University Divinity School

Linda I. Perrotti, PhD
Assistant Professor, Department of Psychology, College of Science, University of Texas at Arlington

Russell K. Portenoy, MD
Chairman, Department of Pain Medicine and Palliative Care, Beth Israel Medical Center; Professor of Neurology and Anesthesiology, Albert Einstein College of Medicine

Lynn R. Rader, MD
Rehabilitation Institute of Chicago

Seddon R. Savage, MD, MS
Director, Dartmouth Center on Addiction Recovery and Education; Pain Consultant, Manchester Veterans Administration Medical Center

Lauren Shaiova, MD
Chief, Department of Pain Medicine and Palliative Care, Metropolitan Hospital Center HHC, and Associate Professor, Departments of Pain Medicine and Rehabilitation Medicine, New York Medical College, Valhalla, New York

Kara Lee Shirley, PharmD, BCPS, BCPP
Department of Pharmacy Practice, Albany College of Pharmacy

Thomas Simopoulos, MA, MD
Instructor, Department of Anesthesiology, Harvard Medical School; Director, Acute and Interventional Pain Services, Beth Israel Deaconess Medical Center

Raymond S. Sinatra, MD, PhD
Professor of Anesthesiology, Yale University School of Medicine

Howard S. Smith, MD
Departments of Anesthesiology, Physical Medicine and Rehabilitation, and Internal Medicine, Albany Medical College

Pamela Squire, MD
University of British Columbia, Vancouver

Shrikant Srivastava, MBBS, MRCPsych, MD
Specialist Registrar in Psychiatry, University of Bristol

Steven Stanos, DO
Medical Director, Chronic Pain Care Center, Rehabilitation Institute of Chicago; Assistant Professor, Department of Physical Medicine and Rehabilitation, Northwestern University Feinberg School of Medicine

Tracy A. Steen, PhD
Charles O'Brien Center for Addiction Treatment, University of Pennsylvania

Jeffery N. Talbot, PhD
Department of Pharmaceutical and Biomedical Sciences, Ohio Northern University College of Pharmacy

Knox H. Todd, MD, MPH
Director, Professor, Pain and Emergency Medicine Institute, Department of Emergency Medicine, Beth Israel Medical Center, Albert Einstein College of Medicine, New York

John R. Traynor, PhD
Department of Pharmacology, University of Michigan Medical School

Todd W. Vanderah, PhD
Assistant Professor of Anesthesiology and Pharmacology, University of Arizona

Louk J. M. J. Vanderschuren, PhD
Rudolf Magnus Institute of Neuroscience, Department of Neuroscience and Pharmacology, University Medical Center Utrecht

Anya Kerith Vice
Pharmacy Practice and Science, University of Kentucky

Lynn R. Webster, MD, FACPM, FASAM
Medical Director, Lifetree Clinical Research and Pain Clinic, Salt Lake City, Utah

Sandra P. Welch, PhD
Department of Pharmacology and Toxicology, Virginia Commonwealth University

Tim M. Williams, MB ChB, MRCPsych
Academic Specialist Registrar in Psychiatry, University of Bristol

Joshua Wootton, MDiv, PhD
Director of Pain Psychology, Arnold Pain Management Center, Beth Israel Deaconess Medical Center, Boston; Assistant Professor, Department of Anesthesia, Harvard Medical School

James P. Zacny, PhD
Department of Anesthesia and Critical Care, University of Chicago

Douglas M. Ziedonis, MD, MPH
Professor and Director, Division of Addiction Psychiatry, Robert Wood Johnson Medical School

Part I
Introduction

1

History of Opioids and Opiophobia

Kenneth L. Kirsh

Anya Kerith Vice

Steven D. Passik

> Among the remedies which it has pleased Almighty God to give to man to relieve his sufferings, none is so universal and so efficacious as opium.
> —Thomas Sydenham, 17th-century pioneer of English medicine

The field of pain management has arrived at a crossroads in history with regard to the topic of opioid analgesics. Over the past several years, one of the most widely used opioid pharmaceuticals, OxyContin, had become a popular alternative to street drugs such as heroin. Called "Hillbilly Heroin" because of its popularity in Appalachia and other rural areas, it is available as an oral preparation, although illicit users tend to crush the tablet to circumvent the sustained release delivery system and then snort it or dissolve it in water to inject the drug (Hancock, 2002). Although the abuse or diversion of this drug was originally thought to have begun in Kentucky and other Appalachian areas, it has spread through other states. It has been most popular east of the Mississippi with the following states having the most prescriptions of OxyContin per capita in the year 2000: West Virginia, Alaska, Delaware, New Hampshire, Florida, Kentucky, Pennsylvania, Maine, Rhode Island, and Connecticut (*Workplace Substance Abuse Advisor,* 2002). As a result of this problem, we have begun to see pullback from this treatment modality and an increase in regulatory pressure and law enforcement scrutiny.

We must view this current trend toward demonizing opioid medications from a historical perspective. Although it is easy to imagine a new, growing pandemic because of these medications, concern over opioid use has been in an ever-changing cycle for quite some time, with marked periods of widespread use followed by rigid control and near-elimination of the drug class by naysayers. This chapter will attempt to recount the historical use of opioids as well as the rise of problems with opiophobia.

The Origins of Opium and Its Early Use

> History is only the register of crimes and misfortunes.
> —Voltaire

For centuries, the opium poppy, or Papaver somniferum, has been revered as the "plant of joy." The earliest uses of the opium-producing poppy plant were for recreation because of the feeling of euphoria to which the user succumbs. It has been evidenced that opium was in use in Mesopotamia as early as 5,000 years ago. By 460 B.C., Hippocrates had deemed opium to have redemptive medicinal purposes for problems such as pain, internal diseases, and illnesses specific to women (Booth, 1996). Opium has been grown primarily in areas of China, Turkey, and what is now labeled Afghanistan. However, opium use spread throughout the world as exploration and new trade markets were opened between foreign allies. When European explorers discovered opium being grown in mass amounts in areas of the Eastern world, they found a new trade and new product that would eventually spread throughout the world.

The Cultural Phenomenon of Opium in Society

> It is difficult to free fools from the chains they revere.
> —Voltaire

Since the beginning of the mass supply and demand of opium, there has been a struggle for the control of the drug. Whether it was tradesmen trying to force fair or unfair trade practices, or lawmakers trying to control the flow and use of opium, there has always been a battle for the power that comes with such a commanding commodity.

In the United States, the use of opium started only as a flicker, mostly used in its manmade forms as laudanum for headaches, fevers, and diarrhea. In the Civil War, countless numbers of soldiers were addicted to morphine, due to the pain and disease they endured and the means by which they were treated. By the end of the war, morphine addiction was referred to in the United States as "the soldier's disease." However, soldiers were not the only ones entrapped by morphine, as many were finding the pleasure that morphine brought to the woes of everyday life.

After the introduction of heroin as a treatment for morphine addiction, the nation found a new and more immediate means for a high. Opium smoking and morphine injection were certainly able to produce a state of euphoria that was acceptable for an addict. With heroin, however, that state could be heightened and achieved much more rapidly.

The Medical Uses of Opium

> It is inhumane, in my opinion, to force people who have a genuine medical need for coffee to wait in line behind people who apparently view it as some kind of recreational activity.
> —Dave Barry

From the inception of its use, there has been knowledge of some healing power in opium, although this did not always prevail as the reason for its use. Different societies and cultures valued opium for various reasons, be it as an analgesic or, as postulated by Galen, as "a cold, earthy drug which worked by impairing the vital heat of the heart and blood... hence it would be most effective for those with too much hot, expansive blood [we might call this condition high blood pressure today]" (Latimer & Goldberg, 1981). Table 1.1 offers a partial timeline of the medical uses of opioids throughout history.

Over time, the advancement of medicine has allowed for the increase in knowledge, not only about the human body and ailments, but also how the pathophysiology of the body is affected by foreign elements introduced into the system, including plant extracts and derivatives. These advancements brought forth mass manufacturing of medications by pharmaceutical companies, especially in Europe. In Germany in 1799, a pharmacist's apprentice derived an active ingredient, an alkaloid, from crude opium. This apprentice later became a scientist, Friedrich Sertürner, and is credited with creating the first batches or what he called morphine (Latimer & Goldberg, 1981).

The use of morphine was willingly accepted by physicians, yet was not as widely popular with users as pure opium. This remained true until another scientist discovered a novel way to deliver medications directly into the bloodstream, thereby speeding up the rate of effectiveness. Dr. Alexander Wood discovered the system that was later perfected by Charles Hunter and what is now known as the hypodermic needle (Latimer & Goldberg, 1981). As with many great inventions, the intent and improvement opened the door for ways in which others could use it for destruction.

It was not long before addicts became aware of the instant high that came with injecting morphine and later heroin. The invention of the hypodermic needle opened a door to many new advances in medical treatment, and without these advances today, we would be still in the dark ages of patient care and the treatment of many ailments. Although the hypodermic needle was a major advance, it was not without its negative consequences. The increased number of opioid addicts due to intravenous drug use created a new medical need: specifically, how to treat opioid addiction.

Some of the first people to test treatments in the 1930s for addiction on human populations were Drs. Harry Anslinger and Lawrence Kolb. Although Dr. Anslinger preferred abstinence and prohibition of opioids to be used as legal maintenance for addiction treatment, Dr. Kolb was often in disagreement and did not feel that overzealous law enforcement was required. Dr. Kolb was associated with the first federal facility to house the testing of addiction treatment at the United States Public Health Service Hospital in Lexington, Kentucky. Both prisoners and addicts were admitted and treated (only the latter received treatment voluntarily) at the facility, which, as one doctor stated, was "more like a prison than a hospital and more like a hospital than a prison" (Courtwright, 1992). It was not until the 1960s that this facility was made into a real hospital, The Addiction Research Center, and began making significant, ethical contributions to the study of pain, addiction, and chemical dependence (Musto, 1996).

Legal Issues With Opium

> Ice-cream is exquisite—what a pity it isn't illegal.
> —Voltaire

By 1903, the rate of heroin addiction in the United States was higher than ever before, and so began the laws of inhibition and prohibition. In 1905, the United States passed a federal drug prohibition to stop importation of opium (Booth, 1996).

In 1914, the U.S. Congress passed the Harrison Narcotics Tax Act. The basis of the act was "to provide for the registration of, with collectors of internal revenue, and to impose a special tax on all persons who produce, import, manufacture, compound, deal in, dispense, sell, distribute or give away opium or coco leaves, their salts, derivatives, or preparations, and for other purposes" (Harrison Narcotics Tax Act, 1914). The goal of this act was to keep narcotics out of the hands of persons with nonmedical need. By the early 1920s, the Narcotics Division of the U.S. Treasury Department had banned legal sale of narcotics, thereby sustaining a thriving black market of heroin sales.

Opioid Concerns in the Modern Era

> It is not a case we are treating; it is a living, palpitating, alas, too often suffering fellow creature.
> —John Brown

In recent decades, tremendous progress has been made in the study and treatment of pain (Berry & Dahl, 2000; SUPPORT Study Principal Investigators, 1995). Efforts have been undertaken to make pain assessment and treatment a priority of medical care and to utilize all of the weapons in our armamentarium to bring relief to the millions of people with chronic pain (Osterweis et al., 1987; Verhaak et al., 1998). This includes the use of opioid therapy for the treatment of both malignant and nonmalignant pain. There is no doubt that hundreds of thousands of pain patients have benefited from this increased willingness to prescribe opioids.

Pain management professionals, however, have cycled through various stages in their beliefs regarding the abuse potential of opioids. The old mythology during the past century stated that addiction was so fearsome and unavoidable that opioids should be withheld until patients were close to death (Musto, 1999; Rock, 1977). This was usually presented sans solid data and research. When the president of the American Medical Association wrote famously in a 1941 editorial that "the use of narcotics in the terminal cancer [patient] is to be condemned if it can possibly be avoided... [because one] of the unfortunate [side] effects is addiction," he was voicing an extreme view on opioids with equally little basis in science (Lee, 1941).

Luckily, a revolution in pain management, along with the use of opioids that began in oncology and spread to all branches of medicine, did away with this false perception. But this myth was replaced by another, one suggesting that chronic pain patients are somehow immune to problems of aberrant drug taking, abuse, or diversion (Friedman, 1990). These conclusions were erroneously based on questionable data, such as in the Boston Collaborative Drug Surveillance Project. In that study, the authors evaluated

Table 1.1. A Medical Timeline of Opium

Date	Event
1200 AD	Ancient Indian treatises *The Shodal Gadanigrah* and *Sharangdhar Samhita* describe the use of opium for sexual dysfunction and diarrhea. The *Dhanvantri Nighantu* also describes the medical properties of opium.
1527	During the height of the Reformation, opium is reintroduced into European medical literature by Paracelsus as laudanum. These "stones of immortality" were made of opium thebaicum, citrus juice, and essence of gold, and were prescribed as painkillers.
1680	English apothecary introduces Sydenham's Laudanum, a compound of opium, sherry wine and herbs. The pills become popular remedies for numerous ailments.
1803	Friedrich Sertürner of Paderborn, Germany, discovers the active ingredient of opium by dissolving it in acid and then neutralizing it with ammonia. The result: alkaloids—*principium somniferum*, or morphine.
1827	The manufacture of morphine begins at E. Merck & Company of Germany.
1843	Injection of morphine with a syringe is tested by Dr. Alexander Wood of Edinburgh. He finds the effects of morphine on his patients instantaneous and three times more potent.
1895	Heinrich Dreser, employed by The Bayer Company of Elberfeld, Germany, dilutes morphine with acetyls and produces a drug without the common side effects. Bayer begins production of diacetylmorphine and coins the name *heroin*. Heroin would not be introduced commercially for another 3 years.
Early 1900s	The Saint James Society, a philanthropic group in the United States, mounts a campaign to supply free samples of heroin through the mail to morphine addicts who are trying give up their habit.
1902	Physicians discuss the side effects of using heroin as a morphine step-down cure. Several physicians would argue that their patients suffered from heroin withdrawal symptoms equal to those caused by morphine addiction.
1906	Physicians experiment with treatments for heroin addiction. Dr. Alexander Lambert and Charles B. Towns tout their popular cure as the most "advanced, effective, and compassionate cure" for heroin addiction. The cure consisted of a 7-day regimen, which included a 5-day purge of heroin from the addict's system with doses of belladonna delirium.
Dec. 17, 1914	The Harrison Narcotics Tax Act passes, which aims to curb drug (especially cocaine but also heroin) abuse and addiction. It requires doctors, pharmacists, and others who prescribed narcotics to register and pay a tax.
1935	The Addiction Research Center, also known as "narcotic farm," opens in Lexington, Kentucky, under supervision of the U.S. Department of Treasury. It held addicts and criminals in the "prison-hospital" and used them to test new methods of addiction treatment.
1941	The president of the American Medical Association wrote that "the use of narcotics in the terminal cancer [patient] is to be condemned if it can possibly be avoided... [because one] of the unfortunate [side] effects is addiction."
July 1, 1973	The Drug Enforcement Administration (DEA) is created under the Justice Department to consolidate virtually all federal powers of drug enforcement in a single agency.
1988	The Anti-Drug Abuse Act of 1988 (P.L. 100–690) established the Office of National Drug Control Policy (ONDCP) in the Executive Office of the President. This authorized funds for federal, state, and local law enforcement, school-based drug prevention efforts and drug abuse treatment with special emphasis on injection drug abusers at high risk for AIDS.
1999	An Oregon physician is disciplined by the state medical board for treating an elderly man who was dying of cancer and in pain with "substantially inadequate amounts of pain medication," contrary to a hospice nurse's request for stronger pain drugs and antianxiety medication.
December 2002	U.K. government health plan makes heroin available free on National Health Service "to all those with a clinical need for it."
October 2003	U.S. Food and Drug Administration (FDA) and Drug Enforcement Administration (DEA) launch special task force to curb surge in Internet-based sales of narcotics from online pharmacies.
January 2004	Consumer groups file a lawsuit against OxyContin maker Purdue Pharma. The company is alleged to have used fraudulent patents and deceptive trade practices to block the prescription of cheap generic medications for patients in pain.
September 2004	The FDA grants a product license to Purdue's pain medication Palladone, a high-dose, extended-release hydromorphone capsule. Palladone is designed to provide "around-the-clock" pain relief for opioid-tolerant users. It is pulled from the market in July 2005 for safety concerns, namely potentially fatal reactions if taken with alcohol.
October 2004	Without announcement, DEA withdraws newly issued guidelines to pain specialists. The guidelines had pledged that physicians wouldn't be arrested for providing adequate pain relief to their patients (i.e., volume and dose of opioids written alone would not lead to investigations). DEA drug-diversion chief Patricia Good earlier stated that the new rules were meant to eliminate an "aura of fear" that stopped doctors from treating pain aggressively. Now, volume of prescriptions and dose strengths will be used to flag clinicians for scrutiny.
December 2004	Pain-treatment specialist Dr. William Hurwitz is sent to prison for allegedly "excessive" prescribing of opioid painkillers, along with inadequacy in chart documentation, to chronic pain patients. Testifying in court, Dr. Hurwitz describes the abrupt stoppage of prescriptions as "tantamount to torture."
2004	The National Consensus Project for Quality Palliative Care states that a risk management plan must now be included when prescribing opioids for dying patients on a long-term basis. This development marks an attempt by the end-of-life care community to monitor themselves before the advent of DEA scrutiny.

Adapted from the following sources: Booth, 1996; FDA: http://www.fda.gov/cder/drug/infopage/palladone/default.htm; NIDA: http://www.nih.gov/about/almanac/organization/NIDA.htm; and Institute of Medicine, *Pathways of Addiction: Opportunities in Drug Abuse Research*, Washington, DC: National Academy Press, 1996; 288–289.

11,882 inpatients who had no prior history of addiction and were administered an opioid while hospitalized; only four cases of addiction could be identified subsequently (Porter & Jick, 1980). The study did not concern chronic pain issues, just acute, and it must be noted that it was never a truly developed study but merely a letter to the editor that well-intending professionals used as a rationale to treat more chronic pain with opioids.

Unfortunately, though, this rhetoric from the pain community had a tendency to trivialize the complexities of opioid treatment (Porter & Jick, 1980). The growing problem of prescription drug abuse has forced the field to take a new look at opioid prescribing and to seek balance in its risks and benefits. Although it is no doubt time to tone down the rhetoric (and replace rhetoric with scientifically based approaches to clinical management), it is not the case that we should abandon the use of these agents and return to the "bad old days." Although it is arguable that the dramatically expanded use of opioids was undertaken with a paucity of long-term data to justify it, it is also the case that the complete avoidance of these drugs was equally unsupported.

Today, all practitioners involved in pain management have the dual mission of relieving suffering while avoiding contributing to drug abuse and diversion. If all practitioners can become better acquainted with the principles of addiction medicine as they apply to the world of pain management, pain management can be kept safe and available for all who need it. The assessment of aberrant behaviors in patients with chronic pain is one key aspect of mastering these principles.

The problem of prescription drug abuse has grown by leaps and bounds over the past 10 years. Although initial reports were optimistic that the increasing production and use of opioids was not accompanied by a growth in the abuse and diversion of these drugs, as time has passed the growth of the problem has become more obvious (Joranson et al., 2000). The media spectacle that has accompanied the misuse of sustained-release oxycodone has been only the most visible of the multitude of stories on misuse of opioids by well-known celebrities and the like (Hancock, 2002).

There is little doubt that much of the reporting of the problem in the popular press has been inaccurate, sensationalized, and unbalanced. The result of this distasteful reporting has been that many physicians were initially dismissive of the problem, as the seriousness of the problem was actually obscured for them by the media circus. However, it has become abundantly clear, regardless of what index one uses to gauge the problem (e.g., the Drug Awareness Warning Network, the Household Survey), that the problem is on the rise (Colliver & Kopstein, 1991; Groerer & Brodsky, 1992; Regier et al., 1984). Prescribers must recognize that there is a deteriorating environment around opioid use engendered by the substantial public concern and follow guidelines carefully.

Opiophobia and Its Effects on the Realm of Health Care

> Diagnosis is not the end, but the beginning of practice.
> —Martin H. Fischer

One factor that has an extraordinarily detrimental effect on pain management in this country is the undertreatment of pain due to opiophobia (Marks & Sacher, 1973; Redmond, 1997; Zacny et al., 2003). Opiophobia can be defined as the fear experienced by prescribing clinicians of the processes and consequences of prescribing opioid analgesics (Cohen, 1980; Morgan, 1986; Shine & Demas, 1984). It is believed that opiophobia may stem from multiple concerns including apprehension about "opening the door" to abuse, incurring regulatory and legal sanction, inducing respiratory depression in vulnerable patients, and ultimately establishing a diagnosable addiction problem (Hill, 1993).

With the increasing pressure of regulatory scrutiny and our duty to treat pain but contain abuse or diversion, clinicians often feel that they must avoid being duped by those abusing prescription pain medications at all costs. Thus, although the differential diagnosis of aberrant drug-related behavior is complex, clinicians will tend to simplify the assessment of this issue to either addiction or not addiction. It is important to note, however, that the clinician attempting to diagnose the meaning of aberrant drug-related behaviors during pain management need not be correct in his or her final assessment. The fear of regulatory oversight makes practitioners feel as if they must be right, that if the aberrant behavior presents even the possibility of drug diversion or abuse, they have to "see through" the patient's or family's denials to guard against the possibility of being duped. Undertreatment and avoidance of prescribing is often the result. Yet that is not what the existing laws or guidelines on prescribing opioids necessitate.

The clinician has an obligation to be thorough, thoughtful, logically consistent, and careful (not to mention humane and caring), but not necessarily right. Indeed, there are multiple possibilities in the "differential diagnosis" of aberrant drug-taking behaviors, with criminal intent or diversion being only one of the more remote possibilities. Clinical management can be tailored for the multiple possibilities that might be giving rise to the behaviors noted in the assessment, and asserting control over prescriptions can be accomplished without necessarily terminating the prescribing of controlled substances entirely.

Addiction and Misdiagnosis: Pseudoaddiction

> The doctor may also learn more about the illness from the way the patient tells the story than from the story itself.
> —James B. Herrick

A large problem in wrongful treatment of pain patients may be a diagnosis of addiction, yet addiction may not always be the answer. If it looks like addiction, is it? A patient with chronic pain who is receiving treatment for his pain issues and is presenting with what would typically be aberrant drug-taking behaviors may be what is termed a pseudoaddict. Pseudoaddiction is "the iatrogenic syndrome of abnormal behavior developing as a direct consequence of inadequate pain management" (Weissman & Haddox, 1989). The actions of legitimate chronic pain patients are generally accepted as being compliant and nonthreatening to the health-care delivery system at hand. However, when patients with chronic pain are left with a small amount of opioids that give pain relief only part of the time, and a feeling that health-care providers do not believe the amount of pain they are in, patients may either acquire medications by their own means (illegally) or become aggressive toward their physician in their request for more medications, thereby instilling the belief that the seeking of drugs is not for pain relief but is aberrant. There has been little study in this area to provide significant scientific proof and diagnosis, yet experts in the field have come to accept it clinically (Fishbain, 2003).

Hyperalgesia in Patients on Opioid Treatment

Poisons and medicine are oftentimes the same substance given with different intents.
—Peter Mere Latham

Another phenomenon in the chronic pain patient that has yet to be fully studied or explained by the medical community is opioid-induced hyperalgesia. There are many studies that focus on the effects of hyperalgesia in mice, and in people when the pain is applied by the researcher (Chu et al., 2006; Holtman & Wala, 2005; Juni et al., 2006). Yet work is still under way to explain the events of hyperalgesia in patients on opioid treatment.

One interesting case report tells the story of a young man with metastatic disease and incredible amounts of pain. As his disease progressed, so did his pain, and it was decided that terminal doses of morphine were appropriate. Yet with the increase of the medication, his pain became increasingly worse. The amounts of opioids in his body should have easily warranted heavy sedation, yet he remained awake and in pain. A suggestion was finally made that the dose be decreased to a very low rate. As the rate was lowered, the pain lessened for the young man. He was finally able to reach a level of comfort after the morphine doses were lowered to standard maintenance-dose levels.

The explanation for this event in which a prescribed dose of opioids should be sedating actually allows for increased pain is opioid-induced hyperalgesia. The "hypersensitivity-type reaction of the patient to morphine" indicates a reaction that is largely misunderstood and grossly understudied (Wilson, 2001). Time and further research will hopefully help us to understand whether hyperalgesia is a rare phenomenon seen in occasional case studies or if it is a dose-dependent inevitability for pain patients. Either way, it must not be used as an excuse to further limit and demonize this therapeutic class of medications.

Conclusion

It is said an Eastern monarch once charged his wise men to invent him a sentence to be ever in view, and which should be true and appropriate in all times and situations. They presented him the words: "And this, too, shall pass away." How much it expresses! How chastening in the hour of pride! How consoling in the depths of affliction!
—Abraham Lincoln, September 30, 1859

As the world of pharmaceuticals grows and develops, and new possibilities and technologies emerge in the treatment of pain, we must continually educate ourselves about the effects of these medications and the outcomes of use. Just as importantly is the need to accurately assess patients and understand the effects of opioids and the laws around prescribing them, so that no patient may suffer needlessly and feel alone in his or her battle with chronic pain. Finally, it is important to understand the history of opioids and appreciate that the pendulum is always swinging between widespread acceptance and fear of this medication class. Keeping this larger perspective in mind can help us to weather the storms of prohibition while also managing attempts to increase the prescribing of opioids for legitimate patients without any sufficient controls or caution.

References

Berry PH, Dahl JL. The new JCAHO pain standards: implications for pain management nurses. *Pain Manag Nurs*, 2000 Mar;1(1):3–12.

Booth M. *Opium: A History*. London: Simon & Schuster Ltd., 1996.

Chu LF, Clark DJ, Angst MS. Opioid tolerance and hyperalgesia in chronic pain patients after one month of oral morphine therapy: a preliminary prospective study. *J Pain*, 2006; 7(1):43–48.

Cohen F. Postsurgical pain relief: patient's status and nurses' medication choices. *Pain*, 1980; 9:265–274.

Colliver JD, Kopstein AN. Trends in cocaine abuse reflected in emergency room episodes reported to DAWN. *Publ Health Rep*, 1991; 106:59–68.

Courtwright DT. A century of American narcotic policy. In DR Gerstein & HJ Harwood (Eds.). *Treating drug problems: volume 2*. Washington, DC: Committee for the Substance Abuse Coverage Study, Institute of Medicine, 1992; 1–62.

Fishbain DA. Chronic opioid treatment, addiction and pseudo-addiction in patients with chronic pain. *Psychiatric Times*, 2003; 20(2):1–7.

Friedman DP. Perspectives on the medical use of drugs of abuse. *Journal of Pain and Symptom Management*, 1990; 5(suppl):2–5.

Groerer J, Brodsky M. The incidence of illicit drug use in the United States, 1962–1989. *Brit J Addiction*, 1992;87:1345.

Hancock CM. OxyContin use and abuse. *Clin J Oncol Nursing*, 2002 (March–April); 6(2):109.

Harrison Narcotics Tax Act. Public Acts of the Sixty-Third Congress of the United States. Dec. 17, 1914. Full text of document available at: http://www.historicaldocuments.com/HarrisonNarcoticsTaxAct.htm. Accessed January 22, 2006.

Hill CS Jr. The barriers to adequate pain management with opioid analgesics. *Semin Oncol*, 1993; 20(2 Suppl 1):1–5.

Holtman JR, Wala EP. Characterization of morphine-induced hyperalgesia in male and female rats. *Pain*, 2005; 114: 62–70.

Joranson D, Ryan K, Gilson A, Dahl J. Trends in Medicaid use and abuse of opioid analgesics. *JAMA*, 2000; 283:1710–1714.

Juni A, Klein G, Kest B. Morphine hyperalgesia in mice is unrelated to opioid activity, analgesia, or tolerance: evidence for multiple diverse hyperalgesic systems. *Brain Res*, 2006 Jan 9: [Epub ahead of print].

Latimer D, Goldberg J. *Flowers in the blood*. New York: Franklin Watts, 1981.

Lee LE Jr. Medications in the control of pain in terminal cancer, with reference to the study of newer synthetic analgesics. *JAMA*, 1941; 116(3):217.

Marks RM, Sacher EJ. Undertreatment of medical inpatients with narcotic analgesics. *Ann Intern Med*, 1973, 78:173–181.

Morgan JP. *American Opiophobia: Customary Underutilization of Opioid Analgesia*. New York: Hawthorne. 1986; 163–173.

Musto DF. Drug abuse research in historical perspective. In Institute of Medicine (Eds.), *Pathways of addiction: opportunities in drug abuse research*. Committee on Opportunities in Drug Abuse Research, Division of Neuroscience and Behavioral Health, 1996; 284–294.

Musto DF. *The American Disease: Origins of Narcotics Control*. New York: Oxford University Press, Inc., 1999.

Osterweis M, Kleinman A, Mechanic D, Eds. Pain and disability: clinical, behavioral, and public policy perspectives. Washington, DC: National Academy Press. [*Report of the Committee on Pain, Disability, and Chronic Illness Behavior*, Institute of Medicine, National Academy of Sciences], 1987.

Porter J, Jick H. Addiction rare in patients treated with narcotics. *N Engl J Med*, 1980; 302:123.

Redmond K. Organizational barriers in opioid use. *Support Care Cancer*, 1997; 5:451–456.

Regier DA, Meyers JK, Dramer M. The NIMH epidemiologic catchment area program. Arch Gen Psychiatry 1984; 41:934–941.

Rock, PE, Ed. *Drugs and Politics*. New Brunswick: Transaction Books, 1977.

Shine D, Demas P. Knowledge of medical students, residents, and attending physicians about opioid abuse. *J Med Educ*, 1984; 59:501–507.

SUPPORT Study Principal Investigators. A controlled trial to improve care for seriously ill hospitalized patients: a study to understand prognoses and preferences for outcomes and risks of treatment (SUPPORT). *JAMA*, 1995; 274(20), 1591–1598.

Verhaak PFM, Kerssens JJ, Dekker J, Sorbi MJ, Bensing JM. Prevalence of chronic benign pain disorder among adults: A review of the literature. *Pain,* 1998; 77:231–239.

Weissman DE, Haddox JD. Opioid pseudoaddiction—an iatrogenic syndrome. *Pain,* 1989; 36(3):363–366.

Wilson GR. Morphine hyperalgesia: a case report. *End of Life Care,* 2001 May.

Workplace Substance Abuse Advisor, May 3, 2002; 16(11).

Zacny J, Bigelow G, Compton P, Foley K, Iguchi M, Sannerud C. College on problems of drug dependence taskforce on prescription opioid nonmedical use and abuse: position statement. *Drug Alcohol Depend,* 2003; 69(3):215–232.

2

The Language of Pain and Addiction

Seddon R. Savage

Language is a prism through which we understand—and communicate our understanding of—the world. Although it is currently common to depreciate the power of words by labeling thoughtful word selection as political correctness, the resonance of words in shaping perceptions at both cognitive and affective levels is clear. Care in the use of language is particularly important in communication related to issues about which there is pervasive misunderstanding, significant controversy, and in which rapid change is occurring. Understanding in such contexts is best served by language that is unambiguous, accurate, and free of emotional resonance or stigma.

The interface of pain, opioid analgesic therapy, and substance use problems demands particular care in communication and language selection; understanding in the three areas is rapidly changing, there is significant misunderstanding of basic concepts, many issues are controversial, and there is enormous stigma associated with substance problems and with opioid medications. Universally accepted nomenclature that is clear and unambiguous is critical, therefore, to effective communication regarding these issues. Unfortunately, nomenclature related to opioids, substance problems, and addiction remains unsettled. The World Health Organization and the American Psychiatric Association are generally viewed as authoritative sources of standardized terminology and diagnostic criteria related to health and human behavior. Their terminologies related to substance use and addiction are widely utilized, in continuing evolution, and reflect the challenges of language in this rapidly changing field. These will be discussed below.

In recent years, numerous organizations have acknowledged the challenges of substance-related language and some have attempted to address them. In the mid-1980s, in response to concerns regarding the confusing nomenclature of addiction, the American Medical Association's Council on Scientific Affairs created the Panel on Alcoholism and Drug Addiction, which convened 80 experts from 20 different organizations in an attempt to reach consensus on the preferred usage and definitions of 50 terms related to substance abuse (Rinaldi et al., 1988). Despite substantive agreement on many key conceptual issues, the definitions generated by the group continued to contain significant ambiguities and inconsistencies. The persistence of such linguistic irregularities in the context of an effort designed to resolve them underscores the challenges (Savage, Joranson, et al., 2003).

In 1995 and 1996, two separate committees of the Institute of Medicine commented on the need for enhanced clarity in language related to addiction (Institute of Medicine, 1996; Rettig & Yarmolinsky, 1995). In 1999, a Liaison Committee on Pain and Addiction (LCPA), noting the deleterious impact of confusing addictions-related terminology on the management of both pain and of substance use problems, began a consensus process between the American Society of Addiction Medicine, the American Pain Society, and the American Academy of Pain Medicine to develop clear, scientifically based language that would consistently serve clinical needs. The results of this process were published (Savage, Joranson, et al., 2003). The specific challenges of addiction-related terminology in the context of pain treatment noted by the LCPA were echoed by the College of Problems of Drug Dependence Task Force on Prescription Drug Abuse in a position statement issued the same year (Zacny et al., 2003).

This chapter will address key language issues that may undermine understanding of the complex issues at the interface of pain and substance use problems and impede effective care of persons with these conditions. Specific foci of discussion will include the following:

- Substance use, misuse, and abuse
- Addiction and dependence
- Opioids, opiates, and narcotics
- Discontinuation, tapering, and detoxification
- Persons with addictive disorders, addicts, and abusers

Substance Use, Misuse, and Abuse

The term *abuse* in reference to misuse of drugs has widely varying meanings when used by different persons in different contexts. Some use the term to indicate substance behaviors that risk harm to self or others, others use it to mean use of a substance to get high or experience reward effects, and still others use it to indicate any illegal use of a substance. In the context of prescribed medications, many use the term *abuse* to mean any use of a substance for purposes other than that intended by the prescriber. This imprecision in usage of the term may lead to misunderstanding and in turn mismanagement of the circumstances that are actually present.

DSM-IV uses the term *substance abuse* to label potentially harmful misuse of substances. To meet criteria for substance abuse, an individual must demonstrate a maladaptive pattern of substance use leading to clinically significant impairment or distress, as reflected in one more of several criteria within a 12-month period. These include the following: failure to fulfill major role obligations at work, school, home; recurrent substance use in situations in which it is physically hazardous; recurrent substance-related legal problems; and/or continued substance use despite having persistent or recurrent social or interpersonal problems caused or exacerbated by the effects of the substance. This formulation is very helpful in identifying persons at risk for harm to self or others due to substance use, but it does not, in the clinical context of pain treatment, assist clinicians in understanding the underlying reasons for substance misuse and does not provide direction for resolving the misuse.

Persons misuse substances, including prescribed medications, for a variety of reasons, among them: to self-medicate depressed or anxious mood, sleep disturbance, or traumatic memories; to experience euphoria or reward (a rush or a high); to satisfy an addictive drive to use; to avoid physiologic withdrawal; or to sell for profit (Savage 1993; Zacny et al., 2003). Fusing these diverse forms of misuse under the term *abuse* does not help distinguish reasons for misuse and therefore imparts no information on which to base appropriate clinical responses. In addition, when medications are misused the object of actual abuse is most often the user, not the drug, so the term is conceptually inaccurate, even amusing. Finally, the term *abuse* has pejorative resonance that does not foster dispassionate and medically focused management of the problem.

Framing medication misuse as "use for..." or "misuse for..." with an indication of the purpose (when known) is more clinically helpful. For example, concerns may arise that a patient is misusing opioid medications when she exhibits frequent requests for early renewals or reports repeated "loss" of meds; on careful evaluation, she may be found to have used extra doses to relieve anxiety related to traumatic memories. Consider the different image and understanding suggested by stating that this patient is "abusing her medications" versus that the patient is "misusing her medications to control PTSD symptoms." The former is stigmatizing and risks omission of important clinical responses to an identified problem, whereas the latter provides a path to appropriate clinical care.

In the absence of a universally accepted understanding of the term *abuse*, and in the presence of associated stigma, a brief statement of the purpose of use or misuse of drugs, including prescribed medications, is likely to be more clinically helpful than use of the broad, imprecise, and somewhat pejorative term "abuse."

Addiction and Substance Dependence

Label Selection

As scientific and clinical understanding of reward and addiction mechanisms have evolved over the past several decades, addiction has become recognized as a chronic medical condition, prone to periods of remission and exacerbation, that engages multiple brain systems in intense preoccupation with substance-induced or behavioral reward effects and that is reflected in fervent seeking of drugs, loss of control over drug use, and/or continued use despite knowledge of harm due to use. Distinct from addiction, physical dependence is recognized as an expected physiologic occurrence that develops due to neurobiologic adaptation to the presence of a drug and is characterized by the development of a drug specific withdrawal syndrome.

Physical dependence occurs to many medications including both those with potential reward (euphorogenic) effects, such as opioids or benzodiazepines, and others such as prednisone, tricyclic antidepressants, and many antihypertensive medications with no reward effects. Physical dependence on opioids develops over a period of 3 to 10 days in most persons who use opioids regularly for therapeutic or other purposes. An opioid withdrawal syndrome may occur when opioids are abruptly discontinued, tapered rapidly, or on administration of an opioid antagonist. Physical dependence may or may not be present in the context of addiction (note, for example, intermittent binge addiction to cocaine without continuous physical dependence but with crescendo/decrescendo craving), but it does not in and of itself indicate addiction. It is often present in pain treatment when opioids are used for a prolonged period.

The term *addiction* was commonly used through the mid-20th century to indicate a compulsive attachment to alcohol, opium, or other substances. Derived from the Latin *addictus* meaning "sentenced, doomed, or enslaved"—a fusion of the Latin *ad* ("to" or "toward") and *dico* ("dedicate," "consecrate," "devote"; Maddux & Desmond, 2000)—the term was used in both medical contexts and common parlance. Many medical writers in the 18th and 19th centuries, however, used other terms as well to refer to specific addictions: *drunkenness*, *inebria*, and *intemperance* commonly referred to chronic recurrent alcohol intoxication, whereas *opium habit, morphia habit, morphinism,* and *morphinomania* were some labels of opiate addiction (Maddux & Desmond, 2000).

As medical interest in addiction has evolved, efforts to refine language to reflect emerging understanding of different conditions related to drug use have also evolved. In 1952, the World Health Organization (WHO) distinguished *addiction* from *drug habituation* with reference to the perceived effects of different drugs. Addiction was understood to occur in response to morphine and morphine-like drugs that "will always produce compulsive craving, dependence, and addiction in any individual" and whose use "cannot be interrupted without significant disturbance, always psychic and sometimes physical." Habituation was understood as a less intense attachment that occurred in response to drugs "which never produce compulsive craving, yet their pharmacologic action is found desirable to some individuals... [who] readily form a habit of administration" (WHO, 1952). In 1957, WHO delineated a distinction between psychic and physical dependence (defining *physical dependence* in terms of the development of an abstinence syndrome on cessation) and defined *addiction* to include both psychic and physical dependence, whereas habituation was characterized primarily by psychological dependence (WHO, 1957a,b).

The term *drug dependence* replaced *addiction* and *habituation* in the WHO lexicon in 1964 (WHO, 1964), and this was subsequently replaced by the term *dependence syndrome* in 1998 (WHO, 1998). In 1993, recognizing confusion between physiologic and maladaptive drug dependence, WHO suggested that use of the term *withdrawal syndrome* replace *physical dependence* (WHO 1993). Reflecting WHO policy, the *International Classification of Diseases* edition 7 (*ICD-7*), published in 1957, used the terms *drug addiction* and *alcoholism* (WHO, 1957), but in 1968, *ICD* adopted the term *drug dependence* (WHO, 1968) and, subsequently in 1992, the term *dependence syndrome* (*ICD*-10; WHO, 1992). This usage persists through the time of publication.

Table 2.1. Challenges in Using *DSM-IV* Criteria to Diagnose Addiction in Opioid Analgesia

Substance Dependence Criteria	Challenges
1. Tolerance	Expected with prolonged analgesic use
2. Physical dependence/withdrawal	Expected with prolonged, regular analgesic use
3. Used in greater amounts or longer than intended	Emergence of pain may demand increase dose or prolonged use
4. Unsuccessful attempts to cut down or discontinue	Emergence of pain may deter dose taper or cessation
5. Much time spent pursuing or recovering from use	Difficulty finding pain treatment may drive time spent seeking analgesics
6. Important activities reduced or given up	(Valid criteria—activity engagement expected to increase, not decline, with pain treatment)
7. Continued use despite knowledge of persistent physical or psychological harm	(Valid criteria—no harm anticipated from analgesic opioid use for pain)

The first edition of the American Psychiatric Association's *Diagnostic and Statistical Manual of Mental Disorders* (*DSM*), published in 1952, used the terms *drug addiction* and *alcoholism*, which were both then subclassifications of sociopathic personality disturbance. After considerable debate (O'Brien, 2006), the APA adopted the term *substance dependence* and created a separate category of conditions, independent of sociopathic personality disturbance, in *DSM-II*, published in 1968. This was intended to reduce stigmatization of the condition of addiction and to be consistent with the emerging WHO and *ICD* definitions and criteria.

Unfortunately use of the term *dependence* has caused ongoing confusion between physical dependence and substance dependence (addiction). Although experts in addiction medicine and pain medicine may use care in discriminating "physical dependence" from "substance dependence," other health-care professionals, patients, and the general public, who may be less familiar with the correct meaning and usage of the terms, often perceive the terms to be interchangeable. This may result in overidentification of addiction in persons who are appropriately using opioid medications for pain and have become physically dependent. Conversely, it may result in trivialization of the disease of addiction when someone actually develops addiction to opioids and may be perceived to be simply physically dependent.

At the time of this printing, there is debate regarding whether the American Psychiatric Association should eliminate the term *dependence* in favor of *addiction* in the next edition of *DSM*. It has been pointed out that, despite the authoritative standards of WHO, *ICD*, and *DSM* that dictate use of the term *dependence*, many respected organizations, such as the American Society of Addiction Medicine and the American Academy of Addiction Psychiatry, and many respected journals in the field, such as *Addiction* and *Journal of Addictive Diseases*, persist in using the term *addiction*, suggesting at a strong subcurrent or resonance that favors use of this term (Maddux & Desmond, 2000). Indeed, numerous published articles on the subject have favored return to the term *addiction* (Heit, 2002; Maddux & Desmond, 2000; O'Brien et al., 2006; Rettig & Yarmolinsky, 1995; Savage, Joranson, et al., 2003; Zacny et al., 2003).

Identification of Addiction

The diagnosis of addiction (substance dependence) using *DSM-IV-TR* requires that an individual meet three of seven defined criteria over a period of 6 months. Five of the seven criteria can easily be met by patients using opioids for the treatment of pain who have no aberrant behaviors that experts would identify as reflecting addiction (Sees and Clark 1993; see Table 2.1). Therefore, it has been recommended that when *DSM-IV-TR* is used to assess for addiction in persons using opioids for pain, only the two criteria that refer to function be used. *DSM-IV-TR* does contain clear notation that the criteria related to physiologic dependence and withdrawal cannot be reliably used with patients using prescription medications that produce these conditions; however, this fine print is not uniformly honored in practice, and many patients are identified as addicted in part based on meeting these criteria (APA, 2000).

The American Society of Addiction Medicine, the American Pain Society, and the American Academy of Pain Medicine (1988) have jointly developed and published a definition of addiction that relies on clear functional criteria to identify addiction. These include impaired control over drug use, continued use despite harm, preoccupation with use, and craving. Many clinicians find that observation for behaviors indicating these criteria is helpful in understanding whether use of opioids prescribed for pain is adaptive and therapeutic, or potentially suggestive of addiction (Table 2.2).

Opioids, Opiates, and Narcotics

Opioid medications are a diverse group of alkaloid drugs that act at opioid receptors in the central and peripheral nervous systems. Opioids have diverse actions including the following: analgesia, inhibition of smooth muscle, shift in CO_2 response with ventilatory depression, and neuroendocrine effects. Some opioids, such as morphine, codeine, and heroin, are naturally occurring derivatives of *Papaver somniferum*, the opium poppy, whereas others, such as hydrocodone and oxycodone, are synthesized from naturally occurring components of opium. Other opioids are entirely synthetic, such as meperidine, fentanyl, propoxyphene, and methadone, and may have relatively little structural similarity to naturally occurring or semisynthetic opiates though they exhibit similar actions on opioids receptors. The term *opioid*, meaning "opiumlike," is an inclusive term, referring to all substances with opiumlike effects. Opioid medications that are derived or synthesized from opium (natural or semisynthetic opioids) are more correctly termed

Table 2.2. Addiction

A primary, chronic, neurobiologic disease with genetic, psychosocial, and environmental factors influencing its development and manifestations characterized by behaviors that include one or more of the following:

ASAM-APS-AAPM Behavioral Criteria	Examples of Specific Behaviors
Impaired control over use, compulsive use	Frequent loss/theft reported, calls for early renewals, withdrawal noted at appointments
Continued use despite harm due to use	Declining function, intoxication, persistently sedated
Preoccupation with use, craving	Nonopioid interventions ignored, recurrent requests for opioid increase in absence of disease progression despite titration

Source: American Society of Addiction Medicine, American Pain Society, American Academy of Pain Medicine, 1998.

opiates, though some agencies—including the U.S. Drug Enforcement Agency (Controlled Substances Act, 2002)—refer to all opioids as "opiates."

The term *narcotic* is derived from the Greek *narkoun* and *narkotikos*, meaning "to make numb or stupefy" (*Webster's Third International Dictionary*, 1993). In a medical context, a "narcotizing" substance is one that induces a state of narcosis, "a state of stupor, unconsciousness, or arrested activity" (Controlled Substances Act, 2002). In a legal and criminal justice context in the United States, "narcotic" refers to a number of illicit substances including heroin and cocaine (Controlled Substances Act, 2002); because of its association with illicit substance use, the term *narcotic* implies illicit or criminal behavior.

The use of the term *narcotics* to refer to "opioid" medications is common but problematic in a number of important ways. First, because "narcotizing" medications are medically expected to cause a stuporous state with reduced activity, the term perpetuates the misperception that appropriately used opioid medications often cause sedation or cognitive blurring; although this is sometimes true on initiation or titration of therapeutic opioids or with their misuse, persons using opioids appropriately on a long-term basis seldom experience persistence of these effects. Opioids are, in contrast, expected to help patients become more active and increase their engagement in valued life functions as a result of pain relief.

Second, because of its association with illicit activities, the use of the term *narcotic* to indicate opioid medications perpetuates stigma by conjuring a sense that the medications are illicit and by logical extension, the persons who use them, criminal. In fact, many patients who use opioids for pain management report that they feel they are often treated with suspicion or disapproval, "like criminals," in many of their encounters with health-care providers.

Finally, the term *narcotic* is frequently used in association with words connoting adverse outcomes, such as "dangerous narcotics," "narcotics addiction," or "narcotics addict." Because these concepts (*dangerous* and *addiction*) often resonate silently when the word *narcotic* is used, the term suggests that clinical harm and addiction may be common outcomes of use. Although inappropriate use of opioids may result in adverse outcomes, when used as prescribed, opioids are generally safe and effective medications.

Opioid is a scientifically accurate term when used to indicate medications that provide analgesia through actions on opioid receptors. The term *opioid* does not inappropriately suggest narcotizing effects and is relatively free of unwarranted connotations of illicitness or danger. The use of the term *narcotic* should be discouraged when reference to opioid medications is intended.

Discontinuation, Tapering, and Detoxification

When the term *detoxification* is used to indicate discontinuation of medications or other drugs, it suggests the substance being discontinued is toxic in some way to the individual using it. This may be appropriate in describing cessation of a substance to which an individual has become addicted and which is, by definition, causing harm or toxicity. The term is misleading, however, to describe elective discontinuation of a medication that was simply not effective for the purpose prescribed and/or to which an individual has developed a physiologic dependency expected as a result of long-term use. Used in the context of therapeutically prescribed opioids, it reinforces the perception that persons who use opioids for treatment and/or who are physically dependent on the medications are necessarily addicted because "detoxification" is the term most often used to describe drug withdrawal in the context of addiction treatment.

Gradual discontinuation, tapering, and *weaning* are terms more commonly used to describe the cessation of other medications, such as beta blockers, antihypertensives, or tricyclics, that cannot be stopped abruptly due to the potential for adverse physiologic effects. Use of these terms is preferred to indicate cessation of opioids in the context of pain treatment when addiction or other toxic states are not present. These terms do not imply the individual is in a state of toxicity, and they do not reinforce the perception of opioids as medications that routinely cause addiction or other toxicity; they simply describe the process of medication cessation.

Persons With Addictive Disorders, Addicts, and Substance Abusers

It is not uncommon, as a type of shorthand, to refer to an individual, or group of individuals, by a single prominent feature. When the reference is to a respected attribute, —such as leader, award-winner, or athlete—there is generally no protest and probably little harm (though overreliance on such labels may distort a realistic perception of the individual). When the attribute reflects a prominent personal challenge, such as a developmental or physical disability or the disease of addiction, use of labels such as *retard*, *quad*, or *addict* may evoke a series of assumptions and images that stigmatize the individual and, in a clinical context, impede appropriate and respectful care. In the medical context, patient labels have been demonstrated to have significant impact on the patient-provider relationship (Deber et al., 2005).

In addition to conjuring only one aspect of the individual, in the context of a more complex persona, the terms *addict* and *abuser* carry a connotation suggestive of illicit drug use and associated crime, which may or may be present in a given medical context. Illicit drug use or criminal behaviors have important clinical implications and should be clearly specified, when present, rather than passively implied. Routine use of the terms *addict* and *abuser* to indicate, respectively, someone with an addictive disorder and someone misusing his or her medications, inappropriately stigmatizes patients, especially those whose addiction or misuse of medications does not include illicit or criminal behavior.

It is medically appropriate to refer to an individual with an addictive disorder as just that—"a person with addiction/addictive disorder/substance use disorder"—or a "person who is misusing medications or drugs." Routine use of the terms *addict* and *abuser* serves to reinforce a generalized image and understanding of individuals with substance use disorders that does not serve individualized and appropriate care of patients.

In summary, debate over the best choices of words to indicate different conditions and behaviors related to medication use and misuse will undoubtedly continue into the future as science and clinical practice modify understanding of these phenomena. Most important is that clinicians consider both the meaning and the complex resonance of the words they use and select their words with care; often as much is communicated by the innuendo of words as by their formally accepted meaning.

References

American Psychiatric Association (1952). *Diagnostic and Statistical Manual of Mental Disorders* [*DSM*]. Washington DC: Author.

American Psychiatric Association (1968). *Diagnostic and Statistical Manual of Mental Disorders*, 2nd ed. [*DSM-II*]. Washington DC: Author.

American Psychiatric Association (2000). *Diagnostic and Statistical Manual of Mental Disorders*, 4th ed. rev. [*DSM-IV-TR*]. Washington DC: Author.

American Society of Addiction Medicine, American Pain Society, American Academy of Pain Medicine (1998). "Public policy statement on definitions related to the use of opioids in pain treatment." *Journal of Addictive Diseases* 17(2): 129–33.

Controlled Substances Act (2002). *Code of Federal Regulations* 21:Chapter 13, Section 802.

Deber RB, Kraetschmer N, Urowitz S, Sharpe N (2005). "Patient, consumer, client, or customer: what do people want to be called?" *Health Expectations* 8(4): 345–351.

Heit, H (2002). "Addiction, physical dependence, and tolerance: precise definitions to help clinicians evaluate and treat chronic pain patients." 1–12.

Institute of Medicine (1996). *Pathways of Addiction*. Washington DC: National Academy Press.

Maddux JF, Desmond DP (2000). "Addiction or dependence?" *Addiction* 95(5): 661–665.

O'Brien CP, VN, Li TK (2006). "What's in a word? Addiction versus dependence in *DSM-IV*." *American Journal of Psychiatry* 163: 764–765.

Rettig RA, Yarmolinsky A. (1995). *Federal Regulation of Methadone*. Washington DC: National Academy Press.

Rinaldi RC, Steindler EM, Wilford B, Goodwin D (1988). "Clarification and standardization of substance abuse terminology." *JAMA* 259(4): 555–557.

Savage, S (1993). "Addiction in the treatment of pain: significance, recognition and treatment." *Journal of Pain and Symptom Management* 8(5): 265–278.

Savage S, Joranson D, et al. (2003). "Definitions related to the medical use of opioids: evolution towards universal agreement." *Journal of Pain and Symptom Management* 26(1): 655–667.

Sees K, Clark W (1993). "Opioid use in the treatment of chronic pain: assessment of addiction." *Journal of Pain and Symptom Management* 8(5): 257–264.

Webster's Third International Dictionary, Unabridged. (1993). Springfield, Mass.: Merriam-Webster.

WHO (1952). 3rd Report. World Health Organization Committee on Addiction Producing Drugs. Geneva: Author.

WHO (1957a). 7th Report. World Health Organization Committee on Addiction Producing Drugs. Geneva: Author.

WHO (1957b). *International Classification of Diseases,* 7th revision [*ICD-7*]. Geneva: Author.

WHO (1964). *13th Report.* World Health Organization Expert Committee on Drug Dependence. Geneva: Author.

WHO (1968). *International Classification of Diseases,* 8th revision [*ICD-8*]. Geneva: Author.

WHO (1992). *International Classification of Diseases,* 10th revision [*ICD-10*]. Geneva: Author.

WHO (1993). *28th Report,* World Health Organization Expert Committee on Drug Dependence. Geneva: Author.

WHO (1998). *30th Report,* World Health Organization Expert Committee on Drug Dependence. Geneva: Author.

Zacny J, Bigelow G, Compton P, Foley K, Iguchi M, Sannerud C (2003). "College on Problems of Drug Dependence, taskforce on prescription opioid non-medical use and abuse: position statement." *Drug & Alcohol Dependence* 69: 215–232.

3

Opioids for Chronic Pain: Historical Notes

Russell K. Portenoy

The opioids comprise a very diverse set of compounds that share interaction with an array of opioid receptors throughout the body (Hammer, 1993; Stein, 1998). Endogenous opioids influence numerous physiological domains, including modulation of noxious input (antinociception), mood, immunity, motor control, and other processes. Exogenous opioids, which include alkaloids derived from the poppy and both semisynthetic and synthetic substances, produce similarly varied effects, among the most important of which is the potential to relieve pain. It is axiomatic among experts in pain management that there is no group of drugs that, overall, offer a broader and more effective means to reduce severe pain. Indeed, if not for the potential to cause serious adverse events, it is very likely that opioids would be first-line treatment for virtually all patients with moderate or greater pain.

Both the powerful medicinal properties of exogenous opioid compounds and their potential for adverse effects have been recognized for millennia. The unique challenges posed by the classes of drugs that evolved from this early use relate to the variation in responses, to pharmacological side effects that can be serious in some cases, and to the specific set of potential adverse effects known generically as abuse and dependence.

Humans exposed to opioid compounds react in dramatically varied ways. Although the potential to relieve pain appears to be shared by almost all, many individuals experience an unfavorable balance between analgesia and side effects. Equally important, a small subpopulation develops an intensely positive mood response, drug craving, and in some cases, a pattern of compulsive drug use that continues despite repeated adverse outcomes. Genetic factors are clearly important in determining some of these outcomes (Kreek et al., 2005), but abuse, like every other effect associated with the opioids, is complex and driven by many factors, including the situational context, psychological state, and ease of access to the substance.

Given the potential of opioid compounds to relieve human suffering on the one hand while becoming the focus of craving intense enough to drive antisocial behavior on the other, it is not surprising that the history of these compounds is replete with profound ambivalence and an impact that extends well beyond clinical medicine. Across countries and populations, and over thousands of years, opioid drugs have elicited a remarkable concatenation of societal, cultural, legal, and medical responses (Davenport-Hines, 2002; Meldrum, 2003; Musto, 1999). The historical context may illuminate the role of these drugs in 21st century America and help clarify the nature of the controversies that continue to surround the use of opioids in medicine.

The Early History of Opium Derivatives

The medicinal use of opium derivatives began millennia ago. A Sumerian ideogram from as long as 8,000 years ago depicted the opium poppy, an element of Papaver somniferum, as "the plant of joy." In a papyrus dated 1552 B.C., Theban physicians were instructed to use these derivatives in hundreds of potions, each addressing a medical need. Egyptian and Roman documents specifically describe the use of opium for pain relief during the 1st century A.D.

In some ancient societies, the consumption of opium alkaloids appeared to become routine. In Greece, for example, Galen observed that political leaders could distinguish the quality of the ingredients of their opioid-containing concoctions and could reduce consumption when necessary to execute their duties.

The ancients also noted the potential for adverse outcomes associated with opium derivatives. Toxicities were recorded by Arab, Greek, and Roman physicians around the 2nd century B.C., and the Roman emperor Nero took the throne from Brittanicus in A.D. 55 by using opium as a poison.

In Europe, derivatives of opium were commonly prescribed by early physicians. In the 16th century, laudanum was commonly administered by German and British physicians for a large number of physical and psychiatric problems, including pain. The highly respected 17th century English physician Thomas Sydenham was a strong proponent of this medical application and is remembered for stating: "Among the remedies which it has pleased Almighty God to give to man to relieve his sufferings, none is so universal and so efficacious as opium."

As the use of opioid compounds in Europe became widespread, medical writings began to voice concerns about their negative effects. Some physicians warned about charlatans for whom opioids became a nostrum for virtually any ill. Others described a range of problems associated with overuse, including the self-administration to alter mood, abstinence phenomena, and the occurrence of an addictive pattern of use.

Demand for opioids to meet both medical and nonmedical needs grew in Europe and other countries. This demand offered financial rewards for those who distributed opium. In the 18th century, British and other commercial interests expanded the opium trade, largely by bringing opium from India to China. This trade became a major revenue generator and offset the trade deficit produced by British imports of Chinese silk and other commodities. With increased access to imported opium, the problem of abuse increased in Chinese cities. The imperial Chinese government became increasingly concerned, and in 1800, the emperor issued a proclamation forbidding opium importation.

The opium trade continued to flourish, however, and privately owned vessels of many countries, including the United States, made huge profits from the growing number of Chinese drug users. By the late 1830s, more than 30,000 chests containing opium derivatives were being imported into China.

The British attempted to obtain more favorable trading rights to increase profits further, but the imperial government refused. The tension between the two governments escalated, and in 1839, Chinese authorities at Canton confiscated and burned opium imports. In response, the British attacked and occupied positions around Canton. The British succeeded militarily, and when the conflict concluded with the Treaty of Nanking in 1842, Hong Kong was formally ceded to Great Britain and many new ports were open to British residence and trade. These arrangements were later extended to the French and the Americans, and the opium trade continued to increase. A second opium war was fought in 1856, and again China was forced to open new ports to trading.

Beyond the extraordinary political and national implications of this early history, this conflict foreshadowed the tension between medical and regulatory issues that persists today: The medical benefits of opioid compounds are obvious, but are balanced by medical misuse, by abuse, and in a relatively small subpopulation, by addiction. The medical demand for these compounds creates legitimate business opportunities, but the subculture surrounding abuse and addiction may drive illegitimate activities. Government, with interest in regulating trade and business, and in protecting the public health by controlling the problems of abuse and addiction, can unintentionally become part of the problem by fomenting drug-related conflict.

Advances in Medical Use and the Growing Problem of Abuse

Pharmaceutical advances during the 19th century augmented the medical utility of opioid compounds, but also added to the potential for serious abuse. In 1805, Friederich Wilhelm Sertürner, an apothecary's assistant in Hanover, Germany, isolated a white crystalline powder from opium that he called *morphium* after the Greek god of dreams and sleep, Morpheus. More than a decade later, the Parisian pharmacist Pierre-Jean Robiquet perfected an extraction process for morphine, and this was soon followed by its promotion as both an analgesic and a cure for opium addiction. Commercial morphine appeared in London in 1821, and wholesale production by the German pharmacist Heinrich Emanuel Merck began a few years later.

With the development of the hypodermic syringe in the mid-19th century, morphine could be injected directly into painful areas, which were often labeled neuralgias. Ironically, the inventor of the hypodermic syringe, Dr. Alexander Wood, an Edinburgh physician, was convinced that injection of morphine, in contrast to oral ingestion, would obviate the growing problem of morphine addiction.

Diacetylmorphine was synthesized during the latter part of the 19th century by the English chemist C. R. Alder Wright. Pharmacologists at Bayer, a German pharmaceutical company, noted the positive effects of this compound, and it was marketed as a cough suppressant under the trade name Heroin. In Great Britain, orally administered and intravenously administered heroin was used by physicians as a means to wean patients who had developed an addictive pattern of morphine use. The prevalence of heroin addiction rose.

Legal and Regulatory Events in the United States

The medical and nonmedical uses of opioid compounds in the 19th century United States paralleled those occurring in Europe. Early in the 20th century, politicians began to react to increasing public concern about this use. In 1906, the federal Pure Food and Drug Act was passed. This law was the first to codify the responsibility of the government to ensure the safety and efficacy of drugs entering the U.S. market, and to regulate their use after commercialization. The regulations generated by this law dramatically changed the development and marketing of pharmaceuticals but, for some politicians, did not adequately address the problem of opioid abuse and addiction.

Just 8 years later, in 1914, Congress passed the Harrison Narcotics Act, which applied specific controls to opioid drugs. Among other features, this law prohibited physicians from prescribing opioid drugs to addicts. At the time, many physicians were prescribing opioids to addicts for the purpose of managing abstinence phenomena and the adverse behavioral consequences associated with addiction, and the law was challenged in court.

In 1919, the Supreme Court upheld the Harrison Narcotics Act in a decision known as *Webb v. United States*. This decision criminalized a large component of opioid prescribing and led to the closure of the opioid dispensing centers that had appeared in some locales. Although the use of opioids for medical indications remained legal, physicians who were alleged to prescribe to addicts could become the object of criminal investigation, and perhaps criminal sanction, and patients or others who were accused of acquiring opioids from either medical or nonmedical sources for the purpose of maintaining an addiction could be arrested as felons. The regulation of opioid drugs was increasingly viewed as being under the purview of the criminal justice system, rather than the health-care system. In 1937, the Marijuana Tax Act outlawed cannabis and heroin, adding further aspects of drug use to the criminal code.

The modern federal regulatory structures applied to opioid drugs was created in 1970, with passage of the federal Controlled Substances Act. This law established the Drug Enforcement Administration; required the registration of manufacturers, dispensers, and prescribers of controlled drugs; and further defined the boundaries of acceptable medical use of opioid drugs. The law categorized potentially abusable drugs into five schedules and stipulated regulations for each. Schedule I drugs, such as marijuana and heroin, were deemed as having no legitimate medical use, and the manufacture or distribution of any of these was drug trafficking by definition. Drugs in Schedule II, such as morphine, could not be prescribed by telephone and could not be refilled without a new written prescription. Although the Drug Enforcement Administration was not permitted to regulate medical practice, the law gave this agency a broad mandate to stem illicit drug use, including any use by physicians that exceeded the limits of these regulations.

During the years that these federal laws were being passed, a complex patchwork of state laws and regulations also was established with identical purposes. Physicians were required to adhere to both federal and state regulations when prescribing opioids and other controlled drugs, and individuals who sought these drugs for the purpose of sustaining an addiction or trafficking for profit could be prosecuted by both state and federal authorities.

Outcomes and Evolution of Medical Practice

The laws that set out to regulate the medical use of opioids and criminalize drug diversion and some aspects of opioid prescribing by professionals were intended to support the appropriate medical use of these drugs and stem the threat to the social fabric perceived to be inherent in drug abuse and addiction. It is very likely that these laws have effectively advanced toward this goal by reducing nonmedical access to opioid drugs and removing criminal elements from the street.

At the same time, however, they have encouraged other, unintended and less favorable, consequences (Meldrum, 2003; Musto, 1999). The criminalization of opioid addiction fostered an illicit drug trade that, in turn, brought organized crime and violent gangs into drug trafficking and promoted the widespread dissemination of lethal diseases, most notably HIV and hepatitis. These phenomena have led to questions about the overall effectiveness of a predominant law enforcement solution to the problem of drug abuse and addiction, and generated controversy about the appropriateness of a harm reduction approach, as epitomized by needle exchange programs.

Equally important, the intense focus on drug abuse has had profound effects on medical practice. These effects have raised concern that laws intended to protect the public health could have unintentionally harmed large populations of patients in need of treatment with opioids and other controlled prescription drugs.

Addiction medicine leaped forward with the discovery by Dole and Nyswander that the scheduled administration of methadone could reduce opioid craving, control aberrant drug-related behavior, and contribute to improved functioning (Dole & Nyswander, 1965). These findings, which have been repeatedly confirmed, were a medical watershed and led to regulations establishing a special medical license for the prescribing of methadone for addiction and the creation of methadone maintenance treatment programs. The broad acceptance of this therapy, which is clearly justified by the science, has been impeded by the stigma associated with drug abuse and a complex regulatory framework that established treatment programs outside of mainstream medicine. Although the potential value of office-based opioid treatment for addiction is now being recognized with the advent of buprenorphine therapy in the United States, access to care is still limited, and drug therapy for addiction remains stigmatized by its historical associations.

The underuse of opioid drugs for the treatment of pain became a major issue in the 1980s, following the publication by the World Health Organization of a model for the treatment of cancer pain known as the "analgesic ladder" (World Health Organization, 1998). Numerous studies yielded strong evidence that opioids were not being appropriately prescribed to cancer patients, for whom opioids were widely considered appropriate, and that prescribers' fear of regulatory scrutiny was one of many factors responsible for this underuse (Weinstein et al., 2000).

Pain specialists began to actively debate the appropriateness of opioid prescribing to the larger population of patients with severe chronic pain, including those with highly prevalent disorders such as low back pain and headache. Although this debate continues to the present, pain specialists reached consensus that opioid drugs are indeed appropriate therapy for a carefully selected subset patients with chronic pain (http://www.ampainsoc.org/advocacy/opioids.htm). The development of this consensus drove a national effort on the part of professional societies and others, which had initially focused on cancer pain and then expanded, to educate physicians about the use of opioids in pain management. Much of this education was underwritten by the pharmaceutical industry and coincided with the release of several long-acting opioid formulations that rapidly became preferred for chronic pain management.

In the 1980s and 1990s, further organized efforts began to reduce the negative legal and regulatory effects on legitimate opioid prescribing. This included the passage of laws in many states that purported to provide a "safe harbor" for physician prescribing in a medical context. Although the effectiveness of these laws in changing physician behavior is in doubt, they made a strong statement about the societal acceptance of opioid therapy for pain. Media reports and the activities of patient advocacy groups furthered the impression that a major change was occurring.

By 2000, the use of opioid drugs to treat chronic pain of all types had begun to increase dramatically. Initially, epidemiological data seemed to suggest that this increase was not associated with any rise in indicators of drug abuse (Joranson et al., 2000). Pain specialists and many in the pharmaceutical industry were relieved by this evidence, which appeared to justify the educational focus on undertreatment, rather than the assessment and management of risk.

Unfortunately, the initial positive impressions were tempered by a growing number of reports highlighting the problem of prescription drug abuse. The abuse of modified-release oxycodone was recognized in endemic regions of the United States, and the media coverage of this problem was intensive and resonant with the historical view of opioids as inherently dangerous to the public health. This media coverage raised an equally intense reaction among politicians and those in the law enforcement and regulatory communities.

To some extent, both the reports of prescription drug abuse and the calls for draconian action on the part of regulators and politicians took pain specialists by surprise. The first reaction was confusion or opposition to plans that were perceived to potentially sacrifice the needs of patients in pain to the goal of reducing illicit access to prescription opioids. Gradually, however, pain specialists and the medical community overall began to acknowledge the need to address the risk of abuse, addiction, and diversion associated with expanded medical use of opioids. With new epidemiological data confirming that prescription drug abuse had indeed increased (Gilson et al., 2004), health professionals recognized the importance of including a more effective approach to risk as a fundamental element in the medical use of opioids.

For some pain specialists and regulators, a new paradigm could be articulated: The public health is best served when a "principle of balance" guides the approach to opioids and other controlled prescription drugs. When applied to opioid drugs at the highest level, this principle implies that those in the regulatory community must explicitly acknowledge the essential medical role for opioid drugs and pursue no policy or regulation that could unintentionally worsen the undertreatment of pain, whereas those in the medical community must recognize the appropriate need for regulation to address the problem of abuse and addiction, and assist in reducing these outcomes. When viewed at a patient care level, balance implies that clinicians must understand that the safe and effective prescribing of opioid drugs requires competencies in *both* the pharmacologic principles of prescribing and in the process of risk management, as guided by the basic principles of addiction medicine.

Events during the past few years may be evaluated against this principle of balance. The goal of balance clearly informed the creation of the excellent Model Guidelines for the Use of Controlled Substances for the Treatment of Pain by the Federation of State Medical Boards (http://www.fsmb.org). This document may be applied both by prescribers and the regulators who assess allegations of inappropriate care. A recent "report card" published by the University of Wisconsin's Pain and Policy Studies Group describes many positive changes at the state level, but demonstrates that there is still considerable room for improvement (http://www.painpolicy.wisc.edu/).

This pursuit of balance by informed medical professionals and regulators is a fragile process. A period of increasing collaboration between the Drug Enforcement Administration and pain specialists, which in 2002 culminated in the publication of a consensus statement endorsing the principle of balance (http://www.ampainsoc.org/advocacy/promoting.htm), recently went awry when the DEA withdrew its support from an educational document ("Frequently Asked Questions") and undertook several high profile physician prosecutions. There is new concern about the federal commitment to the principle of balance and increasing recognition that progress in building consensus about the proper role of opioids in society cannot be taken for granted.

The Future

There is now compelling evidence that opioid drugs are extraordinarily effective therapies for a range of maladies, the most significant of which are unrelieved pain and opioid addiction. The past 25 years has witnessed considerable progress in highlighting the problem of undertreatment and expanding appropriate opioid therapy to new populations. It is still very likely, however, that many patients with pain and many with addiction have not had the opportunity to benefit because of inadequate clinician knowledge, fear of regulatory oversight, and stigma. The medical community must become educated about the appropriate clinical use of the various opioid formulations, fully destigmatize these therapies, and vigorously defend patient access to appropriate care.

For clinicians who treat pain, however, there is a concomitant obligation to accept the need for balance and actively engage in the assessment and management of abuse, addiction, and diversion. Recognizing the potential for abuse and endorsing the need to manage risk does not minimize or exacerbate the problem of undertreatment. It is a necessary step by which undertreatment can be safely and effectively addressed.

References

Davenport-Hines R. *The Pursuit of Oblivion: A Global History of Narcotics.* New York: W. W. Norton & Company; 2002.

Dole VP, Nyswander M. A medical treatment for diacetylmorphine (heroin) addiction: a clinical trial with methadone hydrochloride. *J Amer Med Assoc.* 1965; 193: 646–650.

Gilson AM, Ryan KM, Joranson DE, Dahl JL. A reassessment of trends in the medical use and abuse of opioid analgesics and implications for diversion control: 1997–2002. *J Pain Symptom Manage.* Aug. 2004; 28(2):176–88.

Hammer RP (Ed.): *The Neurobiology of Opiates.* Boca Raton, FL: CRC Press; 1993.

Joranson DE, Ryan KM, Gilson AM, Dahl JL. Trends in medical use and abuse of opioid analgesics. *JAMA.* 2000; 283:1710–4.

Kreek MJ, Bart G, Lilly C, LaForge KS, Nielsen DA. Pharmacogenetics and human molecular genetics of opiate and cocaine addictions and their treatments. *Pharmacol Rev.* 2005; 57(1):1–26.

Meldrum M, ed. *Opioids and Pain Relief: A Historical Perspective* (Progress in Pain Research and Management, Vol. 25). Seattle, WA: IASP Press; 2003.

Musto DF. *The American Disease: Origins of Narcotic Control*, 3rd ed. Oxford, England: Oxford University Press; 1999.

Stein C, ed. *Opioids in Pain Control: Basic and Clinical Aspects.* Cambridge: Cambridge University Press; 1998.

Weinstein SM, Laux LF, Thornby JI, et al. Physicians' attitudes toward pain and the use of opioid analgesics: results of a survey from the Texas Cancer Pain Initiative. *South Med J.* 2000; 93:479–87.

World Health Organization. *Cancer pain relief and palliative care in children.* Geneva, Switzerland: World Health Organization; 1998.

Related Web Sites

http://www.ampainsoc.org/advocacy/opioids.htm
http://www.fsmb.org
http://www.medsch.wisc.edu/painpolicy
http://www.ampainsoc.org/advocacy/promoting.htm

4

The Growth of Prescription Opioid Abuse

Sandra D. Comer

Judy B. Ashworth

Data from various sources suggest that the abuse of prescription opioids has risen dramatically in the United States since the mid-1990s. The National Survey on Drug Use and Health (NSDUH), previously known as the National Household Survey on Drug Abuse, is one such source that surveys the civilian, non-institutionalized population of the United States aged 12 years or older and is designed to determine national estimates of rates of use, numbers of users, and other measures related to illicit drugs, alcohol, and tobacco products. As depicted in Figure 4.1, this survey revealed that the initiation of the nonmedical use of prescription pain relievers has quadrupled, from an incidence of 573,000 in 1990 to an astounding 2.5 million in 2002 (SAMHSA, 2004a). Taken in the larger context of substance abuse, the estimated number of new initiates in 2004 to nonmedical use of pain relievers (2.4 million) exceeded even that of illicit drugs such as marijuana (2.1 million) and cocaine (1 million; SAMHSA, 2005a).

The Monitoring the Future (MTF) project, funded by the National Institute on Drug Abuse and previously known as the National High School Senior Survey, is a serial survey of high school students that has been conducted yearly since 1975 by the University of Michigan Survey Research Center. Initially, the survey sampled only 12th graders, but in 1991 it was expanded to include 8th and 10th graders. The most recent data from the 2005 survey showed high rates of nonmedical use of prescription medications, especially opioid painkillers, despite an otherwise general decline in the abuse of illicit drugs among this population (Johnston et al., 2006).

Additional evidence supporting a growth in prescription opioid abuse comes from the Treatment Episode Data Set (TEDS), which is part of the Substance Abuse and Mental Health Services Administration's Drug and Alcohol Services Information System (DASIS). TEDS provides a compilation of data on the demographic and substance abuse characteristics of admissions to substance abuse treatment and consists of data on almost 2 million admissions reported by over 10,000 facilities in the 50 states, District of Columbia, and Puerto Rico over the 12-month period of a calendar year. The proportion of TEDS admissions for primary opiate abuse increased from 13% in 1993 to 18% in 2003. Although heroin represented 84% of all primary opiate admissions in 2003, non-heroin opiates represented an increasing proportion of admissions for opiate abuse, from 7% in 1993 to 16% in 2003. The admission rate for prescription opioids increased by 233% between 1993 and 2003, from 6 per 100,000 population aged 12 and over to 20 per 100,000. Focusing only on new users, defined as those seeking treatment within 3 years of beginning use, there was a substantial increase in the proportion of new users of prescription opioids, from 26% in 1997 to 39% in 2002 (SAMHSA, 2005b).

The Drug Abuse Warning Network (DAWN) is a public health surveillance system that was established in 1972 to monitor drug-related visits to hospital emergency departments as well as drug-related deaths investigated by medical examiners and coroners. Though a redesign of DAWN in 2003 makes it no longer possible to compare trends from the "old DAWN" with the "new DAWN," trend analysis can be made from 1972 through 2002. From 1995 to 2002, drug abuse-related emergency department visits involving narcotic analgesics increased over 2.5 times, from 42,857 to 108,320 (Figure 4.2). More specifically, there was a 159% increase in hydrocodone mentions, 176% increase in methadone mentions, and 512% increase in oxycodone mentions (SAMHSA, 2004b). In the 2003 DAWN report, opiates/opioid analgesics represented roughly 17% of abuse-related admissions (SAMHSA, 2004c).

Taken together, these data reveal that there is a continuing trend toward increasing abuse of prescription opioids in the United States and that this increase has resulted in sharp rises in morbidity and mortality at the local and national levels.

What Are the Characteristics of Prescription Opioid Abusers?

Age

The prevalence of substance abuse among adolescents and young adults is a source of much concern. In the introduction to the White House's 2004 update on its National Drug Control Policy, an 11% reduction in youth drug abuse over a 2-year span was cited based on 2001–2003 data from Monitoring the Future. This decrease exceeded the president's stated goal of reducing youth drug abuse by 10% in 2 years as noted in his 2002 State of the Union Address. Though this observation was encouraging, it did

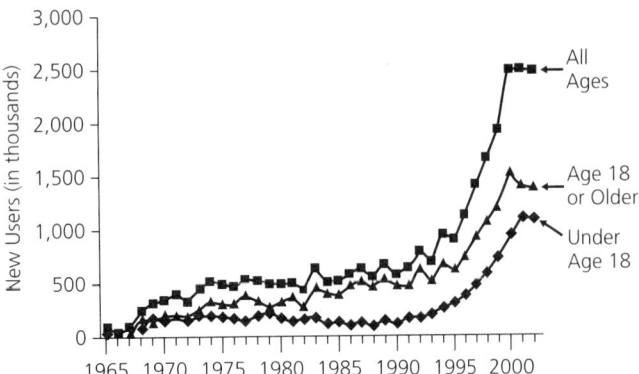

Figure 4.1. Annual numbers of new nonmedical users of pain relievers, 1965–2002. Source: SAMHSA, 2004a.

not acknowledge the fact that in the same time frame, with data collected in the same survey, an increase in youth prescription opioid drug abuse was seen.

In this survey, the lifetime prevalence of abuse of nonheroin opioids among 12th graders, the only grade for which data on prescription opioid abuse was collected, increased from 9.9% in 2001 to 13.2% in 2003. In fact, from 1992 through 2004, a fairly steady increase in the lifetime prevalence of misuse of opiates other than heroin can be seen. Trends in the annual prevalence of these drugs among 12th graders have risen from 3.3% in 1992 to 9.5% in 2004. OxyContin misuse, monitored specifically along with Vicodin since 2002, rose from 4% to 5% in a 2-year span from 2002 through 2004 despite a more modest increase from 9.4% to 9.5% for all nonheroin narcotics combined during the same time period (Johnston et al., 2005). And although the most recent data from the 2005 survey showed a continuing general decline in the abuse of other illicit drugs, high rates of nonmedical use of prescription medications, especially opioid painkillers, were sustained (Johnston et al., 2006).

Data from TEDS also suggest an increase in the abuse of prescription opioids among youth. TEDS data reveal a 61% increase in adolescent admissions (aged 12 to 17) for substance abuse treatment between 1993 and 2003. Though the increase was largely accounted for by the increase in the number of adolescent primary marijuana admissions, the number of adolescent primary nonheroin opiate admissions increased by 860% in this time period, mostly driven by steep increases starting in 1999 (SAMHSA, 2005b).

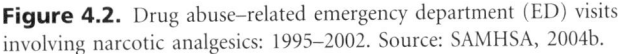

Figure 4.2. Drug abuse–related emergency department (ED) visits involving narcotic analgesics: 1995–2002. Source: SAMHSA, 2004b.

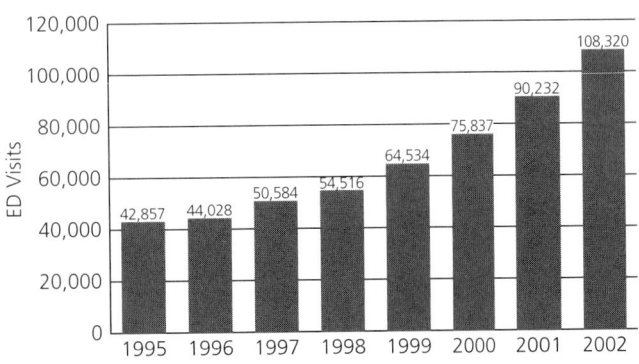

As adolescents enter into young adulthood, their rates of substance abuse also increase, including that of prescription opioids. Data from NSDUH 2004 indicate that the prevalence of lifetime nonmedical use of prescription opioids is highest in the young adult age group (18 to 25 years) at 24.3% compared to 11.4% for the 12–17 age group and 19.2% for the 26 years of age and older group. There is also evidence that in young adults, abuse rates of these products are on the rise. NSDUH 2004 reveals that from 2002 to 2004, there have been increases in lifetime prevalence of use of most prescription opioids (including Vicodin, Lortab, Lorcet; Percocet, Percodan, Tylox, and OxyContin) among 18- to 25-year-olds (SAMHSA, 2005a).

Gender

The 2003 NSDUH report, consistent with prior years, showed that although men were more likely to report current illicit drug use than women (10.0% vs. 6.5%), the rates of nonmedical use of any prescription-type psychotherapeutic, including prescription opioids, were quite similar for males (2.7%) and females (2.6%). Similarly, although boys aged 12 to 17 years had a higher rate of marijuana use than girls (8.6% vs. 7.2%), the rates of nonmedical use of any prescription-type psychotherapeutics were 4.2% for girls and 3.7% for boys, a difference that was not found to be statistically significant (SAMHSA, 2004a).

Trend analysis from TEDS 1993–2003 likewise reveals that although males represented a much larger percentage of admissions for heroin compared to females (67.9% vs. 32.1%, respectively), a much smaller difference was seen in admissions for other opiates (53.3% vs. 46.7%, respectively; SAMHSA, 2005b). Thus, a gender difference in the abuse of prescription opioids appears to be minimal.

Race and Ethnicity

According to data from NSDUH 2004, American Indians and Alaska Natives, grouped together, have the highest rate of lifetime nonmedical use of prescription opioids (18.1%), followed by non-Hispanic Whites (14.6%), Hispanics or Latinos (10.9%), and non-Hispanic Blacks or African Americans (9.0%; SAMHSA, 2005a). The seemingly contradictory low percentage (1.4) of treatment admissions for prescription opioids for American Indians and Alaska Natives found in TEDS 2003 (SAMHSA, 2005b) can be explained by their relatively small population size, estimated to be only 1.5% of the entire U.S. population (U.S. Census Bureau, 2002). Non-Hispanic Whites represented the vast majority of treatment admissions for nonheroin opiates (88.7%) followed by non-Hispanic Blacks (4.8%) and persons of Hispanic origin (3.4%). The lowest rate of lifetime nonmedical use of prescription opioids was seen among Asians at 6.2% (SAMHSA, 2005a).

Geographical Regions

The incidence of abuse and diversion of prescription opioids has been shown to have regional variances, though direct comparisons between states and regions are difficult to make based on the monitoring systems currently available. For instance, records from TEDS indicate where persons entered treatment, not their area of residence. As not all counties have substance abuse treatment facilities, people may seek treatment at an urbanization level different from where they actually live. With this caveat in mind, Figure 4.3, summarizing data from TEDS 2002, illustrates that although treatment admission rates for narcotic painkillers increased between 1992 and 2002 in the United States as a whole and at all levels of urbanization, the increase was smallest in large central metropolitan

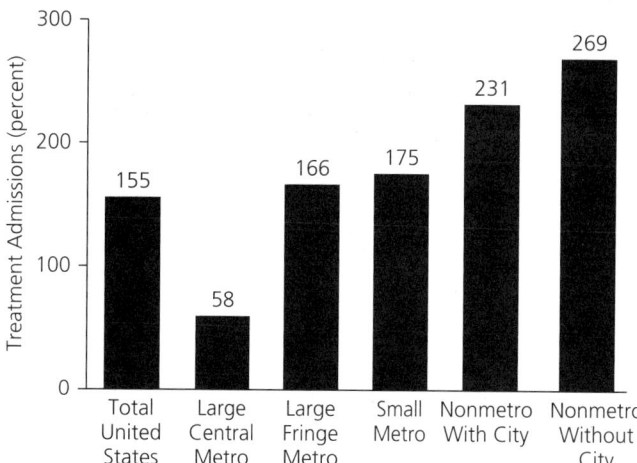

Figure 4.3. Increase in rates of treatment admissions involving narcotic painkillers, by urbanization: 1992–2002. Source: SAMHSA, 2004d.

areas (58%), and greatest in the most rural areas—that is, nonmetropolitan areas without a city (269%; SAMHSA, 2004d).

Data from NSDUH 2002 also suggest that large metropolitan areas have slightly lower rates of prescription opioid abuse than smaller areas. In this survey, it was seen that those living in small metropolitan areas (0.9%) were more likely than persons living in large metropolitan areas (0.5%) or nonmetropolitan areas (0.5%) to be dependent on or have reported past-year use of prescription pain relievers (SAMHSA, 2003a). These findings support the theory that, at least for "hard-core" opioid abusers, variability in prescription opioid abuse is at least in part influenced by the availability, purity, and cost of heroin in a given region. The well-publicized outbreak of OxyContin abuse in the late 1990s in more rural areas of the Appalachians was attributed in part to the lack of high quality, affordable heroin, thus leading to its nickname "hillbilly heroin." In fact, there is a long history of prescription opioid abuse in this region that predates the introduction of OxyContin to the U.S. market.

Nevertheless, in today's information age, regional trends can quickly become nationwide phenomena by a few simple clicks of a mouse. Dedicated Internet forums and chat rooms provide substance abusers worldwide with a means to both seek and give advice on various substances and methods of abuse. Likewise, media attention, even if well intended, can also contribute to the increase in prescription opioid abuse through widely broadcast or published reports on how these products are being abused.

Patient Groups

Although it is widely believed that opioid abuse occurring as a result of pain therapy (iatrogenic opioid abuse) is rare, opioid abuse among pain patients does exist. Chabal and colleagues (1997) found that 34% of all pain patients who were using chronic opiates met at least one criterion for opioid abuse, based on *DSM-III-R* parameters, and 28% met three or more criteria.

Michna and colleagues (2004) also reported high rates of opioid abuse among patients treated at a hospital-based pain management center: Among 145 patients taking opioids for pain, 26% had multiple, unsanctioned dose escalations, 23% reported episodes of lost or stolen medications, 14% made frequent visits to the pain clinic and/or emergency room, and 13% had family members who made contact with the physician to express concern with the patient's use of opioid medications. Katz and colleagues (2003) similarly reported high rates of substance abuse among pain patients chronically treated with opioids: Of 122 patients receiving long-term therapy with opioids, 43% had either one or more aberrant drug-taking behaviors or positive urine toxicologies for an illicit drug, a nonprescribed controlled drug, or ethanol. These data suggest that prescription opioid abuse may be occurring in a significantly higher percentage of chronic pain patients than previously estimated.

Which Prescription Opioids Are Being Abused?

From 2003 to 2004, there were significant increases in the lifetime prevalence of use in several categories of pain relievers among those aged 18 to 25, the group in which prescription opioid abuse is most prevalent. Specific pain relievers with statistically significant increases in lifetime use were Vicodin, Lortab, or Lorcet (from 15.0% to 16.5%); Percocet, Percodan, or Tylox (from 7.8% to 8.7%); hydrocodone products (from 16.3% to 17.4%); OxyContin (from 3.6% to 4.3%); and oxycodone products (from 8.9% to 10.1%; SAMHSA, 2005a). Although hydrocodone products have higher rates of abuse, data from TEDS 2003 (SAMHSA, 2005b) reveal that treatment admissions for which the primary substance was listed as oxycodone (2,587) far outnumbered those listed for hydrocodone (9).

The number of persons reporting use of OxyContin for nonmedical purposes at least once in their lifetime increased from 221,000 in 1999 to 399,000 in 2000 to 957,000 in 2001 (SAMHSA, 2002). Data from DAWN reveal that the number of single-entity oxycodone mentions increased from 100 in 1996 (the year OxyContin was launched) to 14,996 in 2002 (SAMHSA, 2003b). Incidents of diversion of OxyContin from pharmacies were presented in a 2003 report from the Drug Enforcement Administration (DEA) entitled "OxyContin Theft and Loss Incidents" (U.S. DEA, 2003). This report tallied instances of nighttime break-ins, armed robberies, employee pilferage, customer theft, and lost-in-transit. It revealed that in a 2-year period, from 2000 to 2002, the number of such incidents increased from 432 (totaling 218,339 dosage units) to 905 (totaling 506,711 dosage units).

Many factors potentially contributed to the abuse and diversion of OxyContin. Oxycodone itself is a potent opioid analgesic that historically has been shown to be an attractive target for abuse and diversion. The OxyContin controlled-release formulation of oxycodone provided a relatively high dose in a tablet intended to provide 12 hours of pain relief. Unfortunately, given the ease with which the tablet could be tampered, abusers quickly learned how to circumvent the slow-release mechanism and access the entire dose at once. In fact, the original label's safety warning advising patients not to crush the tablets because of the possible rapid release of a potentially toxic amount of oxycodone may have inadvertently alerted abusers to possible methods for misuse.

Why Have Rates of Prescription Opioid Abuse Increased?

There are many potential explanations as to why prescription opioid abuse has undergone such a dramatic increase over the past several years. One is that of availability. Although there was an overall increase in the number of prescriptions written across most drug classes between 1992 and 2002, data analyzed in a special 2005 report from the National Center on Addiction and Drug Abuse at Columbia University on prescription drug abuse showed that the rate of increase in the number of prescriptions written for scheduled drugs was 12 times higher than the rate of increase in the U.S. population itself and three times higher than the rate of increase in the number of prescriptions written for nonscheduled medications.

According to this 2002 report, entitled "Under the Counter: The Diversion and Abuse of Controlled Prescription Drugs in the U.S.," opioids represented the vast majority of these prescriptions (152.8 million), followed by CNS depressants (58.2 million) and CNS stimulants (23.4 million). For opioids, this amounts to a 222% increase from 1992 to 2002 in the number of prescriptions filled (CASA, 2005). On the positive side, this trend reflects efforts and improvements in proper pain management and an acceptance by many practitioners of the appropriate role of opiates in the treatment of nonmalignant pain. On the negative side, the availability of an abusable drug affects its rate of abuse as well as its street value. Those that are widely available, easy to come by, and relatively inexpensive may have higher rates of abuse.

In an analysis by Zacny and colleagues (2003), the ratio of DAWN emergency department mentions for oxycodone to prescriptions dispensed markedly increased in 2000 and 2001 by 39% and 108%, respectively. From 1994 to 1999, this ratio had remained relatively stable. By comparison, the ratio for hydrocodone remained stable over the entire 8-year period with the increase in emergency department mentions rising proportionately with the increase in number of prescriptions dispensed.

There is also some speculation that the media focus on OxyContin abuse in the late 1990s and early 2000s may have exaggerated the situation, which, at the time, was thought to be largely confined to rural areas in Appalachia. Though this media attention no doubt led to a nationwide awareness of the problem of OxyContin abuse, it may also have inadvertently served to inform abusers across the country about this "new craze," in turn contributing to the increase in the abuse of this product.

How Are Prescription Opioids Being Abused and Diverted?

The manner in which prescription opioids are abused has also changed over the last several years. According to data from TEDS 2002, between 1992 and 2002, the route of administration of prescription opioids among prescription opioid abusers who enter treatment showed a general decrease in abuse by injecting and an increase in oral abuse (SAMHSA, 2004d). In 1992, 66% of persons admitted for prescription opioid abuse took the drugs orally, 25% injected them, and 3% inhaled them. By 2002, oral abuse of these drugs had increased to 77%, abuse by injection had fallen to 11%, and abuse by inhaling had increased to 8%.

These shifts in route of administration exhibited regional differences. For instance, in large central metropolitan areas, the proportion of prescription opioid treatment admissions in persons injecting the drugs decreased by 18 percentage points, whereas in fringe and small metropolitan areas, the proportions injecting decreased by only 12 and 15 percentage points, respectively. One explanation for the decrease in the proportion of abusers injecting is the innate danger of contracting HIV or hepatitis. On the other hand, the shift in proportions of routes of abuse from injecting to oral could also be explained by an increase in the attractiveness of oral abuse due the introduction of OxyContin to the market in 1996. These high-dose tablets (10–160 mg of oxycodone) could be easily chewed to circumvent the controlled-release properties of the product. Oral abuse prior to 1996 was limited primarily to ingesting lower-dose, intact tablets.

Despite this apparent shift away from abuse of prescription opioids by injecting, according to the DEA, anecdotal information from across the nation, and especially from the states surrounding Kentucky such as Virginia, Ohio, Indiana, and Pennsylvania, suggests that some OxyContin abusers have switched to heroin in response to a diminished availability of OxyContin in a given region (U.S. DEA, 2006).

The diversion of prescription opioids into the illicit market takes place at all links in the supply chain. Though much attention has been focused on the dishonest patient "doctor shopping" and the rogue physician opening a "pill mill," data gathered from the DEA and analyzed by Joranson (2005) confirmed that much of the diversion of prescription opioids takes place at the level of the pharmacy in the form of burglaries, robberies, and employee and customer theft.

Current Measures to Reduce Abuse

From prescription monitoring programs to public awareness campaigns to physician and patient education and a call for more scientific research, a plethora of actions to curtail the rising rates of prescription opioid abuse have been instituted by various organizations including the Food and Drug Administration, DEA, National Institute of Drug Abuse (Compton & Volkow, 2006), state agencies, medical and academic societies, and others.

In addition to these measures, the pharmaceutical industry has responded by attempting to develop less abusable formulations of their opioid products. These abuse-deterrent or tamper-resistant formulations vary in concept from (1) the addition of ingredients (adding an opioid antagonist like naltrexone or an aversive agent like capsaicin) to (2) changing the physical properties of the tablets to make them either crush-resistant or gel-forming to (3) creating prodrugs that require enzymatic cleavage to release the active drug.

Given the complex nature of the problem of the abuse and diversion of prescription opioids, successful approaches are likely to be multifaceted, combining many of the above elements.

Future Outlook

Though much focus has been directed at our youth with an emphasis on prevention, to "stop abuse before it starts" in order to decrease the number of new initiates to prescription opioid abuse, attention also needs to be given to the aging population. Even if overall rates for new initiates eventually level off or start to decline, we may soon be faced with a new increase in the number of older adults with substance abuse problems due to the aging of the baby boom cohort. Birth cohorts that had high rates of substance abuse in youth have gone on to show higher rates of abuse as they age compared to other cohorts (SAMHSA, 2000a).

A recent regression analysis (Gfroerer et al., 2002) estimated that the number of older adults with substance abuse problems will increase from 2.5 million in 1999 to 5 million in 2020. Many of these individuals will also have painful conditions that will require medical management. In a study by Rosenblum and colleagues (2003), it was found that chronic severe pain, defined as pain that persisted for more than 6 months and was of moderate to severe intensity or that significantly interfered with daily activities, was prevalent in 37% of patients participating in methadone maintenance treatment programs.

Therefore, while attempting to institute programs and policies to minimize rates of substance abuse in younger cohorts, efforts should also be undertaken to prepare for a potential swell of elderly substance abusers in the near future, many of whom will also have comorbid pain conditions that will require treatment with opiates for proper management. The challenge will be to achieve this goal without reversing the progress that has been made over the last decade in improving the quality and accessibility of pain management to patients in need.

As stated in the 2003 position paper from the College on Problems of Drug Dependence (Zacny et al., 2003), we must strive for a balanced approach to the problem of prescription opioid abuse to ensure that the risk-management strategies that are developed in an attempt to prevent and reduce their abuse and diversion do not deter physicians from providing their pain patients with high-efficacy opioids when such medications are indicated.

References

Chabal, C., Erjavec, M.K., Jacobson, L., Mariano, A., Chaney, E., 1997. Prescription opiate abuse in chronic pain patients: clinical criteria, incidence, and predictors. *Clin J Pain* 13(2),150–5.

Compton, W.M., Volkow, N.D., 2006. Major increases in opioid analgesic abuse in the United States: Concerns and strategies. *Drug Alcohol Depend.* 81, 103–7.

Gfroerer, J.C, Penne, M.A., Pemberton, M.R., Folsom, R.E., 2002. The Aging Baby Boom Cohort and Future Prevalence of Substance Abuse. In: Korper, S.P., Council, C.L. (Eds.), *Substance Abuse by Older Adults: Estimates of Future Impact on the Treatment System* (DHHS Publication No. SMA 03–3763, Analytic Series A-21). Rockville, MD: Substance Abuse and Mental Health Services Administration, Office of Applied Studies.

Johnston, L.D., O'Malley, P.M., Bachman, J.G., Schulenberg, J. E., 2005. *Monitoring the Future national results on adolescent drug use: Overview of key findings, 2004* (NIH Publication No. 05–5726). Bethesda, MD: National Institute on Drug Abuse.

Johnston, L.D., O'Malley, P.M., Bachman, J.G., Schulenberg, J.E., 2006. *Monitoring the Future national results on adolescent drug use: Overview of key findings, 2005.* (NIH Publication No. 06–5882). Bethesda, MD: National Institute on Drug Abuse.

Joranson, D.E., 2005. Drug crime is a source of abused pain medications in the United States. *J Pain Symptom Manage.* 30(4), 299–301.

Katz, N.P., Sherburne, S., Beach, M., Rose, R.J., Vielguth, J., Bradley, J., Fanciullo, G.J., 2003. Behavioral monitoring and urine toxicology testing in patients receiving long-term opioid therapy. *Anesth Analg.* 97(4), 1097–102.

Michna, E., Ross, E.L., Hynes, W.L., Nedeljkovic, S.S., Soumekh, S., Janfaza, D., Palombi, D., Jamison, R.N., 2004. Predicting aberrant drug behavior in patients treated for chronic pain: importance of abuse history. *J Pain Symptom Manage.* 28(3), 250–8.

The National Center on Addiction and Substance Abuse (CASA) at Columbia University, 2005. *Under the Counter: The Diversion and Abuse of Controlled Prescription Drugs in the U.S. in 2002.* New York: Author.

Rosenblum, A., Joseph, H., Fong, C., Kipnis, S., Clelend, C., Portenoy, R.K., 2003. Prevalence and characteristics of chronic pain among chemically dependent patients in methadone maintenance and residential treatment facilities. *JAMA* 289(18), 2370–8.

Substance Abuse and Mental Health Services Administration (SAMHSA), Office of Applied Studies, 2000. *Summary of findings from the 1999 National Survey on Drug Use and Health: National Findings* (NHSDA Series H–12, DHHS Publication No. SMA 00–3466). Rockville, MD: SAMSHA.

Substance Abuse and Mental Health Services Administration (SAMHSA), Office of Applied Studies, 2002. *Results from the 2001 National Household Survey on Drug Abuse: Volume I. Summary of National Findings* (NHSDA Series H–17, DHHS Publication No. SMA 02–3758). Rockville, MD: SAMHSA.

Substance Abuse and Mental Health Services Administration (SAMHSA), Office of Applied Studies, 2003a. *Results from the 2002 National Survey on Drug Use and Health: National Findings* (NHSDA Series H–22, DHHS Publication No. SMA 03–3836). Rockville, MD: SAMHSA.

Substance Abuse and Mental Health Services Administration (SAMHSA), Office of Applied Studies, 2003b. *Emergency Department Trends From DAWN: Final Estimates 1995—2002* (DAWN Series D-24, DHHS Publication No. SMA 03–3780). Rockville, MD: SAMHSA.

Substance Abuse and Mental Health Services Administration (SAMHSA), Office of Applied Studies, 2004a. *Results from the 2003 National Survey on Drug Use and Health: National Findings* (NSDUH Series H–25, DHHS Publication No. SMA 04–3964). Rockville, MD: SAMHSA.

Substance Abuse and Mental Health Services Administration (SAMHSA), Office of Applied Studies, 2004b. *The DAWN Report: Narcotic Analgesics, 2002 Update.* Retrieved April 3, 2007, from http://dawninfo.samhsa.gov/old_dawn/pubs_94_02/shortreports/files/DAWN_tdr_NA2002.pdf

Substance Abuse and Mental Health Services Administration (SAMHSA), Office of Applied Studies, 2004c. *Drug Abuse Warning Network, 2003: Interim National Estimates of Drug-Related Emergency Department Visits* (DAWN Series D–26, DHHS Publication No. SMA 04–3972). Rockville, MD: SAMHSA.

Substance Abuse and Mental Health Services Administration (SAMHSA), Office of Applied Studies, 2004d. *Treatment Episode Data Set (TEDS): 1992–2002. National Admissions to Substance Abuse Treatment Services* (DASIS Series: S-23, DHHS Publication No. SMA 04–3965). Rockville, MD: SAMHSA.

Substance Abuse and Mental Health Services Administration (SAMHSA), Office of Applied Studies, 2005a. *Results from the 2004 National Survey on Drug Use and Health: National Findings* (NSDUH Series H-28, DHHS Publication No. SMA 05–4062). Rockville, MD: SAMHSA.

Substance Abuse and Mental Health Services Administration (SAMHSA), Office of Applied Studies, 2005b. *Treatment Episode Data Set (TEDS): 1993–2003. National Admissions to Substance Abuse Treatment Services* (DASIS Series: S-29, DHHS Publication No. SMA 05–4118). Rockville, MD: SAMHSA.

U.S. Census Bureau, 2002. *2000 Census of Population and Housing, Summary Population and Housing Characteristics* (PHC-1–1). Washington, DC: Author.

U.S. Drug Enforcement Administration (DEA), 2003. *OxyContin Theft & Loss Incidents, January 2000 through June.* U.S. Department of Justice. Retrieved April 3, 2007, from www.deadiversion.usdoj.gov/drugs_concern/oxycodone/oxylosses_oct2003_1.pdf

U.S. Drug Enforcement Administration (DEA), 2006. *State Fact Sheets.* U.S. Department of Justice. Retrieved April 3, 2006, from http://www.dea.gov/pubs/states/kentucky.html

Zacny, J., Bigelow, G., Comptom, P., Foley, K., Iguchi, M., Sannerud, C., 2003. College on Problems of Drug Dependence taskforce on prescription opioid non-medical use and abuse: position statement. *Drug Alcohol Depend.* 69, 215–32.

5

Pain Management and the Medical Profession

What Is Our Responsibility?

Richard Payne

[D]uty is the obligation to act from reverence for moral law.... [N]othing in the whole world... can possibly be regarded as good without limitation except a good will.
—Immanuel Kant, *The Metaphysics of Morality*

...am I my brother's keeper?
—Genesis 4:9

...and who is my neighbor?
—Luke 10:29

The quotations above, from the moral philosopher Kant and the New and Old Testaments of the Bible, speak to our obligations to be caring individuals to our neighbors and fellow citizens. I argue that our secular and religious traditions also must influence our behaviors and responsibilities as health-care professionals, and seem particularly relevant to understanding our obligations to relieve pain and suffering. The question posed in the book of Luke (New Testament Bible), "Who is my neighbor?," is a prelude to the parable of the Good Samaritan. This chapter deals with the professional and ethical responsibilities of physicians in the contemporary society, and pleads for reclaiming an ethic of "Good Samaritanism" in 21st-century medicine.

Many recent studies have documented the persistent undertreatment of pain and identified many barriers as causes for this circumstance (Bernabi et al., 1998; Cleeland et al., 1994; SUPPORT Study Principal Investigators, 1995). The commonly listed barriers include the following (Rich, 2000; von Roenn, 1999):

- low prioritization of pain as a clinical problem by clinicians
- lack of knowledge of clinicians regarding the appropriate assessment and management of pain
- the impact of fear of regulatory scrutiny on the use of opioids in pain management
- a lack of medical professionalism and a failure of the health-care system to insist on accountability for appropriate outcomes of pain treatment
- resistance to use opioids by patients and clinicians
- impact of cost constraints on access and quality of pain care

The following case has been reported recently (Payne, 2007) and underscores many of these barriers. This chapter will discuss the factors associated with unsatisfactory and suboptimal pain treatment outcomes, emphasizing the need for realizing the highest ideals of medical professionalism, and highlights the role of physicians as ethical agents in the health-care system. The discussion will point to needed changes in education and training of physicians to produce better patient-centered pain outcomes.

A Case of Sickle-Cell Pain Management: Success and Failure

The patient was a 38-year-old African American physician with sickle-cell disease. He was referred to a pain specialist during his postgraduate training in a highly competitive cardiology program because of persistent pain related to a nonhealing ischemic ulceration of his leg. Pain occurred daily and was usually quite severe (self-reports of daily worst pain typically 7–10/10).

The leg ulceration persisted despite use of disease-modifying antisickling therapy, including administration of hydroxyurea, frequent blood transfusions, and the use of hyperbaric oxygen therapy. When pain was not controlled, the patient slept poorly, was absent from work on several occasions, and often performed less well in patient management tasks. Pain was eventually successfully managed with a combination of transdermal opioids and oral analgesics (for breakthrough pain) titrated to optimal doses over several days. Although his pain regimen varied over time, the initial daily regimen included transdermal fentanyl patches applied every 72 hours and 16 mg hydromorphone every 3 hours prn for breakthrough pain. Later, the fentanyl patches were dropped from his regimen, and he was managed with oral hydromorphone alone, in doses up to 24 mg every 3–4 hours. The patient successfully completed his postgraduate specialty training while on opioid therapy, including performing invasive cardiovascular diagnostic and therapeutic procedures, authoring several manuscripts, and completing neuropsychological examinations, which demonstrated normal psychomotor function.

Following graduation from the training program, the patient moved to another state to start a medical practice. After much debate and controversy, the patient was granted a medical license, but it was subsequently suspended and hospital privileges denied, based in large portion his need to use opioids on a daily basis for pain management. This decision was made despite evidence showing no impairment in his physical or mental abilities to practice medicine, and his voluntary submission to a substance abuse treatment program (as required by the medical board even though there was no evidence of substance use disorder).

Local physicians in his new state were reluctant to prescribe the quantities of opioid medications required for adequate control, necessitating frequent trips of several hundred miles back to a pain treatment center. The patient suspected, but could not prove, that some of these judgments were made because he was African American. He could not remain abstinent from opioid analgesics, as was requested by the medical board as a condition of professional licensure, because attempts to do so were invariably associated with severe recurrences of pain and functional impairment. The patient died related to sepsis complicating a sickle-cell–related vaso-occlusive crisis while in litigation with the medical board.

Professionalism in Medicine

This case is labeled a success because competent and aggressive management of pain was associated with a highly satisfactory patient outcome, including an improved ability to function and, indeed, reduced levels of pain, suffering, and distress by the patient. The case is described as a failure because the tragic events following graduation from his training program highlight incompetent pain management, poor professional behavior on the part of his physicians, lack of compassionate caring by physicians and the healthcare system, and these actions may have indirectly led to his death (see below).

The Accreditation Council for Graduate Medical Education (ACGME) has defined six core competencies that are essential to the practice of medicine (Leach, 2004):

- patient care
- medical knowledge
- practice-based learning and improvement
- interpersonal and communication skills
- system-based practice
- professionalism

Professionalism has been written about and defined in many ways. For example, Rhodes et al. (2004) define medicine as a "socially constructed" profession, and assign two fundamental principles to medical ethics and professionalism: (1) a fiduciary responsibility for physicians to act for the good of their patients and society, especially because medicine deals with people made vulnerable through illness, and (2) a responsibility of physicians to be trustworthy and to be seen as deserving of this trust. This analysis holds that these two fundamental principles directly lead to critical "corollary" values of professionalism: professional competency, caring, confidentiality, nonjudgmental and nonsexual regard of patients, and respect for patient's values. For example, *professional competency* is assigned a corollary (rather than primary) value because "physicians with skills and competency are worthy of trust." Similarly, *caring* is a corollary value because "patients are inclined to trust physicians who genuinely care about their well-being and because caring doctors are likely to fulfill their obligations in the face of conflicting desires" (Rhodes et al., 2004).

Another examination of professionalism in medicine provides a model in which devotion to medical service, public profession of values, and advocacy for patients involving a social contract between physicians and the public occurs (Wynia et al., 1999). Still others have argued that professionalism in medicine must be grounded in specific and virtuous behaviors of physicians and must be based on more than academic theories (Wear & Kuczewski, 2004). Many of these attributes of medical professionalism—competency, caring, nonjudgmental behaviors, devotion to service, and patient advocacy—were breeched in this case, with tragic consequences.

The Physician's Responsibility to Behave Ethically and to Attend to Pain and Suffering

The responsibilities of physicians to treat pain and suffering can be found in ancient documents and writings, and more recently has been stipulated in the American Medical Association's (1996) *Code of Medical Ethics*, which states the following:

> Physicians have the responsibility to relieve pain and suffering and to promote the dignity and autonomy of dying patients in their care. This includes providing effective palliative treatment even though it may foreseeably hasten death.

Of note, the statement emphasizes the obligations to relieve pain and suffering in dying patients, and may have an unintended effect of minimizing these same obligations for chronically but non-terminally ill patients. Sickle-cell anemia is an important case in point. Pain is a cardinal feature of this disease, but is often not managed well (Payne, 1997). Furthermore, pain is an important marker of disease severity. An important natural history study observed that patients with more than three vaso-occlusive crises per year only had a 50% chance of survival to age 55 (Platt et al., 1994). Physical and emotional stresses are among the many possible precipitants of a vaso-occlusive event for sickle-cell patients, and for these reasons. Although admittedly controversial, one might speculate that that the regrettable circumstances experienced by this patient potentially facilitated painful complications of his disease, and thus indirectly led to his death.

The elements of professionalism in pain management involve the practice of evidence-based medicine in a manner that is "patient-centered," in other words, practiced in a way that emphasizes the educational and emotional needs of the patient and focuses on the best health-care outcomes. Clinicians learn the skills required to practice in this way through training programs that have specific standards that certify physicians as qualified after successful completion. Training programs in pain management and palliative medicine were not widely available when this patient was alive, and many publications document the lack of professional education and quality standards of care that compromise professional competency and high-quality pain management (Carver et al., 1999; Cleeland et al., 1998; Galer et al., 1999; Rabow et al., 2000).

Our case raises serious issues regarding professional competency related to pain assessment and management. The failure of physicians to appreciate the wide variability in dose-response relationships associated with opioid pharmacology led to persistent questioning of the validity of the patient's pain complaint and undermined a trusting doctor-patient relationship. A manifestation of this compromised relationship was evidenced in the consistent underdosing of the patient and a refusal to prescribe appropriate amounts of medication. Furthermore, this led to great patient inconvenience and a breech of the caring ethic that the patient expected of his physicians.

The patient believed that some physicians involved in his case lacked the virtue of nonjudgmental and unbiased evaluation of his medical problems, maintaining that his pain complaints were discounted because of accusations that he was "drug seeking," possibly related to racial profiling. This belief on the part of the patient may have some validity, as racial and ethnic biases in pain management have been documented (Green, 2003; Todd, 2000).

Another major aspect of professional incompetence in this case involved the confusion of the phenomenology of pharmacological tolerance, physical dependence, and behavioral syndrome of addiction. Many experienced clinicians and researchers have commented on the need to distinguish pharmacological tolerance from physical dependence, and likewise to distinguish these from the behavioral and psychiatric syndrome of addiction (Portenoy & Payne, 1998). These phenomena are described in detail elsewhere in this book, and further description is beyond the scope of this chapter. However, it is worthwhile to point out that in our case the medical board required the patient to attend a substance abuse program, mistaking opioid tolerance and physical dependence for addiction.

Misperceptions of addictive behavior are particular problems for sickle-cell patients. For example, one study noted that hematologists and emergency department physicians consistently overestimate the prevalence of addiction in sickle-cell patients. In this study, 210 hematologists and 139 emergency department physicians were surveyed by mail (with a 34% response rate). The physicians were asked to respond to questions that reflect their *actual perceptions and practice* relating to sickle-cell patients, and the response rates from the two groups were similar. The study found that when asked about their perceptions of adult sickle-cell patients, 9% of hematologists and 22% of emergency department physicians answered yes to the question: "Are more than 50% of sickle-cell patients addicted?" (Shapiro et al., 1997). When asked about children and adolescents, 46% of emergency department doctors and 4% of hematologists answered yes to the question: "Are more than 10% of children with sickle cell disease addicted?" However, the reality is that retrospective and case-controlled studies of patients with sickle-cell disease indicate an addiction rate of 0.2%–9% (Brozovic et al., 1986; Drayer et al., 1999; Payne, 1989; Vichinski et al., 1982).

It is my contention that the failure to appreciate these distinctions and concepts by practitioners treating sickle-cell patients in which a cardinal feature of the disease is pain, and the relative lack of knowledge of the essential clinical pharmacology of analgesia, testify to the low priority given to pain assessment and management in medical practice. These misbehaviors constitute a breech of high-quality professional behavior.

Ethics and Morals in Modern Medical Practice

> ...I will remember that there is art to medicine as well as science, and that warmth, sympathy, and understanding may outweigh the surgeon's knife or the chemist's drug....
> ...I will remember that I do not treat a fever chart, a cancerous growth, but a sick human being....
> ...I will remember that I remain a member of society, with special obligations to all my fellow human beings, those sound of mind and body as well as the infirm. (Hippocratic Oath, Modern Version; Lasagna, 1964)

The failures of medicine to attend to the pain and suffering for the person described in this case are obvious. In fact, the general lack of advocacy for the well-being of patients in pain by physicians compromises our professional and ethical standing. Despite this, there is universal acknowledgement and overwhelming consensus of all major medical organizations and societies of the ethical imperative of physicians to attend to human pain and suffering (Cassell, 1999). It is my contention that the tragic outcome of this case represents individual failures on the part of clinicians and collective failures of the health-care system, and they are related.

The four cardinal principles of modern bioethics involve: (1) respect for patient autonomy; (2) beneficence (i.e., the obligation to "do good"); (3) nonmalfeasance, the obligation to do "no harm"; and (4) justice (Lo, 1995). The AMA *Code of Medical Ethics* and the bioethics principle of beneficence requires clinicians to act to relieve pain and suffering when patients request our assistance. Furthermore, these contemporary principles of bioethics are quite consistent with principles of moral philosophy and ethics described and accumulated over the centuries of human experience.

For example, the great philosopher Immanuel Kant wrote about a system of ethics, termed deontological ethics, which speak to the ethics of duty. In Kant's words, "Duty is the obligation to act from reverence for moral law...Nothing in the whole world...can possibly be regarded as good without limitation except a good will" (1785). Kant further articulated the concept of a "categorical imperative" as a way to behave or to "act as if the principle from which you act were to become through your will a universal law of nature."

The "categorical imperative" has been called an unconditional moral command and has been said to be a philosophical restatement of the *Golden Rule:* "Do unto others as you would have them do unto you." The Golden Rule is not a distinctly Judeo-Christian concept (Table 5.1). In fact, some version of this statement is found in every major religious tradition.

Do 21st-century clinicians have a responsibility to act as ethical and moral agents, behaving in ways that promote the greatest "good will," and acting in accordance with the professional obligation of duty that categorical imperative and the Golden Rule mandate? Some have criticized these notions of duty and obligation as being too general and essentially meaningless unless placed in a particular context (Wear & Kuczewski, 2004). For

Table 5.1. The Golden Rule in Various Religious Traditions

Religion	Statement
Christianity	"In everything, do to others as you would have them do to you; for this is the law and the prophets." (Jesus, Matthew 7:12)
Buddhism	"Treat not others in ways that you yourself would find hurtful." (The Buddha, Udana-Varga 5.18)
Islam	"Not one of you truly believes until you wish for others what you wish for yourself." (The Prophet Muhammad, Hadith)
Judaism	"What is hateful to you, do not do to your neighbor. This is the whole Torah: all the rest is commentary. Go and learn it." (Hillel, Talmud Shabbath 31a)
Confucianism	"One word which sums up the basis of all good conduct...loving-kindness. Do not do to others what you do not want done to yourself." (Confucius, Analects 15.23)
Unitarianism	"We affirm and promote respect for the interdependent web of all existence of which we are a part." (Unitarian principle)

example, the American Board of Internal Medicine (cited in Wear & Kuczewski, 2004) defines "duty" as the following:

> ...the free acceptance of a commitment to service. This commitment entails being available and responsive... accepting inconvenience to meet the needs of one's patients, enduring unavoidable risks to oneself when a patient's welfare is at stake, advocating the best possible care...and volunteering one's skills and expertise for the welfare of the community.

Accordingly, in this patient narrative, one might ask about the limits of these obligations of duty with respect to practitioners taking risks by forcibly advocating to the medical board to reexamine its policies regarding the aggressive use of opioids in this patient, and the duty to volunteer one's skills and expertise in testifying and participating in discussions with the medical board in advocating for the patient to maintain his medical license. Nevertheless, one can't help but wonder whether the principles of the categorical imperative and the Golden Rule were firmly in mind of the clinicians and regulators—the embodiment of the health-care "system"—in the narrative of this case, and if so, whether the outcome would have been less tragic.

The philosophical and ethical descriptions discussed above point to our *individual and collective* duties and obligations to relieve suffering. Our case illustrates the failures of clinicians to act effectively to meet these professional and ethical requirements to advance individual patient well-being and to effect public policy that is scientifically based, formulated in ways that are just and that advance the greatest "good will" with the intention to relieve individual and collective suffering. For example, many of the physicians involved in this case expressed reluctance to prescribe opioids in appropriate doses because they might be subjected to punishment by medical regulators or law enforcement. This was the attitude and opinion of physicians despite a long-held understanding that the Controlled Substance Act did not impinge on the appropriate medical use of opioids. As stated by Senator Pomerene during the Senate floor debates of the Harrison Narcotics Act on August 15, 1914:

> We must have a cure for the drug habits, but we must not forget the innocent sufferer on his or her bed of sickness and pain. Let us protect the country from the physician or druggist who is encouraging the drug habit for purely commercial purposes: but let us not by too much red tape hinder the physician in the proper practice of his profession. We can prevent the abuse of the drug without unduly hampering its proper use.

Despite this, Portenoy reported that more than 50% of New York State physicians were either "moderately or very concerned" about the possibility of sanctions by state regulators, and these concerns translated into self-imposed restrictions on their prescribing behaviors (Portenoy & Payne, 1998; see Table 5.2).

Most importantly, these observations and reflections would call on us to take a wider view of our clinical responsibilities and professionalism than we currently do, to view ourselves as being accountable as part of the health-care and regulatory systems of the profession and society in which we as physicians are privileged and essential parts.

Although there is universal agreement on the need for clinicians, especially physicians, to attend to pain and suffering in our patients, however, many theologians, moral philosophers and ethicists disagree on *how* physicians and other agents of medical

Table 5.2. Fear of Regulatory Scrutiny by Physicians

"How concerned are you that a drug regulatory agency might some day scrutinize your prescription records?"

Level of Concern	N	%
Not concerned at all	242	19.3
Slightly concerned	315	25.1
Moderately concerned	285	22.7
Very concerned	412	32.8
Missing	3	00.2
Total	1257	100.0

Source: Portenoy RK, Kanner RM. Patterns of analgesic prescription and consumption in a university-affiliated community hospital. Archives of Internal Medicine 1985;145(3):439–41.

care should attend to and manage suffering, and what medicine as a profession should "promise" to individuals and their families.

All experienced clinicians make a distinction between pain and suffering (Cassell, 1999; Cherney et al., 1994). Cassell (1999, p. 513) defines suffering as a "specific state of distress that occurs when the intactness or integrity of the person is threatened or disrupted." The proper assessment of suffering must take into account the person's individual story or narrative, and must include an assessment of the *person*, and not just an assessment of the body or a list of medical problems. The Hippocratic Oath and Cassell assert that caring and attending to suffering requires one to focus on the evaluation of the *person* and not just consider the patient as simply a sum of medical issues in the problem-oriented medical record.

Caring and the Physician

A caring attitude and a devotion to service are, of course, essential elements of medical professionalism. As pointed out by van Hooft (1996), caring can be thought of as a behavior or motivation. Caring as *behavior* implies "looking after another person and seeing to their needs"; caring as *motivation* implies "feeling sympathy or empathy for someone or being concerned with their well-being or having a professional commitment to seeing to their needs" (van Hooft, 1996, p. 83). This author further theorizes that a caring spirit is promoted through an emphasis on "the formation and maintenance of both the integrity of our selves and also of our relationships with others and the world around us."

In our case, the patient's death was associated with much distress and suffering related in part to unrelieved physical pain, an inability to practice in his chosen vocation, and the psychologically devastating effects of discrimination and arbitrary unsympathetic decision making on the part of clinicians and medical regulators. Would a more caring attitude on the part of clinicians and regulators acting on a principle of the categorical imperative, operating with the perspective of creating the greatest good will and compassion for another individual have made a difference in the outcome? What would be required to form more clinicians and regulators in the ways that would promote caring and greater accountability for compassion and professionalism in pain care? Van Hooft's model emphasizes the following:

> ...we realize our selves by reaching out to the world and to others.... If the situation is such that I am in a position to help, my belief that another is suffering is a moral reason for

me to act and will be immediately motivating. The suffering of another typically calls out to us immediately for a response. (We are, of course, free to reject this call, but at a cost to our integrity as self-project and being-for-others.

Concluding Thoughts

In summary, we have a professional, ethical, and moral obligation to assess, attend to, and relieve pain and suffering in individual patients whom we care for. We also have similar responsibilities to behave collectively in ways that promote ethical and compassionate caring throughout the health-care system. These responsibilities mandate that we attend not just to our patients as medical problems, and to pain as a consequence of nociceptive physiology, but that we take a larger worldview, consistent with the clinician as healer and as a "Good Samaritan."

I hypothesize that caring would be more compassionate at individual levels and at the level of the health-care system (which is, after all a creation of the individuals who make up the system) if our education and training were not only scientifically and evidence based, but also done in a way that form clinicians to be more caring. This implies not only rigorous training that emphasizes cognitive skills, but that also allows reflective time for clinicians to understand themselves and their roles relative not only to their individual patients, but to the larger (moral) world. Such patient-centered and socially oriented training would of necessity respect individual and collective patient narratives. In fact, physician training that promotes the highest degree of professionalism requires role modeling, venues for self-awareness, a tolerance and competency in understanding patient narratives, and opportunities for socially relevant community service (Coulehan, 2005). Such training might emphasis how clinicians are formed to contribute to a culture producing the most good will and the greatest sense of caring for the whole person, and how the integrity of the clinician is enhanced by the interactions beyond the individual patient. This could provide meaningful systemic behavioral changes in patients and clinicians to attend to suffering individuals, and to be advocates for our patients within an often unforgiving health-care system.

References

American Medical Association, Council on Ethics and Judicial Affairs of the American Medical Association. *Code of Medical Ethics*. 1996. Chicago: American Medical Association.

Bernabi R, Cleeland CS, Gonin R, et al. Management of pain in elderly patients with cancer. *JAMA* 1998;279:1877–1882.

Brozovic MC, Davies SC, Yarumian A, et al. Pain relief in sickle cell crises. *Lancet* 1986; 1:320–321.

Carver AC, Vicrey BG, Bernat JL, et al. End-of-life care: a survey of U.S. neurologists' attitudes, behavior, and knowledge. *Neurology* 1999;53(2):284–293.

Cassell, EJ. Diagnosing suffering: a perspective. *Ann Intern Med* 1999;131:531–534.

Cherny NI, Coyle N, Foley KM. Suffering in the advanced cancer patient. Part I: a definition and taxonomy. *J Palliat Care* 1994;10:71–79.

Cleeland CS. Undertreatment of cancer pain in elderly patients. *JAMA* 1998;279(23):1914–15.

Cleeland CS, Gonin R, Hatfield A, et al. Pain and its treatment in outpatients with metastatic cancer. *N Engl J Med* 1994;330:592–596.

Coulehan J. Viewpoint: today's professionalism: engaging the mind but not the heart. *Academic Medicine* 2005;80:892.

Drayer RA, Henderson J, Reidenberg M. Barriers to better pain control in hospitalized patients. *J Pain Symptom Manage* 1999;17:434–40.

Galer BS, Keran C, Frisinger M. Pain medicine education among American neurologists: a need for improvement. *Neurology* 1999;52(8):1710–1712.

Green CR, Anderson KO, Baker TA, et al. The unequal burden of pain: confronting racial and ethnic disparities in pain. *Pain Med* 2003;4(3):277–94.

Kant I. *Groundwork for the Metaphysics of Morality*, 1785. Trans. Mary J. Gregor. New York: Cambridge University Press, 1998.

Lasagna, L. Modern Hippocratic Oath. 1964. Retrieved 1/21/08 from http://www.medterms.com/script/main/art.asp?articlekey=20909

Leach DC. Professionalism: the formation of physicians. *American Journal of Bioethics* Spring 2004;4(2):11–12.

Lo B. *Resolving Ethical Dilemmas. A Guide for Clinicians*. Baltimore: Williams & Wilkins; 1995:17–23.

Payne R. Life and death considerations in chronic pain: secular and theological ethical considerations. In: Michael E. Schatman, ed. *Ethical Issues in Chronic Pain Management*. New York: Informa Healthcare; 2007; 33-41.

Payne R. Pain management in sickle cell disease: rationale and techniques. *Ann NY Acad Sci* 1989;565:189–206.

Payne R. Pain management in sickle cell anemia. *Anesthesiology Clinics of North America* 1997;15(2):305–18.

Payne, R. Life and death considerations in chronic pain: secular and theological ethical considerations. In: Schatman M, Grant B, eds. *Ethical Issues in Chronic Pain Management*. In press.

Platt OS, Brambilla DJ, Rosse WF et al. Mortality in sickle cell disease: life expectancy and risk factors for early death. *New Engl J Med* 1994; 330:1639–1644.

Portenoy RK, Payne R, Passik SD. Acute and chronic pain. In: Lowinson JH, Ruiz P, Milman RB, Langrod JG, eds. *Substance Abuse: A Comprehensive Textbook*. 4th ed. Philadelphia: Lippincott Williams & Wilkins; 2005; 863–904.

Rabow MW, Hardie GE, Fair JM, McPhee SSJ. End-of-life care content in 50 textbooks from multiple specialties. *JAMA* 2000;283(6):771–8.

Rhodes R, Cohen D, Friedman E, Muller D. Professionalism in medical education. *The American Journal of Bioethics,* Spring 2004;4(2):20–22.

Rich BA. An ethical analysis of the barriers to effective pain management. *Cambridge Quarterly of Healthcare Ethics* 2000; 9:54–70.

Shapiro BS, Benjamin L, Payne R et al. Sickle cell-related pain: perceptions of medical practitioners. *J Pain Symptom Manage* 1997;14:168–74.

SUPPORT Study Principal Investigators. A controlled trial to improve care for seriously ill hospitalized patients. *JAMA* 1995;274:1591–98.

Todd KH, Deaton C, D'Adamo AP, Goe L. Ethnicity and analgesic practice. *Ann Emerg Med* 2000;35(1):11–16.

van Hooft S. Bioethics and caring. *J Medical Ethics* 1996;22:83–89.

Vichinski EP, Johnson PR, Lubin RB. Multidisciplinary approach to pain management in sickle cell disease. *Am J Pediatr Hematol Oncol* 1982:4: 328–333.

von Roenn JH, Cleeland CS, Gonin R et al. Physician attitudes and practice in cancer pain management: a survey from the Eastern Oncology Group. *Ann Int Med* 1993;119:121–126.

Wear D, Kuczewski MG. The professionalism movement: can we pause? *The American Journal of Bioethics,* Spring 2004;4(2):1–10.

Wynia MK, Latham SR, Koa, AC, Berg JW, Emmanuel LL, Medical professionalism in society, *NEJM* 1999;341:1612–1614.

Part II
Addiction and Related Issues

6

The Basic Science of Addiction

Roberto I. Melendez

Peter W. Kalivas

Drug addiction can be defined as a chronically relapsing behavioral disorder characterized by compulsive, at times uncontrollable, drug craving, seeking, and use that persists even in the face of negative consequences (O'Brien, 2001). Addictive drugs produce their behavioral effects by initiating a cascade of neurochemical events that ultimately makes the organism seek the drug. Thus, addictive drugs have the property of reinforcing or rewarding drug-related behaviors and thereby increasing the probability of a response, which is core to our understanding of the behavioral attributes associated with addiction.

There are two primary features common to addiction. First, the addictive stimulus is a compelling motivator of behavior at the expense of behaviors leading to the acquisition of other rewarding stimuli. Thus, individuals come to orient increasing amounts of their daily activity around the acquisition of the drug(s) to which they are addicted. Second, there is a persistence of seeking for the addictive stimulus, combined with an inability to regulate the behaviors associated with obtaining that stimulus. Thus, years after the last exposure to an addictive stimulus, reexposure to that stimulus or environmental cues associated with that stimulus will elicit behavior aimed at obtaining the reward.

The notion that reward may involve specialized brain systems received its first empirical support from the pioneering work of Olds and Milner (1954). These investigators demonstrated that rats would maintain lever-pressing for the delivery of an electrical stimulus to specific brain sites. Drugs with high addiction potential, including psychostimulants, opiates, and ethanol, have been shown to increase the sensitivity of animals to electrical brain stimulation (Wise and Bozarth, 1982). A theory that has resulted from the early research on intracranial self-stimulation was that the mesolimbic dopamine system served as a "final common neural substrate" for rewards (Wise and Bozarth, 1987). This important concept provided the initial hypothetical backbone upon which much of our current understanding of the biology of addiction is based. Indeed, a major challenge in recent addiction research has been to understand the critical interplay between initial drug action on mesolimbic dopamine and recruitment of other neural substrates by chronic drug use and withdrawal.

As no single technique is ideal, converging evidence from numerous methodological approaches, including stereotaxically directed brain lesions, intracranial self-stimulation, and intracranial microinjections combined with behavioral assessments, as well as in vivo and in vitro electrophysiology, microdialysis of extracellular neurochemicals and molecular techniques, is required to characterize a reward-relevant brain substrate. Consistent with the notion of converging evidence, it has become increasingly evident that the expression of complex behaviors like those sustained by reinforcing drugs engages a much larger complement of neuroanatomical substrates than these originally proposed. For instance, although the mesolimbic dopamine system has been traditionally considered a neurochemical substrate of reward, it may not necessarily impart a sufficient role in reward-mediated behaviors (Salomone et al., 1994; Schultz, 1998). Indeed, the critical role of other transmitters in reward is becoming increasingly clear. Furthermore, the importance of neuroplasticity and the learning processes associated with reinforcement-mediated behavior has become a major consideration. Thus, it is now recognized as imperative to understand not only the anatomical substrates that are involved in the initiation reward but also those that are critical for sustaining the behavior such that it can be reinstated after long periods of abstinence.

The Development of Addiction

The acute administration of all addictive drugs, with the possible exception of the benzodiazepines, stimulates dopamine transmission in the projection from the ventral tegmental area to the nucleus accumbens. This projection is generally referred to as the mesoaccumbens dopamine system. The pharmacological site of action by which different classes of drugs of abuse activate dopamine transmission varies and includes three general cellular mechanisms that encompass all drugs of abuse:

1. Receptors for the drug are on dopamine cell bodies and dendrites, and through these receptors drug administration directly stimulates dopamine neurons. Nicotine and cannabinoids are examples of drugs thought to work in part through this mechanism (Cheer et al., 2000; Nisell et al., 1994).
2. Receptors are located primarily on GABAergic inhibitory afferents to the dopamine cells, and drug binding to these receptors reduces GABA release, thereby disinhibiting dopamine

neuronal activity. Opioids and ethanol produce reward in part by this mechanism (Bunney et al., 2001; Cameron et al., 1997).

3. Drugs can bind to presynaptic receptors to increase the presynaptic release of dopamine without directly altering the activity of dopamine neurons. The primary mechanism in this category is exemplified by amphetamine-like psychostimulants which bind to the dopamine transporter and increase dopamine release by blocking reuptake and/or promoting the release of dopamine via reverse transport (Seiden et al., 1993).

Although mesoaccumbens dopamine has received the most research attention as a "neural message" of acute drug reward, converging evidence places the dopamine system within a broader context of circuits involved. Evidence points to an involvement of several other neurotransmitters including opioid (and peptides), gamma-aminobutyric acid (GABA), glutamate, and serotonin (5-HT) systems. The identification of opioid receptors and their endogenous ligands, the opioid peptides, have immense significance in the development of addiction. A variety of animal models including self-administration, intracranial self-stimulation, and conditioned place preference indicate that opiates have primary reinforcing effects (Bozarth and Wise, 1984). The GABA system provides the brain with inhibitory mechanisms to control neuronal excitation produced by the glutamate system, and neuronal activity associated with reward-mediated behavior may be governed by a balance between inhibitory and excitatory input, with a significant portion of these inputs being mediated through $GABA_A$ and glutamate receptors. Thus, a decrease in inhibition and/or an increase in excitation play an important role in fine-tuning or modulating the proper expression of reward-mediated behaviors.

In recent years, a new emphasis on both 5-HT and cholinergic systems has reemerged. The 5-HT system has long been implicated in various psychiatric disorders including depression, anxiety, and obsessive compulsions. Furthermore, research indicates that 5-HT plays a key modulatory role on reward circuits (Gingrich and Hen, 2001). Enhancing serotonergic activity has been shown to potentiate the rewarding efficacy of various drugs of abuse including morphine (Carboni et al., 1989), cocaine (Loh and Roberts, 1990), and ethanol (Murphy et al., 1992). However, the complexity of the 5-HT system has hampered attempts to achieve better understanding on the role of specific receptors on processes underlying reward.

In relation to cholinergic systems, there are several lines of evidence for the proposition of its involvement in reward-mediated behavior (Dalley et al., 2001). Moreover, cholinergic systems have been suggested to play an important role in the associative mechanisms underlying reward. As indicated by Dalley et al. (2001), cholinergic systems' involvement in aspects of attentional functioning is further superseded by its involvement in detecting shifts in the predictive relationship between instrumental action and reinforcement. Future research is needed to delineate the role of the various cholinergic groups (i.e., cortical versus basal forebrain versus pedunculopontine neurons) on reward-mediated behaviors.

Knowledge about the acute effects of drugs of abuse is not sufficient to explain why when drugs are unavailable for prolonged periods of time, individuals remain vulnerable to cravings and relapse. Indeed, prolonged drug use changes the brain in fundamental ways that appear to last long after the individual has stopped taking drugs (Leshner and Koob, 1999). Upon repeated drug use, reward-mediated behaviors demonstrate a strengthening of the association between the stimulus and the response, which results in numerous brain adaptations. At the level of neurobiology, plasticity from repeated drug use can result from a change in neurotransmitter turnover, neurotransmitter receptors, receptor-mediated signal transduction, and gene expression (Kalivas and Volkow, 2005; Nestler, 2001). Morphological changes may ensue, including the generation of new or the pruning away of preexisting synaptic connections (Hyman and Malenka, 2001). Below, we discuss potential neuroadaptations as they pertain to the pathophysiology of neural circuits that mediate the expression of addictive behaviors, such as craving and relapse.

The Expression of Addiction

Figure 6.1 will be used as a guide for this portion of the chapter and outlines the nuclei and their interconnections that appear critical for the expression of behaviors commonly associated with addiction, such as drug craving and relapse. This circuit has been previously characterized as the motive circuit (Heimer and Alheid, 1991; Mogenson et al., 1993) and contains brain nuclei that are considered critical substrates for drug reward and the development of addiction (as outlined above), such as the dopaminergic neurons in the ventral tegmental area, GABAergic neurons in the nucleus accumbens, and glutamatergic neurons in the prefrontal cortex and basolateral amygdala.

The majority of our recent understanding of how the motive circuit in Figure 6.1 is involved in the expression of addiction is derived from neuroimaging studies in human addicts and animal studies employing the reinstatement model of drug craving. Neu-

Figure 6.1. Hypothesized circuits involved in the development and expression of addiction. A role for these nuclei and interconnections between nuclei in addiction has been revealed using neuroimaging techniques in addicts and/or reinstatement animal models of drug-seeking behavior. Notably, although the motor memory circuit (i.e., PFC–NAc core–VP) is postulated to be involved regardless of stimulus modality, the limbic "priming" circuitry (VTA–BLA–Ext. amygdala) differs between stimuli (e.g., stress, learned associations or an acute drug administration). The arrows illustrate the transition from drug reinforcement processes to addiction. BLA = basolateral amygdala, Ext. amygdala = extended amygdala, NAc core = core of the nucleus accumbens, PFC = prefrontal cortex, VTA = ventral tegmental area, VP = ventral pallidum.

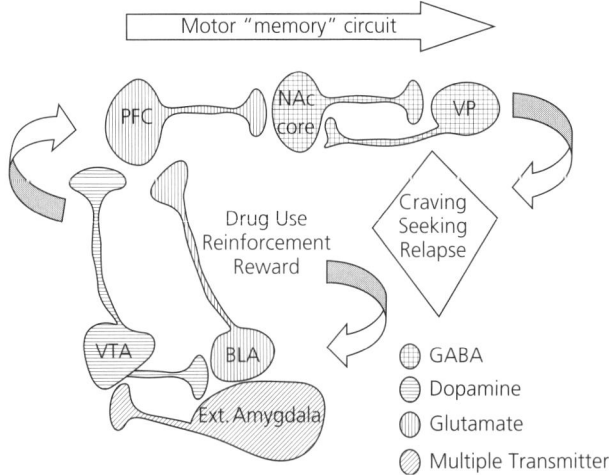

roimaging studies typically involve functional imaging of brain activity in addicts that are exposed to evocative stimuli, such as an injection of a low dose of drug or stimuli (e.g., drug paraphernalia) that the addict associates with drug taking (Volkow and Fowler, 2000). Preclinical studies typically involve animals trained to self-administer drug in a manner akin to human addicts followed by reinstatement of drug-seeking behavior. Thus, once stable self-administration behavior is established, the subjects are put through a period of extinction, whereby the operant response (usually lever pressing) that normally delivers the drug reward is no longer effective. Thereafter, the drug-associated response is reinstated by one of three priming stimuli: (1) administration of a low dose of drug, (2) exposure to a stressful event, or (3) exposure to a cue that was previously paired with the delivery of drug during the maintenance phase of the self-administration protocol (Porrino and Lyons, 2000).

These three priming stimuli are designed to mimic stimuli that are known to elicit craving and relapse in human addicts, including (1) relapse produced by a single dose of drug, (2) relapse arising from a stressful life event, and (3) relapse produced by encountering stimuli that remind the addict of previous drug experiences (O'Brien, 2001). This model is coupled with ex vivo measurements of changes in gene and protein expression and both in vivo and ex vivo indices of neurotransmission. Also, intracranial manipulations can be performed in selected brain nuclei to precisely determine the extent of involvement of a given nucleus in mediating (or inhibiting) drug-seeking behavior.

Neuroimaging studies have clearly identified cortical circuits that are activated by drug-associated stimuli in addicts. This includes areas of the prefrontal cortex, such as the anterior cingulate and the ventral orbital cortex, as well as some allocortical regions including the amygdala (Childress et al., 1999; Grant et al., 1996). In addition, some neuroimaging studies have revealed involvement of the ventral striatum (including the nucleus accumbens), especially in response to a small challenge dose of drug (Breiter et al., 1997). The animal literature has identified homologous cortical and allocortical structures in the reinstatement of drug-seeking behavior. In particular, the basolateral amygdala appears to be critical for cue-induced reinstatement, whereas a number of studies have shown involvement of the dorsal prefrontal cortex and nucleus accumbens, especially the core subcompartment, in drug-primed reinstatement (Everitt et al., 1999; See et al., 2001).

In addition, the animal literature has identified two other brain regions to be critical in models of stress-primed relapse. One area is the ventral tegmental area (McFarland et al., 2004), which, as outlined above, contains dopamine cells projecting to the cortex and nucleus accumbens. The other region that has been associated with stress-induced relapse is the bed nucleus of the stria terminalis and probably the accompanying nuclei of the extended amygdala (Leri et al., 2002). The extended amygdala is a cluster of interconnected nuclei postulated to be a relatively homogeneous functional entity in the execution of motivational behaviors (Leshner and Koob, 1999). The extended amygdala includes the central nucleus of the amygdala and its interconnections with the bed nucleus of the stria terminalis, the shell compartment of the nucleus accumbens, and the ventromedial portion of the ventral pallidum (Zahm and Heimer, 1988).

The ensuing discussion is organized around a growing realization that the expression of addiction is mediated via two circuits, a limbic "priming" circuit and a motor "memory" circuit (see Figure 6.1). The limbic circuit consists of nuclei within the motive circuit including the ventral prefrontal cortex, shell of the nucleus accumbens, ventral tegmental area, and basolateral amygdala. The motor circuit includes the dorsal prefrontal cortex, core of the nucleus accumbens, and dorsolateral ventral pallidum. The notion exists that the limbic circuit activates the motor circuit in response to drug-related stimuli, which essentially leads to the expression of addiction (e.g., drug-seeking behavior). However, the "priming" nuclei involved in activating the motor "memory" circuit is somewhat different depending on stimulus modality. For instance, the ventral tegmental area is integral to various stimuli, whereas the extended amygdala and basolateral amygdala contribute differentially depending on whether the stimulus is a stressor or a drug-associated cue, respectively.

The motor "memory" circuit may be integral to all forms of drug-taking behavior. Priming stimuli access this circuit primarily via the dorsal prefrontal cortex and evoke behaviors organized to obtain drug reward. The motor circuit functions akin to a procedural memory circuit, which when accessed by a priming stimulus, provides a programmed sequence of drug-associated behaviors. Also akin to procedural memory, behaviors elicited by the motor circuit proceed in a nearly unconscious manner and are extremely difficult to disrupt once begun. This latter quality accounts for the extent to which drug-seeking behavior in addicts is resistant to intrusion by executive cognitive thought processing and decision making (Jentsch and Taylor, 1999).

A role in mediating drug-primed reinstatement in animal models has been shown for the projection from the anterior cingulate to the core of the accumbens (McFarland and Kalivas, 2001). Moreover, studies in rodents using immediate early gene expression as markers of neuronal activation show that this projection is activated by presentation of a drug-associated cue (Neisewander et al., 2000; Thomas and Everitt, 2001). Thus, inhibition of the dorsal prefrontal cortex abolishes cocaine-, cue-, or stress-primed reinstatement, and we have recently shown that a rise in glutamate transmission in the core of the accumbens is associated with reinstatement behavior (McFarland et al., 2003). Also, blockade of the AMPA glutamate receptor subtype in the nucleus accumbens inhibits cocaine-induced reinstatement (Cornish and Kalivas, 2000). In turn, GABAergic spiny cells in the nucleus accumbens core innervate the dorsolateral ventral pallidum (Zahm and Heimer, 1988), and reversible or neurotoxic lesions of the ventral pallidum interfere with drug-primed reinstatement (McFarland and Kalivas, 2001). A linkage between the dorsal prefrontal cortex, core of the nucleus accumbens, and the ventral pallidum in cocaine-primed reinstatement was shown by the fact that injection of GABA agonists into the contralateral prefrontal cortex and ventral pallidum disrupted cocaine-primed reinstatement (McFarland and Kalivas, 2001). Thus, the subcircuit from the prefrontal cortex to the ventral pallidum (via a synapse in the nucleus accumbens) must be intact for cocaine-primed reinstatement to occur.

It is important to note that the projection from the nucleus accumbens to the ventral pallidum is GABAergic, and an abundance of literature indicates that activation of GABA transmission in the ventral pallidum inhibits both drug seeking and spontaneous motor activity (Kalivas et al., 1993). However, this projection is also peptidergic and contains enkephalin, substance P, and neurotensin (Zahm and Heimer, 1988). A pivotal role for these peptides in the ventral pallidum has emerged in primed drug-seeking behavior. Tang and colleagues (2005) have recently demonstrated that endogenous enkephalin transmission in the ventral pallidum is a critical mediator of cocaine reinstatement. Because naltrexone, a nonselective mu-opioid antagonist, is effective in reducing relapse in alcoholics (O'Brien, 2001), it is reasonable to propose that the apparent efficacy of naltrexone may result in part from a shared mechanism in the ventral pallidum.

In conclusion, the studies reviewed above point to the possibility of a final common pathway for the expression of addiction, and possibly similar brain circuits between drugs and stimuli that provoke craving and relapse. The extant data support a common role of the motor "memory" circuit shown in Figure 6.1 that consists of the series projection from the prefrontal cortex to nucleus accumbens core to the ventral pallidum. Although the studies outlined above are promising in pointing toward a common site of intervention in the expression of addiction, it is important to note that such a generalization based primarily on work with psychostimulants is premature and requires substantially more research using other classes of drugs, including alcohol, to validate. Similarly, the proposal for a final common "motor" memory pathway mediating craving and relapse induced by different modalities of stimuli is based only on a modest number of neuroimaging studies in addicts and experimental models of relapse. Nonetheless, sufficient supportive data has accrued to postulate a prepotent involvement of the motor "memory" pathway in addiction, especially the glutamatergic projection from regions of the prefrontal cortex including the anterior cingulate and ventral orbital cortex to the core of the nucleus accumbens. These emerging hints and hypotheses pose directions for novel pharmacological therapeutic strategies for ameliorating craving and relapse associated with addiction.

References

Bozarth, MA, and Wise, RA: Anatomically distinct opiate receptor fields mediate reward and physical dependence. *Science* 1984; 224(4648):516–7.

Breiter, HC, Gollub RL, Weisskoff RM, et al.: Acute effects of cocaine on human brain activity and emotion. *Neuron* 1997; 19:591–611.

Bunney, E, Appel S, and Brodie M: Electrophysiological effects of cocaethylene, cocaine, and ethanol on dopaminergic neurons of the ventral tegmental area. *J Pharmacol Exp Ther* 2001; 297(2):696–710.

Cameron, DL, Wessendorf, MW, and Williams, JT: A subset of ventral tegmental area neurons is inhibited by dopamine, 5-hydroxytryptamine and opioids. *Neuroscience* 1997; 77:155–66.

Carboni, E, Imperato, A, Perezzani, L, and Di Chiara, G: Amphetamine, cocaine, phencyclidine and nomifensine increase extracellular dopamine concentrations preferentially in the nucleus accumbens of freely moving rats. *Neuroscience* 1989; 28(3): 653–61.

Cheer, J, Kendall, D, and Marsden, C: Cannabinoid receptors and reward in the rat: a conditioned place preference study. *Psychopharmacology* 2000; 151:(1)25–30.

Childress, AR, Mozley, PD, McElgin, W, et al.: Limbic activation during cue-induced cocaine craving. *Am J Psychiatry* 1999; 156:11–18.

Cornish, JL, and Kalivas, PW: Glutamate transmission in the nucleus accumbens mediates relapse in cocaine addiction. *J Neurosci.* 2000; 20(15): RC89.

Dalley, JW, McGaughy, J, O'Connell, MT, Cardinal, RN, Levita, L, and Robbins, TW: Distinct changes in cortical acetylcholine and noradrenaline efflux during contingent and noncontingent performance of a visual attentional task. *J Neurosci.* 2001; 21(13):4908–14.

Everitt, BJ, Parkinson, JA, Olmstead, MC, et al.: Associative processes in addiction and reward. The role of amygdala-ventral striatal subsystems. *Ann NY Acad Sci* 1999; 877:412–38.

Gingrich, JA, and Hen, R: Dissecting the role of the serotonin system in neuropsychiatric disorders using knockout mice. *Psychopharmacology* 2001; 155(1):1–10.

Grant, S, London, ED, Newlin, DB, et al.: Activation of memory circuits during cue-elicited cocaine craving. *Proc Natl Acad Sci (USA)* 1996; 93: 12040–5.

Heimer, L, and Alheid, GF: Piecing together the puzzle of basal forebrain anatomy. *Adv Exp Med Biol* 1991; 295:1–42.

Hyman, SE, and Malenka, RC: Addiction and the brain: the neurobiology of compulsion and its persistence. *Nat Rev Neurosci.* 2001; 2(10):695–703.

Jentsch, K, and Taylor, J: Impulsivity resulting form frontostriatal dysfunction in drug abuse: implications for the control of behavior by reward-related stimuli. *Psychopharmacol* 1999; 146:373–90.

Kalivas, PW, Churchill, L, and Klitenick, MA: The circuitry mediating the translation of motivational stimuli into adaptive motor responses. In Kalivas, PW, and Barnes, CD (eds.): *Limbic Motor Circuits and Neuropsychiatry*. Boca Raton: CRC Press; 1993:237–87.

Kalivas, PW, and Volkow, ND: The neural basis of addiction: a pathology of motivation and choice. *Am J Psychiatry* 2005; 162(8):1403–13.

Leri, F, Flores, J, Rodaros, D, and Stewart, J: Blockade of stress-induced but not cocaine-induced reinstatement by infusion of noradrenergic antagonists into the bed nucleus of the stria terminalis or the central nucleus of the amygdala. *J Neurosci* 2002; 22(13):5713–8.

Leshner, AI, and Koob, GF: Drugs of abuse and the brain. *Proc Assoc Am Physicians* 1999; 111(2):99–108.

Loh, EA, and Roberts, DC: Break-points on a progressive ratio schedule reinforced by intravenous cocaine increase following depletion of forebrain serotonin. *Psychopharmacol* 1990;101(2):262–6.

McFarland, K, Davidge, SB, Lapish, CC, and Kalivas, PW: Limbic and motor circuitry underlying footshock-induced reinstatement of cocaine-seeking behavior. *J Neurosci* 2004; 24(7):1551–60.

McFarland, K, and Kalivas, PW: The circuitry mediating cocaine-induced reinstatement of drug-seeking behavior. *J Neurosci* 2001; 21:(21)8655–63.

McFarland, K, Lapish, CC, and Kalivas, PW: Prefrontal glutamate release into the core of the nucleus accumbens mediates cocaine-induced reinstatement of drug-seeking behavior. *J Neurosci* 2003; 23(8):3531–7.

Mogenson, GJ, Brudzynski, SM, Wu, M, et al.: From motivation to action: A review of dopaminergic regulation of limbic-nucleus accumbens-pedunculopontine nucleus circuitries involved in limbic-motor integration. In Kalivas, PW, and Barnes, CD (eds.): *Limbic Motor Circuits and Neuropsychiatry*. Boca Raton: CRC Press; 1993:193–236.

Murphy, JM, McBride, WJ, Lumeng, L, and Li, TK: Serotonin and ethanol drinking in the alcohol-preferring (P) rat. *Clin Neuropharmacol* 1992;15 (Suppl 1 Pt A):301A-302A.

Neisewander, JL, Baker, DA, Fuchs, RA, et al.: Fos protein expression and cocaine seeking behavior in rats after exposure to a cocaine self-administration environment. *Neuroscience* 2000; 20:(2)798–805.

Nestler, E: Molecular basis of long-term plasticity underlying addiction. *Nature Rev* 2001; 2:119–28.

Nisell, M, Nomikos, GG, and Svensson, TH: Systemic nicotine-induced dopamine release in the rat nucleus accumbens is regulated by nicotinic receptors in the ventral tegmental area. *Synapse* 1994; 16:36–44.

O'Brien, C: Drug addiction and drug abuse. In Hardman, J, Limbird, L, and Gilman, AG (eds.): *The Pharmacological Basis of Therapeutics*. New York: McGraw-Hill; 2001:621–42.

Olds, J, and Milner, P: Positive reinforcement produced by electrical stimulation of septal area and other regions of rat brain. *J Comp Physiol Psychol* 1954; 47(6):419–27.

Porrino, LJ, and Lyons, D: Orbital and medial prefrontal cortex and psychostimulant abuse: studies in animal models. *Cereb Cortex* 2000; 10:(3) 326–33.

Salamone, J, Cousins, M, McCullough, L, et al.: Nucleus accumbens dopamine release increases during instrumental lever pressing for food but not free food consumption. *Pharmacol Biochem Behav* 1994; 49:25–31.

Schultz, W: Predictive reward signal of dopamine neurons. *Am J Physiol* 1998; 80:1–27.

See, R, Kruzich, P, and Grimm, J: Dopamine, but not glutamate, receptor blockade in the basolateral amygdala attenuates conditioned reward in a rat model of relapse to cocaine-seeking behavior. *Psychopharmacol* 2001; 156:301–10.

Seiden, LS, Sabol, KE, and Ricuarte, GA: Amphetamine: effects on catecholamine systems and behavior. *Ann Rev Pharmacol Toxicol* 1993; 33: 639–77.

Tang, XC, McFarland, K, Cagle, S, and Kalivas, PW: Cocaine-induced reinstatement requires endogenous stimulation of mu-opioid receptors in the ventral pallidum. *J Neurosci* 2005; 25(18):4512–20.

Thomas, KL, and Everitt, BJ: Limbic-cortical-ventral striatal activation during retrieval of a discrete cocaine-associated stimulus: a cellular imaging study with gamma protein kinase C expression. *J Neurosci* 2001; 21:(7)2526–35.

Volkow, ND, and Fowler, JS: Addiction, a disease of compulsion and drive: involvement of the orbitofrontal cortex. *Cereb Cortex* 2000; 10:(3)318–25.

Wise, RA, and Bozarth, MA: Action of drugs of abuse on brain reward systems: an update with specific attention to opiates. *Pharmacol Biochem Behav* 1982; 17:(2)239–43.

Wise, RA, and Bozarth, MA: A psychomotor stimulant theory of addiction. *Psychol Rev* 1987; 94:(4)469–92.

Zahm, DS, and Heimer, L: Ventral striatopallidal parts of the basal ganglia in the rat: I. Neurochemical compartmentation as reflected by the distributions of neurotensin and substance P immunoreactivity. *J Comp Neurol* 1988; 272:516–25.

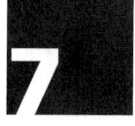

7

Neuroimaging in Addiction

Tim M. Williams

Shrikant Srivastava

Anne R. Lingford-Hughes

David J. Nutt

Dependence on and harmful use of substances have wide reaching public health implications. In 2004, 19.1 million people in the United States (7.9% of the population aged 12 and over) were current illicit drug users, with marijuana being the most commonly used substance (SAMHSA, 2004). Recently there has been a significant increase in the nonmedical use of painkillers among young adults (aged 18–25 years). Alcohol is used regularly by the majority of the population in the United States; however, young adults report the highest prevalence of binge and heavy drinking (41.2 and 15.1%, respectively). Furthermore, 22.5 million people in the United States were classified with past-year substance dependence or abuse (9.4% of the population), 3.8 million of whom had received treatment in the 12 months prior to survey.

Neuroimaging provides measurement of the structure, function, and chemistry of the brain in vivo. Advances in neuroimaging technology have allowed neurobiological theories of addiction to become better defined. Structure of the brain can be measured with computed tomography (CT) or more frequently with the higher resolution of magnetic resonance imaging (MRI). Functional neuroimaging techniques include radiotracer methods, which involve administration of radioactive chemicals, using positron emission tomography (PET) and single photon emission computed tomography (SPECT), and those using functional MRI (fMRI), pharmacological MRI (phMRI), and magnetic resonance spectroscopy (MRS). The radiotracer methods reveal the neurochemistry, blood flow, or metabolism in specific areas of the brain. Functional MRI measures changes in blood flow, reflecting local neuronal activity, and phMRI, when such changes induced by an acute administration of a drug and MRS measures concentrations of chemicals in the brain.

Role of Neurotransmitters in Addiction

This chapter will discuss the role of two major neurotransmitters—dopamine and opioids—as related to addiction, and general findings related to craving for drugs. Further discussion is on neuroimaging studies on individual drugs of abuse, which have been subdivided into structural and functional studies.

Dopamine

Addiction involves a dysfunction in areas mediating pleasure, attention, and emotion. The dopaminergic neurons in ventral tegmental area (VTA) that project to nucleus accumbens and related structures such as limbic cortex, including the orbitofrontal and anterior cingulate cortex, hippocampus, and amygdala, form an important pathway for the reinforcing actions of a number of drugs.

Many drugs of abuse, such as stimulants like cocaine or amphetamine, rather than acting directly on the dopaminergic synapse to increase dopamine levels, modulate the activity of dopaminergic neurons in the VTA, where they are modulated by GABA and opioid systems. GABA receptors are located on dopaminergic neurons and have a tonic inhibitory action, and hence reduce the firing of these dopaminergic neurons. The GABA-ergic neurons themselves express mu-opioid receptors, which when activated inhibit GABA-ergic transmission. The net result of activating the mu-opioid receptors is therefore increased activity of dopaminergic neurons by inhibiting the GABA "brake." This effect is thought to be key in mediating the reinforcing properties of drugs of abuse such as alcohol and opioids.

Opioids

A finding common to many substances of abuse is an increase in opioid receptor availability in early abstinence from dependent substance use. In opioids, it has been shown that there is an increase in opioid receptor levels in patients immediately after detoxification from methadone when compared with nonopioid using controls (Williams et al., 2007). Studies using ^{11}C-carfentanil PET have shown increased levels of the mu-opioid receptors in recently abstinent cocaine dependent subjects, the elevation in receptor level correlating positively with the severity of cocaine craving reported (Gorelick et al., 2005; Zubieta et al., 1996). In alcohol dependence, elevation in mu-opioid receptors persisted up to 5 weeks of abstinence from dependent alcohol use (Heinz et al., 2005a).

The endogenous opioid system has been hypothesized to be involved in the reinforcing action of drugs of abuse by modulating dopamine. Hagelberg et al. (2004) showed evidence of modulation of dopamine pathway by opioids. In the presence of alfentanil, there was higher binding of ^{11}C-FLB457 in medial frontal cortex, dorsolateral prefrontal cortex, superior temporal cortex, anterior cingulate cortex, and medial thalamus. The findings indicate that in the presence of alfentanil, there is reduced synaptic dopamine.

Craving and Anticipation

Craving is a term often used by dependent people to describe difficulty in controlling their drug use, and is implicated in relapse. Craving is a multidimensional phenomenon incorporating a desire to gain a positive feeling (e.g., euphoria), to overcome a negative feeling (e.g., withdrawal), or "urge to use." Cue-exposure paradigms are widely used to study "craving." Areas such as amygdala, anterior cingulate cortex, dorsolateral prefrontal cortex, and orbitofrontal cortex are activated during study paradigms. Amygdala is involved in associative learning (i.e., between cue and drug), the anterior cingulated cortex in emotional processing, and the dorsolateral prefrontal cortex with memory.

It has been observed that that cue exposure generally results in activation of dorsolateral prefrontal cortex and orbitofrontal cortex in nontreatment-seeking individuals and not in those who are in treatment. Wilson et al. (2004) suggest that dorsolateral prefrontal cortex activation reflects generation and maintenance of behavioral goals aimed at obtaining a reward and the orbitofrontal cortex is related to the anticipation of getting the drug.

Anticipation is a related phenomenon to craving, in which knowing that the drug is about to be administered can enhance the effects of the drug (Volkow et al., 2003). Administration of methylphenidate to cocaine users was associated with greater activation in cerebellum and thalamus when the subjects were expecting the drug, but greater activation in orbitofrontal cortex when the subjects were not expecting the drug. The increase in metabolism in the thalamus was correlated positively with subjective feelings of "high." Similarly, in coffee drinkers there is increased binding of ^{11}C-raclopride, signifying release of dopamine, in the thalamus when the subjects were expecting caffeine, as opposed to the time when the subjects were expecting placebo (Kaasinen et al., 2004). The changes seen in orbitofrontal cortex are important owing to its role in impulse control and decision making (Volkow & Fowler, 2000, London et al., 2000).

Opioid Drugs

Opioid drugs are widely abused across the world. Use of heroin produces effects that are strongly reinforcing and causes a potent psychological and physiological dependence. Drug-seeking behavior leads many users to commit acquisitive crime with enormous implications for the individual and society. Continued use is associated with high morbidity and mortality.

Structural Neuroimaging

The technique of voxel-based morphometry has been used to study structural brain changes in opioid-dependent subjects relative to healthy comparison subjects (Lyoo et al., 2006). Decreased gray matter density was found in bilateral prefrontal cortex, bilateral insula, bilateral superior temporal cortex, left fusiform cortex, and right unculus. This may have implications for some of the behavioral and psychological changes seen in the addiction syndrome.

Cerebral Blood Flow and Metabolism

Studies have shown acute doses of opioid agonists result in increased activity in specific brain regions. The effects of fentanyl and remifentanil, selective mu-opioid agonists, on regional cerebral blow flow (rCBF) have been studied using ^{15}O-water PET (Firestone et al., 1996; Wagner et al., 2001). Both opioids resulted in increased rCBF in prefrontal and anterior cingulate areas and decreased activity in the cerebellum. Hydromorphone, another selective mu-agonist, has been shown to increase activity in the anterior cingulate, amygdala, and thalamus using ^{99m}Tc-HMPAO SPECT (Schlaepfer et al., 1998). However, acute morphine administration has shown to reduce glucose utilization throughout the brain, using ^{18}F-FDG PET (London et al., 1990a). The regions identified in these studies are involved in avoidance learning, reward, and pain-related behaviors and help understanding the addictive potential of drugs.

During withdrawal from opioids, a study with ^{99m}Tc-HMPAO SPECT has shown that perfusion deficits persist to 1 week after stopping heroin, but improved after 3 weeks of abstinence, particularly in the frontal and parietal lobes (Rose et al., 1996). Opioid antagonist-assisted withdrawal studies have confirmed decrease in cerebral perfusion, and the severity of withdrawal correlated negatively with perfusion in the anterior cingulate cortex (Van Dyck et al., 1994) and reduced right temporal lobe activity (Krystal et al., 1995).

Cerebral blood flow studies using ^{15}O-water PET have been used to investigate brain regions associated with risk decision making in chronic opioid users, chronic amphetamine users, previously opioid and amphetamine dependent individuals, and healthy comparisons (Ersche et al., 2005). Participants with current or previous dependence on either amphetamines or opioid drugs activated the left orbitofrontal cortex during risky decision making, whereas control participants exhibited relative deactivation in this area. The control participants showed significantly greater activation in the right dorsolateral prefrontal cortex than drug users in response to the task.

Another study of rewards demonstrated increases in rCBF in areas associated with the dopaminergic mesolimbic system in response to monetary rewards in opioid addicts but to both monetary and nonmonetary reward in controls (Martin-Soelch et al., 2001). The lateral orbitofrontal cortex and dorsolateral prefrontal cortex are both associated with response inhibition. The inhibition of responses to risky high-reward choices is thought to be deficient in many drug users.

Craving

Daglish et al. (2001) used a ^{15}O-water PET individualized cue-exposure paradigm and found increased rCBF in the anterior cingulate cortex in response to the salient drug cue, whereas craving itself was associated with activation in the left orbitofrontal cortex. The "urge to use" is correlated strongly with increased rCBF in the inferior frontal and orbitofrontal cortices (Sell et al., 2000).

Neurochemistry

Patients maintained on methadone, when scanned with ^{18}F-cyclofoxy PET, had fewer available opioid receptors in thalamus, amygdala, caudate, putamen, and anterior cingulate cortex, compared to normal controls (Kling et al., 2000). However, a clear dose-response relationship was evident only in caudate and putamen areas. No significant occupancy of opioid receptors by methadone was found in patients on a range substitute methadone doses using ^{11}C-diprenorphine PET, suggesting that very low occupancy is required for clinical efficacy (Melichar et al., 2005).

Stimulants: Cocaine and Amphetamines

Cocaine use is pervasive throughout the world and is recognized as having wide-reaching health consequences. Methamphetamine use is now widespread in the United States and parts of Asia and is an emerging trend in Europe, representing a new public health challenge. Cocaine exerts its effects by competitively blocking uptake of dopamine, noradrenaline, and serotonin. The blockade of dopamine transporter (DAT) leads to increased dopamine in the synapse that stimulates dopamine receptors.

Structural Neuroimaging

Cocaine users have been shown to have structural deficits as compared to drug-naïve controls. Franklin et al. (2002) used voxel-based morphometry of MRI images to compare cocaine-dependent and cocaine-naïve individuals. Reduction in gray matter concentration was seen in ventromedial orbitofrontal, anterior cingulate, anteroventral insular, and superior temporal cortices of cocaine patients in comparison to controls; the average percentage decrease within a region ranged from 5% to 11%. Matochik et al. (2003) showed significantly decreased gray matter density in cocaine users as compared to controls in 10 of 13 small volumes analyzed in the frontal cortex; specifically bilaterally in the anterior cingulate gyrus, medial orbitofrontal cortex, lateral orbitofrontal cortex, and middle/dorsal cingulate gyrus on the right side. Both the above studies did not find any difference in white matter densities between subjects and controls.

Makris et al. (2004) compared cocaine-dependent individuals to matched controls using segmentation-based morphometry. Amygdala volume was significantly reduced in the cocaine-dependent individuals compared to controls, with the decrease of greater magnitude on the right (23%) than the left (13%). In addition, there was loss of normal laterality of amygdala in the addicts. The volume of hippocampi on both sides was less in addicts than controls, but did not reach a statistically significant level.

Cerebral Blood Flow and Metabolism

Cocaine-induced cerebral ischemia is an increasingly common presentation to hospital emergency departments. The mechanism for this is vasospasm of the large cranial arteries and cortical microvasculature. Increased levels of monoamines, principally dopamine, mediate this vasospasm and also reduce blood flow. Chronic use of cocaine has been shown to cause patchy areas of deranged cerebral blood flow and specific decreases in rCBF in the prefrontal cortex when compared to nondrug-using controls using ^{15}O-water PET (Volkow et al., 1988a). High- and low-dose intravenous cocaine administered to cocaine-using subjects causes global and regional cerebral hypoperfusion when compared to placebo injection (Johnson et al., 2005). However a significant dose-dependent effect was seen only in the left sublobar and midbrain regions, areas rich in dopamine projections. The orbitofrontal cortex is a region linked with patterns of drug-using behavior and craving. There are now consistent reports of lower resting orbitofrontal rCBF in cocaine-dependent subjects when compared to nondrug-using controls (Adinoff et al., 2001, 2003; Volkow et al., 1992a).

Reductions in glucose metabolism is also seen with ^{18}F-FDG PET and perfusion as measured with ^{99m}Tc-HMPAO SPECT, with greater reductions associated with increased "rush" (London et al., 1990b, Pearlson et al., 1993). The "rush" following intravenous infusion of cocaine has also been shown to correlate with increased activity in the cingulate and lateral prefrontal cortex on fMRI (Breiter et al., 1997). During withdrawal phase in the first week, there is increased metabolism in orbitofrontal cortex and basal ganglia, which returns to normal levels in 4 weeks (Volkow et al., 1991a). However, reduced metabolism in frontal regions, more on left than right side, is evident up to 4 months of abstinence. This reduction correlates with dose and years of cocaine abuse (Volkow 1992b). These persistent deficits may be responsible for mediating the "urge to use" in cocaine addicts.

Neurochemistry

Cocaine and stimulants act to increase synaptic transmission at the dopamine receptors, thus resulting in the drug's pleasurable and reinforcing effects. Methylphenidate is often used experimentally as a cocaine analogue as it has identical regional distribution, produces the same "high" as cocaine, and competes for the same binding sites, although clearance of methylphenidate is slower, which may account for its lower abuse potential (Volkow et al., 1995). Furthermore, both drugs produced comparable dose-dependent blockade of dopamine transporters (DAT) in animal and human studies (Gatley et al., 1999; Volkow et al., 1999a). The subjective effects of cocaine can be directly attributed to blockade of the DAT and thus an increase in the availability of free dopamine within the brain (Volkow et al., 1997a). The actual release of dopamine in the brain can be measured by its displacement of tracers ^{11}C-raclopride, with PET, and ^{123}I-IBZM, with SPECT. In healthy volunteers, methylphenidate and amphetamine reduce the binding of these tracers, and the greater the displacement of the tracer, the more "rush" is experienced (Volkow et al., 1996a). There is less release of dopamine in more severely cocaine-dependant patients as compared to controls (Volkow et al., 1997b).

Chronic use of a drug results in hypodopaminergic state, particularly during withdrawal and abstinence, and is thought to underlie feelings of dysphoria and irritability. Avoidance of dysphoric mood states may be responsible for the continued use of substance. The neurobiological consequences of prolonged cocaine use have been imaged using 6 fluorodopa (6-FDOPA), an index of dopaminergic presynaptic activity (Wu et al., 1997). Cocaine-dependent subjects who were abstaining for 11–30 days had significantly lower striatal 6-FDOPA uptake compared to normal controls or early abstinence (1–10 days abstinence). The cocaine-dependent subjects showed a significant negative correlation between days off cocaine and striatal 6-FDOPA uptake. This is consistent with the hypothesis of decreasing dopamine synthesis and decreased dopamine concentration during abstinence from cocaine.

There is reduction in number of dopamine D2-type receptors (DRD2) in all addictions (Volkow et al., 2002a, 2004). With cocaine, there is little increase in number of DRD2 receptors even after 4 months of abstinence. Reduced levels of DRD2 in striatum are associated with reduced metabolism in orbitofrontal cortex in cocaine abusers (Volkow et al., 1993a). To determine whether low DRD2 levels are the cause or effect of addiction, Volkow et al. (2002b) administered methylphenidate to healthy volunteers. Those volunteers with low DRD2 numbers experienced liking for the drug, whereas those with high DRD2 levels described methylphenidate as being unpleasant. Using methylphenidate, a DAT blocker, to increase dopamine levels, Volkow et al. (1999b) found that metabolism in the orbitofrontal region was increased, but only in those addicts who reported craving. Thus, simply increasing dopaminergic function is not sufficient to redress hypometabolism in cocaine addicts. Reduced number of striatal DRD2 levels is also reported in methamphetamine addicts that correlated with reduced metabolism in the orbitofrontal cortex. Striatal DAT is also reduced in methamphetamine users (McCann et al., 1998a).

In addition to dopaminergic system, a global decrease in serotonin transporter density in abstinent drug users, as compared to controls, has been reported using $^{11}C(+)$McN-5652 PET scan (Sekine et al., 2006). The authors conclude that protracted use of methamphetamine may reduce the density of the serotonin transporter in the brain.

Craving

Studies using ^{18}F-FDG PET have shown that craving for cocaine correlated with increased activity in the amygdala and dorsolateral prefrontal cortex (Grant et al., 1996), and anterior cingulate cortex (Childress et al., 1999). More recently, fMRI studies have shown activation in similar areas, including the anterior cingulate and prefrontal and orbitofrontal cortices, in response to salient cues (Garavan et al., 2000; Wexler et al., 2001). Breiter et al. (1997) showed that during craving, the nucleus accumbens, right parahippocampal gyrus, and prefrontal cortex were activated.

Sex differences in regional brain activation were seen in a study of script-guided imagery of a stressful and a neutral situation in an fMRI study of abstinent cocaine addicts (Li et al., 2005). Female addicts showed more activation in left middle frontal, anterior cingulate and inferior frontal cortices, and insula and right cingulate cortex during stress imagery. The change of activity in left anterior and right posterior cingulate cortices correlated inversely with the ratings on craving.

Studies using fMRI have shown a relationship between craving and reward pathways implicated in addiction. Risinger et al. (2005) demonstrated when addicts were allowed to self-administer cocaine, the drug-induced "high" correlated negatively with activity in limbic, paralimbic, and mesocortical regions including the nucleus accumbens, inferior frontal/orbitofrontal gyrus, and anterior cingulate, whereas craving correlated positively with activity in these regions. Sinha et al. (2005) compared abstinent cocaine-dependent individuals with normal controls on brief guided imagery and recall of personal stressful and neutral situations. During stress imagery, the patients showed increased activity in the caudate and dorsal striatum region that was significantly associated with craving ratings, and less activation in the anterior cingulate region, left hippocampal-parahippocampal region, right fusiform gyrus, and the right postcentral gyrus, as compared to normal controls.

Abnormalities in opioid receptors have been reported as related to craving. A preliminary study using ^{11}C-carfentanil PET in abstinent cocaine-dependent patients found significant increases in mu-opioid receptor availability 1–4 days after cessation of dependent-cocaine use in the frontal cortex, temporal cortex, anterior cingulate, caudate nucleus, and thalamus (Zubieta et al., 1996). Higher mu-opioid receptor availability was associated with craving for cocaine. In some individuals, mu-opioid receptor availability decreased over time, but in others, this persisted for up to 4 weeks. A follow-up study using similar protocols again identified anterior cingulate and frontal cortex after 1 day and 1 week of abstinence from cocaine (Gorelick 2005).

Ecstasy

Ecstasy (3,4-methylenedioxymethamphetamine; MDMA) is a stimulant drug with mild hallucinatory properties. Its popularity rose as a "club drug" in the 1990s, and its use is second only to cannabis (Condon & Smith, 2003). Ecstasy use results in the release of catecholamines, particularly serotonin, the stores of which are depleted on excessive use. The use of ecstasy has been associated with loss of serotonergic neurons in nonhuman primates and fueled the debate as to the drug's danger; however, whether this loss occurs in humans remains controversial. The main problem in studying ecstasy is that seldom is it the only drug abused; commonly ecstasy forms part of polydrug use.

Structural Neuroimaging

Cowan et al. (2003) employed voxel-based morphometry to study structural brain changes in polydrug users taking ecstasy relative to polydrug users not taking ecstasy. Although several brain regions showed decreased gray matter concentration in the ecstasy group, this group also scored significantly higher on rates of opioid, cocaine, cannabis, PCP, and hallucinogen use. These findings make it difficult to conclude that ecstasy itself resulted in any structural damage to the brain.

A preliminary study (Reneman et al., 2001a) using diffusion and perfusion MRI reported relative higher diffusion coefficient and relative cerebral volume ratios in globus pallidus in ecstasy polydrug users as compared to nonecstasy polydrug users. This increase in the globus pallidus volume was correlated with the extent of previous use of ecstasy.

Cerebral Blood Flow and Metabolism

Schrekenberger et al. (1999) administered ecstasy analogue MDE (3,4-methylene dioxymethamphetamine) to healthy volunteers. PET scan with ^{18}F-FDG showed significantly decreased glucose metabolism in left frontal posterior and right prefrontal superior cortices, and increased metabolism in cerebellum bilaterally and right putamen. In another similar paradigm, Gamma et al. (2000) employed ^{15}O-water PET scan following a single oral dose of ecstasy (1.7 mg/kg) or placebo to 16 MDMA-naive subjects. Ecstasy infusion, as compared to placebo, resulted in increased blood flow in ventromedial frontal and occipital cortex, inferior temporal lobe and cerebellum; and decreased flow in the motor and somatosensory cortex, temporal lobe including left amygdala, cingulate cortex, insula and thalamus. Concomitant with these changes, subjects experienced heightened mood, increased extroversion, slight derealization and mild perceptual alterations.

Chang et al. (2000) used SPECT to compare abstinent with non-users of ecstasy, and did not find any difference in rCBF in both groups of subjects. Ten of the abstinent subjects were given 2 doses of ecstasy, and within 3 weeks after MDMA administration, rCBF remained decreased in the visual cortex, the caudate, the superior parietal and dorsolateral frontal regions compared to baseline rCBF. Two of these subjects, when scanned about 3 months later, showed increased rather than decreased rCBF.

Neurochemistry

The focus of neurochemical imaging studies and ecstasy has been on levels of serotonin (5-hydroxytryptamine or 5-HT) and the 5-HT transporter (5-HTT). Initial studies using the tracers ^{11}C-McN-5652 PET and ^{123}I-beta-CIT SPECT to measure the 5-HTT reported reduced levels throughout the brain in ecstasy users (McCann et al., 1998b; Semple et al., 1999). However, the main limitation of these studies is the inability to discriminate with confidence between the changes produced by use of ecstasy alone as opposed to those produced by other drugs of abuse.

Later studies using the same tracers have reported similar reductions in 5-HTT levels in the thalamus, caudate nucleus, midbrain, and hippocampus of current ecstasy users (Buchert et al.,

2004; Thomasius et al., 2003). These studies are more robust, having included another "control" group of nonecstasy-using polydrug users. Furthermore, it was shown that there is greater reduction of 5-HTT in women than men, and following abstinence (< 1-year duration since last tablet of ecstasy), there was no difference in 5-HTT levels between addicts and controls (Reneman et al., 2001b). The same authors (Reneman et al., 2000c) compared heavy, moderate, and past users with those who had never used ecstasy. The sex difference was apparent again when 5-HTT levels were lower in heavy-using women, but not men, and female past users had higher 5-HTT levels than controls.

Similar results using were obtained by McCann et al. (2005) using ^{11}C-McN56552 and ^{11}C-DASB PET. Comparison of abstinent and nonusers of ecstasy revealed a global reduction in 5-HTT with both ligands. Further exploratory analyses showed that the reduction in 5-HTT was directly related to extent of ecstasy use and on abstinence recovered with time. The N-acetyl content of brain is an indicator of neuronal injury. No difference was discovered in N-acetyl content of ecstasy users and non-users on ^{1}H-MRS scans (Chang et al., 1999). However, there was increased myo-inositol content in the user group, indicative of increased glial content, which correlated with lifetime dose of ecstasy.

Cannabis (Marijuana)

Cannabis, or marijuana, contains over 60 cannabinoid compounds, the most psychoactive of which is delta^9-tetrahydrocannabinol (THC). The differing levels of psychoactive constituents make "dose-effect" studies challenging.

Structural Imaging

There is no conclusive evidence as to whether long-term use of cannabis produces structural changes in the brain. Wilson et al. (2000) reported smaller whole brain, smaller percentage of gray matter, and larger percentage of white matter in subjects with onset of cannabis use before 17 years of age. A voxel-based morphometry study found regional changes in gray and white matter in 11 heavy cannabis users compared to nonusing controls (Matochik et al., 2005). However, other studies report no differences in volumes of gray and white matter between cannabis users and controls (Block et al., 2000a; Tzilos et al., 2005). Importantly, the latter study examined older users of cannabis.

Cerebral Blood Flow and Metabolism

Smoking cannabis produces subjective effects such as depersonalization and changes in time sense, with peak effects seen at approximately 30 minutes. Measures of intoxication, depersonalization, and altered time sense have been characterized in response to intravenous THC and correlated with changes in rCBF and regional cerebral metabolism of glucose (rCMR$_{glu}$), using ^{15}O-water and ^{18}F-FDG PET, respectively.

Significant increases in global perfusion in response to THC have been shown, and in rCBF in the frontal cortex, insula, and anterior cingulate (Mathew et al., 2002). Cannabis intoxication has been shown to be associated with global and rCBF increases that are most notable over the frontal regions (Mathew et al., 1997). Depersonalization in response to THC has been shown to produce a significant positive partial correlation with increase in rCBF in the right anterior cingulate and the right frontal region (Mathew et al., 1999). THC-induced alteration in time sense has been linked to changes in cerebellar rCBF (Mathew et al., 1998).

Acute doses of THC have been shown to cause an increase in normalized cerebellar metabolism. Furthermore, the changes in cerebellar CMR$_{glu}$ correlated with plasma THC levels and ratings of intoxication (Volkow et al., 1991b). Baseline relative cerebellar CMR$_{glu}$ has been shown to be lower in marijuana users than controls but was found to increase in response to THC in all subjects; however, only marijuana users showed rCMR$_{glu}$ increases in orbitofrontal cortex, prefrontal cortex, and basal ganglia (Volkow et al., 1996b).

Neurochemistry

There is a serendipitous case report concerning the effects of marijuana on dopamine release in vivo in man (Voruganti et al., 2001). Smoking marijuana secretly, a medication-free patient with schizophrenia, during an infusion protocol using ^{123}I-IBZM SPECT, showed 20% decrease in striatal DRD2 binding, suggestive of increased synaptic dopamine.

Alcohol

Alcohol is the most commonly abused psychotropic drug. Farrell et al. (2001) showed that 80% of the U.K. population had consumed alcohol within last 12 months, and 5% of the population surveyed was dependent on it. The clinical effects of acute and chronic alcohol and the associated withdrawal phenomena are well described in the literature, but the underlying neurobiology is only just being determined.

Structural Neuroimaging

It is long known that alcohol results in loss of both gray and white matter, and this is clearly shown in a number of CT and MRI studies (see Sullivan & Pfefferbaum 2005). Reduced white matter in the temporal lobes has been related to a history of seizures, but it is not clear whether it is a cause or a consequence (Sullivan et al., 1996). We also know that abstinence promotes recovery, and recent MRS studies are helping us understand this important process. Ende et al. (2005) have shown changes in levels of N-acetyl aspartate and choline that suggest that improved myelination and axonal integrity occur in abstinence.

Cerebral Blood Flow and Metabolism

In social drinkers, alcohol reduces cerebral blood flow within the cerebellum and increases blood flow in the right temporal cortex and prefrontal cortex (Volkow et al., 1988b). Reduced cerebral activity is reported in abstinent alcohol-dependent individuals, particularly within the frontal and parietal lobes and cerebellum, where atrophy might contribute (Gilman et al., 1990; Sachs et al., 1987; Wik et al., 1988). In alcohol-abstinent subjects, administering an intoxicating level of alcohol reduces glucose metabolism in cortical and cerebellar regions, but not in the basal ganglia (Volkow et al., 1990b).

Increasing abstinence from alcohol leads to an increase in brain glucose metabolism, with most improvement seen in frontal lobes (Berglund et al., 1987) and mainly during the first 16 and 30 days of abstinence (Volkow et al., 1994). Metabolism within the frontal, parietal, and temporal cortices was negatively correlated with the number of years of drinking and with age.

Craving

Compared to other substances of abuse, fewer imaging studies have been performed measuring craving for alcohol. Using

⁹⁹ᵐTc-HMPAO SPECT, increased perfusion was found in the right caudate nucleus that correlated with increased desire and craving for alcohol (Modell & Mountz, 1995). Initial fMRI studies reported that cue-induced craving was associated with increased activity in dorsolateral prefrontal cortex and anterior thalamus (George et al., 2001) and in amygdala/hippocampus and cerebellum (Schneider 2001). More recently, however, cue-induced craving has been shown to result in activity in the striatum and medial prefrontal cortex, and this increase relates to relapse rates (Grüsser et al., 2004). In addition, increased activity in the left nucleus accumbens, anterior cingulate, and left orbitofrontal cortex has been shown to significantly correlate with subjective craving ratings in nontreatment-seeking alcoholic individuals but not controls (Myrick et al., 2004).

Neurochemistry

The GABA-BDZ receptor has been studied using ^{11}C-flumazenil PET or ^{123}I-iomazenil SPECT because of similarities between actions of alcohol and benzodiazepines. Three studies are in broad agreement showing reduced levels of the GABA-BDZ receptors in the frontal lobe, particularly in the mediofrontal cortex (Abi-Dargham et al., 1998; Gilman et al., 1996; Lingford-Hughes et al., 1998), which is not attributable in entirety to cerebral atrophy. In addition, reduced sensitivity to benzodiazepines has been shown in alcoholism. The hypnotic effects of midazolam, a benzodiazepine agonist, are attenuated in abstinent alcoholics, but its effects on EEG are not altered (Lingford-Hughes et al., 2005). The mechanisms underlying differential sensitivity to alcohol are as yet unproven in humans, but it is likely that different subtypes of the GABA-BDZ receptor play a role because sensitivity to alcohol depends on the subunit composition.

As already discussed, the dopaminergic system is thought to be crucially involved in the addictive process. Reduced levels of the DRD2 have been reported in abstinent alcohol-dependent patients using ^{11}C-raclopride PET or ^{123}I-IBZM SPECT (Hietala et al., 1994; Volkow et al., 1996c), which persisted for months (Volkow et al., 2002c). By contrast, Guardia et al. (2000) found higher levels of striatal ^{123}I-IBZM uptake during detoxification in patients who were more likely to relapse by 3 months. Such an increase may be due to low endogenous dopamine, which the authors suggest is associated with poorer outcome.

Differing studies have reported normal DAT levels in alcoholics abstinent for over a month, or that acute withdrawal is associated with reduced DAT levels that increase during the first month (Heinz et al., 1998; Volkow et al., 1996c). Tiihonen et al. (1995) differentiated between violent (similar to type 2 alcoholics) and nonviolent (similar to type 1 alcoholics). Compared to control subjects, violent alcoholics had slightly higher DAT levels and nonviolent alcoholics had markedly lower levels.

In addition, there is evidence for involvement of dopamine system in mediating craving. Heinz et al. (2004), using ^{18}F-desmethoxyfallipride PET, showed less availability of DRD2 receptors in ventral striatum correlated with craving severity, and with greater cue-induced activation of medial prefrontal cortex and anterior cingulate cortex as seen with fMRI. In the same subjects, reduced dopamine synthesis in ventral striatum, as measured by blood brain clearance of 6–^{18}F-fluorol-I-dopa, was found to be reduced at follow-up, and correlated inversely with degree of craving (Heinz et al., 2005b).

Using ^{123}I-beta-CIT SPECT, Heinz et al. (1998) reported that alcohol dependence was associated with reduced levels of the 5HTT in the brainstem raphe nucleus that correlated with ratings of depression and anxiety. Notably, this reduction, but not alcoholism, was associated with a particular allelic variation (11) of the 5HT transporter, suggesting that this polymorphism mediates susceptibility to neurotoxicity (Heinz et al., 2000).

Conclusion

The last two decades have seen much advancement in the technology of neuroimaging, which has resulted in better understanding of changes produced in the brain due to addiction. However, questions still remain to be answered with certainty such as are there any particular areas or circuits which predispose to addiction or which lead to relapse? Neuroimaging techniques are constantly providing the clinician with new information towards unraveling the underpinnings of addiction.

References

Abi-Dargham A, Krystal JH, Anjilvel S, et al. Alterations of benzodiazepine receptors in type II alcoholic subjects measured with SPECT and [123I]iomazenil. *Am J Psychiatry* 1998;155(11):1550–5.

Adinoff, Devous MD, Best SE, et al. Limbic responsiveness to procaine in cocaine-addicted subjects. *Am J Psychiatry* 2001;158(3):390–8.

Adinoff B, Devous MD Sr., Cooper DB, et al. Resting regional cerebral blood flow and gambling task performance in cocaine-dependent subjects and healthy comparison subjects. *Am J Psychiatry* 2003;160(10):1892–94.

Berglund M, Hagstadius S, Risberg J, et al. Normalization of regional cerebral blood flow in alcoholics during the first 7 weeks of abstinence. *Acta Psychiat Scand* 1987;75:202–208.

Block RI, O'Leary DS, Ehrhardt SC, et al. Effect of frequent marijuana use on brain tissue volume and composition. *Neuroreport* 2000a;11(3):491–6.

Breiter HC, Gollub RL, Weisskoff RM, et al. Acute effects of cocaine on human brain activity and emotion. *Neuron* 1997;19(3):591–611.

Buchert R, Thomasius R, Wilke F, et al. A voxel-based PET investigation of the long-term effects of "ecstasy" consumption on brain serotonin transporters. *Am J Psychiatry* 2004;161(7):1181–89.

Chang L, Ernst T, Grob CS, Poland RE. Cerebral (1)H MRS alterations in recreational 3,4-methylenedioxymethamphetamine (MDMA, "ecstasy") users. *J Magn Reson Imaging* 1999;10(4):521–6.

Chang L, Grob CS, Ernst T, et al. Effect of Ecstasy [3,4-methylenedioxy-methamphetamine (MDMA)] on cerebral blood flow: a co-registered SPECT and MRI study. *Psychiatry Res* 2000;98(1):15–28.

Childress AR, Mozley PD, McElgin W, et al. Limbic activation during cue-induced cocaine craving. *Am J Psychiatry* 1999;156(1):11–8.

Condon J, Smith N. *Prevalence of drug use: key findings from the 2002/2003 British crime survey*. London: Research Development and Statistics Directorate; 2003.

Cowan RL, Lyoo IK, Sung SM, et al. Reduced cortical gray matter density in human MDMA (ecstasy) users: a voxel-based morphometry study. *Drug Alcohol Depend* 2003;72(3):225–35.

Daglish MRC, Weinstein A, Malizia AL, et al. Changes in regional cerebral blood flow elicited by craving memories in abstinent opiate-dependent subjects. *Am J Psychiatry* 2001;158:1680–86.

Ende G, Welzel H, Walter S, et al. Monitoring the effects of chronic alcohol consumption and abstinence on brain metabolism: a longitudinal proton magnetic resonance spectroscopy study. *Biol Psychiatry* 2005;58(12):974–80.

Ersche KD, Fletcher PC, Lewis SJG, et al. Abnormal frontal activations related to decision-making in current and former amphetamine and opiate dependent individuals. *Psychopharmacology* 2005;180:612–623.

Farrell M, Howes S, Bebbington P, et al. Nicotine, alcohol and drug-dependence and psychiatric morbidity. *Br J Psychiatry* 2001;179:432–437.

Firestone LL, Gyulai F, Mintun M, Adler LJ, Urso K, Winter PM. Human brain activity response to fentanyl imaged by positron emission tomography. *Anesth Analg* 1996;82(6):1247–51.

Franklin TR, Acton PD, Maldjian JA, et al. Decreased gray matter concentration in the insular, orbitofrontal, cingulate and temporal cortices of cocaine patients. *Biol Psychiatry* 2002;51(2):134–42.

Gamma A, Buck A, Berthold T, Liechti ME, Vollenweider FX. 3,4-methylenedioxymethamphetamine (MDMA) modulates cortical and limbic brain activity as measured by [H(2)(15)O]-PET in healthy humans. *Neuropsychopharmacology* 2000;23(4):388–95.

Garavan H, Pankiewicz J, Bloom A, et al. Cue-induced cocaine craving: neuroanatomical specificity for drug users and drug stimuli. *Am J Psychiatry* 2000;157(11):1789–98.

Gatley SJ, Volkow ND, Gifford AN, et al. Dopamine-transporter occupancy after intravenous doses of cocaine and methylphenidate in mice and humans. *Psychopharmacology (Berl)* 1999;146(1):93–100.

George MS, Anton RF, Bloomer C, et al. Activation of prefrontal cortex and anterior thalamus in alcoholic subjects on exposure to alcohol-specific cues. *Arch Gen Psychiatry* 2001;58(4):345–52.

Gilman S, Adams K, Koeppe R, et al. Cerebellar and frontal hypometabolism in alcoholic cerebellar degeneration studied with positron emission tomography. *Ann Neurol* 1990;28:775–85.

Gilman S, Koeppe RA, Adams K, et al. Positron emission tomographic studies of cerebral benzodiazepine-receptor binding in chronic alcoholics. *Ann Neurol* 1996;40(2):163–71.

Gorelick DA, Kim YK, Bencherif B, et al. Imaging brain mu-opioid receptors in abstinent cocaine users: time course and relation to cocaine craving. *Biol Psychiatry* 2005;57(12):1573–82.

Grant S, London ED, Newlin DB, et al. Activation of memory circuits during cue-elicited cocaine craving. *Proc Natl Acad Sci USA* 1996;93,12040–12045.

Grüsser SM, Wrase J, Klein S, et al. Cue-induced activation of the striatum and medial prefrontal cortex is associated with subsequent relapse in abstinent alcoholics. *Psychopharmacology (Berl)* 2004;175(3):296–302

Guardia J, Catafau AM, Batlle F, et al. Striatal dopaminergic D(2) receptor density measured by [(123)I]iodobenzamide SPECT in the prediction of treatment outcome of alcohol-dependent patients. *Am J Psychiatry* 2000;157(1):127–9

Hagelberg N, Aalro S, Kajander J, et al. Alfentanil increases cortical dopamine D2/D3 receptor binding in healthy subjects. *Pain* 2004;20(6):1587–92.

Heinz A, Higley JD, Gorey JG, et al. In vivo association between alcohol intoxication, aggression, and serotonin transporter availability in nonhuman primates. *Am J Psychiatry* 1998;155(8):1023–8.

Heinz A, Jones DW, Mazzanti C, et al. A relationship between serotonin transporter genotype and in vivo protein expression and alcohol neurotoxicity. *Biol Psychiatry* 2000;47(7):643–9.

Heinz A, Reimold M, Wrase J, et al. Correlation of stable elevations of in striatal mu-opioid receptor availability in detoxified alcoholic patients with alcohol craving: a positron emission tomography study using carbon 11-labelled carfentanil. *Arch Gen Psychiatry* 2005a;62(1):57–64.

Heinz A, Siessmeier T, Wrase J, et al. Correlation between dopamine D(2) receptors in the ventral striatum and central processing of alcohol cues and craving. *Am J Psychiatry* 2004;161(10):1783–9.

Heinz A, Siessmeier T, Wrase J, et al. Correlation of alcohol craving with striatal dopamine synthesis and D2/D3 receptor availability: a combined [18F]DOPA and [18F]DMFP PET study in detoxified alcoholic patients. *Am J Psychiatry* 2005b;162(8):1515–20.

Hietala J, West C, Syvalahti E, et al. Striatal D2 dopamine receptor binding characteristics in vivo in patients with alcohol dependence. *Psychopharmacology* 1994;116:285–290.

Johnson BA, Dawes MA, Roache JD, et al. Acute intravenous low- and high-dose cocaine reduces quantitative global and regional cerebral blood flow in recently abstinent subjects with cocaine use disorder. *J Cereb Blood Flow Metab* 2005;25(7):928–36.

Kaasinen V, Aalto S, Nagren K, Rinne JO. Expectation of caffeine induces dopaminergic responses in humans. *Eur J Neurosci* 2004;19(8):2352–6.

Kling MA, Carson RE, Borg L, et al. Opioid receptor imaging with positron emission tomography and [(18)F]cyclofoxy in long-term, methadone-treated former heroin addicts. *J Pharmacol Exp Ther* 2000;295:1070–76.

Krystal J, Woods S, Kosten T, et al. Opiate dependence and withdrawal: preliminary assessment using single photon emission computerized tomography (SPECT). *Am J Drug Alcohol Abuse* 1995;21:47–63.

Li CS, Kosten TR, Sinha R. Sex differences in brain activation during stress imagery in abstinent cocaine users: a functional magnetic resonance imaging study. *Biol Psychiatry* 2005;57(5):487–94.

Lingford-Hughes AR, Acton PD, Gacinovic S, et al. Reduced levels of GABA-benzodiazepine receptor in alcohol dependency in the absence of grey matter atrophy. *Br J Psychiatry* 1998;173:116–22.

Lingford-Hughes AR, Wilson SJ, Cunningham V, et al. GABA-benzodiazepine receptor function in alcohol dependence: a combined 11C-flumazenil PET and pharmacodynamic study. *Psychopharmacology* 2005;80(4):595–606

London ED, Broussolle EPM, Links JM, et al. Morphine-induced metabolic changes in human brain: studies with positron emission tomography and [18F]fluorodeoxyglucose. *Arch Gen Psychiatry* 1990a;47:73–81.

London ED, Cascella NG, Wong DF, et al. Cocaine-induced reduction of glucose utilization in human brain. *Arch Gen Psychiatry* 1990b;47(6):567–74.

London ED, Ernst M, Grant S, Bonson K, Weinstein A. Orbitofrontal cortex and human drug abuse: functional imaging. *Cereb Cortex* 2000;10(3):334–42.

Lyoo IK, Pollack MH, Silveri MM, et al. Prefrontal and temporal gray matter density decreases in opioid dependence. *Psychopharmacology* 2006;184(2):139–44.

Makris N, Gasic GP, Seidman LJ, et al. Decreased absolute amygdala volume in cocaine addicts. *Neuron* 2004;44(4):729–40.

Martin-Soelch C, Chevalley AF, Kunig G, et al. Changes in reward-induced brain activation in opiate addicts. *Eur J Neurosci* 2001a;14(8):1360–8.

Mathew RJ, Wilson WH, Chiu NY, et al. Regional cerebral blood flow and depersonalization after tetrahydrocannabinol administration. *Acta Psychiatr Scand* 1999;100(1):67–75.

Mathew RJ, Wilson WH, Turkington TG, et al. Marijuana intoxication and brain activation in marijuana smokers. *Life Sci* 1997;60(23):2075–89.

Mathew RJ, Wilson WH, Turkington TG, et al. Cerebellar activity and disturbed time sense after THC. *Brain Res* 1998;797(2):183–9.

Mathew RJ, Wilson WH, Turkington TG, et al. Time course of tetrahydrocannabinol-induced changes in regional cerebral blood flow measured with positron emission tomography. *Psychiatry Res* 2002;116(3):173–85.

Matochik JA, Eldreth DA, Cadet JL, Bolla KI. Altered brain tissue composition in heavy marijuana users. *Drug Alcohol Depend* 2005;77(1):23–30.

Matochik JA, London ED, Eldreth DA, Cadet JL, Bolla KI. Frontal cortical tissue composition in abstinent cocaine abusers: a magnetic resonance imaging study. *Neuroimage* 2003;19(3):1095–102.

McCann UD, Szabo Z, Scheffel U, et al. Positron emission tomographic evidence of toxic effect of MDMA ("Ecstasy") on brain serotonin neurons in human beings. *Lancet* 1998b;352(9138):1433–7.

McCann UD, Szabo Z, Seckin E, et al. Quantitative PET studies of the serotonin transporter in MDMA users and controls using [11C]McN5652 and [11C]DASB. *Neuropsychopharmacology* 2005;30(9):1741–50.

McCann UD, Wong DF, Yokoi F, et al. Reduced striatal dopamine transporter density in abstinent methamphetamine and methcathinone users: evidence from positron emission tomography studies with [11C]WIN-35,428. *J Neurosci* 1998a;18(20):8417–22.

Melichar JK, Hume SP, Williams TM, et al. Using [11C]-diprenorphine to image opioid receptor occupancy by methadone in opioid addiction: clinical and preclinical studies. *J Pharmacol Exp Ther* 2005;312(1):309–15.

Modell J, Mountz J. Focal cerebral blood flow change during craving for alcohol measured by SPECT. *J Neuropsychiat Clin Neurosci* 1995;7:15–22.

Myrick H, Anton R, Li X, et al. Differential brain activity in alcoholics and social drinkers to alcohol cues: relationship to craving. *Neuropsychopharmacology* 2004;29(2):393–402.

Pearlson GD, Jeffrey PJ, Harris GJ, et al. Correlation of acute cocaine-induced changes in local cerebral blood flow with subjective effects. *Am J Psychiatry* 1993;150(3):495–97.

Reneman L, Booij J, de Bruin K, et al. Effects of dose, sex, and long-term abstention from use on toxic effects of MDMA (ecstasy) on brain serotonin neurons. *Lancet* 2001a;358(9296):1864–9.

Reneman L, Lavalaye J, Schmand B, et al. Cortical serotonin transporter density and verbal memory in individuals who stopped using 3,4-methylenedioxymethamphetamine (MDMA or "ecstasy"): preliminary findings. *Arch Gen Psychiatry* 2001b;58(10):901–6.

Reneman L, Majoie CB, Habraken JB, den Heeten GJ. Effects of ecstasy (MDMA) on the brain in abstinent users: initial observations with diffusion and perfusion MR imaging. *Radiology* 2001c;220(3):611–7.

Risinger RC, Salmeron BJ, Ross TJ, et al. Neural correlates of high and craving during cocaine self-administration using BOLD fMRI. *Neuroimage* 2005;26(4):1097–1108.

Rose J, Branchey M, Buydens-Branchey L, et al. Cerebral perfusion in early and late opiate withdrawal: a technetium-99m-HMPAO SPECT study. *Psychiat Res Neuroimag* 1996;67:39–47.

Sachs H, Russell JA, Christman DR, Cook B. Alteration of regional cerebral glucose metabolic rate in non-Korsakoff chronic alcoholism. *Arch Neurol* 1987;44(12):1242–51.

SAMHSA (Substance Abuse and Mental Health Services Administration). *Overview of findings from the 2003 National Survey on Drug Use and Health.* Rockville, MD: Office of Applied Studies; 2004.

Schlaepfer TE, Strain EC, Greenberg BD, et al. Site of opioid action in the human brain: mu and kappa agonists' subjective and cerebral blood flow effects. *Am J Psychiatry* 1998;155(4):470–3.

Schneider F, Habel U, Wagner M, et al. Subcortical correlates of craving in recently abstinent alcoholic patients. *Am J Psychiatry* 2001;158(7):1075–83.

Schreckenberger M, Gouzoulis-Mayfrank E, Sabri O, Arning C, Zimny M, Zeggel T. "Ecstasy"-induced changes of cerebral glucose metabolism and their correlation to acute psychopathology. An 18-FDG PET study. *Eur J Nucl Med* 1999;26(12):1572–9.

Sekine Y, Ouchi Y, Takei N, et al. Brain serotonin transporter density and aggression in abstinent methamphetamine abusers. *Arch Gen Psychiatry* 2006;63(1):90–100.

Sell LA, Morris JS, Bearn J, Frackowiak RSJ, Friston KJ, Dolan RJ. Neural responses associated with cue evoked emotional states and heroin in opiate addicts. *Drug Alcohol Depend* 2000;60:207–216.

Semple DM, Ebmeier KP, Glabus MF, O'Carroll RE, Johnstone EC. Reduced in vivo binding to the serotonin transporter in the cerebral cortex of MDMA ('ecstasy') users. *Br J Psychiatry* 1999;175:63–69.

Sinha R, Lacadie C, Skudlarski P, et al. Neural activity associated with stress-induced cocaine craving: a functional magnetic resonance imaging study. *Psychopharmacology (Berl)* 2005;183(2):171–180.

Sullivan E, Pfefferbaum A. Neurocircuitry in alcoholism: a substrate of disruption and repair. *Psychopharmacology (Berl)* 2005;180(4):583–94.

Sullivan, EV, Marsh L, Mathalon DH, Lim KO, Pfefferbaum A. Relationship between alcohol withdrawal seizures and temporal lobe white matter volume deficits. *Alcohol Clin Exp Res* 1996;20: 348–54.

Thomasius R, Petersen K, Buchert R, et al. Mood, cognition and serotonin transporter availability in current and former ecstasy (MDMA) users. Psychopharmacology (Berl) 2003;167(1):85–96.

Tiihonen J, Kiukka J, Bergstrom K, et al. Altered striatal dopamine re-uptake site densities in habitually violent and non-violent alcoholics. *Nature Med* 1995;1:654–657.

Tzilos GK, Cintron CB, Wood JB, et al. Lack of hippocampal volume change in heavy cannabis users. Am J Addict 2005;14(1):64–72.

Van Dyck C, Rosen M, Thomas M et el. SPECT regional cerebral blood flow alterations in naltrexone-precipitated withdrawal from buprenorphine. *Psychiat Res Neuroimag* 1994;55:181–191.

Volkow N, Fowler J, Wolf A, et al. Effects of chronic cocaine abuse on postsynaptic dopamine receptors. *Am J Psychiat* 1990a;147:719–724.

Volkow N, Hitzemann R, Wang GJ, et al. Decreased brain metabolism in neurologically intact healthy alcoholics. *Am J Psychiatry* 1992a;149:1016–22.

Volkow N, Hitzemann R, Wolf A, et al. Acute effects of alcohol on regional brain glucose metabolism and transport. *Psychiat Res Neuroimag* 1990b; 35:39–48.

Volkow N, Mullani N, Gould L, et al. Effects of acute alcohol intoxication on cerebral blood flow measured with PET. *Psychiat Res* 1988b;24(2): 201–9.

Volkow N, Wang G-J, Hitzemann R, et al. Decreased cerebral response to inhibitory neurotransmission in alcoholics. *Am J Psychiatry* 1993b;150: 417–422.

Volkow N, Wang G-J, Hitzemann R, et al. Recovery of brain glucose metabolism in detoxified alcoholics. *Am J Psychiatry* 1994;51:178–183.

Volkow ND, Ding YS, Fowler JS, et al. Is methylphenidate like cocaine? Studies on their pharmacokinetics and distribution in the human brain. *Arch Gen Psychiatry* 1995;52(6):456–63.

Volkow ND, Fowler JS, Wang GJ. The addicted human brain viewed in the light of imaging studies: brain circuits and treatment strategies. *Neuropharmacology* 2004;47(suppl 1):3–13.

Volkow ND, Gillespie H, Mullani N, et al. Brain glucose metabolism in chronic marijuana users at baseline and during marijuana intoxication. *Psychiatry Res* 1996b;67(1):29–38.

Volkow ND, Fowler JS. Addiction, a disease of compulsion and drive: involvement of the orbitofrontal cortex. *Cereb Cortex* 2000;10(3):318–25.

Volkow ND, Fowler JS, Wang GJ, et al. Decreased dopamine D2 receptor availability is associated with reduced frontal metabolism in cocaine abusers. *Synapse* 1993a;14(2):169–77.

Volkow ND, Fowler JS, Wolf AP, et al. Changes in brain glucose metabolism in cocaine dependence and withdrawal. *Am J Psychiatry* 1991a;148(5): 621–26.

Volkow ND, Gillespie N, Mullani L, et al. Cerebellar metabolic activation by delta-9-tetrahydrocannabinol in human brain. A study with positron emission tomography and 18F-2-fluoro-2-deoxyglucose. *Psychiatry Res* 1991b;67(1):29–38.

Volkow ND, Hitzemann R, Wang GJ, et al. Long-term frontal brain metabolic changes in cocaine abusers. *Synapse* 1992b;11(3):184–90.

Volkow ND, Mullani N, Gould KL, Adler S, Krajewski K. Cerebral blood flow in chronic cocaine users: a study with positron emission tomography. *Br J Psychiatry* 1988a;152:641–648.

Volkow ND, Wang GJ, Fischman MW, et al. Relationship between subjective effects of cocaine and dopamine transporter occupancy. *Nature* 1997a; 386(6627):827–30.

Volkow ND, Wang GJ, Fowler JS, et al. Association of methylphenidate-induced craving with changes in right striato-orbitofrontal metabolism in cocaine abusers: implication in addiction. *Am J Psychiatry* 1999b;156(1): 19–26.

Volkow ND, Wang GJ, Fowler JS, et al. Brain DA D2 receptors predict reinforcing effects of stimulants in humans: replication study. *Synapse* 2002b;46(2):79–82.

Volkow ND, Wang GJ, Fowler JS, et al. Decreased striatal dopaminergic responsiveness in detoxified cocaine-dependent subjects. *Nature* 1997b;386(6627):830–832.

Volkow ND, Wang GJ, Fowler JS, et al. Decreases in dopamine receptors but not in dopamine transporters in alcoholics. *Alcohol Clin Exp Res* 1996c; 20:1594–1598.

Volkow ND, Wang GJ, Fowler JS, et al. Methylphenidate and cocaine have a similar in vivo potency to block dopamine transporters in the human brain. *Life Sci* 1999a;65(1):PL7–12.

Volkow ND, Wang GJ, Fowler JS, et al. Role of dopamine in the therapeutic and reinforcing effects of methylphenidate in humans: results from imaging studies. *Eur Neuropsychopharmacology* 2002a;12(6);557–66.

Volkow ND, Wang GJ, Fowler JS, et al. Temporal relationships between the pharmacokinetics of methylphenidate in the human brain and its behavioural and cardiovascular effects. *Psychopharmacology (Berl)* 1996a;123: 26–33.

Volkow ND, Wang GJ, Ma Y, et al. Expectation enhances the regional brain metabolic and the reinforcing effects of stimulants in cocaine abusers. *J Neurosci* 2003;23(36):11461–8.

Volkow ND, Wang GJ, Maynard L, et al. Effects of alcohol detoxification on dopamine D2 receptors in alcoholics: a preliminary study. *Psychiatry Res* 2002c;116(3):163–72.

Voruganti LN, Slomka P, Zabel P, et al. Cannabis induced dopamine release: an in-vivo SPECT study. *Psychiatry Res* 2001;107(3):173–7.

Wagner KJ, Willoch F, Kochs EF, et al. Dose-dependent regional cerebral blood flow changes during remifentanil infusion in humans: a positron emission tomography study. *Anaesthesiology* 2001;94(5):732–9.

Wexler BE, Gottschalk CH, Fulbright RK, et al. Functional magnetic resonance imaging of cocaine craving. *Am J Psychiatry* 2001;158(1):86–95.

Wik G, Borg S, Sjogren I, et al. PET determination of regional cerebral glucose metabolism in alcohol-dependent men and healthy controls using 11C-glucose. *Acta Psychiat Scand* 1988;78:234–241.

Williams TM, Daglish MR, Lingford-Hughes AR, et al. Brain opioid receptor binding in early abstinence from opioid dependence: positron emission tomography study. *Br J Psychiatry* 2007;191:63–69.

Wilson SJ, Sayette MA, Fiez JA. Prefrontal responses to drug cues: a neurocognitive analysis. *Nat Neurosci* 2004;7(3): 211–4.

Wilson W, Mathew R, Turkington T, Hawk T, Coleman RE, Provenzale J. Brain morphological changes and early marijuana use: a magnetic resonance and positron emission tomography study. *J Addict Dis* 2000;19(1):1–22.

Wu JC, Bell K, Najafi A, et al. Decreasing striatal 6-FDOPA uptake with increasing duration of cocaine withdrawal. *Neuropsychopharmacology* 1997; 17(6):402–9.

Zubieta JK, Gorelick DA, Stauffer R, Ravert HT, Dannals RF, Frost JJ. Increased mu opioid receptor binding detected by PET in cocaine-dependent men is associated with cocaine craving. *Nat Med* 1996;2(11):1225–1229.

8

Reward and Addiction

Susan E. Best

Bryon Adinoff

Opiates have been used for the relief of pain and suffering for thousands of years. For almost as long, it has been known that the therapeutic use of opiates for analgesia is complicated by their abuse liability. The writings of the Homer and Virgil indicate that they knew of both the beneficial and addicting properties of opium (Booth, 1996). In the 18th and 19th centuries, addiction to morphine-containing tincture, laudanum, was common (Ballantyne and Mao, 2003). Over the past 10 to 15 years, a gradual increase in the prescription of opiate analgesics has occurred in response to a heightened awareness of the importance of treating pain. Unfortunately, this has been paralleled by a rise in the numbers of individuals addicted to opiate analgesics. Neuroscience seeks to develop synthetic opiates with excellent analgesic qualities but a minimal risk of addiction. Understanding the neurobiological mechanisms underlying the rewarding and addicting properties of opiates may further this research.

At the outset, it is important to distinguish between the concepts of reward and addiction. "Rewards are pleasurable. Addictions hurt" (Adinoff, 2004). In humans, reward is experienced in response to a wide variety of stimuli, providing enjoyment and arousal. Addiction is a persistent, maladaptive pattern of behavior characterized by compulsive use, loss of control, withdrawal, tolerance, and continued use despite adverse consequences. When discussing opiates, it is also important to distinguish between physical dependence (i.e., the development of a characteristic withdrawal syndrome when a steady dose of a drug is suddenly discontinued or an antagonist to that drug is administered) and addiction or substance dependence. Although physical dependence is often seen in conjunction with addiction to opiates, it is neither a necessary nor sufficient criterion by which to establish the diagnosis of addiction.

The differing neurobiology of the rewarding and addicting properties of opiates divides this chapter into two sections. The section on reward will begin by describing the neurobiology of the neural reward circuits, centered on the mesolimbic dopamine system. A great deal of basic research in the addictions has been guided by the concept that the mesolimbic dopamine system represents the final common pathway for the rewarding effects of natural stimuli and drugs of abuse. Because reward circuits initially evolved to mediate natural rewards and were only later co-opted to subserve reward associated with illicit drugs and alcohol, we will first discuss the role of this circuit in the experience of natural reward. Following an introduction to the organization of opiate receptors, the role of each receptor type in mediating opiate reward will be provided. Finally, the implications of these findings for the development of opiate pain medications with limited abuse liability and in the treatment of substance abuse will be discussed. Recent work suggesting a more nuanced role for the mesolimbic dopaminergic system as a mediator of expectation, learning, and novelty will be presented. The section on addiction will then outline the role of several factors that may lead to relapse (priming, drug cues, stress, and neuroadaptation). The section will conclude with a discussion of recent interesting findings regarding the genetic susceptibility to opiate dependence.

Reward

The Mesolimbic Dopamine System

The first evidence that specific brain regions are involved in rewarding processes comes from studies of J. Olds and Milner (1954). These investigators found that rats readily self-administered electrical stimulation into the septum. Extensions of these studies revealed that multiple brain regions support electrical self-stimulation. The neurophysiology and chemistry of other specific brain areas that are involved in reward have been subsequently elucidated. (See Gardner [2004] for a detailed review.)

The mesolimbic pathway originates with A10 dopaminergic cell bodies in the ventral tegmental area (VTA). This pathway primarily projects to the nucleus accumbens (NAc), but there are also projections to the amygdala, bed nucleus of stria terminalis (BNST), lateral septal area, lateral hypothalamus, and frontal cortex (Koob, 1992). Stimulation of VTA cells induces dopamine release in the NAc. Synaptic dopamine in the accumbens binds to G-protein-coupled dopaminergic receptors on postsynaptic neurons. Most drugs of abuse interact either directly or indirectly with the mesolimbic system. Both the VTA and NAc are modulated by rich innervation from GABAergic, glutamatergic, serotonergic, and opioid peptidergic systems. In addition, the VTA receives noradrenergic input from the locus coeruleus.

Enkephalinergic (opioid peptidergic) efferents projecting from the NAc to the ventral palladium (VP) have been shown to be important for opiate self-administration (Hubner and Koob, 1990; Robledo and Koob, 1993). In addition, Carlezon and Wise (1996) have proposed that inhibition of the GABAergic medium spiny output neurons projecting from VTA to NAc may be critical to drug-induced reward. There are many complex reciprocal anatomic connections between the VTA, NAc (especially the NAc shell), VP, amygdala, and the bed nuclei of the medial forebrain bundle, a diffuse structure comprising the "extended amygdala." Gardner (2004) has suggested that the interaction of this complex network is involved in "regulating the functional set point for hedonic tone." This system is shown schematically in Figure 8.1.

Mesolimbic Dopamine System and Natural Rewards

The mesolimbic dopamine system is evolutionarily ancient, as it is involved in promoting behaviors needed for species survival. Thus, dopaminergic neurons in the mesolimbic reward circuit are activated in response to food (Hernandez and Hoebel, 1988a, 1988b; Kiyatkin and Gratton, 1994; Carr, 2002), sexual interaction (Damsma et al., 1992; Lopez and Ettenberg, 2002; Melis and Argiolas, 1995; Pfaus et al., 1995), humor (Mobbs et al., 2003), and other pleasurable activities. For example, genetically engineered dopamine-deficient mice die of starvation in the midst of readily available food (Zhou and Palmiter, 1995). This occurs even though these mice are able to move, find food, and eat, suggesting that a deficiency in dopamine leads to a reduced motivation to obtain reward (Cannon and Bseikri, 2004). The presence of opioid receptor input into food reward is evidenced by work showing suppressed food-induced dopamine release in the NAc shell following the infusion of the opiate antagonist naloxonazine into the VTA (Tanda and Di Chiara, 1998).

NAc dopamine release in response to food is most reliably seen in food-deprived, and not in nondeprived, rats (Bassareo and Di Chiara, 1997; Wilson et al., 1995). Thus, NAc dopamine release is more strongly associated with "incentive salience" (or the magnitude of a reinforcing stimulus [Spanagel and Weiss, 1999]) than with pleasant postconsumption effects of feeding. However, even in well-fed rats, consumption of a novel food item leads to an increase in NAc dopamine release (Bassareo and Di Chiara, 1997). Thus, the presentation of an unexpected reward leads to dopamine release in the NAc. In contrast, consumption of food that is rewarding on a predictable basis, although it is initially associated with dopamine release in NAc, eventually leads to a decline in dopamine release (Schultz, 1997). Taken together, these findings suggest a role for novelty in activation of the mesolimbic dopamine system.

Hollerman and Schultz (1998:304) have further suggested that dopaminergic neurons represent a type of learning signal that codes for an "error in reward prediction." Redgrave et al. (1999) extended this interpretation by hypothesizing that dopamine mediates allocation of cognitive and behavioral resources toward any significant unexpected event. This concept of "behavioral switching" extends the role of dopamine to one of involvement in associative learning. Young et al. (1998) demonstrated that dopamine was even released in the NAc during the associative learning involved in the pairing of two neutral stimuli, neither of which were intrinsically rewarding. Measurements of activity of dopaminergic neurons in primates that were repeatedly presented with small pieces of apple as an incentive showed that initially dopaminergic neurons responded to the consumption of the apple, but with repeated trials the neurons came to respond to the sight of the apple or the opening of the door that hid the apple (Ljungberg et al., 1992). As dopaminergic neurons began to fire in response to predictors of the reward, they ceased to fire in response to the actual consumption of the apple. This work reveals that dopamine release

Figure 8.1. The mesolimbic dopamine system. Simplified diagram showing some of the neural networks involved in opiate-mediated reward. AMYG = amygdala. DA = dopamine. DYN = dynorphin. ENK = enkephalin. FCX = frontal cortex. GABA = gamma-aminobutyric acid. GLU = glutamate. LC = locus coeruleus. NAc = nucleus accumbens. NE = norepinephrine. VP = ventral palladium. VTA = ventral tegmental area. 5HT = 5-hydroxytryptamine.

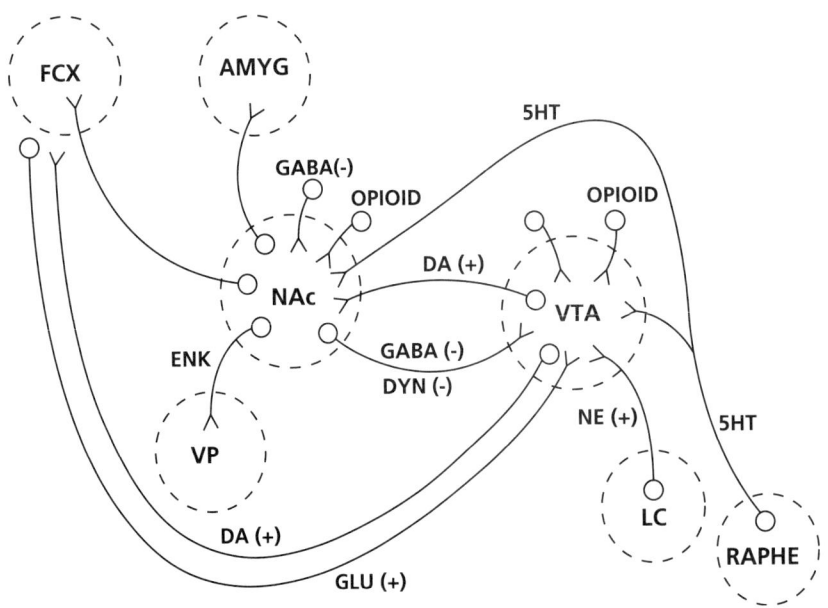

can become associated with the expectation of reward rather than the reward itself.

The Mesolimbic Dopamine System and Opiate-Mediated Reward

Three distinct classes of opiate receptors (μ, δ, and κ) have been described, and each plays a major role in mediating the rewarding effects of opiates. For each of the opiate receptors, Table 8.1 lists the naturally occurring endogenous ligand and a few examples of agonists and antagonists that are specific for that receptor (Shippenberg and Elmer, 1998). (It should be noted that although morphine and naloxone are considered prototypic agonists and antagonists of the μ-opiate receptors, they also bind with low affinity to other opiate receptor subtypes as well.) Modest concentrations of μ and κ receptors are found in the VTA, whereas dense concentrations of μ, δ, and κ receptors are located in the NAc, amygdala, medial prefrontal cortex, and pedunculopontine nucleus (Shippenberg and Elmer, 1998). Recent work studying mRNA colocalization patterns in the NAc shell indicate the presence of mRNA for μ and κ receptors, as well as proenkephalin, prodynorphin, and D1 and D3 receptors. These findings suggest that both opioid and dopaminergic receptor systems are integral to the function of the mesolimbic dopamine system (Akil et al., 1998).

Opiates activate VTA neurons by an indirect mechanism (see Figure 8.1). Some dopaminergic cell bodies in VTA are tonically inhibited by GABAergic neurons intrinsic to the VTA and long GABAergic projections from the NAc. Stimulation of μ and δ receptors in VTA leads to inhibition of GABAergic neurons (Yaksh, 1997) and thus to disinhibition of dopaminergic neurons in VTA and an increase in dopamine release in NAc (Johnson and North, 1992). As predicted by this model, Di Chiara and Imperato (1988) demonstrated that the acute, noncontingent administration of opiates in rodents leads to release of NAc dopamine.

The role of the mesolimbic dopamine system in self-administration paradigms, a model that may be more closely related to addictive behaviors than noncontingent administration, remains debated. Because of their importance to an understanding of opiate-mediated reward, several studies that address this question will be reviewed in some detail. Two of the most commonly used techniques for assessing the rewarding effects of drugs in experimental animals include drug self-administration studies and conditioned place preference (CPP) studies. (Excellent reviews discuss these techniques in detail [Ikemoto and Wise, 2004; Shippenberg and Elmer, 1998; Stolerman, 1992].)

In self-administration studies, an animal is conditioned to give a response (e.g., lever press or nose poke) that leads to administration of the drug of interest. The reinforcing effects of the drug can be gauged by altering the number of responses needed to give a dose of the drug. The more times an animal will perform a specific behavior to obtain a drug, the more reinforcing the drug is thought to be. In cocaine and opiate self-administration studies, experienced animals will press a lever thousands of times to obtain a single dose of drug, and will often self-administer the drug to the exclusion of eating and drinking. In CPP studies, the drug of interest is paired repeatedly with a distinctive environment, and a different environment is paired with the saline state. The animal is then allowed access to both compartments. The amount of time spent in the compartment previously paired with the drug can be taken as a measure of the rewarding nature of the drug.

Self-administration studies often use the intravenous route to allow the reinforcing effect of the drug to be experienced rapidly following the appropriate behavioral response. Animals can be conditioned to self-administer many opiates intravenously. (See van Ree et al. [1999] for an excellent review.) The μ-opiate agonists heroin, morphine, alfentanil, sufentanil, and fentanyl, are all self-administered by animals (Woods et al., 1982). It may take as few as one or two injections for rats to begin to self-administer heroin. In a classic study, Bozarth and Wise (1984) demonstrated that the rewarding effects of morphine do not depend on the relief of withdrawal distress. At the doses used in this study, rats self-administered morphine into the VTA but not into the periventricular gray (PVG). Furthermore, when morphine was continuously infused into either the VTA or PVG for 72 hours, and then naloxone was administered, signs of withdrawal were seen in the rats that had received morphine in the PVG, but not in rats receiving morphine in the VTA. The authors thus concluded that opiates have primary rewarding effects that are not dependent on opiate withdrawal.

Animals will also self-administer δ-agonist peptides (Tortella and Moreton, 1980), but not κ-opiate agonists (Woods and Winger, 1987). Through intracranial microinjection, animals will self-administer μ-opiate agonists directly into the VTA (Bozarth and Wise, 1981; David and Cazala, 1994; Devine and Wise, 1994; Self and Stein, 1993; Welzl et al., 1989), NAc (M. E. Olds, 1982), lateral hypothalamus (LH) (M. E. Olds, 1979), amygdala (David and Cazala, 1994), and hippocampus (Self and Stein, 1993). This work supports the hypothesis that each of these regions is directly involved in opiate reinforcement. Intravenous naloxone, a μ-receptor antagonist, antagonizes the effects of opiates administered directly into VTA, NAc, LH, amygdala, and hippocampus, further suggesting that the reinforcing action of opiates in these areas is mediated by μ-opiate receptors. Fewer studies have addressed intracranial administration of δ-opiates, but one study indicated that animals will self-administer the selective δ-agonist DPDPE into the VTA (Shippenberg et al., 1988). If opiate self-administration were mediated through a dopaminergic mechanism, then giving a dopamine receptor blocker should alter opiate self-administration. Intravenous administration of the D1 antagonist SCH23390, the D2 antagonist pimozide, or the mixed D1/D2 antagonist haloperidol appears to have little effect on intravenous self-administration of opiates. In toto, self-administration studies suggest that opioids directly effect reward in multiple brain regions.

As expected, the administration of μ-opiates successfully induces CPP in rodent models (Bozarth, 1987; Olmstead and Franklin, 1997). In addition, the administration of opioid antagonists into the VTA prevents the development of CPP produced by systemic morphine (Olmstead and Franklin, 1997). Injection of morphine into the periaqueductal gray also produces CPP (Olmstead and Franklin, 1997; van der Kooy et al., 1982). (Interestingly, chronic inflammation of the paw significantly attenuates CPP for morphine in rats [Suzuki et al., 1996], indicating that the presence of chronic pain may decrease the abuse liability of opiates. This

Table 8.1. Opiate Receptors

Receptor	Endogenous Ligand	Selective Agonist	Selective Antagonist
μ	β-endorphin	Morphine DAMGO	Naloxone Naloxonazine
δ	Enkephalin	DPDPE Deltorphin II	Naltrindole BNTX
κ	Dynorphin	U50488H U69593	Nor-binaltorphimine

Adapted from Shippenberg and Elmer (1998).

work is in agreement with the observation that terminal cancer patients rarely exhibit addiction to opiates.)

Although opiates are self-administered into the NAc, studies evaluating the role of NAc in CPP are in conflict. Van der Kooy et al. (1982) demonstrated that morphine produces CPP when injected into NAc, but two other studies (Bals-Kubik et al., 1993; Olmstead and Franklin, 1997) found that neither morphine nor DAMGO (a µ-receptor specific opioid) injected into NAc produced CPP. However, doses of morphine used in the first study were as much as 40 times higher than doses needed to produce CPP when injected into the VTA, and significantly higher than in the two subsequent studies. Results assessing the effect of intrahippocampal administration of µ-opiate agonists are similarly conflicting (Bals-Kubik et al., 1993; Olmstead and Franklin, 1997; van der Kooy et al., 1982), with only a relatively high dose of morphine producing CPP for the opioids.

In contrast to intracranial self-administration studies, the injection of µ-opiate agonists into the amygdala, substantia nigra, caudate/putamen, ventral palladium, pedunculopontine nucleus, and medial prefrontal cortex did not produce reinforcing results as demonstrated by CPP (Bals-Kubik et al., 1993; Baumeister and Hurry, 1993; Olmstead and Franklin, 1997; van der Kooy et al., 1982). CPP has been observed after microinjection of enkephalin (δ-opiate agonist) into VTA (Phillips and LePiane, 1982). In contrast to self-administration study results, intravenous administration of the D1 antagonists SCH23390, SCH23196, and haloperidol decrease CPP to µ-opiates. Intravenous administration of the D2 antagonists sulpiride, spiroperidol and α-flupenthixol have no effect on development of CPP to morphine. In contrast to µ- or δ-agonists, κ-receptor agonists (and mixed agonist-antagonists that bind to κ-receptors) produce marked conditioned place aversion (Iwamoto, 1986). Intracerebroventricular administration of nor-BNI (a κ-opioid receptor antagonist) attenuates the conditioned place aversion produced by U69693 (a κ-opioid agonist), suggesting that the aversive effects produced by κ-opioids are centrally mediated (Bals-Kubik et al., 1989).

Pettit et al. (1984) studied rats that were trained to administer cocaine and heroin on alternating days. Lesions of NAc dopamine terminals with 6-hydroxy-dopamine (6-OHDA, a catecholaminergic neurotoxin) resulted in extinction of the self-administration of cocaine but not of heroin. This work suggests that at least some of heroin's reinforcing actions are independent of the dopaminergic projections to the NAc. In contrast, kainic acid lesions that destroy NAc cell bodies markedly decrease the self-administration of both cocaine and heroin (Zito et al., 1985). Schulteis and Koob (1996: 1440) conclude that "although presynaptic dopamine terminals are not necessary to maintain stable heroin self-administration, cells postsynaptic to these dopamine neurons in the nucleus accumbens do appear to participate in the positive reinforcing effects of heroin."

Taken together, these studies indicate that the reinforcing effects of opiates as measured during self-administration appear to be dopamine independent, whereas the reinforcing effects measured by CPP depend on the functional integrity of mesolimbic dopaminergic neurons. As discussed above, the NAc is rich in µ-opiate receptors, and it has been suggested that the reinforcing effects of opiates during self-administration may be mediated by these receptors (Koob, 1992). Shippenberg and Elmer (1998) point out that CPP studies measure acquisition of the reinforcing effects of drugs of abuse, whereas self-administration studies are usually performed with animals that are experienced in self-administration.

The δ- and κ-Opiate Systems in Reward and Analgesia

Although the µ-opiate system is believed to exert the most significant role in the rewarding and analgesic effects of opiates, the role of the δ- and κ-opiate systems in reward and analgesia is becoming increasingly important in new drug development (Zacny and Galinkin, 1999). δ-opiate agonists are of interest because they have a side effect profile featuring, for example, reduced respiratory depression and decreased gastrointestinal involvement in comparison to µ-opiate agonists (Ahmad and Dray, 2004). Although δ-opiate agonists would not be expected to have decreased abuse liability because they have been shown to be rewarding in animal models, κ-opiate analgesics may have reduced abuse liability because they are neither self-administered nor do they induce CPP when they are administered intracerebrally. Existing agonist/antagonist analgesics (e.g., nalbuphine, butorphanol, and pentazocine) have been observed to be abused in humans, but their abuse liability does appear to be lower than that of the full µ-agonist medications (Preston and Jasinski, 1991).

Unfortunately, the use of the agonist-antagonist medications has been limited by their psychotomimetic side effects (e.g., hallucinations, delusions, and disorientation) and by dysphoria (Millan, 1990). For this reason there is considerable interest in developing κ-opiate analgesics that do not enter the central nervous system. These medications may be particularly useful in treating visceral pain (Riviere, 2004). Medications binding specifically to the κ-opiate receptor are also of potential interest in the treatment of addiction. κ-opiate agonists have been effective in decreasing self-administration and rewarding effects of morphine and psychostimulants in animal models, and thus could be promising medications for the treatment of substance abuse (Heidbreder et al., 1995; Negus et al., 1997; Shippenberg et al., 1996; Suzuki et al., 1992). The same side effect considerations that apply to the use of κ-opiate analgesics apply in this situation.

Addiction and Relapse

The mechanisms underlying the rewarding effects of drugs of abuse differ from those involved in the addictive process. Addiction can be characterized as a chronic relapsing disorder in which periods of sobriety alternate with periods of drug use reinstatement. Self and Nestler (1998) outline a general model for relapse in which drug-associated learning and repeated exposure to drugs leads to neuroadaptations that encompass modulations in neurotransmitters, receptors, signal transduction pathways, and transcription factors. These changes in turn may mediate both proponent processes and opponent processes. Relapse processes involving proponent processes include priming (in which reintroduction of an abused drug leads to relapse to the drug), cue-induced relapse to drug seeking behavior, and stress-related relapse. Relapse involving opponent processes may include tolerance, physical dependence, and withdrawal. In this section, we will discuss some of the neurobiological mechanisms underlying priming, cue-induced, and stress-related relapse as they relate to opiate addiction. Recent research on two transcription factors (CREB and ΔFosB) that may mediate some of the characteristics involved in the development of tolerance and long term neuroadaptation to drug use will also be discussed. An introduction to research on genetic susceptibility to opiate dependence will conclude this section on addiction.

Priming and Relapse

In humans with a history of drug addiction, it is often observed that use of an abused drug on a single occasion can lead to a full relapse to drug taking. In animals trained to self-administer either opiates or stimulant drugs and then allowed to extinguish the behavior, the injection of the previously self-administered drug by an investigator is a powerful stimulus to the reinstatement of drug use (de Wit and Stewart, 1981; Gerber and Stretch, 1975; Slikker et al., 1984). Curiously, opiates can lead to reinstatement of self-administration of cocaine and vice versa (de Wit and Stewart, 1983). This supports the frequently cited clinical injunction that patients in substance abuse treatment should remain abstinent from all drugs of abuse, not just their drug of choice. It also suggests that priming involves a common neurobiological pathway for both opiates and psychostimulants.

Amphetamine infused into the NAc will reinstate use of opiates, whereas microinfusion of morphine into the VTA reinstates use of both heroin- and cocaine-seeking behavior (Stewart et al., 1984; Stewart and Vezina, 1988). These studies suggest that the mesolimbic dopamine system is critically involved in priming in relapse to drugs. Interestingly, Jaeger and van der Kooy (1996) found that the "motivational properties of morphine occur in the absence of detectable subjective effects in animals." Lamb et al. (1991) noted similar findings in detoxified opiate addicted humans who were asked to press a lever on a fixed-rate schedule to obtain an intramuscular dose of morphine (varying from 3.75 mg to 30 mg) or a saline placebo in a single-blind fashion. Subjects responded on the lever for all doses of morphine in spite of the fact that only the highest dose of morphine (30 mg IM) was consistently recognized as "dope" and consistently gave rise to reports of "liking." Subjects did not respond on the lever for placebo. The authors concluded that it is possible that there can be a dissociation of the mechanism underlying the reinforcing effects of morphine in comparison to its euphoric effects.

Cue-Induced Relapse

In humans, exposure to drug-related cues (drug paraphernalia, places previously associated with drug use, etc.) often leads to a relapse to drug use. Di Chiara (1998) has theorized that the repeated use of drugs sensitizes the mesolimbic pathway leading to an association between the substance and its associated drug cues, creating an "addiction memory" (Boening, 2001), which can be activated by drug cues. The amygdala is associated with the acquisition, storage, and expression of emotional memories. Lesions of the amygdala have been shown to decrease the effectiveness of cocaine-related cues in inducing relapse to cocaine-seeking behaviors in animals (Meil and See, 1997). PET and fMRI studies in cocaine-addicted subjects (Breiter et al., 2001; Childress et al., 1999; Grant et al., 1996; Kilts et al., 2001) exposed to drug-related cues show activation of the amygdalar region. In heroin addicts, exposure to heroin-related cues activated a midbrain area (centered on PAG but extending to include the VTA and dorsal raphe) and insula (Sell et al., 1999). Additionally this study showed activation in response to heroin-related cues of the anterior cingulate cortex, amygdala/basal forebrain, and dorsolateral prefrontal cortex but only when activity in the midbrain was high, suggesting that activity in the midbrain modulates the activity of target projection sites. Interestingly, heroin administration itself activated a midbrain area similar to the area activated by heroin-related cues, suggesting overlap in neurobiology mediating response to cues for the drug and to the drug itself.

Stress and Relapse

In a comprehensive review of the role of the limbic-hypothalamic-pituitary-adrenal (HPA) axis in relapse to opiate use, Kreek (2000) hypothesized that an abnormal responsivity of the HPA axis to stressors may lead to continued drug use and relapse to drug use. The HPA axis and the endogenous opioid system are strongly linked. Under normal conditions, exposure to stress leads to the release of corticotropin-releasing factor (CRF) from the hypothalamus. CRF stimulates CR-1 receptors in the anterior pituitary leading to the release of proopiomelanocortin (POMC), the precursor to ACTH and β-endorphin. ACTH in turn stimulates release of cortisol from the adrenal gland. Release of CRF from the hypothalamus and POMC from the anterior pituitary are under negative feedback control from cortisol. Endogenous opiate ligands (and probably particularly dynorphins acting at κ-receptors) also inhibit the HPA axis at the levels of both the hypothalamus and pituitary (Schluger et al., 1998).

Active use of short-acting opiates (heroin or opiate analgesics) leads to suppression of the HPA axis with decreases in ACTH and cortisol (Kreek, 1973; Stimmel and Kreek, 1975), and flattening of the circadian rhythm of cortisol excretion (Kreek et al., 1983). During withdrawal from opiates, the opposite is true: There is abnormal activation of the HPA axis with increases in ACTH and β-endorphin (Kreek et al., 1984). Heroin addicts who are treated with the long-acting opiate methadone and who are abstinent from illicit drugs and alcohol experience normalization of circadian rhythm of release of ACTH, β-endorphins, and cortisol (Stimmel and Kreek, 1975; Kreek et al., 1983). Thus, the disruption of the HPA axis that occurs with intermittent opiate use is normalized by treatment with long-acting opiates (Kreek, 2000).

Studies in animal models are beginning to elucidate interactions between the HPA axis and central mediators of stress. Extrahypothalamic CRF and CRF receptors are found in brain regions typically associated with the stress response including the central nucleus of the amygdala, the bed nucleus of the stria terminalis (BNST), and the locus coeruleus (Swanson et al., 1983; Van Pett et al., 2000). Intracerebrovascular administration of CRF results in behavioral and physiological responses that are typical of the response to stress (Koob and Heinrichs, 1999), and are blocked by CRF antagonists.

Stress interacts with the mesolimbic dopamine system via peripheral release of glucocorticoids that cross the blood brain barrier and bind with glucocorticoid receptors in VTA and elsewhere (Deutch and Bean, 1995; Harfstrand et al., 1986). Glucocorticoids have a permissive effect upon mesolimbic dopamine (Barrot et al., 2000; Marinelli et al., 1998). Thus stress induces release of both extrahypothalamic CRF and glucocorticoids that combine to stimulate neuronal pathways involved in the compulsive drive for substance abuse.

Role of Molecular Neuroadaptation in Relapse

Nestler (2004) has hypothesized that the persistence of addictive behaviors suggests that gene expression plays a role in this process. Drug use is capable of altering gene expression in the brain by altering rates of gene transcription, altering processing of mRNA, translation of mRNA into proteins, and altering the intracellular actions of mature proteins (Nestler et al., 2001). The best studied of these processes is the effect of drugs on the production and action of transcription factors (proteins that act in the nucleus, binding to the regulatory regions of genes and thus controlling the rate of gene transcription). Of the many gene transcription factors that are altered by drugs of abuse, CREB (cAMP response element binding protein) and ΔFosB may have significance for understanding the process of addiction.

Chronic exposure to opiates leads to upregulation of CREB in locus coeruleus and is thought to be involved in the development of opiate physical dependence (Nestler and Aghajanian, 1997). Chronic exposure to cocaine or opiates also leads to neuroadaptations in the NAc cAMP pathway: levels of inhibitory G proteins (Gi and Go) are decreased (these G proteins act to inhibit cAMP formation), whereas levels of adenyl cyclase and protein kinase A (PKA) increased. These changes combine to induce a generalized upregulation of the NAc cAMP pathway (Self and Nestler, 1998). Increased levels of CREB in NAc induce dynorphin production in GABA-containing medium spiny neurons that project from the NAc to VTA (see Figure 8.1). Dynorphin in these neurons suppresses the activity of VTA-NAc reward circuit by binding to κ-opioid receptors on dopaminergic neurons projecting from VTA to NAc, inhibiting release of dopamine in these neurons (Nestler, 2004). Thus, upregulation of the cAMP pathway and CREB in the NAc decreases sensitivity to the rewarding effects of subsequent drug exposures and impairs the response of the reward pathway, creating a type of "motivational tolerance and dependence" mediated by dynorphin (Nestler, 2004a).

ΔFosB is a member of the Fos family of transcription factors. Exposure to most drugs of abuse leads to induction of several Fos proteins in the nucleus accumbens and dorsal striatum (Moratalla et al., 1996; Nye et al., 1995; Nye and Nestler, 1996; Pich et al., 1997). One of these proteins, ΔFosB, is highly stable and, with repeated drug administration, accumulates in the NAc and dorsal striatum (Hiroi et al., 1997) and may be a means by which chronic drug exposure can lead to changes in gene expression that persist long after drug taking ceases (Nestler et al., 2001). Studies in transgenic mice in which ΔFosB can be induced in the NAc (Kelz et al., 1999) show that these animals have an increased sensitivity to the behavioral effects of cocaine and morphine (Colby et al., 2003; Kelz et al., 1999; Nestler et al., 2001). The accumulation of ΔFosB in NAc could mediate a prolonged sensitization to drug exposure (Nestler, 2004a). These results suggest that ΔFosB could be a "sustained molecular switch that helps to initiate and maintain a state of addiction" (Nestler et al., 2004b:215). In contrast to CREB, ΔFosB inhibits the expression of dynorphin in NAc (Chen et al., 2000; McClung and Nestler, 2003).

In summary, CREB accumulates in NAc during chronic drug use. When drug use is stopped, concentrations of CREB decline. Because CREB inhibits dopamine release in VTA-NAc dopaminergic neurons (via action of dynorphin), it appears to mediate the dysphoria or aversive state occurring during the early stages of withdrawal. ΔFosB, which is present in increased concentrations for longer periods after cessation of drug use, may mediate sensitization and be a factor in relapse to drug use (Nestler, 2004).

Genetic Susceptibility to Opiate Addiction

Genetic differences in response to opiates may limit the effectiveness of opiate pain medications and may underlie at least part of an individual's susceptibility to drug addiction. While genetic susceptibility to addiction is likely mediated by multiple genes, the μ-opiate receptor is centrally involved in the euphorigenic effects of opiates and the gene coding for its expression has been the target of recent genetic studies. (See Kreek et al. [2005] and Palmer et al. [2005] for excellent reviews of this subject.)

The most common type of genetic variability is mediated through single-nucleotide polymorphisms (SNPs; Palmer et al., 2005). A SNP results when a single nucleotide in a gene is replaced by an alternate nucleotide, in other words, a "point mutation" occurs. SNPs may have no effect, or they may alter the structure of peptides or the level of gene expression of these peptides. Several SNPs affecting the coding and noncoding regions of the μ-opiate receptor have been identified. The A118G variant and the C17T variants of the μ-opiate receptor have high allelic frequencies (10.5% and 6.6%, respectively; Bond et al., 1998). Functional studies show that β-endorphin binds more strongly to the A118G allele than to the protypic μ-opiate receptor (Bond et al., 1998).

Two studies in well-defined populations (Han Chinese and Swedish, respectively) revealed that the presence of the A118G allele was strongly associated with opiate addiction (Bart et al., 2004; Szeto et al., 2001). Other studies have not been able to replicate these results: Two studies have shown a trend toward an association between presence of the A118G allele and an increased incidence of opiate dependence (Berrettini et al., 1997; Bond et al., 1998), whereas other studies showed no association between the A118G allele and opiate dependence (Franke et al., 2001; Kranzler et al., 1998). The C17T allele does not appear to give rise to a change in function of the μ-opiate receptor (Befort et al., 2001); nevertheless, two studies (Berrettini et al., 1997; Bond et al., 1998) found that the C17T allele was associated with opiate-dependent subjects at a borderline level of significance. Another study (Gelernter et al., 1999) found no association of this variant with cocaine or opiate dependence.

The negative results of some of the genetic studies described above may be due in part to heterogeneity of populations studied. (See Kreek et al. [2005] for further discussion.) In spite of the difficulties inherent in this type of study, the potential to identify individuals at high risk for opiate dependence and customize analgesic regimens based on genetic testing will continue to drive investigations in this area of research.

Conclusion

Some of the substrates underlying the neurobiology of the rewarding effects of opiates have been identified. Elucidation of the role of μ-, δ-, and κ-opioid receptors in the rewarding effects of opiates may suggest strategies for the development of opiate analgesics with low abuse potential. Continued exposure to opiates leads to neurobiological changes that may underlie some of the addicting effects of opiates. Recent insights into the genetics of opiate addiction may lead to an ability to screen individuals for risk of addiction and tailor their treatment to attempt to minimize risk of addiction.

REFERENCES

Adinoff, B. "Neurobiologic Processes in Drug Reward and Addiction." *Harv Rev Psychiatry* 12 (2004): 305–20.

Ahmad, S., and A. Dray. "Novel G Protein-Coupled Receptors as Pain Targets." *Current Opinion in Investigational Drugs* 5 (2004): 67–70.

Akil, H., C. Owens, H. Gutstein, et al. "Endogenous Opioids: Overview and Current Issues." *Drug and Alcohol Dependence* 51 (1998): 127–40.

Ballantyne, J. C., and J. Mao. "Opioid Therapy for Chronic Pain." *New England Journal of Medicine* 349 (2003): 1943–53.

Bals-Kubik, R., A. Ableitner, A. Herz, and T. S. Shippenberg. "Neuroanatomical Sites Mediating the Motivational Effects of Opioids as Mapped by the Conditioned Place Preference Paradigm in Rats." *J Pharmacol Exper Ther* 264 (1993): 489–95.

Bals-Kubik, R., A. Herz, and T. S. Shippenberg. "Evidence That the Aversive Effects of Opioid-Antagonists and Kappa-Agonists Are Centrally Mediated." *Psychopharmacology* 98 (1989): 203–6.

Barrot, M., M. Marinelli, D. N. Abrous, et al. "The Dopaminergic Hyper-Responsiveness of the Shell of the Nucleus Accumbens Is Hormone-Dependent." *Eur J Neurosci* 12 (2000): 973–79.

Bart, G., M. Heilig, K. S. LaForge, et al. "Substantial Attributable Risk Related to Functional Mu-Opioid Receptor Gene Polymorphism in Association with Heroin Addiction in Central Sweden." *Molecular Psychiatry* 9 (2004): 547–49.

Bassareo, V., and G. Di Chiara. "Differential Influence of Associative and Nonassociative Learning Mechanisms on the Responsiveness of Prefrontal and Accumbal Dopamine Transmission to Food Stimuli in Rats Fed Ad Libitum." *J Neuroscience* 17 (1997): 851–61.

Baumeister, A. A., M. Hurry, W. Curtis, et al. "The Antinociceptive and Motivational Effects of Intranigral Injection of Opioid Agonists." *Neuropharmacology* 32 (1993): 1299–303.

Befort, K., D. Filliol, F. M. Decaillot, et al. "A Single Nucleotide Polymorphic Mutation in the Human μ-Opioid Receptor Severely Impairs Receptor Signaling." *J Biol Chem* 276 (2001): 3130–3137.

Berrettini, W. H., M. R. Hoehe, T. N. Ferrada, and E. Gottheil. "Human Mu Opioid Receptor Gene Polymorphisms and Vulnerability to Substance Abuse." *Addiction Biol* 2 (1997): 303–8.

Boening, J. A. "Neurobiology of an Addiction Memory." *J Neural Transm* 108 (2001): 755–65.

Bond, C., K. S. LaForge, M. Tian, et al. "Single Nucleotide Polymorphism in the Human Mu Opioid Receptor Gene Alters Beta-Endorphin Binding and Activity: Possible Implications for Opiate Addiction." *Proc Natl Acad Sci USA* 95 (1998): 9608–13.

Booth, Martin. *Opium: A History*, 18–20. New York: St. Martin's Press, 1996.

Bozarth, M. A. "Neuroanatomical Boundaries of the Reward-Relevant Opiate Receptor Field in the Ventral Tegmental Area as Mapped by the Conditioned Place Preference Method in the Rat." *Brain Res* 414 (1987): 77–84.

Bozarth, M. A., and R. A. Wise. "Anatomically Distinct Opiate Receptor Fields Mediate Reward and Physical Dependence." *Science* 224 (1984): 516–17.

Bozarth, M. A., and R. A. Wise. "Intracranial Self-Administration of Morphine into the Ventral Tegmental Area in Rats." *Life Sci* 28 (1981): 551–55.

Breiter, H. C., I. Aharon, D. Kahneman, et al. "Functional Imaging of Neural Responses to Expectancy and Experience of Monetary Gains and Losses." *Neuron* 30 (2001): 619–39.

Cannon, C. M., and M. R. Bseikri. "Is Dopamine Required for Natural Reward?" *Physiology & Behavior* 81 (2004): 741–48.

Carlezon, W. A. Jr., and R. A. Wise. "Rewarding Actions of Phencyclidine and Related Drugs in Nucleus Accumbens Shell and Frontal Cortex." *J Neuroscience* 16 (1996): 3112–22.

Carr, K. D. "Augmentation of Drug Reward by Chronic Food Restriction: Behavioral Evidence and Underlying Mechanisms." *Physiol Behav* 76 (2002): 353–64.

Chen, J. S., Y. J. Zhang, M. B. Kelz, et al. "Induction of Cyclin-Dependent Kinase 5 in Hippocampus by Chronic Electroconvulsive Seizures: Role of Delta-FosB." *J Neuroscience* 20 (2000): 8965–71.

Childress, A. R., P. D. Mozley, W. McElgin, et al. "Limbic Activation During Cue-Induced Cocaine Craving." *American Journal of Psychiatry* 156 (1999): 11–18.

Colby, C. R., K. Whisler, C. Steffen, et al. "Striatal Cell Type-Specific Overexpression of Delta FosB Enhances Incentive for Cocaine." *J Neuroscience* 23 (2003): 2488–93.

Damsma, G., J. G. Pfaus, D. Wenkstern, et al. "Sexual Behavior Increases Dopamine Transmission in the Nucleus Accumbens and Striatum of Male Rats: Comparison with Novelty and Locomotion." *Behav Neurosci* 106 (1992): 181–91.

David, V., and P. Cazala. "A Comparative Study of Self-Administration of Morphine Into the Amygdala and the Ventral Tegmental Area in Mice." *Behav Brain Res* 165 (1994): 205–11.

Deutch, A. Y., and A. J. Bean. "Colocalization in Dopamine Neurons." In F. E. Bloom and D. J. Kupfer (eds.), *Psychopharmacology: The Fourth Generation of Progress*. New York: Raven, 1995.

Devine, D. P., and R. A. Wise. "Self-Administration of Morphine, DAMGO, and DPDPE Into the Ventral Tegmental Area of Rats." *J Neuroscience* 14 (1994): 1978–84.

de Wit, H., and J. Stewart. "Drug Reinstatement of Heroin-Reinforced Responding in the Rat." *Psychopharmacology* 79 (1983): 29–31.

de Wit, H., and J. Stewart. "Reinstatement of Cocaine-Reinforced Responding in the Rat." *Psychopharmacology* 75 (1981): 134–43.

Di Chiara, G. "A Motivational Learning Hypothesis of the Role of Mesolimbic Dopamine in Compulsive Drug Use." *J Psychopharmacology* 12 (1998): 54–67.

Di Chiara, G., and A. Imperato. "Drugs Abused by Humans Preferentially Increase Synaptic Dopamine Concentrations in the Mesolimbic System of Freely Moving Rats." *Proc Natl Acad Sci USA* 85 (1988): 5274–78.

Franke, P., T. Wang, M. M. Nothen, et al. "Nonreplication of Association Between Mu-Opioid-Receptor Gene (Oprm1) A118g Polymorphism and Substance Dependence." *Am J Med Genet* 105 (2001): 114–19.

Gardner, E. L. "Brain Reward Mechanisms." In J. H. Lowinson, P. Ruiz, R. B. Millman and J. G. Langrod (eds.), *Substance Abuse: A Comprehensive Textbook* (4th ed.). Philadelphia: Lippincott, Williams & Wilkins, 2004.

Gelernter, J., H. Kranzler, and J. Cubells. "Genetics of Two Mu Opioid Receptor Gene (Oprm1) Exon I Polymorphisms: Population Studies, and Allele Frequencies in Alcohol- and Drug-Dependent Subjects." *Molecular Psychiatry* 4 (1999): 476–83.

Gerber, G. J., and R. Stretch. "Drug-Induced Reinstatement of Extinguished Self-Administration Behavior." *Pharmacol Biochem Behav* 3 (1975): 1061–66.

Grant, S., E. D. London, D. B Newlin, et al. "Activation of Memory Circuits During Cue-Elicited Cocaine Craving." *Proc Natl Acad Sci USA* 93 (1996): 12040–45.

Harfstrand, A., K. Fuxe, L. F. Agnati, et al. "Receptor Autoradiographical Evidence for High Densities of 125I-Neuropeptide Y Binding Sites in the Nucleus Tractus Solitarius of the Normal Male Rat." *Acta Physiol Scand* 128 (1986): 195–200.

Heidbreder, C. A., D. Babovic-Vuksanovic, M. Shoaib, et al. "Development of Behavioral Sensitization to Cocaine: Influence of Kappa Opioid Receptor Agonists." *J Pharmacol Exper Ther* 275 (1995): 150–63.

Hernandez, L., and B. G. Hoebel. "Feeding and Hypothalamic Stimulation Increase Dopamine Turnover in the Accumbens." *Physiol Behav* 44 (1988a): 599–606.

Hernandez, L., and B. G. Hoebel. "Food Reward and Cocaine Increase Extracellular Dopamine in the Nucleus Accumbens as Measured by Microdialysis." *Life Sci* 42 (1988b): 1705–12.

Hiroi, N., J. R. Brown, C. N. Haile, et al. "FosB Mutant Mice: Loss of Chronic Cocaine Induction of Fos-Related Proteins and Heightened Sensitivity to Cocaine's Psychomotor and Rewarding Effects." *Proc Natl Acad Sci USA* 94 (1997): 10397–402.

Hollerman, J. R., and W. Schultz. "Dopamine Neurons Report an Error in the Temporal Prediction of Reward During Learning." *Nat Neurosci* 1 (1998): 304–09.

Hubner, C. B., and G. F. Koob. "The Ventral Pallidum Plays a Role in Mediating Cocaine and Heroin Self-Administration in the Rat." *Brain Res* 508 (1990): 20–29.

Ikemoto, S, and R. A. Wise. "Mapping of Chemical Trigger Zones for Reward." *Neuropharmacology* 47 (2004): 190–201.

Iwamoto, E. T. "Place Conditioning Properties of Mu-, Kappa-, and Sigma-Opioid Agonists." *Alcohol Drug Res* 6 (1986): 327–39.

Jaeger, T. V., and D. van der Kooy. "Separate Neural Substrates Mediate the Motivating and Discriminative Properties of Morphine." *Behav Neurosci* 110 (1996): 181–201.

Johnson, S. W., and R. A. North. "Opioids Excite Dopamine Neurons by Hyperpolarization of Local Interneurons." *J Neuroscience* 12 (1992): 483–88.

Kelz, M. B., J. S. Chen, W. A. Carlezon, et al. "Expression of the Transcription Factor Delta-FosB in the Brain Controls Sensitivity to Cocaine." *Nature* 401 (1999): 272–76.

Kilts, C. D., J. B. Schweitzer, C. K. Quinn, et al. "Neural Activity Related to Drug Craving in Cocaine Addiction." *Arch Gen Psychiatry* 58 (2001): 334–41.

Kiyatkin, E. A., and A. Gratton. "Electrochemical Monitoring of Extracellular Dopamine in Nucleus Accumbens of Rats Lever-Pressing for Food." *Brain Res* 652 (1994): 225–34.

Koob, G. F. "Drugs of Abuse: Anatomy, Pharmacology and Function of Reward Pathways." *Trends in Pharmacological Sciences* 131 (1992): 177–84.

Koob, G. F., and S. C. Heinrichs. "A Role for Corticotropin Releasing Factor and Urocortin in Behavioral Responses to Stressors." *Brain Res* 848 (1999): 141–52.

Kranzler, H. R., J. Gelernter, S. O'Malley, et al. "Association of Alcohol or Other Drug Dependence With Alleles of the Mu Opioid Receptor Gene (OPRM1)." *Alcoholism: Clin Exp Ther* 22 (1998): 1359–62.

Kreek, M. J. "Physiologic Implications of Methadone Treatment." Paper presented at the Fifth National Conference of Methadone Treatment, Washington, DC, 1973.

Kreek, M. J. "Methadone-Related Opioid Agonist Pharmacotherapy for Heroin Addiction. History, Recent Molecular and Neurochemical Research and Future in Mainstream Medicine." *Annals of the New York Academy of Science* 909 (2000): 186–216.

Kreek, M. J., G. Bart, C Lilly, K. S. LaForge, and D. A. Nielsen. "Pharmacogenetics and Human Molecular Genetics of Opiate and Cocaine Addictions and Their Treatments." *Pharmacological Reviews* 57 (2005): 1–26.

Kreek, M. J., J. Ragunath, S. Plevy, et al. "ACTH, Cortisol and Beta-Endorphin Response to Metyrapone Testing During Chronic Methadone Maintenance Treatment in Humans." *Neuropeptides* 5 (1984): 277–78.

Kreek, M. J., S. L. Wardlaw, N. Hartman, et al. "Circadian Rhythms and Levels of Beta-Endorphin, ACTH, and Cortisol During Chronic Methadone Maintenance Treatment in Humans." *Life Sci* 33 Suppl. 1 (1983): 409–11.

Lamb, R. J., K. L. Preston, C. W. Schindler, et al. "The Reinforcing and Subjective Effects of Morphine in Post-Addicts: A Dose-Response Study." *J Pharmacol Exper Ther* 259 (1991): 1165–73.

Ljungberg, T., P. Apicella, and W. Schultz. "Responses of Monkey Dopamine Neurons During Learning of Behavioral Reactions." *J Neurophysiology* 67 (1992): 145–63.

Lopez, H. H., and A. Ettenberg. "Sexually Conditioned Incentives: Attenuation of Motivational Impact During Dopamine Receptor Antagonism." *Pharmacol Biochem Behav* 72 (2002): 65–72.

Marinelli, M., B. Aouizerate, M. Barrot, M. LeMoal, and P. V. Piazza. "Dopamine-Dependent Responses to Morphine Depend on Glucocorticoid Receptors." *Proc Natl Acad Sci USA* 95 (1998): 7742–47.

McClung, C. A., and E. J. Nestler. "Regulation of Gene Expression and Cocaine Reward by CREB and Delta-FosB." *Nat Neurosci* 6 (2003): 1208–15.

Meil, W. M., and R. E. See. "Lesions of the Basolateral Amygdala Abolish the Ability of Drug Associated Cues to Reinstate Responding During Withdrawal From Self-Administered Cocaine." *Behav Brain Res* 87 (1997): 139–48.

Melis, M. R., and A. Argiolas. "Dopamine and Sexual Behavior." *Neurosci Biobehav Rev* 19 (1995): 19–38.

Millan, M. J. "Kappa-Opioid Receptors and Analgesia." *Trends in Pharmacological Sciences* 11 (1990): 70–76.

Mobbs, D., M. D. Greicius, E. Abdel-Azim, et al. "Humor Modulates the Mesolimbic Reward Centers." *Neuron* 40 (2003): 1041–8.

Moratalla, R., B. Elibol, M. Vallejo, and A. M. Graybiel. "Network-Level Changes in Expression of Inducible Fos-Jun Proteins in the Striatum During Chronic Cocaine Treatment and Withdrawal." *Neuron* 17 (1996): 147–56.

Negus, S. S., N. K. Mello, P. S. Portoghese, et al. "Effects of Kappa Opioids on Cocaine Self-Administration by Rhesus Monkeys." *J Pharmacol Exper Ther* 282 (1997): 44–55.

Nestler, E. J. "Molecular Mechanisms of Drug Addiction." *Neuropharmacology* 47 Suppl 1 (2004a): 24–32.

Nestler, E. J. "Historical Review: Molecular and Cellular Mechanisms of Opiate and Cocaine Addiction." *Trends in Pharmacological Sciences* 25 (2004b): 210–218.

Nestler, E. J., and G. K. Aghajanian. "Molecular and Cellular Basis of Addiction." *Science* 278 (1997): 58–63.

Nestler, E. J., S. E. Hyman, and R. C. Malenka. *Molecular Basis of Neuropharmacology*. New York: McGraw-Hill, 2001.

Nye, H. E., B. T. Hope, M. B. Kelz, et al. "Pharmacological Studies of the Regulation of Chronic Fos-Related Antigen Induction by Cocaine in the Striatum and Nucleus Accumbens." *J Pharmacol Exper Ther* 275 (1995): 1671–80.

Nye, H. E., and E. J. Nestler. "Induction of Chronic Fos-Related Antigens in Rat Brain by Chronic Morphine Administration." *Molecular Pharmacology* 49 (1996): 636–45.

Olds, J., and P. M. Milner. "Positive Reinforcement Produced by Electrical Stimulation of Septal Area and Other Regions of Rat Brain." *J Comparative Physiology and Psychology* 47 (1954): 419–27.

Olds, M. E. "Hypothalamic Substrate for the Positive Reinforcing Effects of Morphine in the Rat." *Brain Res* 168 (1979): 351–60.

Olds, M. E. "Reinforcing Effects of Morphine in the Nucleus Accumbens." *Brain Res* 237 (1982): 429–40.

Olmstead, M. C., and K. B. J. Franklin. "The Development of a Conditioned Place Preference to Morphine: Effects of Microinjection Into Various CNS Sites." *Behav Neurosci* 111 (1997): 1324–34.

Palmer, S. N., N. M. Giesecke, S. C. Body, et al. "Pharmacogenetics of Anesthetic and Analgesic Agents." *Anesthesiology* 102 (2005): 663–71.

Pettit, H. O., A. Ettenberg, F. E. Bloom, and G. F. Koob. "Destruction of Dopamine in the Nucleus Accumbens Selectively Attenuates Cocaine but Not Heroin Self-Administration in Rats." *Psychopharmacology* 84 (1984): 167–73.

Pfaus, J. G., G. Damsma, D. Wenkstern, and H. C. Fibiger. "Sexual Activity Increases Dopamine Transmission in the Nucleus Accumbens and Striatum of Female Rats." *Brain Res* 693 (1995): 21–30.

Phillips, A. G., and F. G. LePiane. "Reward Produced by Microinjection of (D-Ala2), Met5-Enkephalinamide into the Ventral Tegmental Area." *Behav Brain Res* 5 (1982): 225–29.

Pich, E. M., S. R. Pagliusi, M. Tessari, D. Talabot-Ayer, R. Hooft van Huijsduijnen, and C. Chaimulera. "Common Neural Substrates for the Addictive Properties of Nicotine and Cocaine." *Science* 275 (1997): 83–86.

Preston, K. L., and D. R Jasinski. "Abuse Liability Studies of Opioid Agonist-Antagonists in Humans." *Drug and Alcohol Dependence* 28 (1991): 49–82.

Redgrave, P., T. J. Prescott, and K. Gurney. "Is the Short-Latency Dopamine Response Too Short to Signal Reward Error?" *Trends Neurosci* 22 (1999): 146–51.

Riviere, P. J. "Peripheral Kappa-Opioid Agonists for Visceral Pain." *British J Pharmacology* 141 (2004): 1331–34.

Robledo, P., and G. F. Koob. "Two Discrete Nucleus Accumbens Projection Areas Differentially Mediate Cocaine Self-Administration in the Rat." *Behav Brain Res* 55 (1993): 159–66.

Schluger, J. H., A. Ho, L. Borg, et al. "Nalmefene Causes Greater Hypothalamic-Pituitary-Adrenal Axis Activation Than Naloxone in Normal Volunteers: Implications for the Treatment of Alcoholism." *Alcoholism: Clin Exp Ther* 22 (1998): 1430–36.

Schulteis, G., and G. F. Koob. "Reinforcement Processes in Opiate Addiction: A Homeostatic Model." *Neurochem Res* 21 (1996): 1437–54.

Schultz, W. "Dopamine Neurons and Their Role in Reward Mechanisms." *Curr Opin Neurobiol* 7 (1997): 191–97.

Self, D. W., and E. J. Nestler. "Relapse to Drug-Seeking: Neural and Molecular Mechanisms." *Drug and Alcohol Dependence* 51 (1998): 49–60.

Self, D. W., and L. Stein. "Pertussis Toxin Attenuates Intracranial Morphine Self-Administration." *Pharmacol Biochem Behav* 46 (1993): 689–95.

Sell, L. A., J. Morris, J. Bearn, et al. "Activation of Reward Circuitary in Human Opiate Addicts." *European Journal of Neuroscience* 11 (1999): 1042–48.

Shippenberg, T. S., and A. Herz. "Motivational Effects of Opioids: Influence of D-1 vs. D-2 Receptor Antagonists." *Eur J Pharmacol* 151 (1988): 233–243.

Shippenberg, T. S., and G. I. Elmer. "The Neurobiology of Opiate Reinforcement." *Critical Reviews in Neurobiology* 12, No. 4 (1998): 267–303.

Shippenberg, T. S., A. LeFevour, and C. Heidbreder. "Kappa-Opioid Receptor Agonists Prevent Sensitization to the Conditioned Rewarding Effects of Cocaine." *J Pharmacol Exper Ther* 276 (1996): 545–54.

Slikker, W. J., M. J. Brocco, and K. F. J. Killam. "Reinstatement of Responding Maintained by Cocaine or Thiamylal." *J Pharmacol Exper Ther* 228 (1984): 43–52.

Spanagel, R., and F. Weiss. "The Dopamine Hypothesis of Reward: Past and Current Status." *Trends Neurosci* 22 (1999): 521–7.

Stewart, J., H. de Wit, and R. Eikelboom. "Role of Unconditioned and Conditioned Drug Effects in the Self-Administration of Opiates and Stimulants." *Psychol Rev* 91 (1984): 251–68.

Stewart, J., and P. Vezina. "A Comparison of the Effects of Intra-Accumbens Injections of Amphetamine and Morphine on Reinstatement of Heroin Intravenous Self-Administration Behavior." *Brain Res* 457 (1988): 287–94.

Stimmel, B., and M. J. Kreek. "Pharmacologic Actions of Heroin." In B. Stimmel (ed.), *Heroin Dependency: Medical, Economic and Social Aspects*. New York: Stratton Intercontinental Medical Book Corp., 1975.

Stolerman, I. "Drugs of Abuse: Behavioural Principles, Methods and Terms." *Trends in Pharmacological Sciences* 13 (1992): 170–76.

Suzuki, T., Y. Kishimoto, and M. Misawa. "Formalin- and Carrageenan-Induced Inflammation Attenuates Place Preferences Produced by Morphine, Methamphetamine and Cocaine." *Life Sciences* 59 (1996): 1667–74.

Suzuki, T., Y. Shiozaki, Y. Matsukawa, et al. "The Role of Mu- and Kappa-Opioid Receptors in Cocaine-Induced Place Preference." *Jpn J Pharmacol* 58 (1992): 435–42.

Swanson, L. W., P. E. Sawchenko, J. Rivier, and W. W. Vale. "Organization of Ovine Corticotropin Releasing Factor Immunoreactive Cells and Fibers in the Rat Brain: An Immunohistochemical Study." *Neuroendocrinology* 1983 (1983): 165–86.

Szeto, C. Y., N. L. Tang, D. T. Lee, and A. Stadlin. "Association between Mu Opioid Receptor Gene Polymorphisms and Chinese Heroin Addicts." *Neuroreport* 12 (2001): 1103–06.

Tanda, G., and G. Di Chiara. "A Dopamine-Mu1 Opioid Link in the Rat Ventral Tegmentum Shared by Palatable Food (Fonzies) and Non-Psychostimulant Drugs of Abuse." *Eur J Neurosci* 10 (1998): 1179–87.

Tortella, F. C., and J. E. Moreton. "D-Ala2-Methionine-Enkephalinamide Self-Administration in the Morphine-Dependent Rat." *Psychopharmacology* 69 (1980): 143–47.

van der Kooy, D., R. F. Mucha, M. O'Shaughnessy, and P. Bucenieks. "Reinforcing Effects of Brain Microinjections of Morphine Revealed by Conditioned Place Preference." *Brain Res* 243 (1982): 107–17.

Van Pett, K., V. Viau, J. C. Bittencourt, et al. "Distribution of mRNAs Encoding CRF Receptors in Brain and Pituitary of Rat and Mouse." *J Comp Neurol* 428 (2000): 191–212.

Van Ree, J. M., M. A. F. M. Gerrits, and L. J. M. J. Vanderschuren. "Opioids, Reward and Addiction: An Encounter of Biology, Psychology, and Medicine." *Pharmacological Reviews* 51 (1999): 341–96.

Welzl, H., G. Kuhn, and J. P. Huston. "Self-Administration of Small Amounts of Morphine Through Glass Micropipettes into the Ventral Tegmental Area of the Rat." *Neuropharmacology* 28 (1989): 1017–23.

Wilson, C., GG Nomikos, M Collu, and H. C. Fibiger. "Dopaminergic Correlates of Motivated Behavior: Importance of Drive." *J Neuroscience* 15 (1995): 5169–78.

Woods, J. H., and G. Winger. "Behavioral Characterization of Opioid Mixed Agonist-Antagonists." *Drug and Alcohol Dependence* 20 (1987): 303–15.

Woods, J. H., A. M. Young, and S. Herling. "Classification of Narcotics on the Basis of Their Reinforcing, Discriminative, and Antagonist Effects in Rhesus Monkeys." *Fed Proc* 41 (1982): 221–27.

Yaksh, T. L. "Pharmacology and Mechanisms of Opioid Analgesic Activity." *Acta Anaesthesiologica Scandinavica* 41 (1997): 94–111.

Young, A. M., R. G. Ahier, R. L. Upton, et al. "Increased Extracellular Dopamine in the Nucleus Accumbens of the Rat During Associative Learning." *Neuroscience* 83 (1998): 1175–83.

Zacny, J., and J. L. Galinkin. "Psychotropic Drugs Used in Anesthesia Practice." *Anesthesiology* 90 (1999): 269–88.

Zhou, Q. Y., and R. D. Palmiter. "Dopamine-Deficient Mice Are Severely Hypoactive, Adipsic, and Aphagic." *Cell* 83 (1995): 1197–209.

Zito, K. A., G. Vickers, and D. C. S. Roberts. "Disruption of Cocaine and Heroin Self-Administration Following Kainic Acid Lesions of the Nucleus Accumbens." *Pharmacol Biochem Behav* 23 (1985): 1029–36.

9

Neurobehavioral Mechanisms of Compulsive Drug Seeking

Louk J. M. J. Vanderschuren

Drug addiction is a chronic relapsing disorder characterized by loss of control over drug taking. Whereas drug use starts out as controlled, casual use, during the development of the addiction syndrome, drug seeking and taking escalates into a compulsive mode of behavior. This is reflected by the criteria in *DSM-IV* (American Psychiatric Association, 2000), in which five out of seven symptoms signify that control over drug intake has been lost:

> [Substance dependence is...] a maladaptive pattern of substance use, leading to clinically significant impairment or distress, as manifested by three (or more) of the following, occurring at any time in the same 12-month period:

1. Tolerance
2. Withdrawal
3. The substance is often taken in larger amounts or over a longer period than was intended
4. There is a persistent desire or unsuccessful efforts to cut down or control substance use
5. A great deal of time is spent in activities necessary to obtain the substance, use the substance, or recover from its effects
6. Important social, occupational, or recreational activities are given up or reduced because of substance use
7. The substance use is continued despite knowledge of having a persistent or recurrent physical or psychological problem that is likely to have been caused or exacerbated by the substance

Despite the general awareness that drug addiction is a disorder of the central nervous system (Dackis and O'Brien, 2005; Leshner, 1997; Volkow and Li, 2004) and widespread knowledge of how repeated drug exposure changes brain and behavior (see, for example, Hyman et al., 2006; Kalivas et al., 2005; Kelley, 2004; Koob et al., 2004; Nestler, 2001; Vanderschuren and Kalivas, 2000), there is a great paucity of adequate pharmacotherapies for addiction. One reason for this may be that the neurobiological underpinnings of the compulsive aspects of addiction are not well understood.

In this chapter, I will discuss three processes that have been put forward to contribute to the progression from casual to compulsive drug use. This overview is not meant to be exhaustive; there are other relevant constructs that will be not be discussed here. The processes discussed (incentive sensitization, habit learning, and conditioned aspects of drug seeking) have been a focus of my own work, and other theories of addiction have been discussed in great detail elsewhere (see, e.g., Ahmed, 2005; Bechara, 2005; Jentsch and Taylor, 1999; Koob et al., 2004). At the end of the chapter, I will pinpoint a few possible avenues for development of novel pharmacotherapies for drug addiction.

Incentive Sensitization in Compulsive Drug Use

Since it was first published in 1993, this neuroadaptationist view of addiction (Robinson and Berridge, 1993, 2000, 2001, 2003) has been very influential. The incentive sensitization theory very prominently focuses on drug induced changes in brain function that lead to addiction. Its central idea is that repeated exposure to drugs of abuse leads to a set of adaptations in the neural circuits mediating motivational influences on behavior, most notably the mesoaccumbens dopamine projection. These adaptations render this circuit hypersensitive ("sensitized") to drugs and drug-associated stimuli. Sensitization of the mesoaccumbens dopamine system, which plays a prominent role in attributing incentive salience to stimuli, in other words, the way in which stimuli are perceived as attractive (Berridge and Robinson, 1998), causes drugs and drug-associated stimuli to become excessively "wanted." This exaggerated motivation for drugs, perhaps equivalent to drug craving, then leads to the compulsive pursuit of the drug.

The classic test for behavioral sensitization is an exaggerated psychomotor response to a drug. Drugs of abuse are well known to have characteristic effects on psychomotor activity of laboratory animals. These effects become progressively and persistently enhanced after repeated drug exposure, and this phenomenon has been observed with psychostimulants, opiates, and nicotine as well as alcohol (Robinson and Berridge, 2003; Stewart and Badiani, 1993; Vanderschuren and Kalivas, 2000). The ability to evoke psychomotor sensitization may therefore be a common property of drugs of abuse. The fact that sensitization is very long-lasting (for example, in one set of experiments, a sensitized psychomotor response to amphetamine could be observed for up to 1 year after the last amphetamine pretreatment [Paulson et al., 1991]), fueled the notion that sensitization could be an important factor in some of the persistent features of drug addiction, such as the high risk of relapse, that remains present even after long periods of abstinence. Indeed, there is evidence to support this notion (see below).

Although the neural substrates of drug-induced psychomotor activity and reward overlap (Koob, 1992; Wise and Bozarth, 1987), the measurement of locomotion is at best an indirect measure for the motivational and positive subjective effects of drugs. Moreover, more pertinent animal models are available to investigate these effects of drugs. Therefore, the demonstration that repeated pretreatment with drugs also enhances their capacity to evoke conditioned place preference (Gaiardi et al., 1991; Lett, 1989; Shippenberg and Heidbreder, 1995; Shippenberg et al., 1996) and support self-administration (Covington and Miczek, 2001; Horger et al., 1990, 1992; Piazza et al., 1989, 1990; Valadez and Schenk, 1994) was very important for the relevance of the incentive sensitization theory of addiction.

Perhaps the most convincing set of experiments showing that preexposure to drugs enhances their motivational properties comes from Vezina and colleagues (Lorrain et al., 2000; Suto et al., 2003; Vezina et al., 2002; see also Covington and Miczek, 2001; Mendrek et al., 1998). These authors used a progressive-ratio schedule of self-administration, in which the animal has to perform an increasing amount of work (e.g., lever pressing) for every subsequent reward (Hodos, 1961; Richardson and Roberts, 1996). The maximal number of lever presses that an animal is willing to perform to obtain a single reward (it is no exception that this is hundreds of lever presses) is called "break-point." Vezina and colleagues (2002) found that rats that were pretreated with amphetamine according to a regimen that reliably evoked psychomotor sensitization showed higher break-points when tested for self-administration of amphetamine and cocaine under a progressive ratio schedule. Thus, sensitized animals appeared more motivated to work for a drug reward. Interestingly, not only does sensitizing exposure to drugs enhance their motivational properties, a period of drug self-administration also leads to increased psychomotor responsiveness to drugs (De Vries et al., 1998; Hooks et al., 1994; Phillips and Di Ciano, 1996).

Of course, the most critical demonstration to support the idea that drug use enhances its motivational properties would be to show that drug self-administration (as opposed to experimenter-delivered drugs) also causes incentive sensitization. Indeed, studies from Morgan, Roberts, and colleagues have shown that a period of drug (cocaine or heroin) self-administration leads to increased break-points when these animals are subsequently tested under a progressive ratio schedule of self-administration (Liu et al., 2005a; Morgan et al., 2005, 2006; Ward et al., 2006). One remarkable finding in these studies was that sensitization was most pronounced in animals with limited drug self-administration experience (Morgan et al., 2006) but that sensitized break-points were not found in those animals that had self-administered the highest amounts of cocaine. This is in part consistent with findings from psychomotor sensitization experiments, in which sensitization can be seen after only few drug exposures, and in some cases even a single drug exposure suffices to evoke sensitization (see below). On the other hand, it is known from psychomotor sensitization studies that intermittent exposure is much more effective than chronic or continuous drug treatment in evoking sensitization, but that more aggressive treatment regimens, using prolonged treatment with increasing drug doses (including periods of absence of drug treatment) evokes a sensitization that is stronger and more persistent (e.g., Paulson et al., 1991). It is therefore unexpected that self-administration of high amounts of cocaine does not lead to increased break-points.

Interestingly, there have been demonstrations that prolonged self-administration, or self-administration of high amounts of drugs, does lead to changes in the incentive value of the drug. For example, Deroche et al. (1999) compared two groups of rats, with limited (6 sessions) and extended (29 sessions) cocaine self-administration experience, and found that the extended-experience animals displayed an increased motivation for cocaine. This was assessed in an extinction-reinstatement setup (a well-known animal model to study relapse to drug seeking [Shaham et al., 2003; Shalev et al., 2002]), in which the extended-experience group showed a leftward shift in the dose-response curve for cocaine to reinstate drug seeking. In addition, the animals with extended cocaine experience took less time to traverse a runway reinforced with a cocaine infusion, suggesting that these animals were indeed more motivated for the drug. Interestingly, cocaine-induced conditioned place preference did not differ between these groups, which could indicate that the positive subjective effects of cocaine, in other words, drug "liking" (Robinson and Berridge, 1993), were not changed. However, because place conditioning (which measures approach behavior towards drug-associated stimuli) involves more factors than just drug reward, this latter finding should be interpreted with caution.

In another study from this group (Deroche-Gamonet et al., 2004) that will be discussed in some more detail later, break-points for cocaine appeared to increase with prolonged cocaine self-administration experience (for up to no less than 74 self-administration sessions), but this was found only in a subgroup of animals that also showed characteristics of loss of control over drug use. Consistent with these findings, animals that show escalation of cocaine or heroin intake as a result of long daily access to the drug (this typically entails 6-hr self-administration sessions, as opposed to 1-hr sessions in control groups [Ahmed, 2005; Ahmed and Koob, 1998]) also show increased break-points for the drug under a progressive ratio schedule of self-administration (Ahmed, 2005; Paterson and Markou, 2003; but see Liu et al., 2005b). Remarkably, animals that show escalated cocaine or heroin intake display no (or only marginal) psychomotor sensitization (Ahmed and Cador, 2006; Ben-Shahar et al., 2004, 2005; Ferrario et al., 2005; Lenoir and Ahmed, 2007). These data therefore suggest that increased responsiveness to the psychomotor effects of cocaine and increased motivation for the drug in self-administration settings are not necessarily a manifestation of the same neurobehavioral process.

Ahmed (2005) has suggested that the upward shift in the dose-response curve for cocaine under a progressive ratio schedule in escalated animals (Paterson and Markou, 2003) signifies a down-regulation of brain reward processes, because animals are more motivated to work for all cocaine unit doses. On the other hand, the leftward shift in the dose-response curve for amphetamine seen in sensitized animals (Vezina et al., 2002) may rather indicate enhanced motivation for the drug, because animals only work harder for low-unit doses. This issue clearly warrants further investigation, but also indicates a point of concern. That is, although the standard test for behavioral sensitization is to investigate whether the locomotor response for a drug has increased, the willingness to perform more work for drugs (as studied using a progressive ratio schedule of self-administration) is a more direct way to measure the incentive value of drugs. Because psychomotor sensitization and increased break-points under a progressive ratio schedule can at least be partially dissociated, this raises the question of what behavioral parameter should be used to further investigate the role of incentive sensitization in drug addiction.

The long-lasting character of sensitization suggests that sensitization plays a role in other persistent aspects of addiction, besides a (long-lasting) increase in the motivation for drugs. One such aspect is the risk of relapse to drug abuse, which remains present for years and sometimes even decades in detoxified addicts. The most widely used animal model of relapse is the so-called extinction-reinstatement model. In this setup, animals are trained to self-administer drugs, after which this behavior is extinguished, and attempts are made to reevoke operant behavior, which is interpreted as drug seeking because it is not reinforced in this phase of the experiment. It has been shown that noncontingent exposure to drugs and stress and response-contingent presentation of drug-associated cues can reinstate operant behavior (for reviews, see Shaham et al., 2003; Shalev et al., 2002).

Using a pharmacological approach, it was shown that drugs that evoked a sensitized psychomotor response in morphine-pretreated rats also reinstated heroin seeking, and that drugs that evoked a sensitized psychomotor response in amphetamine- or cocaine-pretreated rats also reinstated cocaine seeking (De Vries et al., 1998, 1999, 2002; Dias et al., 2004; Vanderschuren et al., 1997, 1999b, 1999c). Interestingly, there was considerable overlap between the drugs that reinstated cocaine seeking and heroin seeking, but the pharmacological profile of relapse to psychostimulant and opiate seeking was not identical, suggesting that there is drug-specificity in the neural substrates of relapse. Additional evidence for a relation between sensitization and reinstatement of drug seeking comes from the observation that AMPA receptor stimulation in the nucleus accumbens is important for both processes (Bell and Kalivas, 1996; Cornish et al., 1999; Pierce et al., 1996).

Indeed, rats pretreated with amphetamine and subsequently trained to self-administer cocaine were not only more motivated to work for the drug under a progressive ratio schedule of self-administration (see above; Suto et al., 2003), but also more sensitive to the reinstating effect of intra-accumbens treatment with AMPA (Suto et al., 2004). Furthermore, increased expression of the intracellular signaling protein activator of G-protein signaling (AGS)-3 in the prefrontal cortex is involved in expression of cocaine sensitization as well as relapse to cocaine seeking (Bowers et al., 2004). Together, these data suggest that at least part of the neural changes underlying behavioral sensitization also play a role in relapse to drug seeking. The observation, however, that in animals showing escalated cocaine or heroin intake, the ability of the drug to reinstate cocaine seeking is enhanced but the psychomotor response to the drug is not (Ahmed and Cador, 2006; Ben-Shahar et al., 2004, 2005; Ferrario et al., 2005; Lenoir and Ahmed, 2007; Mantsch et al., 2004), indicates that the neural changes that mediate sensitized psychomotor responsivity to drugs and those that facilitate relapse to drug seeking after extinction of the operant response overlap but are not identical (see also Spanagel et al., 1998; Sutton et al., 2000).

Although the evidence described above clearly shows that the incentive value of drugs can increase after repeated drug exposure, there are two types of observations that argue against the notion that incentive sensitization can explain drug addiction in its entirety. First, it has been shown that a single drug exposure can induce long-lasting behavioral sensitization and associated neuroadaptive changes (Kalivas and Alesdatter, 1993; Magos, 1969; Peris and Zahniser, 1987; Robinson, 1984; Robinson et al., 1982; Vanderschuren et al., 1999a, 2001). Whereas these observations clearly indicate that a single drug exposure may not be without lasting consequences, it would be difficult to maintain that a single episode of drug use leads to compulsive drug use, as drug addiction is the outcome of lengthy periods of intake of great amounts of drugs.

Second, there is a substantial body of evidence that repeated pretreatment with drugs of abuse not only increases the motivational properties of drugs (see above), but also of nondrug reinforcers. Thus, amphetamine-pretreated animals show facilitated sexual behavior (Fiorino and Phillips, 1999a, 1999b) and approach behavior to palatable food (Nocjar and Panksepp, 2002), as well as lever pressing for sucrose (Nordquist et al., 2007). Interestingly, amphetamine-pretreated rats do not consume more sucrose when it is freely available (Nordquist et al., 2007; Vanderschuren, unpublished observations), suggesting that it is the motivation for food ("wanting") rather than its hedonic value ("liking") that is increased in amphetamine-sensitized rats. Sensitizing pretreatment with amphetamine or cocaine also increases acquisition of approach behavior toward food-associated stimuli (Harmer and Phillips, 1998; Taylor and Jentsch, 2001). An important follow-up study (Harmer and Phillips, 1999) showed that not only acquisition of conditioned approach was enhanced in amphetamine-sensitized rats, but that acquisition of conditioned inhibition was accelerated as well. This shows that the increases in conditioned responding can't be explained on the basis of increased locomotor activity in sensitized animals, but that the association between food and conditioned stimuli gains control over behavior faster in sensitized animals. Responding with conditioned reinforcement, in which the animals have to acquire a novel response for presentation of a stimulus that has previously been paired with a reward (in this case, food), was shown to be enhanced after pretreatment with cocaine, amphetamine, or nicotine (Mead et al., 2004; Olausson et al., 2004; Taylor and Horger, 1999). In addition, the potentiation of responding with conditioned reinforcement after either systemic or intra-accumbens injection of amphetamine (Robbins, 1976; Taylor and Robbins, 1984, 1986) was exaggerated in sensitized animals (Mead et al., 2004; Olausson et al., 2004; Taylor and Horger, 1999).

Lastly, the ability of conditioned stimuli to enhance instrumental responding for food (so-called Pavlovian-to-instrumental transfer) was also found to be enhanced after pretreatment with amphetamine (Wyvell and Berridge, 2001). Together, these data show that in behaviorally sensitized animals, the motivation for nondrug reinforcers, as well as the ability of stimuli associated with them to gain control over behavior, is augmented. This suggests that repeated drug exposure causes a general enhancement in the responsiveness of the neural systems involved in motivation, rather than specific increases in the motivation for artificial, drug reinforcers. This is inconsistent with one of the core symptoms of addiction as formulated in *DSM IV* (American Psychiatric Association, 2000), that is, the sacrifice of social and professional activities in favor of drug-related activities, or in other words, the decreased interest in nondrug reinforcers.

Habit Learning in Compulsive Drug Use

In 1990, Tiffany (1990) put forward that automated, habitual behaviors could play a role in the maintenance of addictive behavior. In recent years, this notion has been advocated by Everitt, Robbins, and Dickinson (Everitt et al., 2001; Everitt and Robbins, 2005; Robbins and Everitt, 1999, 2002). The general idea of this theory is as follows. Early on, during acquisition of drug taking (or, in human terms, casual or recreational drug use), this behavior is a willful act, driven by a representation of the outcome, in other words, experiencing a positive subjective effect of the drug. However, after many cycles of drug taking, this behavior becomes dominated by a stimulus-response mechanism, whereby drug seeking becomes an automatic process, being triggered by drug-associated stimuli, beyond the individual's control and insensitive to devaluation of the drug reward (Everitt and Robbins, 2005; Robbins and Everitt, 1999; Tiffany, 1990). This drug-directed form of habitual behavior is a maladaptive form of stimulus-response habit learning (perhaps akin to procedural learning) that is a normal phenomenon with overtraining in many nondrug-associated tasks and contexts (Dickinson, 1985; Packard and Knowlton, 2002; White and McDonald, 2002; Yin and Knowlton, 2006). Thus, acquisition of stimulus-response habit learning is not equivalent to compulsive behavior. Rather, the habit theory of addiction poses that chronic exposure to self-administered drug subverts neural mechanisms of stimulus-response habit learning, causing a maladaptive, drug-directed form of habitual behavior.

The classic way of testing whether responding for a reinforcer occurs according to a stimulus-response (habitual) or action-outcome (goal-directed) associative structure is by evaluating responding for a devalued reinforcer (Adams, 1982; Dickinson, 1985; Killcross and Coutureau, 2003). In the case of ingestive reinforcers (food or fluid), this can be done by either prefeeding the subject with the foodstuff it can subsequently respond for (note that these tests are always done in extinction), or by associating this food with illness (typically by pairing it with lithium chloride). If the animal responds less for the devalued outcome, responding is mediated by an action-outcome process (as the animal appears to have a representation of the outcome, and the devalued outcome is less desirable and therefore merits less work), but if there is no difference between responding for valued and devalued outcomes, behavior is interpreted as mediated by a stimulus-response process.

In studies in which solutions containing drugs (ethanol, amphetamine, or the μ-opioid receptor agonist etonitazene) were offered to rats, and subsequently devalued by adding quinine, it was found that rats with prolonged (> 8 months of intake, plus a 1- to 6-month period of abstinence) drug experience were insensitive to quinine. That is, whereas early on, adding quinine to the drug solution caused their drug intake to decline, their intake levels were no longer modulated by quinine after prolonged periods of drinking. Similar findings were obtained by using social factors (dominance/subordination, social isolation) to influence drug intake (Heyne, 1996; Heyne and Wolffgramm, 1998; Wolffgramm and Heyne, 1995).

Using an instrumental approach, Dickinson et al. (2002) showed that lever pressing for ethanol gained habitual characteristics more quickly than food. Thus, lever pressing for food was markedly suppressed after it had been made aversive by pairing it with lithium chloride. However, when ethanol was paired with lithium, lever pressing did not decline. Likewise, instrumental behavior directed at obtaining a cocaine solution appeared insensitive to devaluation by pairing cocaine with lithium, whereas this was not the case in animals working for a sucrose solution (Miles et al., 2003).

These studies demonstrated that seeking of a drug reinforcer can be habitual under circumstances in which behavior directed at obtaining a natural reinforcer is not. Thus, seeking drugs progresses more readily from a goal-directed action-outcome to a habitual stimulus-response associative structure than seeking natural rewards does.

Using an intravenous self-administration setup, two recent studies have shown that instrumental behavior directed at obtaining cocaine indeed starts off as a flexible, goal-directed form of behavior, but after lengthy drug exposure acquires compulsive characteristics (Deroche-Gamonet et al., 2004; Vanderschuren and Everitt, 2004). In these studies, intravenous injections of cocaine were devalued, not by pairing them with illness, but with aversive stimuli. In the first of these (Vanderschuren and Everitt, 2004), drug seeking in the face of adverse consequences (American Psychiatric Association, 2000) was investigated in rats with a limited or an extended cocaine self-administration history. Cocaine was devalued by letting the animals respond for the drug in a state of conditioned fear. That is, rats were presented with a footshock-associated conditioned stimulus (CS) during cocaine seeking in order to measure conditioned suppression. In animals with limited experience of self-administering cocaine, the aversive CS markedly suppressed cocaine seeking, but in animals with an extended cocaine self-administration history, the footshock-associated CS no longer affected cocaine seeking.

This progression from flexible to inflexible appetitive behavior was specific to drugs, because in rats with an equivalent extended history of sucrose ingestion, the footshock CS still profoundly suppressed sucrose seeking. The differences between groups of animals in conditioned suppression of appetitive behavior was not paralleled by differences in freezing to a different footshock CS, showing that the absence of an effect of the footshock CS on cocaine seeking was not the result of the inability of the animals to encode or express a CS-US association, in other words, display conditioned fear.

In a series of experiments conducted independently (Deroche-Gamonet et al., 2004), it was demonstrated that over an extended period of cocaine self-administration, rats developed three manifestations of behavior reminiscent of symptoms of drug addiction according to *DSM-IV* (American Psychiatric Association, 2000). First, difficulty limiting drug intake was observed as persistence in responding during explicit extinction periods (i.e., when it was clearly indicated to the animal that responding would not result in cocaine delivery). Second, high motivation to obtain cocaine was observed as raised break-points under a progressive ratio schedule with increasing cocaine experience. Lastly, and similar to the study described above (Vanderschuren and Everitt, 2004), they found drug seeking despite adverse consequences, as the suppression of cocaine taking when it was paired with footshock was decreased after a lengthy cocaine-taking history. These symptoms of addiction were seen only in a subset of animals, those that subsequently showed high levels of relapse to cocaine seeking in an extinction-reinstatement setup (Shaham et al., 2003; Shalev et al., 2002). However, the development of these addiction-like behaviors was not correlated with locomotor activity (either in a novel environment or after cocaine infusion), anxiety, or amount of cocaine intake.

Thus, both these studies showed that in animals with a lengthy drug history, cocaine is insensitive to devaluation. Interestingly, both studies also assessed whether the progression of sensitivity to insensitivity to devaluation of the cocaine reinforcer was associated by changes in the incentive value of the drug. By assessing the rate of responding during drug seeking (Olmstead et al., 2000), Vanderschuren and Everitt (2004) found that it was not. In contrast, using the progressive ratio schedule, Deroche-Gamonet et al. (2004) did see increases in the incentive value of cocaine over time. This may be reconciled by close examination of the data, because Deroche-Gamonet et al. (2004) observed an increase in break-point for cocaine at a much earlier stage in the experiment (35 self-administration sessions) than a change in the willingness to endure delivery of footshock together with a cocaine infusion (74 sessions). These findings suggest this increase in the incentive value of the drug does not itself result in persistent drug seeking in the face of adversity. Rather, changes in the incentive value of drugs may precede the more critical changes in behavior that cause drug seeking to become impervious to adversity.

Conditioned Stimuli in Compulsive Drug Seeking

Some of the inflexible characteristics of addiction are caused by the strong control of drug-associated stimuli over behavior. The impact of drug-associated stimuli can be assessed using various ways of drug-stimulus pairing. In the place conditioning paradigm (Bardo and Bevins, 2000; Bardo et al., 1995; Tzschentke, 1998), an animal learns to associate subjective effects of drugs with a particular environment, and the absence of drug effects with a different environment. If, when given the choice between these two environments, animals spend more time in the drug-associated environment, this is called conditioned place preference. This is a Pavlovian conditioning setup, in which the drug is passively administered to the animal, and pairing of the environment with drug effects happens regardless of the animal's behavior. Conditioned place preference can therefore be interpreted as approach behavior toward Pavlovian conditioned stimuli (although this interpretation is not undisputed, see Uslaner et al., 2006). Conditioned place preference has been shown to be remarkably persistent, in other words, resistant to extinction (e.g., Cunningham et al., 1998; Mueller et al., 2002; Mueller and Stewart, 2000; Sakoori and Murphy, 2005), although this is not a general finding (Fuchs et al., 2002; Itzhak and Martin, 2002; Romieu et al., 2004; Sanchez and Sorg, 2001; Szumlinski et al., 2002).

The influence of drug-associated cues on drug seeking and taking has been most widely investigated using operant setups. In this case, drug-associated CSs are paired with delivery of self-administered drugs and the subjective effects of the drug. Alternatively, a drug-associated discriminative stimulus (DS) is not explicitly paired with drug delivery, but signals that the reinforcer is available response-contingently. By acting as conditioned reinforcers, drug-paired CSs as well as DSs can maintain drug seeking (Everitt and Robbins, 2000; Goldberg et al., 1975; Schindler et al., 2002), but only if they are presented response-contingently (Di Ciano and Everitt, 2003; Grimm et al., 2000; Kruzich et al., 2001).

Using a combination of drug-paired DSs and CSs, Weiss et al. (2001) have shown that responding for drug-paired cues was remarkably persistent. In these experiments, rats learned that in the presence of an auditory DS, lever pressing resulted in an intravenous infusion of cocaine and a visual CS. After extinction of operant responding (with neither cocaine, the DS, or the CS present during extinction sessions), presentation of the DS reinstated lever pressing for the cocaine-associated CS, even if cocaine itself was not available during these sessions. The capacity of the DS to reinstate responding for the cocaine-associated CS did not diminish at all over 11 repeated tests, the last test session being performed 18 weeks after the first reinstatement session. These experiments show that the DS and/or the CS supported lever pressing by themselves, being insensitive to presentation in the absence of cocaine. This was subsequently shown to require only one self-administration session, after which the DS remained capable of reinstating responding for the cocaine CS for up to 9 months, when the animals were retested at 3-month intervals (Ciccocioppo et al., 2004). From these experiments, it can't be distinguished whether it was the DS, the CS, or the combination of the two that supported responding and was resistant to extinction.

In the studies described above, the response that had to be made for presentation of the drug CS was the same one that was reinforced with the drug during initial training, making it also difficult to discern whether residual drug-directed behavior contributed to responding during testing, or whether responding was truly directed at obtaining a presentation of the drug-associated CS. To establish that a drug-associated CS can gain reinforcing properties itself, Di Ciano and Everitt (2004) trained animals to perform a new response (lever pressing) for presentations of a CS previously paired with self-administered cocaine, heroin, or sucrose (using nose poking as the operant). Animals readily acquired the lever-press response for presentation of the reinforcer-paired CS.

Remarkably, levels of lever pressing remained stable over more than 9 weeks of repeated testing. Leaving the animals undisturbed for 1 month before acquisition of lever-press responding for the CS, or response (i.e., nose-poke)-contingent presentation of the CS without cocaine before CS-cocaine association, retarded the acquisition of lever pressing for the CS. This is likely the result of spontaneous recovery mitigating the effect of forgetting or extinction, respectively (see Conklin and Tiffany, 2002, for a discussion). Contingent (upon nose poking) or noncontingent presentation of the CS after CS-cocaine training had no effect on lever pressing for the CS. Together, these data (Di Ciano and Everitt, 2004) provide strong evidence for persistence of the ability of drug-associated CSs to underpin drug-seeking responses, suggesting that CS-maintained drug seeking is resistant to extinction of the CS-drug association and may therefore gain a habitual quality.

It was recently shown that human cocaine users will also perform high levels of responding reinforced by a cocaine-associated CS only, in other words, while being aware that responding would not produce cocaine (Panlilio et al., 2005). In an earlier study, in which the effects of extinction were studied in animals responding for cocaine under a second-order schedule of reinforcement (Di Ciano and Everitt, 2002), it was found that nonreinforced exposure to the drug-associated CS did decrease responding when the animals were retested 1 day after the last extinction session, but that prolonged unavailability of the drug and the CS (i.e., the rats were left undisturbed in their home cages for 3 weeks) mitigated this effect. Thus, when extinction of responding was followed by a period of abstinence, the capacity of the drug-associated CSs to support drug seeking spontaneously recovered.

This latter observation (Di Ciano and Everitt, 2002) is reminiscent of a time-dependent increase, or "incubation," of drug seeking. In studies from Shaham and colleagues (Grimm et al., 2001, 2002, 2003; Lu et al., 2004a; Shepard et al., 2004; for review, see Lu et al., 2004b), it was found that drug seeking evoked by reexposure to drug-associated cues, but not the drug itself, increased with prolonged withdrawal in rats previously trained to self-administer cocaine or methamphetamine. Responding was found to increase progressively over the first 3 months of withdrawal, and declined thereafter.

A similar but somewhat less robust time-dependent effect of withdrawal was found in rats responding for sucrose cues (Grimm et al., 2002, 2003, 2005) or responding in extinction in the presence of cues signaling heroin availability (Shalev et al., 2001). The precise psychological mechanism underlying the incubation effect, which also occurs with cues associated with aversive events (see Houston et al., 1999, for a recent example), is unknown. It has been hypothesized that strengthening and generalization of cue-drug associations over time, to include not only the immediate drug-associated cues but also stimuli surrounding them in space and time, might underlie the increases in responding (see Houston et al., 1999, for a discussion).

The persistence of drug-seeking underpinned by drug-associated stimuli suggests that there may be a habitual component to this behavior. Recent analysis of its neural basis suggests that this is indeed the case. Thus, well-established cocaine seeking under a second-order schedule of reinforcement, which depends upon the conditioned reinforcing properties of cocaine-associated stimuli, was accompanied by increased dopamine efflux in the dorsal striatum, but not the nucleus accumbens (Ito et al., 2000, 2002). The importance of dorsal striatal mechanisms for cocaine seeking under a second-order schedule of reinforcement was confirmed by the observation that infusion of a dopamine receptor antagonist or an AMPA/kainate receptor antagonist into the dorsolateral striatum attenuated cue-controlled cocaine seeking (Vanderschuren et al., 2005). Because of the involvement of the dorsal striatum in stimulus-response habit learning, whereby behavior becomes automatic and is no longer driven by an action-outcome relationship (Everitt et al., 2001; Packard and Knowlton, 2002; White and McDonald, 2002; Yin and Knowlton, 2006), these findings suggest that the performance of well-established cocaine seeking may reflect the establishment of a habitual form of responding.

Possibilities for Therapeutic Interventions

The work reviewed above describes recent advances in the behavioral basis of compulsive drug seeking. As stated in the introduction of this chapter, elucidation of the neural underpinnings of compulsive aspects of drug addiction may open new avenues for the development of its pharmacological treatment. The recent explicit demonstration of compulsive drug seeking in laboratory animals (Deroche-Gamonet et al., 2004; Vanderschuren and Everitt, 2004) is an important step in this process. The fact that compulsive aspects of addiction can now be studied in laboratory animals allows for the neural basis of this core feature of addiction to be studied.

Of course, there is a large amount of work that these investigations can build on. Evidence from behavioral neuroscientific animal studies, as well as human functional imaging studies and neuropsychological investigations into the cognitive sequelae of chronic drug abuse has suggested that drug-induced dysfunctions of prefrontal corticostriatal systems underlying adaptive behavior may underlie the development of addiction (for recent reviews, see Bechara, 2005; Everitt and Robbins, 2005; Hyman et al., 2006; Volkow and Li, 2004). These studies have as yet not clearly indicated how compulsive drug use may be treated pharmacologically. The combination of studies into the compulsive aspects of drug seeking and the pharmacological targeting of cessation of drug use and relapse prevention (for reviews, see, e.g., Bossert et al., 2005; Heidbreder and Hagan, 2005) holds promise for the future.

Given the importance of incentive sensitization for addiction, targeting the neural changes underlying sensitization may also be a useful strategy. It is beyond the scope of this chapter to describe the neural basis of drug sensitization in detail (for reviews, see Carlezon and Nestler, 2002; Hyman et al., 2006; Nestler, 2001; Pierce and Kalivas, 1997; Vanderschuren and Kalivas, 2000; Wolf et al., 2004). In recent years, several studies have shown that psychostimulant sensitization can be reversed pharmacologically. Thus, when animals were repeatedly treated with either a dopamine D1 receptor agonist (Li et al., 2000; Shuto et al., 2006), a combination of an NMDA receptor antagonist and a dopamine D2 receptor agonist (Li et al., 2000), a serotonin (5-hydroxytryptamine; 5-HT)$_3$ receptor antagonist (King et al., 2000), a combination of a 5-HT$_3$ receptor antagonist and a dopamine D1/D2 receptor agonist (Zhang et al., 2007), or a selective 5-HT reuptake inhibitor (Kaneko et al., 2007) after cessation of repeated treatment with cocaine or methamphetamine, behavioral sensitization was no longer apparent for up to 3 weeks later. Moreover, treatment with the dopamine D1 receptor agonist (Li et al., 2000; Shuto et al., 2006), the combination of the NMDA receptor antagonist and the dopamine D2 receptor agonist (Li et al., 2000), or the combination of the 5-HT$_3$ receptor antagonist and the D1/D2 receptor agonist (Zhang et al., 2007) also reversed several cellular changes associated with sensitization. Because some of the compounds used in these studies are approved for human use, this may open a possibility for drug development.

Several other interesting advances in this field come from Kalivas and colleagues, who have shown that reversing cocaine-induced neural adaptations can also reverse the drug-hypersensitive phenotype. For example, repeated cocaine exposure causes decreased cystine-glutamate exchange in the nucleus accumbens, which leads to reduced basal extracellular levels of glutamate and increases in glutamate transmission after reexposure to the drug (Baker et al., 2003; Hotsenpiller et al., 2001; McFarland et al., 2003; Pierce et al., 1996). Restoring the decreased cystine/glutamate exchange prevents reinstatement of extinguished cocaine seeking (Baker et al., 2003; Moran et al., 2005). In addition, counteracting the cocaine-induced downregulation of the expression of Homer proteins (which play important roles in calcium signaling, glutamatergic neurotransmission, and synaptic plasticity) in the nucleus accumbens reversed the sensitized psychomotor response to the drug (Szumlinski et al., 2005a). Preventing the cocaine-induced increases in prefrontal cortical AGS-3 expression also prevented the expression of cocaine sensitization and relapse to cocaine seeking (Bowers et al., 2004).

Together, these studies show that by targeting cocaine-induced neuroadaptations, drug-induced changes in brain and behavior can be counteracted or reversed. Although promising, a few remarks should be made here. First, these studies have focused on psychostimulant drugs, in most cases cocaine, so that it remains to be shown whether similar mechanisms also hold for other drugs of abuse. In fact, whereas underexpression of Homer2 in the nucleus accumbens causes hypersensitivity to cocaine, it leads to hyposensitivity to ethanol (Szumlinski et al., 2005a, 2005b). Moreover, whether molecules like Homer, AGS-3, and the cystine-glutamate exchanger represent viable targets for drug development is not known. Last, although behavioral sensitization plays an important role in several aspects of drug addiction, it does not explain addiction in its entirety. Therefore, treating sensitization may not be sufficient to cure addiction.

Targeting the influence of conditioned stimuli on drug seeking is another possibility of treating the persistent aspects of addiction. One way to counteract the effects of conditioned stimuli on drug seeking is by extinguishing the drug-cue association. Although extinction of drug-cue associations is not a straightforward way to prevent drug seeking or relapse in humans (Conklin and Tiffany, 2002), and extinction of drug-cue associations has been particularly difficult in animal studies, too (see above), recent data show that extinction of drug-cue or drug-context associations can be facilitated neuropharmacologically. Thus, systemic or intra-amygdala injections with the muscarinic acetylcholine receptor agonist oxotremorine have been shown to enhance extinction of amphetamine conditioned place preference (Schroeder and Packard, 2004). In addition, postextinction session treatment with D-cycloserine, a partial NMDA receptor agonist that has been shown to enhance extinction of fear in human phobic patients (Ressler et al., 2004), has also been shown to facilitate extinction of a cocaine conditioned place preference (Botreau et al., 2006). The incubation of responding for cocaine-associated cues has been shown to depend on extracellular signal-regulated kinase (ERK) signaling in the amygdala. Thus, inhibition of ERK phosphorylation in the central nucleus of the amygdala decreased cocaine seeking after 30 days of withdrawal from cocaine self-administration, when levels of responding for cocaine cues had markedly increased compared to earlier time points (Lu et al., 2005).

Perhaps the most spectacular demonstrations of the notion that the influence of drug cues on addictive behavior is sensitive to disruption come from reconsolidation studies. Thus, during reactivation, established memory traces may become labile and sensitive to disruption. For example, blockade of protein synthesis in the basolateral amygdala has been shown to disrupt the reconsolidation of a footshock-CS association, so that the influence on behavior of the fear CS became greatly reduced (Nader et al., 2000; for reviews on the notion of reconsolidation and the differences with consolidation and extinction, see Alberini, 2005; Dudai and Eisenberg, 2004; Nader, 2003).

In the context of drug-associated cues, Lee et al. (2005) demonstrated that infusion of a Zif268 antisense oligodeoxynucleotide into the basolateral amygdala blocked reconsolidation of a CS-cocaine association, so that this CS was no longer able to support acquisition of a new response with conditioned reinforcement (Di Ciano and Everitt, 2004). Moreover, blockade of the reconsolidation of this cue-drug association blocked the ability of the cocaine-associated CS to support drug seeking under a second-order schedule of reinforcement, as well as its ability to reinstate extinguished drug seeking (Lee et al., 2006).

Using place conditioning, it was shown that inhibition of phosphorylation of ERK in the core of the nucleus accumbens disrupted reconsolidation of a cocaine-context association (Miller and Marshall, 2005). Consistent with these findings, systemic administration of an ERK activation inhibitor (or a protein synthesis inhibitor) disrupted the reconsolidation of cocaine and morphine conditioned place preference (Valjent et al., 2006). Blockade of protein synthesis, either by systemic treatment, or by injection into the nucleus accumbens, hippocampus, or basolateral amygdala (but not ventral tegmental area) also disrupted reconsolidation of a morphine-context association (Milekic et al., 2006).

Interestingly, whereas in the former three studies (Lee et al., 2005, 2006; Miller and Marshall, 2005) exposure to the cue or environment was sufficient to reactivate the drug-cue/environment association, in the latter two (Milekic et al., 2006; Valjent et al., 2006) it was necessary to expose the animals to the drug-associated environment while under the influence of the drug, suggesting that reactivation of different kinds of associations requires different molecular cascades and neural systems. Together, these data show that reactivation of drug-associated memories is amenable to reconsolidation-disrupting treatment, which may be an interesting therapeutic avenue to counteract the great control that drug-associated memories have over the behavior of addicts.

Indeed, disruption of a drug-context memory suppressed cocaine conditioned place preference for up to 14 days (Miller and Marshall, 2005) and abolished morphine place preference did not return after a single reconditioning session (Milekic et al., 2006), which suggests that blockade of drug-cue memories may have lasting effects. Moreover, disruption of an old cocaine-CS association (i.e., 27 days after the last training session) also attenuated the ability of the CS to support operant behavior (Lee et al., 2006). On the other hand, one should also bear in mind that in human addicts, drug-cue associations may not be simple associations between just one neutral cue and the subjective drug effect. Rather, the conditioned stimuli that drive addicts' behavior are probably complex chains of cues, events, and contexts that may not be easy to abolish, as indirectly reactivated memories have been found not to undergo reconsolidation (Debiec et al., 2006). However, the data published so far indicate that disruption of reconsolidation is an exciting treatment opportunity to be explored.

Conclusion: A Scenario for the Development of Compulsive Drug Seeking

The data reviewed above show that after repeated exposure to drugs, the drugs' reinforcing properties become enhanced. This is the result of a general increase in the sensitivity of the neural systems involved in motivation, not a specific increase in the motivational properties of drugs. Furthermore, after prolonged drug self-administration, drug use becomes inflexible, in that it is less sensitive to interference by aversive stimuli. Increases in the incentive value of drugs seem to precede the development of compulsive drug seeking. Last, drug-associated conditioned stimuli readily gain control over behavior—they can enhance drug seeking and taking, and become attractive themselves. The influence of conditioned stimuli on drug seeking is quite persistent.

Therefore, the progression of casual to compulsive drug seeking could happen as follows. Initial drug use will, under certain circumstances, or in susceptible individuals, lead to incentive sensitization, causing drugs to become more attractive. At the same time, repeated and consistent pairing of the subjective effects of drugs with environmental stimuli (drug paraphernalia, and contextual and social cues) causes these drug-associated stimuli to gain control over behavior. Incentive sensitization causes both drug and nondrug reinforcers to become more attractive, but because drug cues increasingly direct behavior, the likelihood of further drug intake greatly increases. At this stage, the amount of drug intake may escalate, perhaps causing dysfunction of brain reward systems (see Ahmed, 2005, Koob et al., 2004, for a discussion of how hypofunction of brain reward systems may contribute to addiction). Chronic exposure to large amounts of drugs leads to dysfunction of the prefrontal cortex, causing drug seeking to become inflexible. In parallel, prolonged drug exposure results in the recruitment of dorsal striatal mechanisms, causing an aberrant form of stimulus-response habitual behavior to support compulsive drug seeking. Elucidation of the neural basis of these component processes of addiction could open new avenues for the treatment of this disorder.

REFERENCES

Adams CD (1982) "Variations in the sensitivity of instrumental responding to reinforcer devaluation." *Quarterly Journal of Experimental Psychology* 34B: 77–98.

Ahmed SH (2005) "Imbalance between drug and non-drug reward availability: A major risk factor for addiction." *European Journal of Pharmacology* 526: 9–20.

Ahmed SH, Cador M (2006) "Dissociation of psychomotor sensitization from compulsive cocaine consumption." *Neuropsychopharmacology* 31: 563–571.

Ahmed SH, Koob GF (1998) "Transition from moderate to excessive drug intake: change in hedonic set point." *Science* 282: 298–300.

Alberini CM (2005) "Mechanisms of memory stabilization: are consolidation and reconsolidation similar or distinct processes?" *Trends in Neurosciences* 28: 51–56.

American Psychiatric Association (2000) *Diagnostic and statistical manual of mental disorders* (4th ed., text rev.). Washington, DC: American Psychiatric Association.

Baker DA, McFarland K, Lake RW, Shen H, Tang XC, Toda S, Kalivas PW (2003) "Neuroadaptations in cystine-glutamate exchange underlie cocaine relapse." *Nature Neuroscience* 6: 743–749.

Bardo MT, Bevins RA (2000) "Conditioned place preference: what does it add to our preclinical understanding of drug reward?" *Psychopharmacology* 153: 31–43.

Bardo MT, Rowlett JK, Harris MJ (1995) "Conditioned place preference using opiate and stimulant drugs: a meta-analysis." *Neuroscience and Biobehavioral Reviews* 19: 39–51.

Bechara A (2005) "Decision making, impulse control and loss of willpower to resist drugs: a neurocognitive perspective." *Nature Neuroscience* 8: 1458–1463.

Bell K, Kalivas PW (1996) "Context-specific cross-sensitization between systemic cocaine and intra-accumbens AMPA infusion in the rat." *Psychopharmacology* 127: 377–383.

Ben-Shahar O, Ahmed SH, Koob GF, Ettenberg A (2004) "The transition from controlled to compulsive drug use is associated with a loss of sensitization." *Brain Research* 995: 46–54.

Ben-Shahar O, Moscarello JM, Jacob B, Roarty MP, Ettenberg A (2005) "Prolonged daily exposure to IV cocaine results in tolerance to its stimulant effects." *Pharmacology Biochemistry & Behavior* 82: 411–416.

Berridge KC, Robinson TE (1998) "What is the role of dopamine in reward: hedonic impact, reward learning, or incentive salience?" *Brain Research Reviews* 28: 309–369.

Bossert JM, Ghitza UE, Lu L, Epstein DH, Shaham Y (2005) "Neurobiology of relapse to heroin and cocaine seeking: an update and clinical implications." *European Journal of Pharmacology* 526: 36–50.

Botreau F, Paolone G, Stewart J (2006) "D-Cycloserine facilitates extinction of a cocaine-induced conditioned place preference." *Behavioural Brain Research* 172: 173–178.

Bowers MS, Mcfarland K, Lake RW, Peterson YK, Lapish CC, Gregory ML, Lanier SM, Kalivas PW (2004) "Activator of G protein signaling 3: a gatekeeper of cocaine sensitization and drug seeking." *Neuron* 42: 269–281.

Carlezon WA, Jr., Nestler EJ (2002) "Elevated levels of GluR1 in the midbrain: a trigger for sensitization to drugs of abuse?" *Trends in Neurosciences* 25: 610–615.

Ciccocioppo R, Martin-Fardon R, Weiss F (2004) "Stimuli associated with a single cocaine experience elicit long-lasting cocaine-seeking." *Nature Neuroscience* 7: 495–496.

Conklin CA, Tiffany ST (2002) "Applying extinction research and theory to cue-exposure addiction treatments." *Addiction* 97: 155–167.

Cornish JL, Duffy P, Kalivas PW (1999) "A role for nucleus accumbens glutamate transmission in the relapse to cocaine-seeking behavior." *Neuroscience* 93: 1359–1367.

Covington HE, III, Miczek KA (2001) "Repeated social-defeat stress, cocaine or morphine—Effects on behavioral sensitization and intravenous cocaine self-administration 'binges.'" *Psychopharmacology* 158: 388–398.

Cunningham CL, Henderson CM, Bormann NM (1998) "Extinction of ethanol-induced conditioned place preference and conditioned place aversion: effects of naloxone." *Psychopharmacology* 139: 62–70.

Dackis C, O'Brien C (2005) "Neurobiology of addiction: treatment and public policy ramifications." *Nature Neuroscience* 8: 1431–1436.

De Vries TJ, Schoffelmeer ANM, Binnekade R, Mulder AH, Vanderschuren LJMJ (1998) "Drug-induced reinstatement of heroin- and cocaine-seeking behaviour following long-term extinction is associated with expression of behavioural sensitization." *European Journal of Neuroscience* 10: 3565–3571.

De Vries TJ, Schoffelmeer ANM, Binnekade R, Raasø H, Vanderschuren LJMJ (2002) "Relapse to cocaine- and heroin-seeking behavior mediated by dopamine D2 receptors is time-dependent and associated with behavioral sensitization." *Neuropsychopharmacology* 26: 18–26.

De Vries TJ, Schoffelmeer ANM, Binnekade R, Vanderschuren LJMJ (1999) "Dopaminergic mechanisms mediating the incentive to seek cocaine and heroin following long-term withdrawal of IV drug self-administration." *Psychopharmacology* 143: 254–260.

Debiec J, Doyère V, Nader K, LeDoux JE (2006) "Directly reactivated, but not indirectly reactivated, memories undergo reconsolidation in the amygdala." *Proceedings of the National Academy of Sciences of the USA* 103: 3428–3433.

Deroche V, Le Moal M, Piazza PV (1999) "Cocaine self-administration increases the incentive motivational properties of the drug in rats." *European Journal of Neuroscience* 11: 2731–2736.

Deroche-Gamonet V, Belin D, Piazza PV (2004) "Evidence for addiction-like behavior in the rat." *Science* 305: 1014–1017.

Dias C, Lachize S, Boilet V, Huitelec E, Cador M (2004) "Differential effects of dopaminergic agents on locomotor sensitisation and on the reinstatement of cocaine-seeking and food-seeking behaviour." *Psychopharmacology* 175: 414–427.

Di Ciano P, Everitt BJ (2002) "Reinstatement and spontaneous recovery of cocaine-seeking following extinction and different durations of withdrawal." *Behavioural Pharmacology* 13: 397–405.

Di Ciano P, Everitt BJ (2003) "Differential control over drug-seeking behavior by drug-associated conditioned reinforcers and discriminative stimuli predictive of drug availability." *Behavioural Neuroscience* 117: 952–960.

Di Ciano P, Everitt BJ (2004) "Conditioned reinforcing properties of stimuli paired with self-administered cocaine, heroin or sucrose: implications for the persistence of addictive behaviour." *Neuropharmacology* 47 Suppl. 1: 202–213.

Dickinson A (1985) "Actions and habits: the development of behavioural autonomy." *Philosophical Transactions of the Royal Society of London (Biology)* 308: 67–78.

Dickinson A, Wood N, Smith JW (2002) "Alcohol seeking by rats: action or habit?" *Quarterly Journal of Experimental Psychology* 55B: 331–348.

Dudai Y, Eisenberg M (2004) "Rites of passage of the engram: reconsolidation and the lingering consolidation hypothesis." *Neuron* 44: 93–100.

Everitt BJ, Dickinson A, Robbins TW (2001) "The neuropsychological basis of addictive behaviour." *Brain Research Reviews* 36: 129–138.

Everitt BJ, Robbins TW (2000) "Second-order schedules of drug reinforcement in rats and monkeys: measurement of reinforcing efficacy and drug-seeking behaviour." *Psychopharmacology* 153: 17–30.

Everitt BJ, Robbins TW (2005) "Neural systems of reinforcement for drug addiction: from actions to habits to compulsion." *Nature Neuroscience* 8: 1481–1489.

Ferrario CR, Gorny G, Crombag HS, Li Y, Kolb B, Robinson TE (2005) "Neural and behavioral plasticity associated with the transition from controlled to escalated cocaine use." *Biological Psychiatry* 58: 751–759.

Fiorino DF, Phillips AG (1999a) "Facilitation of sexual behavior and enhanced dopamine efflux in the nucleus accumbens of male rats after d-amphetamine-induced behavioral sensitization." *Journal of Neuroscience* 19: 456–463.

Fiorino DF, Phillips AG (1999b) "Facilitation of sexual behavior in male rats following *d*-amphetamine-induced behavioral sensitization." *Psychopharmacology* 142: 200–208.

Fuchs RA, Weber SM, Rice HJ, Neisewander JL (2002) "Effects of excitotoxic lesions of the basolateral amygdala on cocaine-seeking behavior and cocaine conditioned place preference in rats." *Brain Research* 929: 15–25.

Gaiardi M, Bartoletti M, Bacchi A, Gubellini C, Costa M, Babbini M (1991) "Role of repeated exposure to morphine in determining its affective properties: place and taste conditioning studies in rats." *Psychopharmacology* 103: 183–186.

Goldberg SR, Kelleher RT, Morse WH (1975) "Second-order schedules of drug injection." *Federation Proceedings* 34: 1771–1776.

Grimm JW, Fyall AM, Osincup DP (2005) "Incubation of sucrose craving: effects of reduced training and sucrose pre-loading." *Physiol Behav.* 84: 73–79.

Grimm JW, Hope BT, Wise RA, Shaham Y (2001) "Incubation of cocaine craving after withdrawal." *Nature* 412: 141–142.

Grimm JW, Kruzich PJ, See RE (2000) "Contingent access to stimuli associated with cocaine self-administration is required for reinstatement of drug-seeking behavior." *Psychobiology* 28: 383–386.

Grimm JW, Lu L, Hayashi T, Hope BT, Su TP, Shaham Y (2003) "Time-dependent increases in brain-derived neurotrophic factor protein levels within the mesolimbic dopamine system after withdrawal from cocaine: Implications for incubation of cocaine craving." *Journal of Neuroscience* 23: 742–747.

Grimm JW, Shaham Y, Hope BT (2002) "Effect of cocaine and sucrose withdrawal period on extinction behavior, cue-induced reinstatement, and protein levels of the dopamine transporter and tyrosine hydroxylase in limbic and cortical areas in rats." *Behavioural Pharmacology* 13: 379–388.

Harmer CJ, Phillips GD (1998) "Enhanced appetitive conditioning following repeated pretreatment with d-amphetamine." *Behavioural Pharmacology* 9: 299–308.

Harmer CJ, Phillips GD (1999) "Enhanced conditioned inhibition following repeated pretreatment with d-amphetamine." *Psychopharmacology* 142: 120–131.

Heidbreder CA, Hagan JJ (2005) "Novel pharmacotherapeutic approaches for the treatment of drug addiction and craving." *Current Opinion in Pharmacology* 5: 107–118.

Heyne A (1996) "The development of opiate addiction in the rat." *Pharmacology Biochemistry & Behavior* 53: 11–25.

Heyne A, Wolffgramm J (1998) "The development of addiction to d-amphetamine in an animal model: same principles as for alcohol and opiate." *Psychopharmacology* 140: 510–518.

Hodos W (1961) "Progressive ratio as a measure of reward strength." *Science* 134: 943–944.

Hooks MS, Duffy P, Striplin C, Kalivas PW (1994) "Behavioral and neurochemical sensitization following cocaine self-administration." *Psychopharmacology* 115: 265–272.

Horger BA, Giles MK, Schenk S (1992) "Preexposure to amphetamine and nicotine predisposes rats to self-administer a low dose of cocaine." *Psychopharmacology* 107: 271–276.

Horger BA, Shelton K, Schenk S (1990) "Preexposure sensitizes rats to the rewarding effects of cocaine." *Pharmacology Biochemistry & Behavior* 37: 707–711.

Hotsenpiller G, Giorgetti M, Wolf ME (2001) "Alterations in behaviour and glutamate transmission following presentation of stimuli previously associated with cocaine exposure." *European Journal of Neuroscience* 14: 1843–1855.

Houston FP, Stevenson GD, McNaughton BL, Barnes CA (1999) "Effects of age on the generalization and incubation of memory in the F344 rat." *Learning & Memory* 6: 111–119.

Hyman SE, Malenka RC, Nestler EJ (2006) "Neural mechanisms of addiction: the role of reward-related learning and memory." *Annual Review of Neuroscience* 29: 565–598.

Ito R, Dalley JW, Howes SR, Robbins TW, Everitt BJ (2000) "Dissociation in conditioned dopamine release in the nucleus accumbens core and shell in response to cocaine cues and during cocaine-seeking behavior in rats." *Journal of Neuroscience* 20: 7489–7495.

Ito R, Dalley JW, Robbins TW, Everitt BJ (2002) "Dopamine release in the dorsal striatum during cocaine-seeking behavior under the control of a drug-associated cue." *Journal of Neuroscience* 22: 6247–6253.

Itzhak Y, Martin JL (2002) "Cocaine-induced conditioned place preference in mice: Induction, extinction and reinstatement by related psychostimulants." *Neuropsychopharmacology* 26: 130–134.

Jentsch JD, Taylor JR (1999) "Impulsivity resulting from frontostriatal dysfunction in drug abuse: implications for the control of behavior by reward-related stimuli." *Psychopharmacology* 146: 373–390.

Kalivas PW, Alesdatter JE (1993) "Involvement of N-methyl-D-aspartate receptor stimulation in the ventral tegmental area and amygdala in behavioral sensitization to cocaine." *Journal of Pharmacology and Experimental Therapeutics* 267: 486–495.

Kalivas PW, Volkow N, Seamans J (2005) "Unmanageable motivation in addiction: a pathology in prefrontal-accumbens glutamate transmission." *Neuron* 45: 647–650.

Kaneko Y, Kashiwa A, Ito T, Ishii S, Umino A, Nishikawa T (2007) "Selective serotonin reuptake inhibitors, fluoxetine and paroxetine, attenuate the expression of the established behavioral sensitization induced by methamphetamine." *Neuropsychopharmacology* 32: 658–664.

Kelley AE (2004) "Memory and addiction: shared neural circuitry and molecular mechanisms." *Neuron* 44: 161–179.

Killcross S, Coutureau E (2003) "Coordination of actions and habits in the medial prefrontal cortex of rats." *Cerebral Cortex* 13: 400–408.

King GR, Xiong Z, Douglass S, Ellinwood EH, Jr. (2000) "Long-term blockade of the expression of cocaine sensitization by ondansetron, a 5-HT$_3$ receptor antagonist." *European Journal of Pharmacology* 394: 97–101.

Koob GF (1992) "Drugs of abuse: anatomy, pharmacology and function of reward pathways." *Trends in Pharmacological Sciences* 13: 177–184.

Koob GF, Ahmed SH, Boutrel B, Chen SA, Kenny PJ, Markou A, O'Dell LE, Parsons LH, Sanna PP (2004) "Neurobiological mechanisms in the transition from drug use to drug dependence." *Neuroscience and Biobehavioral Reviews* 27: 739–749.

Kruzich PJ, Congleton KM, See RE (2001) "Conditioned reinstatement of drug-seeking behavior with a discrete compound stimulus classically conditioned with intravenous cocaine." *Behavioral Neuroscience* 115: 1086–1092.

Lee JLC, Di Ciano P, Thomas KL, Everitt BJ (2005) "Disrupting reconsolidation of drug memories reduces cocaine-seeking behavior." *Neuron* 47: 795–801.

Lee JLC, Milton AL, Everitt BJ (2006) "Cue induced cocaine seeking and relapse are reduced by disruption of drug memory reconsolidation." *Journal of Neuroscience* 26: 5881–5887.

Lenoir M, Ahmed SH (2007) "Heroin-induced reinstatement is specific to compulsive heroin use and dissociable from heroin reward and sensitization." *Neuropsychopharmacology* 32: 616–624.

Leshner AI (1997) "Addiction is a brain disease, and it matters." *Science* 278: 45–47.

Lett BT (1989) "Repeated exposures intensify rather than diminish the rewarding effects of amphetamine, morphine, and cocaine." *Psychopharmacology* 98: 357–362.

Li Y, White FJ, Wolf ME (2000) "Pharmacological reversal of behavioral and cellular indices of cocaine sensitization in the rat." *Psychopharmacology* 151: 175–183.

Liu Y, Roberts DCS, Morgan D (2005a) "Sensitization of the reinforcing effects of self-administered cocaine in rats: effects of dose and intravenous injection speed." *European Journal of Neuroscience* 22: 195–200.

Liu Y, Roberts DCS, Morgan D (2005b) "Effects of extended-access self-administration and deprivation on breakpoints maintained by cocaine in rats." *Psychopharmacology* 179: 644–651.

Lorrain DS, Arnold GM, Vezina P (2000) "Previous exposure to amphetamine increases incentive to obtain the drug: long-lasting effects revealed by the progressive ratio schedule." *Behavioural Brain Research* 107: 9–19.

Lu L, Grimm JW, Dempsey J, Shaham Y (2004a) "Cocaine seeking over extended withdrawal periods in rats: different time courses of responding induced by cocaine cues versus cocaine priming over the first 6 months." *Psychopharmacology* 176: 101–108.

Lu L, Grimm JW, Hope BT, Shaham Y (2004b) "Incubation of cocaine craving after withdrawal: a review of preclinical data." *Neuropharmacology* 47 Suppl 1: 214–226.

Lu L, Hope BT, Dempsey J, Liu SY, Bossert JM, Shaham Y (2005) "Central amygdala ERK signaling pathway is critical to incubation of cocaine craving." *Nature Neuroscience* 8: 212–219.

Magos L (1969) "Persistence of the effect of amphetamine on stereotyped activity in rats." *European Journal of Pharmacology* 6: 200–201.

Mantsch JR, Yuferov V, Mathieu-Kia AM, Ho A, Kreek MJ (2004) "Effects of extended access to high versus low cocaine doses on self-administration, cocaine-induced reinstatement and brain mRNA levels in rats." *Psychopharmacology* 175: 26–36.

McFarland K, Lapish CC, Kalivas PW (2003) "Prefrontal glutamate release into the core of the nucleus accumbens mediates cocaine-induced reinstatement of drug-seeking behavior." *Journal of Neuroscience* 23: 3531–3537.

Mead AN, Crombag HS, Rocha BA (2004) "Sensitization of psychomotor stimulation and conditioned reward in mice: differential modulation by contextual learning." *Neuropsychopharmacology* 29:249–258.

Mendrek A, Blaha CD, Phillips AG (1998) "Pre-exposure of rats to amphetamine sensitizes self-administration of this drug under a progressive ratio schedule." *Psychopharmacology* 135: 416–422.

Milekic MH, Brown SD, Castellini C, Alberini CM (2006) "Persistent disruption of an established morphine conditioned place preference." *Journal of Neuroscience* 26: 3010–3020.

Miles FJ, Everitt BJ, Dickinson A (2003) "Oral cocaine seeking by rats: Action or habit?" *Behavioural Neuroscience* 117: 927–938.

Miller CA, Marshall JF (2005) "Molecular substrates for retrieval and reconsolidation of cocaine-associated contextual memory." *Neuron* 47: 873–884.

Moran MM, McFarland K, Melendez RI, Kalivas PW, Seamans JK (2005) "Cystine/glutamate exchange regulates metabotropic glutamate receptor presynaptic inhibition of excitatory transmission and vulnerability to cocaine seeking." *Journal of Neuroscience* 25: 6389–6393.

Morgan D, Liu Y, Roberts DCS (2006) "Rapid and persistent sensitization to the reinforcing effects of cocaine." *Neuropsychopharmacology* 31: 121–128.

Morgan D, Smith MA, Roberts DCS (2005) "Binge self-administration and deprivation produces sensitization to the reinforcing effects of cocaine in rats." *Psychopharmacology* 178: 309–316.

Mueller D, Perdikaris D, Stewart J (2002) "Persistence and drug-induced reinstatement of a morphine-induced conditioned place preference." *Behavioural Brain Research* 136: 389–397.

Mueller D, Stewart J (2000) "Cocaine-induced conditioned place preference: reinstatement by priming injections of cocaine after extinction." *Behavioural Brain Research* 115: 39–47.

Nader K (2003) "Memory traces unbound." *Trends in Neurosciences* 26: 65–72.

Nader K, Schafe GE, LeDoux JE (2000) "Fear memories require protein synthesis in the amygdala for reconsolidation after retrieval." *Nature* 406: 722–726.

Nestler EJ (2001) "Molecular basis of long-term plasticity underlying addiction." *Nature Reviews Neuroscience* 2: 119–128.

Nocjar C, Panksepp J (2002) "Chronic intermittent amphetamine pretreatment enhances future appetitive behavior for drug- and natural-reward: interaction with environmental variables." *Behavioural Brain Research* 128: 189–203.

Nordquist RE, Voorn P, De Mooij-van Malsen J.G., Joosten RNJMA, Pennartz CMA, Vanderschuren LJMJ (2007) "Augmented reinforcer value and accelerated habit formation after amphetamine sensitization." *European Neuropsychopharmacology* 17: 532–540.

Olausson P, Jentsch JD, Taylor JR (2004) "Nicotine enhances responding with conditioned reinforcement." *Psychopharmacology* 171: 173–178.

Olmstead MC, Parkinson JA, Miles FJ, Everitt BJ, Dickinson A (2000) "Cocaine-seeking by rats: regulation, reinforcement and activation." *Psychopharmacology* 152: 123–131.

Packard MG, Knowlton BJ (2002) "Learning and memory functions of the basal ganglia." *Annual Review of Neuroscience* 25: 563–593.

Panlilio LV, Yasar S, Nemeth-Coslett R, Katz JL, Henningfield JE, Solinas M, Heishman SJ, Schindler CW, Goldberg SR (2005) "Human cocaine-seeking behavior and its control by drug-associated stimuli in the laboratory." *Neuropsychopharmacology* 30: 433–443.

Paterson NE, Markou A (2003) "Increased motivation for self-administered cocaine after escalated cocaine intake." *NeuroReport* 14: 2229–2232.

Paulson PE, Camp DM, Robinson TE (1991) "Time course of transient behavioral depression and persistent behavioral sensitization in relation to regional brain monoamine concentrations during amphetamine withdrawal in rats." *Psychopharmacology* 103: 480–492.

Peris J, Zahniser NR (1987) "One injection of cocaine produces a long-lasting increase in [^{3}H]-dopamine release." *Pharmacology Biochemistry & Behavior* 27: 533–535.

Phillips AG, Di Ciano P (1996) "Behavioral sensitization is induced by intravenous self-administration of cocaine by rats." *Psychopharmacology* 124: 279–281.

Piazza PV, Deminière J-M, Le Moal M, Simon H (1989) "Factors that predict individual vulnerability to amphetamine self-administration." *Science* 245: 1511–1513.

Piazza PV, Deminière J-M, Le Moal M, Simon H (1990) "Stress- and pharmacologically-induced behavioral sensitization increases vulnerability to acquisition of amphetamine self-administration." *Brain Research* 514: 22–26.

Pierce RC, Bell K, Duffy P, Kalivas PW (1996) "Repeated cocaine augments excitatory amino acid transmission in the nucleus accumbens only in rats having developed behavioral sensitization." *Journal of Neuroscience* 16: 1550–1560.

Pierce RC, Kalivas PW (1997) "A circuitry model of the expression of behavioral sensitization to amphetamine-like psychostimulants." *Brain Research Reviews* 25: 192–216.

Ressler KJ, Rothbaum BO, Tannenbaum L, Anderson P, Graap K, Zimand E, Hodges L, Davis M (2004) "Cognitive enhancers as adjuncts to psychotherapy: use of D-cycloserine in phobic individuals to facilitate extinction of fear." *Archives of General Psychiatry* 61: 1136–1144.

Richardson NR, Roberts DCS (1996) "Progressive ratio schedules in drug self-administration studies in rats: a method to evaluate reinforcing efficacy." *Journal of Neuroscience Methods* 66: 1–11.

Robbins TW (1976) "Relationship between reward-enhancing and stereotypical effects of psychomotor stimulant drugs." *Nature* 264:57–59.

Robbins TW, Everitt BJ (1999) "Drug addiction: bad habits add up." *Nature* 398: 567–570.

Robbins TW, Everitt BJ (2002) "Limbic-striatal memory systems and drug addiction." *Neurobiology of Learning & Memory* 78: 625–636.

Robinson TE (1984) "Behavioral sensitization: characterization of enduring changes in rotational behavior produced by intermittent injections of amphetamine in male and female rats." *Psychopharmacology* 84: 466–475.

Robinson TE, Becker JB, Presty SK (1982) "Long-term facilitation of amphetamine-induced rotational behavior and striatal dopamine release produced by a single exposure to amphetamine: sex differences." *Brain Research* 253: 231–241.

Robinson TE, Berridge KC (1993) "The neural basis of drug craving: an incentive-sensitization theory of addiction." *Brain Research Reviews* 18: 247–291.

Robinson TE, Berridge KC (2000) "The psychology and neurobiology of addiction: an incentive-sensitization view." *Addiction* 95 Suppl. 2: S91-S117.

Robinson TE, Berridge KC (2001) "Incentive-sensitization and addiction." *Addiction* 96: 103–114.

Robinson TE, Berridge KC (2003) "Addiction." *Annual Review of Psychology* 54: 25–53.

Romieu P, Meunier J, Garcia D, Zozime N, Martin-Fardon R, Bowen WD, Maurice T (2004) "The sigma1 (σ1) receptor activation is a key step for the reactivation of cocaine conditioned place preference by drug priming." *Psychopharmacology* 175: 154–162.

Sakoori K, Murphy NP (2005) "Maintenance of conditioned place preferences and aversion in C57BL6 mice: effects of repeated and drug state testing." *Behavioural Brain Research* 160: 34–43.

Sanchez CJ, Sorg BA (2001) "Conditioned fear stimuli reinstate cocaine-induced conditioned place preference." *Brain Research* 908: 86–92.

Schindler CW, Panlilio LV, Goldberg SR (2002) "Second-order schedules of drug self-administration in animals." *Psychopharmacology* 163: 327–344.

Schroeder JP, Packard MG (2004) "Facilitation of memory for extinction of drug-induced conditioned reward: role of amygdala and acetylcholine." *Learning & Memory* 11: 641–647.

Shaham Y, Shalev U, Lu L, De Wit H, Stewart J (2003) "The reinstatement model of drug relapse: history, methodology and major findings." *Psychopharmacology* 168: 3–20.

Shalev U, Grimm JW, Shaham Y (2002) "Neurobiology of relapse to heroin and cocaine seeking: a review." *Pharmacological Reviews* 54: 1–42.

Shalev U, Morales M, Hope B, Yap J, Shaham Y (2001) "Time-dependent changes in extinction behavior and stress- induced reinstatement of drug seeking following withdrawal from heroin in rats." *Psychopharmacology* 156: 98–107.

Shepard JD, Bossert JM, Liu SY, Shaham Y (2004) "The anxiogenic drug yohimbine reinstates methamphetamine seeking in a rat model of drug relapse." *Biological Psychiatry* 55: 1082–1089.

Shippenberg TS, Heidbreder C (1995) "Sensitization to the conditioned rewarding effects of cocaine: pharmacological and temporal characteristics." *Journal of Pharmacology and Experimental Therapeutics* 273: 808–815.

Shippenberg TS, Heidbreder C, Lefevour A (1996) "Sensitization to the conditioned rewarding effects of morphine: pharmacology and temporal characteristics." *European Journal of Pharmacology* 299: 33–39.

Shuto T, Kuroiwa M, Hamamura M, Yabuuchi K, Shimazoe T, Watanabe S, Nishi A, Yamamoto T (2006) "Reversal of methamphetamine-induced behavioral sensitization by repeated administration of a dopamine D_1 receptor agonist." *Neuropharmacology* 50:991–997

Spanagel R, Sillaber I, Zieglgänsberger W, Corrigall WA, Stewart J, Shaham Y (1998) "Acamprosate suppresses the expression of morphine-induced sensitization in rats but does not affect heroin self-administration or relapse induced by heroin or stress." *Psychopharmacology* 139:391–401.

Stewart J, Badiani A (1993) "Tolerance and sensitization to the behavioral effects of drugs." *Behavioural Pharmacology* 4:289–312.

Suto N, Tanabe LM, Austin JD, Creekmore E, Pham CT, Vezina P (2004) "Previous exposure to psychostimulants enhances the reinstatement of cocaine seeking by nucleus accumbens AMPA." *Neuropsychopharmacology* 29: 2149–2159.

Suto N, Tanabe L, Austin JD, Creekmore E, Vezina P (2003) "Previous exposure to VTA amphetamine enhances cocaine self-administration under a progressive ratio schedule in an NMDA, AMPA/kainate, and metabotropic glutamate receptor-dependent manner." *Neuropsychopharmacology* 28: 629–639.

Sutton MA, Karanian DA, Self DW (2000) "Factors that determine a propensity for cocaine-seeking behavior during abstinence in rats." *Neuropsychopharmacology* 22:626–641.

Szumlinski KK, Abernathy KE, Oleson EB, Klugmann M, Lominac KD, He DY, Ron D, During M, Kalivas PW (2005a) "Homer isoforms differentially regulate cocaine-induced neuroplasticity," *Neuropsychopharmacology* 31: 768–777.

Szumlinski KK, Lominac KD, Oleson EB, Walker JK, Mason A, Dehoff MH, Klugman M, Cagle S, Welt K, During M, Worley PF, Middaugh LD, Kalivas PW (2005b) "Homer2 is necessary for EtOH-induced neuroplasticity." *Journal of Neuroscience* 25: 7054–7061.

Szumlinski KK, Price KL, Frys KA, Middaugh LD (2002) "Unconditioned and conditioned factors contribute to the 'reinstatement' of cocaine place conditioning following extinction in C57BL/6 mice." *Behavioural Brain Research* 136: 151–160.

Taylor JR, Horger BA (1999) "Enhanced responding for conditioned reward produced by intra-accumbens amphetamine is potentiated after cocaine sensitization." *Psychopharmacology* 142: 31–40.

Taylor JR, Jentsch JD (2001) "Repeated intermittent administration of psychomotor stimulant drugs alters the acquisition of Pavlovian approach behavior in rats: Differential effects of cocaine, d-amphetamine and 3,4-methylenedioxymethamphetamine ("ecstasy")." *Biological Psychiatry* 50: 137–143.

Taylor JR, Robbins TW (1984) "Enhanced behavioural control by conditioned reinforcers following microinjections of d-amphetamine into the nucleus accumbens." *Psychopharmacology* 84: 405–412.

Taylor JR, Robbins TW (1986) "6-Hydroxydopamine lesions of the nucleus accumbens, but not of the caudate nucleus, attenuate enhanced responding with reward-related stimuli produced by intra-accumbens *d*-amphetamine." *Psychopharmacology* 90: 390–397.

Tiffany ST (1990) "A cognitive model of drug urges and drug-use behavior: role of automatic and nonautomatic processes." *Psychological Reviews* 97: 147–168.

Tzschentke TM (1998) "Measuring reward with the conditioned place preference paradigm: A comprehensive review of drug effects, recent progress and new issues." *Progress in Neurobiology* 56: 613–672.

Uslaner JM, Acerbo MJ, Jones SA, Robinson TE (2006) "The attribution of incentive salience to a stimulus that signals an intravenous injection of cocaine." *Behavioural Brain Research* 169: 320–324.

Valadez A, Schenk S (1994) "Persistence of the ability of amphetamine preexposure to facilitate acquisition of cocaine self-administration." *Pharmacology Biochemistry & Behavior* 47: 203–205.

Valjent E, Corbillé A-G, Bertran-Gonzalez J, Hervé D, Girault J-A (2006) "Inhibition of ERK pathway or protein synthesis during reexposure to drugs of abuse erases previously learned place preference." *Proceedings of the National Academy of Sciences of the USA* 103: 2932–2937.

Vanderschuren LJMJ, De Vries TJ, Wardeh G, Hogenboom FACM, Schoffelmeer ANM (2001) "A single exposure to morphine induces long-lasting behavioral and neurochemical sensitization in rats." *European Journal of Neuroscience* 14: 1533–1538.

Vanderschuren LJMJ, Di Ciano P, Everitt BJ (2005) "Involvement of the dorsal striatum in cue-controlled cocaine seeking." *Journal of Neuroscience* 25: 8665–8670.

Vanderschuren LJMJ, Everitt BJ (2004) "Drug seeking becomes compulsive after prolonged cocaine self-administration." *Science* 305: 1017–1019.

Vanderschuren LJMJ, Kalivas PW (2000) "Alterations in dopaminergic and glutamatergic transmission in the induction and expression of behavioral sensitization: a critical review of preclinical studies." *Psychopharmacology* 151: 99–120.

Vanderschuren LJMJ, Schmidt ED, De Vries TJ, Van Moorsel CAP, Tilders FJH, Schoffelmeer ANM (1999a) "A single exposure to amphetamine is sufficient to induce long-term behavioral, neuroendocrine and neurochemical sensitization in rats." *Journal of Neuroscience* 19: 9579–9586.

Vanderschuren LJMJ, Schoffelmeer ANM, Mulder AH, De Vries TJ (1999b) "Dopaminergic mechanisms mediating the long-term expression of locomotor sensitization following pre-exposure to morphine or amphetamine." *Psychopharmacology* 143: 244–253.

Vanderschuren LJMJ, Schoffelmeer ANM, Mulder AH, De Vries TJ (1999c) "Lack of cross-sensitization of the locomotor effects of morphine in amphetamine-treated rats." *Neuropsychopharmacology* 21: 550–559.

Vanderschuren LJMJ, Tjon GHK, Nestby P, Mulder AH, Schoffelmeer ANM, De Vries TJ (1997) "Morphine-induced long term sensitization to the locomotor effects of morphine and amphetamine depends on the temporal pattern of the pretreatment regimen." *Psychopharmacology* 131: 115–122.

Vezina P, Lorrain DS, Arnold GM, Austin JD, Suto N (2002) "Sensitization of midbrain dopamine neuron reactivity promotes the pursuit of amphetamine." *Journal of Neuroscience* 22: 4654–4662.

Volkow ND, Li T-K (2004) "Drug addiction: the neurobiology of behaviour gone awry." *Nature Reviews Neuroscience* 5: 963–970.

Ward SJ, Lack C, Morgan D, Roberts DCS (2006) "Discrete-trials heroin self-administration produces sensitization to the reinforcing effects of cocaine in rats." *Psychopharmacology* 185: 150–159.

Weiss F, Martin-Fardon R, Ciccocioppo R, Kerr TM, Smith DL, Ben-Shahar O (2001) "Enduring resistance to extinction of cocaine-seeking behavior induced by drug-related cues." *Neuropsychopharmacology* 25: 361–372.

White NM, McDonald RJ (2002) "Multiple parallel memory systems in the brain of the rat." *Neurobiology of Learning & Memory* 77: 125–184.

Wise RA, Bozarth MA (1987) "A psychomotor stimulant theory of addiction." *Psychological Reviews* 94: 469–492.

Wolf ME, Sun X, Mangiavacchi S, Chao SZ (2004) "Psychomotor stimulants and neuronal plasticity." *Neuropharmacology* 47 Suppl 1: 61–79.

Wolffgramm J, Heyne A (1995) "From controlled drug intake to loss of control: the irreversible development of drug addiction in the rat." *Behavioural Brain Research* 70: 77–94.

Wyvell CL, Berridge CW (2001) "Incentive sensitization by previous amphetamine exposure: increased cue-triggered "wanting" for sucrose reward." *Journal of Neuroscience* 21: 7831–7840.

Yin HH, Knowlton BJ (2006) "The role of the basal ganglia in habit formation." *Nature Reviews Neuroscience* 7:464–476.

Zhang X, Lee TH, Davidson C, Lazarus C, Wetsel WC, Ellinwood EH (2007) Reversal of cocaine-induced behavioral sensitization and associated phosphorylation of the NR2B and GluR1 subunits of the NMDA and AMPA receptors. *Neuropsychopharmacology* 32:377–387.

10

Neurochemical Approaches to Addiction Treatment

William R. Millington

Gökhan Göktalay

> Why does an addict get a new habit so much quicker than a junk virgin, even after the addict has been clean for years? I do not accept the theory that junk is lurking in the body all that time... and I disagree with all psychological answers. I think the use of junk causes permanent cellular alteration. Once a junky, always a junky.
> —William S. Burroughs, *Junky*, p. 117, 1977

William S. Burroughs was something of an expert on drug addiction; he was a heroin addict, a "junky" as he put it, for much of his adult life. An offbeat novelist and contemporary of Allen Ginsberg and Jack Kerouac, Burroughs created one of the most eloquent descriptions of opiate addiction we have. *Junky*. In it, he describes the defining components of addiction: the initial euphoria, or "kick," naive users experience, the decline of euphoria and onset of craving that marks the transition from drug use to drug addiction, the overwhelming compulsion to obtain and consume "junk," no matter what the consequences, the intense dysphoria of withdrawal, and the seeming inevitability of relapse. It is this progression of events that addiction research attempts to model, to understand and to treat and it is Burroughs' dictum, "Once a junky, always a junky" that addiction research strives to overturn.

It is easy to see why Burroughs arrived at this pessimistic conclusion. In the 1950s the prospect of treating addiction seemed remote. The only pharmacotherapy available was disulfiram, an aldehyde dehydrogenase inhibitor given to recovering alcoholics as a type of aversive therapy (Kiefer and Mann, 2005). The first real breakthrough came in the mid-1960s with the introduction of methadone as maintenance therapy for opiate addiction (Kreek, 2000). This was a dramatic step forward, not only because it was the first truly effective treatment for opiate dependence, but also because it created a new social paradigm, one that classified addiction as a medical problem rather than moral degeneracy. Maintenance therapy remains the primary treatment for opiate and nicotine dependence, although it is obviously not a cure (Kreek, 2000; Silagy et al., 2004).

One could argue that the current era of addiction therapy began with the introduction of naltrexone to treat alcohol recidivism in 1994 (O'Brien et al., 1996). The idea of using naltrexone was rationally based on evidence that ethanol reward is mediated by opioid neurons (Kiefer and Mann, 2005; O'Brien et al., 1996). It thus provided material proof that basic research on the neural mechanisms responsible for addiction could lead to new treatments. Subsequent FDA approval of acamprosate for the treatment of alcohol addiction reinforced this idea, even though acamprosate's mechanism of action was not completely understood (Scott et al., 2005). The past decade has produced a steady advance in our understanding of the neurobiology of addiction, and an impressive number of potential treatments have emerged, several of which are in clinical trials.

This chapter will review the neurochemistry of addiction and discuss several ways in which pharmacologists have "mined" the reward circuit to devise new treatments for addiction. This objective far exceeds the space allocated to a single chapter, if not an entire book, and so this review will inevitably be incomplete. To compensate, we will focus primarily on newly emerging strategies for addiction therapy and review briefly, if at all, treatments that are already in clinical use or have been reviewed so thoroughly elsewhere as to render any new discussion redundant. To further focus the topic, we will dwell primarily on neurochemical and behavioral data loosely related to drug reward, knowing full well this omits important aspects of addiction and addiction treatment. Fortunately, some topics introduced—or omitted—here will be reviewed in greater detail in subsequent chapters of this volume.

The Neurochemistry of Addiction

Any discussion of the anatomy of addiction must inevitably begin with dopamine. Dopamine neurons in the midbrain ventral tegmental area (VTA) that innervate the nucleus accumbens (NAc) and other corticolimbic areas have long been thought to mediate drug reward and reinforcement (Kalivas and Volkow, 2005). Indeed, virtually all drugs of abuse stimulate dopamine release in the NAc (Nestler, 2005). This, and other evidence, initially led to the concept that dopamine release was closely associated with reward, even pleasure, but we now know the role of dopamine is more subtle. Dopamine neurons are activated not only by pleasure, but also by stressful stimuli and dopamine release is better correlated with environmental cues associated with a reward than with experience of the reward itself (Wise, 2004). Current hypotheses consider dopaminergic activity to be more closely aligned with motivational processes: learning to associate rewarding experiences with environmental cues, for example, to predict reward, or to establish the motivational salience of events (Hyman and Malenka, 2001; Salamone et al., 2005; Wise, 2004).

It has also become increasingly apparent that dopamine neurons are but one component of the reward circuit (see Figure 10.1). The VTA is reciprocally interconnected with the NAc, prefrontal cortex, ventral pallidum, basolateral amygdala, and extended amygdala (Kalivas and Volkow, 2005; Koob, 2003; Nestler, 2005). Neurons in several of these pathways release glutamate as a neurotransmitter. Glutamate neurons in the prefrontal cortex innervate the VTA, where they synapse on dopamine neurons, and the NAc, where they synapse on the same medium spiny neurons that received dopaminergic input from the VTA, for example (Meredith et al., 1999). GABA is the third major neurotransmitter in the reward circuit (Kalivas and Volkow, 2005). GABA neurons, many of which colocalize enkephalin and other neuropeptides, form a dense projection from the NAc to the ventral pallidum, a major output pathway of the reward circuit. The VTA is also innervated by GABA neurons in the NAc, extended amygdala, and ventral pallidum, and GABA interneurons are located in both the VTA and NAc. Adrenergic, serotonergic, cholinergic, and opioid neurons also play an important role in the reward circuit.

Dopamine Neurons

Dopamine neurons play a pivotal role in the reward circuit, and so it would seem that addiction could be controlled rather easily with drugs that block dopamine receptors. Dopamine D_2 receptor antagonists are not particularly effective, however, and the dysphoria and extrapyramidal side effects they produce are problematic for long-term therapy (Grabowski et al., 2000; Heidbreder, 2005). D_1 receptor antagonists are currently under study for the treatment of nicotine and ethanol dependence, but reports that they fail to reduce cocaine craving in human volunteers has dampened enthusiasm for using them to treat psychostimulant abuse (Haney et al., 2001). Dopamine D_3 receptor antagonists are considerably more promising. D_3 receptors are located in the mesocorticolimbic system but not, to a significant extent, in extrapyramidal motor areas (Levant, 1997), which suggests that D_3 receptor blockers may interfere with drug reward without causing the adverse effects associated with D_2 antagonists (Heidbreder et al., 2005; Le Foll et al., 2005).

Figure 10.1. Schematic representation of components of the reward circuit. NAc = nucleus accumbens; VTA = ventral tegmental area; LDT = laterodorsal tegmental area; Arc = arcuate nucleus.

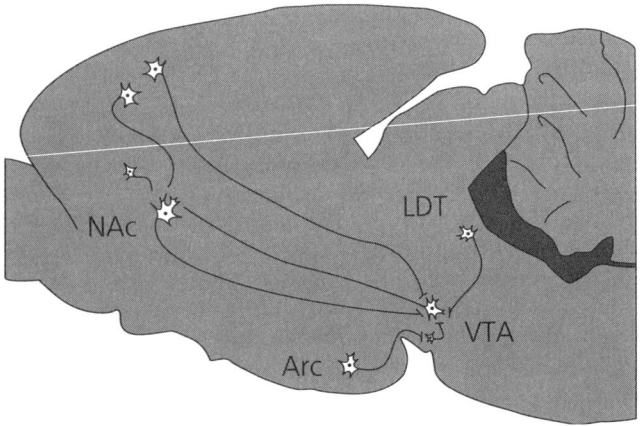

Behavioral experiments with newly developed D_3 receptor selective antagonists support this prediction. Vorel et al. (2002) reported, for example, that the D_3 receptor antagonist SB-277011A prevents acquisition and expression of a conditioned place preference for cocaine. Conditioned place preference is a Pavlovian procedure in which animals learn to associate the hedonic properties of a drug with a specific environment (O'Brien and Gardner, 2005; Tzschentke, 1998). Animals are conditioned with a drug for several days then allowed to choose between the environment in which they experienced the drug and the one in which they received saline. Vorel et al. (2002) showed that SB-277011A prevented acquisition of a place preference to cocaine when it was given to rats before each conditioning session. It also inhibited expression of a preestablished place preference when given to cocaine conditioned rats immediately before testing. Loosely interpreted, these data suggest that SB-277011A prevents drug-naive rats from experiencing the hedonic effects of cocaine and eliminates drug seeking, perhaps even craving, in cocaine conditioned animals. SB-277011A also inhibited acquisition and expression of a place preference to heroin, but not to palatable food, again suggesting that it interferes with a common neural substrate for drug reward but not natural rewards (Ashby et al., 2003; Vorel et al., 2002).

Conditioned place preference has good predictive value (most drugs abused by humans generate place preference in animals; Tzschentke, 1998), but it can be justly criticized for failing to adequately model drug abuse by humans who freely self-administer drugs. Several laboratories have tested whether D_3 receptor antagonists also inhibit intravenous self-administration of cocaine and other drugs, a procedure that more closely resembles human drug seeking. Unexpectedly, initial reports indicated that D_3 antagonists fail to affect cocaine or nicotine self-administration in standard fixed-ratio schedules of reinforcement (Andreoli et al., 2003; Di Ciano et al., 2003). Although these data seem to question whether D_3 antagonists truly inhibit drug reinforcement, subsequent studies showed that SB-277011A is effective when the cocaine dose is reduced, the reinforcement schedule is increased, or a progressive-ratio reinforcement schedule is used, all of which increase the work required for reinforcement (Heidbreder et al., 2005; Xi et al., 2006

The self-administration paradigm has also been widely used to study relapse, a major challenge for the pharmacotherapy of addiction. To study cocaine relapse, for example, animals are trained to self-administer cocaine, the behavior is extinguished by withholding the drug, and self-administration is then reinstated by "priming" animals with a single dose of cocaine. Stress and environmental cues previously associated with the drug also reinstate self-administration in laboratory animals, as they do in humans (Kalivas and McFarland, 2003). Pretreatment with a D_3 receptor antagonist prevents reinstatement of cocaine self-administration provoked by stress (Xi et al., 2004), environmental cues (Gilbert et al., 2005), or a priming dose of cocaine (Xi et al., 2005). Reinstatement of ethanol (Heidbreder et al., 2005) and nicotine (Andreoli et al., 2003) self-administration are also effectively prevented, which, again, indicates that the effectiveness of D_3 receptor antagonists is not restricted to cocaine.

Collectively, these data show that D_3 receptor antagonists interfere with drug-seeking behaviors and attenuate reinstatement in abstinent animals without affecting natural reinforcers, such as palatable food, and without causing an aversive response. It will be interesting to see whether these properties hold up in clinical trials. SB-277011A and other D_3 receptor blockers are currently under investigation for nicotine, alcohol, and psychostimulant dependence (Heidbreder and Hagan, 2005).

GABA Neurons

GABA is released by medium spiny neurons that innervate the ventral pallidum and VTA from the NAc and by interneurons in both the VTA and NAc (Kalivas and Volkow, 2005; see Figure 10.1). Drugs that activate GABA receptors indirectly by stimulating GABA release (gabapentin), inhibiting its metabolism (γ-vinyl GABA) or blocking GABA uptake (tiagabine) are widely used to treat seizure disorders and are already under investigation for alcohol, opiate, and psychostimulant dependence (Heidbreder, 2005). Their clinical availability seems to have circumvented the need for extensive preclinical research, but behavioral experiments with laboratory animals generally support the conclusion that indirect GABA agonists attenuate drug reward (Ashby et al., 2002; Kushner et al., 1999; Paul et al., 2001; Xi and Stein, 2002).

It is often assumed that indirect agonists produce their effects by activating $GABA_A$ receptors, but preclinical data do not support such a simple explanation. Direct $GABA_A$ receptor agonists certainly do inhibit reward-related behaviors (Corrigall et al., 2000; Samson and Chappell 2001; Zarrindast et al., 2004), but so do $GABA_A$ receptor antagonists (Koob, 2004; Nowak et al., 1998; Sahraei et al., 2005). Furthermore, $GABA_A$ receptor agonists and antagonists both stimulate dopamine release in the NAc and induce conditioned place preference when they are administered directly into the VTA (Laviolette and van der Kooy, 2001; Xi and Stein, 1998). This apparent paradox is probably explained by the fact that $GABA_A$ receptors are expressed by both dopamine and GABA neurons in the VTA (Kalivas, 1993). It could also be attributable to regional differences in the function of $GABA_A$ receptors within the VTA (Ikemoto et al., 1997a, 1998). In either case, $GABA_A$ receptor activation does not adequately explain the ability of indirect agonists to inhibit drug reward.

These disparities prompted some investigators to conclude that indirect agonists inhibit drug reward by activating $GABA_B$ receptors (Cousins et al., 2002), which are also expressed by dopamine neurons in the VTA (Wirtshafter and Sheppard, 2001). This idea is supported by a report that the $GABA_B$ receptor agonist baclofen prevents heroin-stimulated dopamine release (Xi and Stein, 1999). Baclofen injection into the VTA also inhibits heroin (Xi and Stein, 1999), nicotine (Corrigall et al., 2000), and cocaine (Brebner et al., 2000) self-administration and blocks acquisition of a place preference to morphine (Tsuji et al., 1996). Moreover, the inhibitory effect of γ-vinyl GABA, an indirect GABA receptor agonist, on heroin self-administration can be eliminated by blocking $GABA_B$, but not $GABA_A$, receptors in the VTA (Xi and Stein, 2000). Baclofen has been found to be effective in clinical trials for nicotine, alcohol, and cocaine dependence, but the sedation and motor impairment it causes are serious liabilities (Cousins et al., 2002). Recently developed allosteric modulators of the $GABA_B$ receptor may lack these adverse effects (Roberts, 2005).

Glutamate Neurons

Historically, the finding that the NMDA glutamate receptor antagonist dizocilpine (MK-801) inhibited morphine tolerance and dependence was an important landmark in the modern era of addiction research (Trujillo and Akil, 1991). The psychotomimetic side effects of dizocilpine and other high affinity NMDA receptor ion channel blockers ultimately made them unsuitable for clinical use. Low affinity channel blockers, like memantine and neramexane, and $glycine_B$ receptor antagonists have also proven effective in preclinical studies but do not produce these deleterious effects in humans (Bienkowski et al., 2001; Papp et al., 2002; Popik and Danysz, 1997; Tzschentke and Schmidt, 1995). NMDA receptor antagonists are already in clinical trials, and this extensive literature has been reviewed in detail elsewhere (Bisaga and Popik, 2000; Krystal et al., 2003; Trujillo, 2000; Tzschentke and Schmidt, 2000).

Metabotropic Glutamate Receptors

Recently, it has become apparent that metabotropic glutamate receptors (mGluR) also play an important role in the reward circuitry. There are three major groups of mGluRs: Group I mGluRs (mGluR1 and mGluR5) are primarily postsynaptic receptors, whereas groups II (mGluR2 and mGluR3) and III mGluRs (mGluR4 and mGluR6–8) are predominantly, although not exclusively, presynaptic (Kenny and Markou, 2004). Group II mGluR agonists inhibit glutamate release in the NAc (Xi et al., 2002) and reduce extracellular dopamine concentrations as well (Greenslade and Mitchell, 2004; Hu et al., 1999). Group I mGluRs, on the other hand, are found on medium spiny output neurons in the NAc (Lu et al., 1999; Tallaksen-Greene et al., 1998) and do not influence dopamine release (Hu et al., 1999). Nevertheless, in theory, one might be able to diminish the output of the reward circuit with drugs that either block group I or activate group II mGluRs.

This prediction is certainly true for the group I receptor, mGluR5 (Kenny and Markou, 2004). Mice deficient in the mGlu5R gene do not readily self-administer cocaine (Chiamulera et al., 2001), and mGluR5 antagonists inhibit cocaine (Paterson and Markou, 2005; Tessari et al., 2004), nicotine (Paterson et al., 2003; Tessari et al., 2004), and alcohol (Cowen et al., 2005; Schroeder et al., 2005) self-administration and suppress morphine-induced conditioned place preference responding (Aoki et al., 2004; Popik and Wrobel, 2002). Although contradictory data have been reported (McGeehan and Olive, 2003), overall, these findings support the conclusion that blockade or deletion of the mGluR5 inhibits drug reward.

Group II receptor agonists are not particularly potent at blocking self-administration, per se (Baptista et al., 2004), but their ability to inhibit glutamate release apparently makes them quite effective in animal models of drug reinstatement (Cornish and Kalivas, 2000; McFarland et al., 2003). Systemic administration of LY379268, an mGluR2/3 agonist, prevents reinstatement of cocaine self-administration (Baptista et al., 2004), and both systemic and intra-VTA LY379268 administration inhibits reinstatement of heroin seeking (Bossert et al., 2004). Together, these findings confirm that mGluRs play an important role in the reward circuit. Moreover, they show that mGluR5 antagonists inhibit multiple components of reward and suggest that mGluR2/3 agonists may be useful for preventing cocaine and opiate relapse.

Other Glutamate-Related Strategies

The mGluR3 is also activated by a peptide, N-acetylaspartylglutamate (NAAG). Actually, NAAG has several mechanisms of action: it inhibits synaptic transmission by inhibiting glutamate release (by activating presynaptic mGluR3s) and by blocking NMDA receptors. At the same time, NAAG is rapidly metabolized to glutamate and so facilitates synaptic transmission by elevating synaptic glutamate concentrations (Neale et al., 2005; Thomas et al., 2000). Consequently, drugs that inhibit the NAAG metabolizing enzyme glutamate carboxypeptidase II (GCPII) interfere with synaptic transmission by simultaneously increasing NAAG and lowering glutamate concentrations (Neale et al., 2005). In theory, GCPII inhibitors should interfere with drug reward. In fact, Slusher et al.

(2001) found that systemic administration of the GCPII inhibitor 2-(phosphonomethyl)-pentanedioic acid (2-PMPA) prevents acquisition and expression of a conditioned place preference to cocaine, 2-PMPA had no effect on place preference responding for a food reward and it did not cause place preference or aversion by itself (Slusher et al., 2001). Popik et al. (2002) later reported similar effects of 2-PMPA on morphine place preference. These intriguing initial findings with GCPII inhibitors certainly warrant further study.

A second strategy for inhibiting glutamate transmission is to use drugs like riluzole or lamotrigine to prevent glutamate release (Bisaga and Popik, 2000). Riluzole is currently used to treat amyotrophic lateral sclerosis and, in theory, it should inhibit reward-related behaviors. Indeed, Tzschentke and Schmidt (1998) reported that riluzole blocks morphine- and amphetamine-induced conditioned place preference completely, and a later study showed that it inhibits morphine tolerance and dependence (Sepulveda et al., 1999). However, preliminary clinical trials revealed that riluzole is not particularly effective at reducing cocaine craving(Ciraulo et al., 2005). Although further study may be in order, these initial data should remind us that it is often difficult to predict clinical efficacy from preclinical evidence.

Cholinergic Neurons

Naturally, nicotinic receptors have been the subject of intense interest due to the addictive power of nicotine. Dopamine neurons in the VTA express a number of different nicotinic receptor subtypes (Wonnacott et al., 2005). GABA neurons in the VTA are more homogenous, and primarily express $\alpha_4\beta_2$ nicotinic receptors. Partial agonists at the $\alpha_4\beta_2$ receptor are currently under evaluation for the treatment of nicotine dependence (Heidbreder, 2005). The $\alpha_3\beta_4$ nicotinic receptor antagonist 18-methoxycoronaridine also blocks the rewarding effects of nicotine and other drugs of abuse, as will be discussed in a later chapter. This extensive literature has been reviewed thoroughly elsewhere (Laviolette and van der Kooy, 2004; Watkins et al., 2000; Wonnacott et al., 2005).

There is growing interest in the role of muscarinic receptors in the reward circuit. Electrical stimulation of the laterodorsal tegmental nucleus (LDT), which provides the main cholinergic innervation of the VTA (Oakman et al., 1995; see Figure 10.1), causes a delayed increase in dopamine release that can be blocked by infusing a muscarinic receptor antagonist into the VTA (Forster and Blaha, 2000). Interestingly, the M_5 muscarinic receptor apparently mediates this response. Although generally present in rather low amounts in brain, the M_5 receptor is the only muscarinic receptor expressed by dopamine neurons (Weiner et al., 1990). Forster et al. (2002) confirmed this by showing that LDT stimulation does not produce a delayed increase in NAc dopamine release in M_5 receptor knockout mice. Morphine-induced dopamine release and place preference responding are also attenuated in M_5 deficient mice (Basile et al., 2002), as is cocaine self-administration (Thomsen et al., 2005), again stressing the importance of M_5 receptors and emphasizing the essential nature of the LDT-VTA pathway in drug reward.

Pharmacological studies tend to support this conclusion. Microinjection of a muscarinic receptor agonist into the VTA induces a conditioned place preference (Yeomans et al., 1985) and, conversely, rats will self-administer the nonselective cholinergic agonist carbachol directly into the VTA (Ikemoto and Wise, 2002). Unfortunately, definitive pharmacological studies await development of selective M_5 receptor antagonists.

Cannabinoids

Endogenous cannabinoids are different from other neurotransmitters: anandamide and 2-arachidonylglycerol are lipids, arachidonic acid derivatives to be specific, and they often act in a retrograde direction—that is, released from postsynaptic neurons, they inhibit transmitter release presynaptically (Mechoulam et al., 1998; Wilson and Nicoll, 2002). Systemic administration of cannabinoids excites dopamine neurons in the VTA and stimulates dopamine release in the NAc (Chen et al., 1990; French, 1997). The mechanism responsible for this is unclear, in part because dopamine neurons do not express cannabinoid-1 (CB_1) receptors (Herkenham et al., 1990; Mailleux and Vanderhaeghen, 1992). One plausible explanation is that cannabinoids activate CB_1 receptors on GABA nerve terminals in the VTA and excite dopamine neurons by inhibiting GABA release (Melis et al., 2004a; Riegel and Lupica, 2004). This simple explanation is complicated by evidence that CB_1 receptors are also located on glutamate nerve terminals in the VTA (Melis et al., 2004b; Riegel and Lupica, 2004) and on both GABA and glutamate terminals in the NAc (Hoffman and Lupica, 2001; Lupica et al., 2004; Szabo et al., 1999).

Despite mechanistic ambiguity, there is compelling evidence that CB_1 receptor antagonists inhibit drug reward (De Vries and Schoffelmeer, 2005; Gardiner, 2005; Le Foll and Goldberg, 2005; Lupica and Riegel, 2005). Rimonabant (SR141716A), a CB_1 receptor antagonist, inhibits acquisition of morphine place preference (Chaperon et al., 1998), for example, and blocks heroin self-administration in fixed and progressive ratio schedules of reinforcement (De Vries et al., 2003). Mice deficient in the CB_1 receptor also fail to acquire a place preference to morphine (Martin et al., 2000) and do not self-administer opiates (Cossu et al., 2001). The effects of rimonabant extend to other drugs of abuse, as well, including ethanol (Gessa et al., 2005; Manzanares et al., 2005; Poncelet et al., 2003) and nicotine (Cohen et al., 2002, 2005; Forget et al., 2005; Le Foll and Goldberg, 2004). The involvement of CB_1 receptors in psychostimulant reward is more controversial. Cocaine reward behaviors are not inhibited by rimonabant or by deletion of the CB_1 receptor gene (Cossu et al., 2001; De Vries et al., 2001; Lesscher et al., 2005; Martin et al., 2000). Contradictory data have been published (Soria et al., 2005), however, and De Vries et al. (2001) reported that rimonabant does prevent reinstatement of cocaine self-administration. Nevertheless, there is considerable interest in rimonabant's therapeutic potential, and clinical trials with rimonabant and other CB_1 antagonists are currently underway for nicotine and alcohol dependence (Heidbreder and Hagan, 2005).

Opioid and "Antiopioid" Neurons

Morphine and other opiates exert their addictive properties primarily by activating mu-opioid receptors expressed by GABA neurons in the VTA. By inhibiting GABA release, opioids disinhibit dopamine neurons and stimulate dopamine release (Herz, 1998). Opioids are also thought to act in the NAc, albeit through a mechanism that does not involve dopamine neurons (Xi and Stein, 2002). It is not entirely clear which endogenous opioid peptides normally activate opioid receptors in the VTA and NAc. Medium spiny neurons that project from the NAc to the ventral pallidum release enkephalin from axon collaterals in the NAc (Meredith, 1999; Zhou et al., 2003), and proopiomelanocortin (POMC) neurons innervate both the VTA and NAc from the arcuate nucleus

(Khachaturian et al., 1985). Clinically, opioid receptor antagonists are used to treat alcohol and opiate dependence, and new opioid antagonists and antagonist dosage forms continue to be developed (Heidbreder, 2005). Nevertheless, there may be other ways to exploit opioid systems to inhibit drug reward.

POMC Derived Peptides

Opioid neurons are multitransmitter neurons, particularly POMC neurons, which synthesize β-endorphin, α-melanocyte-stimulating-hormone (α-MSH), γ_1-MSH and a variety of other peptides (Cone, 2005; Khachaturian et al., 1985). Like opioids, α-MSH and γ_1-MSH stimulate dopamine release in the NAc when microinjected into the VTA (Jansone et al., 2004; Lindblom et al., 2001). Interestingly, the effect of γ_1-MSH can be blocked with γ_2-MSH, which differs from γ_1-MSH by only a single amino acid (Jansone et al., 2004). These responses are probably mediated by melanocortin-3 (MC3) and/or MC4 receptors, both of which are found in the VTA and NAc (Alvaro et al., 1997). Logically, MC3/MC4 receptor antagonists should interfere with drug reward but, surprisingly, this possibility was not investigated until quite recently. Hsu et al. (2005) reported that bilateral injection of the MC3/MC4 receptor antagonist SHU-9119 into the NAc inhibited cocaine-induced self-administration, conditioned place preference, and locomotor sensitization. Cocaine sensitization was completely abolished in MC4 receptor knockout mice, implicating the MC4 receptor in the response to SHU-9119 (Hsu et al., 2005). Certainly, more work with MC4 receptor antagonists is warranted.

It is interesting that β-endorphin and α-MSH both stimulate dopamine release because it is far more common to find the two peptides producing antagonistic responses (Cone, 2005; O'Donohue and Dorsa, 1982). Perhaps this explains why some POMC neurons convert β-endorphin to a series of nonopioid derivatives before it is released (Loh, 1992). One of these peptides, β-endorphin$_{1-27}$, displays opioid receptor antagonist properties and reportedly prevents acquisition of a conditioned place preference to β-endorphin and other opioids (Bals-Kubik et al., 1988). The conversion of β-endorphin$_{1-31}$ to β-endorphin$_{1-27}$ also generates a dipeptide, β-endorphin$_{30-31}$. β-Endorphin$_{30-31}$ inhibits the rewarding effects of morphine, nicotine, and ethanol and attenuates morphine and nicotine withdrawal in dependent animals (Cavun et al., 2005; Göktalay et al., 2006; Resch et al., 2005). Unlike β-endorphin$_{1-27}$, however, it does not block opioid receptors or inhibit morphine analgesia (Owen et al., 2000). Thus, paradoxically, β-endorphin may provide yet another source of novel treatments for drug addiction.

Nociceptin

Other "antiopioid" peptides modulate the rewarding effects of opioids (Mollereau et al., 2005), the most notable of which is nociceptin/orphanin FQ (NOP). NOP is a 17-amino acid peptide that activates a previously cloned opioid receptorlike (ORL1) receptor (Mogil and Pasternak, 2001). Despite its structural homology to opioids, NOP lacks opioid activity (Mogil and Pasternak, 2001). NOP is released by GABA neurons in the VTA (Norton et al., 2002), and ORL1 receptors are expressed by most VTA dopamine neurons (Maidment et al., 2002; Norton et al., 2002). Accordingly, NOP lowers extracellular dopamine concentrations in the NAc when it is injected into the VTA (Murphy et al., 1999) and inhibits the rewarding effects of morphine (Ciccocioppo et al., 2000; Murphy et al., 1999), psychostimulants (Kotlinska et al., 2003; Sakoori and Murphy, 2004) and ethanol (Ciccocioppo et al., 2003; Kuzmin et al., 2003) following central administration. These data might be considered esoteric, however, because peptides as large as NOP are not useable clinically. But recent development of nonpeptide ORL1 agonists, such as R064–61989, may change this pessimistic outlook. R064–61989 inhibits morphine conditioned place preference, as does NOP itself, and inhibits reinstatement of a place preference to morphine (Shoblock et al., 2005) and ethanol (Kuzmin et al., 2003). These findings raise the possibility that ORL1 agonists may ultimately be useful for suppressing craving and lessening the relapse potential of opiates and other drugs of abuse.

Conclusions

Perhaps the most remarkable observation one can make from the preclinical data reviewed here is just how easy it is to interfere with drug reward pharmacologically. A wide variety of neurochemical manipulations inhibit reward-related behaviors, ranging from drugs that block D_3 dopamine and GABA$_B$ receptors, which are critical components of the reward circuit, to peptides like NOP and nonopioid β-endorphin derivatives, which seem more peripheral anatomically but are equally effective. A great deal of progress has been made toward understanding both the neurobiology and neuropharmacology of addiction in a relatively short amount of time. Nevertheless, it remains to be seen which, if any, of the many prospective treatments emerging from preclinical research will prove to be effective therapeutically.

References

Alvaro JD, Tatro JB, Duman RS. Melanocortins and opiate addiction. *Life Sci.* 61:1–9, 1997.

Andreoli M, Tessari M, Pilla M, Valerio E, Hagan JJ, Heidbreder CA. Selective antagonism at dopamine D$_3$ receptors prevents nicotine-triggered relapse to nicotine-seeking behavior. *Neuropsychopharmacology.* 28:1272–1280, 2003.

Aoki T, Narita M, Shibasaki M, Suzuki T. Metabotropic glutamate receptor 5 localized in the limbic forebrain is critical for the development of morphine-induced rewarding effect in mice. *Eur J Neurosci.* 20:1633–1638, 2004.

Ashby CR, Paul M, Gardner EL, Gerasimov MR, Dewey SL, Lennon IC, Taylor SJ. Systemic administration of 1R,4S-4-amino-cyclopent-2-ene-carboxylic acid, a reversible inhibitor of GABA transaminase, blocks expression of conditioned place preference to cocaine and nicotine. *Synapse.* 44:61–63, 2002.

Ashby CR, Paul M, Gardner EL, Heidbreder CA, Hagan JJ. Acute administration of the selective D$_3$ receptor antagonist SB-277011A blocks the acquisition and expression of the conditioned place preference response to heroin in male rats. *Synapse.* 48:154–156, 2003.

Bals-Kubik R, Herz A, Shippenberg TS. β-endorphin-(1–27) is a naturally occurring antagonist of the reinforcing effects of opioids. *N-S Arch Pharmacol.* 338:392–396, 1988.

Baptista MA, Martin-Fardon R, Weiss F. Preferential effects of the metabotropic glutamate 2/3 receptor agonist LY379268 on conditioned reinstatement versus primary reinforcement: comparison between cocaine and a potent conventional reinforcer. *J Neurosci.* 24:4723–4727, 2004.

Basile AS, Fedorova I, Zapata A, Liu X, Shippenberg T, Duttaroy A, Yamada M, Wess J. Deletion of the M$_5$ muscarinic acetylcholine receptor attenuates morphine reinforcement and withdrawal but not morphine analgesia. *Proc Natl Acad Sci USA.* 99:11452–11457, 2002.

Bienkowski P, Krzascik P, Koros E, Kostowski W, Scinska A, Danysz W. Effects of a novel uncompetitive NMDA receptor antagonist, MRZ 2/579 on ethanol self-administration and ethanol withdrawal seizures in the rat. *Eur J Pharmacol.* 413:81–89, 2001.

Bisaga A, Popik P. In search of a new pharmacological treatment for drug and alcohol addiction: N-methyl-D-aspartate (NMDA) antagonists. *Drug Alcohol Depend.* 59:1–15, 2000.

Bossert JM, Liu SY, Lu L, Shaham Y. A role of ventral tegmental area glutamate in contextual cue-induced relapse to heroin seeking. *J Neurosci.* 24:10726–10730, 2004.

Brebner K, Phelan R, Roberts DCS. Intra-VTA baclofen attenuates cocaine self-administration on a progressive ratio schedule of reinforcement. *Pharmacol Biochem Behav.* 66:857–862, 2000.

Burroughs WS. *Junky.* New York: Penguin Books, 1977.

Cavun S, Göktalay G, Millington WR. Glycyl-glutamine, an endogenous β-endorphin-derived peptide, inhibits morphine conditioned place preference, tolerance, dependence and withdrawal. *J Pharmacol Exp Ther.* 315:949–958, 2005.

Chaperon F, Soubrie P, Puech AJ, Thiebot MH. Involvement of central cannabinoid (CB_1) receptors in the establishment of place conditioning in rats. *Psychopharmacology.* 135:324–332, 1998.

Chen JP, Paredes W, Li J, Smith D, Lowinson J, Gardner EL. Delta 9-tetrahydrocannabinol produces naloxone-blockable enhancement of presynaptic basal dopamine efflux in nucleus accumbens of conscious, freely-moving rats as measured by intracerebral microdialysis. *Psychopharmacology.* 102:156–162, 1990.

Chiamulera C, Epping-Jordan MP, Zocchi A, Marcon C, Cottiny C, Tacconi S, Corsi M, Orzi F, Conquet F. Reinforcing and locomotor stimulant effects of cocaine are absent in $mGluR_5$ null mutant mice. *Nat Neurosci.* 4:873–874, 2001.

Ciccocioppo R, Angeletti S, Sali PP, Weiss F, Massi M. Effect of nociceptin/orphanin FQ on the rewarding properties of morphine. *Eur J Pharmacol.* 404:153–159, 2000.

Ciccocioppo R, Economidou D, Fedeli A, Massi M. The nociceptin/orphanin FQ/NOP receptor system as a target for treatment of alcohol abuse: a review of recent work in alcohol-preferring rats. *Physiol Behav.* 79:121–128, 2003.

Ciraulo DA, Sarid-Segal O, Knapp CM, Ciraulo AM, LoCastro J, Bloch DA, Montgomery MA, Leiderman DB, Elkashef A. Efficacy screening trials of paroxetine, pentoxifylline, riluzole, pramipexole and venlafaxine in cocaine dependence. *Addiction.* 100(suppl) 1:12–22, 2005.

Cohen C, Kodas E, Griebel G. CB_1 receptor antagonists for the treatment of nicotine addiction. *Pharmacol Biochem Behav.* 81:387–395, 2005.

Cohen C, Perrault G, Voltz C, Steinberg R, Soubrie P. SR141716, a central cannabinoid (CB_1) receptor antagonist, blocks the motivational and dopamine-releasing effects of nicotine in rats. *Behav Pharmacol.* 13:451–463, 2002.

Cone RD. Anatomy and regulation of the central melanocortin system. *Nat Neurosci.* 8:571–578, 2005.

Cornish JL, Kalivas PW. Glutamate transmission in the nucleus accumbens mediates relapse in cocaine addiction. *J Neurosci.* 20:RC89, 2000.

Corrigall WA, Coen KM, Adamson KL, Chow BL, Zhang J. Response of nicotine self-administration in the rat to manipulations of mu-opioid and γ-aminobutyric acid receptors in the ventral tegmental area. *Psychopharmacology.* 149:107–114, 2000.

Cossu G, Ledent C, Fattore L, Imperato A, Bohme GA, Parmentier M, Fratta W. Cannabinoid CB1 receptor knockout mice fail to self-administer morphine but not other drugs of abuse. *Behav Brain Res.* 118:61–65, 2001.

Cousins MS, Roberts DC, de Wit H. $GABA_B$ receptor agonists for the treatment of drug addiction: a review of recent findings. *Drug Alcohol Depend.* 65:209–220, 2002.

Cowen MS, Djouma E, Lawrence AJ. The metabotropic glutamate 5 receptor antagonist 3-((2-methyl-1,3-thiazol-4-yl)ethynyl)-pyridine reduces ethanol self-administration in multiple strains of alcohol-preferring rats and regulates olfactory glutamatergic systems. *J Pharmacol Exp Ther* 315:590–600, 2005.

De Vries TJ, Homberg JR, Binnekade R, Raaso H, Schoffelmeer AN. Cannabinoid modulation of the reinforcing and motivational properties of heroin and heroin-associated cues in rats. *Psychopharmacology.* 168:164–169, 2003.

De Vries TJ, Schoffelmeer AN. Cannabinoid CB_1 receptors control conditioned drug seeking. *Trends Pharmacol Sci.* 26:420–426, 2005.

De Vries TJ, Shaham Y, Homberg JR, Crombag H, Schuurman K, Dieben J, Vanderschuren LJ, Schoffelmeer AN. A cannabinoid mechanism in relapse to cocaine seeking. *Nat Med.* 7:1151–1154, 2001.

Di Ciano P, Underwood RJ, Hagan JJ, Everitt BJ. Attenuation of cue-controlled cocaine-seeking by a selective D_3 dopamine receptor antagonist SB-277011-A. *Neuropsychopharmacology.* 28:329–338, 2003.

Forget B, Hamon M, Thiebot MH. Cannabinoid CB_1 receptors are involved in motivational effects of nicotine in rats. *Psychopharmacology.* 181:722–734, 2005.

Forster GL, Blaha CD. Laterodorsal tegmental stimulation elicits dopamine efflux in the rat nucleus accumbens by activation of acetylcholine and glutamate receptors in the ventral tegmental area. *Eur J Neurosci.* 12:3596–3604, 2000.

Forster GL, Yeomans JS, Takeuchi J, Blaha CD. M5 muscarinic receptors are required for prolonged accumbal dopamine release after electrical stimulation of the pons in mice. *J Neurosci.* 22:RC190, 2002.

French ED. Δ^9-tetrahydrocannabinol excites rat VTA dopamine neurons through activation of cannabinoid CB1 but not opioid receptors. *Neurosci Lett.* 226:159–162, 1997.

Gardner EL. Endocannabinoid signaling system and brain reward: emphasis on dopamine. *Pharmacol Biochem Behav.* 81:263–284, 2005.

Gessa GL, Serra S, Vacca G, Carai MA, Colombo G. Suppressing effect of the cannabinoid CB_1 receptor antagonist, SR147778, on alcohol intake and motivational properties of alcohol in alcohol-preferring sP rats. *Alcohol Alcohol.* 40:46–53, 2005.

Gilbert JG, Newman AH, Gardner EL, Ashby CR Jr, Heidbreder CA, Pak AC, Peng XQ, Xi ZX. Acute administration of SB-277011A, NGB 2904, or BP 897 inhibits cocaine cue-induced reinstatement of drug-seeking behavior in rats: role of dopamine D_3 receptors. *Synapse.* 57:17–28, 2005.

Göktalay G, Cavun S, Levendusky MC, Hamilton JR, Millington WR. Glycyl-glutamine inhibits nicotine conditioned place preference and withdrawal. *Eur J Pharmacol* 530:95–102, 2006. Grabowski J, Rhoades H, Silverman P, Schmitz JM, Stotts A, Creson D, Bailey R. Risperidone for the treatment of cocaine dependence: randomized, double-blind trial. *J Clin Psychopharmacol.* 20:305–310, 2000.

Greenslade RG, Mitchell SN. Selective action of (-)-2-oxa-4-aminobicyclo (3.1.0)hexane-4,6-dicarboxylate (LY379268), a group II metabotropic glutamate receptor agonist, on basal and phencyclidine-induced dopamine release in the nucleus accumbens shell. *Neuropharmacology.* 47:1–8, 2004.

Haney M, Ward AS, Foltin RW, Fischman MW. Effects of ecopipam, a selective dopamine D1 antagonist, on smoked cocaine self-administration by humans. *Psychopharmacology.* 155:330–337, 2001.

Heidbreder C. Novel pharmacotherapeutic targets for the management of drug addiction. *Eur J Pharmacol.* 526:101–112, 2005.

Heidbreder CA, Gardner EL, Xi ZX, Thanos PK, Mugnaini M, Hagan JJ, Ashby CR. The role of central dopamine D_3 receptors in drug addiction: a review of pharmacological evidence. *Brain Res Brain Res Rev.* 49:77–105, 2005.

Heidbreder CA, Hagan JJ. Novel pharmacotherapeutic approaches for the treatment of drug addiction and craving. *Curr Opin Pharmacol.* 5:107–118, 2005.

Herkenham M, Lynn AB, Little MD, Johnson MR, Melvin LS, de Costa BR, Rice KC. Cannabinoid receptor localization in brain. *Proc Natl Acad Sci USA.* 87:1932–1936, 1990.

Herz A. Opioid reward mechanisms: a key role in drug abuse? *Can J Physiol Pharmacol.* 76:252–258, 1998.

Hoffman AF, Lupica CR. Direct actions of cannabinoids on synaptic transmission in the nucleus accumbens: a comparison with opioids. *J Neurophysiol.* 85:72–83, 2001.

Hsu R, Taylor JR, Newton SS, Alvaro JD, Haile C, Han G, Hruby VJ, Nestler EJ, Duman RS. Blockade of melanocortin transmission inhibits cocaine reward. *Eur J Neurosci.* 21:2233–2242, 2005.

Hu G, Duffy P, Swanson C, Ghasemzadeh MB, Kalivas PW. The regulation of dopamine transmission by metabotropic glutamate receptors. *J Pharmacol Exp Ther.* 289:412–416, 1999.

Hyman SE, Malenka RC. Addiction and the brain: the neurobiology of compulsion and its persistence. *Nat Rev Neurosci.* 2:695–703, 2001.

Ikemoto S, Kohl RR, McBride WJ. GABA$_A$ receptor blockade in the anterior ventral tegmental area increases extracellular levels of dopamine in the nucleus accumbens of rats. *J Neurochem.* 69:137–143, 1997a.

Ikemoto S, Murphy JM, McBride WJ. Self-infusion of GABA$_A$ antagonists directly into the ventral tegmental area and adjacent regions. *Behav Neurosci.* 111:369–380, 1997b.

Ikemoto S, Murphy JM, McBride WJ. Regional differences within the rat ventral tegmental area for muscimol self-infusions. *Pharmacol Biochem Behav.* 61:87–92, 1998.

Ikemoto S, Wise RA. Rewarding effects of carbachol and neostigmine in the posterior ventral tegmental area. *J Neurosci.* 22:9894–9904, 2002.

Jansone B, Bergstrom L, Svirskis S, Lindblom J, Klusa V, Wikberg JE. Opposite effects of γ_1- and γ_2-melanocyte stimulating hormone on regulation of the dopaminergic mesolimbic system in rats. *Neurosci Lett.* 361:68–71, 2004.

Kalivas PW. Neurotransmitter regulation of dopamine neurons in the ventral tegmental area. *Brain Res Rev.* 18:75–113, 1993.

Kalivas PW, McFarland K. Brain circuitry and the reinstatement of cocaine-seeking behavior. *Psychopharmacology.* 168:44–56, 2003.

Kalivas PW, Volkow ND. The neural basis of addiction: a pathology of motivation and choice. *Am J Psychiatry.* 162:1403–1413, 2005.

Kenny PJ, Markou A. The ups and downs of addiction: role of metabotropic glutamate receptors. *Trends Pharmacol Sci.* 25:265–272, 2004.

Khachaturian H, Lewis ME, Schafer, MKH, Watson SJ. Anatomy of CNS opioid systems. *Trends Neurosci.* 8:111–119, 1985.

Kiefer F, Mann K. New achievements and pharmacotherapeutic approaches in the treatment of alcohol dependence. *Eur J Pharmacol.* 526:163–171, 2005.

Koob GF. Neuroadaptive mechanisms of addiction: studies on the extended amygdala. *Eur Neuropsychopharmacol.* 13:442–452, 2003.

Koob GF. A role for GABA mechanisms in the motivational effects of alcohol. *Biochem Pharmacol.* 68:1515–1525, 2004.

Kotlinska J, Rafalski P, Biala G, Dylag T, Rolka K, Silberring J. Nociceptin inhibits acquisition of amphetamine-induced place preference and sensitization to stereotypy in rats. *Eur J Pharmacol.* 474:233–239, 2003.

Kreek MJ. Methadone-related opioid agonist pharmacotherapy for heroin addiction. History, recent molecular and neurochemical research and future in mainstream medicine. *Ann N Y Acad Sci.* 909:186–216, 2000.

Krystal JH, Petrakis IL, Mason G, Trevisan L, D'Souza DC. N-methyl-D-aspartate glutamate receptors and alcoholism: reward, dependence, treatment, and vulnerability. *Pharmacol Ther.* 99:79–94, 2003.

Kushner SA, Dewey SL, Kornetsky C. The irreversible γ-aminobutyric acid (GABA) transaminase inhibitor γ-vinyl-GABA blocks cocaine self-administration in rats. *J Pharmacol Exp Ther.* 290:797–802, 1999.

Kuzmin A, Sandin J, Terenius L, Ogren SO. Acquisition, expression, and reinstatement of ethanol-induced conditioned place preference in mice: effects of opioid receptor-like 1 receptor agonists and naloxone. *J Pharmacol Exp Ther.* 304:310–318, 2003.

Laviolette SR, van der Kooy D. GABA$_A$ receptors in the ventral tegmental area control bi-directional reward signaling between dopaminergic and non-dopaminergic neural motivational systems. *Eur J Neurosci.* 13:1009–1015, 2001.

Laviolette SR, van der Kooy D. The neurobiology of nicotine addiction: bridging the gap from molecules to behaviour. *Nat Rev Neurosci.* 5:55–65, 2004.

Le Foll B, Goldberg SR. Rimonabant, a CB$_1$ antagonist, blocks nicotine-conditioned place preferences. *Neuroreport.* 15:2139–2143, 2004.

Le Foll B, Goldberg SR. Cannabinoid CB$_1$ receptor antagonists as promising new medications for drug dependence. *J Pharmacol Exp Ther.* 312:875–883, 2005.

Le Foll B, Goldberg SR, Sokoloff P. The dopamine D$_3$ receptor and drug dependence: effects on reward or beyond? *Neuropharmacology.* 49:525–541, 2005.

Lesscher HM, Hoogveld E, Burbach JP, van Ree JM, Gerrits MA. Endogenous cannabinoids are not involved in cocaine reinforcement and development of cocaine-induced behavioural sensitization. *Eur Neuropsychopharmacol.* 15:31–37, 2005.

Levant B. The D$_3$ dopamine receptor: neurobiology and potential clinical relevance. *Pharmacol Rev.* 49:231–252, 1997.

Lindblom J, Opmane B, Mutulis F, Mutule I, Petrovska R, Klusa V, Bergstrom L, Wikberg JE. The MC4 receptor mediates alpha-MSH induced release of nucleus accumbens dopamine. *Neuroreport.* 12:2155–2158, 2001.

Loh YP. Molecular mechanisms of ß-endorphin biosynthesis. *Biochem Pharmacol.* 44:843–849, 1992.

Lu XY, Ghasemzadeh MB, Kalivas PW. Expression of glutamate receptor subunit/subtype messenger RNAS for NMDAR1, GLuR1, GLuR2 and mGLuR5 by accumbal projection neurons. *Brain Res Mol Brain Res.* 63:287–296, 1999.

Lupica CR, Riegel AC. Endocannabinoid release from midbrain dopamine neurons: a potential substrate for cannabinoid receptor antagonist treatment of addiction. *Neuropharmacology.* 48:1105–1116, 2005.

Lupica CR, Riegel AC, Hoffman AF. Marijuana and cannabinoid regulation of brain reward circuits. *Br J Pharmacol.* 143:227–234, 2004.

Maidment NT, Chen Y, Tan AM, Murphy NP, Leslie FM. Rat ventral midbrain dopamine neurons express the orphanin FQ/nociceptin receptor ORL-1. *Neuroreport.* 13:1137–1140, 2002.

Mailleux P, Vanderhaeghen JJ. Distribution of neuronal cannabinoid receptor in the adult rat brain: a comparative receptor binding radioautography and in situ hybridization histochemistry. *Neuroscience.* 48:655–668, 1992.

Manzanares J, Ortiz S, Oliva JM, Perez-Rial S, Palomo T. Interactions between cannabinoid and opioid receptor systems in the mediation of ethanol effects. *Alcohol Alcohol.* 40:25–34, 2005.

Martin M, Ledent C, Parmentier M, Maldonado R, Valverde O. Cocaine, but not morphine, induces conditioned place preference and sensitization to locomotor responses in CB1 knockout mice. *Eur J Neurosci.* 12:4038–4046, 2000.

McFarland K, Lapish CC, Kalivas PW. Prefrontal glutamate release into the core of the nucleus accumbens mediates cocaine-induced reinstatement of drug-seeking behavior. *J Neurosci.* 23:3531–3537, 2003.

McGeehan AJ, Olive MF. The mGluR5 antagonist MPEP reduces the conditioned rewarding effects of cocaine but not other drugs of abuse. *Synapse.* 47:240–242, 2003.

Mechoulam R, Fride E, Di Marzo V. Endocannabinoids. *Eur J Pharmacol.* 359:1–18, 1998.

Melis M, Perra S, Muntoni AL, Pillolla G, Lutz B, Marsicano G, Di Marzo V, Gessa GL, Pistis M. Prefrontal cortex stimulation induces 2-arachidonoyl-glycerol-mediated suppression of excitation in dopamine neurons. *J Neurosci.* 24:10707–10715, 2004a.

Melis M, Pistis M, Perra S, Muntoni AL, Pillolla G, Gessa GL. Endocannabinoids mediate presynaptic inhibition of glutamatergic transmission in rat ventral tegmental area dopamine neurons through activation of CB1 receptors. *J Neurosci.* 24:53–62, 2004b.

Meredith GE. The synaptic framework for chemical signaling in nucleus accumbens. *Ann N Y Acad Sci.* 877:140–156, 1999.

Mogil JS, Pasternak GW. The molecular and behavioral pharmacology of the orphanin FQ/nociceptin peptide and receptor family. *Pharmacol Rev.* 53:381–415, 2001.

Mollereau C, Roumy M, Zajac JM. Opioid-modulating peptides: mechanisms of action. *Curr Top Med Chem.* 5:341–355, 2005.

Murphy NP, Lee Y, Maidment NT. Orphanin FQ/nociceptin blocks acquisition of morphine place preference. *Brain Res.* 832:168–170, 1999.

Neale JH, Olszewski RT, Gehl LM, Wroblewska B, Bzdega T. The neurotransmitter N-acetylaspartylglutamate in models of pain, ALS, diabetic neuropathy, CNS injury and schizophrenia. *Trends Pharmacol Sci.* 26:477–484, 2005.

Nestler EJ. Is there a common molecular pathway for addiction? *Nat Neurosci.* 8:1445–1449, 2005.

Norton CS, Neal CR, Kumar S, Akil H, Watson SJ. Nociceptin/orphanin FQ and opioid receptor-like receptor mRNA expression in dopamine systems. *J Comp Neurol.* 444:358–368, 2002.

Nowak K, McBride L, Lumeng J, Li T-K, Murphy JM. Blocking GABA$_A$ receptors in the anterior ventral tegmental area attenuates ethanol intake of the alcohol-preferring P rat. *Psychopharmacology.* 139:108–116, 1998.

Oakman SA, Faris PL, Kerr PE, Cozzari C, Hartman BK. Distribution of pontomesencephalic cholinergic neurons projecting to substantia nigra differs significantly from those projecting to ventral tegmental area. *J Neurosci.* 15:5859–5869, 1995.

O'Brien CP, Gardner EL. Critical assessment of how to study addiction and its treatment: human and non-human animal models. *Pharmacol Ther.* 108:18–58, 2005.

O'Brien CP, Volpicelli LA, Volpicelli JR. Naltrexone in the treatment of alcoholism: a clinical review. *Alcohol.* 13:35–39, 1996.

O'Donohue, TL, Dorsa DM. The opiomelanotropinergic neuronal and endocrine systems. *Peptides* 3:353–395, 1982.

Owen MD, Unal CB, Callahan MF, Triveda K, York C, Millington WR. Glycyl-glutamine inhibits the respiratory depression, but not the antinociception, produced by morphine. *Am J Physiol Regul Integr Comp Physiol.* 279:1944–1948, 2000.

Papp M, Gruca P, Willner P. Selective blockade of drug-induced place preference conditioning by ACPC, a functional NDMA-receptor antagonist. *Neuropsychopharmacology.* 27:727–743, 2002.

Paterson NE, Markou A. The metabotropic glutamate receptor 5 antagonist MPEP decreased break points for nicotine, cocaine and food in rats. *Psychopharmacology.* 179:255–261, 2005.

Paterson NE, Semenova S, Gasparini F, Markou A. The mGluR5 antagonist MPEP decreased nicotine self-administration in rats and mice. *Psychopharmacology.* 167:257–264, 2003.

Paul M, Dewey SL, Gardner EL, Brodie JD, Ashby CR. Gamma-vinyl-GABA (GVC) blocks expression of the conditioned place preference response to heroin in rats. *Synapse* 41:219–220, 2001.

Poncelet M, Maruani J, Calassi R, Soubrie P. Overeating, alcohol and sucrose consumption decrease in CB1 receptor deleted mice. *Neurosci Lett.* 343:216–218, 2003.

Popik P, Danysz W. Inhibition of reinforcing effects of morphine and motivational aspects of naloxone-precipitated opioid withdrawal by N-methyl-D-aspartate receptor antagonist, memantine. *J Pharmacol Exp Ther.* 280:854–865, 1997.

Popik P, Kozela E, Wrobel M, Wozniak KM, Slusher BS. Morphine tolerance and reward but not expression of morphine dependence are inhibited by the selective glutamate carboxypeptidase II (GCP II, NAALADase) inhibitor, 2-PMPA. *Neuropsychopharmacology.* 28:457–467, 2002.

Popik P, Wrobel M. Morphine conditioned reward is inhibited by MPEP, the mGluR5 antagonist. *Neuropharmacology.* 43:1210–1217, 2002.

Riegel AC, Lupica CR. Independent presynaptic and postsynaptic mechanisms regulate endocannabinoid signaling at multiple synapses in the ventral tegmental area. *J Neurosci.* 24:11070–11078, 2004.

Resch GE, Shridharani S, Millington WR, Garris DR, Simpson CW. Glycyl-glutamine in nucleus accumbens reduces ethanol intake in alcohol preferring (P) rats. *Brain Res.* 1058:73–81, 2005.

Roberts DCS. Preclinical evidence for $GABA_B$ agonists as a pharmacotherapy for cocaine addiction. *Physiol Behav.* 86:18–20, 2005.

Sahraei H, Amiri YA, Haeri-Rohani A, Sepehri H, Salimi SH, Pourmotabbed A, Ghoshooni H, Zahirodin A, Zardooz H. Different effects of GABAergic receptors located in the ventral tegmental area on the expression of morphine-induced conditioned place preference in rat. *Eur J Pharmacol.* 524:95–101, 2005.

Sakoori K, Murphy NP. Central administration of nociceptin/orphanin FQ blocks the acquisition of a conditioned place preference to morphine and cocaine, but not conditioned place aversion to naloxone in mice. *Psychopharmacology.* 172:129–136, 2004.

Salamone JD, Correa M, Mingote SM, Weber SM. Beyond the reward hypothesis: alternative functions of nucleus accumbens dopamine. *Curr Opin Pharmacol.* 5:34–41, 2005.

Samson HH, Chappell A. Muscimol injected into the medial prefrontal cortex of the rat alters ethanol self-administration. *Physiol Behav.* 74:581–587, 2001.

Schroeder JP, Overstreet DH, Hodge CW. The mGluR5 antagonist MPEP decreases operant ethanol self-administration during maintenance and after repeated alcohol deprivations in alcohol-preferring (P) rats. *Psychopharmacology.* 179:262–270, 2005.

Scott LJ, Figgitt DP, Keam SJ, Waugh J. Acamprosate. A review of its use in the maintenance of abstinence in patients with alcohol dependence. *CNS Drugs.* 19:445–464, 2005.

Sepulveda J, Astorga JG, Contreras E. Riluzole decreases the abstinence syndrome and physical dependence in morphine-dependent mice. *Eur J Pharmacol.* 379:59–62, 1999.

Shoblock JR, Wichmann J, Maidment NT. The effect of a systemically active ORL-1 agonist, Ro 64-6198, on the acquisition, expression, extinction, and reinstatement of morphine conditioned place preference. *Neuropharmacology.* 49:439–446, 2005.

Silagy C, Lancaster T, Stead L, Mant D, Fowler G. Nicotine replacement therapy for smoking cessation. *Cochrane Database Syst Rev.* CD000146, 2004.

Slusher BS, Thomas A, Paul M, Schad CA, Ashby CR. Expression and acquisition of the conditioned place preference response to cocaine in rats is blocked by selective inhibitors of the enzyme N-acetylated-alpha-linked-acidic dipeptidase (NAALADASE). *Synapse.* 41:22–28, 2001.

Soria G, Mendizabal V, Tourino C, Robledo P, Ledent C, Parmentier M, Maldonado R, Valverde O. Lack of CB1 cannabinoid receptor impairs cocaine self-administration. *Neuropsychopharmacology.* 30:1670–1680, 2005.

Szabo B, Muller T, Koch H. Effects of cannabinoids on dopamine release in the corpus striatum and the nucleus accumbens in vitro. *J Neurochem.* 73:1084–1089, 1999.

Tallaksen-Greene SJ, Kaatz KW, Romano C, Albin RL. Localization of mGluR1a-like immunoreactivity and mGluR5-like immunoreactivity in identified populations of striatal neurons. *Brain Res.* 780:210–217, 1998.

Tessari M, Pilla M, Andreoli M, Hutcheson DM, Heidbreder CA. Antagonism at metabotropic glutamate 5 receptors inhibits nicotine- and cocaine-taking behaviours and prevents nicotine-triggered relapse to nicotine-seeking. *Eur J Pharmacol.* 499:121–133, 2004.

Thomas AG, Vornov JJ, Olkowski JL, Merion AT, Slusher BS. N-Acetylated α-linked acidic dipeptidase converts N-acetylaspartylglutamate from a neuroprotectant to a neurotoxin. *J Pharmacol Exp Ther.* 295:16–22, 2000.

Thomsen M, Woldbye DP, Wortwein G, Fink-Jensen A, Wess J, Caine SB. Reduced cocaine self-administration in muscarinic M_5 acetylcholine receptor-deficient mice. *J Neurosci.* 25:8141–8149, 2005.

Trujillo KA. Are NMDA receptors involved in opiate-induced neural and behavioral plasticity? A review of preclinical studies. *Psychopharmacology.* 151:121–141, 2000.

Trujillo KA, Akil H. Inhibition of morphine tolerance and dependence by the NMDA receptor antagonist MK-801. *Science.* 251:85–87, 1991.

Tsuji M, Nakagawa Y, Ishibashi Y, Yoshii T, Takashima T, Shimada M, Suzuki T. Activation of ventral tegmental $GABA_B$ receptors inhibits morphine induced place preference in rats. *Eur J Pharmacol.* 313:169–173, 1996.

Tzschentke TM. Measuring reward with the conditioned place preference paradigm: a comprehensive review of drug effects, recent progress and new issues. *Prog Neurobiol.* 56:613–672, 1998.

Tzschentke TM, Schmidt WJ. N-methyl-D-aspartic acid-receptor antagonists block morphine-induced conditioned place preference in rats. *Neurosci Lett.* 193:37–40, 1995.

Tzschentke TM, Schmidt WJ. Blockade of morphine- and amphetamine-induced conditioned place preference in the rat by riluzole. *Neurosci Lett.* 242:114–116, 1998.

Tzschentke TM, Schmidt WJ. Blockade of behavioral sensitization by MK-801: fact or artifact? A review of preclinical data. *Psychopharmacology.* 151:142–151, 2000.

Vorel SR, Ashby CR, Paul M, Liu X, Hayes R, Hagan JJ, Middlemiss DN, Stemp G, Gardner EL. Dopamine D_3 receptor antagonism inhibits cocaine-seeking and cocaine-enhanced brain reward in rats. *J Neurosci.* 22:9595–9603, 2002.

Watkins SS, Koob GF, Markou A. Neural mechanisms underlying nicotine addiction: acute positive reinforcement and withdrawal. *Nicotine Tob Res.* 2:19–37, 2000.

Weiner DM, Levey AI, Brann MR. Expression of muscarinic acetylcholine and dopamine receptor mRNAs in rat basal ganglia. *Proc Natl Acad Sci USA.* 87:7050–7054, 1990.

Wilson RI, Nicoll RA. Endocannabinoid signaling in the brain. *Science.* 296:678–682, 2002.

Wirtshafter D, Sheppard AC. Localization of GABA$_B$ receptors in midbrain monoamine containing neurons in the rat. *Brain Res Bull.* 56:1–5, 2001.

Wise RA. Dopamine, learning and motivation. *Nature Rev Neurosci.* 5:1–12, 2004.

Wonnacott S, Sidhpura N, Balfour DJK. Nicotine: from molecular mechanisms to behavior. *Curr Opin Pharmacol.* 5:53–59, 2005.

Xi ZX, Baker DA, Shen H, Carson DS, Kalivas PW. Group II metabotropic glutamate receptors modulate extracellular glutamate in the nucleus accumbens. *J Pharmacol Exp Ther.* 300:162–171, 2002.

Xi ZX, Gilbert J, Campos AC, Kline N, Ashby CR Jr., Hagan JJ, Heidbreder CA, Gardner EL. Blockade of mesolimbic dopamine D$_3$ receptors inhibits stress-induced reinstatement of cocaine-seeking in rats. *Psychopharmacology.* 176:57–65, 2004.

Xi ZX, Newman AH, Gilbert JG, Pak AC, Peng XQ, Ashby CR, Gitajn L, Gardner EL. The novel dopamine D$_3$ receptor antagonist NGB 2904 inhibits cocaine's rewarding effects and cocaine-induced reinstatement of drug-seeking behavior in rats. *Neuropsychopharmacology.* 31:1393–1405, 2006.

Xi ZX, Stein EA. Nucleus accumbens dopamine release modulation by mesolimbic GABA$_A$ receptors-an in vivo electrochemical study. *Brain Res.* 798:156–165, 1998.

Xi ZX, Stein EA. Baclofen inhibits heroin self-administration behavior and mesolimbic dopamine release. *J Pharmacol Exp Ther.* 290:1369–1374, 1999.

Xi ZX, Stein EA. Increased mesolimbic GABA concentration blocks heroin self-administration in the rat. *J Pharmacol Exp Ther.* 294:613–619, 2000.

Xi ZX, Stein EA. GABAergic mechanisms of opiate reinforcement. *Alcohol Alcohol.* 37:485–494, 2002.

Yeomans JS, Kofman O, McFarlane V. Cholinergic involvement in lateral hypothalamic rewarding brain stimulation. *Brain Res.* 329:19–26, 1985.

Zarrindast MR, Ahmadi S, Haeri-Rohani A, Rezayof A, Jafari MR, Jafari-Sabet M. GABA$_A$ receptors in the basolateral amygdala are involved in mediating morphine reward. *Brain Res.* 1006:49–58, 2004.

Zhou L, Furuta T, Kaneko T. Chemical organization of projection neurons in the rat accumbens nucleus and olfactory tubercle. *Neuroscience.* 120:783–798, 2003.

11

Neurobiology of Opioids in Dependency

Linda I. Perrotti

Opiates exert their rewarding effects though actions at μ-opioid receptors (MOR) in the ventral tegmental area (VTA) in the midbrain. Activation of MOR disinhibits GABA neurons, which ordinarily hold VTA dopaminergic neurons in abeyance. This disinhibition increases the release of dopamine (DA) to the major target of the VTA dopaminergic cells, the nucleus accumbens (NAc), as well as other regions of the limbic forebrain.

Chronic exposure to opiates results in neural adaptations that lead to tolerance, sensitization, and dependence. Tolerance is the loss of sensitivity to certain pharmacological affects of the drug that requires higher doses be consumed in order to achieve the desired effects of the drug. Sensitization is a heightened responsiveness to the drug following multiple exposures, and dependence is defined pharmacologically by withdrawal when drug taking ceases. These long-term changes occur because repetitive exposure to the drug activates signaling pathways, which, in turn, alter the rate of gene transcription and result in altered neuronal activity.

The goal of this chapter is to demonstrate how changes in intracellular signaling proteins are important contributors to neural adaptations, which are characteristic of chronic opiate use.

Signal Transduction

Signal transduction is the process whereby neurotransmitter-receptor interactions alter gene expression by activating or deactivating transcription factors. This process produces a wide range of effects on target cells and involves a complex network of intracellular messenger systems involving G proteins, second messengers, and protein phosphorylation. The focus of this chapter will be to examine the role of regulators of G protein signaling (RGS) proteins and two transcription factors (CREB and ΔFosB) involved in opiate dependence.

Opioid receptors belong to the family of G protein-coupled receptors (GPCR) and are sites of opiate actions. There are three major classes of opioid receptors: μ, δ, and κ. Of the three, the μ-opioid receptor (MOR) is established as the main target of opiate analgesics.

Regulators of G Protein Signaling (RGS Proteins)

The MOR is a conventional GPCR in that it is a cell surface protein with seven transmembrane domains. It consists of α, β, and γ subunits, and an effector protein. The G protein functions to amplify a signal received by a transmembrane receptor, transmitting that message to effector proteins within a neuron. Each G protein exists as a heterotrimeric complex that comprises a GTP-hydrolyzing Gα subunit and a Gβγ dimeric partner. The resting G protein exists as the heterotrimer with GDP bound to the α subunit and the Gα subunit bound to the βγ complex.

Opiates induce conformational changes at the MOR and enhance the guanine-nucleotide-exchange activity of the receptor, leading to the release of GDP and subsequent binding of GTP by the Gα subunit. On binding GTP, these conformational changes allow the dissociation of the Gβγ subunit, which allows the freed α subunit to bind with and alter the activity of effector proteins. Freed Gβγ subunits can also modulate effectors. GTPase activity of the α subunit is fundamentally slow; eventually the bound GTP is hydrolyzed to GDP (3–15 seconds). Reassociation of the α subunit-GDP complex with the βγ complex then completes the cycle. The duration of G protein signaling through effectors is controlled by the lifetime of the Gα subunit in the GTP bound form. Thus, the responses mediated by these receptors are generally slow (hundreds of milliseconds to minutes). All α-subunits can hydrolyze GTP on their own, but the rate of this self-inactivation is too slow to account for the rapid shutoff of GPCR signaling seen physiologically. Discovery of the RGS proteins as being critical elements of GPCR signal transduction has helped to explain this timing discrepancy.

Proteins that regulate the signaling activity of GTP-binding proteins are divided into three categories depending upon whether they stimulate GTPase activity (GTPase-activating proteins), inhibit release of GDP (guanine nucleotide dissociation inhibitors), or exchange GTP for GDP (guanine nucleotide exchange factors). RGS proteins serve as GTPase-activating proteins (GAPs) for α subunits of heterotrimeric Gi, Go, Gz, Gt, and Gq proteins. RGS proteins are responsible for the rapid turnoff of G protein–coupled receptor signaling pathways. The major mechanism whereby RGS proteins negatively regulate G proteins is via the GTPase activating protein activity of their RGS domain. Through this mechanism RGS proteins hasten the deactivation of G proteins to reduce GPCR signaling. Thus, RGS proteins are negative regulators of G protein signaling (see Figure 12.1).

To date, over 30 RGS proteins have been identified (Siderovski and Willard, 2005). A few members of this family are abundantly expressed in reward-related brain regions, and this expression has been shown to be regulated by exposure to opiates. Several RGS family members are expressed in the brain, where they show distinct regional and cellular distributions (Gold et al., 1997). In relation to their distribution, expression patterns, and induction by drugs of abuse, RGS9–2, RGS2, and RGS4 have proved to be the most relevant of the RGS proteins (Traynor and Neubig, 2005).

Figure 11.1. Scheme illustrating opiate actions in the locus coeruleus (LC). Opiates acutely inhibit LC neurons by increasing the conductance of an inwardly rectifying K+ channel via coupling with subtypes of Gi/o and by decreasing a NA+ dependent inward current via coupling with Gi/o and the consequent inhibition of adenylyl cyclase. Reduced levels of cAMP decrease protein kinase A (PKA) activity and the phosphorylation of the responsible channel or pump. Inhibition of the cAMP pathway also decreases phosphorylation of numerous other proteins and thereby affects many additional processes in the neuron. For example, it reduces the phosphorylation state of CREB, which may initiate some of the longer-term changes in LC function. Chronic morphine increases levels of types I (ACI) and VIII (ACVIII) adenylyl cyclase, PKA catalytic (C) and regulatory type II (RII) subunits, and several phosphoproteins, including CREB and tyrosine hydroxylase (TH), the rate-limiting enzyme in norepinephrine synthesis. These changes contribute to the altered phenotype of the drug-addicted state. Reprinted with permission from Chao and Nestler 2004.

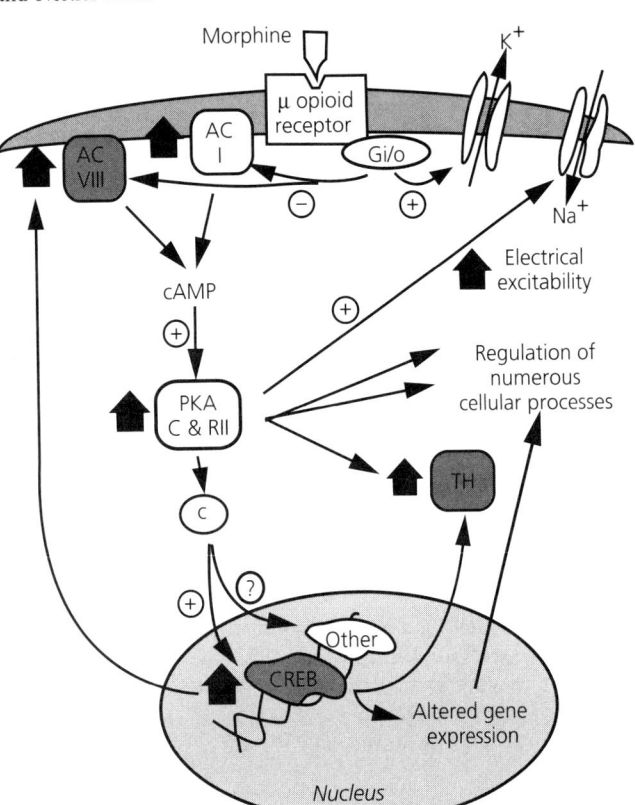

RGS9–2 and RGS4 are implicated in modulating MOR signaling in heterologous expression systems (Chuang et al., 1998; Potenza et al., 1999; Rahman et al., 1999; Traynor and Neubig, 2005) and in vivo (Garzon et al., 2001). They have also been shown to affect opiate-induced neural adaptations such as tolerance and withdrawal (Gold et al., 2003).

RGS9–2 is expressed only in the brain and is highly enriched in the striatum, an area essential for the actions of the rewarding effects of opiates (Gold et al., 1997; Rahman et al., 1999). It is also present at lower levels in regions critical for the analgesic effects of opiates (periaqueductal gray and spinal cord; Koob et al., 1998).

Initial investigations revealed that RGS9–2 negatively modulates MOR function in vitro (Rahman et al., 1999). More recent in vivo work with mice deficient in RGS9 revealed that deletion of the RGS9 gene increases sensitivity to the rewarding effects of morphine, enhances morphine-induced analgesia, delays the development of analgesic tolerance, and results in severe morphine dependence and withdrawal (Zachariou et al., 2003). In concordance, Garzon et al. (2001) showed that RGS9 proteins facilitate analgesic tolerance to μ-opioid agonists by demonstrating that a reduction in RGS9 levels in mice using antisense oligonucleotide leads to an increase in the antinociceptive potency of morphine.

Additionally, RGS9 appears to regulate tonic opioidergic signaling in the brain. Opiate-naïve RGS9 knockout mice are more sensitive to the aversive effects of naloxone then their wild-type littermates (Zachariou et al., 2003). These studies implicate RGS9 as a critical negative regulator of opiate action and outline a potential role for its involvement in cellular adaptations that occur after chronic opiate administration.

The following outlines the evidence that RGS proteins in MOR-containing neurons may contribute to morphine tolerance. A series of experiments by several laboratories mapping the expression and induction of RGS4 protein and mRNA ultimately lead to functional studies describing possible mechanisms for such tolerance.

RGS4 mRNA is basally expressed in the cortex, amygdala, striatum, thalamus, locus coeruleus (LC; Gold et al., 1997, 2003), and dorsal horn of the spinal cord (Garnier et al., 2003). There is some evidence for a potential role of RGS4 after an acute but not chronic morphine regimen in the limbic forebrain (Bishop et al., 2002). Acute morphine treatment increases levels of RGS4 mRNA in the nucleus accumbens, whereas chronic morphine treatment has no effect on RGS4 mRNA in the limbic forebrain (Bishop et al., 2002; Narita et al., 2002). A biphasic regulatory response of RGS4 to acute and chronic morphine treatments is reported in the LC (Bishop et al., 2002). Decreased RGS4 levels are observed after acute morphine administration and would seem to indicate an increase in GPCR signaling, whereas the increases in RGS4 mRNA after a chronic morphine treatment would imply a decrease in signaling (Bishop et al., 2002). Experiments investigating the expression of RGS4 protein levels give better insight into GPCR signaling. Chronic morphine doubles RGS4 protein levels in dopamine cells in the LC, and these protein levels return to basal levels following precipitation of withdrawal (Gold et al., 2003). Functionally, increased levels of RGS4 protein decrease the electrophysiological responsivity of LC neurons to morphine (Gold et al., 2003).

Taken together, these investigations document intricate time-dependent alterations in RGS4 protein and mRNA expression in the LC and support a role for this protein in cellular adaptations, such as tolerance, following chronic morphine administration. The identification of RGS4 expression in dopaminergic cells of the LC indicates that RGS4 could be involved in morphine-induced functional changes in local norepinephrine neurons (Gold et al., 2003). Thus, RGS4 could be one fundamental mechanism causing changes in MOR signaling after chronic opiate administration.

The above discussion illustrates likely roles for RGS proteins—in particular, aspects of opiate pharmacology. Future and ongoing investigations will help to define roles for specific RGS proteins in opioid reward, reward-related behaviors, and the molecular adaptations that accompany long-term exposure to opiates. Given the accumulating evidence for RGS9–2 as a critical contributor to the development of tolerance and dependence on morphine, it is being given much attention as a potential therapeutic target (Traynor and Neubig, 2005).

Transcription Factors

In addition to activation of opioid systems, addictive patterns of opiate use also cause chronic stimulation of dopamine systems. Predictably, such stimulation has been reported to change hundreds of proteins in reward-related brain regions. Among those best studied are the cAMP response element binding protein (CREB) and the Fos family of transcription factors. These transcription factors have repeatedly been demonstrated to play a substantial role in drug-mediated gene regulation.

cAMP-Response-Element-Binding Protein (CREB)

CREB is a member of the bZIP superfamily of transcription factors. It has a basic C-terminal domain that is responsible for binding to DNA and a leucine zipper domain that mediates dimerization with itself or other members of the CREB family of transcription factors. CREB is activated by several signal transduction pathways, which suggests it may be responsible for the integration of signaling information from multiple sources and in this way mediates complex forms of neural plasticity (Bailey et al., 1996; Daniel et al., 1998; Mayr and Montminy, 2001; Nestler, 2001).

CREB is of particular interest in drug addiction because its activation is downstream of the cAMP signaling pathway, whose upregulation has been extensively characterized as an adaptation to chronic exposure to drugs of abuse (Guitart et al., 1992). Investigations into its role in addiction began in cultured neuronal cell lines and, to date, extend to several of the reward-related brain regions in rodents. Together these studies invariably demonstrate that acute exposure to opiates acts to inhibit the production of cAMP, whereas chronic opiate exposure upregulates the cAMP signaling cascade (Nestler and Aghajanian, 1997; Sharma et al., 1975). This biphasic regulation can be viewed as a homeostatic compensatory mechanism to the initial inhibition of the cAMP signaling by opiates. Upregulation of the cAMP pathway mediates several facets of addiction depending upon the specific region of the brain involved (Nestler, 2001). Effects on the locus coeruleus, nucleus accumbens, and ventral tegmental area (VTA) are discussed below.

The locus coeruleus (LC), the main noradrenergic nucleus in the brain, is the best characterized brain region for the cellular adaptations that occur during prolonged activation of MOR (Aghajanian and Wang, 1986; Alreja and Aghajanian, 1993; Ivanov and Aston-Jones, 2001; Nakai et al., 2002; Nestler and Aghajanian, 1997; Figure 11.1). In general, it is important in mediating arousal, attention, and autonomic tone. Additionally, the LC is important in opiate physical dependence and the stresslike effects of withdrawal. Overactivation of cells in the LC is both necessary and sufficient for producing some of the symptoms underlying physical opiate dependence and the behavioral signs of withdrawal (Lane-Ladd et al., 1997; Nestler and Aghajanian, 1997).

Acute administration of opiates inhibits LC neurons by inhibiting the activation of the cAMP pathway (Aghajanian and Wang, 1986; Alreja and Aghajanian, 1993; North et al., 1987). Chronic exposure to opiates results in LC neurons developing tolerance to these acute inhibitory actions. Increases in CREB expression and phosphorylation, and the previously depressed LC neuronal firing rates gradually recover toward preexposure levels (Guitart et al., 1992; Widnell et al., 1994). Administration of an opioid receptor antagonist causes a dramatic increase in firing rates (withdrawal; Guitart et al., 1992; Widnell et al., 1994). Accordingly, mutant mice lacking certain forms of CREB show moderate physical symptoms of morphine withdrawal (Maldonado et al., 1996). However, these same mice display a strong aversion to opiate withdrawal in a conditioned-aversion paradigm despite their attenuated physical withdrawal symptoms, suggesting that the mechanisms of physical dependence may be separate from those mediating the incentive motivational aspects of morphine withdrawal (Walters and Blendy, 2001). Thus, CREB activity appears to play an important role in the molecular adaptations to chronic opiate exposure in the LC. These adaptations imply a homeostatic or compensatory regulatory mechanism.

CREB function within the striatal complex has also been implicated in opiate addiction and associated behaviors. Repeated exposure to morphine upregulates cAMP-PKA activity (Terwilliger et al., 1991) and stimulates CRE-mediated transcription in the NAc (Barrot et al., 2002; Shaw-Lutchman et al., 2002). Similarly, chronic but not acute morphine exposure decreases CREB immunoreactivity in the NAc (Widnell et al., 1996). Functionally, CREB overexpression in the NAc is shown to decrease morphine reward, whereas expression of a mutant form of the protein increases it, suggesting that sustained CREB activation in the NAc could be a mechanism by which drugs of abuse produce tolerance to their rewarding effects. At the cellular level, precipitated opiate withdrawal in primary culture of NAc neurons increases CREB phosphorylation and the expression of CREB-related target genes (Chartoff et al., 2003). Aside from dampening the rewarding effects of drugs of abuse, upregulation of the cAMP pathway and CREB in the NAc contribute to physical signs of early opiate withdrawal (Hyman and Malenka, 2001; Nestler, 2001). Thus, it is plausible that CREB activity in the NAc may also influence this aspect of addiction.

Considering the fact that the ventral tegmental area (VTA) of the midbrain is a prominent structure in brain reward circuitry, it is interesting that only a few studies have investigated the role of CREB here. Studies of CREB-knockdown mice support a role for CREB in regulation of morphine reward via the VTA (Walters et al., 2003). The active form of CREB is present in the VTA after acute opiate exposure (Walters et al., 2003), whereas chronic morphine exposure increases levels of CREB and CRE binding (Widnell et al., 1996). Likewise, CREB-mediated transcription is upregulated in the VTA in response to chronic morphine exposure (Olson et al., 2005). Interestingly, this upregulation has different behavioral consequences depending on the anatomical localization of expression of the gene. Overexpression of CREB in rostral portions of the VTA increases the rewarding properties of morphine, whereas similar changes in caudal portions decrease morphine reward as measured in place conditioning assays (Olson et al., 2005). These data indicate that within VTA differences in neuronal input and output could reflect region-specific signal discrimination through CREB transcription (Mayr and Montminy, 2001).

Overall, exposure to morphine increases CREB function and causes the addictive phenotypes of tolerance and dependence and may contribute to states of dysphoria seen in early withdrawal. Investigations are currently underway to identify the particular CREB target genes that contribute to these behavioral effects. One likely candidate in the NAc is dynorphin, an opioid peptide expressed in a subset of medium spiny neurons in the NAc. Dynorphin is induced in this region after chronic drug exposure (Carlezon et al., 1998; Cole et al., 1995; Daunais and McGinty, 1995; Spangler et al., 1996; Figure 11.2). CREB-mediated increases in dynorphin release from the NAc to the VTA appear to contribute to some of the aversive or depressive effects (dysphoria) involved in opiate withdrawal (Shippenberg and Rea, 1997). Dynorphin binds to κ-opioid receptors on VTA dopamine neuron cell bodies and terminals to inhibit their activity and decrease dopamine release in the NAc (Spanagel et al., 1992). Several other CREB targets have been identified in the NAc (McClung et al., 2004). Future studies are underway to relate CREB-induced changes in the expression of these target genes to the specific processes that contribute to addictive patterns of behavior.

ΔFosB

Long-term drug exposure causes changes in CREB function, but these changes are short-lived and have been implicated in aspects of dependence that are resolved within short periods of abstinence. ΔFosB is a member of the Fos family of transcription factors that are induced rapidly and transiently in response to a wide variety of perturbations, including administration of drugs of abuse. ΔFosB is induced only slightly by an initial stimulation, but begins to accumulate in cells after repeated stimulation. Because of its unusual stability, it appears to be an important means for long-term modifications in the brain.

Figure 11.2. Opiate regulation of CREB. The figure shows a VTA dopamine (DA) neuron innervating a class of NAc GABAergic projection neurons that express dynorphin (DYN). Dynorphin serves a negative feedback mechanism in this circuit: Dynorphin, released from terminals of the NAc neurons, acts on κ-opioid receptors located on nerve terminals and cell bodies of the DA neurons to inhibit their functioning. Chronic exposure to cocaine or opiates regulates the activity of this negative feedback loop via upregulation of the cAMP pathway, activation of CREB, and induction of dynorphin. DR: dopamine receptor; OR: opiate receptor. Reprinted with permission from Nestler, 2004.

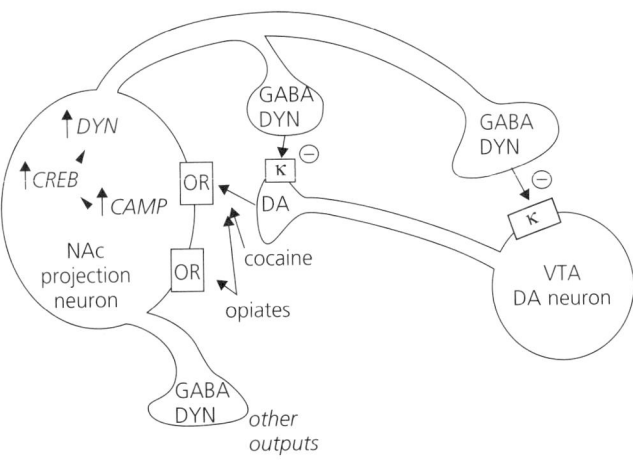

Immediate early genes (IEGs) are a class of genes whose expression is activated transiently and rapidly within minutes of exposure to a stimulus. Of particular interest in the study of addiction are the Fos and Jun families of immediate early genes, which encode transcription factors. The Fos family of transcription factors includes c-Fos, FosB, Fos-related antigens 1 and 2 (Fra-1 and -2), and ΔFosB. ΔFosB is a truncated splice variant of full-length FosB, and lacks a portion of the C-terminal transactivation domain present in other Fos proteins (Mumberg et al., 1991). Fos family members heterodimerize with Jun family transcription factors (c-Jun, JunB, JunD) to form the activator protein-1 (AP-1) complex. The AP-1 complex binds to specific DNA sequences in the promoters of various target genes, with the consensus sequence TGAC/GTCA. AP-1 complexes can act as either a transcriptional inducer or repressor, depending on the specific AP-1 binding site and promoter in question.

Over a decade ago, a broad band of Foslike proteins was identified by immunoblotting as proteins induced exclusively by chronic treatments (Hope et al., 1994, 1992). Additionally, these proteins were shown to persist in the brain for an extended period of time compared with all other known Fos and Jun family members (Figure 11.3).

Acute exposure to drugs of abuse causes the transient induction of the transcription factors c-Fos and FosB (Graybiel et al., 1990; Hope et al., 1992; Young et al., 1991), whereas chronic exposure to virtually all drugs of abuse causes the accumulation of ΔFosB (Hiroi et al., 1997; Hope et al., 1994; Moratalla et al., 1996; Nye et al., 1995; Nye and Nestler, 1996; Pich et al., 1997; Rahman et al., 1999; Young et al., 1991). ΔFosB induction has also been observed with other chronic stimulations, such as chronic stress (Perrotti et al., 2004), repeated seizures (Hiroi et al., 1998; Hope et al., 1994), antipsychotic drug treatment (Andersson et al., 2003; Hiroi and Graybiel, 1996; Kontkanen et al., 2002; Rodriguez et al., 2001; Vahid-Ansari and Leenen, 1998), or even repeated running (Werme et al., 2002). Because of its stability, ΔFosB not only accumulates but also persists long after termination of the stimulus (Nestler, 2001). Chronic alterations in dopamine neurotransmission have long-lasting effects on ΔFosB expression in the striatum (Doucet et al., 1996). ΔFosB accumulation after chronic exposure to opiates has previously been detected in the reward-relevant nucleus accumbens and dorsal striatum (Hiroi et al., 1997; Hiroi and Graybiel, 1996; Hope et al., 1994; Nye et al., 1995; Nye and Nestler, 1996; Pich et al., 1997; Rahman et al., 1999). Prolonged withdrawal from morphine induces ΔFosB in some regions, like locus coeruleus and VTA, where chronic morphine treatment itself, in the absence of withdrawal, does not (Nye and Nestler, 1996; Perrotti et al., 2005).

The functional role of ΔFosB expression in the striatal complex has been characterized by using transgenic mice. Marked effects of ΔFosB on various behavioral responses to morphine have recently been reported (Zachariou et al., 2006). Mutant mice that inducibly overexpress ΔFosB mostly in striatal regions display increased sensitivity to the rewarding effects of morphine, reduced analgesic responses to acute morphine administration, accelerated development of morphine tolerance, and a greater physical dependence on morphine (Zachariou et al., 2006). Moreover, overexpression of a dominant negative mutant form of c-Jun, which antagonizes the transcriptional activating effects of ΔFosB, and all AP-1 mediated transcription, had the opposite effects on all behavioral phenotypes examined (Zachariou et al., 2006). Further, the actions of ΔFosB seem dependent upon its expression in dynorphin positive neurons as these behavioral effects were not

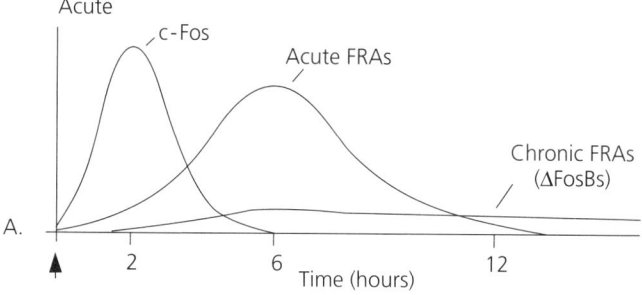

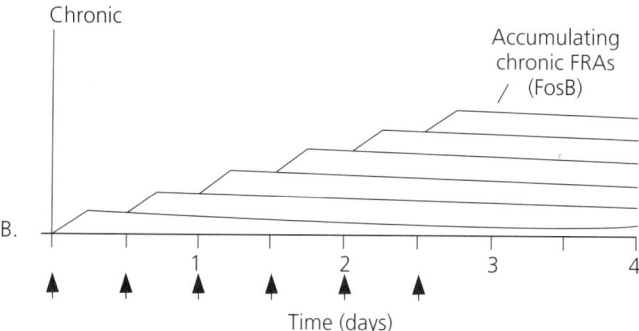

Figure 11.3. Scheme for the gradual accumulation of ΔFosB versus the rapid and transient induction of acute Fos family proteins in the brain (A) Several waves of Foslike proteins are induced in neurons by acute stimuli. c-Fos is induced rapidly and degraded within several hours of the acute stimulus, whereas other "acute FRAs" (Fos-related antigens; e.g., FosB, ΔFosB, FRA-1, FRA-2) are induced somewhat later and persist somewhat longer than c-Fos. The "chronic FRAs" are biochemically modified isoforms of ΔFosB; they, too, are induced (although at low levels) following a single acute stimulus but persist in the brain for long periods. In a complex with Junlike proteins, these waves of FRAs form AP-1 binding complexes with shifting composition over time. (B) With repeated stimulation, each acute stimulus induces a low level of ΔFosB. This is indicated by the lower set of overlapping lines, which indicate ΔFosB induced by each acute stimulus. The result is a gradual increase in the total level of ΔFosB induced with repeated stimuli during a course of chronic treatment. This is indicated by the increasing stepped line in the graph. The increasing levels of ΔFosB with repeated stimulation would result in the gradual induction of significant levels of a long-lasting AP-1 complex, which is hypothesized to underlie persisting forms of neuronal plasticity in the brain. Reprinted with permission from Nestler, 2004.

observed in mice expressing ΔFosB in dynorphin-negative cells. These data support the long-held view that the induction of ΔFosB within dynorphin-containing neurons in the NAc in response to chronic opiate exposure is very important in modulating many of the diverse plastic behavioral adaptations that result from repeated opiate exposure.

Several other target genes of ΔFosB have been established using both a candidate gene approach and an open-ended search measuring the gene expression changes that occur upon ΔFosB expression using DNA microarrays. One candidate gene is GluR2, an AMPA glutamate receptor subunit (Kelz et al., 1999). ΔFosB overexpression in inducible bitransgenic mice selectively increases GluR2 expression in the nucleus accumbens, with no effect on several other AMPA glutamate receptor subunits analyzed. Additionally, GluR2 overexpression via viral-mediated gene transfer increases the rewarding effects of cocaine, much like prolonged ΔFosB overexpression (Kelz et al., 1999). The relevance of the upregulation of GluR2 by ΔFosB warrants further investigation.

Overall, ΔFosB seems both necessary and sufficient for sensitizing animals to opiate reward and might even increase drive for such reward. Additionally, because of its unusual stability (Carle et al., 2007; Ulery, 2005), it may potentially drive such behavioral changes for weeks and months after the last drug exposure (Perrotti et al., 2005). In this way, ΔFosB could be a sustained molecular switch that facilitates the initiation to and maintenance of states of addiction (Nestler, 2001).

Conclusions

The studies described in this chapter substantiate the view that opiates exert changes in brain function that ultimately affect addictive patterns of behavior through a variety of molecular mechanisms. Accumulating evidence for RGS9–2 as a critical contributor to opiate dependence makes it a very attractive candidate as a potential therapeutic target. It is interesting to think of the opposite effects of CREB and ΔFosB on reward mechanisms: CREB inhibits drug reward, whereas ΔFosB enhances it. Further, opiate regulation of the two transcription factors exhibits very different temporal properties in that activation of CREB generally resolves within a few days to a week after drug withdrawal whereas induction of ΔFosB lasts considerably longer. As a result, the actions of the two transcription factors can account for an initial period of dysphoria known to predominate during early phases of drug withdrawal followed by a more sustained period of sensitized responses to the drug and drug-related stimuli.

References

Aghajanian GK, Wang YY (1986) Pertussis toxin blocks the outward currents evoked by opiate and alpha 2-agonists in locus coeruleus neurons. *Brain Res* 371:390–394.

Alreja M, Aghajanian GK (1993) Opiates suppress a resting sodium-dependent inward current and activate an outward potassium current in locus coeruleus neurons. *J Neurosci* 13:3525–3532.

Andersson M, Westin JE, Cenci MA (2003) Time course of striatal δFosB-like immunoreactivity and prodynorphin mRNA levels after discontinuation of chronic dopaminomimetic treatment. *Eur J Neurosci* 17: 661–666.

Bailey CH, Bartsch D, Kandel ER (1996) Toward a molecular definition of long-term memory storage. *Proc Natl Acad Sci USA* 93:13445–13452.

Barrot M, Olivier JD, Perrotti LI, Dileone RJ, Berton O, Eisch AJ, Impey S, Storm DR, Neve RL, Yin JC, Zachariou V, Nestler EJ (2002) CREB activity in the nucleus accumbens shell controls gating of behavioral responses to emotional stimuli. *Proc Natl Acad Sci USA* 99:11435–11440.

Bishop GB, Cullinan WE, Curran E, Gutstein HB (2002) Abused drugs modulate RGS4 mRNA levels in rat brain: comparison between acute drug treatment and a drug challenge after chronic treatment. *Neurobiol Dis* 10:334–343.

Carle TL, Ohnishi YN, Ohnishi YH, Alibhai IN, Wilkinson MB, Kumar A, Nestler EJ (2007) Proteasome-dependent and -independent mechanisms for FosB destabilization: identification of FosB degron domains and implications for ΔFosB stability. *Eur J Neurosci* 25:3009–3019.

Carlezon WA, Jr., Thome J, Olson VG, Lane-Ladd SB, Brodkin ES, Hiroi N, Duman RS, Neve RL, Nestler EJ (1998) Regulation of cocaine reward by CREB. *Science* 282:2272–2275.

Chao J, Nestler EJ (2004) Molecular neurobiology of drug addiction. *Annu Rev Med* 55:113–132.

Chartoff EH, Papadopoulou M, Konradi C, Carlezon WA, Jr. (2003) Dopamine-dependent increases in phosphorylation of cAMP response element binding protein (CREB) during precipitated morphine withdrawal in primary cultures of rat striatum. *J Neurochem* 87:107–118.

Chuang HH, Yu M, Jan YN, Jan LY (1998) Evidence that the nucleotide exchange and hydrolysis cycle of G proteins causes acute desensitization of G-protein gated inward rectifier K+ channels. *Proc Natl Acad Sci USA* 95: 11727–11732.

Cole RL, Konradi C, Douglass J, Hyman SE (1995) Neuronal adaptation to amphetamine and dopamine: molecular mechanisms of prodynorphin gene regulation in rat striatum. *Neuron* 14:813–823.

Daniel PB, Walker WH, Habener JF (1998) Cyclic AMP signaling and gene regulation. *Annu Rev Nutr* 18:353–383.

Daunais JB, McGinty JF (1995) Cocaine binges differentially alter striatal pre-prodynorphin and zif/268 mRNAs. *Brain Res Mol Brain Res* 29:201–210.

Doucet JP, Nakabeppu Y, Bedard PJ, Hope BT, Nestler EJ, Jasmin BJ, Chen JS, Iadarola MJ, St-Jean M, Wigle N, Blanchet P, Grondin R, Robertson GS (1996) Chronic alterations in dopaminergic neurotransmission produce a persistent elevation of deltaFosB-like protein(s) in both the rodent and primate striatum. *Eur J Neurosci* 8:365–381.

Garnier M, Zaratin PF, Ficalora G, Valente M, Fontanella L, Rhee MH, Blumer KJ, Scheideler MA (2003) Up-regulation of regulator of G protein signaling 4 expression in a model of neuropathic pain and insensitivity to morphine. *J Pharmacol Exp Ther* 304:1299–1306.

Garzon J, Rodriguez-Diaz M, Lopez-Fando A, Sanchez-Blazquez P (2001) RGS9 proteins facilitate acute tolerance to mu-opioid effects. *Eur J Neurosci* 13:801–811.

Gold SJ, Han MH, Herman AE, Ni YG, Pudiak CM, Aghajanian GK, Liu RJ, Potts BW, Mumby SM, Nestler EJ (2003) Regulation of RGS proteins by chronic morphine in rat locus coeruleus. *Eur J Neurosci* 17:971–980.

Gold SJ, Ni YG, Dohlman HG, Nestler EJ (1997) Regulators of G-protein signaling (RGS) proteins: region-specific expression of nine subtypes in rat brain. *J Neurosci* 17:8024–8037.

Graybiel AM, Moratalla R, Robertson HA (1990) Amphetamine and cocaine induce drug-specific activation of the c-fos gene in striosome-matrix compartments and limbic subdivisions of the striatum. *Proc Natl Acad Sci USA* 87:6912–6916.

Guitart X, Thompson MA, Mirante CK, Greenberg ME, Nestler EJ (1992) Regulation of cyclic AMP response element-binding protein (CREB) phosphorylation by acute and chronic morphine in the rat locus coeruleus. *J Neurochem* 58:1168–1171.

Hiroi N, Brown JR, Haile CN, Ye H, Greenberg ME, Nestler EJ (1997) FosB mutant mice: loss of chronic cocaine induction of Fos-related proteins and heightened sensitivity to cocaine's psychomotor and rewarding effects. *Proc Natl Acad Sci USA* 94:10397–10402.

Hiroi N, Graybiel AM (1996) Atypical and typical neuroleptic treatments induce distinct programs of transcription factor expression in the striatum. *J Comp Neurol* 374:70–83.

Hiroi N, Marek GJ, Brown JR, Ye H, Saudou F, Vaidya VA, Duman RS, Greenberg ME, Nestler EJ (1998) Essential role of the fosB gene in molecular, cellular, and behavioral actions of chronic electroconvulsive seizures. *J Neurosci* 18:6952–6962.

Hope B, Kosofsky B, Hyman SE, Nestler EJ (1992) Regulation of immediate early gene expression and AP-1 binding in the rat nucleus accumbens by chronic cocaine. *Proc Natl Acad Sci USA* 89:5764–5768.

Hope BT, Nye HE, Kelz MB, Self DW, Iadarola MJ, Nakabeppu Y, Duman RS, Nestler EJ (1994) Induction of a long-lasting AP-1 complex composed of altered Fos-like proteins in brain by chronic cocaine and other chronic treatments. *Neuron* 13:1235–1244.

Hyman SE, Malenka RC (2001) Addiction and the brain: the neurobiology of compulsion and its persistence. *Nat Rev Neurosci* 2:695–703.

Ivanov A, Aston-Jones G (2001) Local opiate withdrawal in locus coeruleus neurons in vitro. *J Neurophysiol* 85:2388–2397.

Kelz MB, Chen J, Carlezon WA, Jr., Whisler K, Gilden L, Beckmann AM, Steffen C, Zhang YJ, Marotti L, Self DW, Tkatch T, Baranauskas G, Surmeier DJ, Neve RL, Duman RS, Picciotto MR, Nestler EJ (1999) Expression of the transcription factor deltaFosB in the brain controls sensitivity to cocaine. *Nature* 401:272–276.

Kontkanen O, Lakso M, Wong G, Castren E (2002) Chronic antipsychotic drug treatment induces long-lasting expression of Fos and Jun family genes and activator protein 1 complex in the rat prefrontal cortex. *Neuropsychopharmacology* 27:152–162.

Koob GF, Sanna PP, Bloom FE (1998) Neuroscience of addiction. *Neuron* 21:467–476.

Lane-Ladd SB, Pineda J, Boundy VA, Pfeuffer T, Krupinski J, Aghajanian GK, Nestler EJ (1997) CREB (cAMP response element-binding protein) in the locus coeruleus: biochemical, physiological, and behavioral evidence for a role in opiate dependence. *J Neurosci* 17:7890–7901.

Maldonado R, Blendy JA, Tzavara E, Gass P, Roques BP, Hanoune J, Schutz G (1996) Reduction of morphine abstinence in mice with a mutation in the gene encoding CREB. *Science* 273:657–659.

Mayr B, Montminy M (2001) Transcriptional regulation by the phosphorylation-dependent factor CREB. *Nat Rev Mol Cell Biol* 2:599–609.

McClung CA, Ulery PG, Perrotti LI, Zachariou V, Berton O, Nestler EJ (2004) DeltaFosB: a molecular switch for long-term adaptation in the brain. *Brain Res Mol Brain Res* 132:146–154.

Moratalla R, Elibol B, Vallejo M, Graybiel AM (1996) Network-level changes in expression of inducible Fos-Jun proteins in the striatum during chronic cocaine treatment and withdrawal. *Neuron* 17:147–156.

Mumberg D, Lucibello FC, Schuermann M, Muller R (1991) Alternative splicing of FosB transcripts results in differentially expressed mRNAs encoding functionally antagonistic proteins. *Genes Dev* 5:1212–1223.

Nakai T, Hayashi M, Ichihara K, Wakabayashi H, Hoshi K (2002) Noradrenaline release in rat locus coeruleus is regulated by both opioid and alpha(2)-adrenoceptors. *Pharmacol Res* 45:407–412.

Narita M, Mizuo K, Shibasaki M, Narita M, Suzuki T (2002) Up-regulation of the G(q/11alpha) protein and protein kinase C during the development of sensitization to morphine-induced hyperlocomotion. *Neuroscience* 111:127–132.

Nestler EJ (2001) Molecular neurobiology of addiction. *Am J Addict* 10:201–217.

Nestler EJ, Aghajanian GK (1997) Molecular and cellular basis of addiction. *Science* 278:58–63.

North RA, Williams JT, Surprenant A, Christie MJ (1987) Mu and delta receptors belong to a family of receptors that are coupled to potassium channels. *Proc Natl Acad Sci USA* 84:5487–5491.

Nye HE, Hope BT, Kelz MB, Iadarola M, Nestler EJ (1995) Pharmacological studies of the regulation of chronic FOS-related antigen induction by cocaine in the striatum and nucleus accumbens. *J Pharmacol Exp Ther* 275:1671–1680.

Nye HE, Nestler EJ (1996) Induction of chronic Fos-related antigens in rat brain by chronic morphine administration. *Mol Pharmacol* 49:636–645.

Olson VG, Zabetian CP, Bolanos CA, Edwards S, Barrot M, Eisch AJ, Hughes T, Self DW, Neve RL, Nestler EJ (2005) Regulation of drug reward by cAMP response element-binding protein: evidence for two functionally distinct subregions of the ventral tegmental area. *J Neurosci* 25:5553–5562.

Perrotti LI, Bolanos CA, Choi KH, Russo SJ, Edwards S, Ulery PG, Wallace DL, Self DW, Nestler EJ, Barrot M (2005) DeltaFosB accumulates in a GABAergic cell population in the posterior tail of the ventral tegmental area after psychostimulant treatment. *Eur J Neurosci* 21:2817–2824.

Perrotti LI, Hadeishi Y, Ulery PG, Barrot M, Monteggia L, Duman RS, Nestler EJ (2004) Induction of deltaFosB in reward-related brain structures after chronic stress. *J Neurosci* 24:10594–10602.

Pich EM, Pagliusi SR, Tessari M, Talabot-Ayer D, Hooft van HR, Chiamulera C (1997) Common neural substrates for the addictive properties of nicotine and cocaine. *Science* 275:83–86.

Potenza MN, Gold SJ, Roby-Shemkowitz A, Lerner MR, Nestler EJ (1999) Effects of regulators of G protein-signaling proteins on the functional response of the mu-opioid receptor in a melanophore-based assay. *J Pharmacol Exp Ther* 291:482–491.

Rahman Z, Gold SJ, Potenza MN, Cowan CW, Ni YG, He W, Wensel TG, Nestler EJ (1999) Cloning and characterization of RGS9-2: a striatal-enriched alternatively spliced product of the RGS9 gene. *J Neurosci* 19:2016–2026.

Rodriguez JJ, Garcia DR, Nakabeppu Y, Pickel VM (2001) FosB in rat striatum: normal regional distribution and enhanced expression after 6-month haloperidol administration. *Synapse* 39:122–132.

Sharma RK, McLaughlin CA, Pitot HC (1975) Cyclin nucleotide binding sites of the smooth endoplasmic reticulum from normal and neoplastic liver in the rat. *Cancer Lett* 1:61–67.

Shaw-Lutchman TZ, Barrot M, Wallace T, Gilden L, Zachariou V, Impey S, Duman RS, Storm D, Nestler EJ (2002) Regional and cellular mapping of cAMP response element-mediated transcription during naltrexone-precipitated morphine withdrawal. *J Neurosci* 22:3663–3672.

Shippenberg TS, Rea W (1997) Sensitization to the behavioral effects of cocaine: modulation by dynorphin and kappa-opioid receptor agonists. *Pharmacol Biochem Behav* 57:449–455.

Siderovski DP, Willard FS (2005) The GAPs, GEFs, and GDIs of heterotrimeric G-protein alpha subunits. *Int J Biol Sci* 1:51–66.

Spanagel R, Herz A, Shippenberg TS (1992) Opposing tonically active endogenous opioid systems modulate the mesolimbic dopaminergic pathway. *Proc Natl Acad Sci USA* 89:2046–2050.

Spangler R, Ho A, Zhou Y, Maggos CE, Yuferov V, Kreek MJ (1996) Regulation of kappa opioid receptor mRNA in the rat brain by "binge" pattern cocaine administration and correlation with preprodynorphin mRNA. *Brain Res Mol Brain Res* 38:71–76.

Terwilliger RZ, Beitner-Johnson D, Sevarino KA, Crain SM, Nestler EJ (1991) A general role for adaptations in G-proteins and the cyclic AMP system in mediating the chronic actions of morphine and cocaine on neuronal function. *Brain Res* 548:100–110.

Traynor JR, Neubig RR (2005) Regulators of G protein signaling and drugs of abuse. *Mol Interv* 5:30–41.

Ulery PG, Rudenko G, Nestler EJ (2006) Regulation of DFosB stability by phosphorylation. *J Neurosci* 26:5131–5142.

Vahid-Ansari F, Leenen FH (1998) Pattern of neuronal activation in rats with CHF after myocardial infarction. *Am J Physiol* 275:H2140-H2146.

Walters CL, Blendy JA (2001) Different requirements for cAMP response element binding protein in positive and negative reinforcing properties of drugs of abuse. *J Neurosci* 21:9438–9444.

Walters CL, Kuo YC, Blendy JA (2003) Differential distribution of CREB in the mesolimbic dopamine reward pathway. *J Neurochem* 87:1237–1244.

Werme M, Messer C, Olson L, Gilden L, Thoren P, Nestler EJ, Brene S (2002) Delta FosB regulates wheel running. *J Neurosci* 22:8133–8138.

Widnell KL, Chen JS, Iredale PA, Walker WH, Duman RS, Habener JF, Nestler EJ (1996) Transcriptional regulation of CREB (cyclic AMP response element-binding protein) expression in CATH.a cells. *J Neurochem* 66:1770–1773.

Widnell KL, Russell DS, Nestler EJ (1994) Regulation of expression of cAMP response element-binding protein in the locus coeruleus in vivo and in a locus coeruleus-like cell line in vitro. *Proc Natl Acad Sci USA* 91:10947–10951.

Young ST, Porrino LJ, Iadarola MJ (1991) Cocaine induces striatal c-fos-immunoreactive proteins via dopaminergic D1 receptors. *Proc Natl Acad Sci USA* 88:1291–1295.

Zachariou V, Bolanos CA, Selley DE, Theobald D, Cassidy MP, Kelz MB, Shaw-Lutchman T, Berton O, Sim-Selley LJ, Dileone RJ, Kumar A, Nestler EJ (2006) An essential role for DeltaFosB in the nucleus accumbens in morphine action. *Nat Neurosci* 9:205–211.

Zachariou V, Georgescu D, Sanchez N, Rahman Z, DiLeone R, Berton O, Neve RL, Sim-Selley LJ, Selley DE, Gold SJ, Nestler EJ (2003) Essential role for RGS9 in opiate action. *Proc Natl Acad Sci USA* 100:13656–13661.

12

The Regulation of Cellular Mechanisms in Antinociception and Dependency

Jeffery N. Talbot

John R. Traynor

Opioid drugs such as morphine and its derivatives are essential clinical tools for the treatment of pain yet are often accompanied by undesirable effects greatly limiting their use in pain management. In addition, the euphoric and dependent properties of these compounds have resulted in widespread abuse of illicit and prescription opioid drugs. More effective treatments for addiction as well as improved therapy for pain depend on increased understanding of the mechanisms regulating opioid signaling. Several important proteins have recently been characterized that regulate opioid signaling in vitro and in vivo, including regulators of G protein signaling (RGS) proteins and arrestins. Together with other interacting/scaffolding proteins, this group of regulatory factors presents new and potentially powerful targets for manipulating specific opioid effects.

Background

The clinically relevant effects of morphine-like drugs occur with a relatively rapid time course. Acute opioid receptor stimulation produces neuronal hyperpolarization and attenuates neurotransmitter release, which leads to numerous physiological effects such as analgesia, euphoria, respiratory suppression, and decreased gastrointestinal transit (Dhawan et al., 1996). However, repeated or chronic exposure to opioid drugs, as for example in the management of chronic pain or in continual abuse, results in long-term adaptive changes. Tolerance, a reduction in drug effect over time, and dependence, requirement for continued drug to prevent symptoms of withdrawal, limit the therapeutic utility of opioids and contribute to their potential for abuse (Kreek et al., 2002).

Opioid drugs target a class of receptors belonging to the superfamily of heptahelical G protein coupled receptors (GPCRs). Pharmacological and molecular biological evidence indicates there are three opioid receptor types, mu, delta, and kappa, which are primarily expressed in the nervous system. Evidence derived from genetic deletion of these genes in transgenic animal models con-

firms that most of the clinically relevant effects of opioids are mediated through the mu receptor (Matthes et al., 1996; Sora et al., 1997).

As GPCRs, opioid receptors transmit extracellular agonist information to intracellular effectors via G protein coupling, a highly conserved signaling system that is utilized by many hormones and neurotransmitters (Hepler and Gilman, 1992). G proteins are comprised of α- and $\beta\gamma$-subunits as a tightly bound heterotrimer. In the basal state, α-subunits exist in a conformation that favors binding of the guanine nucleotide GDP. Activation occurs following agonist binding to GPCRs, which promotes the exchange of GTP for GDP binding to the α-subunit. GTP-Gα then dissociates from its $\beta\gamma$-subunits allowing free Gα and G$\beta\gamma$ to regulate a variety of intracellular signaling pathways, such as adenylyl cyclases (AC), ion channels, and components of the mitogen-activated protein kinase (MAPK) cascade (Law et al., 2000). G protein-mediated signaling is terminated by reassociation of the heterotrimer following GTP hydrolysis to GDP by enzymatic activity of the Gα-subunit (Figure 12.1). In this way, G proteins act as a molecular switch by controlling the duration of G protein-mediated signaling events (Childers, 1991; Gilman, 1987).

Studies investigating the molecular mechanisms underlying opioid dependency have revealed that many important biochemical pathways common to opioids and other addictive drugs are controlled via G protein activation. For example, chronic morphine causes upregulation of the cAMP second messenger pathway, including adenylyl cyclase (AC) and protein kinase A (PKA). This occurs in multiple neuronal cell types and is seen in several brain regions involved in addiction, such as the locus coeruleus, nucleus accumbens, and dorsal striatum (Nestler and Aghajanian, 1997). Also, the activity and/or expression level of multiple transcription factors is altered by chronic opioid exposure. These include the cAMP response element binding protein (CREB) and the immediate early gene ΔfosB, both of which correlate strongly with the behavioral and biochemical changes caused by opioid drug exposure (Guitart et al., 1992; Nye and Nestler, 1996; Unterwald et al., 1993). These drug-induced alterations in protein expression result in a vastly modified neuronal signaling environment and are considered to be important in the underlying molecular basis for behaviors associated with drugs of abuse (Chao and Nestler, 2004).

The authors acknowledge support from NIH grants DA04087 and the Biology of Substance Abuse Training Grant T32 DA007268 during the preparation of this chapter.

Regulation of Mu-Opioid Receptor Signaling

Both the short- and long-term effects of opioid drugs are the direct consequence of opioid receptor-mediated activation of G protein signaling pathways. Several key regulatory mechanisms have been identified that control the activity of opioid receptor signaling at the cellular level, which in turn dictates the overall behavioral response to opioid drugs. Recent evidence suggests that discrete proteins involved in these processes are novel targets for manipulating specific opioid effects in vitro and in vivo.

Regulation of G Protein Signaling Proteins

Regulators of G protein signaling (RGS) proteins are a family of proteins whose primary function is to control the activity of receptor-stimulated, GTP-bound Gα (Figure 12.1). Early work characterizing G protein function revealed that many G protein-regulated signaling responses in a cellular setting were deactivated at a rate that was several hundredfold faster than the GTP hydrolysis promoted by purified Gα in vitro (Gilman, 1987). This suggested that the GTP hydrolase activity of G proteins in vivo must be accelerated by an additional protein or factor. This apparent discrepancy was resolved upon the discovery of RGS proteins. These proteins are characterized by a conserved 120 amino acid "RGS" domain whose primary function is to switch off activated G proteins via direct interaction of the RGS domain with Gα subunits (Hollinger and Hepler, 2002). As a result, RGS proteins act as GTPase accelerating proteins or GAPs that negatively regulate G protein-mediated signaling.

Over 30 RGS proteins have been identified and classified into seven subfamilies according to sequence similarity and structural

Figure 12.1. Involvement of regulatory proteins in opioid signaling. Upon agonist binding, opioid receptors activate heterotrimeric G proteins by stimulating the exchange of GTP for GDP binding to Gα. GTP-Gα and free βγ dissociate and regulate various effectors. Opioid signaling is terminated when GTP is hydrolyzed by Gα leading to the reassociation of the G protein heterotrimer, a process accelerated by RGS proteins. Receptors are desensitized to continued agonist exposure by being internalized to intracellular compartments following association with β-arrestins. Interacting proteins function to modulate various aspects of receptor signaling, including G protein activation and receptor internalization.

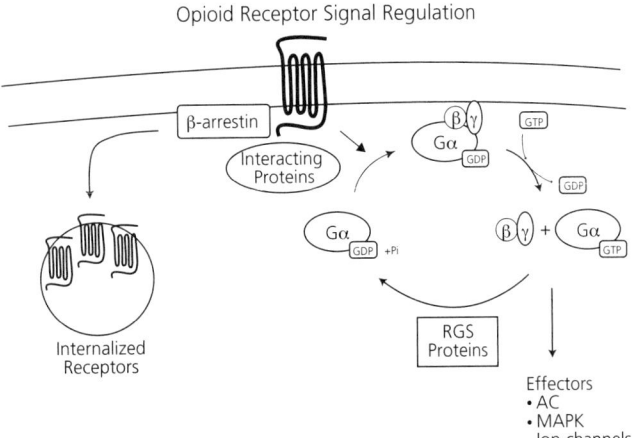

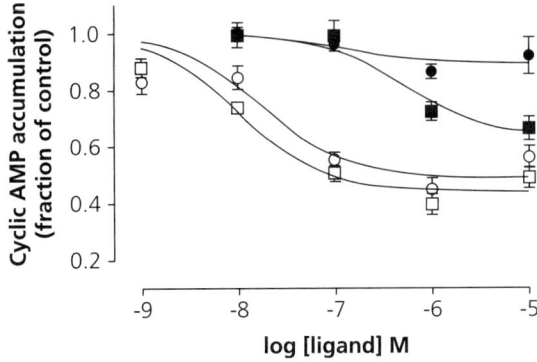

Figure 12.2. Regulators of G protein signaling proteins. Enhanced potency and efficacy of morphine (circles) or DAMGO (squares) in cells expressing the mu opioid receptor and Gαo protein that is either sensitive (filled symbols) or insensitive (open symbols) to the action of endogenous RGS proteins. Both types of Gαo protein are resistant to pertussis toxin, which is used in all cell cultures in order to inhibit endogenous Gαo activity. (Reprinted from Clark et al., 2003, with permission.)

homology (Hollinger and Hepler, 2002). RGS proteins vary extensively in size and domain architecture outside the RGS domain. For example, members of the B/R4 subfamily are mostly small proteins of 20–30 kDa consisting almost entirely of the conserved RGS domain. In contrast, members of the C/R7 subfamily are much larger, possessing multiple domains, such as DEP (disheveled, Egl-10, pleckstrin) and GGL (G protein gamma subunit-like). These motifs participate in interactions with signaling and/or structural proteins and contribute to the stability, localization, and non-GAP related functions of RGS proteins (Siderovski and Willard, 2005).

Recent work has demonstrated that many different RGS proteins alter opioid signaling. Using heterologous in vitro over-expression systems, it has been shown that RGS2 (Potenza et al., 1999), RGS4 (Garnier et al., 2003; Georgoussi et al., 2005; Hepler et al., 1997; Ippolito et al., 2002; Pil and Tytgat, 2003; Ulens et al., 2000), RGS8 (Clark et al., 2003), RGS9 (Xu et al., 2004), and GAIP/RGS19 (Elenko et al., 2003; Ito et al., 2000) manipulate opioid potency and efficacy of coupling to a variety of effectors. These include AC, MAPK, inwardly rectifying potassium channels (GIRKs) and voltage-gated calcium channels (see Xie and Palmer, 2005, for review).

The regulation of opioid signaling by endogenous RGS proteins has been resolved using modified Gα proteins. In this paradigm, the GAP effects of endogenous RGS proteins are silenced via a mutation in the region of Gα that disrupts its association with RGS proteins, without diminishing coupling to effector pathways. Expression of these RGS-insensitive Gαo proteins in C6 glioma cells stably expressing the mu opioid receptor resulted in dramatically enhanced opioid coupling to its effectors. For example, inhibition of AC by DAMGO, an opioid peptide derivative with high selectivity for the mu receptor, was increased in both potency (> tenfold) and efficacy (twofold) in cells expressing mutant Gαo (Figure 12.2). An even more striking effect was observed with morphine, which was converted from a weak partial agonist to a full agonist that was equipotent with DAMGO. Similar results were obtained for opioid stimulation of MAPK (Clark et al., 2003). Consequently, blocking the GAP effects of endogenous RGS proteins resulted in exaggerated signaling through the opioid receptor due to greatly enhanced G protein activity, showing that endogenous RGS proteins strongly influence signaling responses to opioid agonists.

Studies following manipulation of RGS activity have been conducted using animal models of opioid-induced behavior. Knockdown of individual endogenous RGS protein mRNA in mice using i.c.v. injections of antisense oligodeoxynucleotides has shown that specific RGS proteins modulate opioid-induced signaling in vivo. Morphine-induced antinociception was enhanced following knockdown of RGS9–2 and RGS12, whereas knockdown of RGS2 and RGS3 diminished morphine antinociception (Garzon et al., 2001). These findings are supported by studies using mice in which the gene for RGS9–2, the striatal-specific isoform of RGS9, has been deleted (Zachariou et al., 2003). These mice showed markedly enhanced morphine-induced antinociception compared to wild-type controls (Figure 12.3).

As expected, withdrawal behaviors associated with opioid dependence, such as jumps, paw tremors, and wet dog shakes were elevated in the knockout mice. Typically, morphine exhibits profound tolerance, in which its antinociceptive effects are rapidly and significantly reduced following repeated exposure. However, under the experimental paradigm used, RGS9 null mice exhibited almost no tolerance to morphine-induced antinociception relative to animals expressing RGS9 following chronic administration. Importantly, even more dramatic effects were seen when these mice were evaluated in a conditioned place-preference assay, which assesses the rewarding properties of drugs. In this assay, morphine was found to be tenfold more potent in RGS9 knockout mice compared to control animals (Figure 12.4), suggesting that signaling pathways that transmit the rewarding effects of morphine are significantly enhanced in mice lacking RGS9. These altered behavioral responses to morphine in knockout animals indicate that RGS9–2 influences morphine-induced behavior by negatively regulating morphine-mediated G protein activity.

The discovery that RGS proteins regulate opioid-related behaviors in vivo is consistent with studies showing a marked tissue-specific expression. Message for RGS proteins is expressed in brain regions that are rich in opioid receptors and/or are involved in the expression of opioid behaviors, such as the thalamus, striatum, nucleus accumbens, and locus coeruleus (Gold et al., 1997; Ingi and

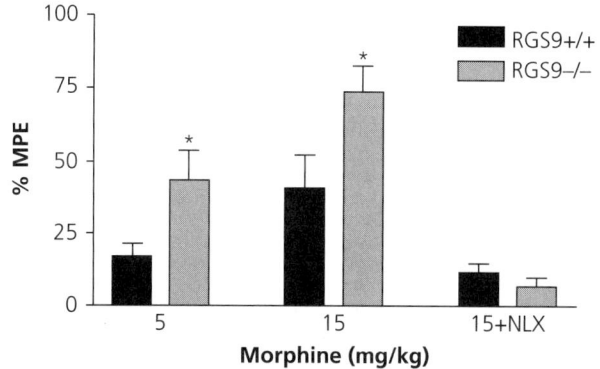

Figure 12.3. Regulators of G protein signaling proteins. Mice lacking RGS9–2 (RGS9-/-) show enhanced antinociceptive responses to morphine in the hot plate test (56°C) compared to wild-type littermates (RGS9+/+). The effect of morphine was completely blocked by the addition of the opioid antagonist naloxone (NLX; 1 mg/kg, s.c.). % MPE = percent maximal effect of morphine compared to the vehicle control. (Reprinted from Zachariou et al., 2003, with permission.)

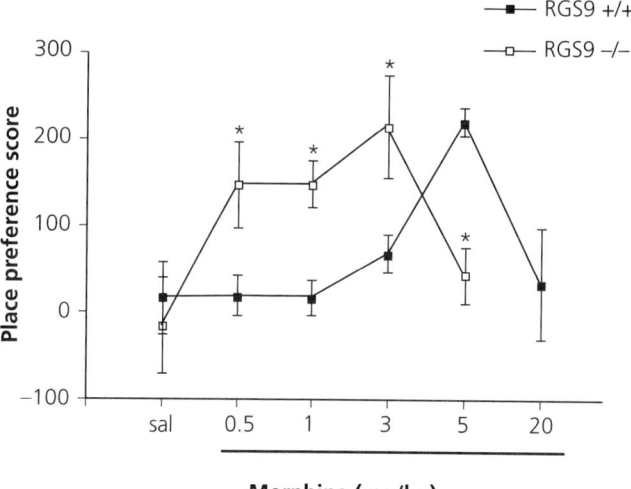

Figure 12.4. Regulators of G protein signaling proteins. RGS9–2 knockout mice (–/–; open squares) show ~ tenfold greater responsiveness to the rewarding effects of morphine (s.c.) compared to wild-type littermates (+/+; filled squares) in a place-preference conditioning assay. Scores are calculated as the difference between times spent in the drug-paired side post- versus preconditioning. (Reprinted from Zachariou et al., 2003, with permission.)

Aoki, 2002). For example, the caudate putamen and nucleus accumbens, regions within the striatum that are involved in mediating the rewarding properties of addictive drugs such as morphine, express RGS2, RGS4, RGS8, and RGS9–2. In contrast, the thalamus, which is a mu opioid receptor-rich relay station for transmitting pain information, contains RGS4, RGS7, and RGS8 but not RGS9–2 or RGS2 (Gold et al., 1997; Grafstein-Dunn et al., 2001). It is possible that the combination of individual RGS proteins provides discrete regulation of opioid signals in brain regions where opioid activation serves distinct roles. It is also important to note that acute and chronic morphine alters message for RGS2, RGS4, and RGS9–2 in the brain regions relevant to opioid signaling (Bishop et al., 2002; Gold et al., 2003; Zachariou et al., 2003).

Taken together, these findings point to an inhibitory role of endogenous RGS proteins in regulating opioid signaling in vitro and in vivo. Moreover, endogenous RGS proteins appear to dramatically alter the expression of opioid drug effects in the whole animal. Opioid coupling to AC and MAPK are strongly regulated by endogenous RGS proteins, whereas DAMGO-stimulated increases in intracellular calcium release are not, suggesting that discrete signaling pathways are more susceptible to RGS protein regulation than others (Clark et al., 2003). RGS specificity at the level of intracellular signaling suggests certain behaviors may be more sensitive to regulation by RGS proteins than others. This gives rise to the exciting possibility that modulating RGS protein activity in vivo may prevent specific, unwanted effects of opioid use without altering the beneficial antinociceptive properties of drugs such as morphine. For example, in mice lacking RGS9–2, morphine was tenfold more potent in the conditioned-place preference assay, was only 2–3 times more effective in assays for antinociception and withdrawal, and showed decreased ability to induce tolerance following chronic treatment (Zachariou et al., 2003). These significant findings give rise to the possibility of RGS proteins as viable targets for potential pain and drug abuse medications (Traynor and Neubig, 2005).

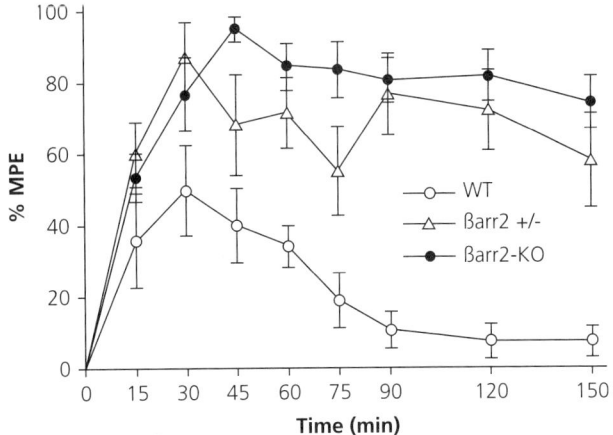

Figure 12.5. Arrestins. Mice deficient in β-arrestin 2 (heterozygous [βarr2 +/−] and knock-out [βarr2-KO] animals) show enhanced and prolonged morphine (10 mg/kg, s.c.) antinociception compared to wild-type (WT) littermate animals in the hot plate assay (56°C). % MPE = percent maximal effect of morphine compared to the vehicle control. (Reprinted from Bohn et al., 1999, with permission.)

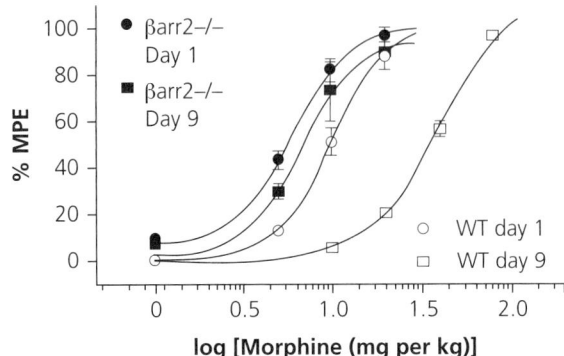

Figure 12.6. Arrestins. In antinociceptive tests (hot plate test—56°C), naïve β-arrestin 2 knockout mice (βarr2-/-) are as responsive to morphine (Day 1, filled circles; ED_{50} 5.9 mg/kg) as when treated chronically (Day 9, filled squares; ED_{50} 6.7 mg/kg), indicating a lack of morphine tolerance in these animals. In contrast, wild-type littermates (WT) expressing endogenous levels of β-arrestin 2 exhibit profound tolerance to morphine as demonstrated by the greater than threefold loss in morphine potency in mice treated chronically (Day 9, open squares; ED_{50} 39.6) compared to naïve animals (Day 1, open circles; ED_{50} 10.1). In this study, morphine was administered s.c. using a cumulative dosing regimen. % MPE = percent maximal effect of morphine compared to the vehicle control. (Reprinted with permission from Bohn et al., 2000.)

Arrestins

Shortly after agonist exposure, GPCRs rapidly lose their ability to respond to further challenges with agonist. This process of converting activated, functional receptors to the inactive state is referred to as desensitization (Gainetdinov et al., 2004), and is the culmination of several different mechanisms. Following agonist activation, receptors are phosphorylated, resulting in the partial uncoupling of the receptor from its cognate G proteins. Receptors are also removed from repeated activation by agonists at the cell surface through sequestration and internalization to intracellular compartments.

Early studies revealed that although phosphorylated receptors showed reduced function, phosphorylation alone was not sufficient for agonist-mediated desensitization. An additional cofactor or "arresting agent" was required to fully suppress receptor function. This activity was later isolated, and named arrestin (Pfister et al., 1985). To date, four arrestins have been characterized: two are associated with the visual system (rod and cone arrestins) and two are characterized as nonvisual or β-arrestins (β-arrestin 1 and β-arrestin 2; Benovic et al., 1987; Pfister et al., 1985).

Mechanistically, arrestin proteins serve at least two functions in GPCR desensitization. First, binding of both visual and nonvisual arrestins to GPCRs serves to terminate G protein-mediated signal transduction. Phosphorylation of the GPCR C-terminal tail by G protein-receptor kinases (GRKs) increases the affinity of arrestins for receptor, which results in the rapid translocation of arrestins from the cytosol to receptors in the plasma membrane. Interaction of arrestins with the mu opioid receptor sterically hinders receptor association with G proteins, which facilitates receptor uncoupling from its cognate G proteins (Ferguson, 2001).

Second, the nonvisual arrestins promote GPCR internalization through scaffolding of the receptor to machinery involved in clathrin-mediated endocytosis. For example, β-arrestin interacts with proteins that function as endocytic regulators, including clathrin (Goodman, et al., 1996), the clathrin adapter protein 2 (AP-2; Laporte et al., 1999), and N-ethylmaleimide-sensitive fusion protein (NSF; McDonald et al., 1999). Functionally, β-arrestin recruitment to the receptor following agonist-mediated phosphorylation leads to the lateral redistribution or sequestration of GPCRs into clathrin-coated pits that are endocytosed. The processes of receptor phosphorylation, uncoupling, and internalization have a compounding effect upon GPCR desensitization, in that receptors are sequestered away from signal transducers/effectors and protected from further exposure to agonist at the cell surface.

The ability of β-arrestin to alter behavioral responses to opioids has been explored using animals that lack β-arrestin 2. These knockout animals exhibited enhanced and prolonged antinociception in response to morphine compared to control animals (Figure 12.5; Bohn et al., 1999), which is consistent with in vitro studies showing that β-arrestins terminate opioid signaling (Claing et al., 2000; Zhang et al., 1998). However, further study revealed that β-arrestin 2 knockout mice exhibited very little tolerance to chronic morphine compared to control animals (Figure 12.6) despite showing a normal profile of morphine withdrawal behavior (Bohn et al., 2000). It has since been determined that genetic deletion of β-arrestin 2 also dramatically limits the respiratory suppression and constipation caused by morphine (Raehal et al., 2005).

These findings provide yet another example of how altering the activity of key regulatory proteins can alter the behaviors induced by opioid drugs. Like RGS proteins, endogenous β-arrestins appear to play an important role in determining the opioid response in vivo. In this role, the β-arrestins are also considered potential targets for drug manipulation in order to discriminate the beneficial and deleterious effects of opioid drugs (Raehal and Bohn, 2005).

Receptor Interacting/Scaffolding Proteins

Recent advances in proteomics technology have made possible the identification and characterization of proteins that interact with GPCRs via unique domain architecture and in many cases provide receptor-selective regulation of signaling (see Brady and Limbird, 2002; Hall and Lefkowitz, 2002; Milligan and White, 2001, for review). Receptor families for which regulation by scaffold/interacting proteins has been demonstrated include, but are not limited to, α_2- and β_2-adrenergic, AT_1-angiotensin, metabotropic glutamate, D_2 and D_3 dopamine, CB_1 cannabinoid, and $5\text{-}HT_{2C}$ serotonin receptors (Hall and Lefkowitz, 2002). Several proteins that interact with the mu opioid receptor have also been identified (Table 12.1). Several of these mu receptor–interacting proteins will be discussed below, including those whose effects have been characterized in vivo.

In vitro studies have shown that mu-interacting proteins regulate various intracellular signaling pathways employed by opioid receptor agonists. For example, periplakin, a structural protein that binds to actin and other cytoskeletal elements, was found to interact with the mu receptor C-terminal tail. Coexpression of periplakin with the mu receptor inhibited mu-stimulated [^{35}S]GTPγS binding but had no effect on agonist-stimulated receptor internalization (Feng et al., 2003). Another actin-associated protein, filamin A, also interacts with the mu receptor C-terminal tail. However, the filamin A/mu receptor interaction had no effect on G protein-mediated signaling of the mu receptor to AC. Rather, in cells lacking filamin A, agonist-induced receptor internalization, desensitization, and downregulation was selectively and completely abolished, suggesting filamin A is required for mu receptor trafficking (Onoprishvili et al., 2003).

These and other studies show that mu-interacting proteins often regulate distinct phases of mu receptor signaling. Yet, the physiologic function of these opioid-receptor-interacting proteins is not yet understood. Nearly all of these proteins have been identified using proteomic-based screening methodology (Guarente, 1993), and the functional consequence of protein-protein interaction with opioid receptors has been investigated almost exclusively using heterologous cell expression systems. More information is needed to determine how these proteins act in an endogenous signaling environment. These studies will undoubtedly yield valuable insight into how opioid signaling is regulated in vivo.

One such example of opioid regulation by mu receptor–interacting proteins in vivo is the protein kinase C-interacting protein (PKCI; Guang et al., 2004). As its name implies, PKCI was originally characterized by its association with and inhibition of the second messenger kinase protein kinase C (PKC). In vitro data indicate that PKCI, which interacts with the mu receptor C-terminus, negatively regulates mu receptor signaling by promoting agonist-induced desensitization of the receptor. These data suggest that PKCI negatively regulates opioid signaling, presumably by facilitating signal termination through enhanced receptor phosphorylation and internalization. Morphine produced a greater antinociceptive response in PKCI knockout mice compared to control animals, which is consistent with PKCI working to suppress opioid effects in vivo (Figure 12.7). However, it is not clear whether the effects of PKCI are the result of a direct action on the mu receptor itself or an indirect effect on other proteins such as PKC. Regardless, these data demonstrate a clear role for PKCI in regulating opioid signaling, not just at the level of intracellular signaling but also in the whole animal.

Another example has been the identification and characterization of the accessory protein RanBP9/RanBPM (RanBPM) as a modulator of mu opioid receptor signaling. RanBPM is a 90 kDa protein that contains multiple protein binding domains, such as the SPRY domain (SP1a/Ryanodine receptor), which mediates protein-protein interactions, the LiSH/CTLH motif (Lissencephaly type-1-like homology/C-terminal to LisH), which is involved in binding to microtubules, and a proline-rich N-terminus that contains multiple putative SH3-domain binding sites. The presence of these unique domains suggests that RanBPM interacts with multiple and potentially diverse groups of signaling and structural proteins. RanBPM was found to interact with the C-terminus of the mu receptor and blocked agonist-induced mu receptor endocytosis, a process that has been suggested to promote opioid tolerance and dependence (von Zastrow et al., 2003), without altering opioid-mediated inhibition of adenylyl cyclase (Talbot et al., 2004, 2005). Importantly, in rats treated with chronic morphine, RanBPM expression is completely abolished in the thalamus and is upregulated in the cortex, two brain regions involved in the manifestation of opioid-mediated behaviors (Berridge and Robinson, 2003; Chao and Nestler, 2004). These data suggest RanBPM may play a central role in regulating mu receptor signaling pathways in vivo. Preliminary data also suggests that RanBPM interacts with both the delta and kappa opioid receptors, implying that

Table 12.1. Mu-Opioid Receptor–Interacting Proteins

Interacting Protein	Site of Interaction	Function	Reference
Calmodulin*	3rd i-loop	Impaired G protein coupling	Wang et al., 1999
Filamin A	C-terminus	Receptor trafficking	Onoprishvili et al., 2003
GASP-1*	C-terminus	Receptor trafficking	Whistler et al., 2002
Periplakin*	C-terminus	Impaired G protein coupling	Feng et al., 2003
PKCI	C-terminus	Receptor desensitization	Guang et al., 2004
PLD2	C-terminus	Receptor endocytosis	Koch et al., 2003
RGS4*	C-terminus	Decreased G protein activity	Georgoussi et al., 2005
RanBPM*	C-terminus	Impaired receptor internalization	Talbot et al., 2004, 2005; Murrin and Talbot 2007

*Interaction with delta opioid receptor also demonstrated (in some cases preferred relative to the mu receptor). "3rd i-loop" indicates that the site of interaction occurs at the 3rd intracellular loop of the receptor.

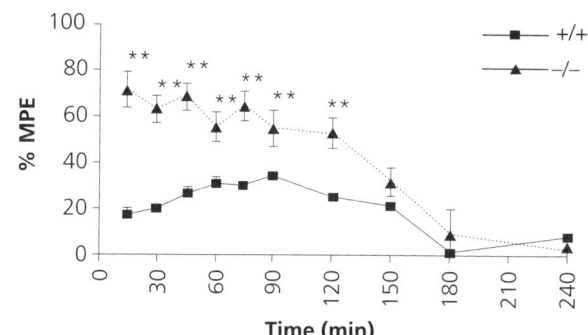

Figure 12.7. Receptor interacting/scaffolding proteins. Genetic deletion of protein kinase C-interacting protein in mice (-/-) results in enhanced but not prolonged antinociception in response to morphine (10 mg/kg, s.c.) compared to wild-type animals (+/+). The antinociceptive effects of morphine were assessed using the hot plate assay (55°C). % MPE = percent maximal effect of morphine compared to the vehicle control. (Reprinted from Guang et al., 2004, with permission.)

RanBPM may regulate the signaling properties of each of the opioid receptors.

As with RGS proteins and β-arrestin, receptor-interacting proteins such as PKCI and RanBPM regulate important aspects of opioid signaling and are potential targets for modifying the in vivo response to opioid drugs. An important property of the receptor-interacting/scaffolding proteins is that nearly all identified to date, including those that modulate the opioid receptors, display some degree of receptor selectivity. In addition, many of these proteins also modulate discrete parts of the receptor signaling pathway. These properties can potentially be exploited such that specific signaling pathways activated by a family of receptors or, in some cases, a receptor subtype can be selectively targeted. This is despite the fact that these receptors utilize redundant signaling machinery, such as those involved in G protein coupling and receptor internalization.

Summary

It is becoming increasingly clear that many beneficial and deleterious behaviors induced by morphine-like drugs, including antinociception, tolerance, dependence, and reward are distinct processes that can be differentiated through pharmacological and/or genetic means. Proteins that regulate opioid signaling such as RGS proteins, arrestins, and receptor-interacting/scaffolding proteins provide a molecular basis for these observations. The possibility of manipulating specific opioid effects may ultimately lead to improved treatments for addiction as well as improved therapy for pain, and highlight the potential of these regulatory proteins as new and potentially powerful drug targets.

References

Benovic JL, Kuhn H, Weyand I, Codina J, Caron MG, and Lefkowitz RJ (1987) Functional desensitization of the isolated beta-adrenergic receptor by the beta-adrenergic receptor kinase: potential role of an analog of the retinal protein arrestin (48-kDa protein). *Proc Natl Acad Sci USA* 84: 8879–8882.

Berridge KC and Robinson TE (2003) Parsing reward. *Trends Neurosci* 26: 507–513.

Bishop GB, Cullinan WE, Curran E, and Gutstein HB (2002) Abused drugs modulate RGS4 mRNA levels in rat brain: comparison between acute drug treatment and a drug challenge after chronic treatment. *Neurobiol Dis* 10:334–343.

Bohn LM, Gainetdinov RR, Lin FT, Lefkowitz RJ, and Caron MG (2000) Mu-opioid receptor desensitization by beta-arrestin-2 determines morphine tolerance but not dependence. *Nature* 408:720–723.

Bohn LM, Lefkowitz RJ, Gainetdinov RR, Peppel K, Caron MG, and Lin FT (1999) Enhanced morphine analgesia in mice lacking beta-arrestin 2. *Science* 286:2495–2498.

Brady AE and Limbird LE (2002) G protein-coupled receptor interacting proteins: emerging roles in localization and signal transduction. *Cell Signal* 14:297–309.

Chao J and Nestler EJ (2004) Molecular neurobiology of drug addiction. *Annu Rev Med* 55:113–132.

Childers SR (1991) Opioid receptor-coupled second messenger systems. *Life Sci* 48:1991–2003.

Claing A, Perry SJ, Achiriloaie M, Walker JK, Albanesi JP, Lefkowitz RJ, and Premont RT (2000) Multiple endocytic pathways of G protein-coupled receptors delineated by GIT1 sensitivity. *Proc Natl Acad Sci USA* 97:1119–1124.

Clark MJ, Harrison C, Zhong H, Neubig RR, and Traynor JR (2003) Endogenous RGS protein action modulates μ-opioid signaling through Gα$_o$. Effects on adenylyl cyclase, extracellular signal-regulated kinases, and intracellular calcium pathways. *J Biol Chem* 278:9418–9425.

Dhawan BN, Cesselin F, Raghubir R, Reisine T, Bradley PB, Portoghese PS, and Hamon M (1996) International Union of Pharmacology. XII. Classification of opioid receptors. *Pharmacol Rev* 48:567–592.

Elenko E, Fischer T, Niesman I, Harding T, McQuistan T, Von Zastrow M, and Farquhar MG (2003) Spatial regulation of Galphai protein signaling in clathrin-coated membrane microdomains containing GAIP. *Mol Pharmacol* 64:11–20.

Feng GJ, Kellett E, Scorer CA, Wilde J, White JH, and Milligan G (2003) Selective interactions between helix VIII of the human μ-opioid receptors and the C terminus of periplakin disrupt G protein activation. *J Biol Chem* 278:33400–33407.

Ferguson SS (2001) Evolving concepts in G protein-coupled receptor endocytosis: the role in receptor desensitization and signaling. *Pharmacol Rev* 53:1–24.

Gainetdinov RR, Premont RT, Bohn LM, Lefkowitz RJ, and Caron MG (2004) Desensitization of G protein-coupled receptors and neuronal functions. *Annu Rev Neurosci* 27:107–144.

Garnier M, Zaratin PF, Ficalora G, Valente M, Fontanella L, Rhee MH, Blumer KJ, and Scheideler MA (2003) Up-regulation of regulator of G protein signaling 4 expression in a model of neuropathic pain and insensitivity to morphine. *J Pharmacol Exp Ther* 304:1299–1306.

Garzon J, Rodriguez-Diaz M, Lopez-Fando A, and Sanchez-Blazquez P (2001) RGS9 proteins facilitate acute tolerance to mu-opioid effects. *Eur J Neurosci* 13:801–811.

Georgoussi Z, Leontiadis L, Mazarakou G, Merkouris M, Hyde K, and Hamm H (2005) Selective interactions between G protein subunits and RGS4 with the C-terminal domains of the mu- and delta-opioid receptors regulate opioid receptor signaling. *Cell Signal*.

Gilman AG (1987) G proteins: transducers of receptor-generated signals. *Annu Rev Biochem* 56:615–649.

Gold SJ, Han MH, Herman AE, Ni YG, Pudiak CM, Aghajanian GK, Liu RJ, Potts BW, Mumby SM, and Nestler EJ (2003) Regulation of RGS proteins by chronic morphine in rat locus coeruleus. *Eur J Neurosci* 17:971–980.

Gold SJ, Ni YG, Dohlman HG, and Nestler EJ (1997) Regulators of G-protein signaling (RGS) proteins: region-specific expression of nine subtypes in rat brain. *J Neurosci* 17:8024–8037.

Goodman OB, Jr., Krupnick JG, Santini F, Gurevich VV, Penn RB, Gagnon AW, Keen JH, and Benovic JL (1996) Beta-arrestin acts as a clathrin adaptor in endocytosis of the beta2-adrenergic receptor. *Nature* 383:447–450.

Grafstein-Dunn E, Young KH, Cockett MI, and Khawaja XZ (2001) Regional distribution of regulators of G-protein signaling (RGS) 1, 2, 13, 14, 16, and GAIP messenger ribonucleic acids by in situ hybridization in rat brain. *Brain Res Mol Brain Res* 88:113–123.

Guang W, Wang H, Su T, Weinstein IB, and Wang JB (2004) Role of mPKCI, a novel mu-opioid receptor interactive protein, in receptor desensitization, phosphorylation, and morphine-induced analgesia. *Mol Pharmacol* 66:1285–1292.

Guarente L (1993) Strategies for the identification of interacting proteins. *Proc Natl Acad Sci USA* 90:1639–1641.

Guitart X, Thompson MA, Mirante CK, Greenberg ME, and Nestler EJ (1992) Regulation of cyclic AMP response element-binding protein (CREB) phosphorylation by acute and chronic morphine in the rat locus coeruleus. *J Neurochem* 58:1168–1171.

Hall RA and Lefkowitz RJ (2002) Regulation of G protein-coupled receptor signaling by scaffold proteins. *Circ Res* 91:672–680.

Hepler JR, Berman DM, Gilman AG, and Kozasa T (1997) RGS4 and GAIP are GTPase-activating proteins for Gq alpha and block activation of phospholipase C beta by gamma-thio-GTP-Gq alpha. *Proc Natl Acad Sci USA* 94:428–432.

Hepler JR and Gilman AG (1992) G proteins. *Trends Biochem Sci* 17:383–387.

Hollinger S and Hepler JR (2002) Cellular regulation of RGS proteins: modulators and integrators of G protein signaling. *Pharmacol Rev* 54:527–559.

Ingi T and Aoki Y (2002) Expression of RGS2, RGS4 and RGS7 in the developing postnatal brain. *Eur J Neurosci* 15:929–936.

Ippolito DL, Temkin PA, Rogalski SL, and Chavkin C (2002) N-terminal tyrosine residues within the potassium channel Kir3 modulate GTPase activity of Galphai. *J Biol Chem* 277:32692–32696.

Ito E, Xie G, Maruyama K, and Palmer PP (2000) A core-promoter region functions bi-directionally for human opioid-receptor-like gene ORL1 and its 5'-adjacent gene GAIP. *J Mol Biol* 304:259–270.

Koch T, Brandenburg LO, Schulz S, Liang Y, Klein J, and Hollt V (2003) ADP-ribosylation factor-dependent phospholipase D2 activation is required for agonist-induced μ-opioid receptor endocytosis. *J Biol Chem* 278:9979–9985.

Kreek MJ, LaForge KS, and Butelman E (2002) Pharmacotherapy of addictions. *Nat Rev Drug Discov* 1:710–726.

Laporte SA, Oakley RH, Zhang J, Holt JA, Ferguson SS, Caron MG, and Barak LS (1999) The beta2-adrenergic receptor/betaarrestin complex recruits the clathrin adaptor AP-2 during endocytosis. *Proc Natl Acad Sci USA* 96:3712–3717.

Law PY, Wong YH, and Loh HH (2000) Molecular mechanisms and regulation of opioid receptor signaling. *Annu Rev Pharmacol Toxicol* 40:389–430.

Matthes HW, Maldonado R, Simonin F, Valverde O, Slowe S, Kitchen I, Befort K, Dierich A, Le Meur M, Dolle P, Tzavara E, Hanoune J, Roques BP, and Kieffer BL (1996) Loss of morphine-induced analgesia, reward effect and withdrawal symptoms in mice lacking the mu-opioid-receptor gene. *Nature* 383:819–823.

McDonald PH, Cote NL, Lin FT, Premont RT, Pitcher JA, and Lefkowitz RJ (1999) Identification of NSF as a beta-arrestin1-binding protein. Implications for beta2-adrenergic receptor regulation. *J Biol Chem* 274:10677–10680.

Milligan G and White JH (2001) Protein-protein interactions at G-protein-coupled receptors. *Trends Pharmacol Sci* 22:513–518.

Nestler EJ and Aghajanian GK (1997) Molecular and cellular basis of addiction. *Science* 278:58–63.

Nye HE and Nestler EJ (1996) Induction of chronic Fos-related antigens in rat brain by chronic morphine administration. *Mol Pharmacol* 49:636–645.

Onoprishvili I, Andria ML, Kramer HK, Ancevska-Taneva N, Hiller JM and Simon EJ (2003) Interaction between the μ opioid receptor and filamin A is involved in receptor regulation and trafficking. *Mol Pharmacol* 64:1092–1100.

Pfister C, Chabre M, Plouet J, Tuyen VV, De Kozak Y, Faure JP, and Kuhn H (1985) Retinal S antigen identified as the 48K protein regulating light-dependent phosphodiesterase in rods. *Science* 228:891–893.

Pil J and Tytgat J (2003) Serine 329 of the mu-opioid receptor interacts differently with agonists. *J Pharmacol Exp Ther* 304:924–930.

Potenza MN, Gold SJ, Roby-Shemkowitz A, Lerner MR and Nestler EJ (1999) Effects of regulators of G protein-signaling proteins on the functional response of the μ-opioid receptor in a melanophore-based assay. *J Pharmacol Exp Ther* 291:482–491.

Raehal KM and Bohn LM (2005) Mu opioid receptor regulation and opiate responsiveness. *AAPS J* 7:E587-E591.

Raehal KM, Walker JK, and Bohn LM (2005) Morphine side effects in beta-arrestin 2 knockout mice. *J Pharmacol Exp Ther* 314:1195–1201.

Siderovski DP and Willard FS (2005) The GAPs, GEFs, and GDIs of heterotrimeric G-protein alpha subunits. *Int J Biol Sci* 1:51–66.

Sora I, Takahashi N, Funada M, Ujike H, Revay RS, Donovan DM, Miner LL, and Uhl GR (1997) Opiate receptor knockout mice define mu receptor roles in endogenous nociceptive responses and morphine-induced analgesia. *Proc Natl Acad Sci USA* 94:1544–1549.

Talbot JN, Toews ML, and Murrin LC (2004) The effects of RanBPM on agonist-mediated endocytosis of the mu opioid receptor. *FASEB J* 18 Abstract #399.13

Talbot JN, Toews ML, and Murrin LC (2005) Regulation of mu opioid receptor internalization by the accessory protein RanBPM. *FASEB J* 19 Abstract # 635.7.

Traynor JR and Neubig RR (2005) Regulators of G protein signaling & drugs of abuse. *Mol Interv* 5:30–41.

Ulens C, Daenens P, and Tytgat J (2000) Changes in GIRK1/GIRK2 deactivation kinetics and basal activity in the presence and absence of RGS4. *Life Sci* 67:2305–2317.

Unterwald EM, Cox BM, Kreek MJ, Cote TE, and Izenwasser S (1993) Chronic repeated cocaine administration alters basal and opioid-regulated adenylyl cyclase activity. *Synapse* 15:33–38.

von Zastrow M, Svingos A, Haberstock-Debic H, and Evans C (2003) Regulated endocytosis of opioid receptors: cellular mechanisms and proposed roles in physiological adaptation to opiate drugs. *Curr Opin Neurobiol* 13:348–353.

Wang D, Sadee W, and Quillan JM (1999) Calmodulin binding to G protein-coupling domain of opioid receptors. *J Biol Chem* 274:22081–22088.

Whistler JL, Enquist J, Marley A, Fong J, Gladher F, Tsuruda P, Murray SR, and von Zastrow M (2002) Modulation of postendocytic sorting of G protein-coupled receptors. *Science* 297:615–620.

Xie GX and Palmer PP (2005) RGS proteins: new players in the field of opioid signaling and tolerance mechanisms. *Anesth Analg* 100:1034–1042.

Xu H, Wang X, Wang J, and Rothman RB (2004) Opioid peptide receptor studies. 17. Attenuation of chronic morphine effects after antisense oligodeoxynucleotide knock-down of RGS9 protein in cells expressing the cloned Mu opioid receptor. *Synapse* 52:209–217.

Zachariou V, Georgescu D, Sanchez N, Rahman Z, DiLeone R, Berton O, Neve RL, Sim-Selley LJ, Selley DE, Gold SJ, and Nestler EJ (2003) Essential role for RGS9 in opiate action. *Proc Natl Acad Sci USA* 100:13656–13661.

Zhang J, Ferguson SS, Barak LS, Bodduluri SR, Laporte SA, Law PY, and Caron MG (1998) Role for G protein-coupled receptor kinase in agonist-specific regulation of mu-opioid receptor responsiveness. *Proc Natl Acad Sci USA* 95:7157–7162.

13

"Impulsology"
A New Paradigm for Addiction

Kara Lee Shirley

Lisa J. Norelli

Howard S. Smith

Every form of addiction is bad, no matter whether the narcotic be alcohol or morphine or idealism.
—Carl Gustav Jung, *Memories, Dreams, Reflections*, 1973, p. 329

Addiction is a chronic relapsing disease in which compulsive seeking and participation persist despite serious negative consequences (Camí et al., 2003). Participation of the addictive behavior often induces euphoria in initiation phase, or may significantly relieve stress (Camí et al., 2003). Continued participation in the addictive behavior can lead to adaptive changes within the central nervous system that can lead to tolerance, physical dependence, sensitization, craving, and relapse (Camí et al., 2003; see Figure 13.1).

Addiction closely resembles other chronic relapsing disease states such as diabetes, asthma, and hypertension (Heilig et al., 2006). Although it is inappropriate to forgo the social and behavioral context of addiction, this is consistent with the therapeutic approach of other chronic relapsing disease states. Unfortunately, addiction is viewed by many to result from deficits in character such as "willpower," not amenable to comprehensive medical care (Heilig et al., 2006). The impulsive nature of addictive behavior renders the disease susceptible to societal judgment of patient character. Character judgment is often based upon the social and legal acceptance of the addictive behavior, rather than the multifaceted consequences of the behavior itself.

> You do anything long enough to escape the habit of living until the escape becomes the habit. (David Ryan, actor)

Impulsivity, as a psychopathological construct, is typically defined along either behavioral or personality lines. Pathological impulsivity can be evident via both discreet acts and interactive patterns such as verbal and physical aggression, hostility, recklessness, risk taking, and sensation seeking.

There is a paucity of data exploring the use of "impulsivity" measurements as predictors for addiction risk assessment, but the neurobiological and psychological underpinnings common to impulsivity, pain, and addiction are strongly suggestive of this as an important and perhaps a key paradigm. Therefore we propose a clinical addiction paradigm inclusive of maladaptive impulsive behaviors that provide the participant with euphoria and or significant relief.

We coin the term of "impulsology" (Smith et al., 2006) to unify the examination of sensation seeking and/or chemical coping behaviors (see Chapter 35, "Chemical Coping: The Clinical Middle Ground," this volume) that yield stress reduction for the participant. As described by Smith and colleagues (2006), reward behaviors inclusive to the spectrum of "impulsology" include, but are not limited to, the following: substance use, chemical dependency, self-starvation, binge eating, compulsive gambling, compulsive shopping, compulsive sexual activity, compulsive working, compulsive Internet use, compulsive video gaming, tics, and self-harm, including self-mutilation. In clinical illustration of impulsology, we will focus upon the screening and evidence-based pharmacotherapy of neuropsychiatric behaviors within our paradigm.

Addiction and Learning

Less than 2 decades ago, dopamine was perceived as a hedonic signal, with dependence and withdrawal for the propulsion of compulsive behaviors (Hyman, 2006). Our brain's dopamine circuitry provides a "common currency" for the evaluation of exogenous as well as endogenous rewards (Hyman, 2005, 2006). Rewards stimulate the release of dopamine from the neurons of the presynaptic ventral tegmental area into the nucleus accumbens, inducing subsequent reinforcement of the behavior (Camí et al., 2003). The primary difference is that the exogenously rewarding impulsive behavior, such as compulsive gambling, shopping, self-harm, and so forth, serves no appropriate biological purpose.

Dopamine appears to mediate the consequences of a reinforcing behavior, self-promoting associative learning about the behavior and its anticipated effects (Camí et al., 2003). Rewards subject to manipulation, such as impulsive drug use, may have an advantage over endogenous stimuli in that they may produce more reward intensity, duration, and frequency (Hyman, 2005, 2006).

Physical as well as emotional stress may also modify the ability of dopamine cells for autoregulation (Marinelli et al., 2006). The potential autoregulation of dopamine-producing cells may enhance their sensitivity to excitation and therefore potential reward response (Marinelli et al., 2006). The emotional and physical stress of chronic pain, and the subsequent vulnerability for impulsive behaviors, may be directly related to alterations in dopamine

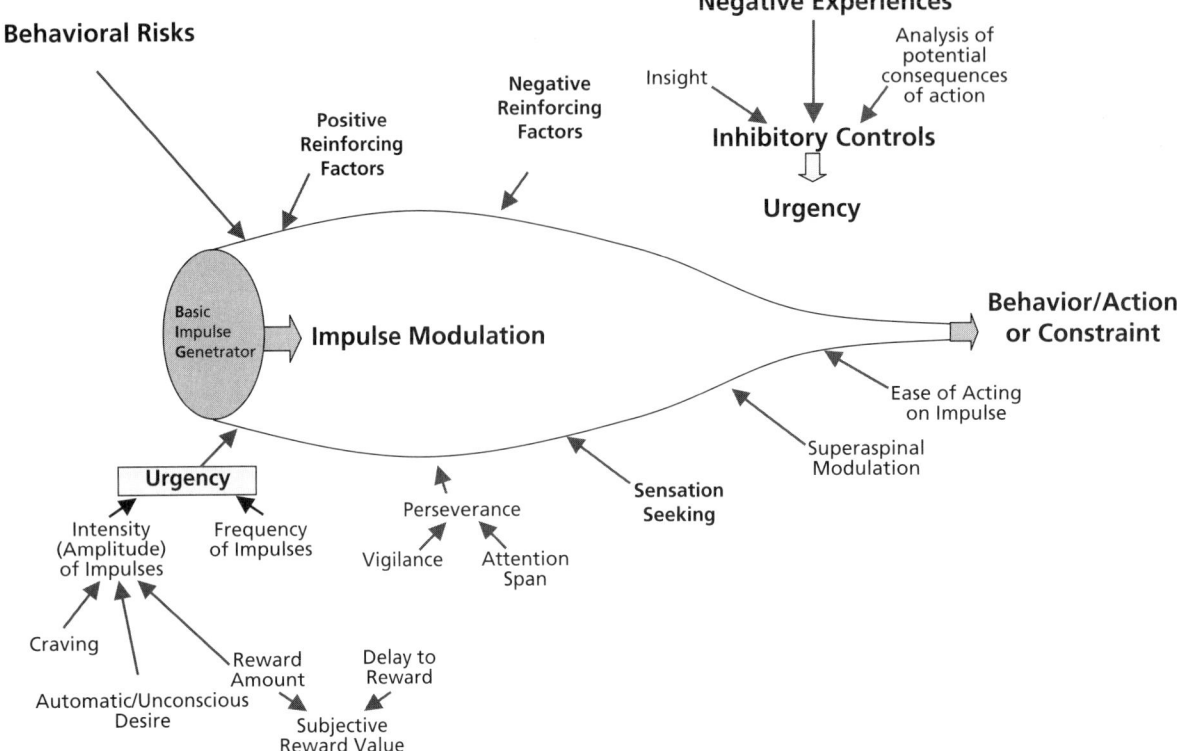

Figure 13.1. Basic impulse generator (BIG).

autoregulation and reward memory. Addiction clearly involves selection-making processes, which gradually narrow down and prioritize the reward-producing behavior (Hyman, 2005, 2006). Our selection-making processes and normal dopamine-related learning are disrupted by addictive behaviors. Addictive behaviors would produce a potent but highly distorted signal, disrupting normal activity within the prefrontal cortex as well as the nucleus accumbens and dorsal striatum (Hyman, 2005, 2006). The precise manner in which substances disrupt dopamine signaling in different circuits, as well as the functional and neuroplastic consequences of the disruption itself, have yet to be fully elucidated (Hyman, 2005, 2006).

In an individual who develops an addiction, excessive dopamine exposure may affect neuronal plasticity such that response to natural cues may diminish and fail to influence healthy goal selection (see Figure 13.1). Worthy of mention is that initial neuroimaging studies of addicted patients have reported abnormal activation patterns within the cingulate cortex and orbital prefrontal cortex (Goldstein et al., 2002; Kaufman et al., 2003; Volkow et al., 2000).

Our current understanding of dopamine's role within reward learning, as well as stimulus action learning, has important implication for the neurodevelopment of addiction (Hyman, 2005, 2006). Availability cues that predict reward become overprioritized through dopamine actions in the nucleus accumbens and prefrontal cortex, perhaps intensifying urgency (Hyman, 2005, 2006). Reward-seeking strategies would be powerfully reinforced within the prefrontal cortex and dorsal striatum by point-to-point excitatory neurotransmission (Hyman, 2005, 2006).

Persistence of addiction is characteristic of synaptic remodeling characteristic of long-term memory (Hyman, 2005, 2006). Substance-induced alteration in gene expression and/or protein translation is a significant theoretical approach for the physical remodeling of dendrites, axons, and synapses (Hyman, 2005, 2006). The longest lived molecular alteration known to occur in response to addictive stimuli is the upregulation of posttranslationally modified forms of delta-Fos-B (ΔFosB; Hyman, 2005, 2006).

Conversely, the activation of dopamine D^1 receptors instigates transient gene expression (minutes to hours) via transcription factors, including that of CREB, or cyclic AMP response element binding protein (Hyman, 2005, 2006). Chronic activation of opioid receptors produces effects opposite to those of acute activation (Camí et al., 2003).

Possibly bridging the gap between short-term and long-term addiction potentiation is the transcription factor CREB. CREB is activated by and can respond to both the cyclic AMP and Ca^{2+} dependent pathways (Hyman, 2005, 2006). The duality of CREB permits its possible function as a "coincidence detector," and as a candidate for both associative memory and long-term potentiation (Hyman, 2005, 2006).

The prodynorphin gene is a CREB-regulated target gene that may be involved in tolerance as well as dependence (Hyman, 2005, 2006). The prodynorphin gene encodes for endogenous opioid peptides, which include kappa opioid receptors agonists (Hyman, 2005, 2006). Cocaine and/or amphetamine administration stimulates dopamine-1 [D^1] receptors within the nucleus accumbens and dorsal striatum, thereby leading to CREB phosphorylation and activation of prodynorphin gene expression. Dynorphin then inhibits the release of dopamine from midbrain terminals, thereby decreasing responsiveness of dopamine systems (Hyman, 2005, 2006). Dynorphin induction may play a key role in certain pain states, substance dependence, and withdrawal development via kappa opioid receptors and other targets (Hyman, 2005, 2006). It is thought that kappa receptor activation via dynorphin production contributes to the negative emotions present during the early phases of abstinence (Camí et al., 2003).

Repeated exposure to endogenous or exogenous addictive chemicals sensitizes laboratory animals to reward response (Camí et al., 2003). Long-lasting alterations within the functional activity of mesocorticolimbic dopamine system occur with behavioral sensitization. These alterations include glutamate and dopamine transmission in the nucleus accumbens (Camí et al., 2003; Hyman, 2005, 2006). Even a single dose of mechanistically unique addictive substances produces similar degrees of enhancement in the strength of glutamate excitatory synapses (AMPA-sensitive glutamate receptors) on dopaminergic neurons within the ventral tegmental area (Camí et al., 2003). Genes expressed downstream from ΔFosB may be candidates for amplifying reward intensity and response to reward-related cues (Hyman, 2005, 2006). Impulsive behaviors that produce an endogenous reward (e.g., opioid peptides), may also induce behavioral sensitization of reward and enhance the learning of addiction (Papageorgiou et al., 2003).

By an indirect mechanism of decreased GABA inhibitory interneurons in the ventral tegmental area of the nucleus accumbens, opioids release dopamine (Camí et al., 2003). The reward and physical dependence of opioids is mediated by the activation of mu receptors because reinforcement is blocked by selective receptor antagonists (Camí et al., 2003).

The level of compulsivity and obsessiveness in opioid-dependent patients has been estimated to exceed 12%, which is over 4 times the rate of obsessive-compulsive disorder in general (Papageorgiou et al., 2003). An intimate relationship exists between opiate receptors and brain dopamine, a neurotransmitter implicated in obsessive-compulsive disorder (OCD) and opiate addiction (Papageorgiou et al., 2003). When compared to healthy controls, adult OCD patients have elevated prodynorphin (dynorphin precursor) serum antibodies (Papageorgiou et al., 2003). Elevated prodynorphin antibodies may infer decreased midbrain dopamine inhibition of addictive behaviors (Mathon et al., 2005; Smith et al., 2006). Neurophysiologic studies indicate that working memory (WM) deficits of the prefrontal cortex may be involved in recreational and clinical opioid dependence as well as OCD (Papageorgiou et al., 2003).

Memory disorders are often thought of as exclusive conditions of loss, rather than dysfunction. However, the brain may integrate too much information, too powerfully, as with patients with posttraumatic stress disorder (PTSD). In fact, it is hypothesized that those with PTSD may have an intrinsic potentiation for reward, due to pathophysiologic involvement of the hypothalamic-pituitary axis (HPA) as well as autoregulation of dopamine and norephinephrine (Yehuda, 2005).

There is a growing body of literature linking noradrenergic activation to the physiologic as well as behavioral consequences of stress (see Chapter 16, "Methadone Pharmacology in Pain and Addiction," this volume; Lee et al., 2004). Yohimbine increases norephinephrine release and firing rate, and is used as a challenge in patients with anxiety disorders such as PTSD (Lee et al., 2004). Yohimbine, an alpha-2 receptor antagonist, is known to be anxiogenic and induce stress-related responses in humans as well as animals (Lee et al., 2004). As shown in one prospective primate investigation, pharmacological blockade of alpha-2 receptors with yohimbine can induce reinstatement of cocaine-seeking behavior and characteristic stress responses (Lee et al., 2004).

"Pathways of Impulsivity"

Behavioral decision-making, consisting of processes involved with the selection of an action/behavior from a set of available options, may be part of a homeostatic process (Paulus, 2007). Impulsivity has been considered to be in the spectrum of behavioral decision-making dysfunction, selecting options that are either nonoptimal or nonhomeostatic (Paulus, 2007). Human behavior decision-making generally only makes sense within a social environment. Social exchange can directly impact the brain's reward system and the normally well-balanced interplay between brain regions that exists in decision-making processing (Sanfrey, 2007). The frontopolar cortex (FPC), the most anterior part of the frontal lobes, appears to form the apex of the executive system for behavioral decision-making. The function and connectivity of the FPC/anterior prefrontal cortex seems efficient in protecting the execution of long-term mental plans from immediate environmental demands and in generating new, possibly more rewarding, behavioral or cognitive sequences (e.g., delayed gratification) (Koechlin, 2007). The dorsolateral prefrontal cortex (DLPFC) appears essential in conflict detection/resolution processes (Mansouri, 2007).

Increased risk-taking behavior in drug addicts, for example, although maladaptive in the generic sense, may actually be considered somewhat "adaptive" for the substance user in a complex, highly unpredictable environment while attempting to resolve conflict and respond to urges and cravings (Stern, 2007).

It appears that there may be multiple pathways by which impulsive behaviors may arise. Normally, when presented with difficult, complex behavioral decisions the subthalamic nucleus initiates a "pause" message to other parts of the brain to allow more time to carefully consider the options. Deep brain stimulation (DBS) appears to interfere with this "pause" signal, potentially leading to hasty choices (Frank, 2007). Alternatively, drugs that boost dopamine levels may trigger impulsivity by interfering with the ability to learn from bad experiences/mistakes (Frank, 2007). Drugs that elevate dopamine levels do not affect the speed of decisions but do reduce the patients' tendency to avoid bad choices that had burned them in the past (e.g., persistent gambling despite repeated losses) (Miller, 2007; Frank, 2007).

Functional Pharmacotherapy of Relief-Seeking Behavior

Published literature of patient-oriented, evidence-based addiction medicine appears to be somewhat proportional to the social acceptability, as well as the medical consequences, of the relief-seeking behavior itself. Currently, the majority of evidence-based pharmacotherapy publications are within the study of nicotine and/or tobacco smoking cessation.

Smoking

Cigarette smoking remains the leading preventable cause of illness and premature death, with a claimed annual mortality rate of 438,000 (Jorenby et al., 2006). Each year, approximately 41% of smokers in the United States try to quit smoking. However, approximately 10% percent of those who try achieve long-term abstinence (Gonzales et al., 2006; Jorenby et al., 1999). Currently there are seven pharmacotherapies approved by the U.S. Food and Drug Administration, five of which are nicotine-replacement products.

Bupropion is an aminoketone antidepressant (Bupropion SR, Zyban SR) that is FDA labeled for the pharmacotherapy of smoking cessation. It is thought that bupropion's dopamine reuptake blocking effect within the mesolimbic dopamine system (reward center) may precipitate resultant increase in smoking cessation. As compared with placebo for long-term abstinence, efficacy odds ratios of bupropion SR ranged from 1.43 to 2.13 according to meta-analyses (Jorenby et al., 2006). With respect to long-term abstinence, bupropion may have greater efficacy, particularly in those patients with comorbid mood disorders (Jorenby et al., 1999). In contrast to bupropion, nicotine replacement therapies therapeutically focus upon the acute or short-term effects of withdrawal itself. Antidepressants, in general, are known to have a long-term effect upon neuroplasticity in patients with mood and anxiety disorders (Hyman, 2005, 2006). Once could also speculate that as an antidepressant, bupropion may address neurochemical mechanisms that result in relapse. Bupropion may accomplish this through its effects on neuroplasticity of midbrain dopaminergic neurons as well as other neurobiological possibilities too numerous for the context of this chapter.

Vareniciline (Chantrix) is our newest FDA-labeled addition to our pharmacotherapy arsenal. Vareniciline is a partial agonist at the alpha-4 beta-2 nicotinic acetylcholine receptor (Jorenby et al., 2006). Nicotine exerts its positive reinforcement by acting on alpha-4 beta-2 nicotinic acetylcholine receptors of the dopamine cells in the ventral tegmental area (Camí et al., 2003). Nicotine may also sensitize alpha-7 nicotinic acetylcholine receptors located on glutamate terminals (Camí et al., 2003). Vareniciline (Chantrix) therefore has the therapeutic potential of reducing withdrawal symptoms as an agonist, as well as reducing the rewarding properties of nicotine as an antagonist (Jorenby et al., 2006). The effects of vareniciline (Chantrix) upon alpha-7 nicotinic receptors located on glutamate terminals have not been published to date; therefore no comment can be made with respect to possible decreased in behavioral sensitization.

A randomized double-blind placebo controlled trial of vareniciline (Chantrix), Bupropion SR, and placebo was conducted at 14 research centers with a 12-week treatment and 52-week follow-up period (Jorenby et al., 2006). As compared against placebo and Bupropion SR, the odds of quitting with vareniciline (Chantrix) were significantly greater than with Bupropion SR (OR = 1.90, CI 95%, $p < .001$) or placebo (OR = 3.85, CI 95%, $p < .001$; Jorenby et al., 2006). The most common adverse effect of vareniciline (Chantrix) was nausea at 29.4%. Tolerability to vareniciline (Chantrix) was comparable to that of Bupropion SR with similar treatment discontinuation rates. Of note, the dropout rate was higher in the placebo group and the overall rate of discontinuation due to adverse events was 10.1%, adding weight to the tolerability of vareniciline (Chantrix; Jorenby et al., 2006).

Impulsive Behavior and Pharmacotherapeutic Strategies

Alcoholism is a major public health problem and, in many ways, closely resembles other chronic relapsing medical conditions (Heilig and Egli, 2006). As with other addictions, at least two pathophysiologic dimensions of its symptomatology are pharmacologically targetable (Heilig and Egli, 2006): (1) early reinforcement and (2) long-term neuroadaptive changes that may potentiate the development of impulsive behaviors into learned addiction (Smith et al., 2006). The objective of any treatment strategy (pharmacotherapy and neurobehavioral) is to modulate the dysregulated motivations and cognitions within methods, which will assist the patient in reclaiming their ability to self-regulate, thereby decreasing his or her physical and emotional vulnerability to addiction (Heilig and Egli, 2006). Treatment development efforts targeting relapse prevention and long-term neuroadaptation are gradually coming to preclinical fruition (Heilig and Egli, 2006).

Preexisting genetic susceptibility factors are clearly present in many addictions (Heilig and Egli, 2006; Smith et al., 2006). Genetic factors are important for the initiation phase of addiction learning and may also contribute to the long-term neuroadaptation associated with the addiction disease process (Heilig and Egli, 2006). As previously mentioned, consumption/behavior frequency may also induce sensitization of neuroexcitability associated with learning and long-term memory. Lastly, the third category of potential treatments lies within the highly complex interactions of stress and reward response.

Our first generation of pharmacotherapy strategies has focused on the prevention of short-term reward from relief-seeking behavior. These modalities include disulfiram and naltrexone, although their mechanisms of action are each quite different. Since the development of disulfiram, we have learned that it does not directly or positively target the core of alcohol dependence and it is viewed as an outdated, even inappropriate, treatment approach (Heilig and Elgi, 2006).

Alcohol administration leads to the release of endogenous opioid peptides and subsequent mesolimbic (reward center) dopamine release. Acute activation of mesolimbic dopamine release positively contributes to reinforcing properties of endogenous and exogenous substances, both involved with relief-seeking behaviors (Kreek et al., 2002; Smith et al., 2006). It has been demonstrated that mice devoid of mu receptors do not self-administer alcohol (Roberts et al., 2000).

Originally developed for the treatment of opioid dependence, naltrexone is an antagonist at opioid receptors with relative selectivity for the mu opioid receptor at lower doses (Heilig and Egli, 2006). Theoretically, naltrexone would be most beneficial to those patients whose disease is predominately characterized by reward craving, although no direct or circumstantial evidence supports this concept (Heilig and Egli, 2006).

Initial efficacy for naltrexone in alcohol addiction was published in 1992 (O'Malley et al., 1992). Clinical evidence for naltrexone has been reproduced in numerous trials, recently reviewed via meta-analysis with unequivocally positive results (Heilig and Egli, 2006; Srisurapont and Jarusurian, 2005). Based upon its mechanism of action (MOA) as well as preclinical data, naltrexone has been examined for relief-seeking behaviors that may be associated with the release of endogenous opioid peptides. Published clinical data currently include, but are not exclusive to, self-harm, self-mutilation, Lesch-Nyhan syndrome, tics and tic disorders, as well as pathological gambling. The potential efficacy of naltrexone in such disorders remains to be determined in additional scientifically rigorous studies.

Our second generation of treatment strategies is focused upon the prevention of long-term neuroadaptation associated with addiction "learning." These treatment modalities include, but are not exclusive to, acamprosate (Campral) and ondansteron (Zofran). Acamprosate is a compound that may modulate acute as well as long-term potentiation via attenuation of NMDA signaling secondary to actions at several glutamatergic sites (Heilig and Egli, 2006). Acamprosate may steady the progression of glutamatergic excitation, which occurs with repeated cycles of intoxication and withdrawal (COMBINE Study Research Group, 2003). Acamprosate alone has not fared well in follow-up COMBINE data (Donovan et al., 2008).

An exquisite illustration of acamprosate's ability to stabilize a glutamatergic state was recently generated (Spanagel et al., 2005). Null-mutation of the "clock gene per 2" results in attenuated expression of a glutamate transporter termed GLAST, resulting in elevated glutamate levels and rodent alcohol consumption (Spanagel et al., 2005). The clinical efficacy of acamprosate is well-documented in meta-analyses of available studies (Mann et al., 2004). Possible limitations for the use of acamprosate include the large doses required, dosage regimen (2 tablets taken 3 times a day), and its narrower pharmacologic focus (Heilig and Egli, 2006).

Ondansetron was initially developed as a preventative antinausea agent, and it was observed preclinically that ondansetron also suppressed several measures of alcohol consumption in laboratory animals (Tomkins et al., 1995). Interestingly, when Johnson and colleagues studied ondansetron pharmacotherapy within an alcohol dependent population, only the early-onset group, not the late-onset group, reported a robust reduction in drinking (Cloninger et al., 1991; Johnson et al., 2000). Within this investigation, drinking correlated with subjective craving, supportive of ondansetron's efficacy via suppression of the learned "reward-craving" response (Heilig and Egli, 2006; Johnson et al., 2000).

Not surprisingly, ondansetron pharmacotherapy has also been examined for possible efficacy in binge-eating disorders, Tourette's syndrome, and other tic disorders, as well as pathological gambling and other relief-seeking behaviors. However, yet again the potential efficacy of ondansetron in such disorders remains to be determined in additional scientifically rigorous studies.

Similar to acamprosate, topiramate (Topamax) has an extremely complex mechanism of action that has not been fully elucidated. Proposed mechanisms of action include, but are not limited to, the following: antagonism of glutamatergic transmission AMPA receptors and potentiation of GABA signaling (Heilig and Egli, 2006). Based upon what we do understand regarding topiramate's MOA, it has been postulated that it may provide neuroprotection against the acute as well as long-term neuromodulation associated with the "learning" of addiction (Heilig and Egli, 2006; Smith et al., 2006). In preliminary investigations, topiramate pharmacotherapy has been shown to show reductions in drinking (in early- as well as late-onset alcoholics), smoking secondary to drinking, and binging/purging with binge eating Disorder (BED; Johnson et al., 2003; 2005; McElroy et al., 2004).

In contrast to agents discussed previously, topiramate offers promise with respect to the pharmacotherapy of acute as well as long-term self-regulation. Not only has it shown initial promise within several types of addictions, it may also be the most patient-accessible with respect to tolerability, cost, and provision of care. However, long-term efficacy and safety of topiramate remain either to be determined or duplicated in additional scientifically rigorous studies. However, topiramate does provide an invaluable clinical illustration for the strategic drug development and the pharmacologic modulation of reward-seeking behaviors.

Strategic development of novel pharmacotherapy is imperative to advance the comprehensive treatment of addictions. At the heart of drug development, discovery of neurobiological underpinnings is essential. We must elucidate the molecular mechanisms by which impulsive relief-seeking behaviors are consolidated into urgency, frequency, persistent and compulsive use, as well as the molecular mechanisms by which impulsive coping cues come to control behavior (Hyman, 2005, 2006).

Clinical Approach

Impulsivity is a complex trait encompassing a range of emotional experience and behavioral expression. This includes subjective emotional experience and reactivity to the environment, relative inhibition or disinhibition of emotional and behavioral responses, and accompanying verbal and physical behaviors. However, in its maladaptive connotation, impulsivity is typically defined as reckless activity without thinking and without regard for consequences.

An individual's relative propensity toward impulsivity is one of the central features of temperament or personality. Traits such as these help define who we are as individuals and shade the range of normal human personality. When traits become maladaptive, the result may be functional interference or violation of societal norms. Maladaptive personality traits, along with their associated emotional states and behaviors, are deemed pathological.

The two most widely used psychiatric classification systems, *The Diagnostic and Statistical Manual for Mental Disorders* (*DSM-IV-TR*; American Psychiatric Association, 2000) and the *ICD-10 Classification of Mental and Behavioural Disorders* (*ICD-10*; World Health Organization, 1992), each contain over 10 disorders with impulsivity as a diagnostic element. For example, impulsivity is a common symptom in psychoactive substance use disorders, bipolar disorders, personality disorders (*DSM-IV-TR*'s antisocial personality disorder, borderline personality disorder, or *ICD-10*'s dissocial personality disorder, emotionally unstable personality disorder), and impulse control disorders in *DSM-IV-TR* or habit and impulse disorders in *ICD-10* (e.g., intermittent explosive disorder, pathological gambling, pyromania). Compared to the general population, individuals with many of these psychiatric disorders possessing impulsivity as a feature have higher rates of comorbid psychoactive substance misuse.

There is evidence that impulsive traits could be additive in these coexisting conditions. For example, Swann et al. (2004) found increased Barratt Impulsiveness Scale scores in bipolar disorder patients between episodes with a comorbid history of substance abuse compared to patients without substance abuse. In addition, patients with substance dependence alone, without a comorbid psychiatric disorder, have higher rates of impulsivity as measured by high tendency toward novelty seeking and a low tendency toward harm avoidance and reward dependence (Bond et al., 2004; Wills et al., 2004).

An extensive discussion of assessing patients with chronic pain and their risk for substance abuse appears in this volume (see Chapter 47, "Screening for the Risk of Substance Abuse in Pain Management"). The general psychosocial risk factors for opioid misuse will help guide the clinician in assessing and monitoring the individual patient. Admittedly, there is a need for more precise predictive tests for screening patients who may develop substance misuse problems. Impulsivity and its related features are common underlying personality characteristics for both addictive and psychiatric disorders alone and in combination. Further investigation is needed to determine whether this construct is a robust predictive marker for those at higher risk for substance dependence.

Current Measures Available for Impulsivity

Several different scales to measure general impulsivity and related constructs such as anger, aggression, and hostility are available to the clinician. They can be utilized to measure impulsive personality traits along with episodes of aggressive behavior, severity of current impulsive behavior, and change in impulsivity over time. Although there is some conceptual overlap, the scales are typically weighted toward assessing either underlying personality characteristics or behavioral aspects of impulsivity. Of the eight instruments described here, seven are self-report questionnaires and one is a semistructured interview. Potential limitations of these measures include various reporting biases, the subjects' lack of insight or understanding into their behaviors, and the tendency of some to exaggerate distress or symptoms and minimize other, socially undesirable, traits. The scales are generally aimed at individuals with normal intellect and are likely to be less helpful in those with significant intellectual dysfunction. As with all such measures, the predictive value is limited and results must be interpreted in context along with other clinical information.

1. The Barratt Impulsiveness Scale, Version 11 (BIS-11; Patton et al., 1995) was developed as a clinical research scale to assess impulsivity in three domains: motor impulsiveness, nonplanning impulsiveness, and attentional impulsiveness. The BIS is a self report measure with 30 items scored on a 4-point scale, taking about 10–15 minutes. It is intended for subjects aged 13 years and older. Although there is a lack of established norms for this scale, in studies it has been able to discriminate between nonimpulsive and impulsive groups. BIS impulsiveness scores have been positively correlated with a range of disorders including addictions, eating disorders, antisocial and borderline personality disorders, and bipolar disorder. The BIS appears to be the most useful instrument currently available for measuring impulsivity traits across diagnostic categories, and may be useful in tracking changes in impulsivity over time, for example, in response to treatment.

2. The Eysenck Impulsiveness Questionnaire (EIQ; Eysenck and Eysenck, 1991) is a measure of the personality traits of impulsiveness and venturesomeness. Eysenck and Eysenck define impulsiveness as risk taking without regard to consequences, whereas venturesomeness is risk taking despite comprehension of potential negative consequences. The EIQ is a 35-item, true/false, self-report questionnaire. This scale was developed to study the links between impulsiveness and various personality dimensions (e.g., neuroticism, extroversion, psychoticism; Eysenck and Eysenck, 1977).

3. The UPPS Impulsive Behavior Scale (Whiteside and Lynam, 2001) is a 44-item self-report inventory that measures four personality pathways to impulsive behavior: urgency, (lack of) premeditation, (lack of) perseverance, and sensation seeking. This instrument was derived through a factor analysis of other previously used impulsivity scales (Whiteside and Lynam, 2001).

4. The Tridimensional Personality Questionnaire (TPG; Cloninger et al., 1991) is a 100 item, self-administered, true/false questionnaire. It is based on C. R. Cloninger's biosocial model for personality that intends to link personality traits to the individual's patterns of response to external stimuli. The original instrument is a three-factor model: novelty seeking (NS), harm avoidance (HA), and reward dependence (RD), and the revised instrument is a four-factor model that splits off the independent dimensions of reward dependence on social attachments (RD) and persistence despite intermittent reinforcement (P). The NS factor measures the subscale dimensions of impulsiveness, exploratory excitability, extravagance, and disorderliness. The HA factor is comprised of four subscales; RD, three subscales; and P, the remaining subscale originally from the RD scale. Of these dimensions, there is more consistent evidence for high NS scores to be associated with, and perhaps even predictive of, a higher risk of substance abuse and other disorders in which poor impulse control is a feature, such as antisocial personality disorder (Howard et al., 1997; Wills et al., 1994). In a sample of healthy volunteers, high HA scores have been correlated with heightened pain responsiveness, and also predicted larger pain relief to morphine treatment (Pud et al., 2004, 2006).

5. The Anger, Irritability, and Assault Questionnaire (AIAQ; Coccaro et al., 1991) was designed to evaluate impulsive aggression by examining the three domains of labile anger, irritability, and assault. This scale was originally designed for neurobiological research. The domains were specifically chosen reflect the serotonergic dysfunction observed in impulsive and aggressive patients. The AIAQ is a self-report measure with 28 questions rated on a 4-point scale, with each question rated on three time frames (past week, past month, and adulthood) for a total of 84 items. The revised AIAQ has additional time frames for childhood (6–10 years) and adolescence (12–18 years). As this instrument has been used mainly in neurobiological research, there are fewer data around applying it to clinical populations. The AIAQ may be of use in assessing clinical severity of impulsivity and aggression and measuring change over time in response to treatment.

6. The Buss-Durkee Hostility Inventory (BDHI; Buss and Durkee, 1957) was developed to assess hostility components in both clinical and research settings. In the BDHI, the term *hostility* has been generally applied as the emotional, attitudinal, and behavioral expression of aggression, but not specifically for impulsivity. The BDHI is a 75-item, self report, true/false instrument that takes about 20 minutes to complete. The inventory produces one total hostility score and eight subscale scores: assault, indirect hostility, irritability, negativity, resentment, suspicion, verbal hostility, and guilt. It may be of clinical use in assessing general traits of aggression in conjunction with other more specific measures of impulsivity.

7. The Overt Aggression Scale-Modified (OAS-M; Coccaro et al., 1991) was designed to assess aggressive behavior in outpatient populations. The scale examines three domains: aggression, irritability, and suicidality; and therefore it reflects some common impulsive behavioral expressions. The OAS-M is a 25-item, semistructured, clinician-administered interview. It has nine subscales rating the three above-named domains. The scale is most useful in assessing levels of behavioral aggression related to impulsivity as part of a comprehensive evaluation. The interview format also allows the clinician to clarify vague or inconsistent answers, an advantage over self-report instruments.

8. The State-Trait Anger Expression Inventory (STAXI; Spielberger et al., 1996) was designed to assess the contribution of components of anger to the development of various medical conditions. This instrument evaluates the individual's propensity to experience anger (trait), the amount of anger he or she experiences at the moment (state), and his or her behavioral expression of anger. Again, although the experience of and reaction to anger is related to impulsivity in many individuals, this instrument is not specifically designed to be a general measure of impulsivity. The STAXI is a 44-item, self-administered instrument from which eight subscale scores can be derived. It is of less use in populations that have a high degree of impulsivity (e.g., antisocial and borderline personality disorders), but may be useful as a general measure of anger susceptibility and expression in other clinical populations.

There is a paucity of data exploring the use of impulsivity measurements as a predictor for future substance abuse risk, but the neurobiological and psychological underpinnings common to impulsivity, pain, and addiction are strongly suggestive of this as an important and perhaps a key paradigm.

Final Comments on "Impulsology"

Coping can be defined as behaviors that minimize the impact of painful and adverse life stressors (Kubany et al., 2003). *Emotion-focused coping* involves placing your focus on finding ways to get immediate relief from the impact of negative life stressors without addressing the underlying problem (Kubany et al., 2003). When emotionally and physically painful situations are perceived as "unsolvable," we are most susceptible to the impulsive behaviors that accompany emotion-focused coping (Kubany et al., 2003; Zarmatten et al., 2005). Learned powerlessness is a powerful adaptation, if in fact the perception of entrapment is a reality. However, when the perception of entrapment is not realistic, impulsive behavior accompanying emotion-focused coping is maladaptive (Kubany et al., 2003). Addiction is often the learned response to chronic impulsivity, whether the physiologic reward is endogenously created via impulsive behaviors or exogenously induced with ingested substances ("sensation seeking" and/or "chemical coping").

Impulsology is a potentially fertile area of clinical research. It would be invaluable for the clinician to accurately screen patients vulnerable to impulsivity and learned addiction when treating chronic pain. Accurate screening would of course allow for a comprehensive as well as a preventative approach to destructive impulse-control behaviors. Specialized neurobehavioral interventions and behaviorally targeted pharmacotherapy would provide patients the opportunity for medically comprehensive rehabilitation.

References

American Psychiatric Association. *Diagnostic and Statistical Manual of Mental Disorders–Text Revision*, 4th ed. rev. Washington, DC: American Psychiatric Association; 2000.

Anton RF, O'Malley SS, Ciraulo DA, et al. Combined pharmacotherapies and behavioral interventions for alcohol dependence: the COMBINE study: a randomized controlled trial. *JAMA*. 2006;17:2003–17.

Bond AJ, Verheyden SL, Wingrove J, Curran HV. Angry cognitive bias, trait aggression, and impulsivity in substance users. *Psychopharmacology*. 2004; 171:331–339.

Buss AH, Durkee A. An inventory for assessing different kinds of hostility. *J Consult Psychol*. 1957;21:343–349.

Cami J, Farre M. Mechanisms of disease: drug addiction. *NEJM*. 2003; 349(10):975–986.

Coccaro EF, Harvey PD, Kupsaw-Lawrence E, et al. Development of neuropharmacologically based behavioral assessments of impulsive aggressive behavior. *J Neuropsychiatry Clin Neurosci*. 1991;3:S44–S51.

Cloninger CR, Przybeck TR, Svrakic DM. The Tridimensional Personality Questionnaire: US normative data. *Psychol Rep*. 1991;69(3 pt 1):1047–57.

COMBINE Study Research Group. Testing combined pharmacotherapies and behavioral interventions for alcohol dependence (the COMBINE study): a pilot feasibility study. *Alcohol Clin Exp Res*. 2003;27:1123–31.

Donovan DM, Anton RF, Miller WR, et al. Combined Pharmacotherapies and Behavioral Interventions for Alcohol Dependence (The COMBINE Study): examination of posttreatment drinking outcomes. *J Stud Alcohol Drugs*. 2008;69:5–13.

Eysenck HJ, Eysenck SPG. *Manual of the Eysenck Personality Scales (EPS Adult)*. London: Hodder and Stoughton; 1991.

Eysenck SBG, Eysenck HJ. The place of impulsiveness in a dimensional system of personality description. *Br J Soc Clin Psychology*. 1977;16:57–68.

Goldstein RZ, Volkow ND. Drug addiction and its underlying neurobiological basis: neuroimaging evidence for involvement of the frontal cortex. *Am J Psychiatry*. 2002; 159: 1642–1652.

Gonzales D, Rennard SI, Nides M., et al. Varenicline, an alpha-2 beta 4 nicotinic acetylcholine receptor partial agonist, vs. sustained release bupropion and placebo for smoking cessation. *JAMA*. 2006;296:47–55.

Heilig M, Egli M. Pharmacological treatment of alcohol dependence: target symptoms and target mechanisms. *Pharmacology & Therapeutics*. 2006. Epub ahead of print.

Howard MO, Kivlahan D, Walker RD. Cloninger's tridimensional theory of personality and psychopathology: applications to substance use disorders. *J Stud Alcohol*. 1997;58(1):48–66.

Hyman SE. Addiction: a disease of learning and memory. *Am J Psychiatry*. 2005;162:1414–1422.

Hyman SE, Malenka RC, Nestler EJ. Neural mechanisms of addiction: the role of reward-related learning and memory. *Annu Rev Neurosci*. 2006; 29:565–98.

Johnson BA, Ait-Daoud N, Akhtar FZ, et al. Use of oral topiramate to promote smoking abstinence among alcohol-dependent smokers: a randomized trial. *Arch Intern Med*. 2005; 165: 1600–1605.

Johnson BA, Ait-Daoud N, Bowden CL, et al. Oral topiramate for treatment of alcohol dependence: a randomized controlled trial. *Lancet*. 2003; 361:1677–1685.

Johnson BA, Roache JD, Javors M., et al. Ondansetron for reduction of drinking among biologically predisposed alcoholic patients: a randomized controlled trial. *JAMA*. 2000 Aug 23–30;284(8):963–971.

Jorenby DE, Leischow SJ, Nides MA, et al. A controlled trial of sustained release bupropion, a nicotine patch or both for smoking cessation. *NEJM*. 1999;340:685–691.

Kaufman JN, Ross TJ, Stein EA, et al. Cingulate hypoactivity in cocaine users during a GO-NOGO task as revealed by event-related functional magnetic resonance imaging. *J Neurosci*. 2003;23:7839–7843.

Koechlin E, Hyafil A. Anterior prefrontal function and the limits of human decision-making. *Science*. 2007;318:594–598.

Kreek MJ, Laforge KS, Butelman E. Pharmacotherapy of addictions. *Nat Rev Drug Discov*. 2003;1:710–726.

Kubany ES, McCaig MA, Laconsay JR. *Healing the Trauma of Domestic Violence: A Workbook for Women*. Vancouver, Canada: Raincoast Books; 2003.

Lee B, Tiefenbacher S, Platt DM, et al. Pharmacological blockade of alpha-2 adrenoreceptors induces reinstatement of cocaine-seeking behavior in squirrel monkeys. *Neuropsychopharmacology*. 2004; 29:686–693.

Mann K, Lehert P, Morgan MY. The efficacy of acamprosate in the maintenance of abstinence in alcohol-dependent individuals: results of a meta-analysis. *Alcohol: Clin Exp Res*. 2004;28:51–63.

Mansouri FA, Buckley MJ, Tanaka K. Mnemonic function of the dorsolateral prefrontal cortex in conflict-induced behavioral adjustment. *Science*. 2007; 318:987–990.

Marinelli M, Rudnick CN, Xu HT, et al. Excitability of dopamine neurons: modulation and physiological consequences. *CNS Neurol Disord Drug Targets*. 2006 Feb;5(1):79–97.

Mathon DA, Ramakers GMJ, Pintar JE, et al. Decreased firing of midbrain dopamine neurons in mice lacking mu opioid receptors. *Eur J of Neuroscience*. 2005;21:2883–2886.

McElroy SL, Shapira NA, Arnold LM, et al. Topiramate in the long-term treatment of binge eating disorder associated with obesity. *J Clin Psychiatry*. 2004;65:1463–1469.

O'Malley, SS, Jaffe AJ, Chang G, et al. Naltrexone and coping skills therapy for alcohol dependence: a controlled study. *Arch Gen Psychiatry*. 1992; 49:881–887.

Papageorgiou C, Rabavilas A, Liappas I, et al. Do obsessive-compulsive patients and abstinent heroin addicts share a common pathophysiologic mechanism? *Neuropsychobiology*. 2003;47:1–11.

Patton JH, Stanford MS, Barrett ES. Factor structure of the Barrett impulsiveness scale. *J Clin Psychol*. 1995;51:768–774.

Paulus MP. Decision-making dysfunctions in psychiatry—altered homeostatic processing? *Science*. 2007;318:602–606.

Pud D, Eisenberg E, Sprecher E, Rogowski Z, Yarnitsky D. The tridimensional personality theory and pain: harm avoidance and reward dependence traits correlate with pain perception in health volunteers. *Eur J Pain*. 2004;8(1):31–38.

Pud D, Yarnitsky D, Sprecher E, Rogowski Z, Adler R, Eisenberg E. Can personality traits and gender predict the response to morphine? An experimental cold pain study. *Eur J Pain.* 2006;10(2):103–112.

Roberts AJ, McDonald JS, Heyser CJ, et al. Mu-opioid receptor knock-out mice do not self-administer alcohol. *J. Pharmacol Exp Ther.* 2000;293;1002–1008.

Sanfrey AG. Social decision-making: insights from game theory and neuroscience. *Science.* 2007;318:598–602.

Smith H, Shirley KL, Norelli L. Impulsology: a new paradigm for addiction. Paper presented at: Stratton VAMC Grand Rounds; September 2006; Albany, NY.

Spanagel R, Pendyala G, Abarca C, et al. The clock gene Per2 influences the glutamatergic system and modulates alcohol consumption. *Nat Med.* 2005; 11:35–42.

Spielberger CD. *State-Trait Anger Expression Inventory: STAXI Professional Manual.* Odessa, FL: Psychological Assessment Resources; 1996.

Srisurapanont M, Jarusurian N. Opioid antagonists for alcohol dependence. *Cochrane Database Sys Rev.* 2005;1:[CD001867].

Swann AC, Dougherty DM, Pazzaglia PJ, Pham M, Moeller FG. *Bipolar Disord.* 2004 Jun;6(3):204–12.

Tomkins DM, Le AD, Sellers EM, et al. Effect of the 5HT-3 antagonist ondansteron on voluntary ethanol intake in rats and mice maintained on a limited-access procedure. *Psychopharmacology* (Berl). 1995;117:479–485.

Volkow ND, Fowler JS. Addiction, a disease of compulsion and drive: involvement of the orbitofrontal cortex. *Cereb Cortex.* 2000;10:318–325.

Wills TA, Vaccaro D, McNamara G. Novelty seeking, risk taking, and related constructs as predictors of adolescent substance abuse: an application of Cloninger's theory. *J Subst Abuse.* 1994;6(1):1–20.

Whiteside SP, Lynam DR. The five-factor model and impulsivity: using a structural model of personality to understand impulsivity. *Personality and Individual Differences.* 2001;30:669–689.

World Health Organization. *International Statistical Classification of Disease and Related Health Problems.* 10th Revision, Vol. 10. Geneva, Switzerland: World Health Organization; 1992.

Yehuda R. Neuroendocrine aspects of PTSD. *Handbook of Exp Pharmac.* 2005(169): 371–403.

Zarmatten A, Van der Linden M, d'Acremont M, et al. Impulsivity and Decision Making. *J of Nervous and Mental Dis.* 2005;193(10):647–650.

14

Natural and Synthetic Ibogamines
A Novel Approach to Treating Opioid Dependency

Stanley D. Glick

Isabelle M. Maisonneuve

Of several alkaloids found in the root bark of the African shrub *Tabernanthe iboga*, ibogaine has certainly attracted the most interest. Although it has a long history of use in Africa, in initiation rites and religious rituals of Bwiti and Mbiri cults, ibogaine became newsworthy in the United States only after it was claimed to be an effective treatment for addiction to a variety of other drugs. Five United States patents (numbers 4,499,096; 4,587,243; 4,857,523; 5,026,697; 5,124,994) issued between 1985 and 1992 claimed that ibogaine could be used to successfully treat opioid (heroin) addiction, stimulant (cocaine and amphetamine) abuse, alcohol dependence, cigarette smoking (nicotine dependence), and polydrug abuse. Ibogaine was said to interfere with the "physiological and psychological aspects" of addiction, abolishing the craving for drugs, and, at least in the case of opioids, abolishing withdrawal symptoms as well.

Studies in animals corroborated some of these claims. In rats, ibogaine was reported to decrease the self-administration of intravenous morphine (Glick et al., 1991) and cocaine (Cappendijk and Dzoljik, 1993; Glick et al., 1994), the oral intake of alcohol (Rezvani et al., 1995) and nicotine (Glick et al., 1998), and several signs of morphine withdrawal (Glick et al., 1992). However, reports of side effects also appeared, in both animals and humans. Aside from well-known stimulant and hallucinogenic effects, ibogaine was shown to have some neurotoxicity (damaging the cerebellar vermis in rats; cf. Molinari et al., 1996; O'Hearn and Molliver, 1993, 1997) and cardiotoxicity (producing a bradycardia; cf. Glick et al., 1999; Hajo et al., 1981).

Although still used outside of the United States, ibogaine's side effects have limited its potential therapeutic utility and made it unlikely to become an approved legal medication. Such considerations led us to pursue a research program focused on the development of safer ibogamine congeners having perhaps even better antiaddictive efficacy. The mechanism of action of such compounds was, of course, of intense interest because knowledge of such a mechanism could lead to further innovations in the development and design of new treatments. Below, we will review our work pertaining to both of these issues.

In addition to neurotoxicity and cardiotoxicity at very large doses ($\geq$ 100 mg/kg), ibogaine has considerable behavioral toxicity at lower doses (20–40 mg/kg). In rats, the most obvious behavioral effects are whole-body tremors and nonspecific suppression of all operant responding. We initially studied other naturally occurring *iboga* alkaloids with the hope of finding one that lacked these side effects of ibogaine, and indeed we had some success in dissociating decreases in drug self-administration from tremorigenic activity. R-ibogamine and R-coronaridine had no tremorigenic effects yet mimicked ibogaine's effects on morphine and cocaine self-administration (Glick et al., 1994). However, similar to ibogaine, acutely, both R-ibogamine and R-coronaridine had nonspecific effects, reducing responding for a nondrug reinforcer (water) during the first 1–2 hours after administration. We next decided to test noribogaine, the major metabolite of ibogaine (Mash et al., 1995). Although noribogaine was not tremorigenic, it also had acute nonspecific effects, reducing responding for water as well as for drugs (morphine, cocaine; Glick et al., 1996b). Our focus then shifted to synthetic ibogamine congeners.

Several synthetic analogues of ibogamine and coronaridine had profiles of activity similar to one or another of the parent compounds (ibogaine, R-ibogamine, R-coronaridine). However, we eventually identified one that was quite different. 18-methoxycoronaridine (18-MC) mimicked ibogaine's effects on morphine and cocaine self-administration without having an acute depressant effect on responding for water (Glick et al., 1996a; Maisonneuve and Glick, 1999). In subsequent studies, 18-MC was found to reduce oral alcohol and nicotine intake as well as intravenous nicotine and methamphetamine self-administration (Glick et al., 2000a; Rezvani et al., 1997); like ibogaine (Glick et al., 1992), 18-MC also attenuated several signs of morphine withdrawal (Rho and Glick, 1998). 18-MC was nontremorigenic (Glick et al., 1996a), had no cerebellar toxicity (Glick et al., 1996a), and produced no bradycardia (Glick et al., 1999). After establishing the efficacy and relative safety of 18-MC, we focused our efforts on elucidating 18-MC's mechanism of action, identifying other novel compounds and treatments having similar profiles of activity, and further characterizing 18-MC's spectrum of behavioral effects.

This research was supported by NIDA grants DA 03817 and DA 016283. We would like to thank the many collaborators who contributed to the work summarized here, including Drs. M. E. Kuehne, L. B. Hough, M. W. Fleck, H. H. Molinari (deceased), M. Teitler, K. Herrick-Davis, D. Deecher, K. K. Szumlinski, C. Pace, and O. Taraschenko.

Mechanism of Action of 18-MC and Related Congeners

Initial mechanistic studies utilized radioligand binding assays to determine how 18-MC differed from ibogaine. Although both drugs had micromolar affinities for several receptors, the spectrum of actions was considerably narrower for 18-MC as compared to ibogaine. Whereas ibogaine interacted with kappa and mu opioid receptors, NMDA receptors, 5HT-3 receptors, muscarinic receptors, sigma-2 sites, sodium channels and the serotonin transporter, 18-MC appeared to act only at opioid receptors (mu, delta, and kappa) and the 5HT-3 receptor (Glick et al., 1999, 2000b). However, all these binding affinities, for both drugs, were low, and it did not seem likely that any of these actions could mediate the putative antiaddictive effects reported. It seemed more probable that the actions of ibogaine not shared by 18-MC might be related to the relative toxicity of the former. In particular, ibogaine's actions at muscarinic receptors and at sodium channels might mediate its effect on heart rate (bradycardia), whereas its action at sigma-2 sites appears to produce its neurotoxicity (Bowen et al., 1995). The hallucinogenic effect of ibogaine can be attributed to a combination of actions: release of serotonin (an effect also not exhibited by 18-MC; cf. Wei et al., 1998) and antagonism of NMDA receptors (Popik et al., 1994).

Functional studies indicated that both ibogaine (Badio et al., 1997; Fryer and Lucas, 1999; Mah et al., 1998) and 18-MC (Glick et al., 2002a; Pace et al., 2004) were relatively potent noncompetitive antagonists at nicotinic $\alpha3\beta4$ receptors. However, 18-MC showed more specificity for this site than did ibogaine; whereas ibogaine had some affinity for nicotinic $\alpha3\beta4$ receptors 18-MC was inactive (at least up to 20 μM) at this site. Several 18-MC derivatives also blocked $\alpha3\beta4$ receptors, and the potencies to do so were positively correlated with their effects on morphine and methamphetamine self-administration (Pace et al., 2004). The (+) and (-) enantiomers of 18-MC were equally potent, both in blocking $\alpha3\beta4$ receptors and in reducing morphine self-administration (Glick and Maisonneuve, 2000b; King et al., 2000). Together, all these data suggested that antagonism at $\alpha3\beta4$ receptors could be the primary mechanism mediating the therapeutic actions of both ibogaine and 18-MC. Moreover, the data suggested a more general novel hypothesis, namely that $\alpha3\beta4$ nicotinic receptors were part of a mechanism modulating drug self-administration.

The above findings indicated that other $\alpha3\beta4$ receptor antagonists should also reduce drug self-administration. But totally selective antagonists of $\alpha3\beta4$ receptors were unavailable. We therefore developed a rationale for using mixed action agents. We reasoned that if two agents had the common action of blocking the $\alpha3\beta4$ site but also had other actions that were unique to each agent, a combination of low doses of such agents (doses ineffective if administered alone) should produce additive effects at the $\alpha3\beta4$ site and reduce drug self-administration without the involvement of other actions that might contribute to side effects.

Six treatments, consisting of all possible two-drug combinations of four drugs, were used to test this prediction. In addition to 18-MC, the treatment drugs included mecamylamine (a nonspecific nicotinic antagonist), dextromethorphan (also known to be an antagonist at NMDA glutamate receptors), and bupropion (also known to be a weak inhibitor of dopamine reuptake). Consistent with our prediction, all of the drug combinations, but none of the drugs administered alone at the same doses, significantly decreased morphine, methamphetamine, and nicotine self-administration in rats while having no effect on responding for water (Glick et al., 2002a, 2002b). The same rationale, using the same drugs, was applied to the study of opioid withdrawal (naltrexone-precipitated withdrawal signs in morphine-dependent rats). The results showed that low doses of dextromethorphan plus mecamylamine, mecamylamine plus bupropion, and a combination of all three drugs significantly attenuated diarrhea and weight loss, whereas none of the agents alone had these effects. We concluded that $\alpha3\beta4$ receptors are involved in the expression of at least two signs of opioid withdrawal (Taraschenko et al., 2005).

Having provided evidence that ibogamines decrease drug self-administration by acting at $\alpha3\beta4$ nicotinic receptors, the next issue to address was how this might occur, in which brain areas, via which pathways. It was well established that the rewarding effects of many drugs of abuse are, to some extent, all mediated by the mesolimbic dopaminergic pathway originating in the ventral tegmental area and innervating the nucleus accumbens. Opioids, stimulants, ethanol, and nicotine all share the common effect of increasing extracellular levels of dopamine in the nucleus accumbens, and with repeated administration, this effect becomes greater, in other words, sensitization occurs.

Substantial evidence suggests that the neuroadaptations mediating sensitization are responsible for drug-seeking behavior and especially for the craving associated with addiction (De Vries et al., 1998, 1999; Robinson and Berridge, 1993, 2001; Vanderschuren et al., 1999). Consistent with 18-MC's effect in an animal model of craving (Glick et al., 1999), as well as with its effects on drug self-administration, 18-MC was found to attenuate sensitization to the dopamine-enhancing effects of both morphine and cocaine (Szumlinksi et al., 2000a, 2000b). However, because relatively low densities of $\alpha3\beta4$ receptors reside in the ventral tegmental area (e.g., Klink et al., 2001), the evidence implicating antagonism of $\alpha3\beta4$ nicotinic receptors as the mechanism of action of 18-MC did not initially appear to be related to 18-MC's effects on the mesolimbic dopamine system. But further research would make this relationship more obvious.

The highest densities of $\alpha3\beta4$ nicotinic receptors in the brain are located in the medial habenula and the interpeduncular nucleus (e.g., Klink et al., 2001; Quick et al., 1999). The medial habenula provides the major input to the interpeduncular nucleus, forming the habenulointerpeduncular pathway. There are multiple routes by which the habenulointerpeduncular pathway can interact with the mesolimbic pathway. For example, the medial habenula receives input from the nucleus accumbens and has efferents to the ventral tegmental area; and the interpeduncular nucleus has efferent connections to the brainstem raphe nuclei and the medial dorsal thalamic nucleus, both of which, directly or indirectly (e.g., via the prefrontal cortex), have connections to the ventral tegmental area. Some evidence of functional interactions between the habenulointerpeduncular and mesolimbic pathways had in fact been demonstrated many years ago (Nishikawa et al., 1986). Accordingly, we pursued the hypothesis that 18-MC acts in the habenulointerpeduncular pathway to mediate its effects on the mesolimbic pathway and on drug self-administration. So far these studies have focused only on morphine.

18-MC (10 μg) was first locally infused into either the medial habenula (MHb) or interpeduncular nucleus (IPN) of morphine self-administering rats. In both cases, 18-MC produced approximately a 40% decrease in intravenous morphine self-administration (Maisonneuve and Glick, 2003; Glick et al., 2006); however, there was no effect of intra-MHb or intra-IPN infusions of 18-MC on oral self-administration of a nondrug reward (15% sucrose). Moreover, intra-MHb or intra-IPN infusions of other nicotinic α3β4 antagonists (mecamylamine, a nonspecific nicotinic antagonist and alpha-conotoxin AuIB, a specific α3β4 nicotinic antagonist) produced similar decreases in morphine self-administration. These effects seemed to be regionally localized to the MHb and IPN because infusions of 18-MC into the ventral tegmental area had no effect on morphine administration.

The effects of localized administration of 18-MC were also assessed in our model of opioid withdrawal (naltrexone-precipitated withdrawal signs in morphine-dependent rats). Besides the MHb and IPN, the locus coeruleus (LC) was examined as well because it is known to be involved in the expression of opioid withdrawal and has moderate densities of nicotinic α3β4 receptors. When infused into the LC, 18-MC reduced "wet dog" shakes, teeth chattering, burying, and diarrhea; infusion into the MHb reduced teeth chattering, burying, and weight loss; whereas infusion into the IPN reduced rearing, teeth chattering, and burying. The findings suggested that 18-MC acts in all three nuclei to suppress various signs of opioid withdrawal (Panchal et al., 2005).

The effects of local brain infusions of 18-MC on morphine-induced increases in nucleus accumbens dopamine levels were examined next. The effects were similar to those previously reported with systemic 18-MC; that is, intra-MHb or intra-IPN infusion of 18-MC (10 μg) was found to attenuate sensitization to the dopamine enhancing effects of repeated morphine (20 mg/kg, i.p.) injections (Taraschenko et al., 2007). Together, all the data collected thus far indicate that 18-MC acts as an antagonist of α3β4 nicotinic receptors in the MHb and/or IPN; this action appears to dampen the dopaminergic mesolimbic pathway's responses to morphine and other addictive drugs and thereby decrease their self-administration. In addition, the LC appears to partially mediate 18-MC's effects on opioid withdrawal signs.

Other Effects of 18-MC and Other Effects It Does Not Have

18-MC appears to have few effects aside from decreasing drug self-administration and attenuating opioid dependence. Unlike ibogaine, which has pronounced effects on motor behavior (tremors, diminished locomotor activity, impaired rotarod performance), 18-MC produced no motoric effects in several kinds of tests (Glick et al., 1996a, 1999; Maisonneuve and Glick, 2003). 18-MC also had no effect on body weight regulation (daily treatment for 2 weeks) and no effect in a commonly used paradigm (Morris water maze) of learning and memory.

In psychotherapeutic screening tests, 18-MC showed no potential for antidepressant efficacy (Porsolt immobility test) and had no effect on one index of anxiety (Vogel conflict test); however, 18-MC was clearly anxiolytic in another test (plus maze), whereas, in contrast, in the same test, ibogaine was anxiogenic (cf. Maisonneuve and Glick, 2003). Mice lacking β4 nicotinic receptor subunits have been found to be anxiolytic in the plus maze but not in other "anxiety" paradigms (Salas et al., 2002). The similarity of the latter findings to the effects of 18-MC suggests that the anxiolytic effect of 18-MC in the plus maze may, like its anti-addictive effects, be mediated by antagonism of α3β4 nicotinic receptors.

Lastly, it should be noted that 18-MC has recently been reported to inhibit HIV-1 infection in human peripheral blood mononuclear cells and monocyte-derived macrophages (Silva et al., 2004); moderate inhibition of HIV-1 reverse transcriptase appeared to partly account for 18-MC's antiretroviral activity. Regardless of the mechanism(s) involved, the anti-HIV-1 activity suggests that 18-MC might be especially useful in treating addictive disorders of HIV-1-infected individuals.

Summary

Our research to date indicates that 18-MC is likely to be a broad spectrum antiaddictive agent having few, if any, side effects. Although optimal dosage regimens have not yet been defined, preclinical data suggest that its antiaddictive efficacy will increase with repeated administration (Glick et al., 1999). 18-MC's mechanism of action is unlike that of any other drug used to treat addiction or being developed to do so. Although not tested as extensively as 18-MC, several related synthetic compounds appear to act similarly, and it is likely that some of these will be more potent than 18-MC (e.g., Kuehne et al., 2003; Pace et al., 2004). Being the lead compound of this series, the development of 18-MC has reached the point at which clinical trials need to be envisioned.

References

Badio B, Padgett WL, Daly JW. Ibogaine: A potent noncompetitive blocker of ganglionic/neuronal nicotinic receptors. *Mol. Pharmacol.* 1997;51:1–5.

Bowen WD, Vilner BJ, Williams W, Bertha CM, Kuehne ME, Jacobson AE. Ibogaine and its congeners are s$_2$ receptor-selective ligands with moderate affinity. *Eur. J. Pharmacol.* 1995;279:R1–R3.

Cappendijk SLT, Dzoljic MR. Inhibitory effects of ibogaine on cocaine self-administration in rats. *Eur. J. Pharmacol.* 1993;241:261–265.

De Vries TJ, Schoffelmeer AN, Binnekade R, Mulder AH, Vanderschuren LJ. Drug-induced reinstatement of heroin- and cocaine-seeking behaviour following long-term extinction is associated with expression of behavioural sensitization. *Eur. J. Neurosci.* 1998;10:3565–3571.

De Vries TJ, Schoffelmeer AN, Binnekade R, Vanderschuren LJ. Dopaminergic mechanisms mediating the incentive to seek cocaine and heroin following long-term withdrawal of IV drug self-administration. *Psychopharmacology* (Berl). 1999;143:254–260.

Fryer JD, Lukas RJ. Noncompetitive functional inhibition at diverse, human nicotinic acetylcholine receptor subtypes by bupropion, phencyclidine, and ibogaine. *J. Pharmacol. Exp. Ther.* 1999;288:88–92.

Glick SD, Kuehne ME, Maisonneuve IM, Bandarage UK, Molinari HH. 18-Methoxycoronaridine, a non-toxic *iboga* alkaloid congener: effects on morphine and cocaine self-administration and on mesolimbic dopamine release in rats. *Brain Res.* 1996a;719:29–35.

Glick SD, Kuehne ME, Raucci J, Wilson TE, Larson D, Keller RW, Jr., Carlson JN. Effects of *iboga* alkaloids on morphine and cocaine self-administration in rats: relationship to tremorigenic effects and to effects on dopamine release in nucleus accumbens and striatum. *Brain Res.* 1994;657:14–22.

Glick SD, Maisonneuve IM. Development of novel medications for drug addiction. The legacy of an African shrub. *Ann. N.Y. Acad. Sci.* 2000b;909:88–103.

Glick SD, Maisonneuve IM, Dickinson HA. 18-MC reduces methamphetamine and nicotine self-administration in rats. *Neuroreport.* 2000a;11:2013–2015.

Glick SD, Maisonneuve IM, Hough LB, Kuehne ME, Bandarage UK. (±)-18-Methoxycoronaridine: A novel *iboga* alkaloid congener having potential anti-addictive efficacy. *CNS Drug Review.* 1999;5:27–42.

Glick SD, Maisonneuve IM, Kitchen BA. Modulation of nicotine self-administration in rats by combination therapy with agents blocking α3β4 nicotinic receptors. *Eur. J. Pharmacol.* 2002b;448:185–191.

Glick SD, Maisonneuve IM, Kitchen BA, Fleck MW. Antagonism of alpha 3 beta 4 nicotinic receptors as a strategy to reduce opioid and stimulant self-administration. *Eur. J. Pharmacol.* 2002a;438:99–105.

Glick SD, Maisonneuve IM, Szumlinski KK. 18-Methoxycoronaridine (18-MC) and ibogaine: comparison of antiaddictive efficacy, toxicity, and mechanisms of action. *Ann. N.Y. Acad. Sci.* 2000b;914:369–386.

Glick SD, Maisonneuve IM, Visker KE, Fritz KA, Bandarage UK, Kuehne, ME. 18-Methoxycoronardine attenuates nicotine-induced dopamine release and nicotine preferences in rats. *Psychopharmacology* (Berl) 1998;139:274–280.

Glick SD, Pearl CM, Cai J, Maisonneuve IM. Ibogaine-like effects of noribogaine in rats. *Brain Res.* 1996b;713:294–297.

Glick SD, Ramirez RL, Livi JM, Maisonneuve IM. 18-Methoxy-coronaridine acts in the medial habenula and/or interpeduncular nucleus to decrease morphine self-administration in rats. *Eur. J. Pharmacol.* 2006; 537:94–98.

Glick SD, Rossman K, Rao NC, Maisonneuve IM, Carlson JN. Effects of ibogaine on acute signs of morphine withdrawal in rats: independence from tremor. *Neuropharmacology.* 1992;31:497–500.

Glick SD, Rossman K, Steindorf S, Maisonneuve IM, Carlson JN. Effects and aftereffects of ibogaine on morphine self-administration in rats. *Eur. J. Pharmacol.* 1991;195:341–345.

Hajo N, Dupont C, Wepierre J. Effects of tabernanthine on various cardiovascular parameters in the rat and dog. *J. Pharmacol.* 1981;12:441–453.

King CR, Meckler H, Herr RJ, Trova MP, Glick SD, Maisonneuve IM. Synthesis of enantiomerically pure (+)- and (−)-18-methoxycoronaridine and their preliminary assessments as anti-addictive agents. *Biorg. Med. Chem. Lett.* 2000;10:473–476.

Klink R, de Kerchove DA, Zoli M, Changeux JP. Molecular and physiological diversity of nicotinic acetylcholine receptors in the midbrain dopaminergic nuclei. *J. Neurosci.* 2001; 21:1452–1463.

Kuehne ME, He L.-W, Jokiel PA, Pace CJ, Fleck MW, Maisonneuve IM, Glick SD, Bidlack JM. Synthesis and biological evaluation of 18-methoxycoronaridine congeners: potential anti-addiction agents. *J. Med. Chem.* 2003; 46:2716–2730.

Mah SJ, Tang Y, Liauw PE, Nagel JE, Schneider AS. Ibogaine acts at the nicotinic acetylcholine receptor to inhibit catecholamine release. *Brain Res.* 1998;797:173–180.

Maisonneuve IM, Glick SD. Attenuation of the reinforcing efficacy of morphine by 18-methoxycoronaridine. *Eur. J. Pharmacol.* 1999;383:15–21.

Maisonneuve IM, Glick SD. Anti-addictive actions of an *iboga* alkaloid congener: a novel mechanism for a novel treatment. *Pharmacol. Biochem. Behav.* 2003;75:607–618.

Mash DC, Staley JK, Baumann MH, Rothman RB, Hearn JL. Identification of a primary metabolite of ibogaine that targets serotonin transporters and elevates serotonin. *Life Sci.* 1995;57:PL 45–50.

Molinari HH, Maisonneuve IM, Glick SD. Ibogaine neurotoxicity: a re-evaluation. *Brain Res.* 1996;737:255–262.

Nishikawa T, Fage D, Scatton B. Evidence for, and nature of, the tonic inhibitory influence of habenulointerpeduncular pathways upon cerebral dopaminergic transmission in the rat. *Brain Res.* 1986;373:324–336.

O'Hearn E, Molliver ME. Degeneration of Purkinje cells in parasagittal zones of the cerebellar vermis after treatment with ibogaine or harmaline. *Neuroscience.* 1993;55:303–310.

O'Hearn E, Molliver ME. The olivocerebellar projection mediates ibogaine-induced degeneration of Purkinje cells: a model of indirect, trans-synaptic excitotoxicity. *J. Neurosci.* 1997;17:8828–8841.

Pace CJ, Glick SD, Maisonneuve IM, He LW, Jokiel PA, Kuehne ME, Fleck MW. Novel *iboga* alkaloid congeners block nicotinic receptors and reduce drug self-administration. *Eur. J. Pharmacol.* 2004;492:159–167.

Panchal V, Taraschenko OD, Maisonneuve IM, Glick SD. Attenuation of morphine withdrawal signs by intracerebral administration of 18-methoxycoronaridine. *Eur. J. Pharmacol.*, 2005; 525: 98–104.

Popik P, Layer RT, Skolnick P. The putative anti-addictive drug ibogaine is a competitive inhibitor of [^{3}H]MK-801 binding to the NMDA receptor complex. *Psychopharmacology* (Berl) 1994;114:672–674.

Quick MW, Ceballos RM, Kasten M, McIntosh JM, Lester RA. α3β4 subunit-containing nicotinic receptors dominate function in rat medial habenula neurons. *Neuropharmacology.* 1999;38:769–783.

Rezvani AH, Overstreet DH, Lee YW. Attenuation of alcohol intake by ibogaine in three strains of alcohol-preferring rats. *Pharmacol. Biochem. Behav.* 1995;52:615–620.

Rezvani AH, Overstreet DH, Yang Y, Maisonneuve IM, Bandarage UK, Kuehne ME, Glick SD. Attenuation of alcohol consumption by a novel nontoxic ibogaine analogue (18-methoxycoronaridine) in alcohol-preferring rats. *Pharmacol. Biochem. Behav.* 1997;58:615–619.

Rho B, Glick SD. Effects of 18-methoxycoronaridine on acute signs of morphine withdrawal in rats. *Neuroreport.* 1998;9:1283–1285.

Robinson TE, Berridge KC. The neural basis of drug craving: An incentive-sensitization theory of addiction. *Brain Res. Rev.* 1993;18:247–291.

Robinson TE, Berridge KC. Incentive-sensitization and addiction. *Addiction.* 2001;96:103–114.

Salas R, Pieri F, Fung B, Dani JA, De Biasi M. Altered anxiety-related responses in mutant mice lacking the β4 subunit of the nicotinic receptor. *J. Neurosci.* 2003;23: 6255–6263.

Silva EM, Cirne-Santos CC, Frugulhetti ICPP, Galvao-Castro B, Kuehne ME, Bou-Habib DC. Anti-HIV-1 activity of the *iboga* alkaloid congener 18-methoxycoronaridine. *Planta Med.* 2004;70: 808–812.

Szumlinski KK, Maisonneuve IM, Glick SD. The potential anti-addictive agent, 18-methoxycoronaridine, blocks the sensitized locomotor and dopamine responses produced by repeated morphine treatment. *Brain Res.* 2000b;864:13–23.

Szumlinski KK, McCafferty CA, Maisonneuve IM, Glick SD. Interactions between 18-methoxycoronaridine (18-MC) and cocaine: dissociation of behavioural and neurochemical sensitization. *Brain Res.* 2000a;871:245–258.

Taraschenko OD, Panchal V, Maisonneuve IM, Glick SD. Is antagonism of α3β4 nicotinic receptors a strategy to reduce morphine dependence? *Eur. J. Pharmacol.* 2005;513:207–218.

Taraschenko OD, Shulan JM, Maisonneuve IM, Glick SD. 18-MC acts in the medial habenula and interpeduncular nucleus to attenuate dopamine sensitization to morphine in the nucleus accumbens. *Synapse* 2007; 61: 547–560.

Vanderschuren LJ, Schoffelmeer AN, Mulder AH, De Vries TJ. Dopaminergic mechanisms mediating the long-term expression of locomotor sensitization following pre-exposure to morphine or amphetamine. *Psychopharmacology* (Berl). 1999;143:244–253.

Wei D, Maisonneuve IM, Kuehne ME, Glick SD. Acute iboga alkaloid effects on extracellular serotonin (5-HT) levels in nucleus accumbens and striatum in rats. *Brain Res.* 1998;800:260–268.

15

Opioid Tolerance

Jianren Mao

Lucy Chen

The development of opioid tolerance is an intrinsic pharmacological phenomenon of opioid receptors following exposure to opioid agonists (O'Brience, 1996; Reisine and Pasternak, 1996). Although the time course and degree of opioid tolerance vary in clinical settings, profound tolerance to opioid analgesics sometimes necessitates an opioid dose escalation in order to achieve the clinical analgesic effect of opioids. Opioid dependence is also an intrinsic phenomenon of opioid receptors, which may or may not be associated with the development of opioid tolerance. This chapter will focus on the clinical features of opioid tolerance, its cellular mechanisms, and clinical management.

Clinical Features

Clinical opioid tolerance may be described as *apparent opioid tolerance*, a term that refers to a loss of opioid analgesic effects after a course of opioid treatment or the need to increase an opioid dose in order to achieve the same analgesic effect (Figure 15.1). There are at least three major contributors to the clinical presentation of apparent opioid tolerance: (1) pharmacological tolerance, (2) opioid-induced hyperalgesia, and (3) worsening pain due to disease progression, among others (Pappagallo, 2000).

Not every demand for opioid dose escalation is attributable to the development of pharmacological opioid tolerance, although pharmacological opioid tolerance is likely to play a significant role in the development of apparent opioid tolerance. Another possible contributor to apparent opioid tolerance is the development of opioid-induced hyperalgesia, which facilitates nociceptive processing and may counteract the analgesic effect of opioids (Mao, 2002; Mao et al., 1995a, 1995b).

The development of apparent opioid tolerance may also be due to disease progression resulting in a worsening pain condition and the need for opioid dose escalation. Of note is that in some cases an increased demand of opioid analgesics may be independent of the major concerns of apparent opioid tolerance. In such cases, possible opioid abuse, addiction, and diversion should also be considered. Although a clinical distinction among potential contributors of apparent opioid tolerance is often difficult, every effort should be made to investigate the underlying causes that lead to increased opioid demand during a course of opioid therapy.

Mechanisms

Over several decades, the cellular mechanisms of opioid tolerance have been explored through extensive basic science and clinical research. To date, several lines of research have shed light on the cellular mechanisms of opioid tolerance and provided some important guidance for its clinical management. The following sections provide a brief discussion about several areas of basic science research regarding opioid tolerance.

Opioid receptors belong to a super family of G-protein coupled receptors. The effect of receptor phosphorylation on opioid receptor uncoupling (desensitization) and internalization has been described for G-protein coupled receptors including opioid receptors. G-protein activation serves as a coupling mechanism between opioid receptors and rectifying K^+ channels, leading to cell membrane hyperpolarization and inhibition under most circumstances. Moreover, the cyclic AMP and protein kinase A system may be upregulated during the development of opioid tolerance and may contribute to the process of opioid withdrawal (Nestler and Aghajanian, 1997). Uncoupling of G-protein from opioid receptors may be an important mechanism of opioid tolerance. More recently, alteration of G-protein signaling (Gintzler and Chakrabarti, 2001) also has been implicated in the mechanisms of opioid tolerance.

β-arrestin is a regulatory protein and has been shown to play a role in the development of opioid tolerance (Bohn et al., 1999, 2000; Whistler and von Zastrow, 1999). In addition, μ-opioid receptor oligomerization and endocytosis have been suggested to be contributory to the development of morphine tolerance (Finn and Whistler, 2001; He et al., 2002). Relatedly, an opioid agonist that facilitates μ-opioid receptor endocytosis has been shown to reduce the development of morphine tolerance (He et al., 2002).

Activation of N-methyl-D-aspartate (NMDA) receptors and protein kinase C as well as regulation of glutamate transporters are also areas of great interest in investigating the cellular mechanisms of opioid tolerance (Mao et al., 1995a, 1999, 2002; Trujillo and Akil, 1991; Xu et al., 2003; Zeitz et al., 2002). Studies conducted over the last decade suggest a link between neuronal plasticity resembling learning and memory and the cellular mechanisms of opioid tolerance. Among three major opioid receptor subtypes, the

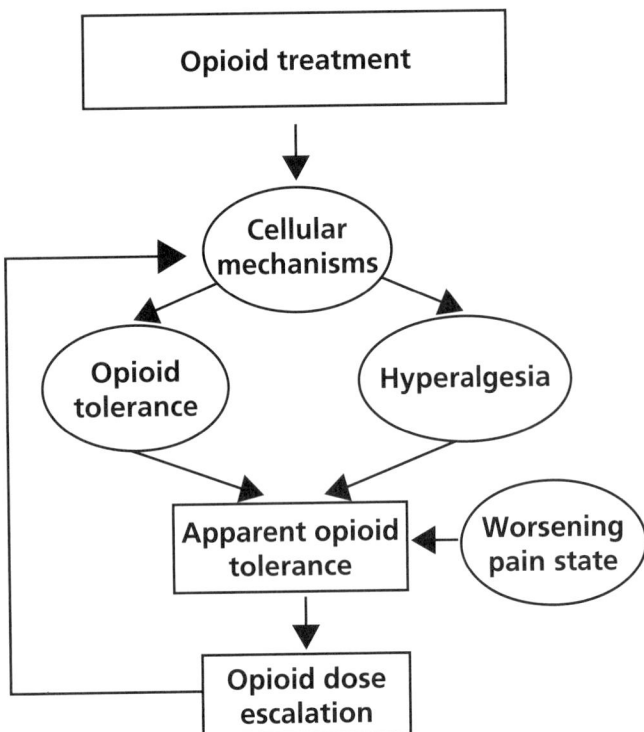

Figure 15.1. The development of opioid-induced hyperalgesia is mechanistically linked to pharmacological opioid tolerance. Both are initiated by opioid administration and could contribute to the clinical presentation of apparent opioid tolerance. It is often difficult to distinguish these two contributors of apparent opioid tolerance, in addition to worsening pain due to disease progression, if the clinical assessment endpoints are simply the opioid consumption and pain scores. However, clinical approaches to resolving apparent opioid

role of NMDA receptors in μ-opioid tolerance has been well established (Elliott et al., 1994a, 1994b).

Opioid actions also may be negatively modulated by cholecystokinin (CCK), an endogenous neuropeptide, in the central nervous system (Watkins et al., 1985). In animal studies, morphine-6-glucuronide (M-6-G) and morphine-3-glucuronide (M-3-G), two active morphine metabolites, may potentiate and reduce the analgesic effects of μ-opioid agonists, respectively.

Most recently, central glucocorticoid receptors have been implicated in the development of opioid tolerance as well (Lim et al., 2005). Of significance is that repeated cycles of morphine exposure have been shown to shorten the onset of opioid tolerance after each cycle of morphine exposure and that central glucocorticoid receptors may serve as a link between previous morphine exposure and the facilitated development of opioid tolerance upon a subsequent morphine exposure (Lim et al., 2005). These findings suggest that previous opioid exposure may have a prolonged influence on the development of opioid tolerance upon future opioid exposure, raising the possibility that the development of opioid tolerance could be facilitated in human subjects who have a history of previous opioid (medical or nonmedical) exposure.

Although extensive basic science research has led to several proposed mechanisms of opioid tolerance, the application of these preclinical findings in clinical settings remains to be seen. Of interest, however, is that investigation into the relationship between opioid tolerance and neuropathic pain has found similarities in the cellular and molecular mechanisms between opioid tolerance and neuropathic pain (Mao et al., 1995a, 1995b) and led to the observation of opioid-induced hyperalgesia or opioid-induced pain sensitivity in both animals and human subjects (Mao, 2002). It is possible that opioid-induced hyperalgesia may be an important contributor to the clinical presentation of apparent opioid tolerance, in addition to pharmacological opioid tolerance (an intrinsic property of opioid receptors) and worsening pain due to the progression of an underlying disease state (Ballantyne and Mao, 2003; Mao, 2002).

Clinical Management

Despite extensive preclinical studies on the cellular mechanisms of opioid tolerance, their implications for preventing and managing opioid tolerance in clinical settings remain unclear. Several clinical approaches have been suggested and are discussed below.

Because the cross-tolerance among subtypes of opioids is often incomplete, opioid rotation may be a useful approach if a substantial increase in one opioid analgesic alone does not provide satisfactory pain relief. Although there is no single formula to follow for opioid rotation, a replacing opioid may be given at 50%–75% of the dose equivalent to the original opioid at the beginning of an opioid rotation. However, patients should be closely followed to ensure that an adequate dose conversion is made between two opioids in order to avoid withdrawal, overdose, or unrelieved pain.

Adjunctive medications such as nonsteroidal antiinflammatory drugs and all others, alpha-adrenergic receptor agonist (e.g., clonidine) may be considered as part pharmacologic regimen along with opioids to reduce the total amount of opioid analgesics.

Because NMDA receptors are implicated in the development of opioid tolerance, it is reasonable to consider a combined treatment of an opioid analgesic and a clinically available N-methyl-D-aspartate receptor antagonist. Several clinically available NMDA receptor antagonists may be considered, including dextromethorphan, methadone, and ketamine. The combined use of opioids and an NMDA receptor antagonist may increase the opioid analgesic efficacy and attenuate the development of tolerance and opioid-induced hyperalgesia (Elliott et al., 1994a, 1994b; Mao, 2002).

Preclinical studies have indicated that the combination of an opioid analgesic and an ultra low dose of opioid receptor antagonist such as naltraxone may improve the opioid analgesic efficacy (Crain and Shen, 1999). The clinical utility of this observation is under investigation.

As discussed earlier, the presence of apparent opioid tolerance in the clinical setting may reflect several elements including pharmacological tolerance, opioid-induced hyperalgesia, and/or worsening pain due to disease progression. However, the clinical management of these elements of apparent opioid tolerance varies (see Fig. 15.1). For example, opioid dose escalation may be a necessary approach to overcome opioid tolerance, whereas opioid tapering may be a positive step toward reducing opioid-induced hyperalgesia and restoring the opioid analgesic effect by minimizing the sensitization process (Mao, 2002). On the other hand, worsening pain due to disease progression may be managed by adding appropriate adjunctive therapies (e.g., radiation therapy to bone lesions in cancer patients) instead of simply increasing an opioid dose.

In summary, adjusting opioid dose should not be made simply based on changes in pain scores (e.g., pain score using visual analog scale), but require consideration of multiple clinical variables. However, the presence of tolerance to and dependence on opioids should not discourage physicians from using opioids in clinical pain management. In general, opioid tolerance can be effectively managed by formulating a thoughtful plan for opioid therapy and by understanding the complexity of apparent opioid tolerance that includes several clinical elements other than pharmacological opioid tolerance.

References

Ballantyne J, Mao J. Opioid therapy for chronic pain. *New Eng J Med.* 2003; 349: 1943–1953.

Bohn LM, Gainestdinov RR, Lin FT, et al. Mu-opioid receptor desensitization by beta-arrestin-2 determines morphine tolerance but not dependence. *Nature.* 2000; 408: 720–723.

Crain S, Shen KF. Antagonists of excitatory opioid receptor functions enhance morphine's analgesic potency and attenuate opioid tolerance/dependence liability. *Pain.* 1999; 82: 1–11.

Elliott KJ, Hynansky A, Inturrisi CE. Dextromethorphan attenuates and reverses morphine tolerance. *Pain.* 1994b; 59: 361–368.

Elliott KJ, Minami N, Kolesnikov YA, et al. The NMDA receptor antagonists, LY274614 and MK-801, and the nitric oxide synthase inhibitor, NG-nitro-L-arginine, attenuate analgesic tolerance to the mu-opioid morphine but not to kappa opioids. *Pain.* 1994a; 56: 69–75.

Finn AK, Whistler JL. Endocytosis of the mu opioid receptor reduces tolerance and a cellular hallmark of opiate withdrawal. *Neuron.* 2001; 32: 829–839.

Gintzler AR, Chakrabarti, S. Opioid tolerance and the emergence of new opioid receptor-coupled signaling. *Mol Neurobiol.* 2001; 21: 21–33.

He L, Fong J, von Zastrow M, Whistler JL. Regulation of opioid receptor trafficking and morphine tolerance by receptor oligomerization. *Cell.* 2002; 108: 271–282.

Lim G, Wang S, Zeng Q, et al. Evidence for a long-term influence of previous morphine exposure on morphine tolerance: a role of central glucocorticoid receptors. *Pain.* 2005; 114: 81–92.

Mao J. NMDA and opioid receptors: their interactions in antinociception, tolerance and neuroplasticity. *Brain Research Review.* 1999; 30: 289–304.

Mao J. Opioid-induced abnormal pain sensitivity: Implications in clinical opioid therapy. *Pain.* 2002; 100: 213–217.

Mao J, Piece, DD, Mayer, DJ. Mechanisms of hyperalgesia and morphine tolerance: a current view of their possible interactions. *Pain.* 1995a; 62: 259–274.

Mao J, Price DD, Phillips LL, Lu J, et al. Increases in protein kinase C gamma immunoreactivity in the spinal cord of rats associated with tolerance to the analgesic effects of morphine. *Brain Res.* 1995b; 677: 257–267.

Nestler EJ, Aghajanian GK. Molecular and cellular basis of addiction. *Science.* 1997; 278: 58–63.

O'Brience CP. Drug addiction and Drug abuse. In: Hardman J.G. et al. (eds.), *Goodman & Gilman's Pharmacological Basis of Therapeutics.* 1996. New York: McGraw-Hill; ch. 24, pp. 557–577.

Pappagallo M, Dickerson ED, Hulka S. Pallative care and hospice opioid dosing guidelines with breakthrough pain (BP) doses. *Am J Hosp Palliat Care.* 2000; 17: 407–13.

Reisine T, Pasternak G. Opioid analgesics and antagonists. In: Hardman J.G. et al. (eds.), *Goodman & Gilman's Pharmacological Basis of Therapeutics.* 1996. New York: McGraw-Hill; ch. 23, pp. 521–556.

Trujillo KA, Akil H. Inhibition of morphine tolerance and dependence by the NMDA receptor antagonist MK-801. *Science.* 1991; 251: 85–87.

Watkins LR, Kinscheck IB, Mayer DJ. Potentiation of morphine analgesia by the cholecystokinin antagonist proglumide. *Brain Res.* 1985; 327: 169–180.

Whistler JL, von Zastrow M. Morphine-activated opioid receptors elude desensitization by beta-arrestin. *Proc Natl Acad. USA.* 1999; 95: 9914–9919.

Xu NJ, Bao L, Fan HP, et al. Morphine withdrawal increases glutamate uptake and surface expression of glutamate transporter GLT-1 at hippocampal synapses. *J Neurosci.* 2003; 23: 4775–4784.

Zeitz KP, Malmberg AB, Gilbert H, et al. Reduced development of tolerance to the analgesic effects of morphine and clonidine in PKCgamma mutant mice. *Pain.* 2002; 94: 245–253.

16

Methadone Pharmacology in Pain and Addiction

Howard S. Smith

Mary Jeanne Kreek

Carrie L. Johnson

Kenneth L. Kirsh

Methadone, a synthetic opioid available in the United States as a racemate, was first synthesized by German chemists at I. G. Farben near the end of World War II while researching "spasmolytics." In 1942 clinical trials began under the name "Amidone." After the war the analgesic effects of methadone became apparent, although this was unexpected because its chemical structure was significantly different from other known opioids. Methadone has been available as an FDA-approved product for almost half a century. It has been used (as a component) for heroin addiction for over 40 years and is currently prescribed daily to probably over 215,000 people in the United States for this purpose (Dole et al., 1966; McCaffrey, 2001). Additionally, methadone has been used for many years as an opioid analgesic for the treatment of chronic cancer and noncancer pain (Hays & Woodrotte, 1999).

Morphine, the "prototype" exogenous mu opioid receptor (MOR) agonist, is considered to be a more suitable analgesic to treat "garden variety" nociceptive perioperative pain compared to methadone. However, in certain situations and certain patients with persistent pain, methadone can conceivably provide better analgesia than other MOR agonists. There is some evidence that this can also be achieved at lower equianalgesic doses (Lynch, 2005; Sandoval et al., 2005).

The clinical differences that set methadone apart from other opioids are not completely understood, but have been primarily attributed to its actions as an antagonist at the N-methyl-D-aspartate (NMDA) receptor complex (Davis & Inturrisi, 1999; Inturrisi, 2002; Sang, 2000). Although this action has been proposed as being weak at usual clinical doses (Chizh et al., 2000), more recent studies reveal that methadone, in concentrations that overlap with its established clinical dosing range, is a functionally significant NMDA antagonist (Callahan et al. 2004). Methadone's modest NMDA antagonist activities have been reported to be similar in potency to ketamine (Ebert et al., 1997) or dextromethorphan (Gorman, 1997).

Methadone is a unique opioid that may be regarded as the "black sheep of the opioid family," and its class has been termed the diphenylheptanes. The chemical name for methadone is dl(SR) 4, 4-diphenyl-6-dimethylamine-3-heptanone. It is structurally dissimilar to standard alkaloid-type ringed-type structures (Bruera & Sweeney, 2002). It is distinguished as being an open-chain (linear-type) molecule. In this sense it is most similar to propoxyphene.

Methadone contains a single chiral carbon atom and so exists as two enantiomers. The l(R)-enantiomer is primarily responsible for analgesia (Kristensen et al., 1996) with a tenfold higher affinity for mu opioid receptors, and up to fifty times the analgesic activity of the d(S)-enantiomer (Scott et al., 1948).

The l(R)-isomer is a potent pure full mu opioid-receptor agonist with low affinity for delta and kappa receptor (Kristensen et al., 1995). Multiple studies with cloned human receptors and with mu knock-out mice with full delta receptors show no significant effective methadone agonist action at delta opioid receptors (Bot et al., 1997). The d(S)-enantiomer, although relatively inactive at the mu opioid receptor, functions as a modest noncompetitive N-methyl-d-aspartate (NMDA) antagonist and also prevents the reuptake of 5-hydroxytryptamine and norepinephrine (Codd et al., 1995). Because of the different properties of the methadone enantiomers, they exhibit different treatment profiles in different pain models. Specifically, in the case of nerve injury pain, l(R)-methadone has been shown to yield greater antiallodynic action when compared against morphine, oxycodone, d(S)-methadone, and dl(SR)-methadone (racemic; Lemberg et al., 2006). Therefore, it has been proposed that methadone may be especially useful as an analgesic in neuropathic pain (Altier et al., 2005; Cortés et al., 2005; Gagnon et al., 2003; Morley et al., 2003; Moulin et al., 2005). Additionally, because N-methyl-D-aspartate receptor antagonist activity may also reverse opioid tolerance, methadone may also function to ameliorate this phenomenon (Davis & Inturrisi, 1999; Moulin, 2003).

Another potential explanation as to why methadone may be less prone to problems with opioid tolerance is that it appears that MOR endocytosis may counteract receptor desensitization and opioid tolerance via inducing fast reactivation and receptor recycling and the more endocytotically potent an opioid is, with methadone having high endocytotic potency, the less likely that receptor desensitization and opioid tolerance occurs (Koch et al., 2005). Kling et al. (2000) compared opioid receptor binding in healthy normal volunteers to that of those who were stabilized methadone-maintained former heroin addicts via positron emission tomography (PET) using tracer amounts of [^{18}F]cyclofoxy as radioligant. ([^{18}F]cyclofoxy is an opioid antagonist that labels mu and kappa opioid receptors). Only 20%–30% of mu-opioid receptors in the five brain regions studied (those with closest

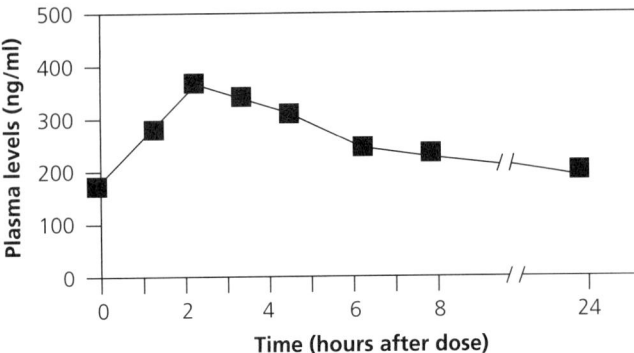

Figure 16.1. Plasma methadone levels in an individual maintained on 100 mg/day. Source: Kreek, M. J. Methadone-related opioid agonist pharmacotherapy for heroin addiction. *Annals of the New York Academy of Sciences*, 2000; 909: 186–216.

relations to pain and addiction) were occupied by methadone (Kling et al., 2000). Conversely, over 65% of primarily mu-opioid receptors apparently remain unoccupied by methadone during chronic methadone pharmacotherapy (Kling et al., 2000).

In the United States methadone is available in racemic form, a 50:50 mixture of two enantiomers, 1 (R)-enantiomer and d(S)-enantiomer. Germany has access to the 1(R)-enantiomer, which exhibits twice the potency of the racemic product (Bruera & Sweeney, 2002; Kristensen et al., 1996).

Methadone Pharmacology

Methadone is a relatively lipophilic basic drug with a pK_a about 9.1 and is available as a hydrochloride salt. Methadone is extremely versatile in terms of routes of administration and has been given via oral (tablet, solution), rectal (using tablets to compound a suppository), parenteral (subcutaneous, intramuscular, intravenous; Mathew and Storey, 1999), spinal (e.g., epidural [Shir et al., 2001], or intrathecal [Jacobson et al., 1990]) routes.

Methadone can be detected in the blood 15–45 minutes after oral administration (Eap et al., 2002). The onset of action of methadone is roughly 0.5 to 1.5 hour after oral administration and about 10–20 minutes after parenteral administration (Davis & Walsh, 2001; Wolff, 1997). The peak effect after parenteral administration is 1–2 hours and 2 to 4 hours after oral administration for analgesia (Davis & Walsh, 2001; Kreek, 2000; Wolff et al., 1997). The duration of action of methadone for the purpose of suppressing opioid withdrawal is substantially longer—24 to 48 hours (Fishman et al., 2002; Gutstein & Akil, 2001; Kreek, 1995).

By 1972 two different groups had developed techniques using gas liquid chromatography to quantitatively measure plasma blood and urine levels of methadone (Inturrisi & Verebely, 1972a, 1972b; Kreek, 1973b). In these studies, it was found that the half-life of racemic methadone in humans as used in the chronic treatment of addiction was 24 hours (see Figure 16.1). In later studies using gas chromatography-chemical ionization mass spectrometry with selective ion monitoring, and with different stable isotope labeling of the two enantiomers of methadone, carried out by the Kreek Laboratory in collaboration with the group of Klein, then at the Argonne National Laboratories, it was found that the active R-enantiomer of methadone has a half-life of 36 to 48 hours, whereas the inactive S-enantiomer has a half-life of only 16 to 20 hours (Hachey et al., 1976, 1977; Kreek, 1973b; Kreek et al., 1979; Nakamura et al., 1982).

The time to peak after oral administration of methadone in solution is 2.5–3 hours and 3–4 hours after oral tablet administration (Davis & Walsh, 2001). Less than 10% of an oral dose is extracted by the liver during first pass (Ripamonti & Bianchi, 2002). The oral bioavailability is approximately 80% with a common range of roughly 70%–85% (about 2–3 times that of morphine)—however, it is highly variable and may range from 40% to 99% (Bruera & Sweeney, 2002). The relative analgesic potency ratio of oral to parenteral methadone is 2:1 as estimated from single dose studies; however, confidence intervals are wide (Foley and Houde, 1998). Methadone is highly bound to plasma proteins (86%), predominantly to α_1—acid glycoprotein (AAG). However, at physiologic pH, multiple proteins may be involved including β globulins and albumin in binding to methadone. Methadone undergoes hepatic biotransformation, primarily via N-demethylation, and is cleared via both urine and feces (Kreek et al., 1976a). The major enzyme for N-demethylation is CYP3A4 (with minor roles for CYP1A2 and CYP2D6) and possibly CYP2B6 (Crettol et al., 2005; Davis & Walsh, 2001).

The role of various cytochrome P450 enzymes in human in vivo methadone disposition is variable and has not been completely elucidated. Kharasch and researchers (2004) attempted to shed some light on this issue in healthy volunteers by utilizing a randomized, balanced, four-way crossover study. Subjects received intravenous (IV) midazolam (to assess CYP3A4 activity) and then simultaneous oral deuterium-labeled and IV unlabeled methadone after pretreatment with rifampin (hepatic/intestinal CYP3A induction), troleandomycin (hepatic/intestinal CYP3A inhibition), grapefruit juice (selective intestinal CYP3A inhibition), or nothing. From this study, the investigators concluded that first-pass intestinal metabolism is a determinant of methadone bioavailability. Additionally, the researchers suggested that intestinal and hepatic CYP3A activity may mildly affect human methadone N-demethylation but not methadone concentrations, clearance, or clinical effects. Finally, after finding greater rifampin effects versus troleandomycin or grapefruit juice effects on methadone disposition, they also suggested a significant role for intestinal transporters and other cytochrome P450 enzymes (i.e., CYP2B6).

Methadone pharmacokinetics follow a biexponential model: α-elimination phase (8–12 hours) and β-elimination phase (30–60 hours; range 9–87 hours in a widely varied population, including opioid-addicted patients, patients taking numerous medications, and patients on "high-dose" opioid therapy with various pain states). The values for methadone's elimination half-life conceivably range from 3 to 130 hours. The α-elimination phase is associated with the duration of analgesia (e.g., 6–8 hours; Inturrisi, 2002). Methadone is redistributed into fat tissues due to being highly lipophilic, with subsequent slow rerelease into plasma resulting in a relatively prolonged elimination phase (Wolff et al., 1997). The plasma level in the β-elimination phase is subanalgesic, but is largely adequate enough to reduce opioid drug craving and abort dramatic withdrawal symptoms in most (Peng et al., 2005). When utilized as an analgesic at low doses (< 60–80 mg/d), methadone is generally administered in 3–4 divided doses per day. However, when utilized for analgesia in doses over 60–80 mg/d, many patients may achieve adequate analgesia with once or twice daily dosing (Garrido & Troconiz, 1999; Inturrisi, 2002). When utilized for methadone maintenance therapy (MMT), once a day dosing > 60mg/d can generally achieve an adequate sustained level, although specific methadone levels depend on the individual.

Methadone is transported across the blood-brain barrier relatively easily, with cerebrospinal fluid concentrations up to 73% of serum concentrations (Rubenstein et al., 1978). However, probably <3% of the methadone dose administered gets into brain cells perhaps due to P-glycoprotein effects (Rodriguez et al., 2004; Wang et al., 2004).

The primary N-demethylation metabolite, 2-ethylidene-1,5-dimethyl-3,3-diphenylpyrrolidine (EDDP), gets further N-demethylated to 2-ethyl-5-methyl-3,3-diphenylpyrroline (EMDP). Both of these are essentially inactive and excreted largely in the urine and feces (Kreek, 1973b; Kreek & Hachey, 1975; Kreek et al., 1979). However, the minor metabolites, methadol and normethadol, exhibit pharmacologic activity similar to methadone (Garrido & Troconiz, 1999).

The pyrrolidine metabolites probably comprise close to 70% of metabolites, with pyrroline metabolites accounting for close to 30% with a small amount of other products. Following oral administration and absorption, methadone is widely distributed in the body. Plasma levels are relatively low, even after a chronic daily maintenance dose of 50 to 100 mg (Inturrisi & Verebely, 1972a; Kreek, 1973b; Sullivan & Blake, 1972). Methadone is metabolized primarily in the liver by the hepatic microsomal drug-metabolizing enzymes. In the major pathway of biotransformation, methadone is first N-demethylated and then undergoes cyclization to form its major pyrrolidine metabolite (Sullivan & Due, 1973). This compound is excreted in urine in amounts approximately equal to those of unchanged methadone (Inturrisi & Verebely, 1972b; Kreek, 1973b; Sullivan & Blake, 1972). It is also the major excretory product in feces (Kreek, 1976a; Kreek & Hachey, 1975). The pyrrolidine metabolite may be metabolized by a second N-demethylation to form a pyrroline. Both the pyrrolidine and pyrroline may be hydroxylated (Sullivan & Due, 1973; see Figure 16.2). Methadone may also be metabolized by several alternate minor pathways to form hydroxymethadone, a pyrrolidine, and various methadol metabolites (Sullivan & Due, 1973). All of these metabolites have been identified in human urine by Dr. Hugh Sullivan and colleagues in early studies at Eli Lilly and Company, and the identification of several have been confirmed by other investigators (Sullivan & Due, 1973).

Lehotay et al. (2005) measured the free biologically active form of methadone and its metabolite (EDDP) and concluded that the large variation/range in methadone dosing may be multifactorial and appears not to be primarily related to pharmacokinetic/metabolic factors. In a healthy individual, roughly 50%–60% of methadone and its metabolites appear in the urine with about 40%–50% appearing in the feces. However, in anuric patients, methadone elimination occurs almost exclusively via the fecal route (Kreek et al., 1980). Additionally, renal excretion of methadone is pH dependent, with low urinary pH levels increasing methadone renal clearance threefold and decreasing the major metabolite-to-methadone ratio (Bellward et al., 1977). Methadone pharmacokinetics are altered in pregnancy. Increased methadone doses may be required during pregnancy in order to achieve effective methadone maintenance due to increased methadone clearance (Pond et al., 1985; Wolff et al., 2005).

The Kreek Laboratory has shown (directly in rabbit perfused liver preparation and indirectly in humans by modeling plus studies in humans with severe hepatic cirrhosis) that "hepatic storage" and release is an essential component of the long-acting properties of methadone in humans (Kreek et al., 1978a). This "spongelike" function is clinically important. Some patients with severe hepatic cirrhosis may actually require more methadone

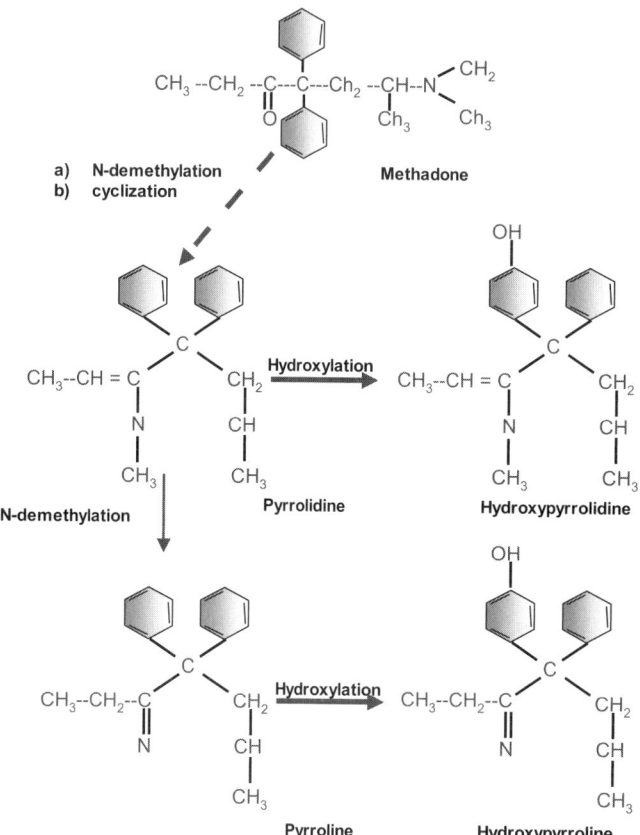

Figure 16.2. Major pathway of *dl*-methadone metabolism in humans. Major products excreted in human urine (methadone, pyrrolidine, pyrroline). Source: Kreek, M. J., et al. Drug interactions with methadone. *Annals of the New York Academy of Sciences*, 1976; 281: 350–370.

despite having poor cytochrome P450 metabolic activity because they lose the "spongelike" hepatic-storage/release function. In other words, the damage to hepatic-drug-metabolizing systems may be offset by damage to the capacity of the liver to store and release unchanged methadone (Novick et al., 1985).

In the management of pain, the conversion from other opioids to methadone is best done by practitioners experienced with this agent. There is no fixed single dose ratio but rather a ratio that increases with higher opioid doses. Patients receiving the highest doses of opioids appear relatively more sensitive to the analgesic effects of methadone and so have the highest dose ratio.

Because there is large interindividual variation, there exists no precise conversion ratio to morphine equivalents, and various suggested conversion guidelines/algorithms may be inconsistent, complex, inexact, and difficult to remember. "Sliding-scale-type" conversion ratios of daily morphine equivalents to methadone have been proposed (e.g., 4:1 for low-dose morphine, <100 mg/d [i.e., 4 mg morphine = 1 mg methadone]; 8:1 for moderate-dose morphine, 100–300 mg/d; 12:1 to 15:1 for high-dose morphine, >300–600 mg/d; 15:1 for 600–800 mg; and 20:1 for >800–1,000 mg; Bruera et al., 1996; Ripamonti et al., 1998). Alternatively, Plonk (2005) devised a linear "rule of 15" equation to convert oral morphine equivalents to estimated methadone. He derived this by extracting average data from five publications and analyzing this with linear regression to describe the "best fit line" (oral methadone per day [mg] = 0.0757 [oral morphine equivalents per day, mg] + 15.82; Plonk, 2005). When simplified and approximated, this equation becomes the following: estimated oral methadone per day (mg) = oral morphine equivalents per day (mg) ÷ 15 + 15 (Plonk, 2005). Higher conversion ratios have been successfully utilized clinically as well for higher morphine doses (Nixon, 2005). In general, it is suggested that nonexpert clinicians should start the opioid-naïve patient on doses not over 40 mg/d of methadone.

Clinicians should be cautious when converting various opioids to methadone. An approach of starting a low dose of methadone in adults with slow titration (not to exceed 10 mg a week) up to efficacy may minimize problems. Various issues to consider when prescribing methadone may include the following: equianalgesic dosing may not apply to repeated dosing of opioids; repetitive (more than one dose per day) analgesic doses of methadone will lead to drug accumulation; significant interpatient variability may exist; when converting from a specific opioid to methadone, the higher the opioid dose, the higher the conversion ratio; and conversion ratios may not be bidirectional (i.e., the morphine-to-methadone conversion ratio may not be the same as the methadone-to-morphine ratio). In short, the use of methadone in a clinical setting requires as much art as science given our present states of knowledge. Careful initial observation of a patient started on methadone, coupled with daily clinic visits conversations during methadone titration, may effectively obviate problems of overdosing or underdosing.

Methadone Drug Interactions

Methadone is primarily a substrate of CYP2C19 (minor), CYP2D6 (minor), and CYP3A4 (major). CYP3A4 inducers (e.g., carbamazepine, phenobarbital) may decrease levels of methadone. CYP3A4 inhibitors (e.g., propofol, verapamil, diclofenac) may increase the levels/effects of methadone. Antiretroviral agents may produce complex interactions when used in conjunction with methadone. For example, nevirapine and efavirenz as well as long-term ritonavir therapy may decrease methadone levels (potentially leading to withdrawal symptoms); methadone may increase the bioavailability of zidovudine and decrease the bioavailability of didanosine and stavudine (Clarke et al., 2001; Fornataro, 1999; Stocker et al., 2004).

Grapefruit juice (which inhibits intestinal CYP3A4) may be associated with a mild–modest increase in methadone bioavailability; however, this is not likely clinically significant in humans (Benmebarek et al., 2004) and has never been a problem in MMT patients.

The clinically significant major drug interactions of methadone include the following: rifampin, phenytoin, barbiturates, and carbamazepine. Rifampin is a CYP3A4 inducer and a drug used in the treatment of tuberculosis. Therefore, rifampin significantly lowers plasma levels of methadone, and this effect is paralleled by the appearance of opioid withdrawal symptoms in previously asymptomatic patients on MMT (Kreek et al., 1976a, 1976b). The mechanism(s) by which rifampin lowers plasma methadone levels remains uncertain, but enhanced microsomal-drug-metabolizing enzyme activities and altered methadone distribution may contribute (Kreek et al., 1976a, 1976b). The antiepileptic drugs phenytoin, phenobarbital, and carbamazepine are inducers of CYP3A4 and, therefore, may diminish methadone concentration in the blood. Phenytoin may cause a reduction in methadone blood levels by roughly half after 3–4 days of concomitant administration (Pond et al., 1985; Saxon et al., 1989). Phenobarbital as well as carbamazepine may increase methadone metabolism, and dose escalation with coadministration of methadone and phenobarbital or carbamazepine may be required to avoid precipitating withdrawal symptoms (Robinson & McDowall, 1979; Saxon et al., 1989).

Although not well studied in humans and of uncertain clinical significance, it appears that methadone has the potential to increase the electrocardiogram QTc interval when dosed at greater than 150 mg per day (Peles et al., 2006). Increasing the QTc interval may lead to torsade de pointes (a potentially fatal polymorphic ventricular arrhythmia; Krantz et al., 2005). These other patient characteristics have been identified that can increase the likelihood of torsade de pointes occurring: abnormal electrolytes (e.g., potassium, magnesium); lower heart rates; concurrent use of illicit drug (e.g., cocaine); large/rapid jumps in methadone dosing; preexisting cardiac dysrhythmias and/or structural heart disease; and concurrent administration of medications such as antiarrhythmics, antidepressants, and antihistaminergics. A list of drugs associated with torsade de pointes can found at http://www.torsades.org, and potentially helpful suggestions when prescribing methadone have been put forth (Sticherling et al., 2005). It may be prudent to obtain an electrocardiogram on patients receiving more than 150 mg per day of methadone and to repeat this periodically as well as monitor for the appearance of any torsades de pointes symptoms (e.g., lightheadedness/dizziness; Peles et al., 2006).

Adverse effects of methadone include typical potential opioid adverse effects such as increased sweating, constipation, urinary retention, anorexia/nausea/vomiting, pruritis, fatigue, dizziness, disturbances of libido/orgasm, confusion/cognitive disturbances, sedation, and respiratory depression. A rare effect perhaps associated with methadone is galactorrhea (Bennett & Whale, 2006).

When considering short-acting opioids to utilize for breakthrough pain in conjunction with methadone in an effort to achieve maximal analgesia with the lowest possible opioid dose (e.g., thereby with hopefully the least adverse effects), one should attempt to take advantage of potential synergistic effects. Therefore the best choice of an opioid analgesic in this situation may be morphine—as it seems to exhibit analgesic synergy with 1(R)-methadone (Bolan et al., 2002). Other opioids including oxymorphone, oxycodone, fentanyl, and meperidine have not found to be synergistic with methadone (Bolan et al., 2002). The combination of 1(R)-methadone and hydromorphone was not studied. Fortunately, although it displayed synergy in analgesic assay, the 1(R)-methadone/morphine combination did not exhibit synergy in the gastrointestinal transit assay (Bolan et al., 2002).

Methadone as an Analgesic

Any health-care provider holding a valid schedule II drug enforcement agency (DEA) license can prescribe methadone for pain, although in some areas it is necessary to write the words "for pain" on the prescription. A special license is required to initiate methadone for the treatment of chemical dependency issues. It is critical that prescribers are aware that they cannot mix these functions (i.e., if you are prescribing methadone for pain, then you cannot also prescribe methadone for addiction in the same patient, regardless of your licenses/qualifications).

Multiple studies have demonstrated the utility of methadone as a therapeutic option in the treatment of cancer-related pain, and extensive reviews on this topic have been published (Nicholson, 2004; Ripamonti & Bianchi, 2002; Soares, 2005). For instance, Bruera and colleagues (2004) compared the effectiveness and tolerability of methadone and morphine as first-line treatment with opioids for cancer pain in a randomized, double-blind study. A total of 103 patients were randomized (49 in the methadone group, 54 in the morphine group) with similar pretreatment symptoms/characteristics (Bruera et al., 2004). Patients receiving methadone had more opioid-related dropouts (11 of 49 [22%]) than those receiving morphine (3 of 54 [6%]; $p = 0.019$). The opioid escalation index at 2 weeks and 1 month was similar between the two groups, and over 75% of patients in both groups reported a reduction in pain intensity of 20% or greater by Day 8. The proportion of patients with pain improvement of 20% or greater at 1 month was similar in both groups. The rates of patient-reported global benefit were nearly identical to the pain response rates and did not differ between the treatment groups (Bruera et al., 2004). Although the researchers suggested that morphine be used as a first-line strong opioid for the treatment of cancer pain, they noted that the study did not meet their accrual goal of 100 assessable patients per study arm and so had only a sufficient power to detect a difference of 30% or greater in the response populations (Bruera et al., 2004).

A review of methadone as an analgesic for cancer pain concluded that the majority of studies involved only single-dose comparisons or short-term use and therefore do not reflect clinical practice (Nicholson, 2004). Thus, conclusions have been limited by variations in trial design, dosing regimens, and limited presentation of primary outcome data. Nicholson (2004) concluded that due to the complex and highly individual pharmacokinetics of methadone, only experienced clinicians should take responsibility for initiating, titrating, and monitoring methadone therapy.

The use of methadone for cancer-related pain appears to be well accepted in clinical practice. The use of methadone for treatment of persistent noncancer pain, however, remains less well-embraced by clinicians. Despite this, its use for noncancer pain appears to have increased significantly over the past decade. In fact, methadone usage as an analgesic for all types of pain has experienced a resurgence of interest. This may be due to it being relatively inexpensive, long-acting, and efficacious. Additionally, it is uninteresting for abuse because of its high degree of binding to plasma proteins, slow delivery to brain during chronic treatment, and its slow onset of action, with steady serum levels and no "on/off" effects (from fluctuating opioid blood levels), as well as relatively reduced reinforcement of opioid craving (unlike short acting opioids such as heroin, morphine, and hydromorphone). Methadone tablet prescriptions in the United States increased from 437,030 in 2001 to 2,609,613 in 2004 (IMS; Dart et al., 2005).

Despite this increase in methadone's clinical use and the growing appreciation of its analgesic benefits, the literature lags behind. Sandoval and colleagues (2005) performed a systematic literature review of oral methadone for chronic noncancer pain and cited only one high-quality study. This was a very small, randomized, crossover, placebo-controlled trial of short duration conducted by Morley and colleagues (2003). They conducted a 20-day evaluation of the analgesic effectiveness and adverse effects of a daily dose of 10 mg or 20 mg of oral methadone in 18 patients with a variety of chronic neuropathic pain syndromes who had had poor responses to traditional analgesic regimens. Ten milligrams of methadone given twice a day resulted in statistically significant ($P = 0.013–0.020$) improvements in maximum pain intensity ratings, average pain intensity, and pain relief versus placebo. Five milligrams of methadone given twice a day also demonstrated analgesic effects versus placebo, but these failed to reach statistical significance. The most common side effects were nausea, vomiting, headache, somnolence, dizziness, and constipation (Morley et al., 2003).

Methadone as Pharmacotherapy for Opioid Dependency

Kreek (2000) has discussed historical events leading to the current system of MMT in the United States. Professor Vincent P. Dole, while at Rockefeller University, turned his attention to pharmacotherapy for the management of heroin addiction, and in late 1963/early 1964 joined forces with Dr. Marie Nyswander, a psychiatrist, and Dr. Mary Jeanne Kreek, then a PGY-2 in internal medicine. Within 6 months, the small team had completed the work to introduce the chronic use of methadone along with behavioral therapy for the maintenance treatment of heroin addiction (Dole et al., 1966). Despite the efforts of this group and others in documenting the safety and efficacy of methadone pharmacotherapy for heroin addiction, federal regulations and societal stigmatization of heroin addicts had impeded treatment implementation for more than 3 decades.

In 1994, the Institute of Medicine of the National Academy of Sciences recommended changing federal regulations to increase medicalization and access to MMT (Rettig & Yarmolinsky, 1995). Three years later, a consensus conference at the National Institutes of Health (NIH) met to consider these recommendations. From this, recommendations were published supporting methadone maintenance treatment for heroin addiction, as well as increased access to and ease of becoming involved in MMT programs (Kreek, 2000). In 1999, the Office of National Drug Control Policy (ONDCP), in conjunction with the Department of Health and Human Services, reinterpreted and published the federal regulations guidelines with respect to the implementation of methadone maintenance programs (Kreek & Vocci, 2002).

MMT is superior to illegal heroin use in part because the extreme highs and lows felt by heroin users (related to the waxing and waning of serum heroin levels) are avoided by the long-acting properties of methadone. The term *agonist blockade* was coined to describe the phenomenon of significantly limited or blunted effects after administration of "usual" doses of mu opioid agonists to subjects on high-dose methadone (e.g., 80–120 mg/day).

In humans, all opiates suppress the hypothalamic-pituitary-adrenal (HPA) axis when given acutely, and this effect persists during chronic, intermittent exposure to short-acting opioids during chronic cycles of heroin addiction (Kreek, 1978b; Kreek et al., 2002). The endogenous mu opioid receptor mediated-opioid system in humans appears to constitutively provide tonic inhibition of the HPA axis (Kreek et al., 2002; Schluger et al., 1998). Thus, administration of mu opioid receptor antagonists to healthy human volunteers leads to activation of the HPA axis (Cohen et al., 1983; King, 2002; Schluger et al., 1998; Volavka et al., 1979). Similarly, the HPA axis is activated in opioid withdrawal, or with administration of mu opioid receptor antagonists to opioid-dependent individuals, or during acute cocaine or alcohol consumption (Culpepper-Morgan et al., 1992; Culpepper-Morgan & Kreek, 1997; King, 2002; Rosen et al., 1996; Schluger et al., 1998).

Kreek and colleagues (Kreek et al., 2002, 2004; Schluger et al., 2001) proposed that the suppression of the HPA axis through administration of intermittent or binge-type short-acting opioids (e.g., heroin) and then with repeated alternating short cycling of suppression (e.g., with heroin administration), followed by activation (e.g., with heroin withdrawal [i.e., just before next dose]) may lead to and/or exacerbate atypical responsivity to stress/stressors as well as addictive-type behavior (with resultant self-administration/relapse). (Incidentally, this atypical stress responsivity that produces the use of abused drugs in some subjects may be on a genetic or acquired basis, thereby predisposing one to addiction.) From this, they reasoned that the administration of an adequate dose of a long-acting opioid (e.g., methadone) may end the repeated suppression/activation cycling of the HPA axis because steady-state equilibrium of opioid could be established, without the peaks and valleys of intermittent short-acting opioid dosing, with the potential beginnings of intermittent early chemical (perhaps subclinical) or symptoms of withdrawal (e.g., drug craving) just before the next opioid dose. In fact, studies have suggested that activation of at least the HPA axis component of stress responsivity may be the earliest event to occur in the spectrum of an opioid withdrawal state, before the onset of overt signs or symptoms (Culpepper-Morgan & Kreek 1997; Culpepper-Morgan et al., 1992).

Adequate methadone maintenance treatment permits normalization of the HPA axis—including response to a chemically induced stress of metyrapone challenge (Kreek 1973a; Kreek et al., 1984). In an optimal situation, stabilized methadone-maintained former heroin addicts treated in high-quality methadone maintenance treatment programs (e.g., associated with psychosocial interventions) with effective methadone doses experience the following: markedly reduced drug craving, reduced or eliminated heroin use, improved or normalized stress-responsive hypothalamic-pituitary-adrenal axis, as well as reproductive, gastrointestinal, and immunologic functions with relatively normal responses to acute pain (Kling et al., 2000; Kreek, 2000).

Multiple studies have demonstrated a benefit of methadone to reduce opioid use and increase retention in treatment as well as to reduce recidivism, criminal activity, and opioid-related mortality (Kayman et al., 2006; Peles et al., 2006; Rich et al., 2005; Tomasino et al., 2001; Villafranca et al., 2005). Researchers (Gearing, 1974; Gearing & Schweitzer, 1974) have published data showing that untreated heroin addicts have a yearly mortality rate of 8.3%, whereas those in methadone treatment programs have a mortality rate of 0.8%. Gronbladh and colleagues (1990) reported a sixfold reduction in mortality in methadone-treated opioid addicts, and Caplehorn and researchers (1996) reported a fourfold reduction in the risk of dying for patients in methadone programs. Optimally, MMT programs should combine psychosocial as well as medical therapy (McLellan et al., 2005).

Trafton and colleagues (2006) prospectively observed a volunteer sample of 222 opioid-dependent U.S. veterans initiating methadone treatment for 1 year as part of the Multi-site Opioid Substitution Treatment (MOST) study. The MOST study was designed to look at outcome differences based on naturalistic characteristics in treatment. In the 168 subjects who achieved heroin abstinence for at least 1 month, the methadone doses ranged from 1.5 mg to 191.2 mg per day (Trafton et al., 2006). Thirty-eight percent of subjects achieved abstinence on less than 60 mg of methadone per day, and 16% received a dosage of over 100 mg per day. Almost half of patients who did not achieve heroin abstinence received the recommended dosage of 60 mg of methadone per day. Among the 168 "abstinent" patients, higher methadone doses were predicted by having a diagnosis of posttraumatic stress disorder or depression, having a greater number of previous opioid detoxifications, living in a region with lower average heroin purity, attending a clinic where counselors discourage dosage reductions, or staying in treatment longer. These factors predicted 42% of the variance in dosage associated with heroin abstinence (Trafton et al., 2006).

Trafton and colleagues (2006) also suggested that several "failed" attempts to stop using methadone may actually increase the need for methadone with respect to long-term maintenance treatment doses. This correlates with proposed theories that excessive neuronal firing during opioid withdrawal facilitates signaling via opioidergic pathways (Ibuki et al., 2003; Jhamandas et al., 1996). This sensitization phenomenon may result in altered spinal cord plasticity and subsequent potential opioid tolerance in the future. Trafton and colleagues (2006) concluded that: (1) effective and ineffective methadone doses overlap substantially; (2) dosing recommendations should concentrate more on processes in order to achieve effective dosage determination (versus suggesting specific doses); and (3) methadone dosages should be skillfully titrated in efforts to achieve optimal effective daily doses.

However, it appears that methadone doses equal to or greater than 60 mg per day (a dose that an National Institutes of Health [NIH] expert panel has regarded as a "best practice" dose) may more effectively and reliably normalize the HPA axis, combat symptoms (e.g., drug craving), and optimize retention in "all comers" to an MMT program (Brady et al., 2005; Kreek & Vocci, 2002). Furthermore, it seems that high methadone dose (175.1 + 42.1 mg/per day) may reduce cocaine use in patients addicted to both heroin and cocaine (Peles et al., 2006). The reduction in cocaine seeking has also been demonstrated in animal models (Leri et al., 2005).

Utilizing a randomized, controlled study design, Schwartz and colleagues (2006) concluded that interim methadone maintenance consisting of individually determined methadone dose and emergency counseling only for up to 120 days results in a significant increase on the likelihood of entry into comprehensive treatment. This was also found to be an effective means of reducing heroin use and criminal behavior among opioid-dependent subjects waiting to gain entry to into a comprehensive methadone maintenance treatment program (Schwartz et al., 2006).

Marsch and colleagues (2005) studied predictors of treatment outcome for opioid-dependent participants in a single-site controlled trial comparing the treatments of methadone, buprenorphine, and levomethadyl acetate (LAAM). They demonstrated that predictors of treatment success were similar in all three study arms and, thus, there were not any factors that would strongly guide selection of one medication over another (Marsch et al., 2005).

In preclinical studies, Negus (2006) suggested that opiate withdrawal increases the relative reinforcing effects of opiate agonists and that full agonist medications (e.g., methadone more effectively than buprenorphine) attenuate withdrawal.

There may be multiple factors associated with retention in MMT programs. Kayman and colleagues (2006) have suggested that the attitudes toward methadone helped predict which subjects were more likely to remain in MMT program. Subjects with favorable opinions regarding methadone were more likely to remain in MMT programs. These researchers suggested utilizing a scale entitled Opinions About Methadone (OAM-5), which is a 5-item scale that may help identify which subjects may be in greatest need of support for remaining in treatment (Kayman et al., 2006).

Genetics in Opioid Dependency

Genetics appear to play a significant role in various opioid dependency states. At least 14 single-nucleotide polymorphisms

(SMPs) of the mu opioid receptor gene (OPRMI) have been identified, with eight variants resulting in different protein sequences of the receptor. The A118G mutation results in an amino acid exchange at position 40 from asparagine to aspartate at the amino terminus of the mu opioid receptor that is involved in the initial binding of opioids (La Forge et al., 2000). The A118G SNP localized at exon 1 on the mu opioid receptor gene is not rare, and occurs with an allelic frequency of about 10.5%. This functional variant binds the endogenous opioid beta-endorphin three times more tightly as well as leads to a roughly three times normal signal transduction via G-protein-coupled potassium inwardly rectifying channels when occupied by a pure agonist (Bond et al., 1998).

Although the potency of morphine is unchanged in patients who carry the A118G mutation and in patients with renal impairment who carry the A118G SNP, the risk for morphine 6-glucuronide (M6G) associated adverse effects was significantly diminished (Lotsch et al., 2002b). Lotsch and colleagues (2006) investigated the central nervous system effects of 0.075 mg levomethadone 9 hours after oral administration in a random sample of 51 healthy volunteers. They concluded that among polymorphisms in OPRM1 (the gene for the mu opioid receptor), ABCB1, and CYP genes previously associated with functional consequences in a different context the major pharmacogenetic factor affecting levomethadone's short-term effects is a polymorphism (OPRM1 118A > G) that modulates mu opioid receptors.

The Kreek laboratory hypothesized that the different binding characteristics and functions of the A118G variant could lead to functionally different physiologic changes in systems affected by the mu opioid receptor (Bond et al., 1998). Kreek and colleagues demonstrated that genetic polymorphism in the mu opioid receptor gene predicts positive response to opioid antagonist treatment of alcoholism (Kreek, 2000; La Forge et al., 2000). Furthermore, Kreek's laboratory demonstrated that A118G polymorphism of the mu opioid receptor gene is significantly associated with both opioid dependency and alcoholism with significant attributable risk (Bart et al., 2004, 2005).

Conclusion

Methadone is a unique drug among the opioid class. A synthetically derived agent, we are still learning many of the intricacies and details for its use some 60 plus years after its creation. Practitioners need to keep in mind its dual use in our society for pain in some patients and as a maintenance drug for addiction in others, as well as the legal implications regarding these different uses. Finally, in the case of pain management, practitioners are cautioned to remember the widely variable conversion ratios that may apply when switching agents in the opioid class either to or from methadone.

References

Altier N, Dion D, Boulanger A, et al. Management of chronic neuropathic pain with methadone: a review of 13 cases. *Clin J Pain.* 2005; 21: 364–9.

Bart G, Kreek MJ, Ott J, LaForge KS, Proudnikov D, Pollak L, Heilig M. Increased attributable risk related to a functional mu-opioid receptor gene polymorphism in association with alcohol dependence in central Sweden. *Neuropsychopharmacology.* 2005 Feb; 30(2): 417–22.

Bellward GD, Warren PM, Harold W, et al. Methadone maintenance: effect of urinary pH on renal clearance in chronic high and low doses. *Clin Pharmacol Ther.* 1977; 22: 92–99.

Benmebarek M, Devaud C, Gex-Fabry M, et al. Effects of grapefruit juice on the pharmacokinetics of the enantiomers of methadone. *Clin Pharmacol Ther.* 2004; 76: 55–63.

Bennett J, Whale R. Galactorrhoea may be associated with methadone use. *BMJ.* 2006; 332: 1071.

Bolan EA, Tallarida RJ, Pasternak GW. Synergy between μ opioid receptor subtypes. *JPET.* 2002; 303: 557–62.

Bond C, LaForge KS, Tian M, Melia D, Zhang S, Borg L, Gong J, Schluger J, Strong JA, Leal SM, Tischfield JA, Kreek MJ, Yu L. Single-nucleotide polymorphism in the human mu opioid receptor gene alters beta-endorphin binding and activity: possible implications for opiate addiction. *Proc Natl Acad Sci USA.* 1998 Aug 4; 95(16): 9608–13.

Bot G, Blake AD, Li S, et al. Opioid regulation of the mouse opioid receptor expressed in human embryonic kidney 293 cells. *Mol Pharmacol.* 1997; 53: 272–81.

Brady TM, Salvucci S, Sverdlow LS, et al. Methadone dosage and retention: an examination of the 60 mg/day threshold. *J Addict Dis.* 2005; 24: 23–47.

Bruera E, Pereira J, Watanabe S, et al. Opioid rotation in patients with cancer pain. *Cancer.* 1996; 78: 852–7.

Bruera E, Palmer JL, Bosnjak S, et al. Methadone versus morphine as a first-line strong opioid for cancer pain: A randomized double-blind study. *J Clin Onc.* 2004; 22: 185–92.

Bruera E, Sweeney C. Methadone use in cancer patients with pain. *J Palliative Med.* 2002; 5: 127–37.

Callahan RJ, Au JD, Paul M, Liu C, Yost CS. Functional inhibition by methadone of N-methyl-D-aspartate receptors expressed in Xenopus oocytes: stereospecific and subunit effects. *Anesth Analg.* 2004 Mar; 98(3): 653–9.

Caplehorn JR, Dalton MS, Haldar F, Petrenas AM, Nisbet JG. Methadone maintenance and addicts' risk of fatal heroin overdose. *Subst Use Misuse.* 1996 Jan; 31(2): 177–96.

Carrasco GA, Van de Kar LD. Neuroendocrine pharmacology of stress. *Eur J Pharmacol.* 2003 Feb 28; 463(1–3): 235–72.

Centeno CC, Sanchez R, Vara F. Methadone for pain syndromes with predominant neuropathic features in cancer patients. *J of Cancer Pain & Symptom Palliation.* 2005; 1(3): 7–10.

Chizh BA, Schlutz H, Scheede M, Englberger W. The N-methyl-D-aspartate antagonistic and opioid components of d-methadone antinociception in the rat spinal cord. *Neurosci Lett.* 2000 Dec 22; 296(2–3): 117–20.

Clarke SM, Mulcahy FM, Tjia J, et al. Pharmacokinetic interactions of nevirapine and methadone and guidelines for use of nevirapine to treat injection drug users. *Clin Infect Dis.* 2001; 33: 1595–7.

Codd EE, Shank RP, Schupsky JJ, et al. Serotonin and norepinephrine up take inhibiting activity of centrally acting analgesics: Structural determinants and role in antinociception. *J Pharmacol Exp Ther.* 1995; 274: 1263–70.

Cohen MR, Cohen RM, Pickar D, et al. High-dose naloxone infusions in normals. Dose-dependent behavioral, hormonal, and physiological responses. *Arch Gen Psychiatry.* 1983; 40: 613–9.

Crettol S, Deglon JJ, Besson, et al. Methadone enantiomer plasma levels, CYP2B6, CYP2C19, and CYP2C9 genotypes, and response to treatment. *Clin Pharmacol Ther.* 2005; 78: 593–604.

Culpepper-Morgan JA, Inturrisi CE, Portenoy RK, Foley K, Houde RW, Marsh F, Kreek MJ. Treatment of opioid-induced constipation with oral naloxone: a pilot study. *Clin Pharmacol Ther.* 1992 Jul; 52(1): 90–5.

Culpepper-Morgan JA, Kreek MJ. Hypothalamic-pituitary-adrenal axis hypersensitivity to naloxone in opioid dependence: a case of naloxone-induced withdrawal. *Metabolism.* 1997 Feb; 46(2): 130–4.

Dart RC, Woody GE, Kleber HD. Prescribing methadone as an analgesic. *Annals of Internal Med.* 2005; 148: 620.

Davis AM, Inturrisi CE. D-Methadone blocks morphine tolerance and N-methyl-D-aspartate-induced hyperalgesia. *J Pharmacol Exp Ther.* 1999; 289: 1048–53.

Davis M, Walsh D, Methadone for the relief of cancer pain: a review of pharmacokinetics, pharmacodynamics, drug interactions and protocols of administration. *Support Care Cancer.* 2001; 9: 73–83.

Dole VP, Nyswander ME, Kreek MJ. Narcotic blockade. *Arch Intern Med.* 1966; 118: 304–9.

Eap CB, Buclin T, Baumann P. Interindividual variability of the clinical pharmacokinetics of methadone: implications for the treatment of opioid dependence. *Clin Pharmacokinet.* 2002; 41: 1153–93.

Ebert B, Mikkelsen S, Thorkildsen C, Borgbjerg FM. Norketamine, the main metabolite of ketamine, is a non-competitive NMDA receptor antagonist in the rat cortex and spinal cord. *Eur J Pharmacol.* 1997 Aug 20; 333(1): 99–104.

Fishman S, Wilsey B, Mahajan G, Molina P. Methadone reincarnated: novel clinical applications with related concerns. *Pain Med.* 2002; 3: 339–48.

Foley KM, Houde RW. Methadone in cancer pain management: individualize dose and titrate to effect. *J Clin Onc.* 1998 Oct; 16(10): 3213–5.

Fornataro K. Methadone and anti-HIV drugs. *Body Posit.* 1999; 12: 13.

Frank MG, Baratta MV, Sprunger DB, Watkins LR, Maier SF. Microglia serve as a neuroimmune substrate for stress-induced potentiation of CNS proinflammatory cytokine responses. *Brain Behav Immun.* 2007 Jan; 21(1): 47–59.

Gagnon B, Almahrezi A, Schreier G. Methadone in the treatment of neuropathic pain. *Pain Res Manag.* 2003 Fall; 8(3): 149–54.

Garrido MJ, Troconiz IF. Methadone: a review of its pharmacokinetic/pharmacodynamic properties. *J Pharmacol Toxicol.* 1999; 42: 61–6.

Gearing FR. Methadone maintenance treatment. Five years later—where are they now? *Am J Public Health.* 1974 Dec; 64 Suppl(0): 44–50.

Gearing FR, Schweitzer MD. An epidemiologic evaluation of long-term methadone maintenance treatment for heroin addiction. *Am J Epidemiol.* 1974 Aug; 100(2): 101–12.

Gorman AL, Elliott KJ, Inturrisi CE. The d- and l-isomers of methadone bind to the non-competitive site on the N-methyl-D-aspartate (NMDA) receptor in rat forebrain and spinal cord. *Neurosci Lett.* 1997; 223: 5–8.

Gronbladh L, Ohlund LS, Gunne LM. Mortality in heroin addiction: impact of methadone treatment. *Acta Psychiatr Scand.* 1990 Sep; 82(3): 223–7.

Gutstein H, Akil H. Opioid analgesics. In Hardman J, Goodman Gilman A, Limbird L, eds. *The Pharmacological Basis of Therapeutics*, 10th ed. New York: McGraw-Hill; 2001: 569–620.

Hachey DL, Kreek MJ, Mattson DH. Quantitative analysis of methadone in biological fluids using deuterium-labeled methadone and GLC-chemical-ionization mass spectrometry. *J Pharm.* 1977; 66: 1579–1582.

Hachey DL, Mattson DH, Kreek MJ. Quantitation of methadone in biological fluids using deuterium labeled internal standards. In Klein ER, Klein PD, eds. *Proceedings of the Second International Conference on Stable Isotopes.* 1976; ERDA-CONF-751027: 518–523. National Technical Information Source. U.S. Dept. of Commerce. Springfield, VA.

Hays H, Woodroffe MA. Use of methadone in treating chronic noncancer pain. *Pain Res Manage.* 1999; 4: 23–7.

Ibuki T, Marsala M, Masuyama T, Yaksh TL. Spinal amino acid release and repeated withdrawal in spinal morphine tolerant rats. *Br J Pharmacol.* 2003 Feb; 138(4): 689–97.

Inturrisi CE. Clinical pharmacology of opioids for pain. *Clin J Pain.* 2002; 18: S3–13.

Inturrisi CE, Verebely K. A gas-liquid chromatographic method for the quantitative determination of methadone in human plasma and urine. *J Chromatogr.* 1972a; 65: 361–369.

Inturrisi CE, Verebely K. The levels of methadone in the plasma in methadone maintenance. *Clin Pharmacol Ther.* 1972b; 13: 633–637.

Jacobson L, Chabal C, Brody MC, et al. Intrathecal methadone: a dose-response study and comparison with intrathecal morphine 0.5 mg. *Pain.* 1990; 43: 141–8.

Jhamandas KH, Marsala M, Ibuki T, Yaksh TL. Spinal amino acid release and precipitated withdrawal in rats chronically infused with spinal morphine. *J Neurosci.* 1996 Apr 15; 16(8): 2758–66.

Kayman DJ, Goldstein MF, Deren S, et al. Predicting treatment retention with a brief "opinions about methadone" scale. *J Psychoactive Drugs.* 2006; 38: 93–100.

Kharasch ED, Hoffer C, Whittington D, et al. Role of hepatic and intestinal cytochrome P450 3A and 2B6 in the metabolism, disposition, and miotic effects of methadone. *Clin Pharmacol Ther.* 2004; 76: 250–69.

King AC. Role of naltrexone in initial smoking cessation: preliminary findings. *Alcohol Clin Exp Res.* 2002 Dec; 26(12): 1942–4.

Kling M, Carson R, Borg L, et al. Opioid receptor imaging with positive emission tomography and [^{18}F]cyclofoxy in long-term, methadone-treated former heroin addicts. *J Pharmacol Exp Ther.* 2000; 295: 1070–76.

Koch T, Wildera A, Bartzsch K, et al. Receptor endocytosis counteracts the development of opioid tolerance. *Mol Pharmacol.* 2005; 67: 280–87.

Krantz MJ, Lowery CM, Martell BA, Gourevitch MN, Arnsten JH. Effects of methadone on QT-interval dispersion. *Pharmacotherapy.* 2005 Nov; 25(11): 1523–9.

Kreek, MJ. Medical complications in methadone patients. *Ann NY Acad Sci.* 1978b; 331: 110–134.

Kreek MJ. Medical safety and side effects of methadone in tolerant individuals. *Journal of the American Medical Association.* 1973a; 223: 665–668.

Kreek MJ. Methadone-related opioid agonist pharmacotherapy for heroin addiction: history, recent molecular and neurochemical research and future in mainstream medicine. *Ann NY Acad Sci.* 2000; 909: 186–216.

Kreek MJ. Pharmacology and medical aspects of methadone treatment. In Rettig RA, Yarmolinsky A, eds. *Federal Regulation of Methadone Treatment.* Washington, DC: National Academy of Sciences, National Academy Press; 1995: 37–60.

Kreek MJ. Plasma and urine levels of methadone. Comparison following four medication forms used in chronic maintenance treatment. *NYS J Med.* 1973b; 73: 2773–2777.

Kreek MJ, Borg L, Zhou Y, et al. Relationships between endocrine functions and substance abuse syndromes: heroin and related short-acting opiates in addiction contrasted with methadone and other long-acting opioid agonists used in pharmacotherapy of addiction. In Pfaff D, ed. *Hormones, Brain and Behavior.* Vol. 5. San Diego, CA: Academic Press; 2002: 781–830.

Kreek MJ, Garfield JW, Gutjahr CL, et al. Rifampin-induced methadone withdrawal. *N Engl J Med.* 1976b; 13: 1104–6.

Kreek MJ, Gutjahr CL, Garfield JW, et al. Drug interactions with methadone. *Ann NY Acad Sci.* 1976a; 281: 350–371.

Kreek MJ, Hachey DL. Use of pentadeuteromethadone in clinical studies of methadone disposition. *Clin Res.* 1975; 23: 571A.

Kreek MJ, Hachey DL, Klein PD. Stereoselective disposition of methadone in man. *Life Sci.* 1979; 24: 925–932.

Kreek MJ, Oratz M, Rothschild MA. Hepatic extraction of long- and short-acting narcotics in the isolated perfused rabbit liver. *Gastroenterology.* 1978a; 75: 88–94.

Kreek, MJ, Ragunath, J, Plevy, S, Hamer, D, Schneider, B, Hartman, N. ACTH, cortisol and beta-endorphin response to metyrapone testing during chronic methadone maintenance treatment in humans. *Neuropeptides.* 1984; 5: 277–278.

Kreek MJ, Schecter AJ, Gutjahr CL, et al. Methadone use in patients with chronic renal disease. *Drug Alcohol Depend.* 1980; 5: 197–205.

Kreek MJ, Schlussman SD, Bart G, LaForge KS, Butelman ER. Evolving perspectives on neurobiological research on the addictions: celebration of the 30th anniversary of NIDA. *Neuropharmacology.* 2004; 47 Suppl 1: 324–44.

Kreek MJ, Vocci FJ. History and current status of opioid maintenance treatments: blending conference session. *J Subst Abuse Treat.* 2002; 23: 93–105.

Kristensen K, Blemmer T, Angelo HR, et al. Stereoselective pharmacokinetics of methadone in chronic pain patients. *Ther Drug Monit.* 1996; 18: 221–7.

Kristensen K, Christensen CB, Christup LL. The mu1, mu2, delta, kappa opioid receptor binding profiles of methadone stereoisomers and morphine. *Life Sci.* 1995; 56: PL45–50.

LaForge KS, Shick V, Spangler R, Proudnikov D, Yuferov V, Lysov Y, Mirzabekov A, Kreek MJ. Detection of single nucleotide polymorphisms of the human mu opioid receptor gene by hybridization or single nucleotide extension on custom oligonucleotide gelpad microchips: potential in studies of addiction. *Am J Med Genet.* 2000 Oct 9; 96(5): 604–15.

Lehotay DC, George S, Etter ML, et al. Free and bound enantiomers of methadone and its metabolite EDDP in methadone maintenance treatment: relationship to dosage? *Clin Biochem,* 2005; 38: 1088–94.

Lemberg K, Kotinen VK, Viljakka K, et al. Morphine, oxycodone, methadone and its enantiomers in different models of nociception in the rat. *Anesth Analg,* 2006; 102: 1768–74.

Leri F, Zhou Y, Goddard B, Cummins E, Kreek MJ. Effects of high dose methadone maintenance on cocaine place conditioning, cocaine self-administration, and mu-opioid receptor mRNA expression in the rat brain. *Neuropsychopharmacology.* 2006; 31: 1462–74.

Lotsch J, Skarke C, Tegeder I, Geisslinger G. Drug interactions with patient-controlled analgesia. *Clin Pharmacokinet,* 2002a; 41(1): 31–57.

Lotsch J, Skarke C, Wieting J, et al. Modulation of the central nervous effects of levomethadone by genetic polymorphisms potentially affecting its metabolism, distribution, and drug action. *Clin Pharmacol Ther.* 2006; 79: 72–89.

Lotsch J, Zimmermann M, Darimont J, et al. Does the A118G polymorphism at the mu-opioid receptor gene protect against morphine-6-glycuronide toxicity? *Anesthesiology.* 2002b; 97: 814–9.

Lu L, Shepard JD, Scott Hall F, Shaham Y. Effect of environmental stressors on opiate and psychostimulant reinforcement, reinstatement and discrimination in rats: a review. *Neurosci Biobehav Rev.* 2003 Aug; 27(5): 457–91.

Lynch ME. A review of the use of methadone for the treatment of chronic noncancer pain. *Pain Res Manage.* 2005; 10: 133–144.

Marsch LA, Stephens MA, Mudric T, et al. Predictors of outcome in LAAM, buprenorphine, and methadone treatment for opioid dependence. *Exp Clin Psychopharmacol.* 2005; 13: 293–302.

Mathew P, Storey P. Subcutaneous methadone in terminally ill patients: manageable local toxicity. *J Pain Symptom Manage.* 1999 Jul; 18(1): 49–52.

McCaffrey BR. Methadone treatment: our vision for the future. *J Addict Dis.* 2001; 20:93–101.

McLellan AT, Weinstein RL, Shen Q, Kendig C, Levine M. Improving continuity of care in a public addiction treatment system with clinical case management. *Am J Addict.* 2005 Oct–Dec; 14(5): 426–40.

Morley JS, Bridson J, Nash TP, et al. Low-dose methadone has an analgesic effect in neuropathic pain: a double-blind randomized controlled crossover trial. *Palliat Med.* 2003; 17: 576–87.

Moulin D. Use of methadone for neuropathic pain. *Pain Res Manage.* 2003; 8: 131–2.

Moulin DE, Palma D, Watling C, Schulz V. Methadone in the management of intractable neuropathic noncancer pain. *Can J Neurol Sci.* 2005; 32: 340–3.

Nakamura K, et al. Quantitation of methadone enantiomers in humans using stable isotope-labeled $^2H_3$, $^2H_5$, $^2H_8$ methadone. *J Pharm.* 1982; 71: 39–43.

Negus SS. Choice between heroin and food in nondependent and heroin-dependent rhesus monkeys: effects of naloxone, buprenorphine, and methadone. *J Pharmacology and Experimental Therapeutics.* 2006 May; 317(2): 711–23.

Nicholson AB. Methadone for cancer pain. *Cochrane Database Syst Rev.* 2004; 2; CD003971.

Nixon AJ. Methadone for cancer pain: a case report. *Am J of Hospice & Palliative Med.* 2005; 22: 337.

Novick DM, Kreek MJ, Arns PA, et al. Effect of severe alcoholic liver disease on the disposition of methadone in maintenance patients. *Alcohol Clin Exp Res.* 1985; 9: 349–54.

Peles E, Bodner G, Kreek MJ, et al. Corrected-QT intervals as related to methadone dose and serum level in Methadone Maintenance Treatment (MMT) patients. *Addiction.* 2006; 102: 289–300.

Peles E, Kreek MJ, Kellogg S, et al. High methadone dose significantly reduces cocaine use in methadone maintenance treatment (MMT) patients. *J of Addictive Diseases.* 2006; 25: 43–50.

Peng WH, Tumber PS, Gourlay D. Review article: perioperative pain management of patients on methadone therapy. *Canadian J of Anes.* 2005; 52: 513–523.

Plonk WM. Simplified methadone conversion. *J Palliat Med.* 2005 Jun; 8(3): 478–9.

Pond SM, Kreek MJ, Tong TG, et al. Altered methadone pharmacokinetics in methadone-maintained pregnant women. *J Pharmacol Exp Ther.* 1985; 233: 1–6.

Rettig RA, Yarmolinsky A, eds. *Institute of Medicine. Federal Regulation of Methadone Treatment.* Washington, DC: National Academy Press, 1995.

Rich JD, McKenzie M, Shield DC, Wolf FA, Key RG, Poshkus M, Clarke J. Linkage with methadone treatment upon release from incarceration: a promising opportunity. *J Addict Dis.* 2005; 24(3): 49–59.

Ripamonti C, Bianchi M. The use of methadone for cancer pain. *Hematol Oncol Clin North Am.* 2002; 16: 543–55.

Ripamonti C, Groff L, Brunelli C, Polastri D, Stavrakis A, De Conno F. Switching from morphine to oral methadone in treating cancer pain: what is the equianalgesic dose ratio? *J Clin Oncol.* 1998 Oct; 16(10): 3216–21.

Robinson AE, McDowall RD. The human distribution of some barbiturate sedatives in combination with miscellaneous CNS-active drugs. *Forensic Sci Int.* 1979; 14: 9–22.

Rodriguez M, Ortega I, Soengas I, et al. Effect of P-glycoprotein inhibition on methadone analgesia and brain distribution in the rat. *J Pharm Pharmacol.* 2004; 56: 367–74.

Rosen MI, McMahon TJ, Hameedi FA, et al. Effect of clonidine pretreatment on naloxone-precipitated opiate withdrawal. *J Pharmacol Exp Ther.* 1996; 276: 1128–1135.

Rubenstein RB, Kreek MJ, Mbawa N, et al. Human spinal fluid methadone levels. *Drug Alcohol Depend.* 1978; 3: 103–6.

Sandoval JA, Furlan AD, Maillis-Gagnon A. Oral methadone for chronic noncancer pain: a systematic literature review of reasons for administration, prescription patterns, effectiveness, and side effects. *Clin J. Pain.* 2005; 21: 503–12.

Sang CN. NMDA-receptor antagonists in neuropathic pain: experimental methods to clinical trials. *J Pain Symptom Manage,* 2000 Jan; 19(1 Suppl): S21–5.

Saxon AJ, Whittaker S, Hawker CS. Valproic acid, unlike other anticonvulsants, has no effect on methadone metabolism: two cases. *J Clin Psychiatry.* 1989; 50: 228–9.

Schluger JH, Borg L, Ho A, Kreek MJ. Altered HPA axis responsivity to metyrapone testing in methadone maintained former heroin addicts with ongoing cocaine addiction. *Neuropsychopharmacology.* 2001 May; 24(5): 568–75.

Schluger JH, Ho A, Borg L, Porter M, Maniar S, Gunduz M, Perret G, King A, Kreek MJ. Nalmefene causes greater hypothalamic-pituitary-adrenal axis activation than naloxone in normal volunteers: implications for the treatment of alcoholism. *Alcohol Clin Exp Res.* 1998 Oct; 22(7): 1430–6.

Schwartz RP, Highfield DA, Jaffe JH, et al. A randomized controlled trial of interim methadone maintenance. *Arch Gen Psychiatry.* 2006; 63: 102–9.

Scott CC, Robbins EB, Chen KK. Pharmacologic comparison of the optical isomers of methadone. *J Pharmacol Exp Ther.* 1948; 93: 282–86.

Shir Y, Rosen G, Zeldin A, et al. Methadone is safe for treating hospitalized patients with severe pain. *Can J Anaesth.* 2001; 48: 1109–13.

Soares LG. Methadone for cancer pain: what have we learned from clinical studies? *Am J Hosp Palliat Care.* 2005 May–Jun; 22(3): 223–7.

Sticherling C, Schaer BA, Ammann P, Maeder M, Osswald S. Methadone-induced torsade de pointes tachycardias *Swiss Med Wkly.* 2005 May 14; 135(19–20): 282–5.

Stocker H, Krause G, Kreckel P, et al. Nevirapine significantly reduces the levels of racemic methadone and (R)-methadone in human immunodeficiency virus-infected patients. *Antimicrob Agents Chemother.* 2004; 48: 4148–53.

Sullivan HR, Blake A. Quantitative determination of methadone concentrations in human blood, plasma, and urine by gas chromatography. *Res Commun Chem Pathol.* 1972; 3: 467–478.

Sullivan HR, Due SL. Urinary metabolites of dl-methadone in maintenance subjects. *J Med Chem.* 1973; 16: 909–913.

Trafton JA, Minkel J, Humphreys K. Determining effective methadone doses for individual opioid-dependent patients. *PLoS Med.* 2006 Feb 7; 3(3): e80.

Villafranca SW, McKellar JD, Trafton JA, Humphreys K. Predictors of retention in methadone programs: A signal detection analysis. *Drug Alcohol Depend.* 2006 Jul 27; 83(3):218–24.

Volavka J, Cho D, Mallya A, et al. Naloxone increases ACTH and cortisol levels in man. *N Engl J Med.* 1979 (letter); 300: 1056–1057.

Wang JS, Ruan Y, Taylor RM, et al. Brain penetration of methadone (R)- and (S)- enantiomers is greatly increased by P-glycoprotein deficiency in the blood-brain barrier of Abcb1a gene knockout mice. *Psychopharmacology* (Berl). 2004; 173: 132–8.

Wolff K, Boys A, Rostami-Hodjegan A, et al. Changes to methadone clearance during pregnancy. *Eur J Clin Pharmacol.* 2005; 61: 763–8.

Wolff K, Rostami-Hodjegan A, Shires S, et al. The pharmacokinetics of methadone in healthy subjects and opiate users. *Br J Clin Pharmacol.* 1997; 44: 325–34.

17

Cannabinoids in Pain and Addiction

Billy R. Martin
Aron H. Lichtman
Sandra P. Welch

Although there is a rich history describing the use of cannabis and its constituents for numerous maladies, pain management represents one of the most prominent indications. However, cannabis and the psychoactive constituent Δ^9-tetrahydrocannabinol (THC) produce a broad spectrum of pharmacological effects in the same dose range. It is this multiplicity of effects that has hampered the clinical usefulness of cannabinoids. Moreover, lack of knowledge regarding the mechanism by which cannabinoids produce their effects has limited the strategies for developing more effective means of controlling pain with this class of drugs. The discovery that THC and related cannabinoids produce their effects via a unique biological pathway, the endocannabinoid system, opens new avenues for exploring the underlying causes of pain, as well as potential for creating new modalities of pain control. This chapter will provide a brief characterization of the endocannabinoid system, evidence it plays a role in pain perception, ways of manipulating it to produce analgesia, and interactions between endocannabinoid and opioid systems in pain control.

The Endocannabinoid System

Research directed at investigating the mechanisms of action underlying marijuana's actions has greatly contributed to the discovery of the endocannabinoid system as well as an impetus to understand the physiological functions of this system. In particular, the endocannabinoid system consists of two G-protein coupled receptors, CB_1 (located in the CNS and periphery; [Matsuda et al., 1990] and CB_2 (localized primarily to the immune system; [Gérard et al., 1991]). Both receptors couple to G-proteins that inhibit adenylyl cyclase (Howlett et al., 2002). Hence, the primary cannabinoid second messenger is cAMP. CB_1 cannabinoid receptors also exert effects on ion channels that include activation of inwardly rectifying potassium channels and inhibition of Q-type calcium channels (Mackie et al., 1995). In addition, they inhibit N-type calcium channels (Mackie & Hille, 1992). These actions on ion channels account for the inhibition of neurotransmitter release, because the CB_1 receptor is predominantly located presynaptically in neural

tissue. In contrast, CB_2 cannabinoid receptors do not act at ion channels (Felder et al., 1995).

Natural ligands, which bind to cannabinoid receptors, have also been identified that include arachidonoylethanolamide (anandamide; [Devane et al., 1992]), 2-arachidonoylglycerol (2-AG; [Mechoulam et al., 1995]), noladin ether; [Hanus et al., 2001], virodhamin [Porter et al., 2002], and N-arachidonoyldopamine [Walker et al., 2002]. These lipid signaling molecules are referred to as endocannabinoids. Multiple enzymes are involved in the biosynthesis and degradation of these lipids (Ueda, 2002). A specific phospholipase D (NAPE-PLD) has been proposed to hydrolyze N-acyl-phosohatidylethanolamine to anandamide (Okamoto et al., 2004). The highest concentrations of this enzyme are found in brain, kidney, and testis of the mouse. Two sn-1-specific diacylglycerol lipases ($DAGL_a$ and $DAGL_b$) has been identified that can hydrolyze diacylglycerol to 2-arachidonoylglycerol (Bisogno et al., 2003). Degradative enzymes include fatty acid amide hydrolase (FAAH) as the enzyme primarily responsible for anandamide catabolism (Cravatt et al., 1996, 2001) and the serine lipase monoacylglycerol lipase (MGL) responsible for 2-AG degradation (Dinh et al., 2002).

Role of the Endocannabinoid System in Pain Perception

The presence of CB_1 receptors in CNS regions associated with pain, such as the periaqueductal gray (PAG) and the dorsal horn of the spinal cord (Herkenham et al., 1991b; Hohmann & Herkenham, 1999a, 1999b), is consistent with the notion that the endocannabinoid system plays a role in modulating pain. Our current understanding of the physiological function of the endocannabinoid system as it pertains to pain is reviewed below.

A commonly used approach to infer whether endocannabinoids are tonically active is to disrupt CB_1 receptor signaling through the employment of knockout mice or receptor antagonists; however, these approaches used alone have generally yielded equivocal findings. For example, administration of the CB_1 receptor antagonist rimonabant (SR 141716) has been found to increase pain sensitivity in the formalin test (Calignano et al., 1998; Strangman et al., 1998), though other studies found no effect of this antagonist on basal pain responses to formalin (Beaulieu et al., 2000; Lichtman et al., 2004a). In addition, intrathecal administration

---

Portions of the research described herein were supported by NIDA grants DA 03672, DA 05274, and DA 09789.

of exceptionally low doses of rimonabant decreased pain thresholds in rats, though the effect failed to occur at higher doses and the duration of the hyperalgesia persisted for only 20 minutes (Richardson et al., 1998), despite the long half-life of this drug (Rinaldi-Carmona et al., 1994).

Compelling evidence supporting a tonic role of endocannabinoids in regulating basal pain thresholds came from an electrophysiological study in which rimonabant dose-dependently enhanced C-fiber activity in anesthetized rats (Chapman, 1999). Nonetheless, in the preponderance of studies, rimonabant has failed to alter nociception across several species, including mice (Compton et al., 1996; Rinaldi-Carmona et al., 1994, 1995), rats (Lichtman & Martin, 1997), and nonhuman primates (Vivian et al., 1998). Similarly, $CB_1^{(-/-)}$ mice generally express normal pain sensitivity (Ledent et al., 1999; Valverde et al., 2000; Zimmer et al., 2001). If the results of the few reports that suggest rimonabant can increase pain sensitivity are subsequently deemed relevant, this basic finding might be attributed to the inverse agonist properties of this drug at the CB_1 receptor, as assessed in in vitro systems (Landsman et al., 1997; Pan et al., 1998). Accordingly, rimonabant would be expected to elicit hyperalgesia, the opposite effect of cannabinoid agonists, without invoking a role for endocannabinoids. Thus, if it is subsequently found that rimonabant elicits a clinically relevant increase in pain sensitivity, it will be difficult to discern whether the effect is due to inverse agonism or blockade of endogenous cannabinoid tone.

The short half-lives of the endocannabinoids (Willoughby et al., 1997) present a significant challenge in investigating their function. However, the identification of fatty acid amide hydrolase (FAAH) as the enzyme primarily responsible for anandamide catabolism (Cravatt et al., 1996, 2001) and the serine lipase monoacylglycerol lipase (MGL) responsible for 2-AG degradation (Dinh et al., 2002) have provided valuable targets to increase endogenous levels of each of these respective endocannabinoids, by using genetically engineered mice devoid of FAAH as well as pharmacological inhibitors of each of these enzymes. As expected, $FAAH^{(-/-)}$ mice have an impaired ability to metabolize anandamide as well as noncannabinoid fatty acid amides. Consequently, they possess highly elevated endogenous levels of these compounds in the CNS and periphery (Clement et al., 2003; Cravatt et al., 2001). $FAAH^{(-/-)}$ mice display a phenotypic hypoalgesia in the tail immersion, hot plate, and formalin tests, which are completely normalized by rimonabant (Cravatt et al., 2001; Lichtman et al., 2004b). $FAAH^{(-/-)}$ mice also exhibit decreased inflammatory responses in the formalin (Lichtman et al., 2004b), carrageenan paw edema (Cravatt et al., 2004; Lichtman et al., 2004b), and DNBS-induced colitis models (Massa et al., 2004), though the mechanism of action of these effects is poorly understood. In one study (Lichtman et al., 2004b), the CB_2 receptor antagonist SR 144528, but not rimonabant, partially attenuated the $FAAH^{(-/-)}$ anti-edema phenotype in the carrageenan model, suggesting some involvement of CB_2 receptors, though in a subsequent study CB_1 and CB_2 antagonists administered separately or in combination failed to block this anti-edema phenotype (Cravatt et al., 2004).

In addition to the issue of receptor mechanism of action, another important question is whether analgesic and antiinflammatory phenotypes of the $FAAH^{(-/-)}$ mouse are mediated through central or peripheral sites of action. This question has been investigated through the use of genetically engineered mice that express FAAH specifically in the nervous system and not in the periphery (FAAH-NS mice; [Cravatt et al., 2004]). As FAAH-NS mice possess wild type levels of fatty acid amides in the CNS and significantly elevated concentrations of these lipids in peripheral tissues, the occurrence of a given phenotype in these mice implies a peripheral site of action, whereas the absence of the phenotype suggests a central site of action. Although these mice exhibit normal pain responses in the tail immersion and hot plate tests, they continue to display an anti-edema phenotype in the carrageenan model (Cravatt et al., 2004). Taken together, these findings indicate that anandamide acting at CB_1 receptors in the CNS mediates the hypoalgesic phenotype of $FAAH^{(-/-)}$ mice, whereas peripheral noncannabinoid fatty acid amides are chiefly responsible for the antiinflammatory phenotype. Through the use of selective receptor antagonists and the FAAH-NS mice, one could also ascertain whether the anandamide/fatty acid amide signaling systems mediate other pain and antiinflammatory phenotypes of the $FAAH^{(-/-)}$ mouse.

Other research has demonstrated that pain can lead to functional adaptations within the endocannabinoid system. For example, spinal nerve ligation in the rat has been found to upregulate CB_1 receptors in the thalamus (Siegling et al., 2001) and spinal cord (Lim et al., 2003). In an analogous study, anandamide levels in the PAG were increased by an injection of formalin into a hind paw (Walker et al., 1999). Moreover, electrical stimulation of the dorsal PAG led to the release of anandamide in this brain region along with a CB_1 receptor mediated analgesia (Walker et al., 1999). Further suggesting that endogenous cannabinoids dampen the impact of prolonged pain was the observation that intraplantar injections of complete Freund's adjuvant, a model of inflammatory pain, led to a significantly enhanced sensitivity to mechanical stimulation in the contralateral paw upon treatment with rimonabant (Martin et al., 1999).

Other research has implicated the involvement of endocannabinoids in stress-induced analgesia, an adaptive response that occurs when an animal perceives itself to be in danger. The first evidence suggesting the involvement of the endocannabinoid system in stress-induced analgesia was that $CB_1^{(+/+)}$ mice, but not $CB_1^{(-/-)}$ mice, exhibited increased latencies in the hot plate test following a 3-minute forced swim in warm water (Valverde et al., 2000). In another study that employed a conditioned fear paradigm, rats exhibited a rimonabant-reversible analgesia as assessed in the hot plate test (Finn et al., 2004a). Finally, an intracerebral injection of rimonabant into the PAG blocked stress-induced analgesia in rats exposed to prolonged foot shock (Hohmann et al., 2005). Foot shock also led to increases in both anandamide and 2-AG levels in this brain region. Additionally, the rostral ventromedial medulla has been implicated in the involvement of stress-induced analgesia (Suplita et al., 2005).

CB$_1$ Receptor Agonists as Analgesics

Activation of CB_1 receptors produces myriad behavioral effects that have been well characterized in both humans and laboratory animals. Unfortunately, blockade of pain perception is merely one of many pharmacological effects that result from CB_1 receptor activation. Anandamide produces many of the same pharmacological effects as THC, including hypomotility, antinociception, catalepsy, and hypothermia in laboratory animals (Fride & Mechoulam, 1993; Smith et al., 1994a). 2-AG also produces the full spectrum of cannabinoid effects, although it is somewhat less potent than anandamide (Mechoulam et al., 1995). However, evaluation of CB_1 cannabinoid receptor agonists in a wide range of animal models has consistently shown them to be antinociceptive, as reviewed previously (Martin & Lichtman, 1998).

As for human studies, Noyes et al. (1975a, 1975b) provided one of the first systematic studies to demonstrate that THC had analgesic properties. They also reported that at effective analgesic doses, it elevated mood, stimulated appetite, produced dizziness, blurred vision, and impaired thinking. Structurally diverse CB_1 receptor agonists have been developed, but none has elicited high analgesic selectivity. More recently, efforts have turned to developing different formulations of CB_1 receptor agonists that might provide greater control over drug delivery and hence fewer side effects. These attempts include rectal suppositories (ElSohly et al., 1991), water-soluble cannabinoids (Pertwee et al., 2000; Martin et al., 2006), and a metered dose inhaler (Wilson et al., 2002).

CB_2 Selective Receptor Agonists as Analgesics

The prevalence of CB_2 receptors in immune cells has directed attention to an array of immunological disorders, including inflammation and pain. Furthermore, initial studies failed to detect CB_2 receptors in the central nervous system, thereby suggesting CB_2 selective agonists would be devoid of CB_1-like behavioral effects. However, CB_2 receptors were recently identified in brain stem neurons, which could be a possible site of action (Van Sickle et al., 2005). In addition, sciatic nerve section or spinal nerve ligation causes an upregulation of CB_2 receptors in the dorsal horn of the spinal cord (Wotherspoon et al., 2005). It is reasonable to speculate that the analgesic and antiinflammatory effects of CB_2 selective agonists result from a combination of actions at both neuronal and immune sites.

A large number of CB_2 selective analogs have been developed (Hanus et al., 1999; Huffman et al., 1999; Malan et al., 2002; Showalter et al., 1996; Valenzano et al., 2005; Wiley et al., 2002). HU-308 was found to have analgesic properties while at the same time being devoid of cannabinoid behavioral effects (Hanus et al., 1999). Extensive studies have been conducted with AM 1241 that has been shown to be active in wide range of pain models that includes neuropathic pain (Malan et al., 2002) and capsacin-induced thermal and mechanical hyperalgesia (Hohmann et al., 2004; Quartilho et al., 2003). GW405833 is a CB_2 selective agonist that is effective in acute pain and inflammatory models but more importantly is efficacious in neuropathic, incisional, and chronic inflammatory pain models at doses that do not produce behavioral effects (Valenzano et al., 2005). Recently, a series of 1-methoxy- and 1-deoxyy-THC derivatives were prepared that also have potential as analgesics devoid of cannabinoid behavioral effects (Marriott et al., 2005).

FAAH and MGL Inhibitors as Analgesics

The fact that manipulation of endocannabinoid levels can alter pain sensitivity has made metabolic enzymes of endocannabinoids attractive therapeutic targets. Both irreversible (e.g., URB597) and reversible (e.g., OL-135) inhibitors of FAAH produce similar pharmacological effects as those observed in $FAAH^{(-/-)}$ mice, including increased brain anandamide levels, increased sensitivity to the pharmacological effects of injected anandamide, and a CB_1-mediated decrease in pain sensitivity in the tail immersion, hot plate, and formalin tests (Kathuria et al., 2003; Lichtman et al., 2004a). URB597 also prevented carrageenan-induced edema, an effect that was completely antagonized by SR 144528 (Holt et al., 2005). Finally, administration of the MGL inhibitor URB602, as well as the FAAH inhibitor URB597, into the PAG prolonged the duration of stress-induced analgesia through a CB_1 receptor mechanism of action (Hohmann et al., 2005).

Anandamide Reuptake Inhibitors

There is strong evidence that anandamide is synthesized and released postsynaptically in order to act in a retrograde manner on presynaptic CB_1 cannabinoid receptors. However, the ultimate fate of anandamide in the synaptic cleft is unclear. There is indirect evidence of a specific transporter that might participate in reuptake of anandamide, a subject surrounded by considerable controversy (Fegley et al., 2004; Hillard & Jarrahian, 2003, 2005). In a recent report, inhibitors of the putative anandamide reuptake transporter did not produce antinociceptive effects when administered alone but were able to potentiate the effects of exogenously administered anandamide (Ligresti et al., 2006). It remains to be established whether these agents will prove to be clinically useful as analgesic agents.

Cannabinoid/Opioid Interactions

Considerable evidence for the interactions of the cannabinoids with opioid systems in the modulation of nociception currently exists and has been reviewed (Corchero, Manzanares, & Fuentes, 2004; Manzanares et al., 1999; Vigano et al., 2005). Cannabinoid-induced antinociception is due to both supraspinal and spinal mechanisms. Anatomical studies have reported a similar distribution of CB_1 cannabinoid and the opioid receptors in the dorsal horn of the spinal cord (Hohmann et al., 1999; Salio et al., 2001) and in several brain structures associated with nociceptive transmission (Herkenham et al., 1991a; Meng et al., 1998; Yaksh et al., 1988). Cannabinoid and opioid receptors are both G-protein-coupled receptors (GPCRs). One of the most extensively reviewed actions of both classes of drugs is the effects of the drugs on adenylyl cyclase, the enzyme responsible for catalyzing the formation of cyclic AMP. Evidence exists that the receptors act via different pools of G-proteins (Childers et al., 1993) and are located in different laminae of the dorsal horn (Hohmann et al., 1999) suggesting that these different populations of receptors could exhibit different signal transduction properties. Both classes of drugs activate numerous signaling pathways that include multiple G-proteins, potassium and calcium channels, as well as numerous kinases, all of which appear to be altered upon development of tolerance and physical dependence.

The pharmacological importance of the role of G-protein activation by the drugs in combination is illustrated by the prevention of tolerance to either drug when low doses of the drugs are combined in vivo. This concept is based on previous studies showing that a low dose of THC greatly enhances the antinociceptive effect of opioids (Cichewicz et al, 1999; Smith et al., 1998) leading to a synergistic interaction (Cichewicz, 2004). The events in morphine tolerance are associated with desensitization of the mu opioid receptor (MOR) and decrease in receptor density (Bernstein & Welch, 1998; Yoburn et al., 1993) and receptor protein (Cichewicz et al., 2001). THC tolerance is associated with cellular events similar to morphine tolerance (Sim-Selley & Martin, 2002). Tolerance does not develop to a low-dose combination of subactive doses of morphine and THC, an effect accompanied by prevention of changes in G-protein activation observed with either drug alone.

Thus, tolerance to the antinociceptive effects is not observed when the doses used do not produce receptor desensitization. Such data support the concept of cannabinoid and opioid activation of distinct pools of G-proteins as previously discussed.

Considerable work has focused on the relationship between cannabinoids and the kappa opioid receptor (KOR) system in the spinal cord. Cannabinoid-induced G_i-protein mediated modulation of cAMP is sensitive to KOR antagonists and bidirectional cross-tolerance of cannabinoid receptor agonists to KOR agonists has been observed in antinociceptive tests. This cross-tolerance suggests that a portion of the antinociceptive effects of cannabinoids is mediated through the KOR (Mason et al., 1999b; Smith et al., 1994b). Dynorphin A is also cross-tolerant to THC (Welch, 1997). Dynorphin A (1–17) levels increase during the onset of THC-induced spinal antinociception, which suggests that THC–mediated release of dynorphin A (1–17) is responsible in part for THC-induced spinal antinociception. In addition, as animals are rendered tolerant to THC, dynorphin A release is elicited only by very high doses of THC. Thus, tolerance to THC involves a decrease in the release of dynorphin A (Mason et al., 1999a). The KOR antagonist, nor-binaltorphimine (nor-BNI), and dynorphin antisera block THC-induced antinociception, but do not block catalepsy, hypothermia, or hypoactivity. Thus, the antinociceptive effects of the cannabinoids can be separated from other effects of the cannabinoids that appear to be less responsive to opioid modulation. However, the effects of nor-BNI antagonism of cannabinoid-induced antinociception are complex and appear to depend on the type of nociceptive stimulus, route of administration, and strain of animal (Gardell et al., 2002), leading to conclusions that a dynorphin-independent mechanism for THC-induced antinociception exists. It has also been shown that in arthritic animals, a model of chronic pain with high levels of dynorphin expression, THC reduces dynorphin levels (Cox & Welch, 2004) via both CB_1- and CB_2-mediated mechanisms. Thus, cannabinoid/opioid interactions in chronic pain states may differ from those in normal animals. A recent review addresses several animal models in order to evaluate the complex cannabinoid/opioid interactions and the neurochemical substrates involved in such interactions (Tanda & Goldberg, 2003).

THC and morphine produce synergistic effects in several antinociceptive models in mice (Cichewicz, 2004; Tham et al., 2005), as well as in normal rats, arthritic rats, and in rats with formalin-evoked chronic pain responses (Finn et al., 2004b). The mechanism for such synergy has been hypothesized to involve THC induction of endogenous opioids (Corchero et al., 2004; Pugh et al., 1996), as well as interactions at the level of second messenger systems, G-proteins, or other intracellular signaling systems as previously described. However, the release of leucine enkephalin and its action at the delta opioid receptor (DOR) is a critical factor in THC/morphine enhancement. Prevention of the metabolism of dynorphin A (1–17) to dynorphin (1–8) or to leucine enkephalin prevents the enhancement of morphine-induced antinociception by THC (Pugh et al., 1996). Functional coupling of the mu/delta and mu/kappa receptors (Miaskowski et al., 1992) or formation of mu/delta heterodimers may explain the enhancement of MOR-mediated analgesia by DOR-specific ligands (Gomes et al., 2002). Thus, the enhancement of morphine analgesia by THC could be occurring not only through the release of endogenous opioids that might interact with proximal receptors but also through a direct stimulation of receptor coupling.

Considerable evidence for the interaction of cannabinoid and opioid systems has recently come from studies of transgenic mice with deletions of cannabinoid receptors, opioid receptors, and endogenous opioid peptide genes (for a review, see Corchero et al., 2004). Most of the acute effects of opioids are unaffected in $CB_1^{(-/-)}$ mice, with the exception of a reduction in morphine's reinforcing activity. Increases in prodynorphin and proenkephalin mRNA have been shown following exposure to THC. In the brain, THC-induced analgesia is reduced in prodynorphin$^{(-/-)}$ mice (Zimmer et al., 2001). Mice lacking opioid receptors develop the same degree of tolerance as wild type mice to THC after chronic administration, showing that the suppression of opioid receptors has no important consequences on the development of cannabinoid tolerance. Cannabinoid-opioid interactions also persist after chronic drug administration (Vigano et al., 2005). Chronic THC increases prodynorphin and proenkephalin gene expression in the rat spinal cord and propiomelanocortin gene expression and proenkephalin mRNA in brain.

Given the mutual control by cannabinoids and opioids in antinociception, it is likely that endogenous opioids and endogenous cannabinoids interact in pain pathways, although the mechanisms of interactions are yet to be determined. Anandamide appears to differ from THC in its lack of interactions with dynorphinergic systems (Welch, 1997). Anandamide fails to enhance the activity of any opioid and does not release dynorphin A. Several elegant reviews have discussed parallel pathways by which the endocannabinoids and endogenous opioids control pain (Mao et al., 2000; Walker & Huang, 2002). The endogenous cannabinoid system appears to play a role in the suppression of chronic pain. It has been shown that in chronic neuropathic pain, an endocannabinoid analog retains the ability to modulate nociception, whereas opioids lose the ability to reduce nociception (Kawasaki et al., 2005). Thus, the endocannabinoid system does not appear to require the opioid system for antinociception in a chronic pain state. Similar results using THC and morphine in chronic intractable pain have led to the conclusion that cannabinoid and opioid pathways are independent in such types of pain and further, that the cannabinoid system may be superior to the opioid system in terms of pain relief (Mao et al., 2000).

Summary

In conclusion, a growing body of evidence suggests that the endocannabinoid system can become functionally activated during chronic pain states as well as by stress-provoking stimuli. The development of cannabinoid CB_1 receptor agonists continue to pose challenges because of their inherent behavioral effects. Although new formulations of current CB_1 receptor agonists may provide increased control over these side effects, development of new CB_1 receptor agonists that have a greater therapeutic/side effect profile is needed. The finding that CB_2 cannabinoid receptor agonists have antinociceptive properties, yet are lacking behavioral effects, holds considerable promise. Furthermore, enzymes such as FAAH and MGL, which are responsible for the rapid degradation of endogenous cannabinoids, may represent attractive therapeutic targets to treat a variety of pain disorders. The discovery of the endocannabinoid system, and its role in pain perception, provides new strategies for development of novel analgesics.

References

Beaulieu, P., Bisogno, T., Punwar, S., Farquhar-Smith, W. P., Ambrosino, G., Di Marzo, V., et al. (2000). Role of the endogenous cannabinoid system in the formalin test of persistent pain in the rat. *Eur J Pharmacol*, 396(2–3), 85–92.

Bernstein, M. A., & Welch, S. P. (1998). Mu-opioid receptor down-regulation and camp-dependent protein kinase phosphorylation in a mouse model of chronic morphine tolerance. *Brain Res Mol Brain Res, 55*(2), 237–242.

Bisogno, T., Howell, F., Williams, G., Minassi, A., Cascio, M. G., Ligresti, A., et al. (2003). Cloning of the first sn1-DAG lipases points to the spatial and temporal regulation of endocannabinoid signaling in the brain. *J Cell Biol, 163*(3), 463–468.

Calignano, A., La Rana, G., Giuffrida, A., & Piomelli, D. (1998). Control of pain initiation by endogenous cannabinoids. *Nature, 394*(6690), 277–281.

Chapman, V. (1999). The cannabinoid CB1 receptor antagonist, SR141716a, selectively facilitates nociceptive responses of dorsal horn neurones in the rat. *Br J Pharmacol, 127*(8), 1765–1767.

Childers, S. R., Pacheco, M. A., Bennett, B. A., Edwards, T. A., Hampson, R. E., Mu, J., et al. (1993). Cannabinoid receptors: G-protein-mediated signal transduction mechanisms. *Biochem Soc Symp, 59*, 27–50.

Cichewicz, D. L. (2004). Synergistic interactions between cannabinoid and opioid analgesics. *Life Sci, 74*(11), 1317–1324.

Cichewicz, D. L., Haller, V. L., & Welch, S. P. (2001). Changes in opioid and cannabinoid receptor protein following short-term combination treatment with delta(9)-tetrahydrocannabinol and morphine. *J Pharmacol Exp Ther, 297*(1), 121–127.

Cichewicz, D. L., Martin, Zachary L., Smith, Forrest L., Welch, Sandra P. (1999). Enhancement of opioid antinociception by oral Δ9- tetrahydrocannabinol: Dose-response analysis and receptor identification. *J Pharmacol Exp Ther, 289*(2), 859–867.

Clement, A. B., Hawkins, E. G., Lichtman, A. H., & Cravatt, B. F. (2003). Increased seizure susceptibility and proconvulsant activity of anandamide in mice lacking fatty acid amide hydrolase. *J Neurosci, 23*(9), 3916–3923.

Compton, D. R., Aceto, M. D., Lowe, J., & Martin, B. R. (1996). In vivo characterization of a specific cannabinoid receptor antagonist (SR141716a): Inhibition of delta 9-tetrahydrocannabinol-induced responses and apparent agonist activity. *J Pharmacol Exp Ther, 277*(2), 586–594.

Corchero, J., Manzanares, J., & Fuentes, J. A. (2004). Cannabinoid/opioid crosstalk in the central nervous system. *Crit Rev Neurobiol, 16*(1–2), 159–172.

Cox, M. L., & Welch, S. P. (2004). The antinociceptive effect of delta9-tetrahydrocannabinol in the arthritic rat. *Eur J Pharmacol, 493*(1–3), 65–74.

Cravatt, B. F., Demarest, K., Patricelli, M. P., Bracey, M. H., Giang, D. K., Martin, B. R., et al. (2001). Supersensitivity to anandamide and enhanced endogenous cannabinoid signaling in mice lacking fatty acid amide hydrolase. *Proc Natl Acad Sci U S A, 98*(16), 9371–9376.

Cravatt, B. F., Giang, D. K., Mayfield, S. P., Boger, D. L., Lerner, R. A., & Gilula, N. B. (1996). Molecular characterization of an enzyme that degrades neuromodulatory fatty-acid amides. *Nature, 384*(7), 83–87.

Cravatt, B. F., Saghatelian, A., Hawkins, E. G., Clement, A. B., Bracey, M. H., & Lichtman, A. H. (2004). Functional disassociation of the central and peripheral fatty acid amide signaling systems. *Proc Natl Acad Sci USA, 101*(29), 10821–10826.

Devane, W. A., Hanus, L., Breuer, A., Pertwee, R. G., Stevenson, L. A., Griffin, G., et al. (1992). Isolation and structure of a brain constituent that binds to the cannabinoid receptor. *Science, 258*(18 December), 1946–1949.

Dinh, T. P., Carpenter, D., Leslie, F. M., Freund, T. F., Katona, I., Sensi, S. L., et al. (2002). Brain monoglyceride lipase participating in endocannabinoid inactivation. *Proc. Natl. Acad. Sci. U.S.A., 99*(16), 10819–10824.

ElSohly, M. A., Stanford, D. F., Harland, E. C., Hikal, A. H., Walker, L. A., Little, T. L., et al. (1991). Rectal bioavailability of d^9-tetrahydrocannabinol from the hemisuccinate ester in monkeys. *J Pharmaceut Sci, 80*(10), 942–945.

Fegley, D., Kathuria, S., Mercier, R., Li, C., Goutopoulos, A., Makriyannis, A., et al. (2004). Anandamide transport is independent of fatty-acid amide hydrolase activity and is blocked by the hydrolysis-resistant inhibitor am1172. *Proc Natl Acad Sci USA, 101*(23), 8756–8761.

Felder, C. C., Joyce, K., Briley, E. M., Mansouri, J., Mackie, K., Blond, O., Lai, Y., et al. (1995). Comparison of the pharmacology and signal transduction of the human cannabinoid CB1 and CB2 receptors. *Mol Pharmacol 48*, 443–450.

Finn, D. P., Beckett, S. R., Richardson, D., Kendall, D. A., Marsden, C. A., & Chapman, V. (2004). Evidence for differential modulation of conditioned aversion and fear-conditioned analgesia by CB1 receptors. *Eur J Neurosci, 20*(3), 848–852.

Finn, D. P., Beckett, S. R., Roe, C. H., Madjd, A., Fone, K. C., Kendall, D. A., et al. (2004). Effects of coadministration of cannabinoids and morphine on nociceptive behaviour, brain monoamines and HPA axis activity in a rat model of persistent pain. *Eur J Neurosci, 19*(3), 678–686.

Fride, E., & Mechoulam, R. (1993). Pharmacological activity of the cannabinoid receptor agonist, anandamide, a brain constituent. *Eur J Pharmacol, 231*, 313–314.

Gardell, L. R., Ossipov, M. H., Vanderah, T. W., Lai, J., & Porreca, F. (2002). Dynorphin-independent spinal cannabinoid antinociception. *Pain, 100*(3), 243–248.

Gérard, C. M., Mollereau, C., Vassart, G., & Parmentier, M. (1991). Molecular cloning of a human cannabinoid receptor which is also expressed in testis. *Biochem J, 279*, 129–134.

Gomes, I., Filipovska, J., Jordan, B. A., & Devi, L. A. (2002). Oligomerization of opioid receptors. *Methods, 27*(4), 358–365.

Hanus, L., Abu-Lafi, S., Fride, E., Breuer, A., Vogel, Z., Shalev, D. E., et al. (2001). 2-arachidonyl glyceryl ether, an endogenous agonist of the cannabinoid CB1 receptor. *Proc Natl Acad Sci USA, 98*(7), 3662–3665.

Hanus, L., Breuer, A., Tchilibon, S., Shiloah, S., Goldenberg, D., Horowitz, M., et al. (1999). Hu-308: A specific agonist for CB(2), a peripheral cannabinoid receptor. *Proc Natl Acad Sci USA, 96*(25), 14228–14233.

Herkenham, M., Lynn, A. B., Johnson, M. R., Melvin, L. S., de Costa, B. R., & Rice, K. C. (1991). Characterization and localization of cannabinoid receptors in rat brain: A quantitative in vitro autoradiographic study. *J Neuroscience, 11*(2), 563–583.

Hillard, C. J., & Jarrahian, A. (2003). Cellular accumulation of anandamide: Consensus and controversy. *Br J Pharmacol, 140*(5), 802–808.

Hillard, C. J., & Jarrahian, A. (2005). Accumulation of anandamide: Evidence for cellular diversity. *Neuropharmacology, 48*(8), 1072–1078.

Hohmann, A. G., Briley, E. M., & Herkenham, M. (1999). Pre- and postsynaptic distribution of cannabinoid and mu opioid receptors in rat spinal cord. *Brain Res, 822*(1–2), 17–25.

Hohmann, A. G., Farthing, J. N., Zvonok, A. M., & Makriyannis, A. (2004). Selective activation of cannabinoid CB2 receptors suppresses hyperalgesia evoked by intradermal capsaicin. *J Pharmacol Exp Ther, 308*(2), 446–453.

Hohmann, A. G., & Herkenham, M. (1999a). Cannabinoid receptors undergo axonal flow in sensory nerves. *Neuroscience, 92*(4), 1171–1175.

Hohmann, A. G., & Herkenham, M. (1999b). Localization of central cannabinoid CB1 receptor messenger RNA in neuronal subpopulations of rat dorsal root ganglia: A double-label in situ hybridization study. *Neurosci, 90*(3), 923–931.

Hohmann, A. G., Suplita, R. L., Bolton, N. M., Neely, M. H., Fegley, D., Mangieri, R., et al. (2005). An endocannabinoid mechanism for stress-induced analgesia. *Nature, 435*(7045), 1108–1112.

Holt, S., Comelli, F., Costa, B., & Fowler, C. J. (2005). Inhibitors of fatty acid amide hydrolase reduce carrageenan-induced hind paw inflammation in pentobarbital-treated mice: Comparison with indomethacin and possible involvement of cannabinoid receptors. *Br J Pharmacol, 146*(3), 467–476.

Howlett, A. C., Barth, F., Bonner, T. I., Cabral, G., Casellas, P., Devane, W. A., et al. (2002). International union of pharmacology. XXVII. Classification of cannabinoid receptors. *Pharmacol Rev, 54*(2), 161–202.

Huffman, J. W., Liddle, J., Yu, S., Aung, M. M., Abood, M. E., Wiley, J. L., et al. (1999). 3-(1,'1'-dimethylbutyl)-1-deoxy-Δ8-THC and related compounds: Synthesis of selective ligands for the CB2 receptor. *Bioorg Med Chem, 7*, 2905–2914.

Kathuria, S., Gaetani, S., Fegley, D., Valino, F., Duranti, A., Tontini, A., et al. (2003). Modulation of anxiety through blockade of anandamide hydrolysis. *Nat Med, 9*(1), 76–81.

Kawasaki, Y., Kohno, T., & Ji, R. R. (2005). Different effects of opioid and cannabinoid on c-fiber-induced ERK activation in dorsal horn neurons in normal and spinal nerve-ligated rats. *J Pharmacol Exp Ther*.

Landsman, R. S., Burkey, T. H., Consroe, P., Roeske, W. R., & Yamamura, H. I. (1997). Sr141716a is an inverse agonist at the human cannabinoid CB1 receptor. *Eur J Pharmacol, 334*(1), R1–2.

Ledent, C., Valverde, O., Cossu, G., Petitet, F., Aubert, J. F., Beslot, F., et al. (1999). Unresponsiveness to cannabinoids and reduced addictive effects of opiates in CB1 receptor knockout mice. *Science, 283*(5400), 401–404.

Lichtman, A. H., Leung, D., Shelton, C. C., Saghatelian, A., Hardouin, C., Boger, D. L., et al. (2004a). Reversible inhibitors of fatty acid amide hydrolase that promote analgesia: Evidence for an unprecedented combination of potency and selectivity. *J Pharmacol Exp Ther, 311*(2), 441–448.

Lichtman, A. H., & Martin, B. R. (1997). The selective cannabinoid antagonist, SR 141716a, blocks cannabinoid-induced antinociception in rats. *Pharmacol Biochem Behav, 57*, 7–12.

Lichtman, A. H., Shelton, C. C., Advani, T., & Cravatt, B. F. (2004b). Mice lacking fatty acid amide hydrolase exhibit a cannabinoid receptor-mediated phenotypic hypoalgesia. *Pain, 109*(3), 319–327.

Ligresti, A., Cascio, M. G., Pryce, G., Kulasegram, S., Beletskaya, I., De Petrocellis, L., et al. (2006). New potent and selective inhibitors of anandamide reuptake with antispastic activity in a mouse model of multiple sclerosis. *Br J Pharmacol, 147*(1), 83–91.

Lim, G., Sung, B., Ji, R. R., & Mao, J. (2003). Upregulation of spinal cannabinoid-1-receptors following nerve injury enhances the effects of win 55,212–2 on neuropathic pain behaviors in rats. *Pain, 105*(1–2), 275–283.

Mackie, K., & Hille, B. (1992). Cannabinoids inhibit n-type calcium channels in neuroblastoma-glioma cells. *Proc Natl Acad Sci USA, 89*(May), 3825–3829.

Mackie, K., Lai, Y., Westenbroek, R., & Mitchell, R. (1995). Cannabinoids activate an inwardly rectifying potassium conductance and inhibit q-type calcium currents in AtT20 cells transfected with rat brain cannabinoid receptor. *J Neurosci, 15*(10), 6552–6561.

Malan, T. P., Ibrahim, M. M., Vanderah, T. W., Makriyannis, A., & Porreca, F. (2002). Inhibition of pain responses by activation of CB(2) cannabinoid receptors. *Chem Phys Lipids, 121*(1–2), 191–200.

Manzanares, J., Corchero, J., Romero, J., Fernandez-Ruiz, J. J., Ramos, J. A., & Fuentes, J. A. (1999). Pharmacological and biochemical interactions between opioids and cannabinoids. *Trends Pharmacol Sci, 20*(7), 287–294.

Mao, J., Price, D. D., Lu, J., Keniston, L., & Mayer, D. J. (2000). Two distinctive antinociceptive systems in rats with pathological pain. *Neurosci Lett, 280*(1), 13–16.

Marriott, K. S., Huffman, J. W., Wiley, J. L., & Martin, B. R. (2005). Synthesis and pharmacology of 11-nor-1-methoxy-9-hydroxyhexahydrocannabinols and 11-nor-1-deoxy-9-hydroxyhexahydrocannabinols: New selective ligands for the cannabinoid CB(2) receptor. *Bioorg Med Chem*.

Martin, B. R., & Lichtman, A. H. (1998). Cannabinoid transmission and pain perception. *Neurobiol Dis, 5*(6 Pt B), 447–461.

Martin, W. J., Loo, C. M., & Basbaum, A. I. (1999). Spinal cannabinoids are anti-allodynic in rats with persistent inflammation. *Pain, 82*(2), 199–205.

Martin, B. R., Wiley, J. L., Beletskaya, I., Sim-Selley, L. J., Smith, F. L., Dewey, W. L., Cottney, J., et al. (2006). Pharmacological characterization of novel water-soluble cannabinoids. *J Pharmacol Exp Ther, 318*(3), 1230–1239.

Mason, D. J., Jr., Lowe, J., & Welch, S. P. (1999a). A diminution of delta9-tetrahydrocannabinol modulation of dynorphin A(1–17) in conjunction with tolerance development. *Eur J Pharmacol, 381*(2–3), 105–111.

Mason, D. J., Lowe, J., & Welch, S. P. (1999b). Cannabinoid modulation of dynorphin A: Correlation to cannabinoid-induced antinociception. *Eur J Pharmacol, 378*(3), 237–248.

Massa, F., Marsicano, G., Hermann, H., Cannich, A., Monory, K., Cravatt, B. F., et al. (2004). The endogenous cannabinoid system protects against colonic inflammation. *J Clin Invest, 113*(8), 1202–1209.

Matsuda, L. A., Lolait, S. J., Brownstein, M. J., Young, A. C., & Bonner, T. I. (1990). Structure of a cannabinoid receptor and functional expression of the cloned cDNA. *Nature, 346*(9 August), 561–564.

Mechoulam, R., Ben-Shabat, S., Hanus, L., Ligumsky, M., Kaminski, N., Schatz, A., et al. (1995). Identification of an endogenous 2-monoglyceride, present in canine gut, that binds to cannabinoid receptors. *Biochem Pharmacol, 50*(1), 83–90.

Meng, I. D., Manning, B. H., Martin, W. J., & Fields, H. L. (1998). An analgesia circuit activated by cannabinoids. *Nature, 395*(September 24), 381–383.

Miaskowski, C., Sutters, K. A., Taiwo, Y. O., & Levine, J. D. (1992). Antinociceptive and motor effects of delta/mu and kappa/mu combinations of intrathecal opioid agonists. *Pain, 49*(1), 137–144.

Noyes, J., R., Brunk, S. F., Avery, D. H., & Canter, A. (1975a). The analgesic properties of d^9-tetrahydrocannabinol and codeine. *Clin Pharmacol Ther, 18*, 84–89.

Noyes, R., Jr., Brunk, S. F., Baram, D. A., & Canter, A. (1975b). Analgesic effect of Δ^9-tetrahydrocannabinol. *J Clin Pharmacol, 15*, 139–143.

Okamoto, Y., Morishita, J., Tsuboi, K., Tonai, T., & Ueda, N. (2004). Molecular characterization of a phospholipase d generating anandamide and its congeners. *J Biol Chem, 279*(7), 5298–5305.

Pan, X., Ikeda, S. R., & Lewis, D. L. (1998). SR 141716a acts as an inverse agonist to increase neuronal voltage-dependent ca^{2+} currents by reversal of tonic CB1 cannabinoid receptor activity. *American Society for Pharmacology and Experimental Therapeutics, 54*, 1064–1072.

Pertwee, R. G., Gibson, T. M., Stevenson, L. A., Ross, R. A., Banner, W. K., Saha, B., et al. (2000). O-1057, a potent water-soluble cannabinoid receptor agonist with antinociceptive properties. *Br J Pharmacol, 129*(8), 1577–1584.

Porter, A. C., Sauer, J. M., Knierman, M. D., Becker, G. W., Berna, M. J., Bao, J., et al. (2002). Characterization of a novel endocannabinoid, virodhamine, with antagonist activity at the CB1 receptor. *J Pharmacol Exp Ther, 301*(3), 1020–1024.

Pugh, J., G., Smith, P. B., Dombrowski, D. S., & Welch, S. P. (1996). The role of endogenous opioids in enhancing the antinociception produced by the combination of Δ^9-tetrahydrocannabinol and morphine in the spinal cord. *J Pharmacol Exp Ther, 279*, 608–616.

Quartilho, A., Mata, H. P., Ibrahim, M. M., Vanderah, T. W., Porreca, F., Makriyannis, A., et al. (2003). Inhibition of inflammatory hyperalgesia by activation of peripheral CB2 cannabinoid receptors. *Anesthesiology, 99*(4), 955–960.

Richardson, J. D., Aanonsen, L., & Hargreaves, K. M. (1998). Hypoactivity of the spinal cannabinoid system results in NMDA-dependent hyperalgesia. *J Neurosci, 18*, 451–457.

Rinaldi-Carmona, M., Barth, F., Heaulme, M., Alonso, R., Shire, D., Congy, C., et al. (1995). Biochemical and pharmacological characterisation of SR141716a, the first potent and selective brain cannabinoid receptor antagonist. *Life Sci, 56*(23–24), 1941–1947.

Rinaldi-Carmona, M., Barth, F., Héaulme, M., Shire, D., Calandra, B., Congy, C., et al. (1994). SR141716a, a potent and selective antagonist of the brain cannabinoid receptor. *FEBS Lett, 350*, 240–244.

Salio, C., Fischer, J., Franzoni, M. F., Mackie, K., Kaneko, T., & Conrath, M. (2001). CB1-cannabinoid and mu-opioid receptor co-localization on postsynaptic target in the rat dorsal horn. *Neuroreport, 12*(17), 3689–3692.

Showalter, V., Compton, D. R., Martin, B. R., & Abood, M. E. (1996). Evaluation of binding in a transfected cell line expressing a peripheral cannabinoid receptor (CB_2): Identification of cannabinoid receptor subtype selective ligands. *J Pharmacol Exp Ther, 278*, 989–999.

Siegling, A., Hofmann, H. A., Denzer, D., Mauler, F., & De Vry, J. (2001). Cannabinoid CB(1) receptor upregulation in a rat model of chronic neuropathic pain. *Eur J Pharmacol, 415*(1), R5–7.

Sim-Selley, L. J., & Martin, B. R. (2002). Effect of chronic administration of r-(+)-[2,3-dihydro-5-methyl-3-[(morpholinyl)methyl]pyrrolo[1,2,3-de]-1,4-benzoxazinyl]-(1-naphthalenyl)methanone mesylae (win55, 212–2) or Δ^9-tetrahydrocannabinol on cannabinoid receptor adaptation in mice. *J Pharmacol Exp Ther, 303*, 36–44.

Smith, F. L., Cichewicz, D., Martin, Z. L., & Welch, S. P. (1998). The enhancement of morphine antinociception in mice by delta-9-tetrahydrocannabinol. *Pharmacol Biochem Behav, 60*(2), 559–566.

Smith, P. B., Compton, D. R., Welch, S. P., Razdan, R. K., Mechoulam, R., & Martin, B. R. (1994). The pharmacological activity of anandamide, a putative endogenous cannabinoid, in mice. *J Pharmacol Exp Ther, 270*, 219–227.

Smith, P. B., Welch, S. P., & Martin, B. R. (1994). Interactions between delta 9-tetrahydrocannabinol and kappa opioids in mice. *J Pharmacol Exp Ther, 268*(3), 1381–1387.

Strangman, N. M., Patrick, S. L., Hohmann, A. G., Tsou, K., & Walker, J. M. (1998). Evidence for a role of endogenous cannabinoids in the modulation of acute and tonic pain sensitivity. *Brain Res., 813*(2), 323–328.

Suplita, R. L., 2nd, Farthing, J. N., Gutierrez, T., & Hohmann, A. G. (2005). Inhibition of fatty-acid amide hydrolase enhances cannabinoid stress-induced analgesia: Sites of action in the dorsolateral periaqueductal gray and rostral ventromedial medulla. *Neuropharmacology, 49*(8), 1201–1209.

Tanda, G., & Goldberg, S. R. (2003). Cannabinoids: Reward, dependence, and underlying neurochemical mechanisms—a review of recent preclinical data. *Psychopharmacology (Berl), 169*(2), 115–134.

Tham, S. M., Angus, J. A., Tudor, E. M., & Wright, C. E. (2005). Synergistic and additive interactions of the cannabinoid agonist cp55,940 with mu opioid receptor and alpha2-adrenoceptor agonists in acute pain models in mice. *Br J Pharmacol, 144*(6), 875–884.

Ueda, N. (2002). Endocannabinoid hydrolases. *Prostaglandins Other Lipid Mediat, 68–69,* 521–534.

Valenzano, K. J., Tafesse, L., Lee, G., Harrison, J. E., Boulet, J. M., Gottshall, S. L., et al. (2005). Pharmacological and pharmacokinetic characterization of the cannabinoid receptor 2 agonist, GW405833, utilizing rodent models of acute and chronic pain, anxiety, ataxia and catalepsy. *Neuropharmacology, 48*(5), 658–672.

Valverde, O., Maldonado, R., Valjent, E., Zimmer, A. M., & Zimmer, A. (2000). Cannabinoid withdrawal syndrome is reduced in pre-proenkephalin knock-out mice. *J Neurosci, 20*(24), 9284–9289.

Van Sickle, M. D., Duncan, M., Kingsley, P. J., Mouihate, A., Urbani, P., Mackie, K., et al. (2005). Identification and functional characterization of brainstem cannabinoid CB2 receptors. *Science, 310*(5746), 329–332.

Vigano, D., Rubino, T., & Parolaro, D. (2005). Molecular and cellular basis of cannabinoid and opioid interactions. *Pharmacol Biochem Behav, 81*(2), 360–368.

Vivian, J. A., Kishioka, S., Butelman, E. R., Broadbear, J., Lee, K. O., & Woods, J. H. (1998). Analgesic, respiratory and heart rate effects of cannabinoid and opioid agonists in rhesus monkeys: Antagonist effects of SR 141716a. *J Pharmacol Exp Ther, 286*(2), 697–703.

Walker, J. M., & Huang, S. M. (2002). Endocannabinoids in pain modulation. *Prostaglandins Leukot Essent Fatty Acids, 66*(2–3), 235–242.

Walker, J. M., Huang, S. M., Strangman, N. M., Tsou, K., & Sanudo-Pena, M. C. (1999). Pain modulation by release of the endogenous cannabinoid anandamide. *Proc Natl Acad Sci USA, 96*(21), 12198–12203.

Walker, J. M., Krey, J. F., Chu, C. J., & Huang, S. M. (2002). Endocannabinoids and related fatty acid derivatives in pain modulation. *Chem Phys Lipids, 121*(1–2), 159–172.

Welch, S. P. (1997). Characterization of anandamide-induced tolerance: Comparison to Δ^9-THC-induced interactions with dynorphinergic systems. *Drug Alc Dep, 45,* 39–45.

Wiley, J. L., Beletskaya, I. D., Ng, E. W., Dai, Z., Crocker, P. J., Mahadevan, A., et al. (2002). Resorcinol derivatives: A novel template for the development of cannabinoid CB(1)/CB(2) and CB(2)-selective agonists. *J Pharmacol Exp Ther, 301*(2), 679–689.

Willoughby, K. A., Moore, S. F., Martin, B. R., & Ellis, E. F. (1997). The biodisposition and metabolism of anandamide in mice. *J Pharmacol Exp Ther, 282,* 243–247.

Wilson, D. M., Peart, J., Martin, B. R., Bridgen, D. T., Byron, P. R., & Lichtman, A. H. (2002). Physiochemical and pharmacological characterization of a delta(9)-THC aerosol generated by a metered dose inhaler. *Drug Alcohol Depend, 67*(3), 259–267.

Wotherspoon, G., Fox, A., McIntyre, P., Colley, S., Bevan, S., & Winter, J. (2005). Peripheral nerve injury induces cannabinoid receptor 2 protein expression in rat sensory neurons. *Neuroscience, 135*(1), 235–245.

Yaksh, T. L., Al-Rodhan, N. R. F., & Jensen, T. S. (1988). Sites of action of opiates in production of analgesia. In H. L. Fields & J. M. Besson (Eds.), *Progress in brain research* (Vol. 77, pp. 371–394).

Yoburn, B. C., Billings, B., & Duttaroy, A. (1993). Opioid receptor regulation in mice. *J Pharmacol Exp Ther, 265*(1), 314–320.

Zimmer, A., Valjent, E., Konig, M., Zimmer, A. M., Robledo, P., Hahn, H., et al. (2001). Absence of delta-9-tetrahydrocannabinol dysphoric effects in dynorphin-deficient mice. *J Neurosci, 21*(23), 9499–9505.

18

Alcohol Use Disorders and Their Treatment

Barbara Flannery
David Newlin

Prevalence, Etiology, and Gender Differences

Alcohol dependence is a chronic, relapsing disorder of the brain (Leshner, 1997, p. 45). It is in this sense similar to dependence/abuse of other drugs and for that matter to most other psychiatric illnesses. Alcohol use disorders (AUDs, which include alcohol dependence and alcohol abuse) are complex diseases that have substantial heritable components ranging from 40% to 60%, which allows for major environmental aspects of their etiologies. Although AUDs appear to be polygenic with many small, additive gene effects, important epistatic (gene-gene interactions) and gene-environment interactions cannot be ruled out at the present time.

The *Diagnostic and Statistical Manual of Mental Disorders*, Fourth Edition–Text Revision (*DSM-IV-TR*; American Psychiatric Association, 2000) is the de facto standard for diagnosing AUDs. The criteria for alcohol abuse include significant problems associated with alcohol and persistent use despite these problems, hazardous use (e.g., intoxicated driving), and/or recurrent legal problems. Importantly, alcohol abuse is diagnosed when the criteria for alcohol dependence have not been met. Alcohol dependence involves a constellation of symptoms associated with significant impairments that include marked tolerance to alcohol's intoxicating effects, withdrawal symptoms, escalating use despite problems, inability to limit use, and/or preoccupation with alcohol. Note that the quantity and frequency of alcohol use are not primary criteria for these diagnoses; they are only inferred from problematic use.

Because not all symptoms must be met to receive these AUD diagnoses, alcohol abuse can be diagnosed with repeated drunken driving episodes as the only positive criterion, and alcohol dependence can be diagnosed without evidence of tolerance or withdrawal. It is important to note that craving for alcohol is not a *DSM-IV-TR* criterion for either disorder, although it is a formal diagnostic criterion for alcohol dependence in the World Health Organization's (WHO) International Classification of Diseases-10th edition (*ICD-10*; WHO, 2003). Consistent with psychiatric practice, AUD diagnoses in *DSM-IV-TR* are categorical in nature. Although a hierarchy of severity is implied by the fact that alcohol abuse is only diagnosed after ruling out alcohol dependence, the *DSV-IV-TR* system does not capture differences in severity of abuse or dependence that are salient to the practicing clinician and researcher. In contrast, psychological traditions of assessment emphasize continuous gradations on dimensional scales that correspond to severity of the disorders (Krueger et al., 2005).

In the United States, about 3 in 10 adults drink at levels that increase their risk for physical, mental health, and social problems (National Institute on Alcohol Abuse and Alcoholism, unpublished data). Alcoholism is associated with heightened risk of hypertension, gastrointestinal bleeding, sleep disorders, major depression, hemorrhagic stroke, pancreatitis, cirrhosis of the liver, and several cancers (Rehm et al., 2003). Although approximately 1 in 4 individuals who are heavy drinkers could be classified as alcohol abusers or alcohol dependent, heavy drinking is often overlooked in primary care settings. It is estimated that alcohol-dependent individuals receive recommended assessment and treatment only about 10% of the time (McGlynn et al., 2003).

The National Institute on Alcohol Abuse and Alcoholism (NIAAA) provides materials for medical personnel, such as the pamphlet "Helping Patients Who Drink Too Much: A Clinician's Guide, Updated 2005 Edition" on their website, http://pubs.niaaa.nih.gov/publications. This brochure includes advice on screening and assessing alcoholism using established instruments, along with suggestions for treatment, epidemiological information, and referral resources. Information also is provided on the three FDA-approved medications used to treat alcohol dependence—disulfiram, naltrexone, and acamprosate. This information includes dosing, mechanisms of action, interactions, and contraindications.

AUDs are by far the most prevalent psychiatric disorders. A recent survey conducted in the United States, the National Epidemiologic Survey on Alcohol and Related Conditions (Grant et al., 2003), used methods very similar to the earlier National Longitudinal Alcohol Epidemiologic Survey, and found the overall 12-month prevalence for alcohol abuse to be 4.65%, and for alcohol dependence, 3.81%. Lifetime prevalence for AUDs is typically about twice those for 12-month prevalence. Men are twice as likely to have an AUD as women, and younger adults have more AUDs than older ones. The data from this survey indicates that the rates of alcohol abuse increased from 1992 to 2002, whereas the prevalence of alcohol dependence decreased over this same 10-year period (Grant et al., 2004).

Given the prevalence of alcohol abuse and dependence in the United States and other countries, it is not surprising that alcohol abuse and dependence has marked deleterious social, medical, and economic effects. WHO (2002) estimated that of the total burden of ill health among men in the developed countries of North America and Europe, approximately 14% was due to alcohol; it was estimated globally at 4%. Considering actual causes of death (for example, the actual cause of death of a chronic smoker with lung cancer would be categorized as smoking rather than cancer) in the United States in 2000, alcohol consumption accounted for approximately 85,000 deaths (Mokdad et al., 2004). This figure does not include medical and psychiatric comorbidities caused or exacerbated by alcohol use that did not lead to death.

Although it is not possible to quantify the suffering associated with alcohol use to the individual, their family, or to the community, the economic cost to society has been estimated at $185 billion dollars per year in the United States alone (Harwood, 2000). For example, preventing a single case of fetal alcohol syndrome (teratogenic effects due to excessive maternal alcohol use during the prenatal period) would save approximately half a million dollars over a 20-year period for a single individual (Klug & Burd, 2003).

The etiology of AUDs is multifactorial and complex. It may be more accurate to think in terms of the etiologies of these disorders, in which causative factors in some individuals may be very different from others. In Cloninger's (1987) classic typology of alcoholics, Type I alcoholism (milieu-limited) is viewed in terms of a genetic-environmental interaction such that mild to moderate genetic predisposition is modified and limited by the social and familial environment. In Type II alcoholism (male-limited), strong genetic determinants are thought to be relatively independent of environmental adversity coupled with a strong predisposition toward antisocial characteristics.

Current thinking concerning the etiology of AUDs emphasizes the developmental trajectories of individuals who are at heightened risk for these disorders by virtue of genetic effects, familial drinking problems, or other drug use, or adverse environmental circumstances (e.g., Sher & Wood, 2005). AUDs typically have adolescent or young adult onset, but often exhibit childhood precursors such as conduct disorder, attention deficit/hyperactivity disorder, or risky, antisocial behaviors. A family history of alcoholism, typically one or more affected first-degree relatives, although most often the father, is thought to increase the probability of an AUD in adulthood by anywhere from two- to fivefold (Sher, 1991) compared to those with no family history of alcoholism.

Although the pervasive assumption in this literature has been that the heightened susceptibility in this group is genetic, it is likely a combination of both genetic and environmental factors (Newlin & Thomson, 1990). In some instances, individuals may carry only a fraction of AUD susceptibility genes, but all have an alcoholic role model in their families and most have adverse familial environments due to the affected family member and compensations made by the rest of the family. The emphasis on family history of alcoholism as a predictor of AUDs is from an era that preceded genomic research in which a number of susceptibility loci have been identified and independently replicated (Uhl et al., 2002).

Due to the recognition of genetic "markers" for alcohol dependence predisposition, it is no longer necessary to rely solely on family history for heightened genetic risk. It is now becoming possible to characterize susceptible individuals based on genomic analyses (Uhl, 2004). With more and more genetic components related to AUDs being identified, it will likely be possible to select on a host of different susceptibility loci to maximize the genetic influence. Of course, selection on genomic criteria would ensure that the increased risk for AUDs was in fact genetic, but would have the limitation of excluding environmental risk factors (Newlin et al., 2000). Another caveat is that it would not be possible to determine which specific susceptibility locus was responsible for the high- and low-risk group differences that were observed.

A critical question in the etiology of AUDs is what psychobiological mechanisms link genetic susceptibility and environmental factors to ultimate development of these disorders (Newlin et al., 2000). The voluminous research on high-risk individuals, based largely upon positive family history of alcoholism, has led to theories of the etiology of alcoholism that emphasize two distinct, but very common, developmental pathways to AUDs: the undercontrolled behavioral pathway and the negative affectivity pathways (Hill et al., 1999; Sher & Wood, 2005; Zucker & Wong, 2005). The undercontrolled pathway is characterized by childhood externalizing disorders such as attention deficit/hyperactivity disorder and conduct disorder, adolescent antisocial behavior such as excessive risk-taking and substance abuse itself, and adult sensation-seeking, antisocial personality disorder, and psychopathy. In contrast, the negative affect pathway to AUDs is characterized by a strong propensity to experience anxiety, fear, and depression (Watson & Clark, 1984). Negative affectivity is a very common vulnerability factor for AUDs, but a less powerful predictor than are antisocial characteristics (e.g., Grant et al., 2004, 2003; Kessler et al., 1996; Robins and Regier, 1991).

These two etiological pathways are not exhaustive, nor do they necessarily map clearly (at this time) to known genomic susceptibility loci, but are thought to encompass a large percentage of heightened vulnerability to AUDs and to manifestation of the disorders.

It has been proposed that women experience more rapid and deleterious physiological brain and other organ system effects in response to chronic alcohol abuse (i.e., the telescoping effect; Randall et al., 1999). A recent computed tomography (CT) imaging study corroborates gender-specific differences in brain and other organ atrophy (e.g., heart, muscle, liver) with women experiencing a faster development of damage compared to men despite shorter durations of alcohol dependence (Mann et al., 2005). Hommer et al. (2001) found more severe ventricular expansion and reduced tissue volumes in the cortices and corpus callosum of female alcoholics, and Agartz and colleagues (1999) reported greater reductions among female alcoholics in hippocampal volumes using imaging techniques with high spatial resolution. The behavioral and imaging data taken together support an increased vulnerability to alcohol among women compared to men. The deleterious effects of alcohol dependence have also been shown in studies of the neurocognitive functioning of abstinent alcoholic men compared to abstinent alcoholic women. Flannery et al. (2007) recently demonstrated that Russian women perform more poorly than men on executive cognitive functioning tasks despite drinking less over a shorter period of time. These data corroborate earlier cognitive performance findings (e.g., Acker 1985, 1986) in women and extend the concept of telescoping to include neurological processes.

Chronic alcoholism also is associated with a high incidence of traumatic brain injuries that typically occur during intoxication. In a recent MRI study, Wilde et al. (2004) found that among patients with traumatic brain injury, those with a positive breath alcohol level and/or a history of moderate to heavy preinjury drinking had increased general atrophy and poorer neurocognitive test performances. In treating patients with alcohol dependence and head injury, Chatham-Showalter and colleagues (1996) found that compared to those without alcohol intoxication at the time of injury, those who were intoxicated required more time on respirators and more days and higher doses of opioids and benzodiazepines.

Neurobiology of Alcohol Dependence

Numerous preclinical and human studies have demonstrated that alcohol, as well as other abused substances, causes both structural and functional neuroadaptations within certain brain structures, specific types of cells, and neurotransmitter (NT) systems. Alcohol's effect on the brain is profound, and damage occurs across widespread areas extending from the prefrontal cortex (PFC) to the cerebellum and cerebellar vermis. Morphometric studies and functional magnetic resonance (fMRI) imaging of the brain of sober alcoholics reveal that alcohol decreases white and gray matter volume within frontal and prefrontal cortical areas (Fein et al., 2002; Jerrigan et al., 1991; Kril et al., 1997; Pfefferbaum et al., 1992), which, in turn, result in deficits in cognitive and emotive functioning (e.g., impaired judgment, blunted affect, poor insight and reduced motivation, as well as social withdrawal, distractibility, and attentional deficits; Oscar-Berman and Hutner, 1993; Parsons et al., 1987; Sullivan et al., 2000).

Neuronal changes also contribute significantly to the maintenance of the compulsive drive to seek and use alcohol and to the development of loss of control over drinking. The neuroadaptations generated by chronic alcohol abuse also lead to physical dependence that involve alterations in the excitability of the central nervous system that is observed during alcohol withdrawal (e.g., anxiety, tremors, seizures) and contributes to the development of tolerance (Hoffman & Tabakoff, 1996). Subcortical changes accompanying alcohol dependence include volume shrinkage within the thalamus (Sullivan, 2003), caudate and putamen (Sullivan & Pfefferbaum, 2005), and hippocampus (Harding et al., 1997; Sullivan et al., 1995), and thinning and atrophy of the corpus callosum (Harper & Kril, 1988; Tarnowska-Dziduszko et al., 1995). Volume reduction within the hippocampus and possibly the cholinergic medial septum may be involved in both Korsakoff's and non-Korsakoff's amnesia (Sullivan & Marsh, 2003). Degeneration within the corpus callosum, pons, and cerebellum are associated with disconnection syndrome, paraplegia, and gait and posture ataxia, respectively (Estruch et al., 1997; Hommer et al., 1996; Pfefferbaum et al., 1996).

Alcohol exerts its neurobiological effects primarily by binding to hydrophobic proteins and modulating their function by changing their three-dimensional structure. Ion channels, neurotransmitter receptors, and enzymes involved in signal transduction are among the proteins affected (Gordis, 1998). Dopamine, serotonin, GABA, glutamate, opioid, adenosine, neuropeptide Y, norepinephrine, cannabinoid receptors, and opioid peptides are among the neurotransmitters and receptors most affected by alcohol (Koob et al., 1998).

The acute effects of alcohol are mediated primarily by the facilitation of inhibitory GABA release coupled with the inhibition of excitatory glutamate neurotransmission. The potentiation of GABA underlies the acute sedative effects produced by alcohol, whereas the long-term adaptive changes within these two NT systems are critical for the development of alcohol dependence. With chronic alcohol consumption, the glutamatergic system becomes upregulated and the GABA system downregulated, resulting in tolerance to alcohol's effects and thus an increase in the amount of alcohol consumed (Grobin et al., 1998). If drinking ceases abruptly, neuronal hyperexcitability develops and is accompanied by arousal, anxiety, sleeplessness, and in some severe instances, the development of delirium tremens. These changes are reversible, albeit slowly, and may contribute to the persistence of craving during alcohol withdrawal and the difficulty in achieving or maintaining abstinence after acute detoxification.

The dopamine (DA) NT system also plays a major role in the development of alcohol dependence. Mesolimbic DA neurons are activated by alcohol consumption, and the release of DA within the limbic system mediates alcohol's positive reinforcing and rewarding effects (Gessa et al., 1985). DA neurons become sensitized to cues that predict or are associated with drinking during the development of alcohol dependence, and this change in reactivity is thought to mediate the increased desirability of alcohol. Alcohol also increases the beta-endorphin stimulation of DA release (Benjamin et al., 1993). Gianoulakis and colleagues (1996) postulate that individual differences in the endogenous endorphins and other opioid peptides may underlie differences in alcohol craving intensity and risk for alcohol dependence. Recent work conducted by Zalewska-Kaszubska and Czarnecka (2005) shows that chronic alcohol consumption leads to a beta-endorphin deficiency and that those with a genetic deficit of beta-endorphins are particularly susceptible to alcoholism. They found that plasma levels of beta-endorphins in individuals at high risk for alcohol abuse show lower basal activity, whereas its release increases significantly after alcohol consumption. Such research not only points to a potential genetic marker for alcohol dependence but also may influence responsivity to naltrexone (a mu-opioid receptor antagonist) pharmacotherapy.

Oslin and colleagues (2003) recently demonstrated that among European Americans treated with naltrexone, those with one or two copies of the Asp40 allele (a polymorphism that produces variations in amino acid sequencing within the terminal domain of the mu-opioid receptor) had significantly lower rates of relapse and took a longer time to return to heavy drinking than those who were homozygous for the Asp40 allele. These findings, although they await replication, are significant in that they represent the first demonstration of a genetic polymorphism related to naltrexone response. Although such genetic research is still in its infancy, understanding of the genetic basis of response to both psychosocial and pharmacologic treatments for alcoholism will allow researchers to develop specific targets for drug discovery and clinicians to tailor treatments to individual patients (Edenberg & Krazler, 2005).

Pharmacologic and Psychosocial Treatments

Benzodiazepines are the treatment of choice for acute alcohol withdrawal and detoxification both during hospitalization and on an outpatient basis (Fuller & Gordis, 1994). Although long-term use of benzodiazepines for alcohol-dependent patients is not suggested, many patients begin benzodiazepine therapy during detoxification and withdrawal and continue taking such medications for long-term symptoms secondary to alcoholism (e.g., anxiety disorders, insomnia). Clinicians must weigh the danger of prescribing a drug with the potential for abuse to an individual with a history of alcohol dependence with the symptom reduction and improved quality of life that benzodiazepine therapy may provide for the abstinent alcoholic (see Lejoyeux et al., 1998, for review of benzodiazepine treatment in alcohol dependence). According to

Lejoyeux et al. (1998), patients who are highly impulsive, have multiple drug dependencies, or have antisocial personality disorder are more likely to develop benzodiazepine dependence. When an opiate analgesic is indicated for injury or disease, clinicians must also be cautious because of the abuse potential and also must inquire whether the patient is taking naltrexone, an opioid antagonist. Higher doses of opioid medication may be indicated when patients are taking naltrexone. When benzodiazepines or opioids are prescribed to alcohol-dependent individuals on an outpatient basis, it should be in small amounts and such patients should be carefully monitored. A recent study conducted in Italy demonstrated that baclofen, a $GABA_B$ agonist, is as effective as diazepam in treating withdrawal symptoms in hospitalized alcohol-dependent patients (Addolorato et al., 2006).

Identification of NTs and receptors that are especially sensitive to alcohol spurs the development of new pharmacotherapies to treat this disorder (Spanagel & Zieglgansberger, 1997). Experimental medications for alcohol dependence include compounds such as baclofen, a $GABA_B$ agonist (Addolorato et al., 2002; Flannery et al., 2004); ondansetron, a selective $5-HT_3$ receptor antagonist (Johnson et al., 2000); topiramate, an antiepileptic agent that enhances GABA and inhibits glutamate kainate receptors (Johnson et al., 2003); as well as anticonvulsants such as gabapetin and vigabatrin as alternatives to benzodiazepine treatment of alcohol withdrawal (Myrick et al., 2001). Combination therapies such as naltrexone and acamprosate (COMBINE Study Research Group, 2003) and ondansetron and naltrexone also are being investigated (Ait-Daoud et al., 2001).

Presently, in the United States there are three FDA-approved pharmacological treatments for alcohol dependence: disulfiram (Antabuse), naltrexone, and acamprosate (Campral). Detailed data on the efficacy of these and the most prominently investigated experimental medications have been presented in several recently published reviews (Buonopane & Petrakis, 2005; Mann, 2005).

Among the FDA-approved medications, disulfiram has been in use the longest—over 50 years—but there is still no unequivocal evidence that it improves abstinence rates (Mann, 2004). Disulfiram blocks the oxidation of alcohol at the acetaldehyde stage and produces sensitivity to alcohol, which results in highly unpleasant symptoms (e.g., headache, respiratory difficulty, nausea, vomiting, sweating) when even small amounts of alcohol are consumed. The limited number of controlled clinical trials of oral disulfiram show modest evidence for its ability to reduce drinking (Garbutt et al., 1999). Poor compliance with oral disulfiram led to the development of a long-acting, implantable form, but studies of this form of disulfiram also have inconsistent findings.

Naltrexone, a mu-opioid receptor antagonist, was approved by the FDA in 1994. Because numerous studies have demonstrated that naltrexone increases abstinence rate and reduces the number of drinks per drinking occasion, it is thought that this medication compared to placebo reduces the pleasurable effects of alcohol and thereby attenuates loss of control over drinking. Some studies report a reduction in self-reported alcohol craving with naltrexone treatment (O'Malley et al., 1992; Vopicelli et al., 1992). Results from more recent trials with larger samples (e.g., Krystal et al., 2001) indicate either a small or no effect of naltrexone compared to placebo on various measures of drinking. In a meta-analysis of placebo-controlled studies conducted between 1992 and 2000, Kranzler and Van Kirk (2001) concluded that naltrexone's effects were modest ranging from 12% to 19% in terms of reduction in drinks per drinking day, percent drinking days, percent abstinent days, and retention in treatment. Of the 19 most recently conducted placebo-controlled naltrexone studies, 13 showed that naltrexone was more effective than placebo (Buonopane & Petrakis, 2005).

Fuller and Gordis (2001) suggest that lack of effect in the negative studies may be due to age, severity, the concomitant psychosocial treatment, and/or unstabilized psychiatric comorbidity. A recently conducted multisite study of a monthly injectable form of naltrexone combined with low-intensity psychosocial therapy found a 25% reduction in rate of heavy drinking among those treated with the 380-mg dose and a 17% reduction in those treated with the 190-mg dose. Men and those abstinent prior to treatment commencement had greater treatment effects (Garbutt et al., 2005).

Although acamprosate's precise mechanism of action is unclear, it may restore the balance between inhibitory and excitatory neurotransmission within the central nervous system. Acamprosate is thought to be effective in blocking conditioned withdrawal-induced craving through its actions on NMDA glutamate receptors (Rossetti & Carboni, 1995) and by decreasing hypersensitivity of calcium channels related to withdrawal (al Qatari et al., 1998). In the United States, one multisite pharmaceutical-sponsored trial has been conducted (Overman et al., 2003) and another NIAAA-sponsored naltrexone and acamprosate trial was recently completed (COMBINE Research Study Group, 2003).

In Europe, where acamprosate has been registered for use in 24 countries since 1996, both preclinical and clinical data support its efficacy in reducing drinking days and increasing length of abstinence (Buonopane and Petrakis, 2005). Both 1.3- and 2.0-g/d acamprosate doses in conjunction with supportive psychotherapy were superior to placebo in more than 2,000 patients in various studies (e.g., Whitworth et al., 1996) as indicated by the outcome variable, cumulative abstinence days. Effect sizes calculated for 11 studies conducted between 1992 and 2000 ranged between 0.07 and 0.13 for cumulative abstinence days, percent abstinent days, and retention (Kranzler and Van Kirk, 2001).

In a recent analysis of psychosocial intervention for alcohol dependence, Andréasson and Öjehagen (2003) found different effect sizes for specific types of therapies: cognitive behavioral therapy (CBT) $d=0.73$, contingency reinforcement or contingency management approach (CMA) $d=0.26$, and educational or bibliotherapy $d=0.19$, all compared to treatment as usual for alcohol dependence. Yet, when specific psychosocial approaches were compared to each other, no statistical differences were found despite considerable differences in theoretical approach. Twelve-step facilitation, CBT, motivational enhancement, psychodynamic psychotherapy, and family therapy produced similar results (Bergin & Garfield, 1994).

In summary, AUDs are complex disorders, often co-occurring with other psychiatric illnesses. The neurobiological effects of AUDs have been well characterized, and extant pharmacologic and psychosocial treatments are effective for some with these disorders. Researchers expect that genetic research may provide additional insights into the factors leading to AUDs that will, in turn, aid in the development of treatments that are more effective in countering the chronic relapsing that is a hallmark of alcohol dependence.

References

Acker C. Performance of female alcoholics on neuropsychological testing. *Alcohol and Alcoholism* 20:379–386; 1985.

Acker C. Neuropsychological deficits in alcoholics: the relative contributions of gender and drinking history. *British Journal of Addictions* 81:395–403; 1986.

Addolorato G, Caputo F, Capristo E, Domenicali M, Bernardi M, Janiri L, et al. Baclofen efficacy in reducing alcohol craving and intake: a preliminary double-blind randomized controlled study. *Alcohol and Alcoholism* 37:504–508; 2002.

Addolorato G, Leggio L, Abenavoli L, Agabio R, Caputo F, Capristo E, Colombo G, Gessa GL, Gasbarrini G. Baclofen in the treatment of alcohol withdrawal syndrome: a comparative study vs diazepam. *American Journal of Medicine* 19(3):276.e13–8; 2006.

Agartz I, Momenan R, Rawlings RR, Kerich MJ, Hommer DW. Hippocampal volume in patients with alcohol dependence. *Archives of General Psychiatry* 56:356–363; 1999.

Ait-Daoud N, Johnson BA, Javors M, Roache JD, Zanca NA. Combining ondansetron and naltrexone treats biological alcoholics: corroboration of self-reported drinking by serum carbohydrate deficient transferrin, a biomarker. *Alcoholism: Clinical and Experimental Research* 25:847–849; 2001.

al Qatari M, Bouchenafa O, Littleton J. Mechanism of action of acamprosate. Part II. Ethanol dependence modifies effects of acamprosate on NMDA receptor binding in membranes from rat cerebral cortex. *Alcoholism: Clinical and Experimental Research* 22:810–814; 1998.

Andréasson S, Öjehagen A. Psychosocial treatment for alcohol dependence. In M Berglund, E Johnson, & S Thelander (eds.). *Treatment of Alcohol and Drug Abuse An Evidence-Based Review*, pp. 43–188. Weinheim, Germany: Wiley-VCH; 2003.

American Psychiatric Association. *Diagnostic and Statistical Manual of Mental Disorders* (4th ed. revised; *DSM-IV-TR*). Washington, DC: American Psychiatric Association; 2000.

Benjamin D, Grant E, Pohorecky LA. Naltrexone reverses ethanol-induced dopamine release in the nucleus accumbens in awake, freely moving rats. *Brain Research* 62:137–140; 1993.

Bergin AE, Garfield SL. Overview, trends, and future issues. In Bergin AE, & Garfield SL (eds.). *Handbook of Psychotherapy and Behavior Change* (4th ed.), pp. 821–830. New York: John Wiley & Sons, Inc.; 1994.

Berglund M. A better widget? Three lesions for improving addiction treatment from a meta-analytical study. *Addiction* 100:742–750; 2005.

Buonopane A, Petrakis IL. Pharmacotherapy of alcohol use disorders. *Substance Use & Misuse*, 40:2001–2020; 2005.

Chathan-Showalter PE, Dubov WE, Barr MC, Rhodes M, Sun JM, Wasser T. Alcohol level at head injury and subsequent psychotropic treatment during trauma critical care. *Psychosomatics* 37:285–288, 1996.

Cloninger CR. Neurogenetic adaptive mechanisms in alcoholism. *Science* 236:410–416, 1987.

COMBINE Study Research Group. Testing combined pharmacotherapies and behavioral interventions in alcohol dependence: rationale and methods. *Alcohol: Clinical and Experimental Research* 27:1107–1122; 2003.

Edenberg HJ, Krazler HR. The contribution of genetics to addiction therapy approaches. *Pharmacology & Therapeutics* 108:86–93; 2005.

Estruch, R, Nicolas, JM, Salamero, M, Aragon, C, Sacanella, E, Fernandez-Soal, J, Urban-Marquez, A. Atrophy of the corpus callosum in chronic alcoholism. *Journal of Neurological Science* 146:145–151; 1997.

Fein, G, Di Sclafani, V, Cardenas, VA, Goldman, H, Tolou-Shams, M, Meyerhoff, DJ. Cortical gray matter loss in treatment-naïve alcohol dependent individuals. *Alcoholism: Clinical and Experimental Research* 26: 558–564; 2002.

Flannery BA, Fishbein DH, Krupitsky E, Langevin D, Verbiskaya E et al. Gender differences in neurocognitive functioning among alcohol-dependent Russian patients. *Alcoholism: Clinical and Experimental Research* 31:745–754; 2007.

Flannery BA, Garbutt, JC, Cody MW, Renn W, Grace K, Osborne M et al. Baclofen for alcohol dependence: a preliminary open-label study. *Alcoholism: Clinical and Experimental Research* 28:1517–1523; 2004.

Fuller R, Gordis E. Naltrexone treatment for alcohol dependence. *The New England Journal of Medicine* 345:1770–1771; 2001.

Fuller RK, Gordis E. Refining the treatment of alcohol withdrawal. *JAMA* 272:557–558; 1994.

Garbutt JC, Kranzler HR, O'Malley SS, Gastfriend DR, Pettinati, HM, et al. Efficacy and tolerability of long-acting injectable naltrexone for alcohol dependence: a randomized controlled trial. *JAMA* 293:1617–1625; 2005.

Garbutt JC, West SL, Carey TS, Lohr KN, Crews FT. Pharmacological treatment of alcohol dependence: a review of the evidence. *JAMA* 281: 1318–1325; 1999.

Gessa GL, Muntoni F, Collu M, Vargiu L, Mereu G. Low doses of ethanol activate dopaminergic neurons in the ventral tegmental area. *Brain Research*, 348:201–203; 1985.

Gianoulakis C. Implications of endogenous opioids and dopamine in alcoholism: human and basic science studies. *Alcohol and Alcoholism* (suppl.) 1:33–42; 1996.

Gordis E. The neurobiology of alcohol abuse and alcoholism: building knowledge, creating hope. *Drug and Alcohol Dependence*, 51:9–11; 1998.

Grant BF, Dawson DA, Stinson FS, Chou SP, Dufour MC, Pickering RP. The 12-month prevalence and trends in DSM-IV alcohol abuse and dependence: United States, 1991–1992 and 2001–2002. *Drug and Alcohol Dependence*, 74:223–234; 2004.

Grant BF, Moore TC, Shepard J, Kaplan K. *Source and accuracy statement: Wave 1 National Epidemiologic Survey on Alcohol and Related Conditions (NESARC)*. Bethesda, MD: National Institute on Alcohol Abuse and Alcoholism; 2003.

Grobin AC, Matthews DB, Devaud LL, Morrow AL. The role of $GABA_A$ receptors in the acute and chronic effects of ethanol. *Psychopharmacology* 139:2–19; 1998.

Harding AJ, Wong A, Svoboda M, Kril JJ, Halliday GM. Chronic alcohol consumption does not cause hippocampal neuron loss in humans. *Hippocampus* 7:78–87; 1997.

Harper, CG, Kril, JJ. Corpus callosal thickness in alcoholics. *British Journal of Addictions* 83:577–580; 1988.

Harwood H. *The economic costs of drug abuse in the United States: 1992–2002*. Report prepared by the Lewin Group for the Office of Drug Control Policy (ONDCP); 2004.

Hill EM, Stoltenberg SF, Burmeister M, Closser M, Zucker RA. Potential associations among genetic markers in the serotonergic system and the antisocial alcoholism subtype. *Experimental and Clinical Psychopharmacology* 7:103–121; 1999.

Hoffman PL, Tabakoff B. Alcohol dependence: a commentary on mechanics. *Alcohol and Alcoholism* 31:331–340; 1996.

Hommer, D, Momeman, R, Kaiser, E, Rawlings, RR. Evidence for a gender-related effect of alcoholism on brain volumes. *American Journal of Psychiatry* 158:198–204; 2001.

Hommer, D, Momenan, R, Rawlings, R, Ragan, P, Williams, W, Rio, D, Eckardt, M. Decreased corpus callosum size among alcoholic women. *Archives of Neurology* 53:359–363; 1996.

Jernigan, TL, Butters, N DiTraglia, G, Schafer, K, Smith, T, Irwin, M, Grant, I, Schuckit, M, Cermak, L. Reduced cerebral grey matter observed in alcoholics using magnetic resonance imaging. *Alcoholism: Clinical and Experimental Research* 15:418–427; 1991.

Johnson BA, Ait-Daoud N, Bowden C, DiClememte CC, Roache JA et al. Oral topiramate for treatment of alcohol dependence: a randomized controlled trial. *The Lancet* 361:1677–1685; 2003.

Johnson BA, Roache JD, Javors MA, DiClemente CC, Cloninger CR et al. Ondansetron for reduction of drinking among biologically predisposed alcoholic patients: a randomized controlled trial. *JAMA* 284:963–971; 2000.

Kessler RC, Nelson CB, McGonagle KA, Edlund MJ, Frank RG, Leaf PJ. The epidemiology of co-occurring addictive and mental disorders. *American Journal of Orthopsychiatry* 66:17–31; 1996.

Kiefer F, Mann K. New achievements and pharmaco-therapeutic approaches in the treatment of alcohol dependence. *European Journal of Pharmacology* 536:163–171; 2005.

Klug MG, Burd L. Fetal alcohol syndrome prevention: annual and cumulative cost savings. *Neurotoxicology and Teratology* 25:736–735; 2003.

Koob GF, Roberts AJ, Schulteis G, Parsons LH, Heyser CJ, et al. Neurocircuitry targets in ethanol reward and dependence. *Alcoholism: Clinical and Experimental Research* 22:3–9; 1998.

Kranzler HR, Van Kirk J. Efficacy of naltrexone and acamprosate for alcoholism treatment: a meta-analysis. *Alcoholism: Clinical and Experimental Research* 25:1335–1341; 2001.

Kril, JJ, Halliday, GM, Svoboda, MD, Cartwright, H. The cerebral cortex is damaged in chronic alcoholics. *Neuroscience* 79:983–998; 1997.

Krueger RF, Markon KE, Patrick CJ, Iacono, WG. Externalizing psychopathology in adulthood: a dimensional-spectrum conceptualization and its implications for DSM-V. *Journal of Abnormal Psychology* 114:537–550; 2005.

Krystal JH, Cramer JA, Krol WF, Kirk GF, Rosenheck RA. Veterans Affairs Naltrexone Cooperative Study 425 Group. Naltrexone in the treatment of alcohol dependence. *New England Journal of Medicine* 345:1734–1739; 2001.

Lejoyeux M, Solomon J, Ades J. Benzodiazepine treatment for alcohol-dependent patients. *Alcohol and Alcoholism* 33:563–575; 1998.

Leshner AI. Addiction is a brain disease, and it matters. *Science* 278:45–47; 1997.

Mann K. Pharmacotherapy of alcohol dependence: a review of the clinical data. *CNS Drugs* 18:485–504; 2004.

Mann K, Achermann B, Croissant B, Mundle G, Nakovics H, Diehl A. Neuroimaging of gender differences in alcohol dependence: Are women more vulnerable. *Alcoholism: Clinical and Experimental Research* 29:896–901; 2005.

Mann K, Agartz I, Harper C, Shoaf S, Rawlings RR et al. Neuroimaging in alcoholism: ethanol and brain damage. *Alcoholism: Clinical and Experimental Research* 25 (suppl. ISBRA):104S–109S; 2001.

McGlynn E, Asch SM, Adams J, Keesey J, Hicks J, DeCristofaro A, Kerr EA. The quality of heath care delivered to adults in the United States. *New England Journal of Medicine* 348:2635–2645; 2003.

Mokdad AH, Marks JS, Stroup DF, Gerberding JL. Actual causes of death in the United States, 2000. *JAMA* 291:1238–1245, 2004.

Myrick H, Brady KT, Malcolm R. New developments in the pharmacotherapy of alcohol dependence. *American Journal of Addictions* 10(suppl.):3–15, 2001.

National Institute on Alcohol Abuse and Alcoholism. Unpublished data from the 2001–2002 National Epidemiologic Survey on Alcohol and Related Conditions (NESARC), a nationwide survey of 43,093 U.S. adults aged 10 or older; 2004.

Newlin DB, Miles D, van den Bree, MBM, Gupman A, Pickens RW. Environmental transmission of DSM-IV substance use disorders in adoptive and step families. *Alcoholism: Clinical and Experimental Research* 24:1785–1794; 2000.

Newlin DB, Thomson, JT. Chronic tolerance and sensitization to alcohol in sons of alcoholics: II. Replication and reanalysis. *Experimental and Clinical Psychopharmacology* 7:235–243; 1990.

O'Malley SS, Jaffe AJ, Change G, Schottenfeld RS, Meyer RE, Rounsaville B. Naltrexone and coping skills therapy for alcohol dependence: a controlled study. *Archives of General Psychiatry* 49:881–887; 1992.

Oscar-Berman M, Hutner N. Frontal lobe changes after chronic alcohol ingestions. In WA Hunt, SJ Nixon (eds.) *Alcohol Induced Brain Damage. NIAAA Monographs #22*, Rockville, MD: National Institutes of Health, pp. 121–156; 1993.

Oslin DW, Berrettini W, Kranzler HR, Pettinati H, Gelernter J, et al. A functional polymorphism of the mu-opioid receptor gene is associated with naltrexone response in alcohol-dependent patients. *Neuropsychopharmacology* 28:1546–1552; 2003.

Overman GP, Teter CJ, Guthrie SK. Acamprosate for the adjunctive treatment of alcohol dependence. *Annals of Pharmacotherapy* 37:1090–1099; 2003.

Parsons, OA, Butters, N, Nathan, PE. *Neuropsychology of alcoholism: implications for diagnosis and treatment*. New York: Guilford Press; 1987.

Pfefferbaum, A, Lim, KO, Desmond, J, Sullivan, EV. Thinning of the corpus callosum in older alcoholic men: a magnetic resonance imaging study. *Alcoholism: Clinical and Experimental Research* 20:752–757; 1996.

Pfefferbaum, A, Lim, KO, Zipursky, RB, Mathalon, DH, Lane, B, Ha, CN, Rosenbloom, MJ, Sullivan, EV. Brain gray and white matter volume loss accelerates with aging in chronic alcoholics: a quantitative MRI study. *Alcoholism: Clinical and Experimental Research* 16:1078–1089; 1992.

Randall CL, Roberts JS, DelBoca FK, Carroll KM, Conners GJ, Mattson ME. Telescoping of landmark events associated with drinking: a gender comparison. *Journal of Studies on Alcohol* 60:252–260; 1999.

Rehm JM, Room R, Graham K, Monteiro M, Gmel G, Sempos CT. The relationship of average volume of alcohol consumption and patterns of drinking to burden of disease: An overview. *Addiction* 98:1209–1128; 2003.

Robins LN, Regier DS (Eds.). *Psychiatric Disorders in America: the Epidemiologic Catchment Area Study*. New York: The Free Press; 1991.

Rossetti ZL, Carboni S. Ethanol withdrawal is associated with increased extracellular glutamate in the rat striatum. *European Journal of Pharmacology* 5:177–183; 1995.

Sher KJ. *Children of alcoholics: a critical appraisal of theory and research*. Chicago: University of Chicago Press; 1991.

Sher KJ, Levenson RW. Risk for alcoholism and individual differences in the stress-response-dampening effect of alcohol. *Journal of Abnormal Psychology* 91:350–367; 1982.

Sher KJ, Wood MD. Subjective Effects of Alcohol II: Individual Differences in M Earleywine (Ed). *Mind-altering drugs: the science of subjective experience*. New York: Oxford University Press; 2005.

Spangel R, Zieglgänsberger W. Anti-craving compounds for ethanol: new pharmacological tools to study addictive processes. *Trends in Pharmacologic Science* 18:37–65; 1997.

Sullivan EV. Compromised pontocerebellar and cerebellothalamocortical systems: speculations on their contributions to cognitive and motor impairment in nonamnesic alcoholism. *Alcoholism: Clinical and Experimental Research* 27:1409–1419; 2003.

Sullivan EV, Marsh L. Hippocampal volume deficits in alcoholic Korsakoff's syndrome. *Neurology* 61(12):1716–1719; 2003.

Sullivan EV, Marsh L, Mathalon DH, Lim KO, Pfefferbaum A. Anterior hippocampal volume deficits in nonamnesic, aging, chronic alcoholics. *Alcoholism: Clinical and Experimental Research* 19(1):110–122; 1995.

Sullivan EV, Pfefferbaum A. Neurocircuitry in alcoholism: a substrate of disruption and repair. *Psychopharmacology* 180:583–94; 2005.

Sullivan EV, Rosenbloom MJ, Pfefferbaum, A. Pattern of motor and cognitive deficits in detoxified alcoholic men. *Alcoholism: Clinical and Experimental Research* 24(5):611–621; 2000.

Tarnowska-Dziduszko E, Bertrand E, Szpak GM (1995) Morphological changes in the corpus callosum in chronic alcoholism. *Folia Neuropathologica* 33(1), 25–29.

Uhl GR. Molecular genetics of substance abuse vulnerability: remarkable recent convergence of genome scan results. *Annals of the New York Academy of Sciences* 1025:1–13; 2004.

Uhl GR, Liu QR, Naiman D. Substance abuse vulnerability loci: converging genome scanning data. *Trends in Genetics* 18:420–425; 2002.

Vopicelli JR, Alterman AI, Hayashida, M, O'Brien CP. Naltrexone in the treatment of alcohol dependence. *Archives of General Psychiatry* 49:876–880; 1992.

Watson D, Clark LA. Negative affectivity: The disposition to experience aversive emotional states. *Psychological Bulletin* 96:465–490; 1984.

Whitworth, AB, Fischer, F, Lesch, OM, et al. Comparison of acamprosate and placebo in long-term treatment of alcohol dependence. *Lancet* 347:1438–1442; 1996.

Wilde EA, Bigler ED, Gandhi PV, Lowry CM, Blatter DD, Brooks J, Ryser DK. Alcohol abuse and traumatic brain injury: quantitative magnetic resonance imaging and neuropsychological outcome. *J Neurotrauma* 21:137–147; 2004.

World Health Organization (WHO). *International Statistical Classification of Diseases and Related Health Problems 10th Revision (ICD-10)*, online 2007; Retrieved 1/8/08 from http://www.who.int/classifications/apps/icd/icd10 online.

World Health Organization (WHO). *World Health Organization Report: Reducing Risks, Promoting Healthy Life*. Geneva: WHO; 2002.

Zalewska-Kaszubska J, Czarnecka E. Deficit in beta-endorphin peptide and tendency to alcohol abuse. *Peptides* 26(4):701–705; 2005.

Zucker RA, Wong, MM. Prevention for children of alcoholics and other high risk groups. *Recent Developments*, 17:299–320, 2005.

19

Benzodiazepines
Misuse, Abuse, and Dependence

Danielle M. Ciraulo

Domenic A. Ciraulo

Inappropriate use of benzodiazepines is an important public health problem. In clinical practice benzodiazepine misuse is generally encountered in one of the three following situations: as part of a complex presentation of polysubstance dependence, in patients who have been prescribed therapeutic doses of benzodiazepines and have difficulty stopping use, and rarely, dependence on benzodiazepines as the primary drug of abuse. Determining the extent of the problem is hindered by various definitions of abuse and dependence. In this chapter, we follow the use of previous publications: "The terms *abuse* and *misuse* refer to the use of a drug in a manner that is not consistent with generally accepted medical practice or social and legal custom, e.g., use without a valid prescription or deliberately to produce intoxication, pleasure or a high" (Ciraulo and Sarid-Segal, 2005, p. 1300). *Misuse* is used to describe patients who use higher than prescribed doses, or obtain medications from a friend or relative for therapeutic purposes.

DSM-IV-TR (American Psychiatric Association, 1994) defines *abuse* as "A maladaptive pattern of substance use leading to clinically significant impairment or distress," which includes continued use in the face of social, legal, or physical problems or in hazardous situations such as driving. *Dependence* in *DSM-IV-TR* adds tolerance and withdrawal as criteria, as well as failed efforts to control use. In addition, it lists criteria reflecting disturbances in psychosocial functioning associated with dependence, including lack of control, escalation of dose, persistent use despite physical or psychological problems, and primacy of drug use over other activities.

We also find the term *physiologic dependence,* as defined by the World Health Organization as "a pathological state brought about repeated administration of a drug that leads to the appearance of a characteristic and specific group of symptoms when the drug is discontinued or the dose is significantly reduced," a useful concept in understanding misuse of benzodiazepines. Convention assigns the use of the term *recreational use* for administration of a drug to "get high" or for its hedonic value. The American Psychiatric Association Task Force on Benzodiazepine Dependence, Toxicity, and Abuse (1990) used the term *discontinuance syndrome* to distinguish an abstinence syndrome that develops in the course of stopping therapeutic agents from one that develops from terminating the use of illicit drugs.

Epidemiology

There are several approaches that have been used to look at the extent of benzodiazepine misuse in the population. These include: The National Survey on Drug Use and Health (NSDUH), The Drug Abuse Warning Network (DAWN), Monitoring the Future (MTF), and the Substance Abuse and Mental Health Services Administration (SAMHSA) publication "Treatment Episode Data Set (TEDS)".

The NSDUH reported that lifetime nonmedical use of clonazepam, alprazolam, and lorazepam increased slightly from 2002 to 2003, with age groups 18–25 showing a significant increase in clonazepam use, whereas both 18–25 and 26 and older age groups showed an increase in the use of the latter drugs (see Figure 19.1; SAMHSA, 2005). The percent of the population using clonazepam for nonmedical purposes increased from 1% to 1.2%, and for alprazolam or lorazepam from 3.5% to 4% from 2002 to 2003.

The NSDUH report indicated that 2.7% of the adult population (12 years old and over) used prescription psychotherapeutics for nonmedical purposes in the month prior to the survey. Of these 6.3 million persons, 4.7 million used prescription pain relievers, 2.1 million used tranquilizers or sedatives, and 1.2 million used stimulants in the month prior to the survey. So, even though nonmedical use of tranquilizers increased during 2001–2003, it occupies an intermediate position between pain relievers and stimulants.

The Drug Abuse Warning Network (DAWN) monitors drug-related hospital emergency department visits and drug-related deaths investigated by medical examiners in 21 metropolitan areas in the United States and estimates the number of patients seeking detoxification services for specific drugs (SAMHSA, 2004). Although not representative of the population in general, trends emerge from an estimated 61,506 drug-related ED visits (as recorded in the third and fourth quarters of 2003). During that period, DAWN had 11,391 reported ED visits requesting detoxification for benzodiazepine use. Because 60% of these visits involve more than one substance of abuse, these data do not provide information on the primary drug of abuse. The percentages of drugs implicated are as follows: cocaine 47%, opioids (hydrocodone/oxycodone) 36%, heroin 25%, benzodiazepines 19%, marijuana 14%, and stimulants 9%.

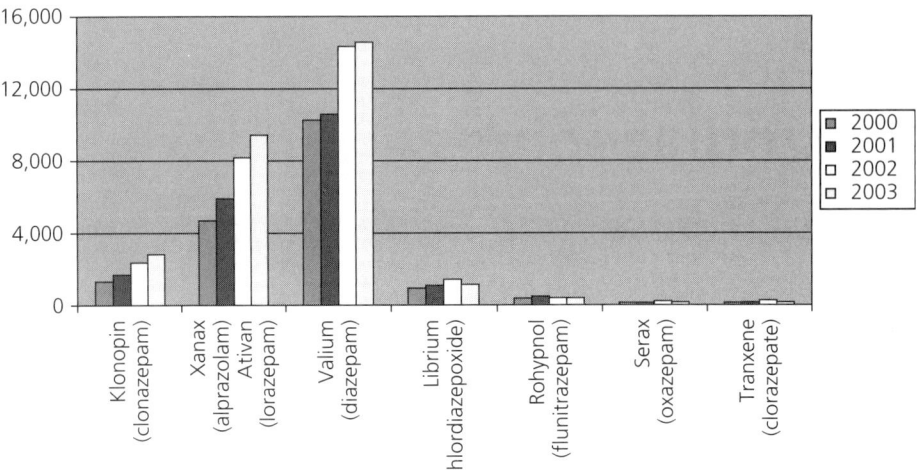

Figure 19.1. Nonmedical use of specific benzodiazepine anti-anxiety agents. Number in thousands. Source: SAMHSA, 2004, 2005.

The Monitoring the Future survey found that after increases in the 1990s, the lifetime, past year, and past month use of tranquilizers in high school students was low, and either declining or stable from 2001 (see Figures 19.2, 19.3, and 19.4; Johnston et al., 2005).

Although benzodiazepines are rarely the primary substance of abuse, SAMHSA's Treatment Episode Data Set (TEDS) reported a 79% increase in patients who reported tranquilizers as their primary substance of abuse, from 4,600 admissions in 1992 to 8,300 in 2002 (SAMHSA, 2005). An additional 32,800 admissions reported benzodiazepines as secondary or tertiary substance of abuse in 2002, most often associated with opiates (46%) and alcohol (30%). Because the TEDS data set includes over 1.8 million admissions, even though there has been a reported increase in tranquilizers as the primary substance of abuse, it represents only 0.4% of admissions.

Conclusions drawn from survey data are limited by the populations studied, the method of interview, reliability and validity of report, and drug classification schemes, yet they are remarkably consistent in establishing that even though benzodiazepines are rarely a primary drug of abuse, their concomitant use with illicit substances is commonplace and clinically important.

Laboratory Models of Abuse

There are several other approaches that have been used to estimate the abuse liability of benzodiazepines. These include both animal models and laboratory studies. Studies in animals universally support that these drugs have minimal reinforcing effects (Woods et al., 1992; Woods and Wigner, 1995). Although a few studies have shown that animals will self-administer benzodiazepines, they are less potent than cocaine, amphetamines, or barbiturates (Griffiths and Ator, 1980).

Two models of human laboratory assessment of abuse liability are commonly used. In the simpler model, doses of the benzodiazepine, a comparator drug, and placebo are administered to subjects with a history of sedative-hypnotic abuse (Jaffe et al., 1983). Subjective ratings of euphoric effect and drug liking are valid and reliable indicators of the drug's potential for misuse. In the second model, the benzodiazepine, comparator drugs, and placebo are offered to subjects with a history of sedative hypnotic abuse as "samples" or priming doses, and then subjects are allowed to self administer the drug of their choice (Griffiths et al., 1980, 1984). Using these models, benzodiazepines have been shown to have lower reinforcing effects than barbiturates or older sedative hypnotics.

Some controversy exists regarding relative abuse liability among the benzodiazepines; however, flunitrazepam (Rohypnol) has consistently been shown to have greater reinforcing effects than other agents in this class (Mintzer and Griffiths, 2005). At the other end of the spectrum, drugs that serve as prodrugs for desmethyldiazepam, such as prazepam or halazepam, may have lower reinforcing effects than alprazolam or diazepam (Ciraulo et al., 1997; Jaffe et al., 1983). A series of studies from Roland Griffiths' laboratory supports lower abuse liability for oxazepam as compared to diazepam (Griffiths et al., 1990, 1997). Although some studies suggest that the nonbenzodiazepines hypnotics such as zolpidem and zopiclone have lower abuse liability than benzodiazepines, case reports suggest that some patients abuse these drugs.

One of the controversies in the human model paradigms is whether self-administration of benzodiazepines or stating that the subject "likes" the effects of the drug is related to drug abuse or to therapeutic effect. It would be expected that both goals (i.e., anxiety reduction or euphoria) would lead to increased self-administration. In an interesting study addressing this issue, Roerhs et al. (2001) found that primary insomniacs consistently chose the hypnotic over placebo, but that the degree of sleep disturbance predicted drug choice and self-administration was related to the drug's efficacy.

Studies in Addiction Treatment Programs

Studies conducted in methadone clinics (Iguchi et al., 1993; Stitzer et al., 1981), indicate that flunitrazepam, diazepam, lorazepam, and alprazolam are more highly valued for the high they produce than are oxazepam, clorazepate, chlordiazepoxide, and phenobarbital. In a study of three addiction treatment centers in the United Kingdom, Jaffe and colleagues (2004) found that three benzodiazepines—diazepam, nitrazepam, and temazepam—were reported by subjects to have greater abuse liability than the comparator agents of antihistamines and antidepressants. They also found that zopiclone and zolpidem were commonly used by addicts to treat insomnia but only about 23% of subjects used

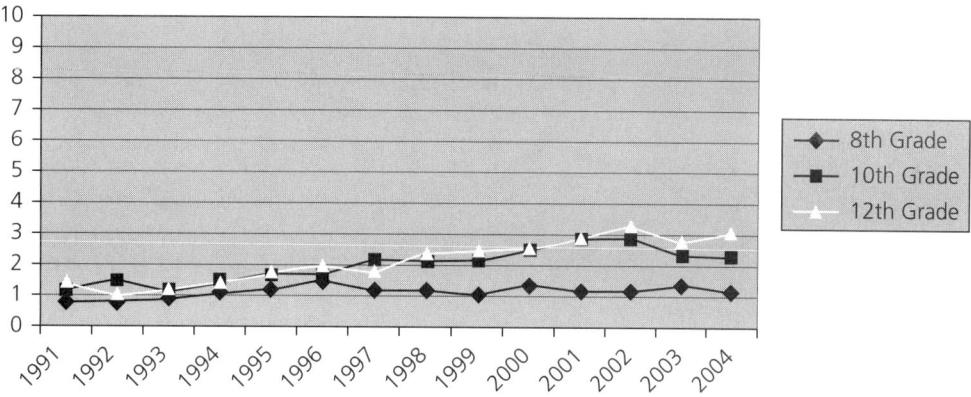

Figure 19.2. Trends (%) in 30-day prevalence of tranquilizer use for 8th, 10th, and 12th graders. Source: Johnston et al., 2005.

these drugs to get high. In comparison, 80.1%, 70.3%, and 71.3 % used diazepam, nitrazepam, and temazepam, respectively, to get high.

In summary, survey and experimental data suggest that benzodiazepines are rarely a primary drug of abuse and that benzodiazepines present a lower risk of abuse than the older sedative hypnotics, such as amobarbital and methaqualone. There is also suggestive evidence that differences exist among the benzodiazepines with flunitrazepam, lorazepam, diazepam, nitrazepam, and temazepam more reinforcing than oxazepam, prazepam, and halazepam. With respect to hypnotics, zopiclone, and zolpidem may have lower abuse liability than benzodiazepines; however, further studies are needed. For clinical purposes, all of these agents should be considered as having potential for abuse in patients at high risk, such as substance abusers.

Benzodiazepine Withdrawal Syndrome

The benzodiazepine withdrawal syndrome was first reported by Leo Hollister in the 1960s (Hollister et al., 1961). It is characterized by disturbances in mood, cognition, sleep, perception, and autonomic arousal (see Table 19.1). The severity of the withdrawal syndrome is increased by higher doses, longer duration of use, rapid rate of drug taper, personality factors, and psychopathology.

The withdrawal syndrome is probably not an important contributing factor to abuse; however, it is very important among some long-term users who want to discontinue the drug but have difficulty doing so because of the appearance of withdrawal symptoms when doses are lowered. Long-term therapeutic users of benzodiazepines are more likely to be older, female, with chronic health problems and high levels of emotional distress (Balter et al., 1984). About 25% of patients prescribed benzodiazepines for anxiety use them for longer than a year, whereas 14% using them as hypnotics take them longer than a year. Long-term therapeutic users rarely increase the dosage without physician authorization, and commonly reduce the dosage.

Clinical management of the withdrawal syndrome involves differentiation of *recurrence, rebound,* and *withdrawal.* "Rebound symptoms are symptoms for which the benzodiazepine was originally prescribed that return in a more severe form (when the benzodiazepine is discontinued)....They have a...rapid onset...and brief duration. Recurrence refers to the return of the original symptoms at or below their original intensity" (Ciraulo and Sarid-Segal, 2005). Rebound anxiety is part of a true withdrawal syndrome and requires pharmacologic treatment. In cases of recurrence, specific treatment of the underlying anxiety disorder is the proper clinical focus, and may involve restarting benzodiazepines or using alternative therapies (e.g., antidepressants, cognitive behavior therapy).

Figure 19.3. Trends (%) in annual prevalence of tranquilizer use for 8th, 10th, and 12th graders. Source: Johnston et al., 2005.

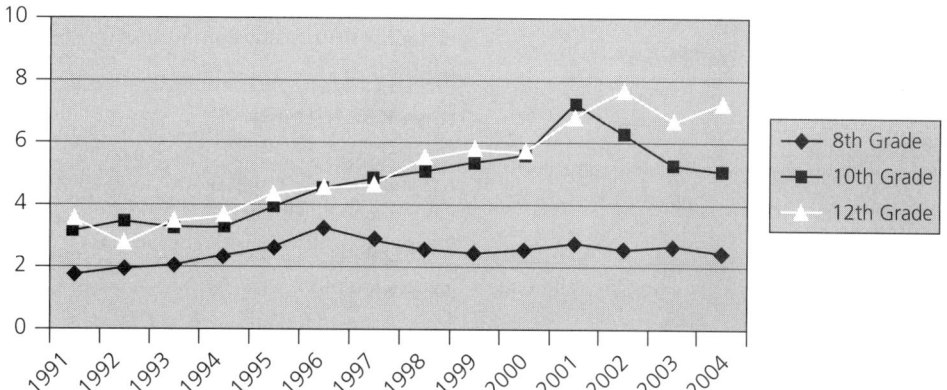

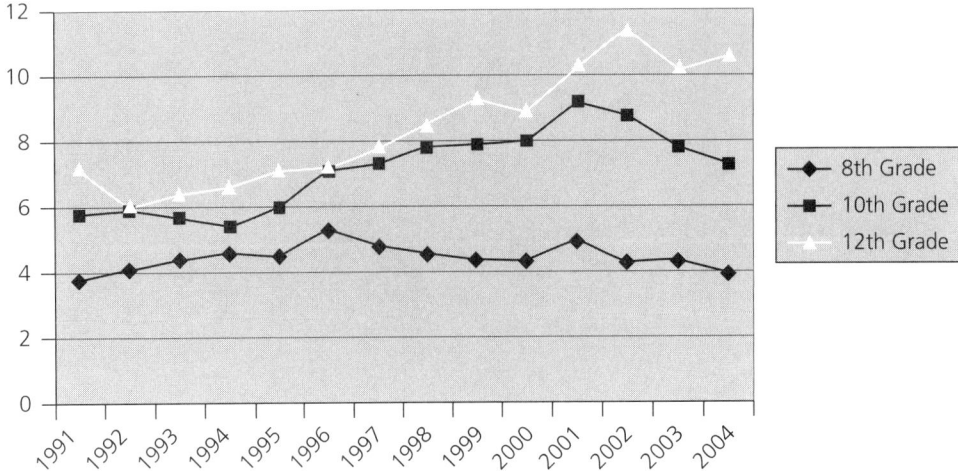

Figure 19.4. Trends (%) in lifetime prevalence of tranquilizer use for 8th, 10th, and 12th graders. Source: Johnston et al., 2005.

Pharmacologic approaches to detoxification vary slightly depending on the clinical situation. Specifically, protocols for discontinuation of therapeutic doses and supratherapeutic doses are different, as is the management of benzodiazepine withdrawal in the context of polysubstance abuse. For discontinuation of therapeutic doses, an initial dose reduction of 10–25% is made, with long-term users requiring the smaller percentage decrease. Symptoms are closely monitored, keeping in mind that discontinuation of short-acting agents without active metabolites (e.g., lorazepam) will be associated with peak withdrawal symptoms rapidly (24–48 hours), whereas abstinence symptoms from stopping long-acting agents (e.g., clonazepam) may be delayed (several days to 2 weeks). Although that is the general rule, an important exception exists. Some patients are exquisitely sensitive to declines in brain levels of the drug, and will experience withdrawal symptoms even when benzodiazepine plasma levels are in the therapeutic range. An additional caution is that many patients tolerate initial decreases without problems, but experience great difficulty in the final stages of withdrawal. Although this may be partly due to psychological factors, some evidence suggests that receptor alterations occur (Miller et al., 1988) during these final dose reductions. In these instances, the taper should be slowed, and/or adjunctive medications added. The evidence for efficacy of adjunctive medication is weak or absent, but clonidine, carbamazepine, valproic acid, gabapentin, topiramate, mirtazapine, trazodone, SSRI, beta blockers, and buspirone all have been used, with inconsistent results.

Table 19.1. Benzodiazepine Withdrawal Syndrome

Changes in Mood, Perception, and Cognition	Physical Signs and Symptoms
○ Anxiety	○ Tachycardia
○ Apprehension	○ Hypertension
○ Dysphoria	○ Hypertension
○ Irritability	○ Tremor
○ Perceptual disturbances (hyperacusis, depersonalization, illusions, visual disturbances, hallucinations)	○ Ataxia
	○ Grand mal seizures
	○ Nausea
	○ Coryza
	○ Diaphoresis

Withdrawal from supratherapeutic doses requires caution because sudden discontinuation is associated with severe consequences including seizures, delirium, and psychosis. In these cases, we prefer to stabilize the patients on an equivalent dose of a long-acting benzodiazepine in a residential setting. The primary reason for using a residential setting is that withdrawal from high doses is almost always accompanied by some discomfort, and without supervision many patients are likely to seek supplementation from other sources. Once stabilized for 2–3 days, 5% daily reductions are made. If this rate of taper is associated with anything greater than mild symptoms, it should be slowed and adjunctive medications added. Some experienced clinicians prefer to use barbiturates in cases of high dose withdrawal.

In cases of polysubstance dependence, the taper strategy depends on the coabused drug. Benzodiazepine abuse is most often seen in the context of alcohol, opiate, and stimulant abuse. It should be remembered that sedative hypnotic withdrawal is associated with the most serious medical consequences and should be the primary focus of treatment. The course and presentation of the alcohol withdrawal syndrome may be altered in the presence of benzodiazepines. Opioid dependence may be managed by stabilization with methadone, followed by taper when the sedative withdrawal syndrome has passed. In patients taking relatively low doses of opioids and benzodiazepines, simultaneous taper may be possible. Some clinicians prefer to use barbiturates in mixed sedative hypnotic dependence. Despite the common cooccurrence of psychostimulant and benzodiazepine abuse, there are no studies to guide the clinician. Primary risks are for psychiatric symptoms, including suicide, however medical problems, such as seizures, and delirium, are also possible.

High-Risk Patients

Clinical experience and research data have identified four groups of patients that are at high risk for long-term use, misuse, and adverse consequences from benzodiazepines: alcoholics, drug addicts, the elderly, and patients with chronic pain.

Alcoholics

Both survey and human laboratory data suggest that alcoholics are at higher risk for benzodiazepine misuse (Ciraulo et al., 1988). In a series of studies, our laboratory found that alprazolam and diazepam produce reinforcing effects in alcoholics but not in nonalcoholic controls (Ciraulo et al., 1997; Sarid-Segal et al., 2000). There is also some evidence to suggest that nonalcoholics with a strong family history of alcoholism (Ciraulo et al., 1996, 1989) and even subjects who are moderate social drinkers experience greater reinforcing effects from benzodiazepines (Evans and Levin, 2002). These findings have raised concern about the therapeutic use of benzodiazepines in abstinent alcoholics (Posternack and Mueller, 2001). Because the cooccurrence of anxiety disorders and alcoholism is not uncommon, this is an important clinical problem (Kessler et al., 1997; Kushner et al., 1990).

The studies of Mueller and colleagues (1996, 2005) addressed the issue of benzodiazepine prescription for patients with anxiety and alcoholism. Following a cohort of subjects with anxiety and "alcohol use disorders (AUD)" over 12 years, these investigators found that prescribed benzodiazepine use remained stable (Mueller et al., 2005). Neither the dosage nor prn usage of a benzodiazepine at intake was associated with AUD onset during follow-up. Five hundred and forty-five subjects reported receiving benzodiazepines in the 12-year follow-up, and 22% ($N = 120$) of those receiving benzodiazepines developed an AUD. Benzodiazepine use did not predict AUD recovery or recurrence. As would be expected from the use of benzodiazepines to treat withdrawal symptoms, there was an increase in the likelihood of receiving a benzodiazepine at the time of AUD onset and a 2% increase in prn usage in the 26 weeks following the onset of AUD. These data strongly support the judicious use of benzodiazepines in alcoholics with anxiety disorders (Ciraulo et al., 1988, Ciraulo and Nace, 2000).

Drug Addicts

Use of benzodiazepines by patients in methadone maintenance clinics is common, ranging from 30% to 90%, with most reports around 50% for current use (Iguchi et al., 1993, Stitzer et al., 1981). The reasons for benzodiazepine use of by methadone-maintained patients (MMP) are complex, and include self-medication of emotional problems, to get high, to treat insomnia, and to suppress withdrawal symptoms (Gelkopf et al., 1999; Noble et al., 2002). Several studies have compared MMPs who take benzodiazepines to those who do not, and have found earlier onset of opioid abuse (Backmund et al., 2005), greater psychopathology (Bleich et al., 1999) and psychological distress (Darke et al., 1994), greater HIV risk-taking behaviors (Metzger et al., 1991), higher incidence of hepatitis C (Van den Hoek et al., 1990), greater criminality (Backmund et al., 2005; Bleich et al., 1999), and higher mortality (Caplehorn et al., 1996) in the group that abuses benzodiazepines.

Heroin users are known to misuse benzodiazepines (Darke, 1994; Ross et al., 1996, 1997), with about 20–25% meeting various criteria for dependence (Ross and Darke, 2000). Concomitant use of heroin and benzodiazepines is associated with a higher risk of overdose (Man et al., 2004), poorer psychosocial functioning (Darke, 1994), and higher utilization of health care services (Darke et al., 2003). Although oral administration of benzodiazepines is most common, intravenous injection is also known to occur as frequently as 13%–17% (past 6 months injection) to 48% (lifetime) of heroin users in some countries (Darke et al., 2002; Ross et al., 1997) and is accompanied by serious health risks, including vascular events.

Comparative abuse liability of the benzodiazepines in opioid dependent patients has been well studied. A consistent finding is that among the benzodiazepines, flunitrazepam is associated with the greatest risk of abuse (Barnas et al., 1992; Farre et al., 1998; Jaffe et al., 2004; Woods and Winger, 1997), although diazepam is also highly valued (Darke et al., 1995). MMPs in the United States, where flunitrazepam is not available legally, report that they use diazepam, alprazolam, and lorazepam to get high and to sell on the street, whereas chlordiazepoxide, oxazepam, and phenobarbital are less likely to be used for these purposes (Iguchi et al., 1993).

Clinical experience suggests that benzodiazepines are commonly used among individuals who abuse cocaine or other psychostimulants, although carefully designed studies have not been reported. In our experience, stimulant abusers report that they use benzodiazepines to self-medicate stimulant-induced anxiety and paranoia, and to terminate a "run." Benzodiazepines are effective anticonvulsants for cocaine-induced seizures. Animal studies have found that diazepam dose-dependently reduces anxiety from cocaine withdrawal (Paine et al., 2002). Benzodiazepines are modulators of the GABA system, and cocaine-abusing subjects demonstrated lower sensitivity to lorazepam in a positron emission tomography study, suggesting that chronic use of cocaine alters the GABA system and the response to benzodiazepines (Volkow et al., 1998). Diazepam had increased anxiolytic effect in animals that were chronically exposed to cocaine for 2 weeks and then withdrawn, although it did not affect diazepam's anticonvulsant activity (Lilly and Tietz, 2000). Alterations in the GABA-A BZD receptor occur during chronic cocaine administration and may account for behavioral toxicity and altered response to benzodiazepines (Suzuki et al., 2000).

Elderly

Long-term benzodiazepine use is common among the elderly, although they are less likely than younger patients to increase the dosage (Soumerai et al., 2003). The greatest clinical concern in the elderly is increased risk of falls (Cumming and Le Couteur, 2003; Landi et al., 2005; Schneeweiss and Wang, 2005) and cognitive impairment (Barker et al., 2004; McAndrews et al., 2000). Most studies suggest that elderly who are prescribed benzodiazepines have significant psychopathology (Petrovic et al., 2002), which appears to be the reason for the prescription, not the consequence of prolonged use (Mattila-Evenden et al., 2001). Other psychotherapeutic agents, such as antidepressants (Ensrud et al., 2003) and antipsychotics (Landi et al., 2005), are also associated with falls in the elderly, so alternative agents must be used cautiously.

It is well established that cognitive changes occur with short-term use of benzodiazepines, including attention and memory problems (Curran, 1998; Rich et al., 2005). For many patients, tolerance develops to the memory disturbance, but in some individuals it may continue to be a problem, especially among the elderly. Whether the cognitive impairment is severe enough to discontinue the benzodiazepine is a matter of clinical judgment. Most authorities do not believe that long-term benzodiazepine use results in persistent cognitive deficits after discontinuation (Salzman et al., 1992), but some studies have reported long-lasting effects (Barker et al., 2005). In our clinical experience, long-term treatment with benzodiazepines in patients with anxiety disorders does not lead to clinically significant impairment upon discontinuation.

People With Chronic Pain

Estimates of benzodiazepine use in chronic pain patients range from 40% to 60% (Fishbain et al., 1992; Hardo and Kennedy, 1991; Hendler et al., 1980; King and Strain, 1990a, 1990b; Kouyanou et al., 1997). Although they have an established role as skeletal muscle relaxants (van Tulder et al., 2003), benzodiazepines are also used as adjunctive medications to treat insomnia and anxiety (Hardo and Kennedy, 1991; Yosselson-Superstine et al., 1985) in patients with chronic pain.

In a study of 125 chronic pain patients in a London pain specialty clinic, 88% were taking medications, including 69.6% opioids, 48% nonopioids analgesics, 25% antidepressants, and 17.6% benzodiazepines (Kouyanou et al., 1997). Using *DSM-III-R* criteria, 4% were abusing benzodiazepines, 3.2% were dependent on benzodiazepines, and 4.8% used them at higher than recommended doses. The percentage taking benzodiazepines in the London clinic is lower than generally reported for patients with chronic pain (King and Strain, 1990a, 1990b), so misuse may be higher with greater drug availability. However, based on available evidence, use of benzodiazepines in chronic pain is common, but does not often lead to abuse or dependence.

Conclusion

Survey data indicate that nonmedical use of benzodiazepines by adults in the United States has increased slightly over the past few years, although use by high school students has remained stable or declined. Benzodiazepines are rarely a primary drug of abuse; they are most often misused in the context of polysubstance abuse involving opioids, alcohol, and cocaine. Long-term prescription use of benzodiazepines is associated with older age, female gender, chronic health problems, and high levels of emotional distress. Elderly patients taking benzodiazepines are at risk for falls and cognitive impairment, and should be closely monitored if these medications are prescribed. Alternative medications should be considered in the elderly, although many psychotherapeutic medications are associated with falls in the elderly. Chronic pain patients are often given benzodiazepines to treat muscle spasms, anxiety, and insomnia, and rates of misuse are low. The benzodiazepine withdrawal syndrome rarely contributes to abuse, but it may make it difficult for some long-term prescription users to discontinue use. There is widespread abuse of benzodiazepines by opioid addicts, both in and out of treatment. Several studies suggest that patients who abuse opioids and benzodiazepines have serious medical and psychological symptoms, and are at high risk for overdose. Individuals with alcohol abuse and dependence also are at high risk for benzodiazepine misuse, but recent studies suggest that when comorbid anxiety is present, judicious use of benzodiazepines may be safe and appropriate.

References

American Psychiatric Association. *Diagnostic and Statistical Manual of Mental Disorders.* 4th ed. rev. Washington, DC: American Psychiatric Association; 1994.

American Psychiatric Association Task Force on Benzodiazepine Dependence, Toxicity, and Abuse. *Benzodiazepine Dependence, Toxicity, and Abuse: A Task Force Report of the American Psychiatric Association.* Washington, DC: American Psychiatric Association; 1990.

Backmund M, Meyer K, Henkel C, et al. Co-consumption of benzodiazepines in heroin users, methadone-substituted and codeine-substituted patients. *J Addict Dis.* 24:17–29, 2005.

Balter MB, Manheimer DI, Mellinger GD, et al. A cross-national comparison of anti-anxiety/sedative drug use. *Curr Med Res Opin.* 8 Suppl 4:5–20, 1984.

Barker MJ, Greenwood KM, Jackson M, et al. Cognitive effects of long-term benzodiazepine use: a meta-analysis. *CNS Drugs.* 18:37–48, 2004.

Barker MJ, Greenwood KM, Jackson M, et al. An evaluation of persisting cognitive effects after withdrawal from long-term benzodiazepine use. *J Int Neuropsychol Soc.* 11:281–289, 2005.

Barnas C, Rossmann M, Roessler H, et al. Benzodiazepines and other psychotropic drugs abused by patients in a methadone maintenance program: familiarity and preference. *J Clin Psychopharmacol.* 12:397–402, 1992.

Blackwell B, Schmidt GL. Drug interactions in psychopharmacology. *Psychiatr Clin North Am.* 7:625–637, 1984.

Bleich A, Gelkopf M, Schmidt V, et al. Correlates of benzodiazepine abuse in methadone maintenance treatment. A 1 year prospective study in an Israeli clinic. *Addiction.* 94:1533–1540, 1999.

Caplehorn JR, Dalton MS, Haldar F, et al. Methadone maintenance and addicts' risk of fatal heroin overdose. *Subst Use Misuse.* 31:177–196, 1996.

Ciraulo AM, Alpert N, Franko KJ. Naltrexone for the treatment of alcoholism. *Am Fam Physician.* 56:803–806, 1997a.

Ciraulo DA, Barnhill JG, Ciraulo AM, et al. Parental alcoholism as a risk factor in benzodiazepine abuse: a pilot study. *Am J Psychiatry.* 146:1333–1335, 1989.

Ciraulo DA, Barnhill JG, Ciraulo AM, et al. Alterations in pharmacodynamics of anxiolytics in abstinent alcoholic men: subjective responses, abuse liability, and electroencephalographic effects of alprazolam, diazepam, and buspirone. *J Clin Pharmacol.* 37:64–73, 1997b.

Ciraulo DA, Knapp CM, LoCastro J, et al. A benzodiazepine mood effect scale: reliability and validity determined for alcohol-dependent subjects and adults with a parental history of alcoholism. *Am J Drug Alcohol Abuse.* 27:339–347, 2001.

Ciraulo DA, Nace EP. Benzodiazepine treatment of anxiety or insomnia in substance abuse patients. *Am J Addict.* 9:276–279; discussion 280–274, 2000.

Ciraulo DA, Sands BF, Shader RI. Critical review of liability for benzodiazepine abuse among alcoholics. *Am J Psychiatry.* 145:1501–1506, 1988.

Ciraulo DA, Sarid-Degal O. Sedative-, hypnotic-, or anxiolytic-related disorders (11.12). Vol. 1. In: Sadock BJ, Sadock VA, eds. *Comprehensive Textbook of Psychiatry.* 8th ed. Philadelphia: Lippincott Williams & Wilkins; 2005.

Ciraulo DA, Sarid-Segal O, Knapp C, et al. Liability to alprazolam abuse in daughters of alcoholics. *Am J Psychiatry.* 153:956–958, 1996.

Cumming RG, Le Couteur DG. Benzodiazepines and risk of hip fractures in older people: a review of the evidence. *CNS Drugs.* 17:825–837, 2003.

Curran HV, Pooviboonsuk P, Dalton JA, Lader MH. Differentiating the effects of centrally acting drugs on arousal and memory: an event-related potential study of scopolamine, lorazepam and diphenhydramine. *Psychopharmacology.* 135:27–36, 1998.

Darke S. Benzodiazepine use among injecting drug users: problems and implications. *Addiction.* 89:379–382, 1994.

Darke S, Topp L, Ross J. The injection of methadone and benzodiazepines among Sydney injecting drug users 1996–2000: 5-year monitoring of trends from the Illicit Drug Reporting System. *Drug Alcohol Rev.* 21:27–32, 2002.

Darke S, Ross J, Teesson M, et al. Health service utilization and benzodiazepine use among heroin users: findings from the Australian Treatment Outcome Study (ATOS). *Addiction.* 98:1129–1135, 2003.

Darke SG, Ross JE, Hall WD. Benzodiazepine use among injecting heroin users. *Med J Aust.* 162:645–647, 1995.

Ensrud KE, Blackwell T, Mangione CM, et al. Central nervous system active medications and risk for fractures in older women. *Arch Intern Med.* 163:949–957, 2003.

Evans SM, Levin FR. The effects of alprazolam and buspirone in light and moderate female social drinkers. *Behav Pharmacol.* 13:427–439, 2002.

Farre M, Teran MT, Roset PN, et al. Abuse liability of flunitrazepam among methadone-maintained patients. *Psychopharmacology* (Berl). 140:486–495, 1998.

Fishbain DA, Rosomoff HL, Rosomoff RS. Drug abuse, dependence, and addiction in chronic pain patients. *Clin J Pain.* 8:77–85, 1992.

Gelkopf M, Bleich A, Hayward R, et al. Characteristics of benzodiazepine abuse in methadone maintenance treatment patients: a 1 year prospective study in an Israeli clinic. *Drug Alcohol Depend.* 55:63–68, 1999.

Griffiths RR, Ator NA. Benzodiazepine self-administration in animals and humans: a comprehensive literature review. *NIDA Res Monogr.* 33:22–36, 1980.

Griffiths RR, Ator NA, Lukas SE, et al. Benzodiazepines: drug discrimination and physiological dependence. *NIDA Res Monogr.* 49:163–164, 1984.

Griffiths RR, Weerts EM. Benzodiazepine self-administration in humans and laboratory animals—implications for problems of long-term use and abuse. *Psychopharmacology* (Berl). 134:1–37, 1997.

Griffiths RR, Wolf B. Relative abuse liability of different benzodiazepines in drug abusers. *J Clin Psychopharmacol.* 10:237–243, 1990.

Hardo PG, Kennedy TD. Night sedation and arthritic pain. *J R Soc Med.* 84:73–75, 1991.

Hendler N, Cimini C, Ma T, et al. A comparison of cognitive impairment due to benzodiazepines and to narcotics. *Am J Psychiatry.* 137:828–830, 1980.

Hollister LE, Motzenbecker FP, Degan RO. Withdrawal reactions from chlordiazepoxide ("Librium"). *Psychopharmacologia.* 2:63–68, 1961.

Iguchi MY, Handelsman L, Bickel WK, et al. Benzodiazepine and sedative use/abuse by methadone maintenance clients. *Drug Alcohol Depend.* 32:257–266, 1993.

Jaffe JH, Bloor R, Crome I, et al. A postmarketing study of relative abuse liability of hypnotic sedative drugs. *Addiction.* 99:165–173, 2004.

Jaffe JH, Ciraulo DA, Nies A, et al. Abuse potential of halazepam and of diazepam in patients recently treated for acute alcohol withdrawal. *Clin Pharmacol Ther.* 34:623–630, 1983.

Jerling M, Bertilsson L, Sjoqvist F. The use of therapeutic drug monitoring data to document kinetic drug interactions: an example with amitriptyline and nortriptyline. *Ther Drug Monit.* 16:1–12, 1994a.

Jerling M, Lindstrom L, Bondesson U, et al. Fluvoxamine inhibition and carbamazepine induction of the metabolism of clozapine: evidence from a therapeutic drug monitoring service. *Ther Drug Monit.* 16:368–374, 1994b.

Johnston LD, O'Malley PM, Bachman JG, et al. *Monitoring the Future: National Survey Results on Adolescent Drug Use: Overview of Key Findings, 2004* (NIH Publication No. 05-5726). Bethesda, MD: National Institute on Drug Abuse, 2005.

Kessler RC, Crum RM, Warner LA, et al. Lifetime co-occurrence of DSM-III-R alcohol abuse and dependence with other psychiatric disorders in the National Comorbidity Survey. *Arch Gen Psychiatry.* 54:313–321, 1997.

King SA, Strain JJ. Benzodiazepine use by chronic pain patients. *Clin J Pain.* 6:143–147, 1990a.

King SA, Strain JJ. Benzodiazepines and chronic pain. *Pain.* 41:3–4, 1990b.

Kouyanou K, Pither CE, Wessely S. Medication misuse, abuse and dependence in chronic pain patients. *J Psychosom Res.* 43:497–504, 1997.

Kushner MG, Sher KJ, Beitman BD. The relation between alcohol problems and the anxiety disorders. *Am J Psychiatry.* 147:685–695, 1990.

Lamberg TS, Kivisto KT, Laitila J, et al. The effect of fluvoxamine on the pharmacokinetics and pharmacodynamics of buspirone. *Eur J Clin Pharmacol.* 54:761–766, 1998.

Landi F, Onder G, Cesari M, et al. Psychotropic medications and risk for falls among community-dwelling frail older people: an observational study. *J Gerontol A Biol Sci Med Sci.* 60:622–626, 2005.

Lilly SM, Tietz EI. Chronic cocaine differentially affects diazepam's anxiolytic and anticonvulsant actions. Relationship to GABA(A) receptor subunit expression. *Brain Res.* 882:139–148, 2000.

Man LH, Best D, Gossop M, et al. Relationship between prescribing and risk of opiate overdose among drug users in and out of maintenance treatment. *Eur Addict Res.* 10:35–40, 2004.

Mattila-Evenden M, Bergman U, Franck J. A study of benzodiazepine users claiming drug-induced psychiatric morbidity. *Nord J Psychiatry.* 55:271–278, 2001.

McAndrews MP, Kayumov L, Phillipson R, Shapiro CM. Self-report of memory and affective dysfunction in association with medication use in a sample of individuals with chronic sleep disturbance. *Hum Psychopharmacol.* 15:583–587, 2000.

McBride WJ, Murphy JM, Lumeng L, et al. Effects of Ro 15-4513, fluoxetine and desipramine on the intake of ethanol, water and food by the alcohol-preferring (P) and -nonpreferring (NP) lines of rats. *Pharmacol Biochem Behav.* 30:1045–1050, 1988.

Meert TF. Effects of various serotonergic agents on alcohol intake and alcohol preference in Wistar rats selected at two different levels of alcohol preference. *Alcohol Alcohol.* 28:157–170, 1993.

Metzger DS, Woody GE, Druley P, et al. Psychiatric symptoms, high risk behaviors and HIV positivity among methadone patients. *NIDA Res Monogr.* 105:490–491, 1991.

Miller LG, Greenblatt DJ, Roy RB, et al. Chronic benzodiazepine administration. II. Discontinuation syndrome is associated with upregulation of gamma-aminobutyric acidA receptor complex binding and function. *J Pharmacol Exp Ther.* 246:177–182, 1988.

Mintzer MZ, Griffiths RR. An abuse liability comparison of flunitrazepam and triazolam in sedative drug abusers. *Behav Pharmacol.* 16:579–584, 2005.

Mueller TI, Goldenberg IM, Gordon AL, et al. Benzodiazepine use in anxiety disordered patients with and without a history of alcoholism. *J Clin Psychiatry.* 57:83–89, 1996.

Mueller TI, Pagano ME, Rodriguez BF, et al. Long-term use of benzodiazepines in participants with comorbid anxiety and alcohol use disorders. *Alcohol Clin Exp Res.* 29:1411–1418, 2005.

Noble A, Best D, Man LH, et al. Self-detoxification attempts among methadone maintenance patients: what methods and what success? *Addict Behav.* 27:575–584, 2002.

Paine TA, Jackman SL, Olmstead MC. Cocaine-induced anxiety: alleviation by diazepam, but not buspirone, dimenhydrinate or diphenhydramine. *Behav Pharmacol.* 13:511–523, 2002.

Petrovic M, Pevernagie D, Mariman A, et al. Fast withdrawal from benzodiazepines in geriatric inpatients: a randomised double-blind, placebo-controlled trial. *Eur J Clin Pharmacol.* 57:759–764, 2002.

Posternak MA, Mueller TI. Assessing the risks and benefits of benzodiazepines for anxiety disorders in patients with a history of substance abuse or dependence. *Am J Addict.* 10:48–68, 2001.

Rich JB, Svoboda E, Brown GG. Diazepam-induced prospective memory impairment and its relation to retrospective memory, attention, and arousal. *Hum Psychopharmacol.* 21:101–108, 2005.

Roehrs T, Bonahoom A, Pedrosi B, et al. Treatment regimen and hypnotic self-administration. *Psychopharmacology* (Berl). 155:11–17, 2001.

Ross J, Darke S. The nature of benzodiazepine dependence among heroin users in Sydney, Australia. *Addiction.* 95:1785–1793, 2000.

Ross J, Darke S, Hall W. Benzodiazepine use among heroin users in Sydney: patterns of use, availability and procurement. *Drug Alcohol Rev.* 15:237–243, 1996.

Ross J, Darke S, Hall W. Transitions between routes of benzodiazepine administration among heroin users in Sydney. *Addiction.* 92:697–705, 1997.

Salzman C. Monoamine oxidase inhibitors and atypical antidepressants. *Clin Geriatr Med.* 8:335–348, 1992.

Sarid-Segal O, Knapp CM, Ciraulo AM, et al. Decreased EEG sensitivity to alprazolam in subjects with a parental history of alcoholism. *J Clin Pharmacol.* 40:84–90, 2000.

Schneeweiss S, Wang PS. Claims data studies of sedative-hypnotics and hip fractures in older people: exploring residual confounding using survey information. *J Am Geriatr Soc.* 53:948–954, 2005.

Silverman G, Braithwaite R. Interaction of benzodiazepines with tricyclic antidepressants. *Br Med J.* 4:111, 1972.

Soumerai SB, Simoni-Wastila L, Singer C, et al. Lack of relationship between long-term use of benzodiazepines and escalation to high dosages. *Psychiatr Serv.* 54:1006–1011, 2003.

Stitzer ML, Griffiths RR, McLellan AT, et al. Diazepam use among methadone maintenance patients: patterns and dosages. *Drug Alcohol Depend.* 8:189–199, 1981.

Substance Abuse and Mental Health Services Administration, Office of Applied Studies. *Drug Abuse Warning Network, 2003: Interim National Estimates of Drug-Related Emergency Department Visits.* DAWN Series D-26, DHHS Publication No. (SMA) 04-3972. Rockville, MD, 2004.

Substance Abuse and Mental Health Services Administration, Office of Applied Studies. *Treatment Episode Data Set (TEDS): 1993–2003. National Admissions to Substance Abuse Treatment Services,* DASIS Series: S-29, DHHS Publication No. (SMA) 05-4118, Rockville, MD, 2005.

Suzuki T, Abe S, Yamaguchi M, et al. Effects of cocaine administration on receptor binding and subunits mRNA of GABA(A)-benzodiazepine receptor complexes. *Synapse.* 38:198–215, 2000.

van den Hoek JA, van Haastrecht HJ, Goudsmit J, de Wolf F, Coutinho RA. Prevalence, incidence, and risk factors of hepatitis C virus infection among drug users in Amsterdam. *J Infect Dis*. 162:823–826, 1990.

van Tulder MW, Touray T, Furlan AD, et al. Muscle relaxants for nonspecific low back pain: a systematic review within the framework of the cochrane collaboration. *Spine*. 28:1978–1992, 2003.

Volkow ND, Wang GJ, Fowler JS, et al. Enhanced sensitivity to benzodiazepines in active cocaine-abusing subjects: a PET study. *Am J Psychiatry*. 155:200–206, 1998.

von Moltke LL, Greenblatt DJ, Schmider J, et al. Midazolam hydroxylation by human liver microsomes in vitro: inhibition by fluoxetine, norfluoxetine, and by azole antifungal agents. *J Clin Pharmacol*. 36:783–791, 1996.

Weller RA, Preskorn SH. Psychotropic drugs and alcohol: pharmacokinetic and pharmacodynamic interactions. *Psychosomatics*. 25:301–303, 305–306, 309, 1984.

Woods JH, Winger G. Current benzodiazepine issues. *Psychopharmacology*. 118:107–115, 1995.

Woods JH, Winger G. Abuse liability of flunitrazepam. *J Clin Psychopharmacol*. 17:1S-57S, 1997.

Woods JH, Winger G, France CP. Use of in vivo apparent pA2 analysis in assessment of opioid abuse liability. *Trends Pharmacol Sci*. 13:282–286, 1992.

Yosselson-Superstine S, Lipman AG, Sanders SH. Adjunctive antianxiety agents in the management of chronic pain. *Isr J Med Sci*. 21:113–117, 1985.

20

Treating Cocaine Dependence

Tracy A. Steen

Charles A. Dackis

Cocaine dependence is a complex disorder with powerful psychological, behavioral, and biological underpinnings. Often viewed as more of a choice than an illness, cocaine dependence is not treated or insured on parity with more traditional medical disorders, despite compelling scientific evidence supporting a *disease concept* based on brain involvement, genetic vulnerability, and a progressive clinical course (Dackis and O'Brien 2005a). Arguably the most addictive of all substances, cocaine is self-administered until death by laboratory animals and produces intense euphoria in humans. The pleasure-reinforced compulsion to use cocaine progresses into addiction with astounding rapidity, leading to alterations in neurochemistry (Dackis and O'Brien, 2005b), plasticity (Thomas, Beurrier, et al. 2001), gene expression (Nestler, 2004), and even brain cell morphology (Robinson and Kolb 2004) in pleasure centers that have evolved to ensure survival by dominating our thoughts, behaviors, and priorities (Dackis and O'Brien, 2001).

Discrete clinical components of cocaine dependence are interwoven into a cycle of addiction that is driven by *euphoria* and *craving* (see Figure 20.1). Addicted patients are typically willing to risk medical complications, family turmoil, financial ruin, imprisonment, and even death for cocaine, but are shielded from these hazards by *denial*, which can be remarkably resilient to logical interventions. Denial and *loss of control*, once thought to be purely psychological, may actually stem in part from disruptions in the prefrontal cortex (PFC) that are increasingly viewed as a core component of cocaine dependence (Dackis and O'Brien, 2005b). Cocaine also produces *withdrawal* symptoms (see Table 20.1) that predict poor clinical outcome (Kampman, Alterman, et al. 2001), despite their brevity, and may identify patients with persistent *hedonic dysregulation*. Neuronal mechanisms that underlie these clinical components are guiding medication development that may dramatically improve the prognosis of cocaine dependence (Dackis and O'Brien, 2005b; Kalivas, 2004; Koob, Ahmed, et al., 2004). However, psychological interventions that engage, motivate, and guide patients into recovery are and will likely remain the mainstay of treatment. This chapter discusses treatment approaches to cocaine-addicted patients that are based on established recovery principles and brain reward function.

Figure 20.1. The clinical components of cocaine dependence drive a cycle of addiction that becomes progressively entrenched and controllable. Pharmacological treatments that effectively target these clinical phenomena should improve treatment outcome.

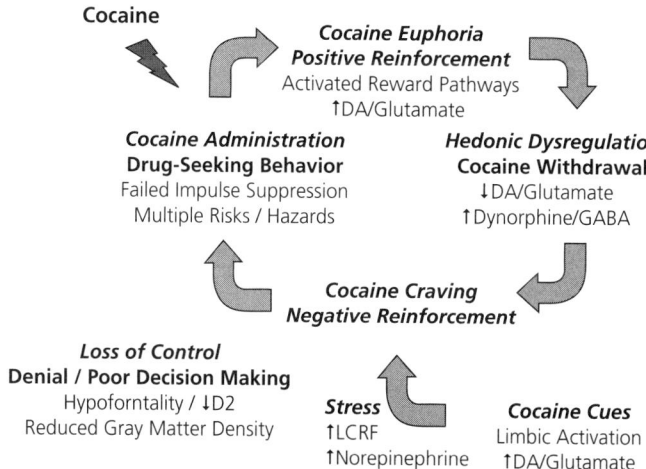

Table 20.1. Clinical Manifestations of Cocaine Intoxication and Cocaine Withdrawal

Cocaine Intoxication	Cocaine Withdrawal
Euphoria	Depression
Increased energy	Anergia
Anorexia	Hyperphagia
Sexual arousal	Reduced sex drive
Racing thoughts	Slowed thoughts
Alertness	Hypersomnia
Grandiosity	Low self-esteem
Hyperactivity	Psychomotor retardation
Vigilance	Poor concentration
Tachycardia	Bradycardia
Diaphoresis	Impotence
Elevated body temperature	
Mydriasis	

Evaluation and Engagement

Cocaine dependence treatment begins with an evaluation of functional impairment, drug use patterns, motivation, and a host of medical and psychiatric complications that are reviewed elsewhere (Dackis and Gold, 1992). A comprehensive evaluation strengthens the therapeutic alliance and can be performed effectively with a multidisciplinary approach that collects pertinent information with or without structured interviews such as the Addiction Severity Index (ASI; McLellan, Luborsky, et al., 1980). It is naïve to assume that cocaine-addicted patients will always provide accurate accounts, and collateral information should be sought from the family, referral sources, past medical records, and laboratory testing. Family members are especially helpful early in the evaluation process when they can relate information about patient strengths as well as external motivating factors for recovery (e.g., "You can't live here if you aren't in treatment"). Inconsistencies in information collected from the various sources are discussed with patients for clarification and assessment of veracity. If a patient has not been wholly truthful, dishonesty is nonjudgmentally framed as addictive behavior, and honesty is discussed as an essential ingredient of recovery.

Patients and families often have unrealistic expectations about addiction treatment and benefit from education during the evaluation period. Cocaine dependence should be described as a chronic, relapsing disease that can be overcome (but not cured) if patients are willing to work hard, make necessary lifestyle changes, and follow treatment recommendations. Discussing the biological basis of cocaine dependence promotes the disease concept, alleviates guilt, and explains why quitting is so difficult.

The patient's insight, openness, and readiness for change are carefully assessed during the evaluation to ensure that the treatment approach is appropriate for their stage of recovery. Patients with massive denial require different interventions from those with insight and determination, and outcome is greatly influenced by the patient's attitude toward recovery. Motivation enhancement techniques have been developed to gauge and enhance commitment to recovery, confidence in success, and readiness to change (Miller and Rollnick, 2002), and some patients are not ready for treatment. Those who are ready receive a comprehensive treatment plan that may include individual, family, and/or group therapy (including self-help groups) as dictated by the clinical situation. Patients often want to negotiate treatment goals they are not yet ready to accept, such as avoiding alcohol, leaving friendships with active users, and attending self-help groups. This dialogue should be encouraged because voiced disagreement is preferable to feigned compliance, and areas of resistance can be identified that will be revisited during ongoing treatment.

Psychological Treatment

A strong therapeutic alliance is essential to maximize retention and form the foundation for future work, but establishing rapport with addicted patients requires balance and sophistication. Confrontational approaches tend to alienate patients, whereas an overly conciliatory stance can undermine the integrity of treatment, which should unambiguously emphasize recovery principles. Helping patients identify and use their personal strengths promotes the therapeutic alliance, whereas an exclusive focus on weaknesses can be demoralizing. Rapport is also established by building self-esteem and confidence in patients through genuine respect, acceptance, and optimism about treatment efficacy.

Initiating Abstinence

Initial attempts at abstinence pit patients against the powerful cycle of euphoria and craving when they are most likely to deny their loss of control, the consequences of their addiction, and the work required to achieve recovery. Early therapeutic interventions counter denial by mobilizing emotions (fear, sadness, guilt, anger) associated with loss of control and the consequences of addiction. Group therapy is an effective means of reducing denial as exposure to other recovering peers provides acceptance, support, and insight into an illness that affects individuals in remarkably similar ways. Denial can also be slowly "chipped away" during individual and family psychotherapy, and its persistence might reflect cocaine-induced cortical dysfunction (Dackis and O'Brien, 2005b).

Cocaine dependence is a disease from which patients may not want to recover, and their attitude toward treatment must be part of the treatment dialogue because it governs clinical outcome. Attitude fluctuates throughout treatment—usually worsening *before* relapse with negativity, cynicism, and reluctance to follow a treatment plan—and these changes provide a useful barometer to perceptive clinicians.

Managing the Lure of Cocaine Euphoria

Even though cocaine euphoria lasts only a few minutes, it becomes indelibly embedded in the memory of addicted patients and should never be underestimated in the clinical setting. Intravenous and intrapulmonary routes of administration produce a particularly intense "rush" of euphoria associated with racing thoughts, bursts of energy, wakefulness, elevated self-esteem, psychomotor activation, gregariousness, and sexual arousal (see Table 20.1). Spontaneous orgasm has been reported by cocaine users (Dackis and Gold, 1985), and there is evidence that cocaine specifically activates sexual reward pathways in the brain (Dackis, 2004). Cocaine euphoria is rapidly replaced by dysphoria and enhanced craving (Jaffe, Cascella, et al., 1989) that amplify the appeal of subsequent doses, as evidenced by the fact that patients with negative baseline mood experience enhanced cocaine euphoria under controlled conditions (Sofuoglu, Brown, et al., 2001). Intensified euphoria combined with heightened craving drives cocaine binges that consume whatever supply is available or attainable, often through desperate behaviors that later engender guilt and shame.

Psychotherapeutic interventions strive to reduce the appeal of cocaine euphoria by linking the pleasure with addiction-related suffering. Its appeal can also be diminished when patients discuss the intense pleasure they derive from cocaine, realize it is irreplaceable, and grieve the loss. This exercise paradoxically increases insight because when patients acknowledge how they miss cocaine euphoria, they often recall specific areas of misery that were clouded by denial.

Emphasizing the Importance of Complete Abstinence

Complete abstinence is the most fundamental goal of treatment, but quitting cocaine is an intimidating objective that is best viewed as a daily goal. Focusing on the difficulty of protracted abstinence can be discouraging ("I will never be able to stop forever so I might as well use now") and should be avoided. Some patients merely want to reduce their intake, but confrontation is seldom effective with these individuals and usually evokes a defensive response that damages the therapeutic alliance. Patients unwilling to accept the need for complete abstinence are best swayed in group therapy, or by paradoxical interventions that simply ask them to give examples of their ability to control the drug. Even patients fully committed to abstinence have difficulty attaining the goal and often underreport their use (Dackis, Kampman, et al., 2005a), necessitating random urine monitoring as a care standard. Patients who cannot quit are encouraged to develop specific abstinence strategies by examining events that preceded their cocaine use. For instance, patients may give themselves permission to use cocaine under certain conditions or recklessly place themselves in situations in which they are inundated with cocaine cues.

Complete abstinence also involves avoiding other addictive substances (e.g., opioids, sedatives, other stimulants, alcohol) that trigger cocaine use or produce concomitant addiction. Patients reluctant to abstain from alcohol can be persuaded after successive cocaine relapses triggered by drinking, especially when predicted by their clinician. The alcohol issue is complicated by the fact that a large number (estimated at 30%–60%) of cocaine dependent patients are also alcoholic (Carroll, Rounsaville, et al. 1993; Heil, Badger, et al., 2001; Higgins, Budney, et al., 1994) and more difficult to treat (Brady, Sonne, et al. 1995), largely because using either substance leads to the other. Patients should know that combining alcohol with cocaine forms cocaethylene, an active metabolite that is associated with significant toxicity (McCance-Katz, Kosten, et al., 1998). Cocaethylene is not only cardiotoxic (Wilson and French, 2002) and more lethal than cocaine (Katz, Terry, et al., 1992), but also 18–25 times more likely to cause sudden death (Andrews, 1997).

Craving Reduction Strategies

Four discrete categories of cocaine craving are analogous to craving for food and sex, illustrating how natural reward function demarcates the clinical manifestations of cocaine dependence. *Baseline craving* can be compared to hunger between meals, whereas *cue-induced craving* is comparable to that recruited by food cues. *Cocaine induced craving* resembles heightened hunger upon eating (try to eat only one potato chip), and *stress-induced craving* is analogous to relieving anxiety with food. Similar analogies exist with sexual desire, which may be even more pertinent because cocaine activates and dysregulates sexual reward pathways (Dackis, 2004). Table 20.2 lists these craving subtypes and proposed neurotransmitter mechanisms, based on current understanding, that identify potential pharmacological treatments for these clinical phenomena.

Psychotherapeutic approaches to craving focus on its identification, avoidance, and reduction. Craving often comes disguised as irritability, boredom, cynicism, or even an impulse to go where cocaine is more available, and unidentified craving is a stealth attack on recovery that should be suspected whenever negative mood states are present. Therapeutic approaches to cue-induced craving emphasize avoidance strategies. Patients first list specific cues that they find most salient and compelling, which often include cash, paraphernalia, active users, and even certain neighborhoods where the drug is available. Strategies are then established to avoid cue exposure by changing habits, routine, and lifestyle. Avoiding cues often requires considerable sacrifice, insight, and resolve, and families should understand and reinforce this cardinal strategy of recovery. Education regarding the biological basis of cue-induced craving (reviewed below) can enhance motivation and promote the disease concept (Dackis and O'Brien, 2005b), providing additional impetus when avoidance is inconvenient (avoiding a bar), time consuming (attending a meeting), or heartbreaking (leaving a spouse).

Patients should be informed that craving is time-limited, does not continue to intensify until satisfied, and can be overcome with specific strategies. Among the most powerful anticraving strategies is simply to talk about cravings at self-help group meetings. Another is distraction, which might involve patients spending a designated number of minutes in an active diversion before submitting to an urge, such as calling a friend, exercising, performing a chore, or even eating a sandwich. Visualization techniques can focus on risky or shameful behaviors associated with using cocaine binges,

Table 20.2. Four Distinct Categories of Cocaine Craving in the Clinical Setting

Baseline Craving	Cocaine-Induced Craving	Cue-Induced Craving	Stress-Induced Craving
Clinical Description			
Craving after cocaine abstinence	↑Craving after a dose of cocaine	Craving when exposed to cocaine cues	Craving during stress
Animal Model			
Cocaine self-administration	Cocaine-induced reinstatement	Cue-induced reinstatement	Stress-induced reinstatement
Proposed Neuronal Mechanism			
↓DA/glutamate↑GABA	↓Baseline levels of glutamate	↑DA↑Glutamate	↑CRF↑Norepinephrine
Food Analogy			
Baseline hunger	↑Hunger upon eating	↑Hunger in response to food cues	↑Hunger in response to stress
Sex Analogy			
Baseline sex drive	↑Sex drive upon sexual activity	↑Sex drive from sex-related cues	↑Sex drive in response to stress
Medication Strategy			
↑DA/glutamate or ↓GABA	↑Glutamate	↓DA↓Glutamate	↓CRF↓Norepinephrine

These four categories have close analogies with the natural rewards of food and sex, illustrating how the effects of cocaine on pleasure centers impact the clinical manifestations of cocaine dependence.

or miserable feelings experienced in the aftermath of cocaine binges. These and other methods of dispelling craving are effective tools of recovery that patients should learn and practice on a daily basis during early recovery.

Relapse Prevention

Once abstinence has been initiated, treatment focus shifts to relapse prevention that continues interventions discussed above (e.g., avoiding cues and stress, utilizing craving reduction strategies) while also addressing life problems associated with early recovery. Patients may enjoy a physical and mental boost during the initial weeks of abstinence, but most experience a subsequent slump as they realize their predicament. Sadness commonly results from contemplating the years of missed opportunities during active addiction, as well as the accumulation of interpersonal, financial, and professional problems. Depression, boredom, and reduced enjoyment of daily activities might also reflect hedonic dysregulation produced by cocaine's long-term effects on brain pleasure centers (Dackis, 2005). Patients must learn new coping mechanisms to replace cocaine, and find satisfying substitutes for exciting aspects of the addicted lifestyle. In this phase of recovery it is critical to help patients explore new ways of building pleasure, engagement, and meaning in their lives. Developing interpersonal relationships, exercising, and seeking new interests or hobbies are encouraged after assessing individual strengths and interests.

Although patients should take responsibility for their addiction, it is important that clinicians dissipate guilt by linking shameful behaviors to the disease process, especially because guilty patients often seek relief by using cocaine ("I am a bad person so I might as well get high"). Group therapy is especially useful in this regard because patients view their own past with more compassion when they realize that other addicted individuals have been similarly affected. Patients can also benefit by writing themselves explicit letters of forgiveness. Therapeutic approaches that reduce guilt promote recovery, self-esteem, and the development of meaningful relationships.

Family therapy helps patients rebuild relationships that have been damaged by a disease that invariably affects the entire support system. Education, open communication, *and* abstinence will usually restore damaged relationships, although patients often complain that significant others are slow to believe and trust them. Such is reality, and patients can be reminded of their manipulations during active addiction. Family members are encouraged to vent their feelings during therapy but ultimately accept that the disease, not the patient, is the root of the problems. Family therapy is particularly indicated when compensatory familial behavioral patterns (e.g., providing money, shelter, excuses) enable active addiction. Addiction seldom occurs in a vacuum, and dysfunctional family patterns must often be changed if treatment is to be successful.

Recovering patients frequently associate happiness with pleasure and benefit from a broader conceptualization of the term (Duckworth, Steen, et al., 2005; Seligman, Steen, et al., 2005). Patients can build happiness into their lives by identifying and using their personal strengths in novel ways (Peterson and Seligman, 2004). Strengths inventories such as the Values in Action Inventory of Strengths (http://www.viasurvey.org) provide concrete feedback about individual character strengths (e.g., courage, perseverance, honesty, creativity, curiosity) that can be recruited to support recovery. Building a sense of purpose and meaning in life by connecting to spiritual or religious faith, relationships, or institutions can also increase happiness and resilience (Haidt, 2005). In addition, patients can be encouraged to pursue activities that create engagement or flow—a sense of time stopping and complete absorption in the present moment—as a satisfying alternative to pleasure (Csikszentmihalyi, Sami, et al., 2005).

Neuronal Mechanisms and Pharmacological Treatments

Despite considerable research over the past 2 decades, there are still no approved medications for cocaine dependence. However, advances in cocaine neurobiology are guiding medication development (see Figure 20.1), and several promising agents are under intense investigation. Pharmacological treatments that target the clinical components of cocaine dependence, when combined with psychotherapeutic approaches, have tremendous potential to improve clinical outcome.

Blocking Cocaine Euphoria

Blocking euphoria is an established pharmacological strategy that follows from an understanding of associated neuronal mechanisms. Cocaine elevates dopamine (DA) levels by blocking the DA transporter (DAT), and its rewarding effect is associated with increased DA neurotransmission in the nucleus accumbens (NAc), PFC, and other reward-related regions (Koob, Ahmed, et al., 2004; Wise, 2004). Human PET studies demonstrate that euphoria is determined by the extent and rate by which cocaine enters the brain and binds the DAT (Volkow, Fowler, et al., 2004), explaining why rapid routes of administration (smoking, injecting) produce more euphoria and, hence, more addiction (Hatsukami and Fischman, 1996). However, cocaine euphoria is not produced by DA receptor agonists (e.g., bromocriptine, pergolide) or blocked by DA antagonists (Dackis, 2004), and the drug is readily self-administered by DAT knockout mice (Rocha, 2003). Therefore, cocaine euphoria cannot be ascribed solely to DA neurotransmission, and several lines of evidence support an important role for glutamate in this critical phenomenon (Dackis and O'Brien, 2003). Indeed, glutamate is probably more important because mGluR5 knockout mice will not self-administer the cocaine, despite elevated DA levels in the NAc (Chiamulera, Epping-Jordan, et al., 2001).

Constitutional, environmental, and psychological factors can dramatically affect the intensity of cocaine euphoria. Normal subjects with low DA D2 receptor availability on PET (↓D2) experience more euphoria from stimulants than subjects with normal D2 availability (Volkow, Fowler, et al., 2004), and it is not surprising that ↓D2 has been demonstrated in cocaine-addicted patients (Martinez, Broft, et al., 2004; Volkow, Fowler, et al., 2004). Cocaine itself can affect D2 availability, since nonhuman primates develop ↓D2 (and increased cocaine intake) when chronically exposed to cocaine (Czoty, Morgan, et al., 2004). Interestingly, these primates also develop ↓D2 after their social rank has been demoted. Also, dysphoric patients report enhanced cocaine-induced euphoria under controlled conditions (Newton, Kalechstein, et al., 2003; Sofuoglu, Brown, et al., 2001; Sofuoglu, Dudish-Poulsen, et al., 2003). These findings suggest that the patient's genetic, psychological, and social state influence the development and perpetuation of cocaine dependence.

Medications that block cocaine euphoria would weaken the addiction cycle and promote recovery. One approach under current investigation is a vaccine that blocks euphoria by slowing the movement of cocaine across the blood/brain barrier (Haney and Kosten, 2004). Despite its association with DA and glutamate neurotransmission, cocaine euphoria is not convincingly blocked by DA or glutamate receptor antagonists (Dackis, 2004), or by γ-amino butyric acid (GABA) agonists that suppress DA/glutamate activity (Lile, Stoops, et al., 2004). In fact, the N-methyl-D-aspartate (NMDA) receptor antagonist, memantine, actually amplifies cocaine euphoria (Collins, Ward, et al., 1998). Furthermore, modafinil (a glutamate-enhancing agent) paradoxically blocked cocaine euphoria in two controlled studies (Dackis, Lynch, et al., 2003; Malcolm, Donovan, et al., 2002) and an open-label outpatient trial (Dackis and O'Brien, 2003).

Craving Reduction Strategies

Human neuroimaging studies and animal models of craving have begun to delineate its underlying neuronal mechanisms and guide the development of anticraving medications. Reinstatement paradigms represent reliable animal models of craving that first train animals to self-administer cocaine and subsequently extinguish self-administration behaviors (lever pressing) by replacing cocaine with saline. Lever pressing can then be reinstated with small doses of cocaine, exposure to cocaine-paired cues, or stress. Medications that block the reinstatement of cocaine-seeking behaviors are candidates to alleviate craving and prevent relapse produced by cues, stress, or cocaine itself.

Cue-induced craving often leads directly to relapse, even after long periods of abstinence, and an effective pharmacotherapy would constitute a major clinical breakthrough. In recent years, a large number of PET and functional magnetic resonance imaging (fMRI) studies of cocaine-dependent patients have consistently demonstrated robust hypermetabolic responses in glutamate-rich regions (e.g., amygdala, orbitofrontal cortex, anterior cingulate cortex) during cue-induced craving (Dackis and O'Brien, 2003; Volkow, Fowler, et al., 2004). These studies firmly establish a neuronal basis of cue-induced craving that stems from hijacked survival-related signaling. It is remarkable that cocaine cues and sexually explicit videos activate overlapping brain regions, reiterating how sexual pleasure centers are subsumed by cocaine addiction (Garavan, Pankiewicz, et al., 2000). It is also interesting that PFC regions that are hypermetabolic during cue-induced craving are hypometabolic at baseline, resulting in a large signal change (Δ metabolism) that might form the neuronal basis of cue *salience* (Dackis, 2004).

Animal models of cue-induced craving link the phenomenon to increased DA and glutamate neurotransmission in the basolateral amygdala, PFC, and NAc (Kalivas and McFarland, 2003), suggesting therapeutic roles for agents that reduce DA/glutamate activity. Cue-induced reinstatement is specifically reduced by GABA agonists (McFarland, Lapish, et al., 2003), agents that block glutamate at the amino-3-hydroxy-5-methyl-4-isoxazole propionate (AMPA) receptor (Di Ciano and Everitt, 2001), and selective DA D1 antagonists. Baclofen, a $GABA_B$ agonist, reduced cue-induced limbic activation and craving in a small pilot study (Brebner, Childress, et al., 2002) and promoted abstinence in a controlled outpatient trial ($n = 35$; 60 mg/day; Shoptaw, Yang, et al., 2003). Likewise, the AMPA antagonist topiramate ($n = 40$; 200 mg/day) promoted abstinence in a controlled outpatient trial (Kampman, Pettinati, et al., 2004). Neuroimaging studies are clearly needed to determine whether these medications reverse cue-induced limbic activation, and to screen other candidate medications to treat cue-induced craving.

Addicted patients typically use cocaine to deal with life stress and are persistently vulnerable to stress-induced craving during recovery attempts. Animal models of stress-induced craving implicate corticotropin-releasing factor (CRF) neurons that project from the central nucleus of the amygdala to the bed of the stria terminalis (BNST; Kalivas, McFarland, et al., 2003). Also implicated are noradrenergic neurons projecting to the BNST and the central amygdala (Kalivas, McFarland, et al., 2003), suggesting therapeutic roles for CRF and noradrenergic antagonists, and possibly explaining why propranolol (a β-adrenergic antagonist) promoted abstinence in a subgroup of cocaine-dependent patients (Kampman, Volpicelli, et al., 2001). Some individuals might be especially vulnerable to stress-induced craving, and more likely to benefit from pharmacotherapy that specifically targets this phenomenon.

A single dose of cocaine produces intense craving that fuels uncontrollable binges, hazardous behaviors, and medical risks. Medications that dampen cocaine-induced craving would reduce drug exposure and weaken the addiction cycle, making full relapse less likely after a cocaine slip. Animal studies demonstrate that N-acetyl-cysteine abolishes cocaine-induced reinstatement by normalizing levels of glutamate that have become depleted by chronic cocaine exposure (Kalivas, 2004). These findings suggest a role for other glutamate-enhancing agents like modafinil, which promoted cocaine abstinence in a recent controlled study ($n = 62$; 400 mg/day).

It has long been hypothesized that baseline cocaine craving is associated with DA dysregulation in reward pathways (Dackis and Gold, 1985), and the extensive evidence supporting DA hypoactivity after chronic cocaine exposure has been recently reviewed (Dackis, 2005; Dackis and O'Brien, 2003). Among the most compelling findings involve PET studies of addicted patients showing reduced DA activity (Wu, Bell, et al., 1997) and markedly suppressed DA responses to stimulants (Volkow, Wang, et al., 1997). Furthermore, neuroendocrine markers of DA hypoactivity predict poor clinical outcome (Patkar, Hill, et al., 2002). Glutamate levels are also depleted by repeated cocaine doses (Kalivas, 2004), whereas GABA levels are elevated (Xi, Ramamoorthy, et al., 2003), suggesting an anticraving role for agents that normalizing DA and/or glutamate activity (Dackis, 2005). Encouraging results have been reported with modafinil (Dackis, Kampman, et al., 2005a), and the DA-enhancing agents amantadine ($n = 61$; 300 mg/day; Kampman, Volpicelli, et al., 2000) and disulfiram ($n = 121$; 250 mg/day; Carroll, Fenton, et al., 2004) promoted abstinence in controlled outpatient trials. Along these lines, the DA antagonist olanzapine ($n = 30$; 10 mg/day) significantly *increased* cocaine use in a recent clinical trial (Kampman, Pettinati, et al., 2003), corroborating prior studies indicating that DA-inhibiting agents are poorly tolerated by patients addicted to cocaine (Dackis and O'Brien, 2002).

Hedonic Dysregulation

At the end of a cocaine binge, when the desperate need for more cocaine has finally passed, users typically feel drained, depressed, and irritable. Symptoms of cocaine withdrawal (see Table 20.1) often follow and are predictive of poor clinical outcome (Kampman, Alterman, et al., 2001). We have hypothesized that the presence of severe cocaine withdrawal identifies patients with persistent hedonic dysregulation that might explain their poor outcome (Dackis and O'Brien, 2001).

Patients anecdotally report diminished enjoyment of life's natural rewards and have been reported to have persistently reduced sex drive (Cocores, Dackis, et al., 1986). However, reliable measures of hedonic function have surprisingly not been developed for humans, and systematic research is lacking in this area. Animal studies demonstrate hedonic dysregulation after chronic cocaine exposure as evidenced by elevated reward thresholds for intracranial self-stimulation (Koob, Ahmed, et al., 2004), which has been linked to increased activity at κ-opioid receptors (Todtenkopf, Marcus, et al., 2004). These receptors are selectively activated by dynorphin, an aversive endogenous opioid that inhibits reward-related DA neurons (Fagergren, Smith, et al., 2003). Autopsies of human cocaine abusers find increased levels of dynorphin and κ-opioid receptors (Mash and Staley, 1999), and animal studies likewise demonstrate dynorphin upregulation after cocaine exposure (Hurd, Svensson, et al., 1999). These findings suggest that hedonic dysregulation might be ameliorated by medications that selectively block κ-opioid receptors or increase DA tone.

Denial

Although traditionally viewed as purely psychological phenomena, denial and loss of control might also reflect PFC dysfunction. Cocaine-addicted patients have hypometabolism and reduced gray matter density in the PFC (Dackis, 2004; Volkow, Fowler, et al., 2004) and show neuropsychological evidence of impaired PFC function (Kaufman, Ross, et al., 2003). As the seat of executive function, the PFC is involved in decision making, risk/benefit assessment, motivation, salience perception, and impulse control, all of which are affected by cocaine dependence. Executive dysfunction in these patients might be reversed by modafinil, which activates the PFC (Ellis, Monk, et al., 1999) and improves PFC task performance (Turner, Robbins, et al., 2003). Whether modafinil or PFC activating agents might improve clinical outcome in cocaine dependence is an important research question that could be assessed by combining clinical trials with neuroimaging studies.

Conclusions

Cocaine dependence is a rapidly progressive disorder associated with significant brain involvement. Neuronal mechanisms underlying discrete clinical components of cocaine dependence are guiding the development of medications that have the potential to improve the prognosis of this devastating illness. Modafinil appears especially promising as a means of blunting cocaine euphoria, reversing cocaine withdrawal symptoms, normalizing DA/glutamate dysregulation, and restoring PFC metabolic activity. However, cocaine dependence cannot be treated solely by medications. Psychotherapeutic approaches outlined in this chapter, which are based on a strong therapeutic alliance, will always be necessary to promote the insight and determination that is required to break the cycle of addiction. The combination of effective pharmacological and psychological treatments is probably the most promising strategy to improve clinical outcome for cocaine-addicted patients.

References

Andrews, P. (1997). "Cocaethylene toxicity." *J Addict Dis* 16(3): 75–84.

Brady, K., S. Sonne, et al. (1995). "Features of cocaine dependence with concurrent alcohol abuse." *Drug and Alcohol Dependence* 39: 69–71.

Brebner, K., A. R. Childress, et al. (2002). "A potential role for GABA(B) agonists in the treatment of psychostimulant addiction." *Alcohol Alcohol* 37(5): 478–84.

Carroll, K., B. Rounsaville, et al. (1993). "Alcoholism in treatment seeking cocaine abusers: clinical and prognostic significance." *Journal of Studies on Alcoholism* 54: 199–208.

Carroll, K. M., L. R. Fenton, et al. (2004). "Efficacy of disulfiram and cognitive behavior therapy in cocaine-dependent outpatients: a randomized placebo-controlled trial." *Arch Gen Psychiatry* 61(3): 264–72.

Chiamulera, C., M. P. Epping-Jordan, et al. (2001). "Reinforcing and locomotor stimulant effects of cocaine are absent in mGluR5 null mutant mice." *Nat Neurosci* 4(9): 873–4.

Cocores, J. A., C. A. Dackis, et al. (1986). "Sexual dysfunction secondary to cocaine abuse in two patients." *J Clin Psychiatry* 47(7): 384–5.

Collins, E. D., A. S. Ward, et al. (1998). "The effects of memantine on the subjective, reinforcing and cardiovascular effects of cocaine in humans." *Behav Pharmacol* 9(7): 587–98.

Csikszentmihalyi, M., A. Sami, et al. (2005). Flow. In: A. J. Elliot and C. S. Dweck (eds.). *Handbook of Competence and Motivation*. New York: Guilford Publications, Inc., pp. 598–608.

Czoty, P. W., D. Morgan, et al. (2004). "Characterization of dopamine D1 and D2 receptor function in socially housed cynomolgus monkeys self-administering cocaine." *Psychopharmacology (Berl)* 174(3): 381–8.

Dackis, C. A. (2004). "Recent advances in the pharmacotherapy of cocaine dependence." *Curr Psychiatry Rep* 6(5): 323–31.

Dackis, C. (2005). "New treatments for cocaine abuse." *Drug Discovery Today* 2(1): 79–86.

Dackis, C. A. and M. S. Gold (1985). "New concepts in cocaine addiction: the dopamine depletion hypothesis." *Neurosci Biobehav Rev* 9(3): 469–77.

Dackis, C. A. and M. S. Gold (1992). *Psychiatric Hospitals for Treatment of Dual Diagnosis*. In: J. H. Lowinson et al. (eds.). *Substance Abuse, A Comprehensive Textbook*. Baltimore: Williams & Wilkins, pp. 467–485.

Dackis, C. A., K. M. Kampman, et al. (2005a). "A double-blind, placebo-controlled trial of modafinil for cocaine dependence." *Neuropsychopharmacology* 30(1): 205–11.

Dackis, C. A., K. M. Kampman, et al. (2005b). "Reply: do self-reports reliably assess abstinence in cocaine-dependent patients?" *Neuropsychopharmacology* 30(12): 2299–300.

Dackis, C. A., K. G. Lynch, et al. (2003). "Modafinil and cocaine: a double-blind, placebo-controlled drug interaction study." *Drug Alcohol Depend* 70(1): 29–37.

Dackis, C. A. and C. P. O'Brien (2001). "Cocaine dependence: a disease of the brain's reward centers." *J Subst Abuse Treat* 21(3): 111–7.

Dackis, C. A. and C. P. O'Brien (2002). "Cocaine dependence: the challenge for pharmacotherapy." *Current Opinion in Psychiatry* 15(3): 261–268.

Dackis, C. and C. O'Brien (2003). "Glutamatergic agents for cocaine dependence." *Ann NY Acad Sci* 1003: 328–45.

Dackis, C. and C. O'Brien (2005a). "Clinical implications of cocaine-induced cortical depression." *Neuropsychopharmacology* 30(5): 1033–5.

Dackis, C. and C. O'Brien (2005b). "Neurobiology of addiction: treatment and public policy ramifications." *Nat Neurosci* 8(11): 1431–6.

Di Ciano, P. and B. J. Everitt (2001). "Dissociable effects of antagonism of NMDA and AMPA/KA receptors in the nucleus accumbens core and shell on cocaine-seeking behavior." *Neuropsychopharmacology* 25(3): 341–60.

Duckworth, A., T. A. Steen, et al. (2005). "Positive psychology in clinical practice." *Annual Review of Clinical Psychology* 1: 629–651.

Ellis, C. M., C. Monk, et al. (1999). "Functional magnetic resonance imaging neuroactivation studies in normal subjects and subjects with the narcoleptic syndrome. Actions of modafinil." *J Sleep Res* 8(2): 85–93.

Fagergren, P., H. R. Smith, et al. (2003). "Temporal upregulation of prodynorphin mRNA in the primate striatum after cocaine self-administration." *Eur J Neurosci* 17(10): 2212–8.

Garavan, H., J. Pankiewicz, et al. (2000). "Cue-induced cocaine craving: neuroanatomical specificity for drug users and drug stimuli." *Am J Psychiatry* 157(11): 1789–98.

Haidt, J. (2005). *The happiness hypothesis: Finding modern truth in ancient wisdom*. New York: Basic Books. New York.

Haney, M. and T. R. Kosten (2004). "Therapeutic vaccines for substance dependence." *Expert Rev Vaccines* 3(1): 11–8.

Hatsukami, D. K. and M. W. Fischman (1996). "Crack cocaine and cocaine hydrochloride. Are the differences myth or reality?" *JAMA* 276(19): 1580–8.

Heil, S., G. Badger, et al. (2001). "Alcohol dependence among cocaine-dependent outpatients: demographics, drug use, treatment outcome and other characteristics." *Journal of Studies on Alcoholism* 62(1): 14–22.

Higgins, S., A. Budney, et al. (1994). "Alcohol dependence and simultaneous cocaine and alcohol use in cocaine-dependent patients." *Journal of Addictive Diseases* 13(4): 177–189.

Hurd, Y. L., P. Svensson, et al. (1999). "The role of dopamine, dynorphin, and CART systems in the ventral striatum and amygdala in cocaine abuse." *Ann NY Acad Sci* 877: 499–506.

Jaffe, J. H., N. G. Cascella, et al. (1989). "Cocaine-induced cocaine craving." *Psychopharmacology* 97(1): 59–64.

Kalivas, P. W. (2004). "Glutamate systems in cocaine addiction." *Curr Opin Pharmacol* 4(1): 23–9.

Kalivas, P. W. and K. McFarland (2003). "Brain circuitry and the reinstatement of cocaine-seeking behavior." *Psychopharmacology (Berl)* 168(1–2): 44–56.

Kalivas, P. W., K. McFarland, et al. (2003). "Glutamate transmission and addiction to cocaine." *Ann NY Acad Sci* 1003: 169–75.

Kampman, K. M., A. I. Alterman, et al. (2001). "Cocaine withdrawal symptoms and initial urine toxicology results predict treatment attrition in outpatient cocaine dependence treatment." *Psychol Addict Behav* 15(1): 52–9.

Kampman, K. M., H. Pettinati, et al. (2003). "A pilot trial of olanzapine for the treatment of cocaine dependence." *Drug Alcohol Depend* 70(3): 265–73.

Kampman, K. M., H. Pettinati, et al. (2004). "A pilot trial of topiramate for the treatment of cocaine dependence." *Drug Alcohol Depend* 75(3): 233–40.

Kampman, K. M., J. R. Volpicelli, et al. (2000). "Amantadine in the treatment of cocaine-dependent patients with severe withdrawal symptoms." *Am J Psychiatry* 157(12): 2052–4.

Kampman, K. M., J. R. Volpicelli, et al. (2001). "Effectiveness of propranolol for cocaine dependence treatment may depend on cocaine withdrawal symptom severity." *Drug Alcohol Depend* 63(1): 69–78.

Katz, J. L., P. Terry, et al. (1992). "Comparative behavioral pharmacology and toxicology of cocaine and its ethanol-derived metabolite, cocaine ethyl-ester (cocaethylene)." *Life Sci* 50(18): 1351–61.

Kaufman, J. N., T. J. Ross, et al. (2003). "Cingulate hypoactivity in cocaine users during a GO-NOGO task as revealed by event-related functional magnetic resonance imaging." *J Neurosci* 23(21): 7839–43.

Koob, G. F., S. H. Ahmed, et al. (2004). "Neurobiological mechanisms in the transition from drug use to drug dependence." *Neurosci Biobehav Rev* 27(8): 739–49.

Lile, J. A., W. W. Stoops, et al. (2004). "Baclofen does not alter the reinforcing, subject-rated or cardiovascular effects of intranasal cocaine in humans." *Psychopharmacology (Berl)* 171(4): 441–9.

Malcolm, R. J., J. L. Donovan, et al. (2002). *Influence of modafinil, 400 or 800 mg/day on subjective effects of intravenous cocaine in non-treatment seeking volunteers.* Quebec City, Canada: College on Problems of Drug Dependence.

Martinez, D., A. Broft, et al. (2004). "Cocaine dependence and d2 receptor availability in the functional subdivisions of the striatum: relationship with cocaine-seeking behavior." *Neuropsychopharmacology* 29(6): 1190–202.

Mash, D. C. and J. K. Staley (1999). "D3 dopamine and kappa opioid receptor alterations in human brain of cocaine-overdose victims." *Ann NY Acad Sci* 877: 507–22.

McCance-Katz, E., T. Kosten, et al. (1998). "Concurrent use of cocaine and alcohol is more potent and potentially more toxic than either alone—a multiple dose study." *Biological Psychiatry* 44: 250–259.

McFarland, K., C. C. Lapish, et al. (2003). "Prefrontal glutamate release into the core of the nucleus accumbens mediates cocaine-induced reinstatement of drug-seeking behavior." *J Neurosci* 23(8): 3531–7.

McLellan, A. T., L. Luborsky, et al. (1980). "An improved diagnostic evaluation instrument for substance abuse patients. The Addiction Severity Index." *J Nerv Ment Dis* 168(1): 26–33.

Miller, W. R. and S. Rollnick (2002). *Motivational Interviewing.* New York: Guilford Press.

Nestler, E. J. (2004). "Historical review: Molecular and cellular mechanisms of opiate and cocaine addiction." *Trends Pharmacol Sci* 25(4): 210–8.

Newton, T. F., A. D. Kalechstein, et al. (2003). "Irritability following abstinence from cocaine predicts euphoric effects of cocaine administration." *Addict Behav* 28(4): 817–21.

Patkar, A. A., K. P. Hill, et al. (2002). "Serum prolactin and response to treatment among cocaine-dependent individuals." *Addict Biol* 7(1): 45–53.

Peterson, C. and M. E. P. Seligman (2004). *Character Strengths and Virtues: A Handbook and Classification.* New York: Oxford University Press and American Psychological Association.

Robinson, T. E. and B. Kolb (2004). "Structural plasticity associated with exposure to drugs of abuse." *Neuropharmacology* 47 Suppl 1: 33–46.

Rocha, B. A. (2003). "Stimulant and reinforcing effects of cocaine in monoamine transporter knockout mice." *Eur J Pharmacol* 479(1–3): 107–15.

Seligman, M. E., T. A. Steen, et al. (2005). "Positive psychology progress: empirical validation of interventions." *Am Psychol* 60(5): 410–21.

Shoptaw, S., X. Yang, et al. (2003). "Randomized placebo-controlled trial of baclofen for cocaine dependence: preliminary effects for individuals with chronic patterns of cocaine use." *J Clin Psychiatry* 64(12): 1440–8.

Sofuoglu, M., S. Brown, et al. (2001). "Depressive symptoms modulate the subjective and physiological response to cocaine in humans." *Drug Alcohol Depend* 63(2): 131–7.

Sofuoglu, M., S. Dudish-Poulsen, et al. (2003). "Association of cocaine withdrawal symptoms with more severe dependence and enhanced subjective response to cocaine." *Drug Alcohol Depend* 69: 273–282.

Thomas, M. J., C. Beurrier, et al. (2001). "Long-term depression in the nucleus accumbens: a neural correlate of behavioral sensitization to cocaine." *Nat Neurosci* 4(12): 1217–23.

Todtenkopf, M. S., J. F. Marcus, et al. (2004). "Effects of kappa-opioid receptor ligands on intracranial self-stimulation in rats." *Psychopharmacology (Berl)* 172(4): 463–70.

Turner, D. C., T. W. Robbins, et al. (2003). "Cognitive enhancing effects of modafinil in healthy volunteers." *Psychopharmacology (Berl)* 165(3): 260–9.

Volkow, N. D., J. S. Fowler, et al. (2004). "The addicted human brain viewed in the light of imaging studies: brain circuits and treatment strategies." *Neuropharmacology* 47 Suppl 1: 3–13.

Volkow, N. D., G. J. Wang, et al. (1997). "Decreased striatal dopaminergic responsiveness in detoxified cocaine-dependent subjects." *Nature* 386 (6627): 830–3.

Wilson, L. D. and S. French (2002). "Cocaethylene's effects on coronary artery blood flow and cardiac function in a canine model." *J Toxicol Clin Toxicol* 40(5): 535–46.

Wise, R. A. (2004). "Dopamine, learning and motivation." *Nat Rev Neurosci* 5(6): 483–94.

Wu, J. C., K. Bell, et al. (1997). "Decreasing striatal 6-FDOPA uptake with increasing duration of cocaine withdrawal." *Neuropsychopharmacology* 17(6): 402–9.

Xi, Z. X., S. Ramamoorthy, et al. (2003). "GABA transmission in the nucleus accumbens is altered after withdrawal from repeated cocaine." *J Neurosci* 23(8): 3498–505.

21

Smoking, Pain, and Addiction

Lara K. Dhingra

Jamie S. Ostroff

Smoking rates among adults with persistent pain are high (30%–64%) compared to the general population (22%). Smokers with persistent pain are likely to be more nicotine dependent and have difficulty quitting smoking. Further, smokers with persistent pain have higher rates of opioid abuse compared to nonsmokers with pain. Smokers with more severe nicotine dependency are more likely to misuse their opioid medications than smokers with lower nicotine dependency. Despite these findings, smoking is an underappreciated risk and poorly understood factor for opioid therapy and functional rehabilitation in pain management. Thus, examining the link between smoking and aberrant drug-taking behavior is critical to clinicians and researchers seeking to understand a patient's potential risk for prescription opioid abuse.

Clearly, the relationship between smoking and aberrant behaviors is complex given that not all smokers are prone to opioid misuse. Thus, by assessing the characteristics of smoking behavior and specific psychosocial risk factors for opioid abuse, pain clinicians can develop effective treatment strategies that address relevant comorbidities and increase a patient's chance of achieving successful pain management outcomes. Although smoking items have appeared on screening tools aimed at assessing a patient's risk potential for opioid misuse, the implications for opioid treatment in smokers are poorly understood. Understanding the behavioral, genetic, and environmental mechanisms that mediate and moderate the smoking–aberrant behavior relationship is critical to improving pain outcomes.

Exploring the link between smoking and aberrant drug-taking behavior is important to pain clinicians treating individuals with pain disorders and to researchers investigating the efficacy of pain interventions for different subgroups. There is little doubt that health-care providers in general, and pain clinicians in particular, should be advising their patients who smoke to quit for their overall health and well-being. However, how should clinicians weigh a history of smoking when considering opioids as a therapeutic option for the patient with persistent pain? How often do pain clinicians employ safeguards in managing smokers as they might patients with other risk factors for opioid therapy? This chapter will review the literature on the increased likelihood of opioid abuse and aberrant drug-taking behaviors among persistent pain patients. Further, it will examine multiple etiologies for the association between smoking and aberrant drug-taking behavior. Finally, this chapter will critically evaluate the clinical significance of smoking in the assessment of the pain patient.

Smoking Among Adults With Persistent Pain

Cigarette smoking is highly prevalent among individuals with comorbid pain. Approximately 21% of adults in the general United States population currently smoke (CDC, 2005). However, the prevalence of smoking among adults with persistent pain is higher, with estimates ranging between 30% and 64% (Deyo et al., 1989; Goldberg et al., 2000; Hahn et al. 2006; Jamison et al., 1991; Oleske et al., 2004; Scott et al., 1999; Sternbach, 1986). With more than 50 million adults in the United States experiencing persistent pain (Louis Harris & Associates, 1999), the projected number of smokers with pain is substantial. Indeed, a meta-analytic review of 38 studies of nonspecific low back pain showed that 69% of men and 85% of women were current smokers (Goldberg et al., 2000). Smoking prevalence is associated with a variety of pain disorders, including nonspecific low back pain, fibromyalgia, and headache disorders (Hahn et al., 2006; Jamison et al., 1991; Payne et al., 1991; Yunus et al., 2002). There is a strong positive association between current smoking status and persistent low back pain (Porter and Hanley, 2001).

Individuals reporting clinically significant persistent pain are more likely to be current smokers (Andersson et al., 1998; Deyo et al., 1989; Goldberg et al., 2000; Hellsing and Bryngelsson, 2000; Porter and Hanley, 2001; Scott et al., 1999; Thomas et al., 1999). In a national survey of pain among 1,254 adults, the prevalence of smoking was 37% for those reporting "unbearable pain" and 27% for those with "slight pain" (Sternbach, 1986). A large cross-sectional study of spinal patients ($N = 25,455$) also concluded that smokers reported greater pain intensity than nonsmokers (Vogt et al., 2002). Among those with low back disorders, smokers (49%) reported more pain-related disability compared to nonsmokers with pain (Oleske et al., 2004). Current smokers are more likely to suffer back pain than nonsmokers (Thomas et al., 1999).

Smokers have reported that they experience a greater need to smoke when their pain increases (Jamison et al., 1991). When stratified into high- and low-pain groups, smokers with more significant pain smoked more in a typical day than smokers without significant pain (Hahn et al. 2006). Greater pain intensity is associated with more cigarette consumption per day (Andersson et al., 1998; Kaila-Kangas et al., 2003). Smokers with persistent pain tend to be heavy smokers. Jamison et al. (1991) observed that 64% of outpatients with low back pain disorders were current smokers, 86% of whom smoked more than 15 cigarettes per day. Among fibromyalgia patients, 22% were current smokers, 61% of whom smoked 1–2 packs per day (Yunus et al., 2002). Among patients treated for recurrent headache disorders ($N = 189$), the mean number of cigarettes per day was 23 (Payne et al., 1991). Hahn and colleagues (2006) found that 66% with various pain disorders smoked less than 1 pack per day and 33% smoked 1 or more packs per day.

Smoking and Aberrant Drug-Taking Behaviors

Current smoking is associated with higher levels of analgesic use (Antonov and Isacson, 1996; Antonov and Isacson, 1998; Corrigall et al., 1992; Jamison et al., 1991) and more aberrant drug-taking behaviors than nonsmoking (Michna et al., 2004). Further, smokers with more severe nicotine dependency are more likely to misuse opioid medication than smokers with lower nicotine dependency (Michna et al., 2004). Michna and colleagues (2004) showed that current smoking status and an index of tobacco dependence (e.g., smokes within 1 hour of waking) were among the most useful predictors of problems with opioid use among persistent pain patients. In this study, 61% of patients at low risk for aberrant drug behaviors and 82% of patients at high risk were current smokers. Hahn and colleagues (2006) found that smokers with persistent pain who smoked more cigarettes per day were less ready to quit than smokers without pain, suggesting that addressing these behaviors in pain patients is a formidable challenge.

Potential Social Learning Mechanisms of Smoking, Aberrant Drug-Taking Behaviors, and Pain

Social learning theory offers a rich perspective for evaluating the relationship between smoking, aberrant drug-taking behaviors (ADTB), and pain. Jamison et al. (1991) speculated that drug effect expectancies derived from utility theory may account for the increased rate of smoking among adults with pain. Because smoking, drinking alcohol, and ingesting other substances are often used as mood regulation strategies for those without pain, their effects on mood may be extremely reinforcing to those in pain (Jamison et al., 1991).

Situational Cues of Smoking and Aberrant Drug-Taking Behaviors

One potential framework for understanding linkages between pain, smoking, and ADTB emphasizes the role of *situational cues* in prompting addictive behaviors (Dhingra et al., 2006; Niaura et al., 2002; Shiffman et al., 2002; Tiffany & Stephen, 1990). Shiffman and colleagues (2002) and Brandon and colleagues (1996) have shown that addictive behaviors are more likely to occur in certain situations with strong contingencies for smoking and substance use. These *situational cues* (e.g., pain intensity, negative affect) prompt smoking and substance use behaviors (Shiffman et al., 2002). Further, specific cues are robust predictors of within- and between-person variation in smoking behavior (Baker et al., 2004; Tennen et al., 2000). Indeed, situational cues account for greater variation in smoking behavior than severity of nicotine dependency.

Smoking and Drug Effect Outcome Expectancies

An additional social learning construct linking pain to addictive behaviors involves *smoking and drug effect outcome expectancies*.

We are currently conducting a prospective evaluation of smoking behavior in pain patients to test the hypothesis that *situation-specific outcome expectancies* (i.e., for pain relief and negative affect regulation) mediate the relationship between smoking and pain (Dhingra et al., 2006). Expectancies are among the most robust predictors of smoking motivation and behavior (Brandon et al., 1999). According to social learning theory (Bandura, 1977; Rotter, 1954), expectancies involve the anticipated effects of a specific behavior on a certain positive outcome (e.g., pain relief). Similarly, beliefs that smoking will reduce pain lead to smoking urges and lapses. Smoking behavior is related to the strength of the expectancies about positive consequences (Brandon et al., 1999).

Smokers who have more favorable expectations about smoking are more likely to initiate smoking, to smoke at a higher rate, to resist attempting to quit smoking, and to have difficulty maintaining abstinence (Brandon and Baker, 1991; Brandon et al., 1999; Copeland et al., 1995; Wetter et al., 1994). Positive outcome expectancies about nicotine effects are also related to overall consumption (Brandon and Baker, 1991; Copeland et al., 1995; Wetter et al., 1994). Heavy smokers have the most positive outcome expectancies (and the least negative outcome expectancies) about smoking, whereas nonsmokers have the least positive expectancies (and the most negative expectancies).

Over time, smokers may consolidate these drug outcome expectancies such that they result in automatized drug use behaviors (Brandon et al., 1999; Oei and Baldwin, 1994; Tiffany, 1990). As such, smoking and substance use become "automatic" behaviors in those with pain. Researchers have recognized the need to identify particular expectancies for drug effects within specific, relevant situations so that we can better understand how certain cues lead to addictive behaviors (Brandon et al., 1996; Leigh, 1989). Understanding the role of pain-specific expectancies in the maintenance of addictive behavior is an area for additional research.

Etiology of Smoking and Aberrant Drug-Taking Behaviors

Individuals commonly report similar reasons for smoking and using substances: to enjoy the psychoactive properties of tobacco and drugs, the social and affiliative consequences of smoking and drugs, the sensory aspects, and to reduce negative affect (Perkins, 2001; Perkins et al., 1999; Piper et al., 2001). Thus, in addition to the role of smoking and drug effect outcome expectancies, most relevant to understanding the linkage between smoking and ADTB are the influential roles of pseudoaddiction (inadequate analgesia), nicotine-induced analgesia, substance use disorders, and chemical coping/self-medication of pain and negative affect (see paragraphs below).

Smoking and the Likelihood of Pseudoaddiction

Weissman and Haddox (1989) posited the iatrogenic phenomenon of pseudoaddiction wherein patients who have inadequate pain relief can be mistaken for addicts in their desperate attempts to find relief. Some of these desperate measures (e.g., using more medication than prescribed, assertive requests for more pain medication) have been subsequently called potentially aberrant drug-taking behaviors (ADTB). The pseudoaddiction concept implies that any of these aberrant behaviors will cease when better analgesia is achieved. This begs the question, are smokers more likely to be pseudoaddicted than other pain patients? And consequently, are smokers more likely to have less adequate analgesia than other pain patients?

Although nicotine is clearly analgesic in studies of acute pain (often in opioid naïve subjects, see below; Flood and Daniel, 2004; Jamner et al., 1998; Perkins et al., 1994), it is not clear that this is the case in the persistent pain scenario. Although Jamison et al. (1991) did find that some patients reported smoking to relieve pain, there are also studies that point to nicotine-opioid interactions that could lead to diminished pain relief in some patients (Zevin and Benowitz, 1999). These findings include, but are not limited to, decreased efficacy of propoxyphene in smokers as compared to nonsmokers (Anonymous, 1973), increased metabolic clearance of pentazocine in smokers (Vaughan et al., 1976), smokers requiring higher doses of pentazocine than nonsmokers (Keeri-Szanto and Pomeroy, 1971), and smoking inducing the metabolism of codeine (Yue et al., 1994). Thus, the smoking–aberrant drug-taking behavior connection could be the result of smokers receiving less analgesia from "routine" doses of opioids than do nonsmokers, and subsequent pseudoaddictive behaviors that are in pursuit of enhanced pain control.

Because of such drug interactions, pain clinicians should be sensitive to the possibility that smokers may require higher doses of opioids while assisting their patients who smoke to quit.

Nicotine-Induced Analgesia

Pain relief is often identified as a consequence of smoking. Interestingly, there is growing evidence that nicotine has analgesic properties and antinociceptive effects (Fertig et al., 1986; Flood and Daniel, 2004; Jamner et al., 1998; Perkins et al., 1994). For example, animal studies suggest that smoking may relieve pain sensations (Han et al., 2005). Wewers et al. (1999) found that the administration of chronic nicotine created antinociception over time. Rat models have also shown that exposure to high levels of cigarette smoke induces antinociceptive effects mediated via nicotinic and mu-opioid pain receptors (Wewers et al., 1999). Recently, clinical research has shown that the nicotine nasal spray has analgesic effects on postoperative pain in women undergoing abdominal surgeries (Flood and Daniel, 2004). Nicotine has also been shown to have mild to moderate analgesic effects in smokers and nonsmokers (Fertig et al., 1986; Jamner et al., 1998; Perkins et al., 1994). Perkins et al. (1994) found that nicotine decreased thermal pain sensitivity in smokers and nonsmokers. Nicotine can have direct antinociceptive effects mediated through endorphinergic mechanisms in the central nervous system (Han et al., 2005; Silverstein, 1982).

Smoking and Substance Use Disorders

The notion that smoking, alcohol, and other substance abuse are positively associated is well-supported by empirical findings. Approximately 50% of adults in the general population report ever smoking (CDC, 2004) compared to 80% of alcohol-dependent (Daeppen et al., 2000; Romberger and Grant, 2004) and 60%–90% of substance abuse patients (Budney et al., 1993; Darke and Hall, 1995; Richter et al., 2002). Approximately 34% of individuals with alcohol disorders and 52% with substance abuse disorders meet full criteria for *DSM-IV* nicotine dependence (Grant et al., 2004; Romberger and Grant, 2004). Heavy drinkers are more likely to be heavy smokers (e.g., smoke more than 1 pack per day; Stotts et al., 2003; Toneatto et al., 1995), and heavy smokers drink more alcohol (e.g., quantity and frequency) than light smokers (Colby et al., 2004; Daeppen et al., 2000). Further research is needed to determine whether relationships between smoking and drinking are unidirectional or bidirectional in nature (Colby et al., 2004). However, smoking and opioid addictive behaviors are likely mediated by similar biological factors and environmental stimuli.

Neurobiological Reward Mechanisms of Nicotine and Opioid Use

Researchers have begun to identify common mechanisms of action in the human brain between nicotine and other drugs of abuse. The mesolimbic-dopaminergic system is the key neurologic system for rewards processes in the brain. The mesolimbic-dopaminergic system provides satisfaction, pleasure, and reduction in stress through a series or "cascade" of neurohormonal release mechanisms. The neurohormonal cascade begins with serotonin, which at the hypothalamus stimulates enkephalin. This subsequently inhibits γ-aminobutyric acid (GABA) at the substantia nigra, which in turn adjusts the amount of dopamine released at the nucleus accumbens or terminal synapse. This stimulation of the dopamine receptor sites (1–5) initiates feelings of reward. This same system also serves as the common pathway for many substances of abuse, including nicotine, alcohol, marijuana, cocaine, glucose, heroin, and opioids. These substances of abuse all have an ability to mediate actions within the neurohormonal reward cascade (Blum et al., 2000).

Neurobiologic theories also suggest that nicotine initiation begins as a pleasure-seeking activity, but as tolerance to nicotine builds and the brain becomes adapted due to maximized upregulation of available dopamine receptors, expected pleasure decreases. Continued smoking may then trigger the smoker to seek out alternate sources of pleasure, weakening inhibitions, initiating the use and abuse of alternate drugs, and consequential aberrant behaviors. How then, do we explain the fact that not all nicotine users become addicted to drugs?

One possible explanation for the link between smoking and other substance abuse involves dysfunction within the neurohormonal reward cascade. Genetic variants may limit the normal effects of dopamine, a hypodopaminergic trait, prompting multiple drug-seeking behaviors in the genetically predisposed population. Current evidence indicates that phenotypic liability may result from polymorphism within dopamine receptor genes. These receptor genes are also linked to obsessive behaviors, alcohol abuse, and other substance abuse disorders, which suggests a common segue way among different addictive behaviors. Hence, genetically predisposed individuals may bypass the threshold for addiction and show a propensity for both smoking and ADTB and subsequent opioid abuse. Although there is no current diagnostic or therapeutic benchmark for such addiction potential, a "diathesis-stress" model of smoking and ADTB would suggest that genetically predisposed smokers may be motivated to seek substances when they experience negative environmental and social stimuli.

In summary, nicotine is known to stimulate the release of norepinephrine (NE) and dopamine (DA; Benwell and Balfour, 1997), and nicotine stimulates dopaminergic activity in the mesolimbic reward/reinforcing system (Corrigall et al., 1992). Furthermore, recent investigations using positron emission tomography show promise in identifying potential sites of nicotine function in the brain, including the hippocampus and the dorsal anterior cingulate (Zubieta et al., 2005). Zubieta et al. (2005) showed that endorphins and enkephalins are released during smoking, and changes in these neurochemicals correlate with prominent behavioral changes in affect, craving, and withdrawal symptoms. From a screening standpoint, smoking may be a more socially acceptable form of substance use to report to a pain clinician than is alcohol or illicit drug use. For some patients, admitting to a history of smoking could be a proxy for other forms of substance use that pain patients might not want to disclose to their prescribing physician. Smokers, particularly heavy smokers, should be screened for the presence of other comorbid substance use disorders.

Smoking and Chemical Coping, Self-Medication, and Negative Affect

Although smokers with comorbid substance use disorders are likely to require referral to an addictions medicine specialist, there is a vast middle ground of persistent pain patients who have problems adhering with the rules of opioid therapy, are very drug focused, and who fail to make progress toward psychosocial goals during pain management. Although many of these patients manifest aberrant drug-taking behaviors, they are unlikely to meet criteria for opioid addiction in that their behavior is not as compulsive, as "out of control," or as obviously and acutely harmful as in substance use disorders. Chambers and colleagues (Chambers et al., 1975) have coined the term "chemical coping" to describe the tendency to rely on psychoactive substances as a means of coping with psychosocial stress. Passik and colleagues have an ongoing effort to develop the *Chemical Coping Inventory*, a measure that also incorporates somatization, alexithymia, and sensation seeking (in progress).

Much attention has been directed toward the development of screening criteria that identify characteristics of patients at risk for engaging in chemical coping. According to the *social stress model* of substance use, individuals use substances as a means of coping with psychosocial stressors. Although the use of alcohol and drugs may temporarily reduce negative affectivity caused by stressors, consistent substance use tends to increase stress over time. Pain sufferers report relying on smoking to reduce their emotional distress and to improve their ability to cope with pain (Jamison et al., 1991). Hence, smoking may be a means of self-medication for stressors related to persistent pain, although this is a detrimental strategy for symptom management long term because of smoking's impact on opioid metabolism, its potential worsening of pain pathophysiology, and function as a maladaptive method of coping.

Thus, patients with tendencies toward chemical coping may require a range of strategies, including management with primarily long-acting drugs (to promote less pill popping), stress management training, behavioral activation, and psychotherapy.

Relatedly, smoking is widely used as a mood regulation strategy to decrease negative affect (e.g., depression, anxiety, and anger) and increase positive affect in those who smoke. Negative affect and mood disorders are common among smokers and those with persistent pain. Specifically, the prevalence of major depressive disorder in patients with chronic low back pain is three to four times greater than base rates in the general population (Sullivan et al., 1992). Across a broad spectrum of smoker subpopulations, negative affect has been identified as one of the primary determinants of smoking initiation, maintenance, and relapse. Thus, the routine practice of depression and anxiety screening as part of the comprehensive pain assessment and the availability of psychosocial interventions for depression and anxiety are critical to reducing barriers to pain management.

Smoking and Pain Management Outcomes

Smoking is an important but understudied risk factor for poor therapeutic outcomes in pain management. Smoking is also associated with other health risk behaviors that compromise the effective self-management of pain. Smokers with pain report more maladaptive and passive pain behaviors including greater use of analgesics and sedatives, higher levels of behavioral deactivation and physical disability (Hellsing and Bryngelsson, 2000; Jamison et al., 1991; Sternbach 1986), and low motivation for self-management of pain (Jensen et al., 2003).

Clinical Implications for Smoking Cessation in Pain Management

Smoking in pain patients is a known risk factor for aberrant drug-taking behaviors. Current smoking is positively associated with the presence of comorbid psychiatric disorders, in particular, substance abuse disorders and mood disorders, and may be implicated in pseudoaddiction phenomena (as described earlier in this chapter). However, multiple behavioral and biological mechanisms may account for the smoking–aberrant drug-taking link.

The evaluation of smoking and aberrant drug-taking behaviors is important to pain clinicians treating individuals with pain disorders and to researchers investigating the efficacy of pain interventions for different subgroups for several reasons reviewed in this chapter. Significantly more individuals with pain disorders report smoking than adults in the general population. Furthermore, smoking can be a prominent barrier to pain management and is known to interfere with the pharmacokinetics of opioid treatment and reduce treatment efficacy. Therefore, the cycle of pain and smoking may continuously interfere with the practice of effective behavioral and pharmacologic strategies for pain on a daily level. Few pain programs offer formal treatments for tobacco dependence. Smoking cessation programs do not routinely tailor interventions to address the needs of pain patients, and there is little information to guide evidence-based treatments for tobacco dependence in this subpopulation. Given the increasing evidence that pain, smoking, and aberrant drug-taking behaviors are linked, it is an opportune time to enhance provider awareness and education about the importance of smoking behavior change in the context of pain management.

References

Andersson, H., Ejlertsson, G., and Leden, I. (1998). Widespread musculoskeletal chronic pain associated with smoking. An epidemiological study in a general rural population, *Scandinavian Journal of Rehabilitation Medicine*, 30 (3), 185–91.

Anonymous (1973). Decreased clinical efficacy of propoxyphene in cigarette smokers, *Clin Pharmacol Ther*, 14 (2), 259–63.

Antonov, K. K., and Isacson, D. D. (1996). Use of analgesics in Sweden—the importance of sociodemographic factors, physical fitness, health and health-related factors, and working conditions, *Social Science & Medicine*, 42 (11), 1473.

Antonov, K. I., and Isacson, D. G. (1998). Prescription and nonprescription analgesic use in Sweden, *The Annals of Pharmacotherapy*, 32 (4), 485.

Baker, T. B., et al. (2004). Addiction motivation reformulated: An affective processing model of negative reinforcement, *Psychol Rev*, 111 (1), 33–51.

Bandura, A. (1977). *Social learning theory* (Englewood Cliffs, NJ: Prentice-Hall, Inc.).

Benwell, M. E., and Balfour, D. J. (1997). Regional variation in the effects of nicotine on catecholamine overflow in rat brain, *Eur J Pharmacol*, 325 (1), 13–20.

Blum, K., Braverman, E. R., Holder, J. M., et al. (2000). Reward Deficiency Syndrome: a biogenetic model for the diagnosis and treatment of impulsive, addictive, and compulsive behaviors. *J Psychoactive Drugs* 32 Suppl:i–iv:1–112.

Brandon, T. H., and Baker, T. B. (1991). The Smoking Consequences Questionnaire: The subjective expected utility of smoking in college students, *Psychological Assessment*, 3 (3), 484–91.

Brandon, T. H., Juliano, L. M., and Copeland, A. L. (1999). Expectancies for tobacco smoking. In Irving Kirsch (ed.), *How expectancies shape experience* (Washington, DC: American Psychological Association), pp. 263–99.

Brandon, T. H., Wetter, D. W., and Baker, T. B. (1996). Affect, expectancies, urges, and smoking: Do they conform to models of drug motivation and relapse? *Experimental & Clinical Psychopharmacology,* 4 (1), 29–36.

Budney, A. J., et al. (1993). Nicotine and caffeine use in cocaine-dependent individuals, *J Subst Abuse,* 5 (2), 117–30.

Chambers, C. D., Inciardi, J. A., and Siegal, H. A. (1975). *Chemical coping: A report on legal drug use in the United States.* New York: Spectrum.

CDC (2004). Cigarette smoking among adults—United States, 2002, *Morb Mortal Wkly Rep,* 53 (20), 427–31.

CDC (2005). Cigarette smoking among adults—United States, 2004, *Morbidity and Mortality Weekly Report,* 54 (44), 1121.

Colby, S. M., et al. (2004). Effects of tobacco deprivation on alcohol cue reactivity and drinking among young adults, *Addict Behav,* 29 (5), 879–92.

Copeland, A. L., Brandon, T. H., and Quinn, E. P. (1995). The Smoking Consequences Questionnaire-Adult: Measurement of smoking outcome expectancies of experienced smokers, *Psychological Assessment,* 7 (4), 484–94.

Corrigall, W. A., et al. (1992). The mesolimbic dopaminergic system is implicated in the reinforcing effects of nicotine, *Psychopharmacology (Berl),* 107 (2–3), 285–9.

Daeppen, J. B., et al. (2000). Clinical correlates of cigarette smoking and nicotine dependence in alcohol-dependent men and women. The Collaborative Study Group on the Genetics of Alcoholism, *Alcohol,* 35 (2), 171–5.

Darke, S., and Hall, W. (1995). Levels and correlates of polydrug use among heroin users and regular amphetamine users, *Drug Alcohol Depend,* 39 (3), 231–5.

Deyo, R. A., et al. (1989). Lifestyle and low-back pain. The influence of smoking and obesity: An epidemiological study of headache in an urban and a rural population in northern Finland, *Spine,* 14 (5), 501–6.

Dhingra, L. K., et al. (2006). Unpublished manuscript.

Fertig, J. B., Pomerleau, O. F., and Sanders, B. (1986). Nicotine-produced antinociception in minimally deprived smokers and ex-smokers, *Addict Behav,* 11 (3), 239–48.

Flood, P., and Daniel, D. (2004). Intranasal nicotine for postoperative pain treatment, *Anesthesiology,* 101 (6), 1417–21.

Goldberg, M. S., Scott, S. C., and Mayo, N. E. (2000). A review of the association between cigarette smoking and the development of nonspecific back pain and related outcomes, *Spine,* 25 (8), 995–1014.

Grant, B. F., et al. (2004). Nicotine dependence and psychiatric disorders in the United States: Results from the national epidemiologic survey on alcohol and related conditions, *Arch Gen Psychiatry,* 61 (11), 1107–15.

Hahn, E. J., et al. (2006). Brief report: Pain and readiness to quit smoking cigarettes, *Nicotine & Tobacco Research,* 8 (3), 473–70.

Han, K. J., et al. (2005). Antinociceptive effect of nicotine in various pain models in the mouse, *Arch Pharm Res,* 28 (2), 209–15.

Hellsing, A. L., and Bryngelsson, I. L. (2000). Predictors of musculoskeletal pain in men: A twenty-year follow-up from examination at enlistment, *Spine,* 25 (23), 3080–6.

Jamison, R. N., Stetson, B. A., and Parris, W. C. (1991). The relationship between cigarette smoking and chronic low back pain, *Addictive Behaviors,* 16 (3–4), 103–10.

Jamner, Larry D., et al. (1998). Pain inhibition, nicotine, and gender, *Experimental & Clinical Psychopharmacology,* 6 (1), 96–106.

Jensen, M. P., Nielson, W. R., and Kerns, R. D. (2003). Toward the development of a motivational model of pain self-management, *Journal of Pain,* 4 (9), 477–92.

Kaila-Kangas, L., et al. (2003). Smoking and overweight as predictors of hospitalization for back disorders, *Spine,* 28 (16), 1860–8.

Keeri-Szanto, M., and Pomeroy, J. R. (1971). Atmospheric pollution and pentazocine metabolism, *Lancet,* 1 (7706), 947–9.

Leigh, B. C. (1989). Attitudes and expectancies as predictors of drinking habits: A comparison of three scales, *J Stud Alcohol,* 50 (5), 432–40.

Louis Harris and Associates (1999). The 1999 National Pain Survey. On behalf of Ortho McNeil.

Michna, E., et al. (2004). Predicting aberrant drug behavior in patients treated for chronic pain: Importance of abuse history, *Journal of Pain and Symptom Management,* 28 (3), 250–58.

Niaura, R., et al. (2002). Response to social stress, urge to smoke, and smoking cessation, *Addict Behav,* 27 (2), 241–50.

Oei, T. P., and Baldwin, A. R. (1994). Expectancy theory: A two-process model of alcohol use and abuse. *Journal of Studies on Alcohol,* 55, 525–34.

Oleske, D. M., et al. (2004). Factors affecting recovery from work-related, low back disorders in autoworkers, *Arch Phys Med Rehabil,* 85 (8), 1362–4.

Payne, T. J., et al. (1991). The impact of cigarette smoking on headache activity in headache patients, *Headache,* 31 (5), 329–32.

Perkins, K. A. (2001). Smoking cessation in women. Special considerations, *CNS Drugs,* 15 (5), 391–411.

Perkins, K. A., Donny, E., and Caggiula, A. R. (1999). Sex differences in nicotine effects and self-administration: Review of human and animal evidence, *Nicotine Tob Res,* 1 (4), 301–15.

Perkins, K. A., et al. (1994). Effects of nicotine on thermal pain detection in humans, *Experimental & Clinical Psychopharmacology,* 2 (1), 95–106.

Piper, M. E., et al. (2001). Gender and racial/ethnic differences in tobacco-dependence treatment: A commentary and research recommendations, *Nicotine Tob Res,* 3 (4), 291–7.

Porter, S. E., and Hanley, E. N., Jr. (2001). The musculoskeletal effects of smoking, *J Am Acad Orthop Surg,* 9 (1), 9–17.

Richter, K. P., et al. (2002). A population-based study of cigarette smoking among illicit drug users in the United States, *Addiction,* 97 (7), 861–9.

Romberger, D. J., and Grant, K. (2004). Alcohol consumption and smoking status: The role of smoking cessation, *Biomed Pharmacother,* 58 (2), 77–83.

Rotter, J. B. (1954). *Social learning and clinical psychology.* Englewood Cliffs, NJ: Prentice-Hall.

Scott, S. C., et al. (1999). The association between cigarette smoking and back pain in adults, *Spine,* 24 (11), 1090–8.

Shiffman, S., et al. (2002). Immediate antecedents of cigarette smoking: An analysis from ecological momentary assessment, *Journal of Abnormal Psychology,* 111 (4), 531–45.

Silverstein, B. (1982). Cigarette smoking, nicotine addiction, and relaxation, *J Pers Soc Psychol,* 42 (5), 946–50.

Sternbach, R. A. (1986). Pain and hassles in the United States: Findings of the Nuprin pain report, *Pain,* 27 (1), 69–80.

Stotts, A. L., Schmitz, J. M., and Grabowski, J. (2003). Concurrent treatment for alcohol and tobacco dependence: are patients ready to quit both? *Drug Alcohol Depend,* 69 (1), 1–7.

Sullivan, M. J., et al. (1992). The treatment of depression in chronic low back pain: Review and recommendations, *Pain,* 50 (1), 5–13.

Tennen, H., et al. (2000). A daily process approach to coping—Linking theory, research, and practice, *American Psychologist,* 55 (6), 626–36.

Thomas, E., et al. (1999). Predicting who develops chronic low back pain in primary care: A prospective study, *BMJ,* 318 (7199), 1662–7.

Tiffany, S. T. (1990). A cognitive model of drug urges and drug-use behavior: Role of automatic and nonautomatic processes, *Psychological Review,* 97 (2), 147–68.

Toneatto, A., et al. (1995). Effect of cigarette smoking on alcohol treatment outcome, *J Subst Abuse,* 7 (2), 245–52.

Vaughan, D. P., Beckett, A. H., and Robbie, D. S. (1976). The influence of smoking on the intersubject variation in pentazocine elimination, *Br J Clin Pharmacol,* 3 (2), 279–83.

Vogt, M. T., et al. (2002). Influence of smoking on the health status of spinal patients: The National Spine Network database, *Spine,* 27 (3), 313–9.

Weissman, D. E., and Haddox, J. D. (1989). Opioid pseudoaddiction—an iatrogenic syndrome, *Pain,* 36 (3), 363–6.

Wetter, D. W., et al. (1994). Smoking outcome expectancies: Factor structure, predictive validity, and discriminant validity, *J Abnorm Psychol,* 103 (4), 801–11.

Wewers, M. E., et al. (1999). The effect of chronic administration of nicotine on antinociception, opioid receptor binding and met-enkephalin levels in rats, *Brain Res,* 822 (1–2), 107–13.

Yue, Q. Y., Tomson, T., and Sawe, J. (1994). Carbamazepine and cigarette smoking induce differentially the metabolism of codeine in man, *Pharmacogenetics*, 4 (4), 193–8.

Yunus, M. B., Arslan, S., and Aldag, J. C. (2002). Relationship between fibromyalgia features and smoking, *Scand J Rheumatol*, 31 (5), 301–5.

Zevin, S., and Benowitz, N. L. (1999). Drug interactions with tobacco smoking: An update, *Clin Pharmacokinet*, 36 (6), 425–38.

Zubieta, J. K., et al. (2005). Regional cerebral blood flow responses to smoking in tobacco smokers after overnight abstinence, *Am J Psychiatry*, 162 (3), 567–77.

Part III
The Problem of Clinical Pain

22

The Pathophysiology of Chronic Pain

Daniel Brookoff

> When pain is chronic, it not only involves the painful area, it involves the entire being.
> —Michel de Montaigne

Life is full of physical pain. Normal pain is a life-sustaining protective mechanism and is not a disease. Dysfunction of normal pain mechanisms can give rise to chronic pain. We are coming to understand that chronic pain is a legitimate medical disorder worthy of medical treatment. This life is full of physical pain, but that doesn't mean that it has to be full of physical suffering. One of the duties with which medical caregivers have been charged since antiquity is the alleviation of suffering. The Hippocratics taught us that it is the suffering individual that physicians must face, not just the pain (Rey, 1995).

It is terribly unfortunate that people seeking relief for chronic pain are often mistaken for drug abusers, when these two conditions are often quite opposite. People with chronic pain who have been shut out from their lives by meaningless physical suffering seek medical treatment in order to rejoin their families and their communities. Substance abusers may take the same drugs in order to escape their families, their communities and—ultimately—their lives, which are filled with existential suffering. Unfortunately, both chronic pain and chronic drug abuse are often accompanied by the same comorbidities, such as depression, anxiety, chronic anger, and despair. It is vital that we remind ourselves that it is not the characteristics of a drug that determines whether its consumption is legitimate or abusive; it is the use to which the drug is being put. When making the judgment about whether a substance is a legitimate medication or a drug of abuse, caregivers have to somehow determine whether the person is using it in order to restore life or diminish it. St. Thomas Aquinas understood this when he wrote that "no *thing* is intrinsically good or evil but its manner of usage may make it so." Fortunately our growing understanding of the pathophysiology of chronic pain is helping us identify sufferers and treat them constructively and humanely. It is also guiding us to remedies that will not be subject to abuse.

A Brief History of Chronic Pain

More than 4,000 years ago, Chinese physicians described a balance of vital energy, the "ch'i," which flowed through the organs and vital structures through a network of bodily conduits called meridians. Disease and pain were thought to be due to an imbalance of two opposing forces, yin and yang, related to obstructions (deficiencies) or outpourings (excesses) in the circulation of the ch'i. This view linked pathology of the visceral organs with dysfunction of somatic structures and abnormal sensations throughout the body such as chronic pain, giving rise to medical treatments designed to restore balance. Among these were the first effective treatments for chronic pain, including the precursors for many of the medications and techniques that we use to this day (Ness, 1995).

Without the concept of "underlying disease," the Hippocratic physicians did not view pain as an alarm or a sentinel or a prodrome of illness—they regarded it as the illness itself. The Hippocratics had not conceived of the positive value of pain and taught that pain predisposed a part of the body to attract and invoke disease. Their observation that artificially induced pain was sharper than naturally occurring pain and could provide relief led to their use of painful remedies such as blistering agents, rubifacients, and moxibustion, an adaptation of traditional Chinese therapy that consisted of burning a fabric or vegetable material on the skin in order to create a diversionary point (Rey, 1995). In addition to painful therapies, the physicians of antiquity promoted the use of narcotic plants such as mandrake, hyocyamus (henbane), nightshade, and opium poppies (Moisan, 1978). In the first century a.d., Dioscorides described the formulation of a strong pain medication in *De Materia Medica:* the juice of the plant papaver nigrum was dried in the sun and then kneaded into small cakes, which he termed *opium*.

With the Age of Enlightenment, Western medicine began to appreciate the usefulness and the value of pain. Pain was seen as a warning or alarm, diverting us from harmful lifestyles. Pain also took on a diagnostic value. Differentiation among the various types of pain led to diagnoses of underlying pathology. As Western medicine strengthened its ties to religion, a link was established between pain and the concept of divine punishment. Pain relief came to be opposed on religious grounds. Pain and illness were seen as an apprenticeship of the functioning of the human spirit (Double, 1805). Chronic pain and suffering took on a redemptive value. Church literature discussed how suffering brought the individual closer to Christ. The concept of the usefulness of medically inflicted pain paralleled the rise of surgery. Postoperative pain was seen as sign that healing was underway. This led to an antipathy toward anesthesia and the contention that "those operations in which sedatives have been used with the aim of sparing the sick some pain have been less successful" (Double, 1805).

The 17th century saw a divergence between physicians who promoted "natural healing" and those who aggressively promoted the interventional "art of medicine." The former included British physicians like Thomas Sydenham (the "English Hippocrates"), who drew attention to observing "the course of nature" in illness. Sydenham felt that it was medically important to treat pain. He revived and publicized the use of opium-containing compounds that had been held in disrepute by other contemporary physicians. He wrote that "so necessary an instrument is opium in the hand of a skillful man that medicine would be a cripple without it" (Latham, 1848). He was also the first modern physician to discuss dosing analgesics for children. Sydenham was credited with popularizing the use of analgesics and with developing the formulation for laudenum.

Sydenham's Recipe for Laudenum
  Sherry wine—1 pint
  Opium—2 ounces
  Saffron—1 ounce
  Cinnamon—1 stick, powdered
  Clove—1 powdered
  Mix and simmer over a vapor bath for 2 to 3 days until the tincture has the proper consistency. (Latham, 1848)

The conflict between the surgeons and physicians over the proper course of European medicine continued on into the end of the 18thcentury. In 18th century Britain surgery, with its qualities of manual labor and technical proficiency, was considered a skilled craft rather than a profession. Its practitioners were considered separate from and subordinate to the gentlemen physicians (hence the distinction between the gentleman "doctor" and the surgical "mister"). With the success of the Revolution, Americans began to bridle against British tradition and searched for uniquely "American" ways of doing things. Hence, the practice of surgery in the United States was elevated and came to be considered heroic.

A major advocate of this change was Dr. Benjamin Rush, a signer of the Declaration of Independence and a founder of America's first medical school who is considered the "father of American medicine" as well as the founder of the field of psychiatry. Although his predecessors had sought to balance "depletive therapies" (bloodletting, purging, emetics, mercury) with "restorative treatments" or "tonics" (e.g., chinchona, opium, alcohol), Rush eschewed the tonics and championed the universal deployment of harsh depletive remedies and their "heroic administration" in massive doses (Pernick, 1985). Rush's teachings dominated American medicine well into the 1830s and reverberate to this day. Rush maintained that without the heroic intervention of the Medical Art most illnesses would naturally worsen, terminating in death (Pernick, 1985). Rush felt that the first duty of the physician was "heroic action to fight disease" rather than to provide comfort. In opposition to the Hippocratic credo of "do no harm"—which at that time had been retranslated to "*first of all*, do no harm" (Holmes, 1891)—Rush regarded the physician who killed the patient through overdosing as merely zealous, whereas the physician who allowed a patient to die through insufficiently vigorous therapy was both a murderer and a quack (Rush, 1947).

A Modern—and Ancient—View of Chronic Pain

In light of recent advances in our understanding of anatomy and physiology, today may be a good time to revisit the concept of yin and yang. We can now regard pain as an expression of the function of a very complex and delicately balanced *nociceptive system*. When this system functions properly, it protects us from injury, promotes healing, protects us from further trauma, and sustains life. In this way, it is analogous to the other balanced healing systems that keep us alive, such as the coagulation system. The analogy even extends to the way the two subjects are taught because current medical teaching about pain mimics the teaching on coagulation that was promulgated up until 30 years ago.

For hundreds of years, we knew only about the procoagulant parts of the coagulation system. The fact that blood coagulated in response to injury was considered a miracle. Later, we began to understand that the real miracle was that our blood wasn't clotting all the time. Eventually, we understood that there was a complex counterbalancing anticoagulation system that was activated as soon as coagulation was triggered. Because of the relationship between these counterbalancing systems, coagulation is localized in time and place, maintaining a meaningful relationship to trauma and promoting survival. When coagulation and anticoagulation maintain this balance, we are healthy. When this balance is disrupted, we have a group of diseases collectively termed the coagulopathies, clinically expressed as inappropriate thromboembolism or hemorrhage. When faced with a patient with a coagulopathy, we don't institute treatment aimed at obliterating clotting, we seek to restore the balance and promote healthful coagulation.

The nociceptive system is similarly balanced by a complex antinociceptive system that allows pain to perform its life-sustaining functions. These include acute pain, which functions as an alarm warning us about injury; the development of transient hypersensitivity, which protects the injured area from further injury; a link to memory, which teaches us to avoid future injury; and the activation of natural pain relievers, which ensure that the pain resolves so that we can continue functioning. When the pain system functions effectively, it promotes life. When pain becomes disconnected from meaning due to an imbalance of its nociceptive and antinociceptive functions, it becomes a disease, chronic pain, and diminishes life. Chronic pain is pain that has lost its purpose.

A comparison of the physiology of normal pain and the pathophysiology of chronic pain reveal important neurochemical differences that support the contention that chronic pain is indeed a medical disorder. Or rather, like the coagulopathies, the term *chronic pain* describes a group of medical disorders with identifiable pathophysiologies whose understanding should guide us to rational treatments. Ultimately, these treatments won't be aimed at "killing pain" but rather at restoring balance, promoting function, and alleviating suffering. This should even be reflected in the words we choose to describe what we do. Many Western words for *pain* come from the Latin root *doles*, which is an objective word that can have an inanimate object, such as *caput doles*, which translates to "my head feels pain" or "I have a headache." In distinction, the Latin root for suffering, *suffere*, means to bear, to endure, or to allow. It is a verb that requires an active subject, in other words, a person. This brings us back to the Hippocratics, who taught us that "pain happens to a body and suffering happens to a person."

What Does the Pain Feel Like?

The understanding that there are different types of pain goes back to antiquity. The Hippocratics taught that the patient had an obligation to disclose and describe his pain. It was the patient's duty to recall what he experienced and the physician's duty to listen. Hippocrates warned that the physician who strayed from this belief would not favor the right frame of mind and would stray from the truth (Rey, 1995). In the early classifications of pain, when the imbalance of humours was seen as a more important generator of disease than the dysfunction of organs, details about the type and intensity of the pain prevailed over location. Books on diagnostics focused on the semiotics of illness and encouraged attention to the minutiae of descriptions because "the mode of the pain indicates the judgement which should be made about the illness" (Landre-Beauvais, 1813). For example, differentiation of various types of "inflammation of the chest" allowed physicians to distinguish among different conditions with different outcomes. "The pain is tearing and superficial and increases with movements of the arms or trunk in inflammation of the chest wall. Pain is lancinating in pleurisy, it is deeper and often gravitative in peripneumonia; it is more general, more widely prevalent and duller in catarrh" (Landre-Beauvais, 1813). These days, patients in chronic pain are still asked, "What does the pain feel like?" but modern culture and linguistics often limit the response. As Virginia Woolf wrote, "The merest schoolgirl, when she falls in love, has Shakespeare or Keats to speak her mind for her; but let a sufferer try to describe a pain in his head to a doctor and language at once runs dry" (Woolf, 1930).

Galen was one of the first to conceptualize the physiology of nociception when he described pain as a response to events that occurred outside the body. He said that there were three necessary conditions for the perception of pain: an organ to receive an outside impression, a connecting passageway, and an organizational center to transform the sensation into a conscious perception (Darmberg, 1856). With the development of the field of pathological anatomy, the identity of the affected area or the damaged organ assumed increasing importance. However, postmortem examinations often found no trace of damage and such pain was often termed "functional" rather than "structural."

A current basis for discriminating among different types of pain depends on the physiologic generator of the pain. Injury to peripheral tissues such as skin, muscle, or fascia gives rise to *somatic* pain. Pain generated by visceral tissues is not always related to injury and gives rise to sensations that can distinctly be identified as *visceral pain*. Injury, stimulation, or regrowth of nerves can give rise to various forms of *neuropathic pain,* which is often characterized by dysesthetic sensations such as burning, painful numbness, or electrical sensations with lancinations. Recognition that these generators give rise to different sensory experiences reinforces the Hippocratic exhortation to listen to our patients' descriptions.

Somatic Pain: A Part of Healing

> We can recollect that we suffered but in no way remember the particular quality of the pain which we suffered. (Boerhaave, *Aphorisms of Surgery*, 1753)

For most people, including physicians, the model of "normal pain" is that of pain linked temporally and topographically to injury to superficial connective tissue. Most of the acute pain that we experience in our lifetimes is somatic pain related to minor trauma to skin, muscle, or fascia. This type of pain has several functions. It acts as an alarm that is localized in time and place. Its most intense component has a fast onset after the injury and is typically dampened long before the injury heals. The injured area is left with a persistent hypersensitivity, which protects against trauma and promotes healing. Another important function of the pain is that it is rapidly integrated into memory to help us avoid repeated injuries. For example, children with attention deficits or learning disorders are found to be at risk for repeat injuries even though they can sense pain adequately (McGrath, 2004). Timely relief of the pain is another function of the nociceptive system that is just as important to normal function as is the ability to sense pain (Apkarian, 1995). Although the memory of injuries is typically profound and evocative, recalling the injury generally does not involve reexperiencing the sensation of pain. Under normal circumstances, we are supposed to remember and learn from our pain but we are not supposed to keep reliving it. In a neurochemical sense, patients with chronic pain are often reexperiencing past injuries.

Somatic Pain and the Process of Inflammation

Even minor disruption of tissue causes the release of chemical mediators from lysosomes and cell membranes, giving rise to a chemically cascading inflammatory reaction triggering electrical signals in sensory nerves that carry the message of pain to the brain (Levine and Taiwo, 1994). Because of the self-augmenting nature of this inflammatory reaction, an intense pain signal can be rapidly generated by a minor injury. The analogy I use when describing this to patients is that of smoke alarms, which we program to give off the loudest blare with the first hint of smoke (i.e., the signal is out of proportion to the stimulus).

The chemical reactions that link the release of cellular elements to pain have much in common with other cascading healing processes such as coagulation and wound healing. They even share some of the same mediators such as the serine protease kallikreins, which cleave high and low molecular weight kinninogens to form the kinins, the peptides bradykinin and kallidin. Bradykinin, which works through the activation of specific B_1 and B_2 receptors, is one of the most important chemical mediators of acute pain. Activation of B_2 receptors stimulates excitatory currents in specific populations of sensory neurons called nociceptors, which carry the electrical signal of pain to the dorsal horn of the spinal cord. Postactivation hyperpolarization limits ability of these nociceptors to fire repetitively, and the initial excitatory effects of bradykinin are transient due to this rapid desensitization. This can account for the short-lived "intensely sharp" element of acute somatic pain. Activation of B_1 receptors on mast cells and macrophages provokes the elaboration of other inflammatory mediators such as cytokines, histamine, and nitric oxide and amplifies the inflammatory reaction. Activation of B_1 receptors on vascular cells cause increase in permeability of blood vessels (Rang and Perkins, 1997).

Injuries to cells will also cause release of a group of cell membrane phospholipids, collectively known as eicosanoids, which are metabolized by the arachadonic acid pathway to prostaglandins and thromboxanes or via the lipooxygenase pathway to leukotrienes ($LT-D_4$ and $LT-B_4$) and "slow reacting-substance" (SRS), all of which are potent mediators of inflammation (Kumazawa, 1996). Activation of the enzyme phopholipase A, which is stimulated by bradykinin acting through the B_1 receptor on inflammatory cells, triggers the arachadonic acid pathway resulting in the production of prostaglandins, most prominently $PG-I_2$ but also $PG-D_2$, $PG-E_1$, and PG-E$_2$. These prostaglandins do not primarily evoke a pain impulse, but they modify B-2 receptors on sensory neurons and sensitize nociceptors terminals to mechanical and thermal stimuli, setting up persistent hypersensitivity of the injured area (hyperalgesia) and the perception of pain in response to mechanical or thermal stimuli that were not painful in the uninjured state (allodynia). These delayed excitatory effects of bradykinin are specifically inhibited by cyclooxygenase inhibitors (Steranka et al., 1988).

Other mediators of delayed-onset pain include leukotriene LT-B$_4$, which exerts its effects through its action as a chemoattractant for leukocytes, which in turn release a factor called 8R,15S-diHETE, which acts at a specific receptor on afferent nerves that is distinct from the prostaglandin receptor (Levine et al., 1986). Other mediators of inflammation including adenosine and mast-cell activators come from the lysosomal contents of injured cells. Adenosine activates the A-2 receptor on nociceptors. Activation of mast cells leads to the release of platelet activating factors, which lead to release of serotonin. Serotonin enhances the response of nociceptors to bradykinin and directly activates 5-HT3 and 5-HT1A receptors on nociceptive afferents (Taiwo and Levine, 1992).

Persistent inflammation can also lead to local tissue acidosis, which contributes to pain and hyperalgesia through the generation of protons. Protons can also selectively activate nociceptors and sensitize nociceptors to mechanical stimuli. Leukocytes attracted by inflammatory mediators and the actions of peripheral nerves elaborate interleukins, which promote inflammation. Interleukin-1 (IL-1) stimulates the activity of phospholipase-C, which promotes the production of prostaglandin-E. Interleukin-8 (IL-8) produces sympathetic-dependent hyperalgesia that is independent of the action of prostaglandins (Cunha et al., 1991). Specific inflammatory factors may be related to specific disease states. For example, certain cancers such as prostate tumors can elaborate high concentrations of endothelin-1 which can primarily activate populations of afferent nerves causing severe pain (Mantyh et al., 2003).

A Role for Nerves in Peripheral Inflammation

Pain-transmitting nerve cells, specifically nonmyelinated C fibers and small-caliber myelinated A-delta fibers, appear to play a dual role in translating trauma into pain. Not only do these cells carry electrical signals from the periphery to the spinal cord, but they are also secrete inflammatory mediators. In response to stimulation of their distal endings by kinins, these nerves release proinflammatory chemicals such as calcitonin-gene related peptide (CGRP) and substance P, both of which promote inflammation and which, with prolonged secretion, can promote the growth of pain nerves possibly contributing to chronic pain states (McMahon, 1996). This efferent function for nociceptive nerves was first suggested over 70 years ago, when it was ascertained that these peripheral fibers mediated the "flare reaction" surrounding acute cutaneous injuries that did not require a connection to the spinal cord (Lewis, 1937).

It has long been noted that cutaneous nerves generally contain more than a fourfold higher number of small nonmyelinated pain fibers than larger myelinated tactile fibers (McMahon and Koltzenburg, 1990) even though electrical activity concerning tactile stimulation is much more frequent than sensory transmissions related to pain. This suggests that the effector functions of these nerves may be as important as their afferent function. These peripheral fibers may play an important role in the efferent control of healing by regulating blood flow and vascular permeability in peripheral tissues, maintaining the integrity of skin, and controlling certain immunologic functions such as emigration of leukocytes (Nilsson et al., 1985).

If inflammation persists, factors that promote nerve growth may be released, prolonging inflammation and setting the stage for the establishment of chronic pain. The source can be immune cells (mast cells, macrophages, lymphocytes), fibroblasts, or Schwann cells in inflamed tissue. In skin, the main source of nerve growth factors are basal keratinocytes. Peripheral concentrations of nerve growth factors are increased in models of chronic inflammation such as the human synovium in arthritis (Aloe et al., 1992) or the bladder wall in interstitial cystitis (Lowe et al., 1997).

Peripheral Hyperalgesia and Allodynia

Peripheral inflammation will not only give rise to acute pain, it will also induce hyperalgesia and allodynia. Hyperalgesia is a sensitized state in which a mildly painful stimuli will cause exaggerated pain. Allodynia describes a state where a normally nonnoxious stimulus, such light touch or movement, will be perceived as painful. An example of this would be an area of skin that has suffered a burn. Not only will that area of skin hurt, but a normally nonpainful stimulus such as light touch will also be painful. Interleukin-1 is important in the initiation of hyperalgesia (McMahon et al., 1995). The release of nerve growth factors such as substance P activating NK-1 receptors on inflammatory cells are often important for the maintenance of the allodynic state, which is often a key feature of chronic pain. Sympathetic activation and release of norepinephrine can also produce hyperalgesia but only in the presence of tissue injury. In these cases, norepinephrine may potentiate pain by stimulating the production of prostaglandins and activating phospholipase C (Gonzales et al., 1989).

Chemosensitive afferent nerves may become so sensitized by persistent pain that a low-intensity stimulus will provoke hyperalgesia, the perception of high-intensity pain. In certain syndromes, unremitting pain signals may activate usually quiet mechanosensitive afferent nerves, called "silent afferents," that are present in synovial tissue and in all viscus organs (McMahon and Koltzenburg, 1994). Once activated, even slight movement or minimal deformity of surrounding tissues can generate pain. This type of allodynia is common in chronic degenerative arthritis, low back pain, and severe irritable bowel syndrome and other chronically painful conditions.

In addition to causing local pain at the site of an injury, bradykinin can also act in the brain and spinal cord to cause global hyperalgesia. This may account for the diffuse myalgias that often accompany infections and other inflammatory states. In animal models, this can be induced by intracerebral injection of bacterial lipopolysaccharides, which globally enhance nociceptive transmission thereby amplifying all pains. Lipopolysaccharides are thought to act by inducing immune cells to secrete interleukin-1beta, resulting in the stimulation of vagal afferents via the tract solitarius which connects to descending pathways from the raphe magnus that synapse with the descending spinal cord tracts that cause diffuse hyperalgesia (Levine and Taiwo, 1994).

Maintaining the Balance: Natural Antiinflammatories

As with other balanced chemical reactions in the body, tissue trauma results in the release of a mix of agonists and antagonists of inflammation. Angiotensin-converting enzyme and other peptidases inactivate bradykinin and other kinins. Another natural antiinflammatory compound is beta endorphin, which is released by peripheral leukocytes. Through their action on opiate receptors on nerve fibers, endorphins inhibit the release of proinflammatory mediators (such as substance P from peripheral sensory nerve endings), reducing peripheral vasodilatation. Opioid receptors are upregulated on cutaneous nerves in inflamed tissue, though this can be undermined by nerve damage (e.g., ligation of the sciatic nerve). Corticotropin-releasing factor (CRF), a major secretagogue for opioid peptides from leukocytes and the pituitary, is locally produced in inflamed tissue. Corticosteroids inhibit phospholipase A2—preventing the generation of arachidonic acid (Stein et al., 1997). IL-1 elaborated by immune cells, usually thought of as a potent mediator of inflammation, can do the same. In studies, locally applied IL-1 and CRF produce antinociceptive effects in inflamed but not in noninflamed tissues (Shafer et al., 1996).

Visceral Pain

In 1628, a nobleman and his son went hunting with the king of England. The boy was thrown from his horse and injured his chest, tearing open his rib cage and exposing his heart and lungs. The King summoned his physician, William Harvey, who probed the exposed viscera with his dagger and noted that the boy, though fully awake, could not detect the pricking or pinching of his heart and lungs. Harvey concluded that these organs were insensate (Bonica, 1991). Visceral tissue will release inflammatory mediators in response to injury, but the pain response differs from that in somatic tissue. The viscera do not have the same protective apparatus signaling tissue damage as do connective tissues. For example, there are no specific nociceptors found in the heart and bradykinin doesn't elicit pain when injected into the coronaries or pericardial sac (Cervero, 1995).

Most visceral organs are invested with high threshold afferents that are triggered by intense contractions of the hollow viscus. The nerves that carry these signals are large-diameter myelinated fibers, which synapse with the posterior columns of the spinal cord, a pattern of input that parallels that for proprioception from the limbs and the trunk (Aidar et al., 1952). Prolonged stimulation or injury leads to a unique form of peripheral sensitization that is dependent on activation and recruitment of silent nociceptors, which respond mostly to mechanical stimuli and may eventually become activated by normal functioning. These two sets of nerves—high threshold contraction receptors and intensity-coding silent afferents—can generate pain in the absence of injury or abnormal mechanical activity. This appears to be the case in irritable bowel syndrome, in which normal activity of the gastrointestinal tract becomes painful. Different organs are invested with a unique palette of receptors that respond to stretch, pressure, and inflammatory chemicals (Sengupta and Gebhart, 1994a). Some visceral organs (e.g., the esophagus) do have nerves with specific receptors for bradykinin. In addition, bradykinin released from injured viscera can trigger vagal impulses (Cervero, 1994).

Typically, pain emanating from the viscera is diffuse and poorly localized. This reflects differences in innervation between somatic and visceral tissue. Somatic connections are precisely located at the spinal cord and the brain, whereas afferent viscerosensory fibers overlap each other and converge at several levels within the central nervous system. Because of this pattern of innervation, visceral injury is often accompanied by motor and autonomic reflexes, and these may be the major generators of the perceived pain related to visceral injury. Of the afferent fibers that innervate the viscera, C-fibers and A-delta fibers make up less than 30%, compared to over 80% in skin and connective tissue (Sengupta and Gebhart, 1994b). Nearly 80% of visceral afferents are silent mechanosensitive afferents.

Although specific areas of the skin and connective tissue are neurologically mapped to single areas of the spinal cord, much of the viscera, such as the gut, have dual sensory circuits, with splanchnic nerves innervating the entire gut projecting to the thoracolumbar spine and vagal afferents projecting from the proximal gut to the sigmoid colon. The close overlap of brain centers concerned with processing visceral afferent information, autonomic function, and arousal account for the distinct reflexive and affective components of visceral pain. This results in a higher degree of visceral-autonomic integration in visceral pain and the recruitment of endocrine function by the time sensation reaches consciousness, usually via stimulation of the vagal fibers—over 85% of which are afferent (Malliani, 1994).

Visceral Pain Is Not a Reliable Alarm Like Somatic Pain

The differences in somatic and visceral neural architecture invest somatic and visceral pains with different meanings.

> Somatosensory pathways consist of an intricate system of afferents, ascending tracts and processing centers in the spinal cord and in the brain that accurately relay bodily encounters with different types of stimuli. The system enables the individual to sense the stimulus, filter it and perceive it at will. Consequently, the individual can often choose the encounter or avoid it if he controls the agent. The motor system is always available to execute his will (i.e., he can find a comfortable bodily position). Viscerosensory mechanisms are different. The individual does not control any of the components involved. The stimuli are not avoidable and the autonomic nervous system is not commonly mastered. (Al Chaer et al., 1998)

Misunderstandings about the differences between the mechanisms of somatic and visceral pain may promote overreliance on visceral pain as a harbinger of injury. Osler wrote extensively about the unreliability of chest pain as an indicator of cardiac injury. He noted that "in acute endocarditis, pain is rarely present, and that ulceration of valves or of the wall may proceed to a most extreme degree without any sensory disturbance" (Osler, 1910).

This is certainly an important issue when a patient's perception of pain is used as a clinical endpoint in the guidance of treatment. For example, compared to the body's response to somatic injury, angina is a relatively late manifestation of myocardial ischemia. One-fourth of documented myocardial infarctions are "silent." In fact, most infarctions are preceded by silent ischemia, which means that only a minority of ischemic cardiac episodes are experienced as angina. This may relate to the individual patient's overall pain threshold (e.g., it is related to sensitivity to electrically induced dental pain). It is well known that silent myocardial infarctions are more frequent in diabetics. This may be due to neuropathy blocking or depressing autonomic activation. It has also been documented that people who secrete more endorphins during exercise, such as athletes, will have more silent ischemia than nonathletes. Because of this, opioid-antagonists like naloxone are sometimes used as a pretreatment in the exercise testing of athletic patients thought to have coronary artery disease (Canon, 1995).

Visceral Hyperalgesia

Because of its neurologic mapping and reflex involvement, chronic visceral pain, such as irritable bowel syndrome (IBS), is often expressed as "a functional disorder". Such syndromes often feature extra-organ involvement, such as sexual dysfunction, sleep disruption, and fibromyalgialike symptoms (Nabiloff et al., 1993). It will often feature a prominent affective component, such as anxiety and depression. In fact, the chemical changes in the spinal cord and peripheral nerves in IBS and other functional visceral disorders bear a striking resemblance to the disordered processing of serotonin in the brain that is associated with depression. IBS affects up to 22% of U.S. population. The majority of these patients report "hypersensitive stomachs" or "mild bowel dysfunction" dating back to childhood, though many do not connect this to their diagnosis of IBS. There is probably a genetic predisposition to IBS (Locke et al., 1996). There also appears to be an association between IBS and a history of major traumatic events (physical or sexual abuse) or major losses during childhood (Talley et al., 1998). This may relate to a specific period of intense neural modeling during childhood. Approximately one-third of IBS patients develop their symptoms following acute gastrointestinal infections, though these patients often have other risk factors. This suggests that in susceptible individuals, enteric infections and other causes of mucosal inflammation can precipitate ongoing IBS symptoms, which can persist long after the infection or inflammation is gone (Nabiloff et al., 1993).

Peripheral Nociceptors

Progressing from the level of peripheral somatic and visceral tissues to the peripheral nervous system, there are two types of specialized nociceptors, poorly myelinated A-delta fibers and unmyelinated C-fibers. A-delta fibers are faster transmitters and mediate "first pain," which usually has sharp or acute pricking characteristics. There are two types of A-delta fibers: type I are activated in heat and burn injury, and type II are activated by substance P and moderate heat.

C-fibers, which are activated by bradykinin and other mediators, are responsible for the delayed, dull, aching and burning components of the pain sensation. One group (type I) can secrete neuropeptide neurotransmitters such as substance P, CGRP and express the TrkA receptor for nerve growth factor (NGF). The other group (type II) depends on local glial cell-derived growth factors and is sensitized by protons. Most C-fibers are polymodal in that they can respond to a broad range of stimuli including thermal, mechanical, and chemical stimulation. One of the most important interfaces between the tissue injury and the nerve impulse is the vanilloid receptor 1 (VR-1) on nociceptive nerve cells. Activating VR-1 opens a calcium channel in the nerve cell. This can be directly activated by capsaicin, heat, protons (H+ ions), lipids (e.g., cell breakdown products), and substance P. Some C-fibers also have channels that respond directly to cold via CMR-1 receptors, which is thought to be the "cold counterpart" and close molecular cousin to VR-1. These receptors can be also triggered directly by chemicals such as menthol and peppermint, and this activation can cause a "cooling" sensation. Other C-fibers can respond directly to mechanical pressure via an apparatus that is localized in the cell membrane (Koltzenburg, 1999).

The two types of C-fibers connect to different areas of the dorsal horn of the spinal cord. C-I fibers synapse with cells in the superficial dorsal horn, and C-II fibers go to the deeper substantia gelatinosa. C-fibers subserving different tissues of the body have their own unique pattern of connection to the spinal cord. C-fibers from the skin terminate in highly topographic fashion in the substantia gelatinosa, whereas nociceptive inputs from the viscera connect in a more diffuse, less topographic pattern.

In chronic pain states, peripheral nociceptors can undergo a broad range of changes. Individual fibers can become more responsive to a given stimulus (a condition termed *wind-up*), firing at lower thresholds and generating more signals for a given stimulus. High-threshold nociceptors may also reduce their thresholds and thus become recruited into the generation of the pain signal, making it a more complex and intense input than it had been originally. This peripheral sensitization is mediated by several factors, which include the persistent generation of bradykinin, high concentrations of protons (which are part of the inflammatory milieu), and neurotrophic factors such as NGF released by mast cells and fibroblasts (Mendell et al., 1999).

Nerve Growth Factors

Nerve growth and maintenance are ongoing processes in normal tissue. Peripheral tissues have to maintain their complement of nociceptors by secreting nerve growth factors. Nerve growth factors influence the growth, survival, and even the phenotype of peripheral sensory nerves. These factors include nerve growth factor-1 (NGF), which is critical to the development and maintenance of both C-fibers and A-delta type nociceptors. Hypersecretion of NGF may also be responsible for the maintenance of chronic pain states. NGF also mediates the hyperalgesia—for example, sensitivity to touch—of injured tissue. Therapeutic trials of NGF in the treatment of diabetic neuropathy have resulted in persistent fibromyalgialike syndromes (Apfel, 2000). Because NGF doesn't cross the blood-brain barrier, this was attributed to actions on peripheral nerves (Apfel, 2002).

In addition to NGF, the family of neurotrophins includes brain-derived neurotrophic factor (BDNF) and neurotrophin-3 (NT-3). Glial-derived neurotrophic factor (GDNF) may have a specific role in maintaining the state of chronic pain. GDNF interacts with type II C-fibers. The different neurotrophins act through a family of specific receptors that activate tyrosine kinase, the Trk receptors. NGF interacts with TrkA, BDNF with TrkB, and NT-3 with TrkC.

Nerves in the Balance: The Ecology of Peripheral Nerve Bundles

Peripheral sensory nerves, both nociceptive and nonnociceptive, exist in a balance within their nerve bundles, which is regulated by the secretion of various neurotrophins. Disruption of this balance can lead to abnormal growth of one population. If one population of nerves is injured, another population may become activated. This is invoked as one of the many mechanisms of nerve-damage derived pain (neuropathic pain).

In an experimental model that reflects clinical experience, resection of the sciatic nerve causes the destruction of the C-fiber terminals where they synapse in the pain-sensing areas of the superficial dorsal horn of the spinal cord. The loss of these connections causes the endings of large myelinated A-fibers to become activated. A-fibers are not nociceptors but rather nerves that carry the sensation of touch. The endings of these large fibers can now invade the superficial dorsal horn region. These large nerves, which are activated by touch, now carry a signal to an area that interprets the incoming signal as pain. That patient will now experience pain to the noninjurious stimulus of touch.

This type of allodynia is commonly seen in patients with chronic back pain who have undergone surgery and may be part of the explanation of "post-laminectomy syndrome." It is easy to assess clinically but does not show up on CT scans, MRIs, EMGs, or nerve conduction studies. Not only do these cells mediate allodynia, but they are relatively resistant to the inhibiting effects of endorphins or opioid medications because A-fibers do not produce opioid receptors. This may also be part of the mechanism of the agonizing pain of reflex sympathetic dystrophy and explain its relative insensitivity to opioid medications (Baron, 2000).

Loss of tactile A-fibers due to destruction by persistent hyperglycemia can result in a different pain syndrome characterized as the "mononeuritis multiplex" seen in diabetics. In this syndrome, C-fibers remain intact. The oligodendrocytes that form the myelin sheath around the dying A-fibers migrate and insulate the pain fibers, which can now transmit their signals with greater efficiency and deliver their signals to the spinal cord unopposed. These patients will experience a loss of tactile function and experience a worsening sensation of "painful numbness." Biopsies of the affected areas show dropout of tactile A-fibers and abnormal myelination of C-fibers. In experimental models that appear to bear close resemblance to what we see in the clinic, damage to motor or sensory nerves in one dermatome (mimicking that caused by back surgery or rhizotomy) can lead to spontaneous activity among nociceptors in adjacent dermatomes. Schwann cells can then be stimulated to proliferate in peripheral nerve Remak bundles causing abnormal myelination (and hyperefficiency) of uninjured peripheral nociceptors (Dyck and Gianni, 1996).

Damage to Pain Nerves Can Cause Pain

Most of what we learned in medical school about the peripheral nervous system is based on motor nerves. Because of this, many of us have come to subscribe to a simple model of the peripheral nervous system—hardwired, unchanging, with a discrete partitioning between the motor and sensory systems. Understanding pain and pain-related disorders will necessitate a reconsideration of the role and actions of the sensory nervous system. The sensory nervous system features constant messages, interactions with motor fibers and neuroplasticity, which is the key to understanding chronic pain. Nerves that carry persistent signals will "learn" how to carry these signals more efficiently (hypersensitization), eventually acquiring the ability to transmit messages independent of peripheral stimuli. They may eventually recruit other nerves that weren't involved in the response to the initial stimulus to start firing. Ultimately, some of these activated sensory nerves may "cross the line" between afferent and efferent.

An important "new" concept that is vital to the understanding of chronic pain is that nerves can heal after injury. The idea that chronic pain can result from injury to nerves and abnormal healing is not really new, but it is still not yet widely accepted. In the 19th century the idea of "pain without lesion," the neuralgias, were first described by Francois Chaussier, a professor at the Ecole de Santé in Paris who is credited with coining the term *tic douloureux* and describing the characteristics of neuropathic pain. He associated this type of pain with damage to a nerve trunk or with disruption of branches of nerves. He observed this type of pain in instances in which tumors compressed nerves or in wounds severing nerves. He described a type of pain that persisted after healing was complete. He noted that a distinctive sign of neuralgia was that sectioning of the nerve "stopped the pain for a certain length of time though it *inevitably returned*—often in a more serious form" (Mitchell, 1874).

One would expect that nerve damage would result in lack of function. Certainly if one cuts a motor nerve, it results in persistent paralysis. That used to be interpreted to mean that the motor nerve had died. For hundreds of years, the same was thought to be true for nociceptive fibers. For hundreds of years, physicians have been treating people in pain by cutting or damaging pain nerves, in the hope that they would reduce or eliminate the ability to feel the pain. Many surgeries and procedures that are done for pain—ranging from occipital neurectomies for chronic headaches to many of the back surgeries that used to be performed to hysterectomies for poorly defined pelvic pain—involve neurodestruction. Some of these procedures do give relief—but often the relief is only temporarily and is followed by a worsening of the previous pain, often with characteristics that clinicians won't believe.

Patients seeking medical care for neuropathic pain syndromes, such as postsurgical neuropathies or reflex sympathetic dystrophy or causalgia, have long been met with confusion, disbelief, and even suspicion (Schott, 2001). Faced with symptoms out of proportion to injury, anatomically "impossible" patterns of pain and lacking a defined pathogenesis or a set of diagnostic criteria, many physicians have been quick to call these pains psychogenic (Zyluk, 1999). Eventually, even neurologically "impossible" findings will find an explanation. Recent advances in research into the mechanisms underlying posttraumatic neuropathic pain are allowing us to look at the sensory nervous system in a completely new way that will help us explain many of the findings characteristic of neuropathic pain.

Until recently, many clinicians and investigators attributed chronic neuropathic pain to personality disorders such as hypochondriasis (Drucker et al., 1959; Holden, 1948). Others, such as Dr. John Bonica, showed that the abnormalities in personality and behavior that were associated with chronic neuropathic pain disappeared after the pain was relieved, strongly suggesting that these abnormalities were the sequelae of the terrible pain and not the cause (Bonica, 1979). Even abnormalities commonly found on psychological testing of patients with pain due to nerve damage, such as those on the MMPI—which was once thought to be an indelible fingerprint of personality—were found to normalize when the pain was relieved (Sternbach and Timmermans, 1975).

Reactive Gliosis as a Generator of Chronic Pain

The most exciting recent insights into the mechanism of neuropathic pain relate to the role played by glial cells, a group of nonneuronal cells that are vital to the maintenance, growth, and repair of the nervous system. There are three major types of glial cells in the central nervous system: astrocytes, microglia, and oligodendrocytes. Astrocytes surround synapses and can sense synaptic activity. They regulate the utilization of neurotransmitters and glucose at the synapse. Microglia are mediators of CNS inflammation and are a rich source of proinflammatory cytokines. Oligodendrocytes are the myelin-forming cells that ensheath nerve axons.

Each nociceptive cell body in a dorsal root ganglion (DRG) is encapsulated by a layer of glial cells with a basement lamina separating neighboring glially encapsulated neuronal cell bodies (Sakuma et al., 2001). Glial cells regulate neuronal activity in the DRG and the availability of extracellular glutamate, aspartate, and the glutamate-precursor glutamine (Duce and Keen, 1983; Kai-Kai and Howe, 1991). The glial cells can communicate with each other via gap junctions (Said and Hontebeyrie-Joskowicz, 1992). They can release proinflammatory cytokines and growth factors when stimulated by peripheral nerve injury. The glia's ability to respond to neurotransmitters allows them to continuously monitor the physiologic integrity of their microenvironment and react rapidly in the event of disturbances.

Injury to the central nervous system often results in the degeneration of neurons and oligodendrocytes (Chen et al., 2005). The destruction of oligodendrocytes and the resultant demyelination after trauma both appear to be mediated by the activation of NMDA receptors on these cells (Micu et al., 2005). Trauma to neural tissue also causes postlesional inhibition of oligodendrocyte growth and replication (Schwab et al., 2005).

In contrast, trauma within the nervous systems triggers the growth of astrocytes and microglia in a process termed *reactive gliosis*, which is analogous to the posttraumatic inflammation seen in peripheral tissues that are subject to injury. Reactive gliosis is a prominent consequence of most pathological processes in the central nervous system and has been associated with the promotion of abnormal pain. The hyperalgesia, allodynia, and many of the "anatomically impossible" features of neuropathic pain become explicable when seen as part of a neuroinflammatory process mediated by glial cells.

Astrocytes and Pain

Astrocytes surround synapses and regulate synaptic activity by adjusting the concentration of neurotransmitters in the synaptic clefts. Under normal conditions, astrocytes remove excess glutamate and aspartate from synaptic spaces and store it. Astrocytes are similar to nerve cells in that they have receptors for neurotransmitters and that they communicate with each other and with neural cells via intercellular gap junctions. In a sense, astrocytes form a second nervous system serving the neural nervous system (Szatkowski et al., 1990).

One of the most important functions of astrocytes is to integrate neuronal inputs and regulate the neurotransmitters that modulate synaptic sensitivity. Under certain conditions, astrocytes can release their stored neurotransmitters into the synapse, initiating or amplifying a pain signal. Astrocytes have their own AMPA and NMDA receptors for glutamate, and stimulation of these receptors or sensitization of the cell by prostaglandins will trigger the release of stored neurotransmitters (Szatkowski et al., 1990).

Astrocytes enwrap pre- and postsynaptic terminals. A single astrocyte can have contact with and be depolarized by multiple neurons (Ventura and Harris, 1999). The excitability of astrocytes is mediated by calcium fluxes. Stimulation of astrocytes by glutamate (Porter and McCarthy, 1996), norepinephrine (Muyderman et al., 1998), histamine, or other inflammatory mediators can trigger the propagation of a "calcium wave." Calcium waves can pass between disconnected astrocytes as long as the gap between them does not exceed 120 microns. These gap junctions are regulated by a number of mediators including glutamate, interleukin-1, and alpha-1 adrenergic agonists (Bezzi et al., 1998; Enkvist and McCarthy, 1994; Rouach et al., 2000). These calcium oscillations can be transmitted to distant astrocytes via gap junctions, causing distant glial cells to release glutamate and aspartate (Vernadakis, 1996), thus depolarizing neurons in a different dermatome (Rose and Konnerth, 2001). This can result in a pain signal that appears to be coming from a nontraumatized area.

Microglia and Abnormal Pain

Microglia mediate the response to injury in the central nervous system as the resident immunocompetent and phagocytic cells. The term *microglia* was coined by Dr. Pio del Rio Hortega in 1919 (Rezaie and Male, 2002), who found that these cells were of a distinct cell type apart from astrocytes and oligodendrocytes (del Rio Hortega, 1993). There was a 20-year period of widespread doubt in the scientific community about the nature and even the existence of microglia in the mid-20th century. Since that time, these cells have been found to play important roles in a variety of neurological illnesses including Alzheimer's disease, Parkinson's disease, and multiple sclerosis (Kim and Vellis, 2005).

Microglia, the nervous system's immune cells, are the most important mediators of CNS inflammation and are a rich source of proinflammatory cytokines, such as IL-1, IL-6, and tumor necrosis factor alpha (TNF). TNF can increase neuronal excitability by inserting into lipid membranes to form a porelike region that becomes a novel voltage-dependent sodium channel (Kagan et al., 1992; Leen and Bove, 2002). TNF can also interact with endogenous sodium and calcium channels on nerve membranes to increase membrane conductance (Van Der Goot et al., 1999; Wilkinson et al., 1996). IL-1 and IL-6 can enhance conduction of these ion channels (Qui et al., 1998; Schettini et al., 1988; Winkelstein et al., 2001). TNF also acts on neuronal TNFR1 receptors to increase exposure of glutamate receptors, thus increasing excitatory synaptic strength. TNF also causes endocytosis of neuronal GABA-A receptors, desensitizing these cells to pain-relieving inputs (Stellwagen et al., 2005). In addition, TNF also reduces glutamate uptake activity by astrocytes (Aoki et al., 1991). IL-1 and IL-6 can also cause hyperexcitability of nociceptors and release of inflammatory mediators such as substance P and histamine from immune cells in peripheral tissues. In addition to cytokines, microglial cells can release short-lived cytotoxic factors such as nitric oxide and superoxide radicals (Thery et al., 1993).

Chemokines and Pain

Components of the nerve cell itself can promote neural inflammation and generate chronic pain. Strong nociceptive activation will release fractaline from the neuron's external surface (Chapman et al., 2000). Fractaline is a member of the immune-related family of proinflammatory proteins called chemokines that activate glial cells and other immune cells. Fractaline receptors are expressed by glial cells in the dorsal horn of the spinal cord. Blocking fractaline receptors can block nerve damage-induced ipsilateral and mirror-image allodynia. Conversely, intrathecal injections of fractaline can induce mechanical allodynia. Fractaline cleavage can be induced by glutamate (Boddeke, 2001). The finding that fractaline is expressed on neurons and sensory afferents and that its receptor is predominantly expressed on microglia imply that fractaline plays a role in neuron-to-glia communication (Johnston et al., 2004).

Evidence of Neural Inflammation in Neuropathic Pain

Peripheral nerve lesions can cause activation of mitogen-associated protein kinases (p38 MAPK) in microglia in the spinal cord, leading to the elaboration of inflammatory mediators that sensitize dorsal horn neurons. Activity of dorsal horn neurons, in turn, enhances activation of spinal glia. This positive feedback mechanism can enhance and prolong neuropathic pain even in the absence of ongoing peripheral external stimulation or injury (Ji and Strichartz, 2004). Abnormal neuronal-glial signaling in neuropathic pain may result in the increased sensitivity to pain that patients experience in body regions other than those originally affected by the inciting injury. It may also mediate the "mental fatigue," which affects many patients with chronic pain (Hansson and Ronnback, 2004).

Both human and animal studies provide evidence of prolonged localized release of proinflammatory cytokines in body regions affected by severe neuropathic pain (Jeanjean et al., 1995). For example, one study showed that IL-1 and IL-6 (but not TNF) were increased in the spinal fluid of patients with reflex sympathetic dystrophy (Alexander et al., 2005). In animal models of posttraumatic neuralgias, blockade of IL-1 (Sommer et al., 1999) or TNF (Illich et al., 1997) after nerve injury reduces thermal hyperalgesia and mechanical allodynia.

Abnormal Spinal Cord Processing: The Case of Mirror-Image Pain

One clinical feature of some cases of severe neuropathic pain is "mirror-image pain" (Maleki et al., 2000). Mirror-image pain arises from the healthy body region contralateral to the actual site of trauma or inflammation. Mirror-image pain is generally characterized as mechanical allodynia (Baron, 2000) and does not involve contralateral nociceptor activity. Rather, it arises from altered spinal processing of incoming sensory information (Koltzenburg et al., 1999). An animal model for mirror-image allodynia is sciatic inflammatory neuropathy (SIN), which develops after microinjection of immune activators around one healthy sciatic nerve at the midthigh level in rats. Low-level immune activation produces unilateral ipsilateral allodynia. More intense immune activation produces bilateral allodynia. Allodynia of both sides can be reversed by intrathecal injection of fluorocitrate, a glial metabolic inhibitor. Allodynia and other signs of advanced neuropathic pain can also be prevented and reversed by intrathecal injection of CNI-1493, an inhibitor of p38 MAPK kinase, or by intrathecal injection of cytokine antagonists specific for IL-1, IL-6, or TNF. These will reverse both the ipsilateral and contralateral allodynia, even if the inflammatory stimulus to the sciatic nerve is maintained (Milligan et al., 2003).

Animal studies provide important evidence that ipsilateral and mirror-image allodynia are mediated through the actions of glial cells and proinflammatory cytokines. In one study, IL-1 antagonist was able to relieve mirror-image pain that had been established for 2 weeks, suggesting that spinal proinflammatory cytokines not only trigger pathological pain but that they are critical for its maintenance as well (Milligan et al., 2003). In a separate study, carbenoxolone, a chemical that disrupts gap junctions, reversed mirror-image pain in the same animal model (Spatero et al., 2004). Mirror-image allodynia is not affected by inhibitors to NMDA or dynorphin. There is, however, a separate syndrome of mirror-image thermal hyperalgesia that is mediated by substance P, NMDA receptors, non-NMDA receptors, and dynorphin (Chen et al., 2000; Malan et al., 2000).

Damage to tactile nerves can cause neuropathic pain syndromes that are relatively insensitive to suppression by the antinociceptive system. In patients who have had a stroke or spinal cord injury, for example, the nerves that carry touch signals may be destroyed. If enough pain-carrying fibers regenerate, tissues presumed to be anesthetic can generate considerable pain if reinjured or inflamed. This "deafferentation pain," as it is called, is most common among patients with spinal cord injuries. Although they may have no normal sensation below the waist, surgery on decubitus ulcers or even a simple bladder infection can be extremely painful. Without the interference of continuous tactile inputs, some patients with spinal cord injuries can discriminate between different types of pain to the point at which they can identify what type of bacteria is infecting their bladder by "the way it feels." This type of pain is also seen in postoperative pain syndromes (e.g., postthoracotomy pain), in which a common finding is pain accompanied by an area of tactile hypesthesia (Ji and Woolf, 2001).

Sympathetically Maintained Pain

Over a hundred years ago, the observation that there was often an overlap of body regions exhibiting pain and autonomic dysfunction (sweating, temperature, and blood flow abnormalities) led to the hypothesis that some cases of chronic neuropathic pain were due to disorders of the sympathetic nervous system (Stanton-Hicks, 2000). Recently, the term *sympathetically maintained pain* (SMP; Roberts, 1986) has come into use to describe a group of specific symptoms that may be associated with certain cases of reflex sympathetic dystrophy and causalgia (Baron et al., 1996). The types of pains most commonly related to SMP are constant burning pain, touch-evoked allodynia, and cold allodynia. Numbness, dysesthesia, paroxysmal pain, and heat-evoked allodynia are generally not associated with sympathetically maintained pain.

Operationally, SMP is defined as pain that is relieved with sympathetic blocks, regional application of guanethidine (Hannington-Kiff, 1974), or intravenous phentolamine (Arner, 1991). Guanethidine injected intravenously into an extremity affected by SMP initially elicits transient pain generated by norepinephrine release (Blumberg and Janig, 1982). Pain relieved by sympatholytic treatment can often be rekindled when alpha-agonists are locally applied via iontophoresis or subcutaneous injection (Davis et al., 1991). An early approach to SMP was surgical resection of sympathetic ganglia. A study showed that pain that was relieved in this manner could be rekindled by stimulating surgically decentralized thoracic sympathetic ganglia (Walker and Nulsen, 1948). In one study of reflex sympathetic dystrophy, sympathectomy not only relieved pain in affected limb, but it also relieved mirror-image pain (Shir and Seltzer, 1991).

One possible mechanism for SMP depends on changes in primary nociceptors. Under normal circumstances, nociceptors do not generate pain signals in response to sympathetic stimulation or to application of catecholamines. In fact, in the absence of local inflammation, sympathetic outflow suppresses C-nociceptor responses to brief noxious stimuli. This is apparently mediated by beta-2 receptors, which are the main catecholamine receptors expressed by normal C-fibers. Most primary nociceptors can develop heightened sensitivity to catecholamines after an injury (Perl, 1994). Nerve lesions can also evoke de novo expression of alpha-2 receptors in a subset of dorsal root ganglion cells (Nishiyama et al., 1993).

A neuroinflammatory mechanism for SMP postulates that nerve damage can induce signals transmitted retrograde up sympathetic fibers into the dorsal root ganglion (DRG), causing activation (Woodham et al., 1989) and proliferation of glial cells (Daemen et al., 1998). Macrophages are then recruited into the DRG (Lu and Richardson, 1993). These glial cells and macrophages release proinflammatory cytokines into the extracellular space of the DRG, which stimulate the growth of sympathetic fibers. These sympathetic fibers form basketlike terminals around the satellite cells that surround neuronal cell bodies (Ramer, 1999; Ramer et al., 1998). Activation of alpha-2 adrenergic receptors on these sympathetic terminals triggers the synthesis of prostaglandins by the satellite cells. Prostaglandins then sensitize nociceptor terminals (Gonzales et al., 1991), which become sensitive to norepinephrine (Sato et al., 1993).

Under normal conditions, catecholamines are antiinflammatory in the skin, acting via beta-2 adrenergic receptors on immune cells and inhibiting the production and release of proinflammatory cytokines (Heijnen et al., 1996). These cells do not express alpha-1 receptors under basal conditions (Kavelaars et al., 1998). In states of chronic inflammation, however, immune cells downregulate beta receptors and express alpha-1 receptors (Haydon, 2001). With increased expression of alpha-1 receptors on immune-competent cells (e.g., synoviocytes, endothelium, Langerhans, fibroblasts), sympathetic activity promotes sustained inflammation in the skin and soft tissues (Poole et al., 1999). Studies show that there is increased alpha-1 expression in skin regions affected by reflex sympathetic dystrophy (Drummond et al., 1996). This norepinephrine responsiveness generally disappears when the local inflammation resolves. Although SMP is most commonly associated with reflex sympathetic dystrophy and causalgia, it can be seen in other pain syndromes. For example, injection of epinephrine around chronic nerve-end neuromas can elicit pain (Chabal et al., 1992). Sympathetically maintained pain can also be demonstrated in some cases of herpes zoster, metabolic neuropathies, and phantom limb pain (Boas, 1996).

Endogenous Pain Relief

Just as clotting is accompanied by anticoagulation, the complex nociceptive system is balanced by an equally complex antinociceptive system. Pain signals arriving from peripheral tissues stimulate the release of endorphins in the periaqueductal gray matter of the brain and enkephalins in the nucleus raphe magnus of the brainstem. Endorphins inhibit the propagation of pain signals by binding to mu-opioid receptors on the presynaptic terminals of nociceptors and postsynaptic surfaces of dorsal horn cells. Enkephalins bind to delta-opioid receptors on inhibitory interneurons in the substantia gelatinosa of the dorsal horn, causing release of gamma-aminobutyric acid (GABA) and other mediators that dampen pain signals in the spinal cord. The endogenous pain control system in the brain is widespread and it is generally localized in the rostral ventromedial medulla (RVM; Tavares and Lima, 2002). This system not only mediates endogenous pain relief but also probably plays a role in the action of nonpharmacological pain relievers, including exercise and placebos. Of note, the pain relief generated by a placebo can be inhibited by pretreatment with opioid antagonists like naloxone.

Dysfunction of this natural pain-relieving mechanism has been invoked to explain certain chronic pain states, such as the chronic daily headaches that sometimes develop in chronic migraineurs. Functional MRI studies of these patients often show iron deposition in the periaqueductal gray matter, which is said to be indicative of fibrosis of endorphin-producing cells (Woolf and Salter, 2000). There appear to be several analgesic centers in the brain, one of which can mediate "stress-induced" analgesia, which is an activated, "goal oriented" state that can cause profound global analgesia and that is not inhibited with opioid antagonists (Willer, 1981). Pharmacologic agonists of this system may include ketamine and phencyclidine, both of which are "dissociative" anesthetics.

Spinal interneurons release dynorphin, which activates kappa-opioid receptors and leads to closure of N-type calcium channels in the spinal cord cells that normally relay pain signals to the brain. Following the release of enkephalins, spinal cord cells release other small molecules, including norepinephrine, oxytocin and relaxin, that can also inhibit the transmission of pain signals (Furst, 1999).

Enkephalin is particularly notable in that it binds to delta-opioid receptors that are selectively exposed on nociceptors that are actively transmitting a pain signals. These receptors are usually localized on presynaptic vesicles storing neurotransmitters. After the neurotransmitters are released, the receptors are incorporated into the presynaptic cell membrane. Active nociceptors thus become more sensitive than inactive nociceptors to both endogenous and exogenous opioids, which can explain how certain opioid analgesics can relieve ongoing pain without impairing the ability to sense pain caused by new injuries.

The natural pain-relieving system may be as important to normal functioning as the pain-signaling system. Because we have the capacity to naturally suppress pain, minor injuries—such as a stubbed toe or a cut finger—make us dysfunctional for only a few minutes, not for a few days, as might be the case if the pain persisted and intensified until the wound completely healed. Just as disorders of the pain-sensing system can give rise to illness and dysfunction, it is very likely that disorders of the pain-relieving system can do the same.

Central Sensitization and the Role of the NMDA Receptor

If pain signals are continuously transmitted to the spinal cord, the central nervous system itself will undergo physiochemical changes resulting in hypersensitivity to pain, increased pain with repeated stimuli ("windup") and resistance to antinociceptive (e.g., pain relieving) inputs. Ultimately the pain signal can be become embedded in the central nervous system like a painful memory, without the need for peripheral input. The analogy to memory is especially fitting because the generation of hypersensitivity in the spinal cord and the development of memory in the brain both share a common chemical pathway involving NMDA (N-methyl-D-aspartate) receptors.

The physical changes that accompany this sensitization process are first seen on the cell membranes of the dorsal horn cells that receive signals from nociceptors. The main chemical mediator used by nociceptors synapsing with the dorsal horn of the spinal cord is glutamate, which can bind to several different types of receptors. AMPA (α-amino-3-hydroxy-5-methylisoxazole-4-propionic-acid) receptors are sodium-potassium channels on postsynaptic afferent nerve terminals in the dorsal horn and mediate the transmission of acute pain. Activation of these receptors triggers a transient activating current that generates a signal to the brain via the spinothalamic tract.

NMDA receptors are a separate class of receptors for glutamate on dorsal horn cells which, when activated, open a channel for the influx of calcium into the spinal cord afferents. In the resting state, this calcium channel is blocked by a magnesium ion. With persistent or intense release of glutamate, due to severe or chronic pain, activation of AMPA receptors results in a change in the charge of the cell membrane and the magnesium ion is said to "pop out" of the calcium channel like a cork popping out of a champagne bottle. The NMDA receptor has now become activated. In a biochemical sense, this conformational change in the NMDA receptor marks a central transition from acute to chronic pain (Bennett, 2000).

Calcium ions flowing into the dorsal horn cell activate protein kinase C, which triggers the production of nitric oxide (NO) by nitric oxide-synthase. NO, which is in essence a very short range neurotransmitter, diffuses back across the synaptic cleft and into the nociceptor, stimulating guanyl-synthetase induced closure of potassium channels. Many of these potassium channels are opioid receptors and the nociceptor is thus rendered insensitive (i.e. tolerant or resistant) to opioid-induced suppression of the pain signal by endorphins, enkephalins, and opioid medications (Riedel and Neeck, 2001). This explains the clinical observation that one of the most important mediators of opioid tolerance is unremitting pain, rather than the use of opioid medications. In clinical studies, NMDA inhibitors such as ketamine or dextromethorphan can reverse opioid tolerance, demonstrating that opioid tolerance in people with chronic pain is more a biochemical phenomenon than a characterologic disorder.

If the pain signal is allowed to persist, NO eventually stimulates the release of substance P from the nociceptors which, by binding to the NK-1 receptors in the dorsal horn membrane, triggers the expression of *c-fos* oncogene, promoting neural remodeling and further hypersensitization. It is interesting to note that the one chemical abnormality repeatedly documented in controlled studies of patients with fibromyalgia syndrome (a condition that many clinicians continue to consider factitious) is an elevated level of substance P in the spinal fluid (Russell, 2002).

Activation of NMDA receptors has many consequences for nerves in the spinal cord, which can ultimately include cell damage and cell death. NMDA receptors are now being implicated in some of the cell damage that occurs in the brain during strokes, in which injured presynaptic cells release torrents of glutamate, literally "burning out" and killing postsynaptic cells. One of the most intriguing avenues in stroke research currently is the therapeutic use of NMDA receptor inhibitors to limit brain damage in the setting of an acute stroke (Costigan and Woolf, 2000).

Activation of the NK-1 receptor triggers production of *c-fos* oncogene product, a protein that, in many respects, can be regarded as a biochemical footprint of chronic pain. In animal models of chronic pain the *c-fos* oncogene protein can be detected in afferent spinal cord cells that are receiving pain signals. As chronic pain persists, the *c-fos* oncogene protein will become detectable in cells higher up the spinal cord, appearing outside the dermatome in which the original painful stimulus occurred. This protein will eventually become detectable in the thalamus itself and, at this point, the pain will be virtually untreatable.

C-fos oncogene protein may be a marker for the acquisition of hypersensitivity to pain signals by these different areas of the spinal cord. This would explain why many patients who have persistent pain find that, after months and years of undertreatment, the pain begins to spread to organs other than the one originally involved (for example, patients with long-standing proctitis due to irritable bowel syndrome will often develop noncardiac chest pain if their chronic pain goes untreated) or the pain will spread outside dermatomal boundaries. Unfortunately, when this happens, physicians who are not familiar with the concept of neural plasticity will think that the abnormal area affected by the pain is not "physiologic" and therefore come to the conclusion that the patient is either mentally ill or faking.

Stimulation of opioid receptors and other inhibitory receptors on peripheral neurons or at the presynaptic terminal in the spinal cord can slow or stop the synaptic release of glutamate and the generation of the pain signal and may prevent subsequent neural remodeling. This explains the unique utility of small doses of intrathecal opioids delivered via an implanted pump in selected pain syndromes. This type of therapy can often provide impressive relief in intractable pain syndromes and works in a complementary fashion with systemically administered opioid medications, which also trigger supraspinal antinociceptive pathways. It is interesting to note that opioids don't have much presynaptic inhibitory activity on normal peripheral nerves but do inhibit the release of glutamate from inflamed nerves.

Afferent Becomes Efferent: Dorsal Root Reflexes

Although medical school taught us that neuronal cells transmit signals in only one direction, either toward (afferent) or away (efferent) from the brain, we now know that many neurons can carry signals in both directions. With the prolonged generation of pain signals, a pathologic phenomenon called a *dorsal root reflex* can become established in which afferent cells in the dorsal horn of the spinal cord release mediators that stimulate nociceptors to fire action potentials antidromically (i.e., backward). When this happens, packets of chemicals located at the peripheral terminals of the nociceptors are released. These chemicals include nerve growth factor and substance P, which is not only a neurotransmitter but also a potent inflammatory agent. Pain signals from peripheral nerves are thus heightened, and the cycle of chronic pain continues. Calcitonin-gene related peptide (CGRP) released in the periphery causes vasodilatation, extravasation of proteins, release of bradykinin from vascular endothelial cells, and degranulation of mast cells with release of histamines and serotonin, which result in a long-lasting lowering of nociceptive thresholds. Other peripheral mediators of neurogenic inflammation probably include nitric oxide (NO) and vasoactive intestinal peptide (VIP; Pinter and Szolcanyi, 1995).

Neurogenic Inflammation

The release of substance P and nerve growth factor into the periphery causes a tissue reaction termed *neurogenic inflammation*. In contrast to the classic inflammatory response to tissue trauma or immune-mediated cell damage, neurogenic inflammation is driven by events in the central nervous system and does not depend on the usual drivers of peripheral inflammation, such as granulocytes or lymphocytes. Substance P causes degranulation of mast cells, and its effects on the vascular endothelium induce the release of bradykinin and production of nitric oxide, a potent vasodilator. Biopsy specimens from neurogenically inflamed tissues—for example, the synovium in certain forms of chronic arthritis, the bladder in interstitial cystitis, or the colon in severe irritable bowel syndrome—typically show vasodilatation, plasma extravasation, abnormal sprouting of peripheral nerve terminals, and an accumulation of mast cells.

Dorsal root reflexes apparently occur only under circumstances in which there has been prolonged and unsuppressed nociception. This model of central nervous system control over peripheral inflammation explains why many painful conditions do not respond to standard "end-organ oriented" treatments, including disorders such as long-standing rheumatoid arthritis, reflex sympathetic dystrophy, certain cases of chronic headache, severe instances of irritable bowel syndrome, and noncardiac chest pain. Similar findings are commonly seen in inflammatory disease of gastrointestinal tract, such as in ulcerative colitis and Crohn's disease, and other chronic inflammatory states, such as psoriasis and chronic arthritis (Dvorak et al., 1992; Hukkanen et al., 1991; McKay and Bienenstock, 1994; Naukkarinen et al., 1991; Yonei, 1987). In some sense, many of these diseases could thus be regarded as "pain disorders." This mechanism explains why we have to treat and suppress certain inflammatory conditions, such as rheumatoid arthritis, within a limited time frame. If we don't, the inflammatory process escapes control by the traditional, peripherally acting, antiinflammatory medications. This is because these medications are active against immunogenic inflammation and not neurogenic inflammation.

What Is Chronic Pain?

The aim of this superficial review has been to show that the perception of injury is mediated by a complex nociceptive system. Nociception is a vital bodily function, without which we cannot survive. Dysfunction of any one of many steps in the nociceptive process can give rise to chronic pain, which can be a destructive and progressive disorder. These dysfunctions can occur either in the peripheral or in the central nervous system. By expanding our view of chronic pain, we can frame certain illnesses previously identified with their involved "end organs" as disorders of the nociceptive system much in the same way that we have come to understand that certain cardiovascular and neurologic illnesses may really reside in dysfunction of the coagulation system rather than a defect in the heart or the brain.

A unifying theme for the basis of most chronic pain syndromes is the development of hypersensitivity—a disordering change in the normal relationship between a painful stimulus and response. It also implies that the ideal agents for the treatment of chronic pain will be "antihypersensitivity" agents rather than analgesic or antinociceptive drugs (Mannion and Woolf, 2000). Current analgesic therapies, along with the introduction of new therapies aimed at generators of hypersensitivity, such as recently introduced antagonists to NMDA, VR-1, and NK-1 receptors, should allow us to help most of our patients with chronic pain to safely regain control over their illness and restore their lives without increasing the risk of drug abuse (Attal, 2000).

References

Aidar O, Geohegan WA, Uingewitter LH. (1952) Splanchnic afferent pathways in the central nervous systems. *J Neurophysiology*, 15:131–138.

Al Chaer ED, Feng Y, Willis WD. (1998) Visceral pain: a disturbance in the sensorimotor continuum. *Pain Forum*, 7:117–125.

Alexander GM, van Rijn MA, van Hilten JJ, Perreault MJ, Schwartzman RJ. (2005) Changes in cerebrospinal fluid levels of pro-inflammatory cytokines in CRPS. *Pain*, 116:213–219.

Aloe L, Tuveri MA, Carcassi U, Levi-Montacalcini R. (1992) Nerve growth factor in the synovial fluid of patients with chronic arthritis. *Arthritis Rheum*, 35:351–355.

Aoki E, Semba R, Kashiwamata S. (1991) Evidence for the presence of L-arginine in the glial components of the peripheral nervous system. *Brain Res*, 559:159–162.

Apfel SC. (2000) Neurotrophic factors and pain. *Clin J Pain*, 16:S7–S11.

Apfel SC. (2002) Nerve growth factor for the treatment of diabetic neuropathy. *Int Rev Neurobiol*, 50:393–413.

Apkarian AV. (1995) Functional imaging of pain: new insights regarding the role of the cerebral cortex in human pain perception. *Semin Neurosci*, 7:279–293.

Arner S. (1991) Intravenous phentolamine test: diagnostic and prognostic use in reflex sympathetic dystrophy. *Pain*, 46:17–22.

Attal N. (2000) Chronic neuropathic pain: mechanisms and treatment. *Clin J Pain*, 16:S118-S130.

Baron R. (2000) Peripheral neuropathic pain: from mechanisms to symptoms. *Clin J Pain*, 16(suppl): S12-S20.

Baron R, Blumberg H, Janig W. (1996) Clinical characteristics of patients with complex regional pain syndrome in Germany with special emphasis on vasomotor function. In: Janig W, Stanton-Hicks M, eds. *Reflex Sympathetic Dystrophy: A Reappraisal*. Seattle: IASP Press; pp. 25–48.

Bennett GJ. (2000) Update on the neurophysiology of pain transmission and modulation: focus on the NMDA-receptor. *J Pain Symptom Manage*, 19:S2–6.

Bezzi P, Carmignoto G, Pasti L, Vesce S, Rossi D, Rizzini BL, Pozzan T, Volterra A. (1998) Prostaglandins stimulate calcium-dependent glutamate release in astrocytes. *Nature*, 391:281–285.

Blumberg H, Janig W. (1982) Activation of fibers via experimentally produced stump neuromas of skin nerves: ephaptic transmission orretrograde sprouting? *Exp Neurol*, 468–482.

Boas RA. (1996) Complex regional pain syndromes: symptoms, signs and differential diagnosis. In: Janig W, Stanton-Hicks M, eds. *Reflex Sympathetic Dystrophy: A Reappraisal*. Seattle: IASP Press; pp. 79–92.

Boddeke EW. (2001) Involvement of chemokines in pain. *Eur J Pharmacol*, 429:115–119.

Boerhaave H. (1753) *Aphorisms de Chirurgie*. Paris: Vve Cavalier & Fil.

Bonica JJ. (1979) Causalgia and other reflex sympathetic dystrophies. In: Bonica JJ, Liebeskind JC, Albe-Fessard DG, eds. *Proceedings of the Second World Congress on Pain, Advances in Pain Research and Therapy, Vol. 3*. New York: Raven Press, pp. 141–166.

Bonica JJ. (1991) The history of pain concepts and pain therapy. *Mt Sinai J Med*, 58:191–202.

Brower V. (2000) New paths to pain relief. *Nature Biotechnology*, 18:387–383.

Canon RO. (1995) Cardiac pain. In: Gebhart GF, ed. *Visceral Pain*. Seattle: IASP Press, pp. 373–389.

Cervero F. (1994) Sensory innervation of the viscera: peripheral basis of visceral pain. *Physiol Rev*, 74:95–138.

Cervero F. (1995) Mechanisms of visceral pain: Past and present. In: Gebhart GF, ed. *Visceral Pain*. Seattle: IASP, pp. 25–40.

Chabal C, Jacobson L, Russell LC, Burchiel KJ. (1992) Pain responses to perineuronal injection of normal saline, epinephrine and lidocaine in humans. *Pain*, 49: 9–12.

Chapman GA, Moores K, Harrison D, Campbell CA, Steward BR, Strijbos PJLM. (2000) Fractaline cleavage from neuronal membranes represents an acute event in the inflammatory responses to excitotoxic brain damage. *J Neurosci*, 20:1–5.

Chen HS, Chen J, Sun YY. (2000) Contralateral heat hyperalgesia induced by unilaterally intraplantar bee venom injection is produced by central changes: a behavioral study in the conscious rat. *Neurosci Lett*, 284: 45–48.

Chen J, Leong SY, Schachner M. (2005) Differential expression of cell fate determinants in neurons and glial cells of adult mouse spinal cord after compression injury. *Eur J Neurosci*, 22:1895–906.

Costigan M, Woolf CJ. (2000) Pain: molecular mechanisms. *J Pain*, 3:35–44.

Cunha FQ, Lorenzetti BB, Poole S, Ferreira SH. (1991) Interleukin-8 as a mediator of sympathetic pain. *Brit J Pharmacol*, 104:765–767.

Daemen MARC, Kurvers HAJM, Kitslaar PJEHM. (1998) Neurogenic inflammation in an animal model of neuropathic pain. *Neurol Res*, 20:41–45.

Darmberg C. (1856) *Galen: On the Uses of the Parts of the Body of Man*. Paris: Ballieres, pp. 539–540.

Davis KD, Treede RD, Raja SN, Meyer RA, Campbell JN. (1991) Topical application of clonidine relieves hyperalgesia in patients with sympathetically maintained pain. *Pain*, 47:309–317.

del Rio Hortega P. (1993) Art and artifice in the science of histology 1933. *Histopathology*, 22:515–25.

Double FJ. (1805) A memorandum on the semiotics and practical considerations concerning pain. *Journal Generale de Medecine* (Paris), 3:359.

Drucker WB, Hubay CA, Holden WD, Bukovnic JA. (1959) Pathogenesis of posttraumatic sympathetic dystrophy. *Am J Surg*, 97:454–464.

Drummond PD, Skipworth S, Finch PM. (1996) Alpha-1 adrenoreceptors in normal and hyperalgesic human skin. *Clin Sci*, 91:73–77.

Duce IR, Keen P. (1983) Selective uptake of tritiated glutamine and tritiated glutamate in neurons and satellite cells of dorsal root ganglia in vitro. *Neuroscience*, 8:861–866.

Dvorak AM, McLeod RS, Onderdonk AB. (1992) Human gut mucosal mast cells. *Int Arch Allergy Immunol*, 98:150–68.

Dyck PJ, Giannini C. (1996) Pathologic alterations in the diabetic neuropathies of humans: a review. *J Neuropathol Exp Neurol*, 55:1181–1193.

Enkvist KO, McCarthy KD. (1994) Astroglial gap junction communication is increased by treatment with either glutamate of high potassium concentration. *J Neurochem*, 62:489–495.

Furst S. (1999) Transmitters involved in antinociception in the spinal cord. *Brain Res Bull*, 48:129–41.

Gonzales R, Goldyne ME, Taiwo YO, Levine JD. (1989) Production of hyperalgesic prostaglandins by sympathetic preganglionic neurons. *J Neurochemistry*, 53:1595–1598.

Gonzales R, Sherbourne CD, Goldyne ME, Levine JD. (1991) Noradrenaline-induced prostaglandin production by sympathetic postganglionic neurons is mediated by alpha-2 adrenergic receptors. *J Neurochem*, 57:1145–1150.

Hannington-Kiff JG. (1974) *Pain Relief*. Philadelphia: Lippincott.

Hansson E, Ronnback L. (2004) Altered neuronal-glial signaling in glutaminergic transmission as a unifying mechanism in chronic pain and mental fatigue. *Neurochem Res*, 29:989–996.

Haydon PG. (2001) Glia: listening and talking to the synapse. *Nature Rev Neurosci*, 2:185–193.

Heijnen CJ, Roupe Van Der Voort C, Wulffrat N, Van Der Net J, Kuis W, Kavelaars A. (1996) Functional alpha-1 adrenergic receptors on leukocytes of patients with polyarticular juvenile rheumatoid arthritis. *J Neuroimmunol*, 71:223–226.

Holden WD. (1948) Sympathetic dystrophy. *Arch Surg*, 57:373–384.

Holmes OW. (1891) *Medical Essays 1842–1882*. Boston: Houghton Mifflin.

Hukkanen M, Gronblad M, Rees R. (1991) Regional distribution of mast cells and peptide-containing nerves in normal and adjuvant arthritic rat synovium. *J Rheumatol*, 18:177–183.

Illich PA, Martin D, Castro GA, Clatworthy AL. (1997) TNF binding protein attenuates thermal hyperalgesia but not guarding behavior following loose ligation of rat sciatic nerve. *Soc Neurosci Abstr*, 23:166.

Jeanjean AP, Moussaoui SM, Maloteaux JM, Laduron PM. (1995) Interleukin-1 beta induces long-term increase of axonally transported opiate receptor and substance P. *Neuroscience*, 68:151–157.

Ji RR, Strichartz G. (2004) Cell signaling and the genesis of neuropathic pain. *Science* (Signal Transduction Knowledge Environment), 252:14–16.

Ji RR, Woolf CJ. (2001) Neuronal plasticity and signal transduction in nociceptive neurons: implications for the initiation and maintenance of pathologic pain. *Neurbiol Dis*, 8:1–10.

Johnston IN, Milligan ED, Wiesler-Frank J, Frank MG, Zapata V, Campisi J, Langer S, Martin D, Green P, Fleshner M, Leinwand L, Maier SF, Watkins LR. (2004) A role for proinflammatory cytokines and fractaline in analgesia, tolerance and subsequent pain facilitation induced by chronic intrathecal morphine. *J Neuroscience*, 24:7353–7365.

Kagan BL, Baldwin RL, Munoz D, Wisnieski BJ. (1992) Formation of ion-permeable channels by tunor necrosis factor-alpha. *Science*, 255:1427–1430.

Kai-Kai MA, Howe R. (1991) Glutamate-immunoreactivity in the trigeminal and dorsal root ganglia and intraspinal neurons and fibres in the dorsal horn of the rat. *Histochem J*, 23:171–179.

Kavelaars A, De Jong- De Vos Van Steenwijk T, Kuis W, Heijnen CJ. (1998) The reactivity of the cardiovascular system and immunomodulation by catecholamines in juvenile chronic arthritis. *Ann NY Acad Sci*, 840:698–704.

Kim SU, de Vellis J. (2005) Microglia in health and disease. *J Neurosci Res*, 81:302–313.

Koltzenburg M. (1999) The changing sensitivity in the life of the nociceptor. *Pain*, 6:S93–102.

Koltzenburg M, Wall PD, McMahon SB. (1999) Does the right side know what the left is doing? *Trends Neurosci*, 22:122–127.

Kumazawa T. (1996) Sensitization of polymodal nociceptors. In: Belmonte C, Cervero F., eds. *Neurobiology of Nociceptors*. Oxford: Oxford University Press, pp. 325–345.

Landre-Beauvais AJ. (1813) *Semiotics and the Features of Illness*. Paris: Brosson, p. 315.

Latham RG. (1848) *The Works of Thomas Sydenham* London: The Thomas Sydenham Society

Leen JG, Bove GM. (2002) Mid-axonal tumor necrosis factor-alpha induces ectopic activity in a subset of slowly conducting cutaneous and deep afferent neurons. *J Pain*, 3:45–49.

Levine J, Taiwo Y. (1994) Inflammatory pain. In: Wall PD, Melzack R. eds. *Textbook of Pain*. London: Churchill Livingstone.

Levine JD, Lam D Taiwo Y. (1986) Hyperalgesic properties of 15-lipooxygenase products of arachadonic acid. *Proc Natl Acad Sci*, 83: 5331–5334.

Lewis T. (1937) The nocisensor system of nerves and its reactions. *Brit Med J*, 3:431–435.

Locke GR, Talley NJ, Zinmaster AR. (1996) The irritable bowel syndrome and functional dyspepsia: functional disorders. *Gastroenterology*, 110:A26.

Lowe EM, Anand P, Terenghi G. (1997) Increased nerve growth factor levels in the urinary bladder with idiopathic sensory urgency and interstitial cystitis. *Br J Urol*, 79:572–577.

Lu X, Richardson PM. (1993) Responses of macrophages in rat dorsal root ganglia following peripheral nerve injury. *J Neurocytol*, 22:334–341.

Malan TP, Ossipov MH, Gardell LR, Ibrahim M, Bian D, Lai J, Porreca F. (2000) Extraterritorial neuropathic pain correlates with multisegmental elevation of spinal dynorphin in nerve-injured rats. *Pain*, 86:185–194.

Maleki J, LeBel AA, Bennett GJ, Schwartzman RJ. (2000) Patterns of spread in complex regional pain syndrome I. *Pain*, 88:259–266.

Malliani A. (1994) The conceptualization of cardiac pain as a nonspecific and unreliable alarm system. In: Gebhart GF, ed. *Visceral Pain*. Seattle: IASP Press, pp. 63–74.

Mannion RJ, Woolf CJ. (2000) Pain mechanisms and management: a central perspective. *Clin J Pain*, 16:S144-S156

Mantyh PW Nelson CD, Sevick MA, Luger NM and Sabino MA. (2003) Molecular mechanisms that generate and maintain cancer pain. In: Dostrovsky JO, Carr D, Koltzenburg M, eds. *Proceedings of the 10th World Congress on Pain*. Seattle: IASP Press, pp. 663–681.

McGrath PJ. (2004) Psychosocial and psychiatric aspects of pain in children. In: Dworkin R, Breitbart W, eds. *Psychosocial Aspects of Pain*. Seattle: IASP Press.

McKay DM, Bienenstock J. (1994) The interaction between mast cells and nerves in the gastrointestinal tract. *Immunol Today*, 15:533–538.

McMahon SB. (1996) NGF as a mediator of inflammatory pain. *Philos Trans R Soc Lond Biol Sci*, 351:431–440.

McMahon SB, Dmitrieva N, Koltzenburg M. (1995) Visceral pain. *Brit J Anesth*, 75:132–144.

McMahon SB, Koltzenburg M. (1990) Novel classes of nociceptors. *Trends in Neuroscience*, 13:199–201.

McMahon SB, Koltzenburg M. (1994) Silent afferents and visceral pain. In: Fields HL, Liebeskind JC, eds. *Progress in Pain Research and Management*. Seattle: IASP Press, pp. 11–30.

Mendell LM, Albers KM, Davis BM. (1999) Neurotrophins, nociceptors and pain. *Microsc Res Tech*, 45:252–261.

Micu I, Jiang O, Coderre E, Ridsdale A, Zhang L, Woulfe J, Yin X, Trapp BD, McRory JE, Rehak R, Zamponi GW, Wang W, Stys PK. (2005, December 21) NMDA receptors mediate calcium accumulation in myelin during chemical ischemia. *Nature*—E published ahead of print

Milligan ED, Twining C, Chacur M, Biedenkapp J, O'Connor K, Poole S, Tracey K, Martin D, Maier SF, Watkins LR. (2003) Spinal glia and proinflammatory cytokines mediate mirror-image neuropathic pain in rats. *J Neuroscience*, 23:1026–39.

Mitchell SW. (1874) *Lesions of Nerves and Their Consequences*. Paris: Masson, p. 70.

Moisan M. (1978) *Narcotic Plants in the Hippocratic Collections*. Paris: Belles Lettres.

Muyderman H, Nilsson M, Blomstrand F, Khatibi S, Olsson T, Hansson E, Ronnback L. (1998) Modulation of mechanically induced calcium waves in hippocampal astroglial cells. Inhibitory effects of alpha-1 adrenergic stimulation. *Brain Res*, 793:127–135.

Nabiloff B, Lembo A, Mayer EA. (1993) Abdominal pain in irritable bowel syndrome. *Current Review of Pain*, 3:144–152.

Naukkarinen A, Harvima IT, Aalto ML. (1991) Quantitative analysis of contact sites beween mast cells and sensory nerves in cutaneous psoriasis. *Arch Dermatol Res*, 283:433–437.

Ness T. (1995) Historical and clinical perspectives In: Gebhart GF, ed. *Visceral Pain*. Seattle: IASP Press, pp. 3–.

Nilsson J, von Euler AM, Dalsgaard CJ. (1985) Stimulation of connective tissue cell growth by substance P and substance K. *Nature*, 315:61–63.

Nishiyama K, Brighton BW, Bossut DF, Perl ER. (1993) Peripheral nerve injury enhances alpha-2 adrenergic receptor expression by some DRG neurons. *Soc Neurosci Abstracts*, 19:499.

Osler W. (1910) Angina pectoris. *Lancet*, 1:839–844.

Perl ER. (1994) Causalgia and sympathetic dystrophy revisited. In: Boivie J, Hansson P, Lindblom U, eds. *Touch, Temperature and Pain in Health and Disease: Mechanisms and Assessments*. Seattle: IASP Press; pp. 231–248.

Pernick M. (1985) *A Calculus of Suffering*. New York: Columbia University Press

Pinter E, Szolcanyi J. (1995) Plasma extravasation in the skin and pelvic organs evoked by antidromic stimulation of the lumbosacral dorsal roots in the rat. *Neuroscience*, 68:603–614.

Poole S, Cunha FQ, Ferreira SH. (1999) Hyperalgesia from subcutaneous cytokines. In: Watkins LR, Maier SF, eds. *Cytokines and Pain*. Berlin: Birkhauser; pp. 89–132.

Porter JT, McCarthy KD. (1996) Hippocampal astrocytes *in situ* respond to glutamate released from synaptic terminals. *J Neurosci*, 16:5073–5081.

Qiu Z, Sweeney DD, Netzeband JG, Gruol DL. (1998) Chronic interleukin-6 alters NMDA receptor-mediated membrane responses and enhances neurotoxicity in developing CNS neurons. *J Neurosci*, 18:10445–10456.

Ramer MS, Murphy PG, Richardson PM, Bisby MA. (1998) Spinal nerve lesion-induced mechanoallodynia and adrenergic sprouting in sensory ganglia are attentuated in interleukin-6 knockout mice. *Pain*, 78:115–121.

Ramer MS, Thompson SW, McMahon SB. (1999) Causes and consequences of sympathetic basket formation in dorsal root ganglia. *Pain*, 6(suppl): S111-S120.

Rang HP, Perkins MN. (1997) The role of bradykinin receptors in inflammatory pain. In: Borsook D, ed. *Molecular Neurobiology of Pain*. Seattle: IASP Press.

Rey, R. (1995) *The History of Pain*. Cambridge MA: Harvard University Press.

Rezaie P, Male D. (2002) Mesoglia and microglia: a historical review of the concept of mononuclear phagocytes within the central nervous system. *J Hist Neurosci*, 11:325–374.

Riedel W, Neeck G. (2001) Nociception, pain and antinociception: current concepts. *Z Rheumatol*, 60:404–415.

Roberts WJ. (1986) A hypothesis on the physiological basis for causalgia and related pains. *Pain*, 24:297–311.

Rose CR, Konnerth A. (2001) Exciting glial oscillations. *Nature Neurosci*, 4:773–774.

Rouach N, Glowinski J, Giaume C. (2000) Activity-dependent neuronal control of gap–junctional communication in astrocytes. *J Cell Biol*, 149: 1513–1526.

Rush B. (1947) *Selected Writings*. DD Runes, ed. New York: Philosophical Library.

Russell LJ. (2002) The promise of substance P inhibitors in fibromyalgia. *Rheum Dis Clin North Amer*, 28:2–10.

Said G, Hontebeyrie-Joskowicz M. (1992) Nerve lesions induced by macrophage activation. *Res Immunol*, 19:589–599.

Sakuma E, Wang HJ, Asai Y, Tamaki D, Amano K, Mabuchi Y, Herbert DC, Soji T. (2001) Gap junctional communication between the satellite cells of rat dorsal root ganglia. *Kaibogaku Zasshi*, 76:297–302.

Sato J, Suzuki S, Iseki T, Kumazawa T. (1993) Adrenergic excitation of cutaneous nociceptors in chronically inflamed rats. *Neurosci Lett*, 164: 225–228.

Schettini G, Meucci O, Florio T, Scala G, Landolfi E, Grimaldi M. (1988) Effect of interleukin 1 beta on transducing mechanisms in 235-I clonal pituitary cells. Part II Modulation of calcium fluxes. *Biochem Biophys Res Commun*, 155:1097–1104.

Schott GD. (2001) Reflex sympathetic dystrophy. *J Neurol Neurosurg Psychiatry*, 71:291–295.

Schwab JM, Bernard F, Moreau-Fauvarque C, Chedotal A. (2005) Injury reactive myelin/oligodendrocyte-derived growth inhibition in the adult mammalian central nervous system. *Brain Res Rev*, 49:295–299.

Sengupta JN, Gebhart GF. (1994a) Mechanoreceptive afferent fibers in the gastrointestinal and lower urinary tract. In: Gebhart G, ed. *Visceral Pain*. Seattle: IASP Press, pp. 75–98.

Sengupta IN, Gebhart GF. (1994b) Gastrointestinal afferent fibers and sensation. In: Johnson LR, ed. *Physiology of the Gastrointestinal Tract*. New York: Raven Press, pp. 483–519.

Shafer M, Mousa SA Zhang Q. (1996) Expression of corticotropin-eleasing factor in inflamed tissue is required for peripheral opioid analgesia. *Proc Natl Acad Sci*, 93:6096–6100.

Shir Y, Seltzer Z. (1991) Effects of sympathectomy in a model of causalgiform pain produced by partial sciatic nerve injury in rats. *Pain*, 45:309–320.

Sommer C, Petrausch S, Lindenlaub T, Toyka KV. (1999) Neutralizing antibodies to interleukin-1 receptor reduce pain associated behavior in mice with experimental neuropathy. *Neurocis Lett*, 270:25–28.

Spatero LE, Sloane EM, Milligan ED, Wiesler-Frank J, Schoniger D, Jekich BM, Barrientos RM, Maier SF, Watkins LR. (2004) Spinal gap junctions: potential involvement in pain facilitation. *J Pain*, 5:392–405.

Stanton-Hicks M. (2000) Complex regional pain syndrome (type I RSD; type II causalgia): controversies. *Clin J Pain*, 16(suppl):S33-S40.

Stein C, Shafer M, Cabot PJ, Zhang Q, Zhou L and Carter L. (1997) Opioids and Inflammation. In: Borsook D, ed. *Molecular Neurobiology of Pain*. Seattle: IASP Press, pp. 25–37.

Stellwagen D, Beattie EC, Seo JY, Malenka RC. (2005) Differential regulation of AMPA receptor and GABA receptor trafficking by Tumor Necrosis Factor-alpha. *J Neuroscience*, 25:3219–3228.

Steranka LR, Manning DC, De Haas CJ. (1988) Bradykinin as a pain mediator. *Proc Natl Acad Sci*, 85:3245–3249.

Sternbach RA, Timmermans G. (1975) Personality changes associated with the reduction in pain. *Pain*, 1:177–181.

Szatkowski M, Barbour B, Atwell D. (1990) Non-vesicular release of glutamate from glial cells by reversed electrogenic glutamate uptake. *Nature*, 348:443–446.

Tabira T, Shibasaki H, Kuroiwa Y. (1983) Reflex sympathetic dystrophy (causalgia) treatment with guanethidine. *Arch Neurol*, 40:430–432.

Taiwo Y, Levine J. (1992) Mediation of serotonin hyperalgesia by the cAMP second messenger system. *Neuroscience*, 48:479–483.

Talley NJ, Boyce PM, Jones M. (1998) Is the association between irritable bowel syndrome and abuse explained by neuroticism? *Gut*, 42:47–53.

Tavares I, Lima D. (2002) The caudal ventrolateral medulla as an important inhibitory modulator of pain transmission in the spinal cord. *J Pain*, 3:337–346.

Thery C, Chamak B, Mallat M. (1993) Neurotoxicity of brain macrophages. *Clin Neuropathol*, 12:288–290.

Van Der Goot FG, Pugin J, Hribar M, Fransen L, Dunant Y, Dunant Y, De Baetselier P, Bloc A, Lucas R. (1999) Membrane interaction of TNF is not sufficient to trigger increase in membrane conductance n mammalian cells. *FEBS Lett*, 460:107–111.

Ventura R, Harris KM. (1999) Three-dimensional relationships between hippocampal synapses and astrocytes. *J Neurosci*, 19:6897–6906.

Vernadakis A. (1996) Glia-neuron intercommunications and synaptic plasticity. *Prog Neurobiol*, 49:185–214.

Walker AE, Nulsen F. (1948) Electrical stimulation of the upper thoracic portion of the sympathetic chain in man. *Arch Neurol Psychiatr*, 59:559–560.

Wilkinson MF, Earle ML, Triggle CR, Barnes S. (1996) Interleukin-1 beta, tumor necrosis factor-alpha and LPS enhance calcium channel current in isolated vascular smooth muscle cells of rat tail artery. *FASEB J*, 10:785–791.

Willer JC. (1981) Stress-induced analgesia in humans: endogenous opioids and naloxone-reversible depression of pain reflexes. *Science*, 212:689–690.

Winkelstein BA, Rutkowski MD, Sweitzer SM, Pahl JL, Deleo JA. (2001) Nerve injury proximal or distal to the DRG induces similar spinal glial activation and selective cytokine expression but differential behavioral responses to pharmacologic treatment. *J Comp Neurol*, 439:127–139.

Woodham P, Anderson PN, Nadim W, Turmaine M. (1989) Satellite cells surrounding axomotised rat dorsal root ganglion cells increased expression of a GFAP-like protein. *Neurosci Lett*, 98:8–12.

Woolf CJ, Salter MW. (2000) Neuronal plasticity: increasing the gain in pain. *Science*, 288:1765–1768.

Woolf, V. (1930) *On Being Ill*. London: Hogarth Press, p. 6.

Yonei Y. (1987) Autonomic nervous alterations and mast cell degranulation in the exacerbation of ulcerative colitis. *Japan J Gastroenterol*, 84:1045–1056.

Zyluk A. (1999) Are mental disorders the cause of reflex sympathetic dystrophy: a review. *Wiad Lek*, 52:500–507.

23

Opioid Pharmacology for Pain

Charles E. Inturrisi

The increased availability of opioid maintenance treatment through office-based practice means that many chemically dependent individuals will require pain management in a primary care setting (Alford et al., 2006). This management will include the use of opioid analgesics because these drugs remain the most effective and commonly used modality for the alleviation of moderate to severe pain (Inturrisi, 2002). The issues, problems, and approaches that are to be used for pain management in chemically dependent patients, regardless of the setting, are discussed throughout this volume. The purpose of this chapter is to focus on the pharmacological properties of opioids that form the basis for their use in pain management. The most effective use of these drugs requires consideration of these properties regardless of whether or not the patient in pain is chemically dependent.

During the past 20 years there has been a dramatic increase in our knowledge of the sites and mechanisms of action of opioids (Gutstein and Akil, 2001). The development of analytical methods has also been of great importance by facilitating pharmacokinetic studies of the disposition and fate of opioids in patients. These studies have begun to offer us a better understanding of some of the sources of interindividual variation in the response to opioids and to suggest ways to minimize some of their adverse effects (Inturrisi, 2002). Although there are gaps in our knowledge of opioid pharmacology, the rational and appropriate use of these drugs is based on the knowledge of their pharmacological properties derived from well-controlled clinical trials (American Pain Society, 2003).

Opioid Analgesics

The opioid analgesics are characterized by their important pharmacological differences that are derived from their complex interactions with three opioid receptor types (mu, delta, and kappa). These opioid receptors belong to the G protein-coupled receptor (GPCR) family and they signal via a second messenger, cyclic adenosine monophosphate (cAMP) or an ion channel (Gutstein and Akil, 2001). Alterations in the levels of cAMP and the transcription factor, CREB (cAMP response element binding protein)

during chronic morphine treatment are associated with a number of cellular changes, including the development of tolerance and physical dependence (Nestler, 2004). Molecular genetic approaches have used gene-targeting (knockout) technology to disrupt the gene that codes for each of the three opioid receptors. Mice that lack the mu receptor (MOR-deficient mice) do not respond to morphine with analgesia, respiratory depression, constipation, physical dependence, reward behaviors, or immunosuppression (Kieffer and Gaveriaux-Ruff, 2002). These results confirm and extend previous pharmacological and receptor binding studies and demonstrate that the mu receptor mediates the analgesic and adverse effects of morphine.

Pharmacological evaluation of the effects of the microinjection of morphine and other opioids has been combined with anatomic characterization of the distribution of opioid receptors to provide insight into the sites of action of morphine and other clinically used mu opioids. Thus, mu opioid receptors (MOR) are found in the periphery (following inflammation), at pre- and postsynaptic sites in the spinal cord dorsal horn and in the brain stem, thalamus, and cortex, in what constitutes the ascending pain transmission system (Terman and Bonica, 2001). In addition, MOR is found in the midbrain periaqueductal gray, the nucleus raphe magnus, and the rostral ventral medulla, where they comprise a descending inhibitory system that modulates spinal cord pain transmission (Terman and Bonica, 2001). At a cellular level, opioids decrease calcium ion entry, resulting in a decrease in presynaptic neurotransmitter release (e.g., substance P release from primary afferents in the spinal cord dorsal horn). They also enhance potassium ion efflux, resulting in the hyperpolarization of postsynaptic neurons and a decrease in synaptic transmission. A third mode of opioid action is to inhibit GABAergic transmission in a local circuit, for example, in the brain stem, where GABA acts to inhibit a pain inhibitory neuron. This disinhibitory action of the opioid has the net effect of exciting a descending inhibitory circuit.

The opioid receptors are part of an endogenous opioid system that includes a large number of endogenous opioid peptide ligands. Based on cloning, three distinct families of classical opioid peptides, the enkephalins, endorphins, and dynorphins, have been identified (Gutstein and Akil, 2001). The physiological roles of the endogenous opioid peptides are not completely understood. They appear to function as neurotransmitters, neuromodulators, and in

---

Dr. Inturrisi is supported in part by NIDA grants DA001457, DA000198 and DA005130.

some cases, as neurohormones (Kieffer and Gaveriaux-Ruff, 2002). They play a role in some forms of stress-induced analgesia and in the analgesia produced by electrical stimulation of discrete brain areas such as the periaqueductal gray (Gutstein and Akil, 2001; Terman and Bonica, 2001).

Animal studies suggest that the reinforcing and rewarding properties of opioids (e.g., euphoria) that are associated with opioid abuse involve the mesolimbic dopamine system and appear to be distinct from those supraspinal systems most prominently involved in the production of analgesia and physical dependence (Gutstein and Akil, 2001).

The morphine-like agonist drugs represent one end of a spectrum. They bind predominantly to the mu opioid receptor and produce analgesia. The opioid antagonists, such as naloxone, represent the other end of the spectrum. Between these two groups are the mixed agonist-antagonist drugs, which, depending on the patient circumstances (see below), can demonstrate agonist (at the kappa receptor) or antagonist (at the mu receptor) properties.

Morphine-like Agonists

Morphine is the prototype and standard of comparison for opioid analgesics. The morphine-like agonists (Table 23.1) share with morphine a similar profile of desirable and undesirable pharmacodynamic effects. However, they differ in factors critical for dosage selection, in other words, relative analgesic potency and oral to parenteral (im/po) analgesic potency (see Table 23.1). They also differ in pharmacokinetics (e.g., elimination half-life; see Table 23.2) and biotransformation to pharmacologically active metabolites (see Inturrisi, 2002; Inturrisi and Hanks, 1993). These latter characteristics are of particular importance when opioid administration is continued beyond one or two days. Much of this information is summarized in Table 23.1 (and also detailed in American Pain Society, 2003).

Morphine

Although its oral bioavailability varies from 35 to 75%, its plasma half-life (2–3.5 hours) is somewhat shorter than its duration of analgesia (4–6 hours), which limits accumulation. Furthermore, with repetitive administration, its pharmacokinetics remain linear and there does not appear to be autoinduction of biotransformation even following large chronic doses (Inturrisi and Hanks, 1993). These pharmacokinetic properties contribute to the safe use of morphine. Morphine-6-glucuronide (M-6-G) is an active metabolite of morphine that appears to contribute to the analgesic activity of morphine (Lotsch, 2005; Portenoy et al., 1992). M-6-G is eliminated by the kidney and will accumulate relative to morphine in patients with renal insufficiency (Tiseo et al., 1995). The degree to which this accumulation of M-6-G contributes to the incidence and severity of adverse effects experienced by these patients has not been conclusively demonstrated (Lotsch, 2005; Tiseo et al., 1995). In a survey that measured steady-state morphine and M-6-G levels and adverse effects in 109 cancer patients, the presence of myoclonus or cognitive impairment was not associated with M-6-G accumulation (Tiseo et al., 1995). For a subset of the 20 patients with the highest M-6-G levels (> 2000ug/ml), the M-6-G level and concurrent organ failure was associated with the most severe toxicity (respiratory depression and/or obtundation; Tiseo et al., 1995). It is appropriate to consider an alternate opioid for a patient receiving morphine who experiences a decrease in renal function and a concomitant increase in undesirable effects. Morphine-3-glucuronide (M-3-G), the predominate metabolite of morphine in humans, is devoid of opioid activity but has excitatory effects in animals after direct injection into the CNS. This has led to the suggestion that M-3-G may be responsible for the neuroexcitatory effects sometimes seen with large chronic morphine dosing (Smith, 2000).

Based on single-dose studies in patients with either acute or chronic pain, the relative potency of intramuscular to oral morphine is 1:6. However, with repeated administration, when patients are dosed on a regular schedule (around the clock), the im/po ratio is reduced to 1:2 or 1:3 (Table 23.1). Thus, for patients with acute pain who are being titrated using a prn schedule, the 1:6 ratio should be used initially with a lower ratio expected, if dosing continues and a steady state develops.

The delayed-release morphine preparations provide analgesia with a duration of 8 to 12 hours (MS-Contin, Roxanol-SR) or 24 hours (Kadian) and allow the cancer patient a greater freedom from repetitive dosing especially during the night. Patients may be titrated using the immediate-release morphine and once stabilized, convert to the delayed-release preparation according to either an 8-hour or a 12-hour dosing schedule. To manage acute "breakthrough" pain, "rescue" medication (immediate-release morphine) should be made available to the patient receiving delayed-release preparations.

Table 23.1 lists other morphine-like agonists that may be substituted for morphine. An alternative opioid to morphine may be selected based on the need with a particular patient to overcome an adverse effect of morphine (e.g., vomiting or sedation). Other reasons include the cost, a patient's favorable prior experience with another opioid, or even local availability of other morphine-like opioids. It must be emphasized that there is no evidence to suggest that any opioid has greater analgesic efficacy than morphine.

Hydromorphone

Hydromorphone is a short half-life opioid used as an alternative to morphine by the oral and parenteral routes. It is more soluble than morphine and available in a concentrated dosage form at 10 mg/ml. This preparation is intended for parenteral administration to the opioid-tolerant patient or cachectic patient when the volume of the opioid solution to be injected must be limited.

Levorphanol

Levorphanol, which is a longer half-life opioid (Table 23.2), is also a useful alternative to morphine but it must be used cautiously to prevent accumulation. For patients who are unable to tolerate morphine and methadone, levorphanol represents a useful medication with a good oral to parenteral potency ratio of 1:2.

Oxymorphone

Oxymorphone, a congener of morphine, has had a limited but important role in the management of pain. It is available in suppository form and infrequently used parenterally on a chronic basis, Oxymorphone has recently become available for oral administration as immediate release (Opana) and Opana ER, an extended release formulation intended for twice-daily dosing. Opana and Opana ER are not intended for opioid naive patients or for as needed (prn dosing). These dosage forms are contraindicated in patients with severe hepatic impairment and should not be crushed or chewed. Like most extended release opioids, alcohol should not be coadministered with Opana ER as it increases the bioavailability of the opioid.

Methadone

Methadone's bioavailability is 85% and from single dose studies its oral to parenteral potency ratio is 1:2. Its plasma half-life averages

Table 23.1. Opioid Analgesics Commonly Used for Severe Pain

Name	Equianalgesic im Dose[a]	im/po Potency	Starting Oral Dose Range (mg)	Comments	Precautions
a. Morphine-like agonists					
Morphine	10	6[b]	30–60[b]	Standard of comparison for opioid analgesics. Sustained-release preparations (MS Contin, OramorphSR, and Kadian)	Lower doses for aged patients; impaired ventilation; bronchial asthma; increased intracranial pressure; liver failure
Hydromorphone (Dilaudid)	1.5	5	4–8	Slightly shorter acting. HP im dosage form for tolerant patients	Like morphine
Methadone (Dolophine)	Variable[c]	2	5–10	Good oral potency; long plasma half-life	Like morphine; may accumulate with repetitive dosing causing excessive sedation
Levorphanol (Levo-Dromoran)	2	2	2–4	Like methadone	Like methadone
Oxymorphone (Opana)	1	5	5	available orally in immediate and extended release preparations; available as a rectal suppository	Like morphine
Oxycodone	20	—	10–20	Immediate-release (Roxicodone and OxyIR) and sustained-release (Oxycontin) forms. Also lower doses in combination with nonopioids for less severe pain	Like morphine
Meperidine (Demerol)	75	4	Not recommended	Slightly shorter acting; used orally for less severe pain	Normeperidine (toxic metabolite) accumulates with repetitive dosing causing CNS excitation; not for patients with impaired renal function or receiving monoamine oxidase inhibitors[d]
Codeine	130	1.5	(see comments)	Used orally for less severe pain	Like morphine
Fentanyl	0.1	—	—	Transdermal fentanyl (Duragesic); also oral transmucosal fentanyl citrate for breakthrough pain	Transdermal creates skin reservoir of drug—12-hour delay in onset and offset. Fever increases absorption
b. Mixed Agonist-Antagonists					
Pentazocine (Talwin)	60	3	(see comments)	Used orally for less severe pain; mixed agonist-antagonist	May cause psychotomimetic effects; may precipitate withdrawal in opioid dependent patients; not for myocardial infarction
Nalbuphine (Nubain)	10	(see comments)	(see comments)	Not available orally; like im pentazocine but not Scheduled	Incidence of psychotomimetic effects lower than with pentazocine
Butorphanol (Stadol)	2	(see comments)	(see comments)	Not available orally. Like im nalbuphine	Like nalbuphine
c. Partial Agonists					
buprenorphine (Buprenex)	0.3	(see comments)	(see comments)	Not available orally; only parenteral form approved in United States for pain; does not produce psychotomimetic effects	May precipitate withdrawal in opioid-dependent patients; not readily reversed by naloxone; avoid in labor

For these equianalgesic im doses (also see comments), the time of peak analgesia in nontolerant patients ranges from 1/2 to 1 hour and the duration from 4 to 6 hours. The peak analgesic effect is delayed and the duration prolonged after oral administration. im = intramuscular; po = oral.

[a]These doses are recommended starting im doses from which the optimal dose for each patient is determined by titration and the maximal dose limited by adverse effects. For single iv bolus doses, use half the im dose.

[b]A value of 3 is used when calculating an oral dosage regimen of q4h around the clock.

[c]Pereira J, Lawlor P, Vigano A, et al. Equianalgesic dose ratios for opioids: a critical review and proposals for long-term dosing. J Pain Symptom Manage. 2001; 22: 672–87.

[d]Irritating to tissues on repeated administration.

Table 23.2. Plasma Half-Life Values for Opioids and Their Active Metabolites

	Plasma Half-Life (hours)
1. Shorter Half-Life Opioids	
Morphine	2–3.5
Morphine-6-glucuronide	2
Hydromorphone	2–3
Oxycodone	2–4
Fentanyl	3.7
Codeine	3
Meperidine	3–4
Pentazocine	2–3
Butorphanol	2.5–3.5
Buprenorphine	3–5
Nalbuphine	5
2. Longer Half-Life Opioids	
Oxymorphone	7.5–9.5
Levorphanol	12–16
Propoxyphene	12
Normeperidine	14–21
Methadone	13–50
Norpropoxyphene	30–40

24 hours but may range from 13 to 50 hours (Table 23.2), whereas the duration of analgesia is often only 4 to 8 hours. Repetitive analgesic doses of methadone lead to drug accumulation because of the discrepancy between its plasma half-life and the duration of analgesia. Sedation, confusion, and even death can occur when patients are not carefully monitored, and dosage adjusted during the accumulation period that can last from 5 to 10 days. However, it is a useful alternative to morphine but requires greater sophistication in its clinical use as compared with morphine. Initial doses should be titrated carefully and the as-needed (prn) mode of dosing used during the titration period.

Ripamonti et al. (1998) reported a prospective study of 38 consecutive cancer patients who were switched from morphine to oral methadone and titrated to effect so that the equianalgesic dose ratio (morphine/methadone) could be estimated. The dose ratio increased as a function of the prior morphine dose so that no single dose ratio was appropriate for naive patients or patients who were receiving various doses of morphine at the time they were switched to methadone. The data indicate that those patients who were receiving the highest doses of morphine were relatively more sensitive to the analgesic effects of methadone, in other words, they had the highest dose ratio. This unidirectional variability in the dose ratio may reflect incomplete cross-tolerance between morphine and methadone and further emphasizes the need for individualization of dose and careful titration to effect when switching to methadone (Foley and Houde, 1998).

The dosage form of methadone that is used clinically in most countries, including the United States, is a racemic mixture of equal amounts of the l-isomer, an opioid, and the d-isomer, which lacks opioid activity (Davis and Inturrisi, 1999). However, both the l- and the d-isomers of methadone bind to the NMDA receptor and the d-isomer has functional NMDA receptor antagonist activity in animals, including antihyperalgesic activity and the ability to prevent the development of morphine tolerance (Davis and Inturrisi, 1999; Inturrisi, 2002).

Meperidine

Studies of meperidine in cancer patients have demonstrated that repetitive dosing can lead to accumulation of its toxic metabolite, normeperidine, resulting in central nervous system hyperexcitability (Kaiko et al., 1983). This is characterized initially by subtle mood effects followed by tremors, multifocal myoclonus, and occasionally seizures. This CNS hyperexcitability occurs commonly in patients with renal disease but it can occur following repeated administration in patients with normal renal function (Kaiko et al., 1983; Szeto et al., 1977).

Oxycodone

Oxycodone is available both as immediate release and a continuous release (8–12 hour duration) preparation (Oxycontin), and these dosage forms can be used for moderate to severe pain. However, lower doses (e.g., 5 mg) in combination with nonopioids (aspirin, acetaminophen) are frequently used for mild to moderate pain. The fixed-dose oxycodone combinations should not be used chronically in large doses for more severe pain because of the risk of dose-related toxicity from the nonopioid ingredients.

Fentanyl

Fentanyl is estimated to be approximately 80 to 100 times as potent as morphine (American Pain Society, 2003; Gutstein and Akil, 2001). It is a highly lipophilic drug with shorter duration of action than parenteral morphine. Fentanyl is used for the management of postoperative pain by the intravenous and epidural routes of administration, a transdermal patch device is used for chronic pain requiring opioid analgesia, and a transmucosal dosage form is used for breakthrough pain in tolerant patients (American Pain Society, 2003).

Agonist-Antagonist Analgesics

The mixed agonist-antagonist analgesics (Table 23.1) include pentazocine, butorphanol, and nalbuphine. They produce analgesia in the nontolerant patient but may precipitate withdrawal in patients who are dependent as a result of repeated exposure to a morphine-like drug. Therefore, they are not appropriate choices for patients who have been receiving a morphine-like agonist drug for pain management or for the maintenance treatment of chemical dependency. There is a ceiling effect on the ability of the mixed agonist-antagonists to produce respiratory depression and they have a significantly lower abuse liability than the morphine-like drugs. In therapeutic doses, they may produce certain self-limiting psychotomimetic effects in some patients, with pentazocine the most common drug associated with these effects.

These drugs play a very limited role in the management of persistent pain because the incidence and severity of the psychotomimetic effects increase with dose escalation and because they are not currently available in convenient oral dosage forms. Thus, nalbuphine is available only for parenteral use and the oral preparation of pentazocine is marketed in combination with naloxone. Butorphanol is available for both parenteral and intranasal use. Following its introduction, the intranasal dosage was found to have a significantly higher abuse liability than anticipated, primarily in migraine patients (Loder, 2006). This formulation, as requested by the manufacturer, is now in a more restricted prescribing category (DEA Schedule IV). Single-dose studies in an oral surgery model indicate that women may derive more pain relief than males from kappa opioid analgesics (Gear et al., 1996), and this may stimulate the development of new kappa opioids that can be administered by routes (oral, transdermal) that are appropriate for the management of persistent pain.

Partial Agonist Analgesics

The partial agonist buprenorphine (Table 23.1) has less abuse liability than the morphine-like drugs but like the mixed agonist-antagonists, it may also precipitate withdrawal in some patients who have received repeated doses of a morphine-like agonist and developed physical dependence. However, it does not produce the psychotomimetic effects seen with the mixed agonist-antagonists and is available in both a sublingual and parenteral form. Only the parenteral dosage form (Buprenex) is currently approved for pain management in the United States. The sublingual form alone (Subutex) and in combination with naloxone (Suboxone) is approved in the United States for the treatment of opioid dependence. Buprenorphine's respiratory depressant effects are reversed only by relatively large doses of naloxone (Gal, 1989). It has been studied in cancer patients with pain and is useful for moderate to severe pain requiring an opioid analgesic. However, it should be used before the morphine-like agonists are introduced. Its use in the maintenance treatment of opioid dependence is discussed elsewhere in this book.

Opioid Pharmacokinetics

As noted above, the opioids differ significantly in one measure of drug elimination, the plasma half-life value (Table 23.2). Thus, although morphine and hydromorphone are short half-life opioids that on repeated dosing reach steady state in 10 to 12 hrs, levorphanol and methadone are longer half-life opioids that on the average may require 70 to 120 hours, respectively, to achieve steady state. During dose titration, the maximal (peak) effects produced by a change dose of a short half-life opioid will appear relatively quickly, whereas the peak effects resulting from a change in the dose of a long half-life opioid will be achieved after a longer accumulation period. For example, a patient who reports adequate pain relief following the initial doses of methadone may experience excessive sedation if this dosage is fixed and not modified as required during the accumulation period of 5 to 10 days.

Also, note that the active (toxic) metabolites normeperidine and norpropoxyphene have much longer plasma half-life values than their corresponding parents (meperidine and propoxyphene) so that administration of the parent on a schedule designed to produce continued pain relief results in accumulation of the metabolite. Opioid pharmacokinetics are altered by certain drug and/or disease interactions (see Inturrisi and Hanks, 1993).

Route of Administration

Opioids are available in dosage forms for use by a number of routes of administration. These include oral, transdermal, intramuscular, intravenous (bolus, continuous infusion, and patient controlled), subcutaneous infusion, rectal, epidural, intrathecal, intranasal, and transmucosal. The rationale for each route of administration and the dosage forms and range of doses are detailed in the American Pain Society guidelines (American Pain Society, 2003).

Opioid Rotation

Opioid rotation (OR) involves switching the opioid a patient is receiving to another opioid with the objective of reducing limiting adverse effects and/or increasing analgesia. Surveys as well as a great deal of anecdotal evidence suggest that OR can "open the therapeutic window" by reducing limiting adverse effects (Indelicato and Portenoy, 2002). When using the values in Table 23.1 for OR, it becomes important to recognize that the equianalgesic dose estimates are based on the single-dose studies and they represent a useful reference point for the initiation of dose titration. They do not take into account incomplete cross-tolerance and therefore are not meant to be used with every patient (Inturrisi, 2007). The overarching consideration in selecting a dosing schedule for opioid rotation is first to limit the risk of overdose as one opioid is discontinued and the substitute is introduced (see Indelicato and Portenoy, 2002; Inturrisi, 2007).

Scheduled Opioid Administration

The schedule of opioid administration should be individualized for each patient. In general, patients with persistent pain should receive opioids on a regular schedule once the patient's dosage has been established by titration using an as-needed (prn) schedule. This approach is especially important when the dose titration involves a long half-life opioid such as methadone or levorphanol, as discussed above. A regular, around-the-clock schedule of opioid administration can prevent severe pain from recurring and may allow for a reduction in the total opioid required per day. For some patients, a prn order for a supplemental opioid dose (rescue) between the regularly scheduled doses may be required to provide adequate pain relief.

Adverse Effects of Opioids

There are a number of side effects associated with the use of opioid analgesics that can, depending upon the circumstances, be categorized as desirable or undesirable. The mechanisms that underlie these various adverse effects are only partly understood and appear to depend upon a number of factors including the patient's age, extent of disease and organ dysfunction, concurrent administration of certain drugs, prior opioid exposure, and the route of drug administration. The most common adverse effects are sedation, nausea and vomiting, constipation, and respiratory depression. But there are other adverse effects including confusion, hallucinations, nightmares, urinary retention, multifocal myoclonus, dizziness, dysphoria, and hyperalgesia that have been reported by patients receiving these drugs (Bruera and O'Pereira, 1997).

Respiratory Depression

Respiratory depression is potentially the most serious adverse effect. The morphine-like agonists act on brainstem respiratory centers to produce, as a function of dose, increasing respiratory depression to the point of apnea. In humans, death due to overdose of a morphine-like agonist is nearly always due to respiratory arrest. Therapeutic doses of morphine may depress all phases of respiratory activity (rate, minute volume, and tidal exchange). However, as CO_2 accumulates, it stimulates central chemoreceptors, resulting in a compensatory increase in respiratory rate, which masks the degree of respiratory depression. At equianalgesic doses, the morphine-like agonists produce an equivalent degree of respiratory depression.

For these reasons, individuals with impaired respiratory function or bronchial asthma are at greater risk of experiencing clinically significant respiratory depression in response to usual doses of these drugs. Respiratory depression and CO_2 retention result in cerebral vasodilation and an increase in cerebrospinal fluid pressure unless PCO_2 is maintained at normal levels by artificial ventilation. When respiratory depression occurs, it is usually in opioid-naive patients following acute administration of an opioid and is associated with other signs of central nervous system depression including sedation and mental clouding. Tolerance develops rapidly to this effect with repeated drug administration, allowing the opioid analgesics to be used in the management of chronic pain without significant risk of respiratory depression. If respiratory depression occurs, it can be reversed by the administration of the specific opioid antagonist naloxone. In patients chronically receiving opioids who develop respiratory depression, naloxone diluted 1:10 should be titrated carefully to prevent the precipitation of severe withdrawal symptoms while reversing the respiratory depression. An endotracheal tube should be placed in the comatose patient before administering naloxone to prevent aspiration-associated respiratory compromise with excessive salivation and bronchial spasm. In patients receiving meperidine chronically, naloxone may precipitate seizures by blocking the depressant action of meperidine and allowing the convulsant activity of the active metabolite, normeperidine, to be manifest. If naloxone is to be used in this situation, diluted doses slowly titrated with appropriate seizure precautions are advised.

The mixed agonist-antagonists and the partial agonist (buprenorphine) appear to differ in the dose-response characteristics of their respiratory depression curves from that of the morphine-like drugs, so that although therapeutic doses of pentazocine produce respiratory depression equivalent to that of morphine, increasing the dose does not ordinarily produce a proportional increase in respiratory depression. Whether this apparent ceiling to respiratory depression offers any clinical advantage remains to be determined. Also, the clinical symptoms of a large overdose of these drugs, with particular respect to respiratory depression, have not been well defined (Gal, 1989).

Nausea and Vomiting

The opioid analgesics produce nausea and vomiting by an action on the medullary chemoreceptor trigger zone. The incidence of nausea and vomiting is markedly increased in ambulatory patients, suggesting that these drugs also alter vestibular sensitivity. The ability of opioid analgesics to produce nausea and vomiting appears to vary with drug and patient so that some advantage may result from opioid rotation. Alternately, an antiemetic may be used in combination with the opioid. For some patients, initiating treatment by the parenteral route and then switching to the oral route may reduce the emetic symptoms (Foley, 1996).

Sedation

The opioid analgesics produce sedation and drowsiness. Although these effects may be useful in certain clinical situations (e.g., preanesthesia), they are not usually desirable concomitants of analgesia, particularly in ambulatory patients. The CNS depressant actions of these drugs can be expected to be at least additive with the sedative and respiratory depressant effects of sedative-hypnotics such as alcohol, the barbiturates, and the benzodiazepines.

Although it has been suggested that methadone produces more sedation than morphine, this has not been supported by single-dose controlled trials or surveys in hospitalized patients (Foley, 1996). However, the half-life of methadone is substantially longer than morphine and can result in cumulative CNS depression after repeated doses. A reduction in dose and interval so that a lower dose is given more frequently may counteract excessive sedation. In addition, other CNS depressants including sedative-hypnotics and antianxiety agents that potentiate the sedative effects of opioids should be discontinued. Concurrent administration of dextroamphetamine in 2.5–5.0 mg oral doses twice daily has been reported to reduce the sedative effects of opioids. Tolerance usually develops to the sedative effects of opioid analgesics within the first several days of chronic administration.

Constipation

The most common adverse effect of the opioid analgesics is constipation. These drugs act at multiple sites in the gastrointestinal tract and spinal cord to produce a decrease in intestinal secretions and peristalsis, resulting in a dry stool and constipation. Tolerance develops very slowly to the smooth muscle effects of opioids so that constipation will persist when these drugs are used for chronic pain. At the same time that the use of opioid analgesics is initiated, provision for a regular bowel regimen, including cathartics and stool softeners, should be instituted to diminish this adverse effect.

Urinary Retention

Because the opioid analgesics increase smooth muscle tone, they can cause bladder spasm and an increase in sphincter tone leading to urinary retention. This is most common in the elderly patient. Attention should be directed at this potential side effect and catheterization may be necessary to manage this transient side effect.

Multifocal Myoclonus

At high doses, all of the opioid analgesics can produce multifocal myoclonus (Foley, 1996). This complication is most prominent with the use of repeated administration of large parenteral doses of meperidine (e.g., 250 mg or more per day). As previously discussed, accumulation of normeperidine is responsible for this toxicity.

The Opioid Tolerant Patient

Tolerance develops when a given dose of an opioid produces a decreasing effect, or when a larger dose is required to maintain the original effect. Some degree of tolerance to analgesia appears to develop in most patients receiving opioid analgesics chronically (McQuay, 1999). The hallmark sign of the development of tolerance is the patient's complaint of a decrease in the duration of effective analgesia. The rate of development of tolerance varies greatly among cancer patients so that some will demonstrate tolerance within days of initiating opioid therapy, whereas others will remain well controlled for many months on the same dose (Kanner and Foley, 1981). A sudden dramatic increase in opioid requirements may represent a progression of the disease rather than the development of tolerance per se. In these patients, objective evidence of progression of disease is sought and pain management techniques reevaluated accordingly (Kanner and Foley, 1981). With the development of tolerance, increasing the frequency and/or increasing the dose of the opioid are required to provide continued pain relief. Because the analgesic effect is a logarithmic function of the dose of opioid, a doubling of the dose may be required to restore full analgesia. There appears to be no limit to the development of tolerance and with appropriate adjustment of dose patients can continue to obtain pain relief. Recent studies, discussed elsewhere in this book, support the concept that the decrease in opioid sensitivity seen with repeated opioid administration may result, at least in part, from opioid-induced neuroplastic changes that result in hyperalgesic states (Mao, 2002). Further, this latent hyperalgesia may contribute to increased pain sensitivity in patients receiving opioid maintenance therapy (Alford et al., 2006).

Combinations of opioids with nonopioids that enhance analgesia not only provide additive analgesia but because tolerance does not develop to the nonopioid component of the mixture, the overall result is a slower rate of development of tolerance. From the start, a nonopioid (e.g., acetaminophen) should be used with the opioid. Cross-tolerance among the opioid analgesics appears not to be complete, and therefore advantage is gained by opioid rotation and selecting some fraction (1/10 to 1/2) of the predicted equianalgesic dose (see Table 23.1) as the starting dose for the alternate opioid (Inturrisi, 2007). The use of bolus or continuous epidural local anesthetics in patients with localized pain, for example, perineal pain, can dramatically reduce the need for systemic opioids and thus diminish opioid tolerance.

The Opioid-Dependent Patient: Definitions and Misconceptions

Psychological and Physical Dependence

The properties of the opioid analgesics that are most likely to lead to their being misused, or the patient mistreated, are effects mediated in the central nervous system and seen following chronic administration, including psychological dependence and physical dependence. It must be emphasized that although the development of physical dependence and tolerance are predictable pharmacologic effects seen in humans and laboratory animals in response to repeated administration of an opioid, these effects are distinct from the behavioral pattern seen in some individuals and described by the terms psychological dependence or addiction (O'Brien, 2001). Psychological dependence is used to describe a pattern of drug use characterized by a continued craving for an opioid that is manifest as compulsive drug-seeking behavior leading to an overwhelming involvement with the use and procurement of the drug. Within these definitions, most, but not all, individuals who are addicted to opioids will have acquired some degree of physical dependence. However, the converse is not true, so that an individual can be physically dependent on an opioid analgesic without being addicted. Fear of addiction is a major concern limiting the use of appropriate doses of opioids in hospitalized patients in pain.

Physical dependence is the term used to describe the phenomenon of withdrawal when an opioid is abruptly discontinued or if an opioid antagonist is administered. The severity of withdrawal is a function of the dose and duration of administration of the opioid just discontinued (i.e., the patient's prior opioid exposure). The administration of an opioid antagonist to a physically dependent individual produces an immediate precipitation of the withdrawal syndrome. Patients who have received repeated doses of a morphine-like agonist to the point at which they are physically dependent may experience an opioid withdrawal reaction when given a mixed agonist-antagonist. Prior exposure to a morphine-like drug can be shown to greatly increase a patient's sensitivity to the antagonist component of a mixed agonist-antagonist. Therefore, when used for chronic pain, the mixed agonist-antagonist opioids should be tried prior to initiating prolonged administration of a morphine-like agonist.

The abrupt discontinuation of an opioid analgesic in a patient with significant prior opioid experience will result in signs and symptoms characteristic of the opioid withdrawal or abstinence syndrome (O'Brien, 2001). The time course of the withdrawal syndrome is a function of the elimination half-life of the opioid to which the patient has become dependent. Abstinence symptoms will appear within 6–12 hours and reach a peak at 24–72 hours following cessation of a short half-life drug such as morphine, whereas onset may be delayed for 36 to 48 hours with methadone, a long half-life drug. Therefore, it is important to emphasize that even in a patient in whom pain has been completely relieved by a procedure (e.g., a cordotomy), it is necessary to slowly decrement the opioid dose to prevent withdrawal.

Experience indicates that the usual daily dose required to prevent withdrawal is equal to approximately one-fourth of the previous daily dose. This detoxification dose, for want of a better term, is given in four divided doses. The initial detoxification dose is given for 2 days and then decremented by one-half (administered in 4 divided doses) for 2 days until a total daily dose of 10 to 15 mg per day (in morphine equivalents) is reached and after 2 days on this dose the opioid can be discontinued. Thus, a patient who had been receiving 240 mg per day of morphine for pain would require an initial detoxification dose of 60 mg given as 15 mg every 6 hours. Alternately, the patient may be switched to the equieffective oral analgesic dose of methadone, using one-fourth of this dose as the initial detoxification dose and proceeding as described above.

Summary

The fundamental concept that underlies the appropriate and successful management of pain by the use of opioid analgesics is individualization of analgesic therapy. This concept entails an understanding of the clinical pharmacology of the opioids to provide the information necessary for the selection of the right analgesic, administered in the right dose and on the right schedule so as to maximize pain relief and minimize adverse effects. The analgesic efficacy of the opioids does not appear to have a conventional dose related ceiling; rather, dose escalation is usually limited by the incidence and severity of adverse effects. Therefore, individual titration of the dose combined with measures to reduce the adverse effects is key to optimizing the management of pain with these drugs.

References

Alford DP, Compton P, Samet JH (2006) Acute pain management for patients receiving maintenance methadone or buprenorphine therapy. *Ann Intern Med* 144:127–134.

American Pain Society (2003) *Principles of Analgesic Use in the Treatment of Acute Pain and Cancer Pain,* 5th ed. Glenview, IL: American Pain Society.

Bruera E, O'Pereira J (1997) Neuropsychiatric toxicity of opioids. In: Jensen TS, Turner JA, Wiesenfeld-Hallin Z, eds. *Proceedings of the 8th World Congress on Pain,* pp. 717–738. Seattle: IASP Press.

Davis AM, Inturrisi CE (1999) d-Methadone blocks morphine tolerance and N-methyl-D-aspartate-induced hyperalgesia. *J Pharmacol Exp Ther* 289:1048–1053.

Foley KM (1996) Problems of overarching importance which transcend organ systems. In: Bennett JC, Plum F, eds. *Cecil's Textbook of Medicine.* Philadelphia: Saunders.

Foley KM, Houde RW (1998) Methadone in cancer pain management: individualize dose and titrate to effect. *J Clin Oncol* 16:3213–3215.

Gal TJ (1989) Naloxone reversal of buprenorphine-induced respiratory depression. *Clin Pharmacol Ther* 45:66–71.

Gear RW, Miaskowski C, Gordon NC, Paul SM, Heller PH, Levine JD (1996) Kappa-opioids produce significantly greater analgesia in women than in men. *Nat Med* 2:1248–1250.

Gutstein HB, Akil H (2001) Opioid analgesics. In: Hardman JG, Limbird LE, eds. *Goodman & Gilman's The Pharmacological Basis of Therapeutics*, 9th ed., pp. 569–619. New York: McGraw-Hill.

Indelicato RA, Portenoy RK (2002) Opioid rotation in the management of refractory cancer pain. *J Clin Oncol* 20:348–352.

Inturrisi CE (2002) Clinical pharmacology of opioids for pain. *Clin J Pain* 18:S3-S13.

Inturrisi CE (2007) Opioid rotation. In: Schmidt RF and Willis WD, eds. *Encyclopedia of Pain*, pp. 1561–1564. Berlin: Springer.

Inturrisi CE, Hanks GWC (1993) Opioid analgesic therapy. In: Doyle D, Hanks GWC, MacDonald N, eds. *Oxford Textbook of Palliative Medicine*, pp. 166–182. Oxford: Oxford University Press.

Kaiko RF, Foley KM, Grabinski PY, Heidrich G, Rogers AG, Inturrisi CE, Reidenberg MM (1983) Central nervous system excitatory effects of meperidine in cancer patients. *Ann Neurol* 13:180–185.

Kanner RM, Foley KM (1981) Patterns of narcotic drug use in a cancer pain clinic. *Ann NY Acad Sci* 362:161–172.

Kieffer BL, Gaveriaux-Ruff C (2002) Exploring the opioid system by gene knockout. *Prog Neurobiol* 66:285–306.

Loder E (2006) Post-marketing experience with an opioid nasal spray for migraine: lessons for the future. *Cephalalgia* 26:89–97.

Lotsch J (2005) Opioid metabolites. *J Pain Symptom Manage* 29:S10–24.

Mao J (2002) Opioid-induced abnormal pain sensitivity: implications in clinical opioid therapy. *Pain* 100:213–217.

McQuay H (1999) Opioids in pain management. *Lancet* 353:2229–2232.

Nestler EJ (2004) Molecular mechanisms of drug addiction. *Neuropharmacology* 47 Suppl 1:24–32.

O'Brien C (2001) Drug addiction and drug abuse. In: Hardman JG, Limbird LE, eds. *Goodman & Gilman's The Pharmacological Basis of Therapeutics*, 9th ed., pp. 621–642. New York: McGraw-Hill.

Portenoy RK, Thaler HT, Inturrisi CE, Friedlander-Klar H, Foley KM (1992) The metabolite morphine-6-glucuronide contributes to the analgesia produced by morphine infusion in patients with pain and normal renal function. *Clin Pharmacol Ther* 51:422–431.

Ripamonti C, Groff L, Brunelli C, Polastri D, Stavrakis A, De Conno F (1998) Switching from morphine to oral methadone in treating cancer pain: what is the equianalgesic dose ratio? *J Clin Oncol* 16:3216–3221.

Smith MT (2000) Neuroexcitatory effects of morphine and hydromorphone: evidence implicating the 3-glucuronide metabolites. *Clin Exp Pharmacol Physiol* 27:524–528.

Szeto HH, Inturrisi CE, Houde R, Saal S, Cheigh J, Reidenberg MM (1977) Accumulation of normeperidine, an active metabolite of meperidine, in patients with renal failure of cancer. *Ann Intern Med* 86:738–741.

Terman GW, Bonica JJ (2001) Spinal mechanisms and their modulation. In: Loeser JD, Butler SH, Chapman CR, Turk DC, eds. *Bonica's Management of Pain*, 3rd ed., pp. 73–152. Philadelphia: Lippincott Williams and Wilkins.

Tiseo PJ, Thaler HT, Lapin J, Inturrisi CE, Portenoy RK, Foley KM (1995) Morphine-6-glucuronide concentrations and opioid-related side effects: a survey in cancer patients. *Pain* 61:47–54.

24

Opioids for Pain

Howard S. Smith

Todd W. Vanderah

Gary McCleane

Nature of Pain

Pain is described as an unpleasant sensation associated with a specific part of the body (Melzack & Katz, 2006). It is produced by processes that either damage, or are capable of damaging, the tissues. Such damaging stimuli are called "noxious" and are detected by specific sensory receptors called "nociceptors" (Sherington, 1906). Nociceptors are identified as C-fibers and Aδ-fibers. By definition, nociceptors respond selectively to noxious stimuli. These nociceptors are free nerve endings with cell bodies in the dorsal root ganglia and terminate in the superficial layers of the dorsal horn of the spinal cord. Here they relay messages by releasing neurotransmitters such as glutamate (Jeftinija et al., 1991), substance P, and calcitonin gene-related peptide (CGRP; Lawson et al., 1997, 2002). These "pain" neurotransmitters will result in the activation of the second-order neuron via their corresponding receptor. The second-order neuron crosses the spinal cord to the contralateral side and travels up the spinothalamic tract until it reaches the thalamus. From there, the third-order neuron is activated, traveling from the thalamus to the somatosensory cortex, which allows for the perception of pain. It should be mentioned that at the level of the spinal cord, second-order neurons result in the direct activation of lower motor neurons in the ventral horn of the spinal cord which provokes a reflex withdrawal from the noxious stimulus. Likewise, there are interneurons at the level of the spinal cord that will modulate the incoming pain information.

Neural Processing of Pain Signals

Several steps can be identified in the neural processing of noxious signals that can lead to the experience of pain. The four major processes leading to the pain experience include: transduction, transmission, modulation, and perception.

1. *Transduction* is the process by which noxious stimuli are converted to electrical signals in the nociceptors. Unlike other sensory receptors, nociceptors are not specialized from the structural point of view (in contrast to, e.g., Pacinian corpuscles or Merkel's disks), but rather exist as free nerve endings. Nociceptors readily respond to different noxious modalities such as thermal, mechanical, or chemical stimuli, but *nociceptors do not respond to nonnoxious stimuli*. Also in contrast to other types of sensory receptors, *nociceptors do not adapt*. That is, continued stimulation results in continuous or repetitive firing of the nociceptor and, in some cases, continued stimulation results in a decrease in the threshold at which the nociceptors respond (i.e., sensitization of nociceptors; Kilo et al., 1994; LaMotte et al., 1982; Meyer & Campbell, 1981).

Nociceptive afferent fibers are typically pseudounipolar neurons, with a peripheral terminal and a central terminal. Neurotransmitters that are produced within the cell body (i.e., in the dorsal root ganglia) are the same at both the central and peripheral ends of the nerve fiber. The neurotransmitters are released at both ends, participating in producing the pain signal peripherally, as well as promoting events that lead to pain perception centrally. The release of neurotransmitters from the peripheral terminals of the afferent fibers is actually an "efferent" function of these afferent neurons. Peripheral release of neurotransmitter substances leads to the classic *axon reflex*. This reflex leads to peripheral changes that are recognized as indicators of pain—redness, swelling, and tenderness (Schmelz & Petersen, 2001).

The pain produced can result from *activation* of the peripheral nociceptors by the released neurotransmitters and inflammatory mediators, as well as decreases in the threshold of response of the nociceptive fiber and surrounding nociceptors (nociceptor *sensitization*). In addition, "sleeping" or "silent" nociceptors that are normally not active are recruited after tissue injury has occurred and may then respond to a variety of stimulus modalities (Handwerker et al., 1991; Meyer et al., 1991). When these previously silent nociceptors become activated, they respond to noxious stimuli more vigorously (i.e., the same stimulus now produces more pain), this is called *hyperalgesia*. Curiously, normally nonnoxious stimuli can also produce pain, a phenomenon called *allodynia*.

More importantly, opioid receptors located on the peripheral nerve endings, when activated by either endogenous or exogenous opioids (i.e., administration of morphine), show inhibition of afferent firing. Morphine acting at these mu opioid receptors (G-protein coupled receptors) results in the *indirect* opening of potassium channels. Potassium with its positive charge flows out of the nociceptor leaving the inside of the neuron with a more negative charge. The enhanced intracellular negative charge hyperpolarizes the nociceptor, resulting in a decrease in nociceptor activity (i.e., analgesia).

2. *Transmission* is the second stage of processing of noxious signals. Information from the periphery is relayed to the spinal cord, then to the thalamus, and finally to the cortex. Noxious information is relayed mainly via two different types of primary afferent nociceptive neurons, C-fibers and A-delta fibers, which conduct at different velocities.

C-fibers are nonmyelinated fibers that conduct in the range of 0.5–2 m/sec. Nociceptive C-fibers transmit noxious information from a variety of modalities including mechanical, thermal, and chemical stimuli—for this reason, they are termed *C-polymodal nociceptors*.

A-delta fibers are thinly myelinated fibers that conduct in the range of 2–20 m/sec. All A-delta fibers respond to high intensity mechanical stimulation and are therefore termed *high threshold mechanoreceptors*. Some, but not all, fibers also respond to thermal stimuli, termed *mechanothermal receptors* (see Meyer et al., 2006, for review).

These afferent fibers then synapse on a second-order neuron in the superficial layer of the spinal cord. This second-order neuron will send its axon across the midline and form the ascending spinothalamic tract that leads to the thalamus. It is in the thalamus that the second-order cell synapses with the third-order cell that projects to the sensory cortex.

An ascending system that complements the classical spinothalamic tract—which provides afferent input regarding the sensory-discriminative aspects of pain—is the spinobulbar pathway, which may contribute afferent input regarding the affective-motivational components of pain. Lamina I projection neurons that express neurokinin-1 (NK1) project to the brainstem, including the parabrachial area, the periaqueductal gray, and the thalamic/limbic system (areas of the central nervous system associated with affective and cognitive functions; Bester et al., 2000; Todd, 2002). Selective partial destruction of these NK1-expressing neurons in the superficial dorsal horn with the use of substance P-saporin yielded animals with significant deficits in behavioral hyperalgesia response to nerve ligation and irritant hind paw injection but normal acute nociceptive responses (Nicols et al., 1999).

Similar results were seen after spinal administration of the 5HT3-receptor antagonist ondansetron, which blocks the activity of the serotonergic descending pain facilitory bulbospinal pathway from the RVM (Suzuki et al., 2002). Another ascending pathway originating from NK1 expressing cells of spinal cord dorsal horn, lamina I may not contribute significantly to acute "physiologic" nociception; however, it may play a role in certain chronic "pathologic" pain states.

Some NK1-expressing neurons of lamina I project to lamina V, where they may excite wide dynamic range (WDR) neurons of the postsynaptic dorsal column (PSDC) pathway—and many of these PSPC neurons terminate in the nucleus gracilis (Cheunsuang & Morris, 2000). Although these neurons typically mediate light touch and vibration, it is conceivable that a sensitized PSDC projection to the nucleus gracilis (NG) may contribute to the NG becoming hyperresponsive to mechanical sensory input from large-diameter Aβ primary afferent fibers (Bennett et al., 1983).

The second-order cells in the spinal dorsal horn also have the capacity to change their response patterns in the circumstance of sustained discharge of afferent fibers (as would occur in the setting of an injury). Under circumstances of "afferent nociceptive barrage," these cells respond at lower thresholds and form inputs over a broader area in the periphery—expanding their "receptive fields," in other words, the second-order cells become "sensitized." This is termed *central sensitization* and also contributes to the phenomena of hyperalgesia and allodynia (LaMotte et al., 1991).

Once the nociceptive afferents have terminated in the dorsal horn of the spinal cord, they transmit the signal from the periphery by releasing specific neurotransmitters associated with pain. One of the most important neurotransmitters for pain and the primary afferent is glutamate, which can interact with both NMDA-type and non-NMDA excitatory amino acid receptors. Another important transmitter associated with the transmission of pain is an 11-amino acid peptide called *substance P*, which interacts with the tachykinin receptor family (G-protein coupled receptors).

3. *Modulation* is a third and critically important aspect of the processing of noxious stimuli. This process represents changes that occur in the nervous system in response to noxious stimuli and allows noxious signals received at the dorsal horn of the spinal cord to be selectively *inhibited* so that the transmission of the signal to higher centers is modified. An endogenous pain modulation system consisting of well-defined *intermediate neurons* within the superficial layers of the spinal cord and *descending neural tracts* can inhibit transmission of the pain signal (Yaksh, 2006). Endogenous and exogenous opioids can act on the presynaptic terminal of the primary afferent nociceptor via the mu opioid receptor by *indirectly* blocking voltage gated calcium channels as well as opening potassium channels. The inhibition of calcium entry into the presynaptic terminal as well as the efflux of potassium (hyperpolarization) results in the inhibition of pain neurotransmitter release from the primary afferent fibers, hence analgesia. Opioids have a second site of action at the level of the spinal cord. When activated by an opioid, opioid receptors on the postsynaptic nerve (the second-order neuron) *indirectly* open potassium channels resulting in hyperpolarization of the nerve (see Figures 24.1 and 24.2.).

a. *Descending modulatory inhibitory systems:* Activation of the descending system by endorphins occurs through specific receptors called *opioid receptors*. These systems are activated in and around the periaqueductal gray (PAG) region of the midbrain. Such neurons then project to sites in the medullary reticular formation and the locus ceruleus (the major source of norepinephrine cells in the brain) through uncertain circuitry where other neurons are activated (probably through disinhibition, an inhibition of a tonically active inhibitory interneuron). These descending fibers then pro-

Figure 24.1. Opioids inhibit noxious input.

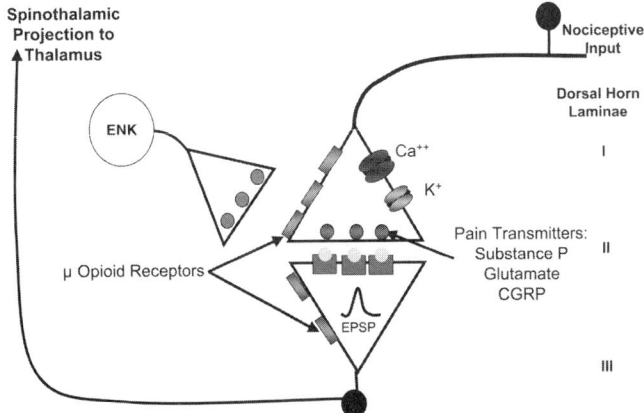

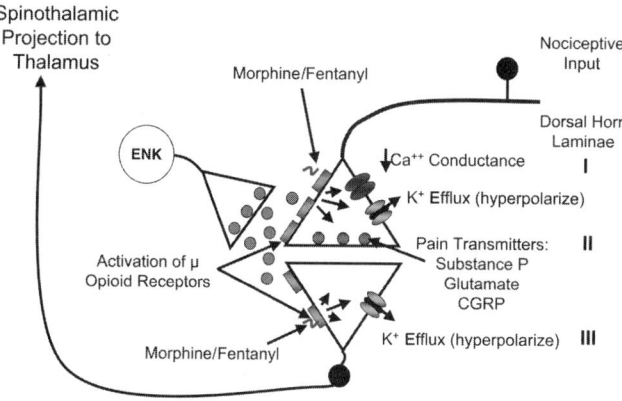

Figure 24.2. Opioids inhibit noxious input.

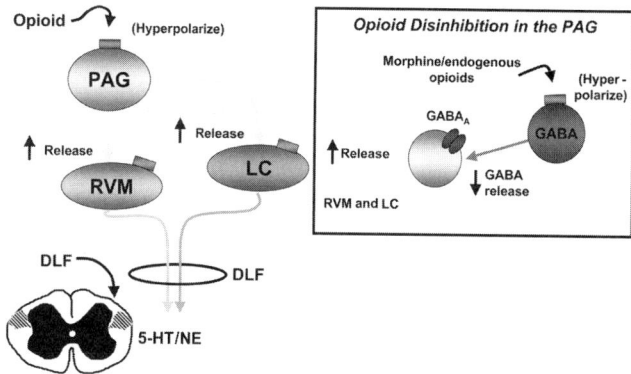

Figure 24.4. Descending modulation of spinal nociceptive input.

ject to the dorsal horn of the spinal cord along a tract called the dorsolateral funiculus (located in the dorsolateral portion of the spinal cord) to synapse with either the incoming primary afferent neuron, the second-order pain transmission neuron, or interneurons (see Figure 24.3). These descending pain modulatory neurons either release neurotransmitters in the spinal cord, especially serotonin (5HT) and norepinephrine (NE), or activate small opioid-containing interneurons in the spinal dorsal horn to release opioid peptides (again through disinhibition; see Figure 24.4). The released NE and 5HT act to directly inhibit the release of pain transmitters from the incoming nociceptive afferent signal, and to inhibit the second-order pain transmission cell. Activation of the descending pain modulatory system is a good example of why subjects report not feeling pain at all under conditions of stress, or perhaps other situations, when even though the pain is felt, the degree appears to be greatly modulated (Boivie & Meyerson, 1982; Fields et al., 1991; Mayer & Price, 1976).

b. *Descending modulatory excitatory (facilitating) systems:* There exist neural pathways emanating from the rostral ventral medulla (RVM) that not only inhibit nociception, but also may facilitate nociceptive input (Gebhart, 2004). These descending facilitatory pathways appear to be serotonergic in nature with 5-HT3 receptors terminating on NK1-expressing neurons in lamina I (see Figure 24.5; Smith, 2006a). Cholecystokinin (CCK) in the RVM appears to facilitate pain as well as antagonize the actions of opioids, and noxious stimulus-induced CCK elevation may contribute to engaging descending facilitatory pathways (Ossipov & Porreca, 2005). Bulbospinal-descending facilitatory pathways travel from the RVM to the dorsal horn of the spinal cord, where the upregulation of spinal dynorphin is promoted (Ossipov & Porreca, 2005). Lesions of the dorsolateral funiculus or dermorphin-saporin microinjection into the RVM prevented both the behavioral manifestations of neuropathic pain and upregulation of spinal dynorphin (Gardell et al., 2004).

4. *Perception:* The final perception of pain in the human brain is a highly complex and incompletely understood process. However, it seems to involve a combination of the nociceptive information that reaches various parts of the brain, brain modulation of nociceptive information, and perhaps a network of ancillary processes from higher CNS centers involved in the interaction of this "fetal perception" of pain. Other factors (e.g., mood, cognition, memory/past history, attention, anxiety, punishment, culture, and environment), as well as other processes, may promote the development and maturation of this fetal perception—leading to of a finalized individual patient pain perception.

Summary of sites of opioid action: We can identify four sites where opioids can act to relieve pain. When you give morphine or other opiates to patients you are doing the following:

Figure 24.3. Descending pain pathways.

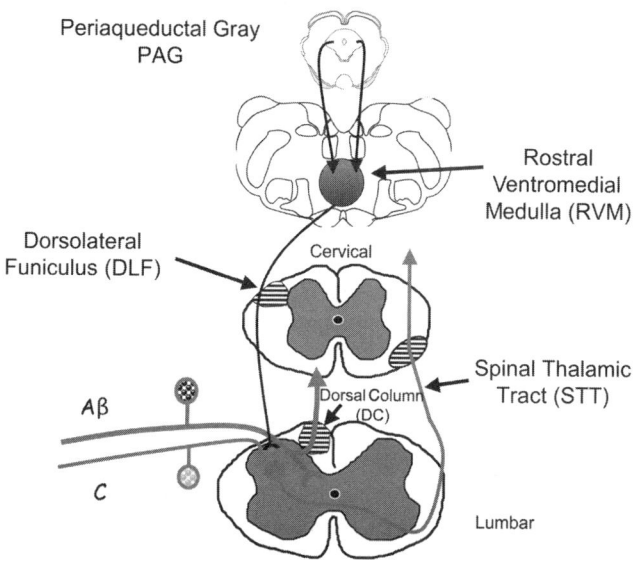

Figure 24.5. Potential supraspinal/spinal modulation of nociception.

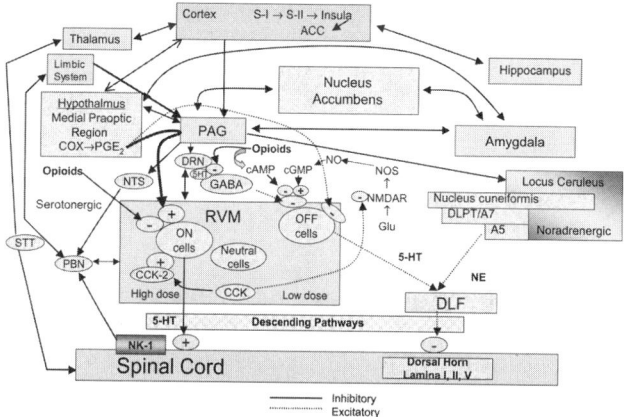

1. Activating the opioid receptors in the midbrain and "turning on" the descending systems (through disinhibition). Activation of the cortical descending inhibitory neural system is thought to involve the supraspinal release of neurotransmitters including beta-endorphins and enkephalins (Fields & Levine, 1984). These peptides represent two families of endogenous peptides which are believed to produce pain relief, mainly under situations of stress. It is important to realize that analgesia results from exogenous opioids (e.g., morphine sulfate), mimicking the actions of these endogenous neurotransmitters.
2. Activating opioid receptors on the second-order pain transmission cells to prevent the ascending transmission of the pain signal.
3. Activating opioid receptors at the central terminals of C-fibers in the spinal cord.
4. Activating opioid receptors in the periphery to inhibit the activation of the nociceptors as well as inhibit cells that may release inflammatory mediators (see Figure 24.6).

Intracellular Mechanisms of Opioid Analgesia

Recent cloning has identified three distinct genes for the mu, delta, and kappa opioid receptors (Chen et al., 1993; Evans et al., 1992; Kieffer et al., 1992; Yasuda et al., 1993). All three receptors belong to the G-protein coupled receptor (GPCR) family. Agonist binding to opioid receptors leads to a conformational change in the opioid receptor itself. This change results in the activation of an intracellular protein called a G-protein. The G-protein is made up of three separate protein subunits termed alpha, beta, and gamma. The alpha portion of the G-protein in an unactivated state associates with GDP, hence earning the name G-protein. Typically, the alpha portion with its GDP will bind with the beta and gamma subunits and exist as an intracellular trimeric protein. Although there are over 100 different types of G-protein coupled receptors, it is thought that the diversity of the G-protein subunit combinations offer diversity among agonist intracellular messages.

When an opioid binds to an opioid receptor, the conformational change in the opioid receptor results in the exchange of the GDP for a GTP on the Gα subunit. It is this exchange of GDP for GTP that activates the G-protein complex. Opioid receptors typically couple to a Gαi subunit and once the exchange of GDP for GTP has occurred, the αi subunit will dissociate from the $\beta\gamma$ subunit and inhibit the activity of adenylyl cyclase, a nearby membrane-bound enzyme. Under resting conditions, adenylate cyclase converts ATP into cAMP at some basal rate. cAMP acts as a second messenger within the cell resulting in several events including the activation of protein kinases and gene transcription proteins. Opioid receptor activation by an opioid will result in the activation of the Gαi subunit and inhibit adenylate cyclase enzyme, hence significantly decreasing intracellular basal levels of cAMP. This opioid via opioid receptor-induced decrease in cAMP indirectly results in the inhibition of voltage dependent calcium channels on presynaptic neurons.

These voltage-dependent calcium channels are important in the release of neurotransmitter and transduction of neuronal communication. Opioid receptors located on the presynaptic terminals of the nociceptive C-fibers and Aδ-fibers, when activated by an opioid agonist, will indirectly inhibit these voltage dependent calcium channels via decreasing cAMP levels, hence blocking the release of pain neurotransmitters such as glutamate, substance P, and calcitonin gene-related peptide (CGRP) from the nociceptive fibers, resulting in analgesia.

In addition to the indirect inhibition of voltage-gated calcium channels by opioid receptors, the $\beta\gamma$ subunit of the G-protein will open inward rectifying potassium (GIRK) channels, allowing K^+ to flow down its concentration gradient and out of the cell carrying its (+) charge. This results in a more negatively charged environment within the cell, termed hyperpolarization (see Figure 24.7; Smith, 2006b). This opioid-induced hyperpolarization results in a decrease in cell excitability, hence attenuating neuronal transmission (Jordan & Devi, 1998).

Free $G_{\beta\gamma}$ subunits bind and regulate multiple target proteins within the cell, including the following: phospholipase C (PLC), $\beta 2$, PLC $\beta 3$, phosphoinositide 3 kinase (PI3K) γ, adenylyl cyclase, N-type Ca^{2+} channels, and inwardly rectifying K^+ channels—as well as mediate physiologic processes (Cabrera-Vera et al., 2003; Clapham & Neer, 1997). Scott et al. (2001) identified a series of peptides that bind to a single preferred protein-protein interaction surface ("hot spot") on $G_{\beta\gamma}$. One of these peptides, known as SIRK (SIRK ALNILGYPDYD), blocked $G_{\beta\gamma}$-dependent regulation of type I adenylyl cyclase of N-type Ca^{2+} channels, thereby revealing the potential for selective targeting of $G_{\beta\gamma}$ signaling (Bonacci et al., 2006). Bonacci et al. (2006) hypothesized that small organic molecules may similarly lead to selective modulation of $G_{\beta\gamma}$-target interactions. Highly specific actions of M119 (a small organic compound with a high apparent affinity for $G_{\beta\gamma}$) may modulate certain G protein subunit functions, because if M119 were "globally blocking" $G_{\beta\gamma}$ subunit functions, attenuation of morphine-induced antinociception would have been expected (Bonacci et al., 2006). One can speculate that it is conceivable in the future that potential combination products of opioids and small organic molecules may yield more effective analgesia in humans than opioids alone.

Future potential "combo-opioid" products (in addition to morphine and NMDA antagonists or morphine and "ultra-low dose" mu-opioid receptor antagonists) that may be worthwhile studying could conceivably include morphine and cholecystokinin antagonists, morphine and selective neuropeptide FF receptor antagonists (e.g., RF9), morphine and 5HT3 antagonists (5HT3 antagonists may be useful for nausea and at least intrathecally may facilitate analgesia), morphine and small organic molecules (e.g., M119), morphine and glial modulators, morphine and delta-opioid receptor modulators, morphine and beta-2-adrenergic receptor blockers, or morphine and baclofen.

Figure 24.6. Locations of μ opioid receptors for analgesia.

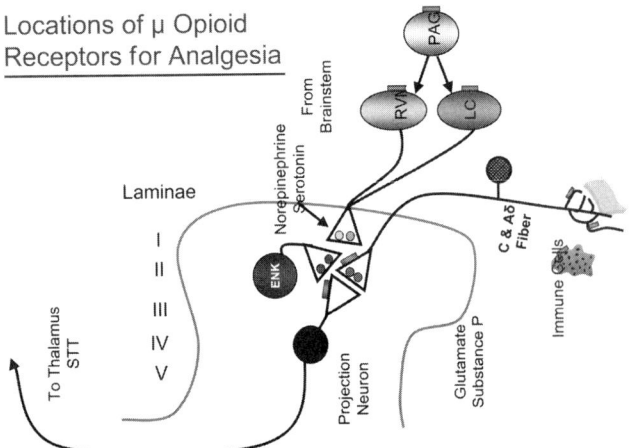

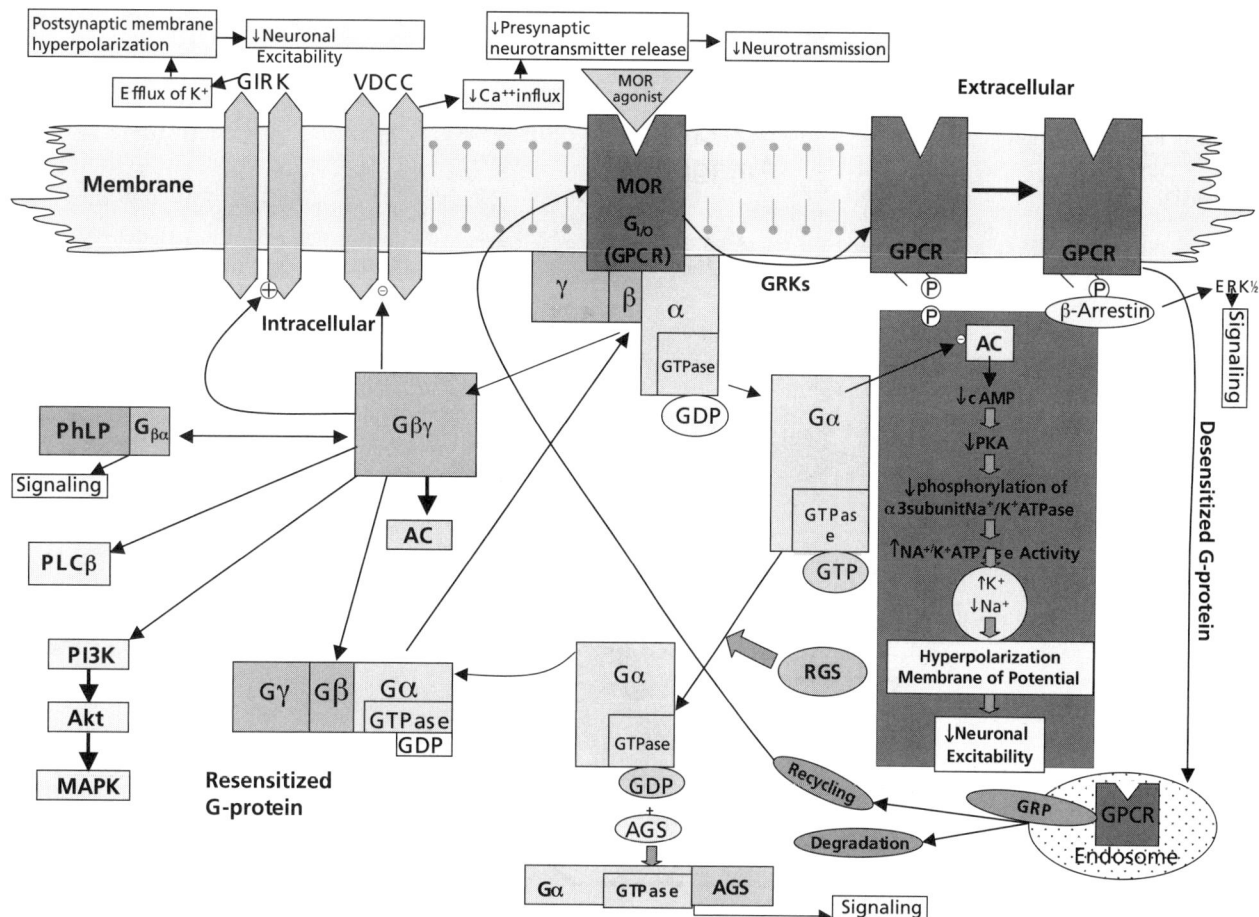

Figure 24.7. Acute MOR agonist-mediated signaling.

Opioid-induced hyperalgesia, which may involve similar mechanisms of opioid tolerance, is a phenomenon characterized by increased sensitivity to noxious stimuli and/or increased clinical reports of pain from patients treated with opioids that are proposed to occur secondary to the opioid. The clinical observation that only a small subset of subjects appears to be susceptible to this phenomenon strongly implicates a genetic influence.

Liang et al. (2006), utilizing in silico techniques to murine genetic studies, provide data supporting a role for beta 2-adrenergic receptor stimulation in the phenomenon of opioid-induced hyperalgesia (OIH). Using the administration of the selective beta-2-adrenergic receptor antagonist butoxamine, produced a dose-dependent reversal of OIH in mice (Liang et al., 2006). Deletion of the beta-2-adrenergic receptor gene sharply reduced the mechanical allodynia present after morphine treatment in the wild-type mouse strain (Liang et al., 2006). Liang and colleagues (2006) concluded that genetic variants of the beta-2-adrenergic receptor gene (especially single nucleotide polymorphisms) potentially explain some part of the difference between various strains of mice to develop OIH.

If it is found that beta-2-adrenergic receptor blockade may reduce OIH in human subjects, then the addition of a beta-2-adrenergic receptor blocker to long-term opioid therapy may improve long-term efficacy of treatment (at least in a subset of patients).

Glial cells have been shown to contribute to and/or facilitate various pain states (Watkins, 2007). Opioids such as morphine can diminish pain but may also activate glial cells (likely via agonist activity at the toll-like receptor 4 (TLR4), which may be counterproductive in terms of analgesia (Hutchinson, 2007). Activation of TLR4 results in downstream signaling factor including: the adaptor protein MyD88, IL-1 receptor-associated protein kinases (IRAKs), TRAF6, and TAK1 (TRAF6 and TAK1 need to be ubiquitinated in order to be active). The polyubiquitination of TRAF6 recognizes TAK1 binding subunit 2 (TAB2) with subsequent recruitment and formation of the TAB 2/TAB 1/TAK 1 complex where the kinase activity of TAK1 leads to phosphorylation of I [kappa] B Kinase complex (IKK) and subsequent activation of nuclear factor kappa B (NF-kB) (Keating, 2007), potentially leading to transcription of inducible nitric oxide synthase (iNOS), cyclooxygenase 2 (COX 2), and various cytokines (TNF, IL-1, IL-6). Additionally, the NADPH oxidase (NOX) protein (associated with TLR4) transfers electrons from NADPH to O_2 to generate superoxide anion free radicals (e.g., reactive oxygen species [ROS]), which are rapidly converted to hydrogen peroxide and oxygen in cells. Hutchinson demonstrated that selective acute antagonism of TLR4 [e.g. by (+)− and(−)-isomer opioid antagonists] may lead to antiallodynia/neuropathic pain palliation and potentiation of opioid analgesia (Hutchinson, 2007). Moreover, activated glia may contribute to opioid tolerance as well as opioid dependence/withdrawal (see Figure 24.8).

Ibudilast (AV-411), a nonselective phosphodiesterase inhibitor known to suppress glial cell activation, appears to essentially

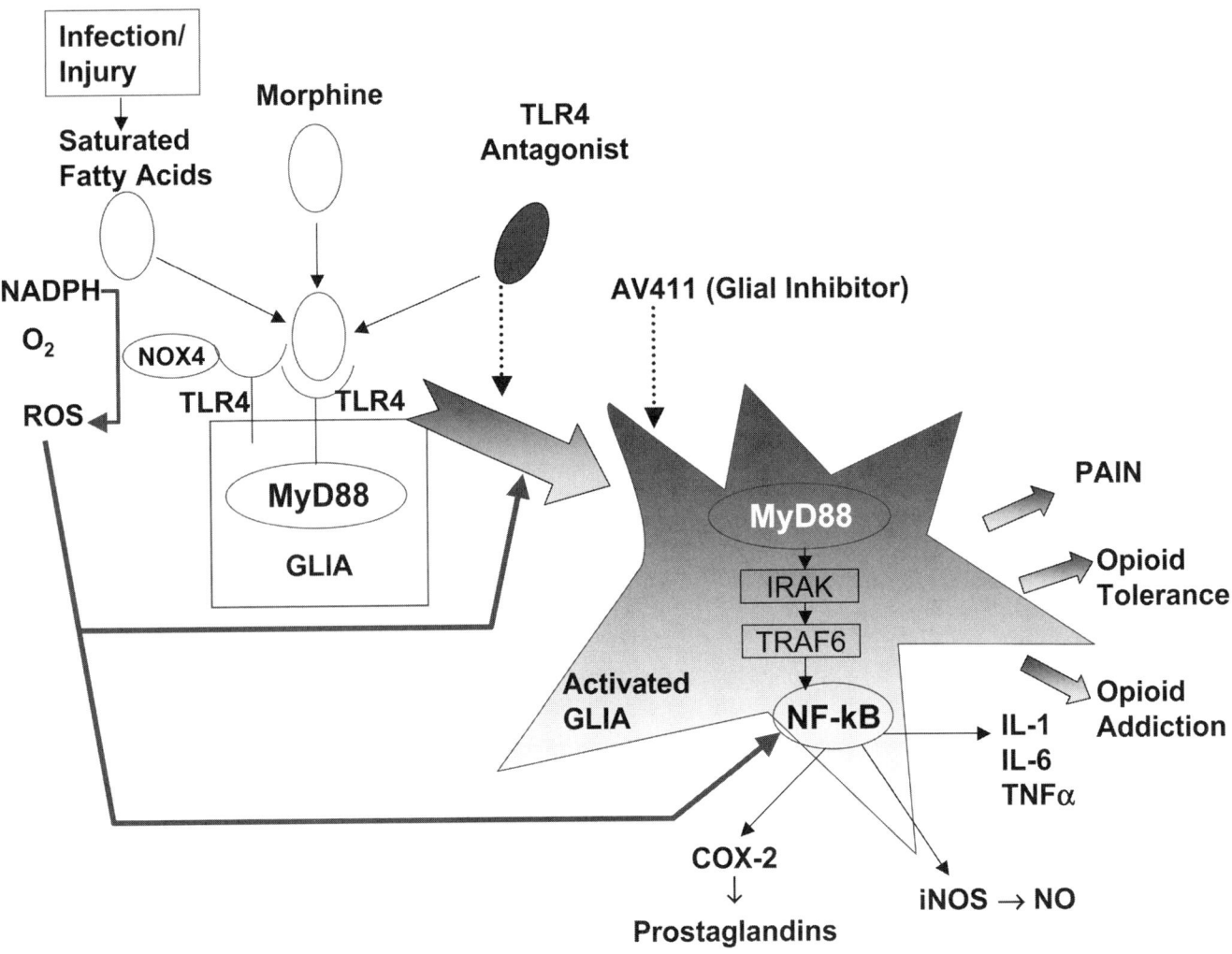

Figure 24.8

block morphine's direct effects on glia but not on neurons. Rats injected with both AV411 and morphine exhibited increased analgesia as well as less tolerance (i.e., over time morphine better retained its analgesia) compared to rats injected with morphine alone.

Furthermore, to check for a link between glia and morphine addiction, Watkins and Hutchinson tested whether blocking morphine's effects on glial cells would keep rats in one location and not in another (e.g., conditioned place preference). Animals receiving morphine alone tended to return to the morphine area over and over, spending most of their time there. However, rats given AV411 in the AV411-plus-morphine group wandered around rather than returning to the morphine area. Combinations of opioids with TLR4 antagonists or glial inhibitors may be potentially useful in the future.

Still another combination that may have potential utility is that of morphine and amitriptyline. Amitriptyline preserves morphine's antinociceptive effect by regulating the glutamate transporter GLAST and G LT-1 trafficking onto glial cell surfaces, thereby enhancing excitatory amino acid (e.g., glutamate) uptake from the synaptic cleft and reducing spinal cerebrospinal fluid glutamate levels (Tai, 2007).

Additionally, opioids may in part promote painful HIV-related neuropathy by (a) upregulation of the expression of the chemokine receptors CCR3 and CCR5, which may promote viral binding and trafficking of HIV-1 infected cells (Mahajan, 2005b); (b) enhancing the cytotoxicity of HIV-1 viral envelope protein gp120 via mechanisms that involve intracellular calcium modulation with subsequent direct glial effects (Mahajan, 2005a); and (c) glial activation with upregulation of TNF, IL-1, and IL-6 (Tai, 2006; Smith, 2007). gp120 is thought to activate glia at least in part by interacting with CD4 and CXCR4/CCR5, and increased CCR5 may lead to further glial activation as well as more TNF-α interacting with neurons, potentially leading to neuronal apoptosis (Smith, 2007).

Clinical Opioid Therapy

In 1871 William Dale, a noted physician of the time in the United Kingdom, wrote: "Opium is... our chief medicine for relieving pain and procuring sleep, our right hand in practice, suffering humanity owes much to its virtues, and the physician could ill spare it in his battle with disease and pain. Its effects are often wonderful, translating the poor patient from a state of the most intolerable torture to one of comparative ease and comfort" (Dale, 1871). That same year, he also wrote, again referring to opium: "This remedy like every good thing is being abused" (Dale, 1871). Therefore, he may have laid the framework for the so-called concept of balance.

Since 1871, the pendulum of "opiophobia" versus "opiophilia" has swung back and forth for health-care providers. Periods are marked by opiophobia, in which opioids were withheld from terminally ill cancer patients because of irrational fears of addiction, as well as opiophilia periods, marked by increased opioid abuse and diversion coexisting with an increase in the medical use of opioids for persistent noncancer pain (PNCP). Recent times have seen a swing toward more extensive use of opioids. Opioid therapy for chronic pain was described as an "extension of the basic principles of good medical practice" in a consensus statement jointly published by the American Pain Society and the American Academy of Pain Medicine (American Academy of Pain Medicine & American Pain Society, 2004).

Studies on the use of long-acting oral opioids for chronic noncancer pain, though still relatively small, have begun to foster more accepting attitudes from mainstream American medicine regarding the use of opioids for PNCP (Chou et al., 2003). However, the "opioid controversy" continues to the present. Portenoy (2004) has illustrated various opiophobic versus opiophilic views in his comments predicting responses of American physicians to the recommendation for the appropriate use of opioids published by the United Kingdom's Pain Society and Royal Colleges of Anaesthetists, General Practitioners, and Psychiatrists (Pain Society et al., 2004). Kalso et al. (2003) and Trescot et al. (2006) have also published recommendations for using opioids in chronic non-cancer pain.

Practicing in the "middle of the road" by employing the appropriate use of opioids in the context of good medical practice, as well as appropriate attention to the risk assessment and management of opioid abuse (being cognizant of potential abuse, addiction, and diversion), has become known as "balance" (Drug Enforcement Administration with 21 health organizations, 2004; World Health Organization, 2000; Zacny, 2003a).

Although opioids have been a mainstay of treatment for acute pain and cancer-related pain, issues surrounding their use for persistent noncancer pain remain somewhat controversial. Although Turk et al. (1994) published their article of physicians' attitudes on prescribing opioids over a decade ago, it still seems to hold true today that physicians tend to disagree regarding multiple issues surrounding the prescription of opioids for the treatment of persistent noncancer pain (). Factors that may influence the decision to prescribe opioids for PCNP may include the physician's medical specialty, geographic region of practice, and patient factors (e.g., age, diagnosis [as well as documentation of diagnosis], and prognosis). Scanlon and Chugh's (2004) report surveyed a total of 125 physicians (63 family physicians [FPs] and 62 specialists in the Calgary Health Region [CHR], Calgary, Alberta) in efforts to explore attitudes regarding the use of LTOT (long-term opioid therapy) for PNCP. A minority of physicians FPs and specialists reported "that they could handle" hydromorphone (36.7% and 13.3% respectively), fentanyl patch (30.6% and 11.1% respectively), and methadone (0% and 6.7% respectively; Scanlon & Chugh, 2004). Scanlon and Chugh concluded that FPs in the CHR need to increase their level of comfort level toward opioids in general so they can adequately manage chronic noncancer pain (Scanlon & Chugh, 2004).

Although there are no easy answers to the opioid controversies, a moderate balanced approach with oversight by a qualified interdisciplinary pain team may be optimal at the current time. "There appears to be a select subpopulation of patients with chronic pain that can achieve sustained partial analgesia from opioid therapy without the occurrence of intolerable side effects or the development of aberrant drug-related behaviors" (Portenoy, 1996). This statement appears to stand the test of time after roughly a decade. Furthermore, there are patients that appear to do well for many years on the same dose of opioid with having their primary care physician following them and writing their prescriptions. However, as the "select population" expands somewhat, the statement may need to be qualified some to include that administration of LTOT. This is optimally achieved in conjunction with a multidisciplinary multimodal approach to the evaluation and management of pain by an interdisciplinary team of pain specialists in conjunction with a risk management plan.

There appears to be general agreement that when a patient is managed by a well-coordinated multidisciplinary team (e.g., pain specialists), compliance is better and risk of loss of control as well as complications are less than when a single doctor (especially if the doctor is not a pain specialist) is managing the patient (Breivik, 2005). However, this may not always be possible. Additionally, close follow-up and reassessment in multiple domains is essential and should guide continuation, or discontinuation, of opioid therapy. It is important to convey to patients and health-care providers unfamiliar with pain management that opioids do not necessarily equate with pain relief. Some people seem to believe that opioids are really the only analgesics that work, that they are fine to use in most or all situations as sole analgesics and should be continually increased if pain is still experienced. However, pain is extremely complex and differs for each individual.

Opioids, when appropriate, may be used in conjunction with many other pharmacologic, behavioral, and physical medicinal approaches, as well as neuromodulation techniques and other various analgesic strategies. Not all patients do well on opioids, and subpopulations of patients may be improved when they are taken off these drugs (Rome et al., 2004). In fact, when given the option to discontinue opioid therapy, more than 50% of patients abandoned opioid therapy voluntarily, predominantly due to intolerable side effects or suboptimal efficacy (Cowan et al., 2003; Kalso et al., 2004).

The Clinical Usage of Opioids

Cowan and colleagues (2005) performed a randomized, double-blind, placebo-controlled, cross-over pilot study to assess the effects of long-term opioid drug consumption and subsequent abstinence in chronic non-cancer pain patients receiving controlled-released morphine. Ten patients with PNCP taking an average daily dose of 40mg controlled-release morphine sulfate (mean 40, range 10–90, SD 21 mg), for an average of two years (mean 2.175, range 2–2.25, SD 0.2 years) had their morphine substituted with placebo for 60-hour periods. Pharmacokinetic data demonstrated compliance with abstinence on all patients. Three patients (30%) reported opioid withdrawal symptoms. Cowan and colleagues (2005) had concluded their results suggested the existence of a group of PNCP patients whose long-term opioid consumption can be beneficial and remain moderate without them suffering from consequences of problematic opioid use.

Kalso and colleagues (2004) analyzed data from 1,145 patients initially randomized in 15 placebo-controlled trials of potent opioids used in the treatment of severe pain for efficacy and safety in chronic noncancer pain. Four studies tested intravenous opioids in neuropathic pain in a crossover design with 115 of 120 patients completing the protocols. Using either pain intensity difference or pain relief as the endpoint, all 4 intravenous studies reported average pain relief of 30%–60% with opioid. Eleven studies (1025 patients) compared oral opioids with placebo for 4 days to 8 weeks. Six of the 15 trials that were included had an open-label follow-up of 6–24 months. The mean decrease in pain intensity in most studies was at least 30% with opioids and was comparable in neuropathic and musculoskeletal pain. Roughly 80% of patients noted at least one adverse effect. The most common adverse effects were constipation (41%), nausea (32%), and somnolence (29%). Only 44% of 388 patients on open-label treatments were still on opioids after therapy for between 7 and 24 months. Adverse effects and lack of efficacy were two common reasons for discontinuation (Kalso et al., 2004).

Watson and colleagues (2004) surveyed 102 patients with PNCP in a neurological practice followed by a neurologist every 3 months for 1 year or more (median 8 years, range 1–22 years). They reported that approximately one-third of patients (34 out of 102) had a change in their pain status from either severe of moderate pain, as measured by a 0 to 10 numerical rating scale (NRS; mild = 1–3, moderate = 4–7, severe = 8–10); by category scale (absent, mild, moderate, severe, very severe); and by considering pain with movement. They queried patients as to whether they were satisfied with pain relief despite adverse events. Forty-five patients (44%) answered that they were satisfied, and 57 (56%) replied that they were not satisfied with their pain relief. However, of the 86 patients assessed for disability, 47 (54%) patients had significant improvement in their disability status on opioids. Also, there was some pain improvement on opioids in 78 (91%) of 102 patients and the patients chose to continue opioid therapy for some analgesia despite adverse effects (Watson et al., 2004).

Dworkin and colleagues (2003) have reviewed randomized clinical trials of various analgesic agents (including five double-blind randomized trials of oral opioids) and proposed five potential analgesics (gabapentin, 5% lidocaine patch, opioids, tramadol hydrochloride, tricyclic antidepressants) as first-line agents in their evidence-based approach to the initial treatment of neuropathic pain.

Eisenberg and colleagues (2005) examined 22 studies that met inclusion criteria and were classified as short-term (less than 24 hours; $n = 14$) or intermediate-term (median = 28 days; range = 8–56 days; $n = 8$) trials. They reported that the short-term trials had contradictory results. However, all 8 intermediate-term trials demonstrated opioid efficacy for spontaneous neuropathic pain. A fixed-effects model meta-analysis of 6 intermediate-term trials showed mean posttreatment visual analog scale scores of pain intensity after opioids to be 14 units lower on a scale from 0 to 100 than after placebo (95% confidence interval [CI]; −18 to −10; $P < 0.001$). As the mean initial pain intensity recorded from four of the intermediate-term trials ranged from 46–69, this 14-point difference was considered to correspond to a 20%–30% greater reduction with opioids than with placebo (Eisenberg et al., 2005).

Analysis of data from large randomized clinical trials has revealed that a roughly 30% reduction in pain intensity may be the threshold for patients to describe a reduction in chronic pain as meaningful (Farrar et al., 2000, 2001). When the number needed to harm (NNH) is considered, the most common adverse event was nausea (NNH, 3.6; 95% CI, 2.9–4.8), followed by constipation (NNH, 4.6; 95% CI, 3.4–7.1), drowsiness (NNH, 5.3; 95% CI, 3.7–8.3), vomiting (NNG, 6.2; 95% CI, 4.6–11), and dizziness (NNH, 6.7; 95% CI, 4.8–10.0; Eisenberg et al., 2005). Eisenberg and colleagues (2005) concluded that although short-term studies provide only equivocal evidence regarding the efficacy of opioids in reducing the intensity of neuropathic pain, intermediate-term studies demonstrate significant efficacy of opioids over placebo for neuropathic pain. They also concluded that further randomized controlled trials are needed in efforts to establish the long-term efficacy of opioids for neuropathic pain, the safety of long-term opioids (including addiction potential), and their effects on quality of life.

Controlled-release oxycodone hydrochloride has been evaluated in postherpetic neuralgia (PHN; Watson & Babul, 1998) and diabetic peripheral neuropathy (Gimbel et al., 2003; Watson et al., 2003). Watson and Babul (1998) reported that a maximum dosage of 60mg/day of morphine equivalents significantly relieved pain, disability, and allodynia for patients with PHN. Watson and (2003) colleagues also reported that overall pain, sleep, as well as health-related quality of life assessments were significantly improved compared with placebo at a mean daily dose of 40.0 + 18.5 mg for controlled-release oxycodone. Gimbel et al. (2003) demonstrated that a maximum dosage of 120 mg/day of morphine equivalents significant improved pain, the performance of daily activities, and sleep. Furthermore, Raja and colleagues (2002) reported that treatment with opioids and tricyclic antidepressants (TCA) resulted in greater pain relief (38% and 32%, respectively) compared with placebo (11%; $p < 0.001$). Patients who completed the study preferred opioids over TCA treatment (54% versus 30%, $P = 0.02$), however, more patients dropped out of the study during or after opioid treatment than during or after opioid TCA therapy (20 patients versus 6 patients).

Therefore, although opioids have been touted as being "the nectar of the gods," only a minority of patients in these studies decided to go on to long-term management with opioids even though all were given that opportunity. The small number of patients and short duration of follow-up did not permit conclusions regarding issues of tolerance and addiction (Kalso et al., 2004). In a survey of patients ($N = 104$) prescribed opioids for mean duration of treatment 14.1 months for severe chronic noncancer pain at a pain clinic within a National Health Service Hospital in London, United Kingdom, a total of 90 (86.5%) patients reported stopping opioid therapy at some point and, of these, 59 (65%) had ceased opioid therapy permanently. This voluntary abandonment of opioids occurred despite that 72.5% of all patients initially derived some benefit from opioids, (although 77% of all patients reported opioid side effects; Cowan et al., 2003).

A significant positive correlation between pain relief during intravenous opioid testing and open-label follow-up of pain relief from oral opioids were not consistently demonstrated in all four studies (Attal et al., 2002; Dellemijn et al., 1997, 1998; Huse et al., 2001). However, in three studies (Attal et al., 2002; Dellemijn et al., 1997, 1998), intravenous opioid testing appeared reasonable at identifying those patients who did not achieve adequate analgesia from opioids. In other words, if patients responded poorly to the analgesic effects of intravenous opioids, they also tended to respond poorly to the analgesic effects of oral or transdermal opioids.

Gustorff (2005) reported on the use of intravenous remifentanil testing in a randomized placebo-controlled crossover study in 24 patients suffering from severe noncancer pain. Using an ascending infusion of remifentanil and placebo titrated against endpoints, he found that the remifentanil testing allowed a distinction between 11 opioid responders and 13 nonresponders. A rapid and complete recovery to the pretesting baseline state occurred by

25 minutes in all patients. Gustorff (2005) concluded that remifentanil testing is rapid, being generally completed in 1 hour or less, and so it has potential to be used as a routine screening process in an ambulatory setting. Subsequent oral or transdermal doses that were used to achieve analgesia after intravenous testing were usually lower than equivalent intravenous doses. Therefore, in most cases intravenous opioid testing should not be used to titrate to the patients' equivalent "long-term" oral or transdermal dose in persistent noncancer pain.

Chou and colleagues performed a systematic review of the comparative efficacy and safety of long-acting oral opioids for chronic noncancer pain and determined that there was insufficient evidence to demonstrate that one long-acting opioid was better than another, nor was there evidence to determine differences in efficacy between long-acting and short-acting opioids (although they reported that no randomized trials were rated as good; Chou et al., 2003). Clinically, it appears that it is not rare that patients may respond to one opioid reasonably well and another opioid poorly. Currently there is no way to predict this, so efforts to attempt to find the opioid with maximal analgesic efficacy for an individual patient are more a matter of trial and error. There was also insufficient evidence to prove that different long-acting opioids are associated with different safety profiles (Chou et al., 2003); however, it appears that long-acting fentanyl is associated with less constipation than long-acting morphine.

The literature appears to support the analgesic efficacy of opioids (at least in the short term) for some patients with chronic noncancer pain (especially with chronic low back pain); however, results are inconsistent regarding the effect of opioid therapy on functional status or quality of life (Bartleson, 2002; Moulin et al., 1996; Rashig et al., 2003). Furthermore, large, multicenter, well-designed studies for over a decade do not exist.

There appears to be less data and more controversy surrounding the use of LTOT for various nonneuropathic PNCP, especially as pertains to chronic headaches, chronic musculoskeletal disorders, and fibromyalgia syndrome. Rowbotham et al. (2003) demonstrated a dose-dependent analgesic effect in patients with mixed neuropathies and reported that high-dose levorphanol yielded significantly more pain relief than lower doses of levorphanol. In a randomized, controlled trial of controlled-release morphine in complex regional pain syndrome (CRPS), Harke et al. (2001) reported there was no difference in pain reduction compared with placebo after 8 days of use.

The National Ambulatory Medical Care Survey (NAMCS) is a nationally representative yearly survey that collects information about outpatient office visits in the United States conducted by the National Center for Health Statistics (NCHS) of the Centers for Disease Control. Caudill-Slosberg and colleagues (2004) analyzed visits and prescriptions from patients of all ages for the treatment of musculoskeletal pain using NAMCS data from 1980 to 1981 ($n = 89,000$ visits) and 1999 to 2001 ($n = 45,000$ visits) obtained from public files on the NCHS website (2002)). They found that the use of potent opioids for the management of chronic musculoskeletal pain has dramatically increased in the United States from roughly 2% in 1980 to around 9% in 2000 (Caudill-Slosberg et al., 2004). During this 2-decade period, NSAID prescriptions increased for both acute (19% vs. 33%, $RR = 1.74$; 95% CI; 1.52–1.95) and chronic (25% vs. 29%, $RR = 1.16$; 95% CI, 0.97–1.35) musculoskeletal pain visits. In 2000, one-third of the NSAID prescriptions were for COX II agents. Opioids increased for acute pain (8% vs. 11%; $RR = 1.38$; 95% CI, 0.92–1.83) and doubled for chronic pain (8% vs. 16%; $RR = 2.0$, 98% CI, 1.52–2.48). The use of more potent opioids (hydrocodone, oxycodone, and morphine) for chronic musculoskeletal pain increased from 2% to 9% of visits ($RR = 4.5$, 95% CI, 2.18–6.187). This significant increase translates into 5.9 million visits in which potent opioids were prescribed in 2000, which is 4.6 million visits more than in 1980 assuming the total number of outpatient visits was roughly constant from 1980 to 2001; (Caudill-Slosberg et al., 2004).

A subset of patients who experience severe and disabling pain while taking opioid therapy can experience significant improvement in pain severity and disability as well as improvement in physical and emotional functioning while participating in a pain rehabilitation program that incorporates opioid withdrawal (Rome et al., 2004).

In a study by Rome and colleagues (2004), 274 study patients who completed a stay at the pain rehabilitation center, as well as pre- and poststay questionnaires, were divided into two groups based on their prestudy "baseline" medications. One group of 99 patients was taking daily opioids, and one group of 175 patients was not taking daily opioids. All patients taking any opioids underwent a gradual structured opioid withdrawal over 2 to 3 weeks, and all 274 patients completed a 3-week multidisciplinary rehabilitation program based on a cognitive-behavioral model. On admission to the program, 37.9% of patients were taking daily opioids with a mean daily dose of 78.4 mg of morphine equivalent (range 3.5–780.0 mg). Patients taking less than the median dose (41.0 mg) were taking a mean (SD) daily morphine equivalent of 25.1 mg (13.69), and patients taking more than the median does were taking a mean (SD) daily morphine equivalent of 137.48 mg (116.8; Rome et al., 2004).

At the completion of the program, patients taking lower opioid doses, higher doses, or no opioids at all prior to the program all reported significantly reduced pain severity ($P < 0.001$), interference due to pain ($P < 0.001$), affective distress ($P > 0.001$), depression ($P < 0.001$), and catastrophizing ($P > 0.001$), as well as increased perceived life control ($P < 0.001$) and general activity ($P < 0.001$). Patients taking higher opioid doses reported significantly greater catastrophizing at discharge than the nonopioid group (mean difference, −2.8; SE; 1.1; $P = 0.03$). Patients taking higher opioid doses also reported greater pain severity at the completion of the program than the nonopioid group; however, this difference was not statistically significant (mean difference, −4.3; SE; 1.9; $P = 0.05$; Rome et al., 2004). Although significant limitations that exist with this study preclude clinicians to generalize the study findings, it does illustrate that at least certain patients can come off opioids and actually do better functionally as well as have less pain. Ballantyne and Mao (2003), in an attempt to utilize the least opioid dose necessary to achieve adequate analgesia, have suggested using a cautious approach to opioid titration.

Unfortunately, the current state of affairs in terms of the clinical use of LTOT for PNCP may be more related to the individual training, experiences, comfort, preferences, and the practice styles of individual prescribers (e.g., opioid generous clinicians [OGCs] vs. opioid stingy clinicians [OSGs]; Smith, 2003a) than to evidence and specific clinical circumstances.

However, there does appear to be some common ground among pain specialists. The following is based on an informal verbal survey conducted with 68 certified pain specialists (unpublished). The majority of pain physicians would probably feel comfortable initiating and maintaining an 82-year-old woman with severe pain and dysfunction on long-term opioid therapy with a long-acting morphine sulfate preparation in a dose of 15 mg orally every 12 hours, assuming the patient was agreeable and satisfied, had no significant adverse effects, and experienced good pain relief and improved function as evidenced by her playing golf again (which she had stopped playing secondary to pain). Contrariwise, the majority of pain physicians may not feel comfortable initiating and maintaining a 22-year-old male who is complaining only of severe lower back pain but has no other significant complaints, an entirely negative physical examination with completely nonsignificant diagnostic testing and imaging studies, on long-term opioid therapy with a long-acting morphine sulfate preparation in a dose of 900 mg orally every 8 hours if the patient had no changes in quality of life, function, mood, sleep, or socializing but did note that his "pain level" decreased from 9/10 to 8/10.

Opioids: Clinical Background

Opioids are broad-spectrum analgesics, utilized for the treatment of nociceptive and neuropathic pain. Although no ideal analgesics exist and opioids are far from perfect, they may be among the best broad-spectrum analgesics currently available for many patients.

Some have held the view that there should be no difference between the treatment approaches to acute pain, cancer pain, and persistent noncancer pain. (For the purposes of this chapter, persistent noncancer pain will be arbitrarily used to refer to any pain that persists over 3 months in patients without a diagnosis of cancer and without a diagnosis of some advanced chronic illness that would potentially qualify them as "terminal" or "palliative care" patients with a prognosis of less than 3 years of life expectancy.) However, this does not seem to be the case for all clinicians. One key difference may be the timing of when to initiate opioid therapy, if indicated. In acute pain, cancer pain, and persistent noncancer pain (with the possible exception of end-of-life care), a careful history and physical examination should be performed before "just throwing analgesics at pain." Otherwise, conditions such as compartment syndrome (acute pain), or deep vein thrombosis may be missed. In acute pain and cancer pain that is severe, regardless of whether the etiology of the pain is apparent or not, potent opioids for severe pain should be considered as part of the treatment plan at the initial visit.

In persistent noncancer pain, clinicians generally attempt to do their best to evaluate patients comprehensively, including appropriate diagnostic testing and imaging in efforts to identify a precise "pain diagnosis" or ascertain "pain generator(s)." Once this workup has been largely completed, a treatment approach may be formulated to attempt to optimally match the patient's diagnosis, situation, and concomitant comorbidities. Opioid therapy for persistent noncancer pain may be initiated early in this process, later in this process, or not at all. However, if a patient has 3 months to live or has just had major surgery performed, most clinicians would institute opioid therapy at the initial consult and would not withhold opioid therapy in an attempt to find a precise "pain generator."

Another issue in which PNCP differs from acute or cancer pain is related to pain assessment. Some clinicians feel that a significant percentage of patients with PNCP on LTOT should not be managed solely on the basis of their report on the NRS-11 scale response regarding pain intensity. Although unidimensional assessments (such as the NRS-11 scale) seem satisfactory (although perhaps not optimal) for pain assessment of most patients with acute or cancer pain, multidimensional assessment tools may be especially preferred for patients with PNCP on LTOT. Additionally, other multidomain assessment tools/instruments may potentially be helpful as well (Smith, 2005a, 2006c). Nevertheless, each individual patient needs to be treated according to his or her specific situation and so management strategies should not strictly adhere to any rigorous algorithms, maximal doses, or rigid protocols.

Pain may be classified in many ways (Smith, 2005b). One approach to the classification of pain is to categorize pain according to its responsiveness to a particular treatment (Smith, 2005b). Utilizing this approach, pain many be divided into opioid responsive pain (ORP), moderately opioid responsive pain (MORP), and poorly opioid responsive pain (PORP). ORP refers to pain with a very significant response (e.g., good-to-excellent analgesia) to opioids (usually with low-to-moderate doses of opioids), MORP refers to pain with a modest response to opioids (usually with moderate-to-high doses of opioids), and PORP refers to pain that responds poorly to high-dose opioid therapy. ORP and MORP may remain as such over many years or may wane over time (e.g., OPR becoming MORP or PORP, and MORP becoming PORP). Currently, there is no way to predict which patients may respond well to opioids. Furthermore, different opioids may yield significantly different analgesic responses in the same patient.

Pud et al. (2006) provided further data suggesting gender differences in the analgesic response to opioids and also suggested that personality traits may help predict analgesic responses to morphine. Pud and colleagues (2006) suggested that high harm avoidance (HA) personality trait is associated with better responsiveness to morphine treatment than other personality types (e.g., reward dependence, novelty seeking). Using data from a previously published crossover trial of opioid and tricyclic antidepressants in postherpetic neuralgia, Edwards and colleagues (2006) suggested that pretreatment assessment of heat pain sensitivity may be potentially helpful in identifying a subset of patients with persistent pain who are most likely to gain analgesic benefit from opioids.

The old teachings of nonsteroidal antiinflammatory drugs (NSAIDs) having an analgesic ceiling effect and acting peripherally, whereas opioids have no ceiling effect and act centrally, are somewhat inaccurate. It appears that opioids (like NSAIDs) work both centrally and peripherally (Dirig et al., 1997, 1998; Malmberg & Yaksh, 1995; Obara et al., 2004; Perrot et al., 1999; Samad et al., 2001; Stein, 2003,; Stein et al., 1998, 2001, 2003; Zhou et al., 1998). Also, opioids do not yield significant analgesic effects in all patients with various painful states. In certain patients, increasing the opioid dose after some point does not yield all that much analgesic bang for the buck. In other words, there exists no ceiling dose for opioids; in some patients, by increasing the opioid dose, pain relief appears to "asymptotically approach" some "effective or functional" analgesic ceiling.

Issues for LTOT for PNCP

In spite of available opioids therapy guidelines, controversies persist. LTOT for persistent noncancer pain is an area that is not easily amenable to algorithms and "black-and-white" doctrines; rather, this "gray zone" is better approached with individualized sound clinical judgment, balanced and appropriate approaches, and common sense.

LTOT should optimally be undertaken in conjunction with the following:

a. Appropriate interdisciplinary medical care and documentation
b. Other appropriate pharmacologic approaches
c. Any appropriate physical medicine approaches

d. Any appropriate behavioral medicine approaches
e. Attention to comorbidities
f. Appropriate clinician-patient relationship
g. Appropriate monitoring and follow-up

The use of long-term opioid therapy (LTOT) for persistent noncancer pain (PNCP) remains one of the most controversial topics in the field of pain medicine. Although it would appear that an overwhelming majority of pain specialists agree with and/or utilize LTOT for PNCP, decisions surrounding initiating LTOT, assessing LTOT, ancillary documentation (e.g., opioid contracts, urine drug testing [UDT]), titration strategies as well as when to cease opioid dose escalation in a particular patient and situations warranting withdrawal of LTOT, and specific treatment goals (if any) continue to be controversial and may vary dramatically from clinician to clinician.

LTOT Management Issues in PNCP

There are many issues surrounding LTOT for PNCP. One way of classifying various issues that may be practical (although artificial and not precise) is to categorize issues into three phases (analogous to the three phases of delivering an anesthetic—induction, maintenance, and emergence): (1) initiation (induction), (2) maintenance, and (3) reassessment (increase dose, continue same dose, decrease dose, or taper to off [emergence]).

Decisions regarding the timing of initiation and whether to initiate LTOT for PNCP must be made on a case-by-case basis. The various factors that may enter into the clinician's decision-making process may include the following: the patient's age, prognosis, documentation of diagnosis, previous treatments, willingness to be involved in his or her treatment (e.g., to help him- or herself), willingness to change (e.g., behavior), pain duration and intensity, history of substance use and mental health issues, patient/clinician goals, and the particular physician-patient relationship.

It is crucial that the clinician has a reasonable dynamic picture of the intensity of the patient's pain, as well as its impact on social domain (e.g., family, relationships, and recreational activities), emotional domain (e.g., mood) and functional domain (e.g., physical functioning, activities of daily life, and occupational issues) before the start of opioid therapy. It is also vital that the clinician continues to evaluate the patient's status in each of these domains. If, in fact, the patient does not improve or deteriorates during LTOT, it may be appropriate at some point to change to a different opioid or taper the patient slowly to a lower dose of LTOT or completely off opioids and attempt different treatments.

Initiation of LTOT

Issues that surround the initiation (and/or maintenance) phase of LTOT for PNCP include the following: the use of opioid contracts, the use of goal-directed therapy agreements (Smith, 2006d), the use of a substance abuse history and/or screening tool(s) for substance misuse, the use of urine testing, and optimally some form of psychological assessment (which could be an informal assessment by the provider), as well as some sense of the doctor-patient relationship. Many of these issues will be dealt with in separate chapters.

Goal-Directed Therapy Agreements

Perhaps one of the most important principles as a clinician in initiating and maintaining LTOT for PNCP is to "know where you are and where you are going." Goal-directed therapy agreements (GDTAs) may be helpful when initiating LTOT for PNCP (Smith, 2006d). Clinicians are sometimes faced with patients in whom opioids were started and/or exculpated in efforts to achieve analgesia without clearly defined endpoints. This may yield patients remaining with severe pain on relatively high-dose opioids. In efforts to clarify patient and clinician expectations and attempt to make expected treatment outcomes more finite and concrete, the use of some form of GDTAs may possess potential utility. As with opioid treatment agreements, GDTAs are not necessarily advocated for all patients or all practices, but merely suggested in situations in which clinicians deem them appropriate to utilize.

GDTAs should be tailored to each individual patient, should be clear and concise, should be reasonable for the patient to attain over a finite period of time, and optimally should be agreed upon by both patient and clinician. Examples may include the following: increasing daily ambulation by a defined amount, increasing social/recreational activities by a defined amount, and so forth. By utilizing GDTAs before instituting opioid therapy, clinicians can set defined criteria that need to be met in order to continue opioid therapy. In this manner, patients may be expected to reach certain reasonably attainable functional goals (which may need to be documented by their physical and/or behavioral therapist) in order to continue opioid therapy. The specific defined goals should be clearly stated in the GDTA. It appears optimal to institute the GDTA prior to instituting opioid therapy. The GDTA is essentially felt to be a contractually agreed-upon realistic target of translational analgesia (Smith, 2006d) which should be realized in order to continue therapy as is.

It is hoped that with the use of GDTAs in certain patients or circumstances, a closer match between both patient and clinician treatment expectations and outcome can be established (Smith, 2006d).

Psychological Assessment

Although prior to LTOT, there may not be any specific need for psychological/psychiatric evaluations or psychological testing, it seems prudent that clinicians should "know" a patient and have an established provider-patient relationship before initiating LTOT. Wasan and colleagues (2005) reported that high levels of psychopathology (comprised mainly of depression, anxiety, and high neuroticism) are associated with diminished opioid analgesia in patients with discogenic low back pain. Furthermore, brief assessment tools exist [SOAPP (Butler, 2004), ORT (Webster, 2005)] which attempt to screen risk potential for opioid-related aberrant behaviors among patients with PNCP.

Maintenance/Reassessment of LTOT

Issues that surround the maintenance of LTOT for PNCP include the following: continued documentation, side effects, tolerance, discontinuation of LTOT, and deviant drug using.

Although for many patients the maintenance phase may be very smooth, there are other patients who will experience "turbulence" during the LTOT maintenance phase for PNCP. There are many possible contributing factors, including increased pain, increased side effects, new pain, new adverse effects, and behavioral issues (alterations, changes, in patient's goals/expectations, and aberrant drug behaviors). Increased pain, increased side effects, new pain, new side effects should prompt a comprehensive history and physical examination in efforts to search for new etiologies of pain and/or side effects. Other considerations include: progression of disease (which may lead to the phenomenon of pseudoaddiction), opioid-induced hyperalgesia and pain, analgesic tolerance, noncompliance or "dyscompliance" (e.g., taking the medicine prescribed but not in the exact manner prescribed), and increased function and physical activity.

With the addition of a collection of various instruments—the NOSE (Numeral Opioid Side Effect assessment tool; Smith, 2006e), GDTAs (Smith, 2006d), SAFE (Social, Analgesia, Function, Emotional scale; Smith, 2005a), TAS (Translational Analgesic Score; Smith, 2002), and PADT (Pain Assessment and Documentation Tool; Passik et al., 2004; each clinic may choose their own collection and uses)—to the mix of data/tools already utilized for following patients on LTOT for PCNP, it is hoped that clinicians may "have a more complete picture" regarding trends in the overall functioning status of their patients on LTOT longitudinally and perhaps even contribute to clinicians feeling more comfortable with making future treatment/management decisions (Smith, 2006f).

Opioid Analgesic Agents

There is significant variability in the responses of different patients to different opioids. Patient factors that may have an impact on opioid activity include body fat content, body mass, organ function, age, volume of distribution, and presence and activity of various metabolic enzymes. Additional factors may include gender, genetics, opioid receptor subtype mix (quantity, distribution, and intrinsic affinity), previous medication/drug history/recreational alcohol use, and status/environment history of nociceptive pathways/ receptors.

The cancer unit of the World Health Organization (WHO) convened an expert committee in 1986 and proposed a useful approach to cancer pain known as the WHO three-step analgesic ladder that relied heavily on the use of potent opioids for severe cancer pain.

Opioids can be categorized into different families:

- Phenanthrenes
- Benzomorphans
- Phenylpiperidines
- Diphenylheptanes

The phenanthrenes have a five-ringed structure and include morphine, codeine, hydromorphone, buprenorphine, nalbuphine, and butorphanol. The 6-OH group on morphine may lead to side effects such as nausea. Phenanthrenes that lack the 6-OH group (e.g., oxycodones, hydromorphone, hydrocodone) may be better tolerated in patients with nausea from morphine. If a patient cannot tolerate a dehydroxylated phenanthrene, it will not be worthwhile giving the patient a trial of a hydroxylated phenanthrene. The benzomorphans have a three-ringed structure, and the prototype is pentazocine. The phenylpiperidines have a two-ringed structure and include meperidine, fentanyl, sufentanil, alfentanil, and remifentanil. The diphenylheptanes are unlike the other groups in that they can be considered somewhat linear in structure.

In general, agents such as the agonist-antagonist group (agents such as nalbuphine and pentazocine, which are antagonists at the mu opioid receptor and agonists at the kappa opioid receptor), meperidine, and propoxyphene have little to no role in the long-term management of persistent noncancer pain.

Morphine sulfate (considered by some the "prototype opioid") is the best known and most commonly used opioid for pain relief in the world. Morphine belongs to the phenanthrene opioid class; absorption post–oral administration is approximately 20%–30% (Janicki & Parris, 2003). After intramuscular administration of morphine sulfate, the analgesic onset is about 10–20 minutes, the time to peak analgesia is roughly 30–60 minutes, the analgesic duration is about 3–5 hours, and the elimination half-life is 203 hours (Janicki & Parris, 2003). It is a relatively hydrophilic opioid with slow elimination from the brain compartment relative to plasma. The oral-to-parental ratio for long-term dosing is 3:1. When initiating therapy, it may be as high as 6:1. The major metabolic pathways of morphine are in the liver via glucuronidation. Although there may be a small unmetabolized fraction present, some of the metabolites of morphine include morphine-6-glucuronide (M6G; 10%), morphine-3-glucuronide (M3G; 60%), morphine-3-sulfate (5%), normorphine (4%), and morphine 3,6 diglucuronide (< 1%; Janicki & Parris, 2003).

M6G possesses analgesic qualities and when administered intrathecally as an infusion to humans, is more potent than morphine (Grace & Fee, 1996). There is dramatic delay in the rate of the rise of M6G plasma concentrations probably resulting from slow and incomplete transfer of M6G through the blood-brain barrier. This could conceivably help explain the increased analgesic efficacy occasionally encountered over the initial titration period of morphine.

M3G is devoid of analgesic activity (Hewett et al., 1993), however, intracerebroventricular or intraperitoneal M3G has been reported to induce allodynia and hyperalgesia, with higher doses potentially leading to behavior excitation, myoclonus, and seizures (Gong et al., 1992; Igawa et al., 1993). These efforts may occur via "nonopioid" mechanisms, perhaps involving the NMDA receptor. Additionally, M3G may actually antagonize the analgesic effects of morphine, perhaps partly via nonopioid mechanisms (e.g., facilitating dynorphin actions and/or direct or indirect effects on the NMDA receptor complex; Janicki & Parris, 2003). It is conceivable that patients' analgesic response to morphine may be related to their M3G-to-M6G ratio (Janicki & Parris, 2003). However, Goucke and colleagues (1994) reported that the M3G-to-M6G ratios in 11 patients with "morphine-resistant pain receiving long-term morphine were similar to published values in patients with well-controlled pain". Clearly, there are no easy answers in attempts to explain opioid analgesic efficacy, but it is hoped that in the future the more that clinicians appreciate the various pharmacokinetic/ pharmacodynamic differences among opioids and patients, the better equipped they may be to approaches issues of suboptimal opioid analgesia.

If a patient has abnormal differential induction and/or function of the various uridine glucuronosyltransferase (UGT) enzymes, conceivably this could lead to M3G-to-M6G ratios and resultant inadequate analgesia. Furthermore, if a patient on high doses of morphine exhibits hyperalgesia, agitation, and/or myoclonus, this could conceivably be due to M3G, and opioid rotation (switching) to the use of non–UGT-metabolized opioids (e.g., methadone) should be considered. Morphine glucuronides are eliminated from the body via urinary excretion. In patients with renal failure, the retention of plasma M6G induces a progressive accumulation of this active metabolite in cerebrospinal fluid; this accumulation may contribute to the increased susceptibility and increased side effects (e.g., respiratory depression, sedation, vomiting) to morphine in patients with renal failure (Janicki & Parris, 2003).

Hydromorphone (Dilaudid) is a phenanthrene-derivative structural analog of morphine; it is essentially "dehydroxylated morphine." It may be produced in the body by N-demethylation of hydrocodone. The oral bioavailability is roughly 30%–40% (Janicki & Parris, 2003). After intramuscular administration of hydromorphone, the analgesic onset is about 10–20 minutes, the time to peak analgesic effect a is roughly 30–60 minutes, the analgesic duration is about 3–5 hours, and the elimination half-life is roughly 2–3 hours (Janicki & Parris, 2003). Hydromorphone has a strong affinity for the mu opioid receptor and is as relatively hydrophilic as morphine sulfate. The oral-to-parental ratio is about 5:1 and when administered parenterally, roughly 1.5 mg of hydromorphone is equivalent to 10 mg of morphine.

The major metabolic pathways of hydromorphone are similar to morphine and predominantly in the liver via glucuronidation (e.g., hydromorphone-3-glucuronide [H3G], hydromorphone-6 glucuronides [H6G]). H3G is similar to M3G, being devoid of analgesic activity and potentially leading to a range of dose-dependent neuroexcitatory side effects (e.g., allodynia, myoclonus, seizures). Hydromorphone appears to be especially well-suited to use cautiously renal failure.

Fentanyl is a synthetic phenylpiperidine mu opioid receptor agonist. It is roughly 80 times more potent than morphine, is highly lipophilic, and binds avidly to plasma proteins. After intramuscular administration of fentanyl citrate, the analgesic onset time is roughly 7–15 minutes, the time to peak analgesia may be extremely variable but could be approximated by 15–45 minutes, the analgesic duration is about 1–2 hours, and the elimination half-life is about 2–4 hours (Janicki & Parris, 2003). Fentanyl is largely metabolized by piperidine N-dealkylation to norfentanyl via hepatic microsomal CYP3A4 (Janicki & Parris, 2003). Amide hydrolysis to desproprionyl fentanyl and alkyl hydroxylation to hydroxyfentanyl are relatively minor pathways (Janicki & Parris, 2003). Hydroxynorfentanyl is a minor, secondary metabolite arising from N-dealkylation of hydroxyfentanyl (Janicki & Parris, 2003).

Oral transmucosal fentanyl citrate (OTFC), a candied matrix formulation administered orally as a palatable lozenge on a stick. It is applied against the buccal mucosa, as it dissolves in saliva a portion of the drug diffuses across the oral mucosa with the rest being swallowed and partially absorbed in the stomach and intestine. The bioavailability is about 50%. OTFC appears to be particularly well-suited for breakthrough pain (which is present in roughly two-thirds of cancer patients with pain) due to its rapid onset. Meaningful analgesia may occur between 5 to 10 minutes after initiating OTFC use. Peak plasma concentrations are achieved at 20 minutes, and the duration of analgesia is roughly 2 hours (Lichtor et al., 1999). The U.S. Food and Drug Administration (FDA) issued an approvable letter for Fentora (Fentanyl buccal tablet) in June 2006. Fentanyl effervescent buccal tablets enhance buccal delivery of fentanyl utilizing the OraVescent drug delivery system (Durfee et al., 2006; Pather et al., 2001).

Oxycodone is a phenanthrene, which, like hydromorphone, lacks the 6-hydroxyl group of morphine and is generally well-tolerated. After oral administration of oxycodone, the analgesic onset is about 30–60 minutes, the time to peak analgesic effect (median tTmax) is roughly 60 minutes, the analgesic duration may be about 3–6 hours but can be variable, and the elimination half-life may vary but is usually about 2–3 hours (Poyhia et al., 1992, 1993). The bioavailability of oral relative to intramuscular oxycodone is 60% (Poyhia et al., 1992).

The metabolism of oxycodone is extensive (about 95%) and complex with many "minor" routes. Oxycodone and its phase I metabolites produced by O-demethylation, N-demethylation, 6-ketoreduction, and N-oxidation yield oxymorphone, noroxycodone, noroxymorphone, 6-oxycodol, nor-6-ocycodol, oxycodone-N-oxide, and 6-oxycodol-N-oxide. Phase II conjugates of several of these compounds with glucuronic acid are present in the urine as well as the N-oxidized derivative of 6-oxycodol and an O-glucuronide of this compound (Baldacci et al., 2004). Ten percent (range 8–14%) of the administered dose is excreted essentially unchanged (conjugated or unconjugated) in the urine (Poyhia et al., 1992).

The O-demethylation pathway represents a relatively minor metabolic pathway for oxycodone, with cytochrome P450 enzyme CYP2D6 being the major O-demethylase most likely accounting for 79% to 90% of O-demethylase activity in human hepatic microsomes (Lalovic et al., 2004). Significant individual variation in oxycodone metabolism may account for wide variability in clinical responses (Heiskanen et al., 2000). Genetic polymorphism in the expression of CYP3A5 may be a significant issue that contributes to the intersubject variability of CYP3A activity in vivo (Lamda et al., 2002). Thus, CYP3A expression and activity may be major determinants of oxycodone clearance in vivo, and inhibitors of or inducers of CYP3A expression and/or activity may significantly affect the activities/actions of oxycodone.

Oxymorphone, a 3-0-demethylation metabolite of oxycodone, is a potent opioid that has a 3 to 5 times higher mu opioid receptor affinity than morphine (Childers et al., 1979). Oxymorphone has been studied for postsurgical pain in an oral immediate-release formulation and appears to be effective (Gimbel & Ahdieh, 2004). It has also been studied as an oral extended-release formulation, and it appears that oxymorphone may be effective for moderate to severe pain secondary to osteoarthritis (Matsumoto et al., 2005). In June 2006, the FDA approved Opana (oxymorphone hydrochloride) tablets (5 mg, 10 mg), and Opana (oxymorphone hydrochloride) extended-release tablets (5 mg, 10 mg, 20 mg, 40 mg). It also seems that oxymorphone extended-release may be equianalgesic to oxycodone controlled-release at half the milligram daily dosage (with comparable safety; Gabrail et al., 2004; Hale et al., 2005) and may be more potent than morphine at equianalgesic doses (Sloan et al., 2005). Oxymorphone extended-release uses a TIMERx delivery system (Penwest Pharmaceuticals, 2005) to provide pharmacokinetic characteristics consistent with 12-hour dosing (Adams & Ahdieh, 2004). Major metabolites of oxymorphone include 6-OH-oxymorphone-3-glucuronide. It appears that oxymorphone extended-release dose not affect CYP2C9 or CYP3A4 metabolic pathways (Adams & Ahdieh, 2005). Noroxymorphone demonstrated a 3- and 10-fold higher affinity for the mu opioid receptor than oxycodone and noroxycodone, respectively (Lalovic et al., 2004).

Drug Interactions With Opioids

The majority of significant pharmacokinetic drug interactions appear to involve drug metabolism or protein binding. Codeine is metabolized to morphine (which is the "active" analgesic agent) via the CYP2D6. Codeine has essentially no analgesic activity in people lacking CYP2D6 (up to roughly 27% of Caucasians) or in people taking CYP2D6 inhibitors (e.g., quinidine; Smith, 2003b). Acceleration of methadone metabolism due to induction of CYP3A4 by antiretroviral drugs or rifampin has led to methadone withdrawal symptoms (Smith, 2003b). Additionally, alkylating agents that may impair α_1-acid glycoprotein synthesis may significantly affect the protein binding and therefore the activity of methadone (Smith, 2003b).

Chemotherapeutic agents could result in altered transmembrane transport of morphine, methadone, or fentanyl secondary to inhibition of P-glycoprotein (Smith, 2003b). However, the clinical significance of this is uncertain.

The epidemiology and relative clinical significance of opioid tolerance and opioid-induced hyperalgesia remains uncertain.

Tolerance may exist as a wide clinical spectrum (being barely perceptible to dramatic, both in its severity as well as in its time course). Although it is easy to produce and appreciate tolerance in animal studies (Compton et al., 2003; DeConno et al., 1991; Devulder, 1997; Guignard et al., 2000; Heger et al., 1999; Hood et al., 2003; Ossipov, 2003; Parisod et al., 2003; Sjogren et al., 1993; 1994; Vanderah et al., 2000, 2001a, 2001b; Z. Wang et al., 2001; Woolf, 1981; Yaksh et al., 1986, 1988), some investigators doubt that it is clinically significant in humans, because it can be difficult to clearly demonstrate and reproduce (Galer et al., 2005), although this may be due to inadequate power. Evidence exists that suggests that opioid-induced hyperalgesia and tolerance may occur within 1 month of initiating opioid therapy in some patients (Chu et al., 2006). After performing a small, prospective, preliminary study with chronic low back pain patients, Chu and colleagues suggested that opioid tolerance and opioid-induced hyperalgesia do occur within 1 month of initiating opioid therapy. If administered as the sole analgesic agent, this has the potential to limit the clinical utility of opioids in controlling persistent pain (Chu et al., 2006). Furthermore, Pud et al. (2005) suggest that they discovered evidence of opioid-induced hyperalgesia in the opioid addict population. However, Reznikov et al. (2005) suggest that the administration of "commonly used" dosages of opioids do not generally lead to abnormal pain sensitivity.

Portenoy (2004) has commented on the consensus statement of the UK Pain Society, the Royal College of Anaesthetists, General Practitioners, and Psychiatrists (Pain Society et al., 2004) stating that their "recommendations properly emphasize that tolerance seems to be a minor problem in practice." Although the authors agree with this statement for patients with a limited lifespan, the authors believe that there exists a subpopulation of patients with persistent noncancer pain on LTOT in whom tolerance represents a significant clinical challenge.

Intrathecal Long-Term Opioid Therapy

Opioids have been administered by most routes, including oral, rectal, transdermal, intratracheal, oral transmucosal, sublingual, intranasal, subcutaneous, intramuscular, subcutaneous, intravenous, epidural, and intrathecal. Although morphine is the only opioid approved for intrathecal use in a continuous pump, many other opioids have been used intrathecally in various clinical circumstances (e.g., fentanyl, hydromorphone).

Intraspinal drug infusion is an available option that may be used for the treatment of intractable persistent pain that is unresponsive to less invasive approaches. In efforts to review current literature, revise the algorithm for drug selection developed in 2000, and develop current guidelines among other goals, the Polyanalgesic Consensus Conference 2003 was organized. Opioids have been and continue to be a mainstay agent for intraspinal therapy. In fact, the guidelines developed at the Polyanalgesic Consensus Conference 2003 suggest that the first-line intraspinal agent should be an opioid alone such as morphine sulfate or hydromorphone (switching from one agent to another if the maximum dose is reached or side effects occur; Hassenbusch et al., 2004). If a maximum dose of 15 mg/day of morphine and/or maximum concentration 30 mg/ml for morphine (or alternatively for hydromorphone 10 mg/d and/or maximum concentration of 30 mg/ml) is reached (or perhaps in selected cases of "predominant" neuropathic pain), the guidelines would suggest that the clinician could proceed to "step 2" (the addition of bupivacaine or clonidine to the opioid) of the six-step algorithm (Hassenbusch et al., 2004). In 2007, the algorithm was updated and Ziconofide became a first-line agent (Deer et al., 2007). Intrathecal catheter-tip inflammatory masses may infrequently occur (Hassenbusch et al., 2002).

Smith and colleagues evaluated 202 patients with life-limiting cancer and pain scores consistently over 5/10 despite 200 mg of morphine or more daily in a multicenter, multinational, randomized, controlled study of comprehensive medical management versus drug delivery systems. They concluded that implantable intrathecal drug delivery systems (IDDS) reduced pain, significantly relieved common drug toxicities, and was possibly associated with improved survival in patients with refractory cancer pain (TJ Smith et al., 2002). One criticism (Davis et al., 2003) of the study by Smith and colleagues was that the authors arbitrarily defined refractory cancer pain for purposes of patient eligibility as pain with a score of $\geq 5/10$ despite 200 mg per day of oral morphine or the equivalent, which did not seem to be an especially high dose of opioids (at least by oncology standards).

Smith et al. further evaluated IDDS in a 6-month clinical trial of IDDS as well as comprehensive medical management versus comprehensive medical management alone (TJ Smith et al., 2005a). Smith et al. concluded that IDDS improved clinical success, reduced pain scores, alleviated analgesic toxicities, and potentially contributed to improved survival for the duration of the 6-onth trial (TJ Smith et al., 2005a). Smith and Coyne (2005b) went onto describe 30 patients who crossed over from unsuccessful comprehensive medical management to implantable drug delivery systems; they concluded that it is possible for even the most refractory of cancer pain patients to potentially derive clinically important pain relief, as well as relief of drug toxicities, by crossing over from comprehensive medical management to an intrathecal implantable drug delivery system. Burton et al. (2004) also found spinal analgesia effective in treating refractory cancer pain.

Opioid Side Effects

Increasing evidence suggests a useful analgesic effect when a variety of strong opioids are used in the treatment of neuropathic and nonneuropathic pain. That said, they are neither universally effective nor universally well-tolerated by patients. Although, some investigators have referred to common opioid side effects as generally benign, they appear to be significantly unpleasant and quite severe to at least some patients and they may contribute to discontinuation of opioid therapy in a significant number of patients. Therefore, it may be useful to have patients fill out an assessment tool (e.g., the NOSE Assessment; Smith, 2006e) in the waiting rooms in efforts to longitudinally follow opioid effects so as to be in a better position to attempt proactive strategies to combat opioid side effects. Common opioid side effects may include nausea and vomiting, pruritus, sedation, and constipation. Potential future agents such as methylnaltrexone or alvimopan may offer promise in the management of opioid-associated constipation without the risk of opioid withdrawal or reversal of opioid analgesic effects.

Opioids and/or opioid-like substances have been used for many centuries; however, various effects of specific agents are only recently becoming appreciated (e.g., buprenorphine hepatotoxicity [Berson et al., 2001; Herve et al., 2004] and codeine phosphate-induced hypersensitivity syndrome [Enomoto et al., 2004]).

Opioids appear to exhibit a relatively good safety profile compared to other medications. Although overall gross clinical safety of usual doses of opioids over years is appreciated, it is conceivable that there may be subtle changes induced by doses of morphine equivalents more than several grams/day over many decades that are not fully appreciated (however, a similar scenario may be true of many other medications). After many decades of use, the association of high-dose methadone and the potential for QT_c prolongation, with possible Torsade de Pointes, has first been noted in this past decade (Krantz et al., 2002). There are no known overt organ toxicities secondary to treatment with opioids. However, it is conceivable (if animal data can be applied to humans [Atici et al., 2005; Todaka et al., 2005; Zhang et al., 2004]) that morphine (or other opioids) and its metabolites (e.g., morphinone; Todaka et al., 2005), over many decades in certain predisposed patients, may (via the risk of increased lipid peroxidation) potentially facilitate certain subtle previously unrecognized subclinical changes in normal organ structure and/or function (e.g., theoretical microalbuminuria). Clearly, there is a need to study potential subtle changes due to the administration over many decades of relatively high doses of opioids as well as other medications.

The biologic consequences of other effects of opioids are also incompletely elucidated. Immunologic effects of opioids appear to differ: different opioid agents (Martucci et al., 2004) with short-term versus long-term administration (Martucci et al., 2004), as well as with the state of the organism (presence of inflammation versus absence of inflammation, presence of pain versus absence of pain).

Although a number of strong opioid preparations have been introduced over the last few years, these tend to be new formulations rather than new compounds. For example, oxycodone, fentanyl, and buprenorphine have a long pedigree as analgesics. The new aspect of them is their presentation, as a controlled-release preparation in the case of oxycodone, and as transdermal preparations in the case of fentanyl and buprenorphine. It is arguable whether any individual opioid offers significant analgesic benefit over the other members of this class. They do, however, differ to a certain extent in the incidence and frequency of side effects associated with their use. For example, Staats and colleagues (2004) retrospectively studied 1,836 patients receiving treatment with transdermal fentanyl, sustained-release oxycodone and sustained-release morphine. Those receiving transdermal fentanyl had a lower risk of developing constipation than those taking either of the other two strong opioids (3% as opposed to a 6% risk with oxycodone and 5% with morphine; Staats et al., 2004). The incidence these authors quote for the occurrence of constipation is significantly lower than other others report with transdermal fentanyl.

Milligan and colleagues (2001) found that in an open-label trial of transdermal fentanyl in which 301 patients continued use for 12 months, constipation was noted as a side effect in 19%. Menten and colleagues (2002) suggest that in terms of patients treated with transdermal fentanyl for cancer-related pain, the incidence of constipation is related not to the dose of transdermal fentanyl used, but rather to the amount of morphine used as a rescue analgesic.

Van Seventer and colleagues (2003) give support to the impression of a lower risk of constipation with transdermal fentanyl. They enrolled 131 patients and commenced them on transdermal fentanyl or controlled-release morphine. Doses were titrated until effect was apparent. The quality of analgesia achieved in both groups was equal. Constipation was less common in those treated with fentanyl: At the end of 1 week, 27% in the fentanyl group reported constipation, as opposed to 57% in the controlled-release morphine group. In general terms, other side effects were more common or severe in the morphine group. Of the patients enrolled in the study, 36% in the controlled-release morphine group withdrew because of side effects, as opposed to only 4% in the transdermal fentanyl group. Of those who continued with the trial, 14% in the fentanyl group reported troublesome side effects, as opposed to 36% in the morphine group (Van Seventer et al., 2003).

Quigley (2002) has reviewed the available studies that examine the use of hydromorphone in the treatment of cancer and non-cancer pain. He concludes that of the limited number of studies available, hydromorphone differs little in its effect or side effect profile to the other strong opioid analgesics (Quigley, 2002).

When incomplete relief or unacceptable side effects are apparent with opioid therapy, substitution to another opioid is suggested as an option. Although this approach has gained popularity, Quigley (2004), in his systematic review of available studies published up until January 2003, concludes that the evidence for this strategy is "...largely anecdotal or based on observational and uncontrolled studies."

A variety of issues influence the tolerability of opioids. Well-known side effects such as nausea, vomiting, constipation, and cognitive impairment can all reduce their tolerability in the short term to the extent that sustained use is impracticable without the development of tolerance. Efficacy and incidence of side effects seems to be, at least in part, dose-related (Rowbotham et al., 2003). Furthermore, the incidence of side effects decreases with sustained-use tolerance usually develops to most opioid side effects often, with the notable exception of constipation (Mystakidou et al., 2003). With extended-release preparations, these side effects may be more gradual in onset, as may be their initial analgesic effect. That said, Watson and colleagues (2003) studied patients with painful diabetic neuropathy. Patients were treated for 4 weeks with controlled-release oxycodone or placebo. The only side effects that occurred on a statistically more significant basis in the oxycodone treated group were dry mouth and constipation (Watson et al., 2003).

A recurrent anxiety associated with chronic strong opioid administration is its effect on cognition and motor tasks as exemplified by driving safety. Schindler and colleagues (2004) examined this issue in opioid addicts (not with chronic pain) using an Austrian standard test battery for measurement of performance related to driving ability, the Act and React Test (ART) system. Subjects were taking either methadone or buprenorphine and were compared to healthy controls. They found that those taking these strong opioids did not differ significantly in comparison with the healthy controls in the majority of the ART standard tests (Schindler et al., 2004).

Jamison and colleagues (2003) examined the psychomotor effects of long-term opioid (oxycodone and fentanyl) use in 144 patients with low back pain. They measured the results of two neuropsychological tests (Digit Symbol and Trail Making Test–B) on all subjects prior to institution of the strong opioid and again 90 and 180 days after opioid commencement. They found that sustained use was not associated with impairment of the neuropsychological variables measured. Indeed, memory, incidental learning, and psychomotor performance were improved in many of the subjects. They also noted that a minority of patients had a decrease in performance. This tended to occur in older patients and in those with lower pretreatment pain scores. There were no differences in neuropsychological performance between patients taking oxycodone or transdermal fentanyl (Jamison et al., 2003).

Tassain and colleagues (2003) studied 28 patients with chronic noncancer pain in whom sustained-release morphine was prescribed. Eighteen stayed on this therapy; the other 10 discontinued treatment because of unacceptable side effects and acted as a control group. They found that when baseline, pretreatment neuropsychological variables were compared in these patients with results obtained after 3, 6, and 12 months of treatment, there were no significant differences. Indeed, in two measures of information processing (the Stroop interference score and the digit symbol test), the results were actually better after 6 and 12 months of treatment. The most frequent side effects with treatment were gastrointestinal in nature with almost 50% of patients still reporting constipation after 12 months of morphine therapy (Tassain et al., 2003).

Similarly, Sabatowski and colleagues (2003) measured attention, reaction, visual orientation, motor coordination, and vigilance in 30 subjects using a stable dose of transdermal fentanyl for noncancer pain and compared them to 90 healthy volunteers. None of the results from the measures differed significantly between the fentanyl treated and volunteer subjects, and they concluded that in patients treated with stable doses of transdermal fentanyl, the threshold for fitness to drive did not differ significantly between the groups (Sabatowski et al., 2003).

In contrast, when morphine and controlled-release oxycodone (OxyContin) are administered on a one-off basis to volunteers and compared to placebo, both morphine and OxyContin produce effects on psychomotor performance, and these effects are dose-related (Zacny & Gutierrez, 2003b).

Longer term administration may be complicated by other factors that can influence their long-term tolerability. For example, acute administration of opioids increases prolactin, growth hormone, thyroid-stimulating hormone, and ACTH while inhibiting luteinizing hormone (LH) release (Grossman, 1983; Paice et al., 1994; Su et al., 1987). When administered on a long-term basis, different endocrine results are observed. Abs and colleagues (2000) have extensively investigated 73 patients receiving an average duration of 26 months of intrathecal opioids for chronic nonmalignant pain. Decreased libido and impotence was present in 23 of the 24 men studied. Nine of the men had a significantly reduced testosterone level, and most had a decreased LH level. All of the premenopausal females had either amenorrhea or an irregular cycle, with ovulation in only 1 patient, as well as decreased LH and FSH level when compared to controls. The 24-hour urinary cortisol excretion was significantly lower than controls in 14 of the 73 patients. Fifteen percent of all patients developed growth hormone deficiency. Therefore, in patients receiving intrathecal opioids on a long-term basis, the majority of men and all women developed hypogonadotrophic hypogonadism, 15% developed central hypocorticism, and about 15% developed growth hormone deficiency (Abs et al., 2000).

A variety of miscellaneous potential opioid adverse effects may have clinical significance. It appears that sleep-disordered breathing (e.g., sleep apnea) may be associated with long-term opioid therapy (Farney et al., 2003; Wang et al., 2005). A single case report highlights a different possible side effect of fentanyl use. Kokko and colleagues (2002) report apparent inappropriate antidiuretic hormone (ADH) release in a patient with a known lung tumor treated with fentanyl. Withdrawal of fentanyl terminated the ADH release, whereas reinstitution of fentanyl at a latter date triggered of a further inappropriate ADH release (Kokko et al., 2002).

Summary

Overall, the use of LTOT for PNCP may provide significant analgesia patients with minimal side effects for many years. However, the following must be kept in mind:

a. LTOT may not be optimal for all patients.
b. LTOT does not provide good or excellent analgesia in all patients.
c. LTOT is not devoid of side effects.
d. LTOT should be monitored in efforts to assess efficacy, side effects, and aberrant drug behavior.
e. LTOT can be successfully withdrawn in selected patients who may do better without opioids.
f. Prescribing LTOT for PNCP remains very much an art that may be used successfully alone or in conjunction with other therapeutic options but typically not as a first-line agent for patients who have not tried previous treatments.

References

Abs R, Verhelst J, Maeyaert J, Van Buyten J-P, Opsomer F, Adriaensen H, Verlooy J, Van Havenbergh, Smet M, Van Acker K. Endocrine consequences of long term intrathecal administration of opioids. *J Clin Endocrinol Metab.* 2000; 85: 2215–22.

Adams MP, Ahdieh H. Pharmacokinetics and dose-proportionality of oxymorphone extended release and its metabolites: results of a randomized crossover study. *Pharmacotherapy.* 2004; 24: 468–76.

Adams MP, Ahdieh H. Single- and multiple-dose pharmacokinetic and dose-proportionality study of oxymorphone immediate-release tablets. *Drugs R D.* 2005; 6: 91–9.

American Academy of Pain Medicine, American Pain Society. *The use of opioids for the treatment of chronic pain.* http://www.painmd.org/productpub/statements/pdfs/opioids.pdf. Accessed August 4, 2004.

Atici S, Cinel I, Cinel L, et al. Liver and kidney toxicity in chronic use of opioids: an experimental long term treatment model. *J Biosci.* 2005; 30: 245–52.

Attal NA, Guirimand F, Brasseur L, et al. Effects of IV morphine in central pain. A randomized placebo-controlled study. *Neurology.* 2002; 58: 554–63.

Baldacci A, Caslavska J, Wey AB, et al. Identification of new oxycodone metabolites in human urine by capillary electrophoresis—mu stage iontrap mass spectrometry. *J Chromatogr A.* 2004; 1051: 273–82.

Ballantyne JC, Mao J. Opioid therapy for chronic pain. *N Eng J Med.* 2003; 349: 1943–53.

Bartleson JD. Evidence for and against the use of opioid analgesics for chronic nonmalignant low back pain: A review. *Pain Med.* 2002; 3: 260–71.

Bennett GJ, Seltzer Z, Lu GW, et al. The cells of origin of the dorsal column postsynaptic projection in the lumbosacral enlargements of cats and monkeys. *Somatosens Res.* 1983; 1: 131–49.

Berson A, Fau D, Fornacciari R, et al. Mechanisms for experimental buprenorphine hepatotoxicity: major role of mitochondrial dysfunction versus metabolic activation. *J Hepatol.* 2001; 34: 261–9.

Bester H, Chapman V, Besson JM, et al. Physiological properties of the lamina I spinoparabrachial neurons in the rat. *J Neurophysiol.* 2000; 83: 2239–59.

Boivie J, Meyerson BA. A correlative anatomical and clinical study of pain suppression by deep brain stimulation. *Pain.* 1982; 13: 113–26.

Bonacci TM, Mathews JL, Yuan C, et al. Differential targeting of $G_{\beta\gamma}$-subunit signaling with small molecules. *Science.* 2006; 312: 443–46.

Breivik H. Opioids in chronic non-cancer pain, indications and controversies. *Eur J Pain.* 2005; 9: 127–30.

Burton AW, Rajagopal A, Shah HN, et al. Epidural and intrathecal analgesia is effective in treating refractory cancer pin. *Pain Med.* 2004; 5: 235.

Butler SF, Budman SH, Fernandez K, et al. Validation of a screener and opioid assessment measure for patients with chronic pain. *Pain.* 2004; 112: 65–75.

Cabrera-Vera TM, Vanhauwe J, Thonmas TO, et al. Insights into G protein structure, function, and regulation. *Endocr Rev.* 2003; 24: 765–81.

Caudill-Slosberg MA, Schwartz LM, Woloshin S. Office visits and analgesic prescriptions for musculoskeletal pain in U.S.: 1980 vs. 2000. *Pain.* 2004; 109: 514–9.

Chen Y, Mestek A, Liu J, Hurley J, Yu L. Molecular cloning and functional expression of a mu-opioid receptor from rat brain. *Molecular Pharmacology.* 1993; 44: 8–12.

Cheunsuang O, Morris R. Spinal lamina I neurons that express neurokinin 1 receptors: morphological analysis. *Neuroscience.* 2000; 97: 335–45.

Childers SR, Creese I, Snowman AM, et al. Opiate receptor binding affected differentially by opiates and opioid peptides. *Eur J Pharmacol.* 1979; 55: 11–8.

Chou R, Clark E, Helfan M, et al. Comparative efficacy and safety of long-acting oral opioids for chronic non-cancer pain: a systematic review. *J Pain Symptom Manage.* 2003; 26: 1026–48.

Chu LF, Clark DJ, Angst MS. Opioid tolerance and hyperalgesia in chronic pain patients after one month of oral morphine therapy: a preliminary prospective study. *J Pain.* 2006; 7: 43–8.

Clapham DR, Neer EJ. G Protein beta gamma subunits. *Annu Rev Pharmacol Toxicol.* 1997; 37: 167–203.

Compton P, Athanasos P, Elashoff D. Withdrawal hyperalgesia after acute opioid physical dependency in non addicted humans: a preliminary study. *J Pain.* 2003; 4: 511–9.

Cowan DT, Wilson-Barnett J, Griffiths P, et al. A survey of chronic noncancer pain patients prescribed opioid analgesics. *Pain Med.* 2003; 4: 340–51.

Cowan DT, Wilson-Barnett J, Griffiths P, et al. A randomized, double-blind, placebo-controlled, cross-over pilot study to assess the effects of long-term opioid drug consumption and subsequent abstinence in chronic noncancer pain patients receiving controlled-release morphine. *Pain Med.* 2005; 6: 113–21.

Dale W. On pain, and some of the remedies for its relief. *Lancet.* 1871; (13 May): 641–642; (20 May): 679–690; (3 June): 739–741; (17 June): 816–7.

Davis, MP, Walsh D, Lagman R, et al. Randomized clinical trial of an implantable drug delivery system. *J Clin Oncol.* 2003; 21: 2800–1.

DeConno F, Caraceni A, Martini C, Spoldi E, Salvetti M, Ventafridda V. Hyperalgesia and myoclonus with intrathecal infusion of high-dose morphine. *Pain.* 1991; 47: 337–9.

Deer T, Krames ES, Hassenbusch SJ, et al. Polyanalgesic Consensus Conference 2007: Recommendations for the management of pain by intrathecal (intraspinal) drug delivery: report of an interdisciplinary expert panel. *Neuromodulation.* 2007; 10: 300–328.

Dellemijn PLI, van Duijn H, Vanneste JAL. Prolonged treatment with transdermal fentanyl in neuropathic pain. *J Pain Symptom Manage.* 1998; 16: 220–9.

Dellemijn PLI, Vanneste JAL. Randomized double-blind active-placebo-controlled crossover trial of intravenous fentanyl in neuropathic pain. *Lancet.* 1997; 349: 753–8.

Devulder J. Hyperalgesia induced by high-dose intrathecal sufentanil in neuropathic pain. *J Neurosurg Anesthesiol* 1997; 9: 146–8.

Dirig DM, Isakson PC, Yaksh TL. Effect of COX-1 and COX-2 inhibition on induction and maintenance of carrageenan-evoked thermal hyperalgesia in rats. *J Pharmacol Exp Ther.* 1998; 285: 1031–8.

Dirig DM, Konin GP, Isakson PC, et al. Effect of spinal cyclooxygenase inhibitors in rat using the formalin test and in vitro prostaglandin E2 release. *Eur J Pharmacol.* 1997; 331: 155–60.

Drug Enforcement Administration with 21 health organizations. *Promoting pain relief and preventing abuse of pain medications: a critical balancing act.* http://www.medsch.wisc.edu/painpolicy/Consensus 2.pdf. Accessed August 4, 2004.

Durfee S, Messina J, Khankari R. Fentanyl effervescent buccal tablets: enhanced buccal absorption. *Am J Drug Deliv.* 2006; 4: 1–5.

Dworkin RH, Backonja M, Rowbotham MC, et al. Advances in neuropathic pain: diagnosis, mechanisms, and treatment recommendations. *Arch Neurol.* 2003; 60: 1524–34.

Edwards RR, Haythornthwaite JA, Tella P, et al. Basal heat pain thresholds predict opioid analgesia in patients with postherpetic neuralgia. *Anesthesiology.* 2006; 104: 1243–8.

Eisenberg E, McNicol ED, Carr DB. Efficacy and safety of opioid agonists in the treatment of neuropathic pain of nonmalignant origin: systematic review and meta-analysis trials. *JAMA.* 2005; 293: 3043–52.

Enomoto M, Ochi M, Teramae K, et al. Codeine phosphate-induced hypersensitivity syndrome. *Ann Pharmacother.* 2004; 38: 799–802.

Evans CJ, Keith DE Jr., Morrison H, Magendzo K, Edwards RH. Cloning of a delta opioid receptor by functional expression. *Science.* 1992; 258: 1952–5.

Farney RJ, Walker JM, Cloward TV, et al. Sleep-disordered breathing associated with long-term opioid therapy. *Chest.* 2003; 123: 632–9.

Farrar JT, Portenoy RK, Berlin JA, et al. Defining the clinically important difference in pain outcome measures. *Pain.* 2000; 88: 287–94.

Farrar JT, Young JP Jr., LaMoreaux L, et al. Clinical importance of changes in chronic pain intensity measured on an 11-point numerical pain rating scale. *Pain.* 2001; 94: 149–58.

Fields HL, Heinricher MM, Mason P. Neurotransmitters in nociceptive modulatory circuits. *Annual Review of Neuroscience.* 1991; 14: 219–45.

Fields HL, Levine JD. Placebo analgesia-a role for endorphins? *Trends in Neurosciences.* 1984; 7:271–3.

Gabrail NY, Dvergsten C, Ahdieh H. Establishing the dosage equivalency of oxymorphone extended release and oxycodone controlled release in patients with moderate to severe cancer pain. *Curr Med Res Opin.* 2004; 20: 911–8.

Galer BS, Lee D, Ma T, et al. MorphiDex (morphine sulfate/dextromethorphan hydrobromide combination) in the treatment of chronic pain: three multicenter, randomized, double-blind, controlled clinical trials fail to demonstrate enhanced opioid analgesia or reduction in tolerance. *Pain.* 2005; 115: 284–95.

Gardell LR, Ibrahim M, Wang R, et al. Mouse strains that lack spinal dynorphin upregulation after peripheral nerve injury do not develop neuropathic pain. *Neuroscience.* 2004; 123: 43–52.

Gebhart GF. Descending modulation of pain. *Neurosci Biobehav Rev.* 2004; 27: 729–37.

Gimbel J, Ahdieh H. The efficacy and safety of oral immediate release oxymorphone for postsurgical pain. *Anesth Analg.* 2004; 99: 1472–7.

Gimbel JS, Richards P, Portenoy RK. Controlled-release oxycodone for diabetic neuropathy: a randomized controlled trial. *Neurology.* 2003; 60: 927–34.

Gong QL, Hedner J, Bjorkman R, et al. Morphine-3-glucuronide may functionally antagonize morphine-6-glucuronide induced antinociception and ventilatory depression in the rat. *Pain.* 1992; 48: 249–55.

Goucke CR, Hackett LP, Ilett KF. Concentrations of morphine, morphine-6-glucuronide and morphine-3-glucuronide in serum and cerebrospinal fluid following morphine administration to patients with morphine-resistant pain. *Pain.* 1994; 56: 145–9.

Grace D, Fee JP. A comparison of intrathecal morphine-6-glucuronide and intrathecal morphine sulfate as analgesics for total hip replacement. *Anesth Analg.* 1996; 83: 1055–9.

Grossman A. Brain opiates and neuroendocrine function. *Clin Endocrinol Metab.* 1983; 12: 725–46.

Guignard B, Bossard AE, Coste C, et al. Acute opioid tolerance: intraoperative remifentanil increases postoperative pain and morphine requirement. *Anesthesiology.* 2000; 93: 409–17.

Gustorff B. Intravenous opioid testing in patients with chronic non-cancer pain. *Eur J Pain.* 2005; 9: 123–5.

Hale ME, Dvergsten C, Gimbel. Efficacy and safety of oxymorphone extended release in chronic low back pain: results of a randomized, double-blind, placebo- and active-controlled phase III study. *J Pain.* 2005; 6: 21–8.

Handwerker HO, Kilo S and Reeh PW. Unresponsive afferent nerve fibers in the sural nerve of the rat. *Journal of Physiology.* 1991; 435: 229–42.

Harke H, Gretenkort P, Ladleif HU, et al. The response of neuropathic pain and pain in complex regional pain syndrome to carbamazepine and sustained-release morphine in patients pretreated with spinal cord stimulation: a double-blinded randomized study. *Anesth Analg.* 2001; 92: 488–95.

Hassenbusch S, Burchiel K, Coffey RJ, et al. Management of intrathecal catheter-tip inflammatory masses: a consensus statement. *Pain Med.* 2002; 3: 313–23.

Hassenbusch SJ, Portenoy RK, Cousins M, et al. Polyanalgesic Consensus Conference 2003: an update on the management of pain by intraspinal drug delivery—report of an expert panel. *J Pain Symptom Manage.* 2004; 27: 540–63.

Heger S, Maier C, Otter K, et al. Morphine induced allodynia in a child with brain tumour. *BMJ.* 1999; 319: 627–9.

Heiskanen TE, Ruismaki PM, Seppala TA, et al. Morphine or oxycodone in cancer pain? *Acta Oncol.* 2000; 39: 941–7.

Herve S, Riachi G, Noblet C, et al. Active hepatitis due to buprenorphine administration. *Eur J Gastroenterol Hepatol.* 2004; 16: 1033–7.

Hewett K, Dickenson AH, McQuay HJ. Lack of effect of morphine-3-glucuronide on the spinal antinociceptive actions of morphine in the rat: an electrophysiological study. *Pain.* 1993; 53: 59–63.

Hood DD, Curry R, Eisenach JC. Intravenous remifentanil produces withdrawal hyperalgesia in volunteers with capsaicin-induced hyperalgesia. *Anesth Analg.* 2003; 97: 810–5.

Huse E, Larbig W, Flor H, et al. The effect of opioids on phantom limb pain and cortical reorganization. *Pain.* 2001; 90: 47–55.

Hutchinson MR, Bland ST, Johnson KW, et al. Opioid-induced glial activation: mechanisms of activation and implications for opioid analgesia, dependence, and reward. *ScientificWorld Journal.* 2007; 7: 98–111.

Igawa Y, Westerling D, Mattiasson A, et al. Effects of morphine metabolites on micturition in normal, unanesthetized rats. *Br J Pharmacol.* 1993; 110: 257–62.

Jamison RN, Schein JR, Vallow S, Ascher S, Vorsanger GJ, Katz NP. Neuropsychological effects of long-term opioid use in chronic pain patients. *J Pain Symptom Manage.* 2003; 26: 913–21.

Janicki PK, Parris WC. Clinical pharmacology of opioids. In: Smith HS, ed. *Drugs for Pain.* Philadelphia, PA: Hanley and Belfus; 2003: 97–118.

Jeftinija S, Jeftinija K, Liu F, Skilling SR, Smullin DH, Larson AA. Excitatory amino acids are released from rat primary afferent neurons in vitro. *Neuroscience Letters.* 1991; 125(2): 191–4.

Jordan B, Devi LA. Molecular mechanisms of opioid receptor signal transduction. *British Journal of Anaesthesia.* 1998; 81: 12–9.

Kalso E, Allan L, Dellemijn PL, et al. Recommendations for using opioids in chronic non-cancer pain. *Eur J Pain.* 2003; 7: 381–6.

Kalso E, Edwards JE, Moore RA, McQuay HJ. Opioids in chronic non-cancer pain: a systematic review of efficacy and safety. *Pain.* 2004; 112: 372–80.

Keating SE, Maloney GM. Moran EM, Bowie AG. IRAK-2 participates in multiple toll-like receptor signaling pathways to NF kB via activation of TRAF6 ubiquitination. *J Biol Chem.* 2007; 282: 33435–43.

Kieffer B, Befort K, Gaveriaux-Ruff C and Hirth C. The delta opioid receptor: isolation of a cDNA by expression cloning and pharmacological characterization. *Proceedings of the National Academy of Sciences (USA).* 1992; 89: 12048–52.

Kilo S, Schmelz M, Koltzenburg M, Handwerker HO. Different patterns of hyperalgesia induced by experimental inflammation in human skin. *Brain.* 1994; 117: 385–96.

Kokko H, Hall PD, Afrin LB. Fentanyl associated syndrome of inappropriate antidiuretic hormone secretion. *Pharmacotherapy.* 2002; 22: 1188–92.

Krantz MJ, Lewkowiez L, Hays H, et al. Torsade de pointes associated with very high-dose methadone. *Ann Intern Med.* 2002; 137: 501–4.

LaMotte RH, Shain CN, Simmone DA and Tsai EF. Neurogenic hyperalgesia: psychophysical studies of underlying mechanisms. *Journal of Neurophysiology.* 1991; 66:190–211.

LaMotte RH, Thalhammer JG, Torebjork HE, Robinson CJ. Peripheral neural mechanisms of cutaneous hyperalgesia following mild injury by heat. *Journal of Neuroscience.* 1982; 2: 765–81.

Lalovic B, Phillips B, Risler LL, et al. Quantitative contribution of CYP2D6 and CYP3A to oxycodone metabolism in human liver and intestinal microsomes. *Drug Metab Dispos.* 2004; 32: 447–54.

Lamda JK, Lin YS, Schuetz EG, et al. Genetic contribution to variable human CTP3A-mediated metabolism. *Adv Drug Deliv Rev.* 2002; 54: 1271–94.

Lawson SN, Crepps BA, Perl ER. Relationship of substance p to afferent characteristics of dorsal root ganglion neurons in guinea-pigs. *Journal of Physiology.* 1997; 505: 177–91.

Lawson SN, Crepps BA, Perl ER. Calcitonin gene related peptide immunoreactivity and afferent receptive properties of dorsal root ganglion neurons in guinea-pigs. *Journal of Physiology.* 2002; 540: 989–1002.

Liang DY, Liao G, Wang J, et al. A genetic analysis of opioid-induced hyperalgesia in mice. *Anesthesiology.* 2006; 104: 1054–62.

Lichtor JL, Sevarino FB, Joshi GP, et al. The relative potency of oral transmucosal fentanyl citrate compared with intravenous morphine in the treatment of moderate to sever post-operative pain. *Anesth Analg.* 1999; 89: 732–8.

Mahajan SD, Aalinkeel R, Reynolds JL, et al. Morphine exacerbates HIV-1 viral protein gp120 induced modulation of chemokine gene expression in U373 astrocytoma cells. *Curr HIV Res.* 2005a; 3: 277–88.

Mahajan SD, Schwartz SA, Aalinkeel R, et al. Morphine modulates chemokine gene regulation in normal human astrocytes. *Clin Immunol.* 2005b; 115: 323–32.

Malmberg AB, Yaksh TL. Cyclooxygenase inhibition and the spinal release of prostaglandin E2 and amino acids evoked by paw formalin injection: a microdialysis study in unanesthetized rats. *J Neurosci.* 1995; 15: 2768–76.

Martucci C, Panerai AE, Sacerdote P. Chronic fentanyl or buprenorphine infusion in the mouse: similar analgesic profile but different effects on immune responses. *Pain.* 2004; 110: 385–92.

Matsumoto AK, Babul N, Ahdieh H. Oxymorphone extended-release tablets relieve moderate to severe pain and improve physical function in osteoarthritis: results of a randomized double-blind, placebo- and active-controlled phase III trial. *Pain Med.* 2005; 6: 357–66.

Mayer DJ, Price DD. Central nervous system mechanisms of analgesia. *Pain.* 1976. 2: 379–404.

Melzack, R, Katz J. Pain assessment in adult patients. In: McMahon S, Koltzenberg M, eds. *Wall and Melzack's Textbook of Pain.* 5th ed. New York: (Elsevier) Churchill Livingstone; 2006: 291–304.

Menten J, Desmedt M, Lossignol D, Mullie A. Longitudinal follow up of TTS-fentanyl use in patients with cancer-related pain: results of a compassionate use study with special focus on elderly patients. *Curr Med Res Opin.* 2002; 18: 488–98.

Meyer RA, Campbell JN. Myelinated nociceptive afferents account for the hyperalgesia that follows a burn to the hand. *Science.* 1981; 213: 1527–9.

Meyer RA, Davis KD, Cohen RH, Treede RD, Campbell JN. Mechanically insensitive afferents (MIAs) in cutaneous nerves of monkey. *Brain Research.* 1991; 561: 252–61.

Meyer RA, Matthias R, Campbell JN and Raja SN. Peripheral mechanisms of cutaneous nocicepetion. In: McMahon S, Koltzenberg M, eds. *Wall and Melzack's Textbook of Pain.* 5th ed. New York: (Elsevier) Churchill Livingstone; 2006: 3–34.

Milligan K, Lanteri-Minet M, Borchert K, et al. Evaluation of long-term efficacy and safety of transdermal fentanyl in the treatment of chronic noncancer pain. *J Pain.* 2001; 2: 197–204.

Moulin DE, Iezzi A, Amireh R, et al. Randomized trial of oral morphine for chronic non-cancer pain. *Lancet.* 1996; 347: 143–7.

Mystakidou K, Parpa E, Tsilika E, et al. Long-term management of noncancer pain with transdermal therapeutic system-fentanyl. *J Pain.* 2003; 4: 298–306.

Nicols ML, Allen BJ, Rogers SD, et al. Transmission of chronic nociception by spinal neurons expressing the substance P receptor. *Science.* 1999; 286: 1558–61.

Obara I, Przewlocki R, Przewlocka B. Local peripheral effects of mu-opioid agnostics in neuropathic pain in rats. *Neurosci Lett.* 2004; 360: 85–9.

Ossipov MH, Lai J, Vanderah TW, et al. Induction of pain facilitation by sustained opioid exposure: relationship to opioid antinociceptive tolerance. *Life Sci.* 2003; 73: 783–800.

Ossipov MH, Porreca F. Descending modulation of pain. In: Mersky H, Loeser JD, Dubner R, eds. *The Paths of Pain 1975–2005.* Seattle, WA: IASP Press, 2005.

Paice JA, Penn RD, Ryan WG. Altered sexual function and decreased testosterone in patients receiving intraspinal opioids. *J Pain Symptom Manage.* 1994; 9: 126–31.

Pain Society, London, the Royal College of Anaesthetists, the Royal College of General Practitioners, and the Royal College of Psychiatrists. *Recommendations for the appropriate use of opioids for persistent non-cancer pain.* London: The Pain Society; March 2004. http://www.painsociety.org/pdf/opioids_doc_2004.pdf. Accessed August 9, 2004.

Passik SD, Kirsh KL, Whitcomb LA, Portenoy RK, Katz N, Kleinman L, Dodd S, Schein J. A new tool to assess and document pain outcomes in chronic pain patients receiving opioid therapy. *Clinical Therapeutics,* 2004; 26(4): 552–61.

Parisod E, Siddall PJ, Viney M, McClelland JM, Cousins MJ. Allodynia after acute intrathecal morphine administration in a patient with neuropathic pain after spinal cord injury. *Anesth Analg.* 2003; 97: 183–6.

Pather SI, Siebert JM, Hontz J, et al. Enhanced buccal delivery of fentanyl using the OraVescent drug delivery system. *Drug Deliv Tech.* 2001; 1: 54–7.

Penwest Pharmaceuticals. TIMERx control release delivery systems. Available at http://www.penwest.com/timerx.html. Accessed January 10, 2005.

Perrot S, Guilbaud G, Kayser V. Effects of intraplantar morphine on paw edema and pain-related acute inflammation. *Pain.* 1999; 83: 249–57.

Portenoy RK. Opioid therapy for chronic nonmalignant pain: a review of the critical issues. *J Pain Symptom Manage.* 1996; 11: 203–17.

Portenoy RK. Appropriate use of opioids for persistent non-cancer pain. *Lancet.* 2004; 364: 739–40.

Poyhia R, Seppala T, Olkkola KT, et al. The pharmacokinetics and metabolism of oxycodone after intramuscular and oral administration to healthy subjects. *Br J Clin Pharmacol.* 1992; 33: 617–21.

Poyhia R, Vainio A, Kalso E. A review of oxycodone's clinical pharmacokinetics and pharmacodynamics. *J Pain Symptom Manage.* 1993; 8: 63–7.

Pud D, Cohen D, Lawental E, et al. Opioids and abnormal pain perception: New evidence from a study of chronic opioid addicts and healthy subjects. *Drug Alcohol Depend.* 2005; Oct 13.

Pud D, Yarnitsky D, Sprecher E, et al. Can personality traits and gender predict the response to morphine? An experimental cold pain study. *Eur J Pain.* 2006; 10(2): 103–12.

Quigley C. Hydromorphone for acute and chronic pain. *Cochrane Database Syst Rev.* 2002; 1: CD003447.

Quigley C. Opioid switching to improve pain relief and drug tolerability. *Cochrane Database Syst Rev.* 2004; 3: CD004847.

Raja SN, Haythornwaite JA, Pappagallo M, et al. Opioids versus antidepressants in post herpetic neuralgia: A randomized placebo-controlled trial. *Neurology.* 2002; 59: 1015–21.

Rashig S, Koller M, Haykowsky M, et al. The effect of opioid analgesia on exercise test performance in chronic low back pain. *Pain.* 2003: 106: 199–25.

Reznikov I, Pud D, Eisenberg E. Oral opioid administration and hyperalgesia in patients with cancer or chronic nonmalignant pain. *Br J Clin Pharmacol.* 2005; 60(3): 331–8.

Rowbotham MC, Twilling L, Davies PS, Reisner L, Taylor K, Mohr D. Oral opioid therapy for chronic peripheral and central neuropathic pain. *N Engl J Med.* 2003; 348: 1223–32.

Rome JD, Townsend CO, Bruce BK, et al. Chronic noncancer pain rehabilitation with opioid withdrawal: comparison of treatment outcomes based on opioid use status at admission. *Mayo Clinic Proc.* 2004; 79: 759–68.

Sabatowski R, Schwalen S, Rettig K, Herberg KW, Kasper SM, Radbruch L. Driving ability under long-term treatment with transdermal fentanyl. *J Pain Sympt Mange.* 2003; 25: 38–47.

Samad TA, Moore KA, Sapirstein A, et al. Interleukin-1 beta-mediated induction on COX-2 in the CNS contributes to inflammatory pain hypersensitivity. *Nature.* 2001; 410: 471–5.

Scanlon MN, Chugh U. Exploring physicians' comfort level with opioids for chronic noncancer pain. *Pain Res Manag.* 2004; 9: 195–201.

Schindler SD, Ortner R, Peternell A, Eder H, Opgenoorth E, Fischer G. Maintenance therapy with synthetic opioids and driving aptitude. *Eur Addict Res.* 2004; 10: 80–7.

Schmelz M, Petersen LJ. Neurogenic inflammation in human and rodent skin. *News in Physiological Sciences.* 2001; 16: 33–7.

Scott JK, Huang SF, Gangadhar BP, et al. Evidence that a protein-protein interaction "hot spot" on heterotrimeric G protein betagamma subunits is used for recognition of a subclass of effectors. *EMBO J.* 2001; 20: 767–76.

Sherington CS. *The Integrative Action of the Nervous System.* New York: Scribner; 1906.

Sjogren P, Jensen N-K, Jensen TS. Disappearance of morphine induced hyperalgesia after discontinuing or substituting morphine with other opioid analgesics. *Pain.* 1994; 59: 313–6.

Sjogren P, Jonsson T, Jensen N-K, Drenck N-E, Jensen TS. Hyperalgesia and myoclonus in terminal cancer patients treated with continuous intravenous morphine. *Pain.* 1993; 55: 93–7.

Sloan P, Slatkin N, Ahdieh H. Effectiveness and safety of oral extended-release oxymorphone for the treatment of cancer pain: a pilot study. *Support Care Cancer.* 2005; 13: 57–65.

Smith HS. Taxonomy of pain syndromes. In: Pappagallo M, ed. *The Neurological Basis of Pain.* New York: McGraw-Hill Companies, Inc.; 2005b: 289–300.

Smith HS. Goal-directed therapy agreements. *Journal of Cancer Pain and Symptom Palliation.* 2006d; 1: 11–3.

Smith HS. Introduction. In: Smith HA, ed. *Drugs for Pain.* Philadelphia, PA: Hanley and Belfus; 2003a: 1–8.

Smith HS. Mechanisms and modulation of mu-opioid receptor agonist signaling. *J of Cancer Pain and Symptom Palliation.* 2006b; 1: 3–13.

Smith HS. The Numerical Opioid Side Effect (NOSE) Assessment Tool. *Journal of Cancer Pain and Symptom Palliation.* 2006e; 1: 3–6.

Smith HS. Perspectives in persistent noncancer pain. *Journal of Cancer Pain and Symptom Palliation.* 2006f; 1: 31–2.

Smith HS. Potential analgesic interactions. In: Smith HS, ed. *Drugs for Pain.* Philadelphia, PA: Hanley and Belfus; 2003b: 453–63.

Smith HS. Supraspinal mechanisms of prostanoids involved in nociceptive processing. *J of Cancer Pain and Symptom Palliation.* 2006a; 2: 17–18.

Smith HS. Translational analgesia and translational analgesia score. *Journal of Cancer Pain and Symptom Palliation.* 2006c; 1: 15–19.

Smith HS. Treatment considerations in HIV-related neuropathy. *Journal of Cancer Pain and Symptom Palliation.* 2007; In Press.

Smith HS, Audette J, Witkower A. Assessing analgesic therapeutic outcomes. In: Smith HA, ed. *Drugs for Pain.* Philadelphia, PA: Hanley and Belfus; 2003.

Smith HS, Audette J, Witkower A. Playing it "SAFE." *J Cancer Pain Symptom Palliation.* 2005a; 1: 3–10.

Smith TJ, Coyne PJ. Implantable drug delivery systems (IDDS) after failure of comprehensive medical management (CMM) can palliate symptoms in the most refractory cancer pain patients. *J Palliat Med.* 2005b; 8: 736–42.

Smith TJ, Coyne PJ, Staats PS, et al. An implantable drug delivery systems (IDDS) for refractory cancer pain provides sustained pain control, less drug-related toxicity, and possibly better survival medical management (CMM). *Ann Oncol.* 2005a; 16: 825–33.

Smith TJ, Staats PS, Deer T, et al. Randomized clinical trial of an implantable drug delivery system compared with comprehensive medical management for refractory cancer pain, drug-related toxicity, and survival. *J Clin Oncol.* 2002; 20: 4040–9.

Staats PS, Markowitz J, Schein J. Incidence of constipation associated with long-acting opioid therapy: a comparative study. *South Med J.* 2004; 97: 129–34.

Stein C. Opioid receptors on peripheral sensory neurons. *Adv Exp Med Biol.* 2003; 521: 69–76.

Stein C, Machelska H, Binder W, et al. Peripheral opioid analgesia. *Curr Opin Pharmacol.* 2001; 1: 62–5.

Stein C, Millan MJ, Yassouridas A, et al. Antinociceptive effects of mu- and kappa- agonists in inflammation are enhanced by a peripheral opioid receptor-specific mechanism. *Eur J Pharmacol.* 1988; 155: 255–64.

Stein C, Schafer M, Machelska H. Attacking pain at its source: new perspectives on opioids. *Nat Med.* 2003; 9: 1003–8.

Su CF, Liu MY, Li MT. Intraventricular morphine produces pain relief, hypothermia, hyperglycemia and increased prolactin and growth hormone levels in patients with cancer pain. *J Neurol.* 1987; 235: 105–8.

Suzuki R, Morcuende S, Webber M, et al. Superficial NK1 expressing neurons control spinal excitability by activation of descending pathways. *Nat Neurosci.* 2002; 5: 1319–26.

Tai YH, Wang YH, Wang JJ, et al. Amitriptyline suppresses neuroinflammation and upregulates glutamate transporters in morphine-tolerant rats. *Pain.* 2006; 124: 77–86.

Tai TH, Wang YH, Tsai RY, et al. Amitriptyline preserves morphine's antinociceptive effect by regulating the glutamate transporter GLAST and GLT-1 trafficking and excitatory amino acids concentration in morphine-tolerant rats. *Pain.* 2007; 129: 343–54.

Tassain V, Attal N, Fletcher D et al. Long term effects of oral sustained release morphine on neuropsychological performance in patients with chronic non-cancer pain. *Pain.* 2003; 389–400.

Todaka T, Ishida T, Kita H, et al. Bioactivation of morphine in human liver: isolation and identification of morphinone, a toxic metabolite. *Biol Pharm Bull.* 2005; 28: 1275–80.

Todd AJ. Anatomy of primary afferents and projection neurons in the rate spinal dorsal horn with particular emphasis on substance P and the neurokinin 1 receptor. *Exp Physiol.* 2002; 87: 245–9.

Trescot AM, Boswell MV, Atluri SL, et al. Opioid guidelines in the management of chronic non-cancer pain. *Pain Physician.* 2006; 9: 1–39.

Turk, DC, Brody MC, Okifuji EA: Physicians' attitudes and practices regarding the long-term prescribing of opioids for non-cancer pain. *Pain.* 1994; 59: 201–8.

Vanderah TW, Gardell LR, Burgess SE, Ibrahim M, Dogrul A, Zhong C-M, Zhang E-T, Malan TP, Ossipov MH, Lai J, Porreca F. Dynorphin promotes abnormal pain and spinal opioid antinociceptive tolerance. *J Neurosci.* 2000; 20: 7074–9.

Vanderah TW, Ossipov MH, Lai J, Malan TP, Porreca F. Mechanisms of opioid induced pain and antinociceptive tolerance: descending facilitation and spinal dynorphin. *Pain.* 2001a; 92: 5–9.

Vanderah TW, Suenaga NM, Ossipov MH, Malan TP, Lai J, Porreca F. Tonic descending facilitation from the rostral ventromedial medulla mediates opioid induced abnormal pain and antinociceptive tolerance. *J Neurosci.* 2001b; 21: 279–86.

Van Seventer R, Smit JM, Schipper RM, Wicks MA, Zuurmond WW. Comparison of TTS-fentanyl with sustained-release oral morphine in the treatment of patients not using opioids for mild-to-moderate pain. *Curr Med Res Opin.* 2003; 19: 457–69.

Wang D, Teichtahl H, Drummer O, et al. Central sleep apnea in stable methadone maintenance treatment patients. *Chest.* 2005; 128: 1348–56.

Wang Z, Gardell LR, Ossipov MH et al. Pronociceptive actions of dynorphin maintain chronic neuropathic pain. *J Neurosci.* 2001; 21: 1779–86.

Wasan AD, Davar G, Jamison R. The association between negative affect and opioid analgesia in patients with discogenic low back pain. *Pain.* 2005; 177: 450–61.

Watkins LR, Hutchinson MR, Milligan ED, et al. "Listening" and "talking" to neurons: Implications of immune activation for pain control and increasing the efficacy of opioids. *Brain Res Rev.* 2007; 148–69.

Watson CP, Babul N. Efficacy of oxycodone in neuropathic pain: A randomized trial in post herpetic neuralgia. *Neurology.* 1998; 50: 1837–41.

Watson CP, Moulin D, Watt-Watson J, Gordon A, Eisenhoffer J. Controlled-release oxycodone relieves neuropathic pain: a randomized controlled trial in painful diabetic neuropathy. *Pain.* 2003; 105: 71–8.

Watson CP, Watt-Watson JH, Chipman ML. Chronic noncancer pain and the long term utility of opioids. *Pain Res Manag.* 2004; 9: 19–24.

Webster LR, Webster RM. Predicting aberrant behaviors in opioid-treated patients: preliminary validation of the Opioid Risk Tool. *Pain Med.* 2005; 6: 432–42.

Woolf CJ. Intrathecal high dose morphine produces hyperalgesia in the rat. *Brain Res.* 1981; 209: 491–5.

World Health Organization. *Achieving Balance in Nation Opioids Control Policy: Guidelines for Assessment.* Geneva: WHO; 2000.

Yaksh TL. Central pharmacology of nociceptive transmission. In: McMahon S, Koltzenburg M, eds. *Wall and Melzack's Textbook of Pain.* 5th ed. Philadelphia, PA: Elsevier/Churchill Livingstone; 2006: 371–414.

Yaksh TL, Harty GJ. Pharmacology of the allodynia in rats evoked by high dose intrathecal morphine. *J Pharmacol Exp Ther.* 1988; 244: 501–7.

Yaksh TL, Harty GJ, Onofrio BM. High dose of spinal morphine produce a non-opiate receptor mediated hyperesthesia: clinical and theoretical implications. *Anesthesiology.* 1986; 64: 590–7.

Yasuda K, Raynor K, Kong H, Breder C, Takeda J, Reisine T, Bell G. Cloning and functional comparison of kappa and delta opioid receptors from mouse brain. *Proceedings of the National Academy of Sciences (USA).* 1993; 90: 6736–40.

Zacny J, Bigelow G, Compton P, et al. College on problems of drug dependence task force on prescription opioid non-medical use and abuse: position statement. *Drug Alcohol Depend.* 2003a; 69: 215–32.

Zacny JP, Gutierrez S. Characterizing the subjective, psychomotor, and physiological effects of oral oxycodone in non-drug abusing volunteers. *Psychopharmacology.* 2003b; 170: 242–54.

Zhang YT, Zheng QS, Pan J, et al. Oxidative damage of biomolecules in mouse liver induced by morphine and protected by antioxidants. *Basic Clin Pharmacol Toxicol.* 2004; 95: 53–8.

Zhou L, Zhang Q, Stein C, et al. Contribution of opioid receptors on primary afferent versus sympathetic neurons to peripheral opioid analgesia. *J Pharmacol Exp Ther.* 1998; 286: 1000–6.

25

Adjuvants for Pain

Craig K. Chang

Marco Pappagallo

An adjuvant for pain is a pharmacological agent that is added to a primary analgesic agent, for example, an opioid, to increase or aid its effect (see Table 25.1). Although adjuvants usually have treatment indications other than pain, advances in molecular biology and neuroscience have generated new strategies to treat pain with these medications.

The major rationale for introducing adjuvants is to better balance efficacy and adverse effects. The following scenarios should prompt the use of adjuvants:

1. The toxic limit of a primary analgesic has been reached.
2. The therapeutic benefit of a primary analgesic has plateaued (e.g., true efficacy limit, tolerance).
3. The primary analgesic is contraindicated (e.g., substance abuse, aberrant behavior, organ failure, allergy).
4. Subjective and qualitative symptoms demand broader coverage. Patients often convey that different medications will impart distinct analgesic benefits.
5. Presence of disabling, nonpainful complaints and need to manage symptoms such as insomnia, depression, anxiety, and fatigue that all cause worsening of the patient's quality of life and function. Indeed, the treatment outcome in pain management is both satisfactory pain relief and improvement in function.

Physicians have also been drawn to the adjuvants secondary to new realities of clinical practice. Aversion to addiction and diversion remains a potent force that shapes prescribing profiles. Fear of scrutiny by regulatory agencies has shifted the focus of pain management toward maximizing the efficacy of "nonabusable" drugs.

Traditional and Emerging Analgesic Adjuvants: Theory and Practice

Chronic pain, whether having neuropathic, visceral, or skeletal origin, is, more often than commonly thought, the result of a mixture of pain mechanisms. Pain syndromes that turn out to be clinical challenges to standard pharmacological therapies, in other words, treatments based on traditional analgesics such as antiinflammatory drugs and opioids, can be labeled difficult pain syndromes. Many drugs from a variety of pharmacological classes and with a variety of therapeutic indications can be classified as adjuvants and used "off-label" in the management of patients with chronic, intractable pain. In many cases, the mechanisms supporting this analgesic enhancement are still unknown.

The multiple theoretical mechanisms by which an adjuvant may "boost" an analgesic drug include the following:

1. Drug-drug interactions that raise serum drug levels.
2. Additivity, which occurs when a drug confers an additive analgesic effect to the primary analgesic, in other words, the effects of the drugs simply summate. Therefore the adjuvant confers only the amount of effect that it can generate on its own.
3. Potentiation, which is an "enabling response" that is present only when one compound acts concurrently with another.
4. Synergism, when the combined effect of two agents exceeds that predicted by the individual actions of the compounds (the resulting effect is more than additive).

At present, pharmacological synergism is heavily studied in pain research, given interest in the sequence of dissimilar targets in pain transmission. Analyzing the effect of all sorts of analgesic permutations has shed light on drug mechanisms and new ways of optimizing pain control (Tallarida, 2001).

Clinical trials seeking to validate opioid and adjuvant combination treatments illustrate not only the need for optimized analgesia, but also the challenge of defining the role adjuvants play in opioid-based regimens. Synergism can be assayed with careful measurement of dose-effect rapport between two medications using isobolograms (Black & Sang, 2005; Laska et al., 1994). In the laboratory, dose-effect curves can be studied in great detail; however, the dose-effect rapport of either drug cannot always be established in clinical trials secondary to logistical constraints.

Beside synergism, combination study designs should also address practical questions. For instance, a study that shows that combination therapy is even modestly additive but more tolerable when compared to a single-agent therapy may be clinically valuable.

At present, the evidence that traditional adjuvants and emerging adjuvants may possess analgesic properties derives mostly from preliminary clinical investigations and observations. This chapter will review the most commonly employed adjuvants in the

Table 25.1. Common Mechanisms of Action for Adjuvants

Target	Medications	Actions
Serotonin and norepinephrine synaptic reuptake mechanisms in CNS	TCAs, SSRIs, SNRIs	Enhance descending inhibition in CNS by blocking serotonin and norepinephrine reuptake
Na+ channels (e.g., TTXr),	Lidocaine, mexiletine, lamotrigine, carbamazepine, phenytoin, amitriptyline, and other TCAs	Frequency-dependent blockade of depolarization; action on nociceptive DRG neurons
N-type Ca++ channels ($\alpha 2\delta$ subunit)	Gabapentin, pregabalin	Suppress ectopic discharges in nociceptive DRG and dorsal horn neurons
GABA-B receptor	Baclofen	Agonist at the GABA-B receptors; enhance intraspinal inhibitory neurons
α-2 adrenoreceptors	Clonidine, tizanidine	Agonists at α-2 adrenoreceptors inhibit neuropeptides release and ascending spinal pain transmission
NMDA receptors	D-methadone, memantine, ketamine	Antagonist at NMDA receptors, inhibit glutamate-mediated nociceptive transmission and prevent central sensitization
Macrophages and osteoclasts	Bisphosphonates (e.g., pamidronate, clodronate, zolendronate, ibandronate)	Decrease inflammatory cytokines by promoting apoptosis and inhibition of macrophages and osteoclasts
Glucocorticoid receptor (GR)	Prednisone, methylprednisolone, dexamethasone	Agonist at peripheral intracellular GR; inhibit nociceptive immune mediators and inflammatory cell recruitment
Cannabinoid receptors	Dronabinol	Agonist at cannabinoid receptors; inhibit transmission at DRG
TRPV1 receptors	Capsaicin	Agonist at TRPV1; C-fibers neurotoxin; inactivation of capsaicin-responsive nociceptors
Somatostatin (SST)	Octreotide	Agonist on SST receptors; reduces vascular and nociceptive components of inflammation

Additional abbreviations used: CNS = central nervous system; DRG = dorsal root ganglion; GABA = γ-aminobutyric acid; NMDA = N-methyl-D-aspartate; TCA = tricyclic antidepressant; SNRI = serotonin and noradrenaline reuptake inhibitor; SSRI = selective serotonin reuptake inhibitor; TRPV1 = transient response potential vanilloid-1; TTXr = tetrodotoxin-resistant sodium channel.

treatment of difficult pain syndromes. For the purpose of this discussion, we will focus on scenarios that befit add-on therapy.

Adjuvants for Neuropathic Pain Syndromes

Management of severe neuropathic pain can be a challenge, and a combination of therapies employing agents from a variety of pharmacological classes represents the contemporary standard approach.

Antiepileptic Drugs

The application of antiepileptic drugs (AEDs) for pain stems from the shared pathophysiology of neuropathic pain and epilepsy. Neuronal hyperexcitability characterizes both conditions. Neuropathic pain is characterized by reduced thresholds (sensitization) and ectopic discharges at the spinal dorsal horn and/or dorsal root ganglion (DRG) pain-signaling neurons due to, for example, the upregulation of Na+ and Ca++ membrane channels (Scholz & Woolf, 2005).

AEDs are becoming the most promising agents for the management of neuropathic pain, given their propensity to dampen neuronal excitability. These qualities have made some AEDs first-line treatment in neuropathic conditions. The gabapentinoid anticonvulsants gabapentin and pregabalin have both established such efficacy for neuropathic pain. Therefore, when used specifically for neuropathic pain, these drugs should be considered primary analgesics and no longer adjuvants (Backonja et al., 1998; Rice et al., 2001; Rowbotham et al., 1998).

Gabapentin and pregabalin act on neither γ–aminobutyric acid (GABA) receptors nor sodium channels. In fact, they modulate cellular calcium influx into nociceptive neurons by binding to voltage-gated calcium channels, in particular to the $\alpha 2\delta$ subunit of the channel (Matthews & Dickenson, 2001). Gabapentin has been regarded as the first-line treatment for neuropathic pain syndromes, likely because of its favorable toxicity profile and lack of major drug interactions (Bennett & Simpson, 2004).

Trigeminal neuralgia, a neuropathic condition characterized by brief and excruciating lancinating pains, responds extremely well to carbamazepine, whereas another AED, lamotrigine, has shown some efficacy for carbamazepine-resistant trigeminal neuralgia (Zakrzewska et al., 1997). The efficacy of lamotrigine may be owed to its blocking tetrodotoxin-resistant Na+ channels (TTXr; Brau et al., 2001). Topiramate has been anecdotally used in the treatment of CRPS type 1 (Pappagallo, 1998). Several new AEDs (levetiracetam, zonisamide, oxcarbazepine, tiagabine) have become available for medical use, and some of these, along with topiramate, may have analgesic effect in primary headaches and perhaps in neuropathic pain (Pappagallo, 2003; Shi et al., 2005).

Of interest, in a recent randomized, double-blind, active placebo-controlled, crossover trial, patients with neuropathic pain received lorazepam (active placebo), controlled-release morphine, gabapentin, and a combination of gabapentin and morphine, each treatment given orally for 5 weeks. The study indicated that the best analgesia was obtained from the gabapentin/morphine combination, with each medication given at a lower dose than when given as a single agent (Gilron et al., 2005).

Other studies have demonstrated that the concomitant administration of gabapentin reduces opioid requirements in the postoperative setting (Eckhardt et al., 2000; Turan et al., 2004). Some putative mechanisms for synergy include morphine increasing gabapentin levels and combined inhibitory action in the brain, spinal cord, and periphery (Carlton et al., 1998; Singh et al., 1996). These studies, however, have not adequately substantiated the use of anticonvulsants for acute pain.

Antidepressants

Antidepressants also play an important role in the treatment of chronic pain. They are comparable in efficacy to AEDs (Saarto & Wiffen, 2005; Sindrup et al., 2005). Antidepressants display a wide variety of interactions with the pain-related neuraxis: monoamine modulation, opioid interactions, descending inhibition, and ion-channel blocking (Sindrup et al., 2005).

A collective review of randomized control trials (RCTs) has demonstrated that the tricyclic antidepressants (TCAs), such as amitriptyline, nortriptyline, and desipramine, are effective for most neuropathic conditions. Though not approved by the Food and Drug Administration (FDA) to treat neuropathic pain, amitriptyline has shown to have efficacy in the treatment of PDN, PHN, and central pain (Saarto & Wiffen, 2005).

Of note, TCAs such as amitriptyline, doxepin, and imipramine have been found to have local anesthetic properties. Amitriptyline appears to be more potent than bupivacaine as a Na+ channel blocker (Sudoh et al., 2003). The use of TCAs should be closely monitored for relatively frequent, poorly tolerated adverse effects, including cardiotoxicity, confusion, urinary retention, orthostatic hypotension, nightmares, weight gain, drowsiness, dry mouth, and constipation.

In animal models, combined reuptake inhibition of two monoamines appears to bestow greater antinociceptive qualities than inhibition of a single monoamine pathway. Serotonin and norepinephrine acting on multiple receptor subtypes lead to increased activation of descending inhibitory neurons (Pedersen et al., 2005).

The pharmacological profiles of the newer antidepressants are defined by both their unique monoamine receptor affinities and their effect on synaptic levels of monoamines.

Duloxetine and venlafaxine represent the serotonin and noradrenaline reuptake inhibitors (SNRIs) that lack the anticholinergic and antihistamine effects of the TCAs (Grothe et al., 2004; Marchand et al., 2003; Rowbotham et al., 2004). Venlafaxine has been shown to modulate allodynia and pinprick hyperalgesia in human models and to relieve neuropathic pain in breast cancer—perhaps by broadening its monoamine coverage by inhibiting the presynaptic uptake of serotonin, norepinephrine, and, to a lesser extent, dopamine. Duloxetine has recently been approved by the FDA for the treatment of pain secondary to diabetic neuropathy. Another atypical antidepressant, bupropion, which inhibits the reuptake of norepinephrine and dopamine, has shown early evidence to be effective for the treatment of neuropathic pain (Semenchuck et al., 2001).

Selective serotonin reuptake inhibitors (SSRIs), such as paroxetine and fluoxetine, are effective antidepressants, but relatively ineffective analgesics. Although used for the management of comorbidities such as anxiety, depression, and insomnia, which frequently affect patients with chronic neuropathic pain, SSRIs have not shown the same efficacy as the TCAs in the treatment of neuropathic pain (Max et al., 1992).

Studies have not shown antidepressants to be helpful in pain due to HIV-related polyneuropathy (Wiffen et al., 2005).

Local Anesthetics

The local anesthetics operate on the principle of decreasing neuronal excitability at the level of Na+ channels that propagate action potentials. This channel blockade has an effect on both spontaneous pain and evoked pain (Cummins & Waxman, 1997). An interesting point is that the analgesic properties occur at subanesthetic doses—lidocaine suppresses the frequency rather than the duration of Na+ channel opening (Rowbotham et al., 1991). In addition, rat models suggest that both topical and central anesthetics may exhibit synergism with morphine (Kolesnikov et al., 2000; Saito et al., 1998).

The FDA has approved transdermal lidocaine for postherpetic pain (Galer et al., 1999). In a controlled clinical trial, the transdermal form of 5% lidocaine relieved pain associated with PHN without significant adverse effects (Rowbotham et al., 1996). There is also early evidence to suggest that the patch provides benefit for other neuropathic pain states (Devers & Galer, 2000), including diabetic neuropathy (Hart-Gouleau et al., 2002), CRPS, postmastectomy pain, and HIV-related neuropathy (Berman et al., 2002).

Systemic local anesthetics can have a role in the treatment of central pain states (Boas et al., 1982; Tremont-Lukats et al., 2005; Wallace, 2000). Intravenous lidocaine suppresses neuronal ectopic discharges sodium channel blockade in the spinal cord (Woolf & Wiessenfeld-Hallin, 1985). This central action may also be augmented by decreasing N-methyl-D-aspartate (NMDA) and neurokinin (NK) receptor-mediated postsynaptic depolarizations (Nagy & Woolf, 1996).

Although intravenous lidocaine cannot be sustained indefinitely, the oral antiarrhythmic local anesthetic mexiletine has been shown to have analgesic properties for neuropathic pain similar to those of some AEDs (e.g., lamotrigine, carbamazepine; Awerbuch & Sandyk, 1990; Ichimata et al., 2001; Nakamura & Atsuta, 2005). Mexiletine is contraindicated in the presence of second- and third-degree atrioventricular conduction blocks. Unfortunately the incidence of gastrointestinal side effects (e.g., diarrhea, nausea) is quite high in patients taking mexiletine.

Sodium channel blocking properties are found not only in the traditional local anesthetics, but also in several antiepileptic drugs, such as carbamazepine, oxcarbazepine, and lamotrigine, and in the tricyclic antidepressants, such as amitriptyline, doxepin, and imipramine (Lai et al., 2003).

α-2 Adrenergic Agonists

α-2 adrenergic agonists are known to have a spinal antinociceptive effect via α-2B/C receptor subtypes (Khasar et al., 1995). Clonidine, an α-2 adrenergic agonist, produces a synergistic antinociceptive effect with opioids (Yaksh & Malmberg, 1994). In addition to being a primary analgesic if given intrathecally in the postoperative period, clonidine potentiates the analgesic benefit of opioids (Goudas et al., 1998; Plummer et al., 1992).

Tizanidine is a relatively short-acting, oral α-2 adrenergic agonist with a much lower hypotensive effect than clonidine. Tizanidine has been mostly used for the management of spasticity. However, animal studies and clinical experience indicate the usefulness of tizanidine for a variety of painful states, including neuropathic pain disorders (Fogelhom et al., 1992; Fromm et al., 1993; Semenchuk et al., 2000).

Capsaicin

Capsaicin is the natural substance present in hot chili peppers. Capsaicin, along with heat and acidification, activates the recently cloned transient receptor potential vanilloid-1 (TRPV1; Caterina et al., 1997; Knotkova & Pappagallo, 2005). After an initial depolarization, a single administration of a large dose of capsaicin appears to produce a prolonged deactivation of capsaicin-sensitive nociceptors. The analgesic effect is dose-dependent and may last for several weeks. Over-the-counter creams must be applied several times a day for many weeks. Controlled studies at low capsaicin concentrations (0.075% or less) have shown mixed results, possibly due to noncompliance. However, when capsaicin is compounded at high concentrations (> 1%) and administered as a single application under local or regional anesthesia, the analgesic benefit appears to last for several weeks (Robbins et al., 1998). At the present time, preparations of injectable capsaicin and local anesthetics are being developed for site-specific, moderate to severe pain. These preparations should provide pain relief in patients with postsurgical, neuropathic, and musculoskeletal pain conditions for weeks or months after a single treatment. Phase 2 clinical trials (http://www.corgentech.com) with injectable capsaicin are currently underway for Morton's neuroma, tendonitis, postsurgical pain following a variety of surgeries, including bunionectomy, hernia repair, total knee replacement, and cholecystectomy.

NMDA Antagonists

Animal experiments show that central and peripheral N-methyl-D-aspartate (NMDA) receptors play an important role in hyperalgesia and chronic pain (Bennett et al., 2000). Glutamate, the dominant excitatory neurotransmitter in the mammalian central nervous system, is released in the spinal cord after stimulation of peripheral nociceptors (Ueda et al., 1994), and several lines of evidence indicate that central sensitization is mediated by NMDA receptors in the spinal cord (Dickenson, 1997).

Dextromethorphan, methadone, memantine, amantadine, and ketamine all antagonize the NMDA receptor. Aside from their other actions, these medications have benefited from this unique property in the management of hyperalgesic neuropathic states poorly responsive to opioid analgesics (Bennett et al., 2000). Ketamine, when used as an adjuvant to opioids, appears to increase pain relief by 20%–30% and allows opioid dose reduction by 25%–50% (Fitzgibbon & Viola, 2005; Lossignol et al., 2005). However, ketamine has a narrow therapeutic window and can cause intolerable side effects, such as hallucinations and memory impairment.

Of novel interest is the possibility that NMDA antagonists, such as D-methadone, memantine, and dextromethorphan may prevent or counteract opioid analgesic tolerance (Davis & Inturrisi, 1999; Price et al., 2000).

Cannabinoids

The main therapeutic use of cannabinoids in humans is in the prevention of nausea and vomiting caused by chemotherapy. In patients with cancer or AIDS, delta(9)-trans-tetrahydrocannabinol (Δ-9-THC) can be used to increase appetite and treat weight loss. Evidence from animal studies and clinical observations indicate that cannabinoids have analgesic properties (Richardson, 1998; Karst et al., 2003; Richardson, 2000). Interestingly, the addition of inactive doses of cannabinoids to low doses of opioid mu agonists appears to potentiate opioid antinociception. Moreover, cannabinoids appear to have a predominant antiallodynic/antihyperalgesic effect, which may act via inhibition at the cannabinoid 2 receptor (CB2R) of the DRG (Beltramo, 2006; Sagar et al., 2005).

Δ-9-THC is the most widely studied cannabinoid. Analgesic sites of action have been identified in brain areas, in the spinal cord, and in the periphery. Cannabinoids appear to have a peripheral antiinflammatory action and induce antinociception at lower doses than those obtained from effective CNS concentrations. In contrast to the strong preclinical data, good clinical evidence on the efficacy of cannabinoids is lacking. CNS depression seems to be the predominant limiting adverse effect. In chronic neuropathic pain, 1',1'-dimethylheptyl-Δ-8-tetrahydrocannabinol-11-oic acid (CT-3), a THC-11-oic acid analogue, at a dose of 40 mg/d, was shown to be more effective than placebo and without major unfavorable side effects (Karst et al., 2003).

Neuroimmunomodulatory Agents

Several lines of evidence indicate that tumor necrosis factor-α (TNF-α), as well as other proinflammatory interleukins, play a key role in the mechanism of inflammatory neuropathic pain (Boddeke, 2001; Marchand et al., 2005; Opree & Kress, 2000). Historically, glucocorticoids, such as prednisone and methylprednisolone, have been employed empirically to blunt the inflammatory response to tissue damage and, hence, pain. Aside from their disease-modifying actions (e.g., limiting tissue damage in autoimmune disorders or altering tumor behavior/size), glucocorticoids provide analgesia through several mechanisms, the most important including switching off several inflammatory genes (Barnes, 1998). The net effect is a reduction in pronociceptive mediators, such as cytokines and prostaglandins, and a curtailment of further immune cell recruitment.

The fact that these initial inflammatory phases can promote central sensitization (Deleo et al., 1996) and neuropathic edema and extravasation (Kingery et al., 2001) has inspired several trials with glucocorticoids in the prevention of inflammatory neuropathic pain states. At this point, however, there is no clear consensus for their use (Pasqualucci et al., 2000; van Wijzck et al., 2006).

The landscape of immune mediators in pain is crowded and intimidating. TNF-α, IL-1-beta, nerve growth factor (NGF), IL-6, leukemia inhibitory factor (LIF), histamine, bradykinin, and prostaglandin E2 can all produce pain when exogenously administered (Marchand et al., 2005). Neutralizing antibodies to TNF-α and interleukin-1 receptor may become an important therapeutic approach for severe inflammatory pain resistant to nonsteroidal antiinflammatory drugs (NSAIDs), as well as for forms of neuropathic inflammatory pain (Schafers et al., 2001). Infliximab, a monoclonal antibody to TNF-α used for the treatment of rheumatoid arthritis, has been shown in an animal model of sciatica to downregulate brain-derived neurotrophic factor (BDNF; Onda et al., 2000). BDNF has been shown to play a key role in inflammatory and neuropathic pain (Coull et al., 2005). Thalidomide has been shown to prevent hyperalgesia caused by nerve constriction injury in rats (Sommer et al., 1998; Ribeiro et al., 2000), and thalidomide is known to inhibit TNF-α production. TNF-α antagonists or newly developed thalidomide analogues with a better safety profile may play a relevant role in the prevention and treatment of otherwise intractable painful disorders (George et al., 2000). Finally, specific inhibitors of CNS microglia activation and of the transcription factor known as NF-κB are being explored and these lines of research may open new exciting treatment avenues (D'Acquisto et al., 2002).

GABA Agonists

Baclofen is an analogue of the inhibitory neurotransmitter gamma-aminobutyric acid (GABA) and has a specific action on the GABA-B receptors. It has been used for many years as an effective spasmolytic agent. Baclofen also has shown anecdotal evidence of effectiveness in the treatment of trigeminal neuralgia (Sindrup & Jensen, 2002). Clinical experience supports the use of low-dose baclofen to potentiate the antineuralgic effect of carbamazepine for trigeminal neuralgia. Baclofen also has been used intrathecally to relieve intractable spasticity, and it may have a role as an adjuvant when added to spinal opioids for the treatment of intractable neuropathic pain and spasticity. The most common side effects of baclofen are drowsiness, weakness, hypotension, and confusion. It is important to note that discontinuation of baclofen always require a slow tapering in order to avoid the occurrence of seizures and other severe neurological manifestations.

Adjuvants for Bone Pain Syndromes

Immunohistochemical studies have revealed an extensive network of nerve fibers in the vicinity of and within the skeleton, not only in the periosteum but also in cortical and trabecular bone, as well as in the bone marrow (Lerner, 2002). Thinly myelinated and unmyelinated peptidergic sensory fibers, as well as sympathetic fibers, occur throughout the bone marrow, mineralized bone, and the periosteum. Although the periosteum is the most densely innervated tissue, when the total volume of each tissue is considered, the bone marrow receives the greatest total number of sensory nerve fibers (Mach et al., 2002). These sensory fibers express multiple signaling molecules, including neuropeptides and neurotrophins. The presence of receptors for some neuropeptides (e.g., calcitonin gene-related protein [CGRP] and substance P) on osteoclasts and osteoblasts and the capacity of these receptors to regulate osteoclast formation, bone formation, and resorption have recently been described. As nerve growth factor (NGF) has been shown to modulate inflammatory neuropathic pain states, in most recent animal models of cancer bone pain, NGF antibody antagonist therapy also has been shown to produce significant reduction in both ongoing and movement-related pain behavior. This treatment was more effective than morphine (Sevcik et al., 2005).

There are numerous options for treatment of bone pain. Metastasis to bone is the most common cause of bone pain in cancer patients (Banning et al., 1991). Bone pain is usually associated with direct tumor invasion of the bone, and is often severe and debilitating. Tumors that metastasize to bone most commonly originate in the breast, lung, prostate, thyroid, and kidney.

Bisphosphonates

Bisphosphonate therapy has proven highly valuable in the management of numerous bone-related conditions, including hypercalcemia, osteoporosis, multiple myeloma, and Paget's disease. Bisphosphonates, synthetic analogues of pyrophosphate, bind with a high affinity to the bone hydroxyapatite crystals and reduce bone resorption by inhibiting osteoclastic activity. Earlier bisphosphonates, such as etidronate, have been largely replaced by the use of second-generation bisphosphonates, including pamidronate, as well as third generation bisphosphonates, including zoledronic acid and ibandronate. Multiple studies have demonstrated the efficacy of second and third generation bisphosphonates in pain reduction for bone metastases (Mystakidou et al., 2005; Smith, 2004; Wardley et al., 2005). Zoledronic acid and ibandronate provide significant and sustained relief from metastatic bone pain, improving patient functioning and quality of life.

Of note, bisphosphonate treatment (e.g., pamidronate, clodronate) has been reported to be efficacious not only in bone cancer pain, but also in the treatment of complex regional pain syndrome (CRPS), a neuropathic inflammatory pain syndrome (Cortet et al. 1997; Varenna et al., 2000).

The bisphosphonate analgesic effect is poorly understood. It may be related to the inhibition and apoptosis of activated phagocytic cells such as osteoclasts and macrophages. This leads to a decreased release of proinflammatory cytokines in the area of inflammation. In animal models of neuropathic pain (sciatic nerve ligature), bisphosphonates reduced the number of activated macrophages infiltrating the injured nerve, reduced Wallerian nerve fiber degeneration, and decreased experimental hyperalgesia (Liu et al., 2000).

One adverse event that has recently emerged in a small number of oncological patients treated with the most potent bisphosphonates is osteonecrosis of the jaw. The disorder affects patients with cancer on bisphosphonate treatment for multiple myeloma or bone metastasis from breast, prostate, or lung cancer. Risk factors include prolonged duration of bisphosphonate treatment (i.e., monthly intravenous administration for more than 1–2 years), poor oral hygiene, and a history of recent dental extraction.

Calcitonin

Calcitonin may have several pain-related indications in patients who have bone pain, including osseous metastases. The most frequent routes of absorption are intranasal and subcutaneous injection. Calcitonin reduces resorption of bone by inhibiting osteoclastic activity and osteolysis (Szanto et al., 1992) and by an unknown central analgesic mechanism (Braga, 1978).

Adjuvants for Visceral Pain Syndromes

The management of unrelenting visceral pain warrants recognition of several unique features to visceral nociception:

1. Pain can be diffuse and poorly localized.
2. Pain may be accompanied by motor and autonomic reflexes (vomiting, diaphoresis, and peristalsis).
3. Pain may manifest viscerosomatic convergence (referred pain).

All of these features, and especially the secremotor reflexes, may unduly influence the affective components of visceral pain (Cervero & Laird, 1999; Ripamonti et al., 2000).

Like somatic neurons, spinal cord visceral neurons exhibit central sensitization that may be regulated by NMDA receptors (Willert et al., 2004). In animal and human models, ketamine, an NMDA receptor antagonist, attenuates visceral pain (Strigo et al., 2005).

Other adjuvants include somatostatin analogs and cannabinoids. Somatostatin appears to exhibit an antiinflammatory (Szolcsanyi et al., 1998) and antinociceptive effect (Helyes et al., 2000). Somatostatin has been shown to downmodulate immune reactivity (ten Bokum et al., 2000). Octreotide, an octapeptide analog of somatostatin, has been used to treat carcinoid tumors. Octreotide has also been used off-label for visceral pain. This is a clinical extrapolation from animal studies, in which octreotide was shown to inhibit pain-related behavior (Carlton et al., 2001, 2004; Karalis et al., 1994).

Currently, dronabinol, a synthetic Δ-9-THC, has been approved for cancer and AIDS patients. Dronabinol is a cannabinoid-1 receptor (CB1R) agonist that acts via a G-protein coupled receptor to inhibit adenylyl cyclase and to reduce cellular cAMP levels. The beneficial effects of CB1R activation in animal models include reduction of transient lower esophageal sphincter relaxations, increased compliance of the stomach, reduced acid secretion, reduction of GI transit, reduced large intestinal propulsive activity, and reduced intestinal fluid secretion in response to secretogogues (Hornby & Prouty, 2004).

Conclusion

Management of severe neuropathic, bone, and visceral pain often represents a difficult treatment challenge. Combination therapy today illustrates the interrelation of molecular biology and the treatment of pain.

The number and variety of adjuvants can be confusing even for physicians specializing in the treatment of pain. Physicians must know how to titrate the dose appropriately while assessing the pain and managing drug-related side effects. Patients suffering from difficult pain syndromes need to have treatment plans tailored to their individual problems. Foremost, the treating physician needs to balance efficacy, safety, and tolerability of several drugs, many being employed "off-label."

The physician who wishes to utilize adjuvants should keep abreast of the predominant mechanisms underlying difficult pain syndromes. Though the pathophysiology of these conditions remains to be fully elucidated, treating multiple targets will likely be the standard of care. As our knowledge of pain expands, so, too, will our arsenal of treatments.

References

Awerbuch GI, Sandyk R. Mexiletine for thalamic pain syndrome. *Int J Neurosci* 1990; 55(2–4):129–133.

Backonja M, Beydoun A, Edwards KR, et al. Gabapentin for the symptomatic treatment of painful neuropathy in patients with diabetes mellitus: a randomized controlled trial. *JAMA* 1998; 280:1831–1836.

Banning A, Sjogren P, Henriksen H. Pain causes in 200 patients referred to a multidisciplinary cancer pain clinic. *Pain* 1991; 45:45–48.

Barnes PJ. Anti-inflammatory actions of glucocorticoids: molecular mechanisms. *Clin Sci (Lond)* 1998; 94(6):557–72.

Beltramo M, Bernardini N, Bertorelli R, et al. CB2 receptor-mediated antihyperalgesia: possible direct involvement of neural mechanisms. *Eur J Neurosci.* 2006; 23:1530–1538.

Bennett GJ. Update on the neurophysiology of pain transmission and modulation: focus on the NMDA-receptor. *J Pain Symptom Manage* 2000; 9:S2–S6.

Bennett M, Simpson K. Gabapentin in the treatment of neuropathic pain. *Palliative Medicine* 2004; 18:5–11.

Berman SM, Justis JV, HO M, et al. Lidocaine patch 5% (Lidoderm) significantly improves quality of life (QOL) in HIV-associated painful peripheral neuropathy [abstract]. *Program and Abstracts of the IASP 10th World Congress of Pain.* Seattle, WA: IASP, 2002.

Black DR, Sang CN. Advances and limitations in the evaluation of analgesic combination therapy. *Neurology* 2005; 65(12 Suppl 4):S3–6.

Boas RA, Covino BG, Shahnarian A. Analgesic response to i.v. lignocaine. *Br J Anaesth* 1982; 54:501–505.

Boddeke, EW. Involvement of chemokines in pain. *Eur. J. Pharmacol* 2001; 429, 115–119.

Braga P, Ferri S, Santagostino A, Olgiati VR, Pecile A. Lack of opiate receptor involvement in centrally induced calcitonin analgesia. *Life Sciences* 1978; 22:971.

Brau ME, Dreimann M, Olschewski A, Vogel W, Hempelmann G. Effect of drugs used for neuropathic pain management on tetrodotoxin-resistant NaC currents in rat sensory neurones. *Anesthesiology* 2001; 94:137–144.

Carlton SM, Zhou S. Attenuation of formalin-induced nociceptive behaviors following local peripheral injection of gabapentin. *Pain* 1998; 76:201–207.

Carlton SM, Du J, Davidson E, Zhou S, Coggeshall RE. Somatostatin receptors on peripheral primary afferent terminals: inhibition of sensitized nociceptors. *Pain* 2001; 90(3):233–244.

Carlton SM, Zhou S, Du J, Hargett GL, Ji G, Coggeshall RE. Somatostatin modulates the transient receptor potential vanilloid 1 (TRPV1) ion channel. *Pain* 2004; 110(3):616–627.

Caterina MJ, Schumacher MA, Tominaga M, et al. The capsaicin receptor: a heat-activated ion channel in the pain pathway. *Nature* 1997; 389:816–824.

Cervero F, Laird JM. Visceral pain. *Lancet.* 1999; 353:2145–2148.

Cortet B, Flipo RM, Coquerelle P, et al. Treatment of severe, recalcitrant reflex sympathetic dystrophy: assessment of efficacy and safety of the second generation bisphosphonate pamidronate. *Clin Rheumatol* 1997; 16:51–56.

Coull JA, Beggs S, Boudreau D, Boivin D, Tsuda M, Inoue K, Gravel C, Salter MW, De Koninck Y. BDNF from microglia causes the shift in neuronal anion gradient underlying neuropathic pain. *Nature* 2005; 38(7070):1017–1021.

Cummins TR, Waxman SG. Downregulation of tetrodotoxin-resistant sodium currents and upregulation of a rapidly repriming tetrodotoxin-sensitive sodium current in small spinal sensory neurons after nerve injury. *J Neurosci* 1997; 17(10):3503–3514.

Davis AM, Inturrisi CE. d-Methadone blocks morphine tolerance and N-methyl-D-aspartate-induced hyperalgesia. *J Pharmacol Exp Ther* 1999; 289:1048–1053.

Deleo JA, Colburn RW, Nichols M, Malhotra A. Interleukin-6-mediated hyperalgesia/allodynia and increased spinal IL-6 expression in rat mononeuropathy model. *J Interferon Cytokine Res* 1996; 16:695–700.

D'Acquisto F, May MJ, Ghosh S. Inhibition of nuclear factor kappa B (NF-B): an emerging theme in anti-inflammatory therapies. *Mol Interv* 2002; (1): 22–35.

Devers A, Galer BS. Topical lidocaine patch relieves a variety of neuropathic pain conditions: an open-label study. *Clin J Pain* 2000; 16:205–208.

Dickenson AH. Mechanisms of central hypersensitivity: excitatory amino acid mechanisms and their control. In: *The pharmacology of pain: handbook of experimental pharmacology* (Dickenson AH, Besson JM, eds.). Berlin: Springer Verlag, 1997; 167–210.

Eckhardt K, Ammon S, Hofmann U, Riebe A, Gugeler N, Mikus G. Gabapentin enhances the analgesic effect of morphine in healthy volunteers. *Anesth Analg* 2000; 91(1):185–191.

Fitzgibbon EJ, Viola R. Parenteral ketamine as an analgesic adjuvant for severe pain: development and retrospective audit of a protocol for a palliative care unit. *J Palliat Med* 2005; 8: 49–57.

Fogelholm R, Murros K. Tizanidine in chronic tension-type headache: a placebo controlled double-blind cross-over study. *Headache* 1992; 32:509–513.

Fromm GH, Aumentado D, Terrence CF. A clinical and experimental investigation of the effects of tizanidine in trigeminal neuralgia. *Pain* 1993; 53:265–271.

Galer BS, Rowbotham MC, Perander J, et al. Topical lidocaine patch relieves postherpetic neuralgia more effectively than a vehicle topical patch: results of an enriched enrollment study. *Pain* 1999; 80:533–538.

George A, Marziniak M, Schafers M, et al. Thalidomide treatment in chronic constrictive neuropathy decreases endoneurial tumor necrosis factor-alpha, increases interleukin-10 and has long-term effects on spinal cord dorsal horn met-enkephalin. *Pain* 2000; 88:267–275.

Gilron I, Bailey JM, Tu D, et al. Morphine, gabapentin, or their combination for neuropathic pain. *N Engl J Med* 2005; 352:1324–1334.

Goudas LC, Carr DB, Filos KS, Laurijssens BE, Kream RM. The spinal clonidine-opioid analgesic interaction: from laboratory animals to the postoperative ward. A review of preclinical and clinical evidence. *Analgesia* 1998; 3:277–290.

Grothe DR, Scheckner B, Albano D. Treatment of pain syndromes with venlafaxine. *Pharmacotherapy* 2004; 24:621–629.

Hart-Gouleau S, Gammaitoni A, Galer B, et al. Open label study of the effectiveness and safety of lidocaine patch 5% (Lidoderm) in patients with painful diabetic neuropathy [abstract]. *Program and Abstracts of the IASP 10th World Congress of Pain.* Seattle, WA: IASP, 2002.

Helyes ZS, Than M, Oroszi G, Pinter E, Nemeth J, Keri GY, and Szolcsanyi J. Anti-nociceptive effect induced by somatostatin released from sensory nerve terminals and by synthetic somatostatin analogues in the rat. *Neurosci Lett* 2000; 278:185–188.

Hornby PJ, Prouty SM. Involvement of cannabinoid receptors in gut motility and visceral perception. *Br J Pharmacol* 2004; 141(8):1335–1345.

Ichimata M, Ikebe H, Yoshitake S, Hattori S, Iwasaka H, Noguchi T. Analgesic effects of flecainide on postherpetic neuralgia. *Int J Clin Pharmacol Res* 2001; 21(1):15–19.

Karalis K, Mastokaros G, Chrousos GP, and Tolis G. Somatostatin analogues suppress the inflammatory reaction in vivo. *J Clin Invest* 1994; 93:2000–2006.

Karst M, Salim K, Burstein S, et al. Analgesic effect of the synthetic cannabinoid CT-3 on chronic neuropathic pain: a randomized controlled trial. *JAMA* 2003; 290:1757–1762.

Khasar SG, Green PG, Chou B, Levine JD. Peripheral nociceptive effects of alpha 2-adrenergic receptor agonists in the rat. *Neuroscience* 1995; 66(2):427–432.

Kingery WS, Guo T, Agashe GS, Davies MF, Clark JD, Maze M. Glucocorticoid inhibition of neuropathic limb edema and cutaneous neurogenic extravasation. *Brain Res* 2001; 913(2):140–148.

Knotkova H, Pappagallo M. Pharmacology of pain transmission and modulation. II. Peripheral mechanisms. In: Pappagallo M, ed. *The Neurological Basis of Pain.* New York: McGraw-Hill, 2005; 53–60.

Kolesnikov YA, Chereshnev I, Pasternak GW. Analgesic synergy between topical lidocaine and topical opioids. *J Pharmacol Exp Ther* 2000; 295(2):546–551.

Lai J, Hunter J C, Porreca F. The role of voltage-gated sodium channels in neuropathic pain. *Curr Opin Neurobiol* 2003; 13:291–297.

Laska EM, Meisner M, Siegel C. Simple designs and model-free tests for synergy. *Biometrics* 1994; 50:834–841.

Lerner UH. Neuropeptidergic regulation of bone resorption and bone formation. *J Musculoskelet Neuronal Interact* 2002; 2:440–447.

Liu T, van Rooijen N, Tracey DJ. Depletion of macrophages reduces axonal degeneration and hyperalgesia following nerve injury. Pain 2000; 86:25–532.

Lossignol DA, Obiols-Portis M, Body JJ. Successful use of ketamine for intractable cancer pain. *Support Care Cancer* 2005; 13:188–193.

Mach DB, Rogers SD, Sabino MC, et al. Origins of skeletal pain: sensory and sympathetic innervation of the mouse femur. *Neuroscience* 2002; 113:155–166.

Marchand F, Alloui A, Pelissier T, et al. Evidence for an antihyperalgesic effect of venlafaxine in vincristine-induced neuropathy in rat. *Brain Res* 2003; 980:117–120.

Marchand F, Perretti M, McMahon SB. Role of the immune system in chronic pain. Nat *Rev Neurosci* 2005; 6(7):521–532.

Matthews EA, Dickenson AH. Effects of spinally delivered N- and P-type voltage-dependent calcium channel antagonists on dorsal horn neuronal responses in a rat model of neuropathy. *Pain* 2001; 92:235–246.

Max MB, Lynch SA, Muir J, et al. Effects of desipramine, amitriptyline, and fluoxetine on pain in diabetic neuropathy. *N Engl J Med* 1992; 326:1250–1256.

Mystakidou K, Katsouda E, Stathopoulou E, et al. Approaches to managing bone metastases from breast cancer: The role of bisphosphonates. Cancer Treat Rev 2005; 31:303–311.

Nagy I, Woolf CJ. Lignocaine selectively reduces C fibre-evoked neuronal activity in rat spinal cord in vitro by decreasing N-methyl-d-aspartate and neurokinin receptor-mediated postsynaptic depolarizations: implications for the development of novel centrally acting analgesics. *Pain* 1996; 64:59–70.

Nakamura S, Atsuta Y. Effect of sodium channel blocker (mexiletine) on pathological ectopic firing pattern in a rat chronic constriction nerve injury model. *J Orthop Sci* 2005; 10(3):315–320.

Onda A, Murata Y, Rydevik B, Larsson K, Kikuchi S, Olmarker K. Infliximab attenuates immunoreactivity of brain-derived neurotrophic factor in a rat model of herniated nucleus pulposus. *Spine* 2004; 29(17):1857–1861.

Opree A, Kress M. Involvement of the proinflammatory cytokines tumor necrosis factor-alpha, IL-1, and IL-6 but not IL-8 in the development of heat hyperalgesia: effects on heat-evoked calcitonin gene-related peptide release from rat skin. *J Neurosci* 2000; 20:6289–6293.

Pappagallo M. *Preliminary experience with topiramate in the treatment of chronic pain syndromes.* Poster presented at the 17th Annual Meeting, American Pain Society, San Diego, CA, 1998.

Pappagallo M. Newer antiepileptic drugs: possible uses in the treatment of neuropathic pain and migraine. *Clin Ther* 2003; 25:2506–2538.

Pasqualucci A, Pasqualucci V, Galla F, De Angelis V, Marzocchi V, Colussi R, Paoletti F, Girardis M, Lugano M, Del Sindaco F. Prevention of postherpetic neuralgia: acyclovir and prednisolone versus epidural local anesthetic and methylprednisolone. *Acta Anaesthesiol Scand* 2000; 44(8):910–918.

Paterson AHG. The potential role of biphosphonates as adjuvant therapy in the prevention of bone metastases. Cancer supplement 2000; 88(12):3038–46.-8.

Pedersen LH, Nielsen AN, Blackburn-Munro G. Anti-nociception is selectively enhanced by parallel inhibition of multiple subtypes of monoamine transporters in rat models of persistent and neuropathic pain. *Psychopharmacology (Berl)* 2005; 182(4):551–561.

Plummer JL, Cmielewski PL, Gourlay GK, Owen H, Cousins MJ. Antinociceptive and motor effects of intrathecal morphine combined with intrathecal clonidine, noradrenaline, carbachol or midazolam in rats. Pain 1992;49:145–152.

Price DD, Mayer DJ, Mao J, et al. NMDA-receptor antagonists and opioid receptor interactions as related to analgesia and tolerance. *J Pain Symptom Manage* 2000; 19:S7-S11.

Ribeiro RA, Vale ML, Ferreira SH, et al. Analgesic effect of thalidomide on inflammatory pain. *Eur J Pharmacol* 2000; 391:97–103.

Rice AS, Maton S. Gabapentin in postherpetic neuralgia: a randomised, double blind, placebo-controlled study. *Pain* 2001; 94:215–224.

Richardson JD. Cannabinoids modulate pain by multiple mechanisms of action. *J Pain* 2000; 1(1):2.

Richardson JD, Aanonsen L, Hargreaves KM. Antihyperalgesia effects of spinal cannabinoids. *Eur J Pharmacol*. 1998; 345:145–153.

Ripamonti C, Mercadante S, Groff L, et al. Role of octreotide, scopolamine butylbromide, and hydration in symptom control of patients with inoperable bowel obstruction and nasogastric tubes: a prospective randomized trial. *J Pain Symptom Manage* 2000; 19:23–34.

Robbins WR, Staats PS, Levine J, et al. Treatment of intractable pain with topical large-dose capsaicin: preliminary report. *Anesth Analg.* 1998; 86:579–583.

Rowbotham MC, Reisner-Keller LA, Fields HL. Both intravenous lidocaine and morphine reduce the pain of postherpetic neuralgia. *Neurology* 1991; 41(7):1024–1028.

Rowbotham MC, Davies PS, Verkempinck C, et al. Lidocaine patch: double-blind controlled study of a new treatment method for post-herpetic neuralgia. *Pain* 1996; 65:39–44.

Rowbotham M, Harden N, Stacey B, et al. Gabapentin for the treatment of postherpetic neuralgia: a randomized controlled trial. *JAMA* 1998; 280:1837–1842.

Rowbotham MC, Goli V, Kunz NR, et al. Venlafaxine extended release in the treatment of painful diabetic neuropathy: a double-blind, placebo-controlled study. *Pain* 2004; 110:697–706.

Saarto T, Wiffen PJ. Antidepressants for neuropathic pain. *Cochrane Database Syst Rev* 2005; (3):CD005454.

Sagar DR, Kelly S, Millns PJ, O'Shaughnessey CT, Kendall DA, Chapman V. Inhibitory effects of CB1 and CB2 receptor agonists on responses of DRG neurons and dorsal horn neurons in neuropathic rats. *Eur J Neurosci* 2005; 22(2):371–379.

Saito Y, Kaneko M, Kirihara Y, Sakura S and Kosaka Y. Interaction of intrathecally infused morphine and lidocaine in rats (part I): synergistic antinociceptive effects. *Anesthesiology* 1998; 89:1455–1463.

Sanger GJ. Neurokinin NK1 and NK3 receptors as targets for drugs to treat gastrointestinal motility disorders and pain. *Br J Pharmacol* 2004; 141(8):1303–1312.

Schafers M, Brinkhoff J, Neukirchen S, et al. Combined epineurial therapy with neutralizing antibodies to tumor necrosis factor-alpha and interleukin-1 receptor has an additive effect in reducing neuropathic pain in mice. *Neurosci Lett* 2001; 310:113–116.

Scholz J, Woolf CJ. Mechanisms of neuropathic pain. In: Pappagallo M, ed. *The Neurological Basis of Pain.* New York: McGraw-Hill, 2005; 71–94.

Semenchuk MR, Sherman S. Effectiveness of tizanidine in neuropathic pain: an open-label study. *J Pain* 2000; 1(4):285–292.

Semenchuk MR, Sherman S, Davis B. Double-blind, randomized trial of bupropion SR for the treatment of neuropathic pain. *Neurology* 2001; 57:1583–1588.

Sevcik M A, Ghilardi J R, Peters C M, et al. Anti-NGF therapy profoundly reduces bone cancer pain and the accompanying increase in markers of peripheral and central sensitization. *Pain* 2005; 115:128–141.

Shi W, Liu H, Zhang Y, et al. Design, synthesis, and preliminary evaluation of gabapentin-pregabalin mutual prodrugs in relieving neuropathic pain. *Arch Pharm (Weinheim)* 2005; 338: 358–364.

Sindrup SH, Jensen TS. Pharmacotherapy of trigeminal neuralgia. *Clin J Pain* 2002; 18(1):22–27.

Sindrup SH, Otto M, Finnerup NB, Jensen TS. Antidepressants in the treatment of neuropathic pain. *Basic Clin Pharmacol Toxicol* 2005; 96(6):399–409.

Singh L, Field MJ, Ferris P, et al. The antiepileptic agent gabapentin (Neurontin) possesses anxiolytic-like and antinociceptive actions that are reversed by D-serine. *Psychopharmacology (Berl)* 1996; 127:1–9.

Smith MR. Osteoclast-targeted therapy for prostate cancer. *Curr Treat Options Oncol* 2004; 5:367–375.

Sommer C, Marziniak M, Myers RR. The effect of thalidomide treatment on vascular pathology and hyperalgesia caused by chronic constriction injury of rat nerve. *Pain* 1998; 74:83–91.

Strigo IA, Duncan GH, Bushnell MC, Boivin M, Wainer I, Rodriguez Rosas ME, Persson J. The effects of racemic ketamine on painful stimulation of skin and viscera in human subjects. *Pain* 2005;113(3):255–64.

Sudoh Y, Cahoon EE, Gerner P, Wang GK. Tricyclic antidepressants as long-acting local anesthetics. *Pain* 2003; 103(1–2):49–55.

Szanto J, Ady N, Jozsef S. Pain killing with calcitonin nasal spray in patients with malignant tumors. *Oncology* 1992; 49:180–182.

Szolcsanyi J, Helyes ZS, Oroszi G, Nemeth J, and Pinter E. Release of somatostatin and its role in mediation of the anti-inflammatory effect induced by antidromic stimulation of sensory fibres of the rat sciatic nerve. *Br J Pharmacol* 1998; 123:936–942.

Tallarida RJ. Drug synergism: its detection and applications. *J Pharmacol Exp Ther* 2001; 298(3):865–72.

ten Bokum AM, Hofland LJ, van Hagen PM. Somatostatin and somatostatin receptors in the immune system: a review. *Eur Cytokine Netw* 2000; 11(2): 161–76.

Tremont-Lukats IW, Challapalli V, McNicol ED, Lau J, Carr DB. Systemic administration of local anesthetics to relieve neuropathic pain: a systematic review and meta-analysis. *Anesth Analg* 2005; 101(6):1738–49.

Turan A, Karamanlioglu B, Memis D, Hamamcioglu MK, Tukenmez B, Pamukcu Z, Kurt I. Analgesic effects of gabapentin after spinal surgery. *Anesthesiology* 2004; 100(4):935–8.

Ueda M, Kuraishi Y, Sugimoto K, and Satoh M. Evidence that glutamate is released from capsaicin-sensitive primary afferents in rats: study with on-line continuous monitoring of glutamate. *Neurosci Res* 1994; 20:231–237.

van Wijck AJ, Opstelten W, Moons KG, van Essen GA, Stolker RJ, Kalkman CJ, Verheij TJ. The PINE study of epidural steroids and local anaesthetics to prevent postherpetic neuralgia: a randomised controlled trial. *Lancet* 2006; 367(9506):219–24.

Varenna M, Zucchi F, Ghiringhelli D, et al. Intravenous clodronate in the treatment of reflex sympathetic dystrophy syndrome. A randomized, double blind, placebo controlled study. *J Rheumatol* 2000; 27:1477–1483.

Wallace MS. Calcium and sodium channel antagonists for the treatment of pain. *Clin J Pain* 2000; 16:S80-S85.

Wardley A, Davidson N, Barrett-Lee P, et al. Zoledronic acid significantly improves pain scores and quality of life in breast cancer patients with bone metastases: a randomised, crossover study of community vs. hospital bisphosphonate administration. *Br J Cancer* 2005; 92:1869–1876.

Wiffen, P. Collins, S. McQuay, H. Carroll, D. Jadad, A. Moore, A. Anticonvulsant drugs for acute and chronic pain. *Cochrane Database Syst Rev* 2005; (3):CD001133.

Willert RP, Woolf CJ, Hobson AR, Delaney C, Thompson DG, Aziz Q. The development and maintenance of human visceral pain hypersensitivity is dependent on the N-methyl-D-aspartate receptor. *Gastroenterology* 2004; 126(3):683–92.

Woolf CJ, Wiesenfeld-Hallin Z. The systemic administration of local anaesthetics produces a selective depression of C-afferent fibre evoked activity in the spinal cord. *Pain* 1985; 23:361–74.

Yaksh Tl, Malmberg AB. Interaction of spinal modulatory receptor systems. In: *Pharmacological Approaches to the treatment of Chronic Pain: New Concepts and Critical Issues. Progress in Pain Research and Management* (Vol. 1). Seattle, IASP Press, 1994; 151–71.

Zakrzewska JM, Chaudhry Z, Nurmikko TJ, et al. Lamotrigine (Lamictal) in refractory trigeminal neuralgia: results from a double-blind, placebo controlled, crossover trial. *Pain* 1997; 73:223–230.

26

Behavioral Medicine Approaches to Pain Management

Akiko Okifuji

Chronic pain is one of the most prevalent physical conditions accounting for long-term disability (Von Korff et al., 2005). Unlike transitory or acute pain that either remits spontaneously or responds to fairly simple intervention, chronic pain persists beyond an expected period for which healing of the initial injury completes despite treatments. The average duration of pain noted for patients treated at clinics specializing in the treatment of chronic pain typically exceeds 7 years with pain duration of 20 to 30 years (Flor, Fydrich, & Turk, 1992).

In noncancer, musculoskeletal chronic pain, pain does not seem to have any obvious pathophysiology that can account for the presence and extent of pain complaints. However, pain that is chronic or recurrent can significantly compromise quality of life and, if unremitting, may actually produce physical harm by suppressing the body's immune system. The current conceptualization of chronic pain rejects the traditional dualism, in which pain is considered as a direct consequence of either organic pathology alone or psychiatric disturbance. Rather, given the complexity of the problem, chronic pain often requires multidimensional conceptualization, and accordingly, multimodal approaches to help patients reduce pain and resume productive lives seem critical. Accumulated research in the past 3 decades strongly suggests that multimodal interventions that include cognitive-behavioral therapy modalities is beneficial and cost-effective (Okifuji, 2003; Turk, 2002).

Assumptions of Cognitive-Behavioral Treatment

The main theme of the cognitive-behavioral perspective focuses upon the integration of cognitive and behavioral factors with the physical and somatic conditions to determine the overall subjective experience of pain patients. In the model, each patient is considered as an active processor of external cues that get blended in with his/her internal state; the cognitive-behavioral model incorporates many of the psychological variables such as anticipation, avoidance, and contingencies of reinforcement, but suggests that cognitive factors, in particular, expectations rather than conditioning factors are of central importance. The critical factor for the cognitive-behavioral model, therefore, is not just patients' responses to actual events, but also learned responses to predict and to summon appropriate reactions to predicted events. It is the individual patient's processing of information that results in anticipatory anxiety and avoidance behaviors.

There are five central assumptions that characterize the cognitive-behavioral perspective on pain management (see Box 26.1). The first assumption is, as noted above, that all people are active processors of information rather than passive reactors to what the environment or physical condition dictates. People attempt to make sense of the situation by filtering information through a well-developed cognitive map that results from their prior learning histories and by general strategies that guide the processing of information.

A second assumption of the cognitive-behavioral perspective is that one's cognitive attributions, beliefs, and expectancies can elicit or modulate affect and physiological arousal, both of which may serve as impetuses for behavior. Conversely, affect, physiology, and behavior can instigate or influence one's thinking processes. This cycle is dynamic and continuous, and it becomes a moot exercise to identify what is causal and results. Causal priority may be less of a concern in this view of an interactive process that

---

Box 26.1. Basic Assumptions of Cognitive-Behavioral Treatment

1. People are active processors of information rather than passive reactors to environmental contingencies.
2. Thoughts (for example, appraisals, attributions, expectancies) can elicit or modulate physiological and affective responses, both of which may serve as impetuses for behavior. Conversely, affect, physiology, and behavior can instigate or influence one's thinking processes.
3. Behavior is reciprocally determined by both the environment and the individual.
4. Idiosyncratic habit of how people think and evaluate the world around them need to be carefully evaluated and if found to be maladaptive, then successful interventions designed to alter behavior should focus on each of these maladaptive thoughts, feelings, physiology, and behaviors, and not one to the exclusion of the others.
5. In the same way that people are instrumental in the development and maintenance of maladaptive thoughts, feelings, and behaviors, they can, are, and should be considered active agents of change of their maladaptive modes of responding.

extends over time with the interaction of thoughts, feelings, physiological activity, and behavior.

Unlike the treatment modality that is based strictly on environmental/behavioral contingencies, the cognitive-behavioral perspective focuses on the reciprocal effects of the individual on the environment as well as the influence of environment on behavior. The third assumption of the cognitive-behavioral perspective, therefore, is that behavior is reciprocally determined by both the environment and the individual. Individuals not only passively respond to their environment but elicit environmental responses by their behavior. In a very real sense, people create their environments. The patient who becomes aware of a physical event (symptoms) and decides the symptom requires attention from a health-care provider initiates a set of circumstances different from the individual with the same symptom who chooses to self-medicate.

A fourth assumption is that if people have learned maladaptive ways of thinking, feeling, and responding, then successful interventions designed to alter behavior should focus on each of these maladaptive thoughts, feelings, physiology, and behaviors, and not one to the exclusion of the others. There is no expectancy that changing thoughts, feelings, or behaviors will necessarily result in the other two following suit.

The final assumption of the cognitive-behavioral perspective is that in the same way as people are instrumental in the development and maintenance of maladaptive thoughts, feelings, and behaviors, they can, are, and should be considered active agents of change of their maladaptive modes of responding. Patients with chronic pain, no matter how severe, despite their common beliefs to the contrary, are not helpless pawns of fate. They can and should become instrumental in learning and carrying out more effective modes of responding to their environment and their plight.

Cognitive-Behavioral Therapy (CBT): Self-Management of Pain

One of the practical methods of CBT is to combine patient education, self-regulatory training, and specific behavioral skill training. A typical CBT for pain management often begins with helping patients understand their own stress response system. Specifically, patients can learn to monitor situational factors that tend to trigger their pain/stress (left column in Table 26.1) and what they actually experience emotionally, behaviorally, and physically when they have pain/stress (right column). The middle column is reserved to help patients monitor and understand their own processes that mediate the relationship between the situation and the consequential experience. There are a number of potential processes that can be discussed; however, it is important for patients to learn what they actually have control over. For example, neurochemical activities in the central nervous system are undoubtedly one of the prominent processes that occur as people go about their lives. However, the amount of direct control that people can have is quite limited. The emphasis is given to the cognitive processing that people can learn to become more aware and self-regulate if desired.

Through collaborative discussion about factors associated with patients' own pain and stress responses, specific treatment approaches and goals are likely to emerge. For example, if patients' pain and stress responses tend to be triggered after being in a crowded place, certain environmental modifications can be con-

Table 26.1. Cognitive-Behavioral Framework for Stress/Pain Management

Stressors	Processes	Stress Response
What triggers stress/pain cycle	Modulating processes mediating between stressors and stress responses	What experientially happens to a person in response to stressors • Physiological • Behavioral • Emotional

sidered to reduce the probability of having to place oneself in a situation as such. Procrastination and interpersonal situations are also common triggers. Time management and communication skill training may aid reduce the potency of these factors as stressors.

However, it is important to be realistic that no matter how the situational factors are improved, stress is a part of life. It is essential for patients to acquire counterstress skills that help them reregulate physiological and emotional responses via behavioral manipulations. These techniques include behavioral therapeutic interventions such as relaxation, imagery, distraction, problem solving, and pacing.

Intervention in the cognitive process, such as cognitive restructuring, is also critical. As the basis of CBT depends upon the thesis that how patients appraise their plight determines the overall psychophysiological consequences, it is essential for patients to learn their own cognitive system and acquire optional cognitive skills.

People with persistent pain often have negative expectations about their own ability and responsibility to exert any control over their pain. Moreover, they often view themselves as helpless. Such negative, maladaptive appraisals about their condition, situation, and their personal efficacy in controlling their pain and disability associated with pain reinforce their experience of demoralization, inactivity, and overreaction to stressors. These cognitive appraisals are posited as having an effect on behavior, leading to reduced effort, reduced perseverance in the face of difficulty, and reduced activity and increased psychological distress. Many handbooks are available to guide the acquisition of cognitive techniques to adequately monitor to identify relationship among thoughts, mood, and behavior.

Behavioral Medicine as a Part of Interdisciplinary Treatment

One of the critical requirements for successful rehabilitation for chronic pain is a paradigm shift in how patients conceptualize themselves in relation to the health-care system, from the traditional passive patient model to an active, participatory model. Rehabilitation often requires a careful review on patients' lifestyle and modifications in how they behave and think. Another critical dimension in functional restoration is physical conditioning, which requires significant commitment from patients.

Even for healthy individuals, compliance with regular physical exercise does not come easy. Every year, a flux of individuals sign up with health clubs and gyms as a part of a New Year's resolution, only to see 50% of them dropping out in 6 months (U.S. Department of Health and Human Services, 1996). Applied to chronic pain patients who suffer from unremitting pain, mood disturbance, sleep problems, and fatigue, it is hardly surprising that many patients find it difficult to adopt an active lifestyle. Even when cognitive-behavioral therapy to improve coping is added, many patients prematurely terminate their participation. Furthermore, long-term treatment success seems to depend on regular adherence to recommended self-care regimens for people suffering from chronic pain conditions (Turk & Rudy, 1991).

When patients show little commitment or willingness to comply with the regimen, the health-care system typically turns its back to them. "You can lead a horse to water but you can't make it drink" is often used to describe the framework in which clinicians operate. However, as we work more with chronic health problems that are closely tied with people's lifestyle issues, helping patients comply with functional regimen has become a critical clinical issue.

Transtheoretical Model of Behavior Change

The attempt to better understand how motivation impacts adherence to health-care regimens has prompted growing attention to the transtheoretical model of behavior change. The transtheoretical model of change offers an integrative framework describing the process of behavior change (Prochaska & DiClemente, 1984) and has been used to understand how people change their health-related behaviors. The basic assumptions underlying the model are the notions that people differ in their readiness to take on behavioral change needed for better health outcome and that there are certain processes of change that facilitate the advancement of one's readiness. The model is organized around a major construct, stages of change, and suggests that individuals attempting to change health-related behavior move through a series of stages of change. Movement through these stages often occurs in a nonlinear fashion because several attempts at behavior change may be needed before

Box 26.2. Stages of Change

1. *Precontemplative stage:* Patient does not perceive a need to change and actively resists change.
2. *Contemplation stage:* Patient begins to see a need for change and may consider making a change in the future.
3. *Preparation stage:* Patient feels ready to change and takes a first concrete (behavioral) change.
4. *Action stage:* Patient actively engages in behaviors consistent with regimen.
5. *Maintenance stage:* Patient executes plans to sustain the changes made.
6. *Relapse stage:* Some patients fail to sustain the effort.

attaining their goals. Relapse is not viewed as a distinct stage in the change process. Rather, knowledge that someone has been regularly active in the past and is not regularly active now provides important information about that individual's exercise history. The description of each stage is listed in Box 26.2.

There are three critical parameters of the model that determines the likelihood of advancing one's readiness. *Processes of change* are one parameter of the transtheoretical model that enables us to understand *how* shifts in behavior occur. Change processes are covert and overt activities and experiences that individuals engage in when they attempt to modify problem behaviors. Each process is a broad category encompassing multiple techniques, methods, and interventions traditionally associated with disparate theoretical orientations. Ten processes cluster into two groups: cognitive-experiential processes and behavioral processes (Table 26.2). As can be seen, it is an eclectic collection of strategies to target each process.

Table 26.2. Processes of Change

Processes	Definition	Therapeutic Strategies That May Help Targeting the Process
Cognitive-Experiential Processes		
Consciousness raising	Increasing information about self and problem	Observations, confrontations, interpretations, bibliotherapy
Self-reevaluation	Assessing how one feels and thinks about oneself with respect to a problem	Value clarification, imagery, corrective emotional experience
Dramatic relief	Experiencing and expressing feelings about one's problem and solutions	Role playing, psychodrama, grieving losses
Environmental reevaluation	Assessing how one's problems affect the physical environment	Empathy training, documentaries
Social liberation	Increasing alternatives for nonproblem behaviors available in society	Advocating for rights of repressed, empowering, policy interventions
Behavioral Processes		
Counterconditioning	Substituting alternatives for problem and anxiety-related behaviors	Relaxation, desensitization, assertion, positive self-statements
Helping relationships	Being open and trusting about problems with someone who cares	Therapeutic alliance, social support, self-help groups
Reinforcement management	Rewarding oneself or being rewarded by others for making changes	Contingency contracts, overt and covert reinforcement, self-reward
Stimulus control	Avoiding stimuli that elicit problem behaviors	Adding stimuli that encourage alternative behaviors, restructuring one's environment, avoiding high-risk cues, fading techniques
Self-liberation	Choosing and committing to act or believe in ability to change	Decision-making therapy, resolution

The model incorporates two additional parameters. *Self-efficacy* is defined as personal confidence in the ability to change across problem situations. Finally, there is *decisional balance*, which is defined as a personal "balance sheet" of gains and losses for changing and not changing their behaviors. People are likely to advance their change stages when they perceive that they have adequate skills to cope and feel confident in executing those skills (high efficacy belief), and when they perceive more gains of changing and losses of not changing than more losses of changing and gains of not changing (decisional balance). The transtheoretical model of change has been applied to various health-related behaviors, particularly helping people to adopt regular exercise. Targeting three components of the model (processes of change, self-efficacy, and decisional balance) seems to improve the readiness to adopt regular exercise (Bock, Marcus, Pinto, & Forsyth, 2001; Marcus et al., 1998; Steptoe, Kerry, Rink, & Hilton, 2001).

Multidisciplinary rehabilitation for chronic musculoskeletal pain typically places greater emphasis on the behavioral strategies such as counterconditioning and stimulus control. This approach may leave patients with a low level of readiness behind because these patients require experiential strategies to facilitate their readiness levels (Prochaska, Velicer, DiClemente, Guadagnoli, & Rossi, 1991). However, baseline levels of self-efficacy vary and there is a linear relationship between the baseline and posttreatment level of self-efficacy (Buckelew et al., 1996), suggesting that those who begin the treatment with low levels of self-efficacy may not achieve optimal benefit from conventional CBT alone.

Motivation Enhancement Therapy (MET)

MET, developed by William Miller and his colleagues (Miller, 1983; Miller & Rollnick, 1991), is one of the therapeutic methods that target motivation. It shares the assumption with the transtheoretical model that people vary in their readiness to adhere to the treatment regimen. MET is a problem-focused, therapist-directed approach with the aim of helping patients enhance their motivation for treatment. MET offers a collection of therapeutic techniques to help patients (1) clearly recognize their problems, (2) perform decisional balance work (personal cost-benefit analysis of staying with pain and disability vs. undergoing rehabilitation), (3) produce self-motivational statements, and (4) internalize those motivational statements via improved self-efficacy.

MET has been tested for facilitating change to reduce problem behaviors, such as smoking (Town et al., 2000; Velasquez et al., 2000), problem drinking (Brown, Saunders, Bobula, & Lauster, 2000; Handmaker, Miller, & Manicke, 1999), problem gambling (Hodgins, Currie, & el-Guebaly, 2001), eating disorders (Feld, 2001), and high-risk sexual behaviors (Carey, 2000; Kalichman, Cherry, & Browne-Sperling, 1999). MET has also been shown to increase healthy behaviors such as promoting exercise with myocardial infarction patients (Song & Lee, 2001), adherence to glucose control regimen in diabetes (Smith, Heckemeyer, Kratt, & Mason, 1997), and mammography screening (Bernstein, Mutschler, & Bernstein, 2000).

Evidence also exists showing that MET enhances adherence to treatments that require patients' commitment for significant behavioral changes (Zweben & Zuckoff, 2002).

Readiness for Treatment in Chronic Pain

Recently, Kerns, Rosenberg, Jamison, Caudill, and Haythornthwaite (1997) developed a self-report inventory to assess patients' readiness to adopt a self-management approach for chronic pain. The subsequent study suggests that readiness is related to attrition in rehabilitative programs to treat chronic pain patients (Biller, Arnstein, Caudill, Federman, & Guberman, 2000; Kerns & Rosenberg, 2000). Similarly, low level of readiness in arthritis patients predicts the diminished likelihood of patients' involvement in treatment (Keefe et al., 2000). Improving patients' readiness for treatment is likely to enhance clinical benefit of the treatment in rehabilitation for chronic pain.

Motivation Enhancement Techniques

MET places a strong emphasis on specific clinician-patient interactions. MET is based on the assumption that people vary in their degree of readiness for change. Specific intervention strategies are organized to help a patient move from one stage to a more desirable stage or to keep the person in the action and maintenance stage. According to Miller and Rollnick (1991), there are several key components in MET that aid in the process of moving patients' readiness forward:

- *Empathetic listening:* Judgmental attitudes and responses, either verbally or behaviorally, by therapist are counterproductive.
- *Reality check:* Identification of specific discrepancy between what the patient wants from therapy (e.g., "I want to get well") and what he or she is doing (e.g., "I can't do my exercise because I am not well"). This should help patients realize that their maladaptive behaviors are actually preventing them from obtaining their goal of getting better.
- *Rolling with resistance:* Therapist and patient should remain on the same side, not arguing against each other. Do not let the patient present a counterargument for why he or she should NOT engage in therapeutic effort.

Concluding Comments

Managing patients with chronic pain can be a daunting task for many clinicians because of the complexity of the condition. Past research has consistently demonstrated that the adequate adaptation and maintenance of quality of life for chronic pain patients depends largely on how patients perceive and process pain and related stressors. Cognitive-behavioral approaches are commonly included as a part of a treatment package for chronic pain patients, aiming at helping patients attain adaptive coping.

Another behavioral medicine approach that significantly enhances treatment benefits from rehabilitation is to help patients become ready to commit to the intervention and comply with the regimen. The motivation enhancement approach has been successfully implemented to help patients become more active and responsible for their own self-management for various habit disorders and chronic illness.

Because patients' own commitment and active participation to modify their life habits is critical to the successful rehabilitation, the role that behavioral medicine specialists play is significant. It is hardly an overstatement to assert that the effectiveness and cost-effectiveness of rehabilitative approach may depend upon how effectively behavioral medicine can be incorporated in the overall treatment plan. Research evaluating the clinical benefit and cost-effectiveness of multidisciplinary interventions strongly suggests this; further research is warranted to identify the key factors of behavioral medicine approaches that enhance the clinical benefit of multimodal interventions for chronic pain.

References

Bernstein, J., Mutschler, P., & Bernstein, E. (2000). Keeping mammography referral appointments: motivation, health beliefs, and access barriers experienced by older minority women. *J Midwifery Women's Health, 45*(4), 308–313.

Biller, N., Arnstein, P., Caudill, M. A., Federman, C. W., & Guberman, C. (2000). Predicting completion of a cognitive-behavioral pain management program by initial measures of a chronic pain patient's readiness for change. *Clin J Pain, 16*(4), 352–359.

Bock, B. C., Marcus, B. H., Pinto, B. M., & Forsyth, L. H. (2001). Maintenance of physical activity following an individualized motivationally tailored intervention. *Ann Behav Med, 23*(2), 79–87.

Brown, R. L., Saunders, L. A., Bobula, J. A., & Lauster, M. H. (2000). Remission of alcohol disorders in primary care patients. Does diagnosis matter? *J Fam Pract, 49*(6), 522–528.

Buckelew, S. P., Huyser, B., Hewett, J. E., Parker, J. C., Johnson, J. C., Conway, R., et al. (1996). Self-efficacy predicting outcome among fibromyalgia subjects. *Arthritis Care Res, 9*(2), 97–104.

Carey, M. P., Braaten, L. S., Maisto, S. A., Gleason, J. R., Forsyth, A. D., Durant, L. E., et al. (2000). Using information, motivational enhancement, and skills training to reduce the risk of HIV infection for low-income urban women: a second randomized clinical trial. *Health Psychol, 19*(1), 3–11.

Feld, R., Woodside, D. B., Kaplan, A. S., Olmsted, M. P., Carter, J. C. (2001). Pretreatment motivational enhancement therapy for eating disorders: a pilot study. *Int J Eat Disord, 29*(4), 393–400.

Flor, H., Fydrich, T., & Turk, D. C. (1992). Efficacy of multidisciplinary pain treatment centers: a meta-analytic review. *Pain, 49*(2), 221–230.

Handmaker, N. S., Miller, W. R., & Manicke, M. (1999). Findings of a pilot study of motivational interviewing with pregnant drinkers. *J Stud Alcohol, 60*(2), 285–287.

Hodgins, D. C., Currie, S. R., & el-Guebaly, N. (2001). Motivational enhancement and self-help treatments for problem gambling. *J Consult Clin Psychol, 69*(1), 50–57.

Kalichman, S. C., Cherry, C., & Browne-Sperling, F. (1999). Effectiveness of a video-based motivational skills-building HIV risk-reduction intervention for inner-city African American men. *J Consult Clin Psychol, 67*(6), 959–966.

Keefe, F. J., Lefebvre, J. C., Kerns, R. D., Rosenberg, R., Beaupre, P., Prochaska, J., et al. (2000). Understanding the adoption of arthritis self-management: stages of change profiles among arthritis patients. *Pain, 87*(3), 303–313.

Kerns, R. D., & Rosenberg, R. (2000). Predicting responses to self-management treatments for chronic pain: application of the pain stages of change model. *Pain, 84*(1), 49–55.

Kerns, R. D., Rosenberg, R., Jamison, R. N., Caudill, M. A., & Haythornthwaite, J. (1997). Readiness to adopt a self-management approach to chronic pain: the Pain Stages of Change Questionnaire (PSOCQ). *Pain, 72*(1–2), 227–234.

Marcus, B. H., Emmons, K. M., Simkin-Silverman, L. R., Linnan, L. A., Taylor, E. R., Bock, B. C., et al. (1998). Evaluation of motivationally tailored vs. standard self-help physical activity interventions at the workplace. *Am J Health Promot, 12*(4), 246–253.

Miller, W. (1983). Motivational interviewing with problem drinkers. *Behav Psychother, 11*, 147–172.

Miller, W., & Rollnick, S. (1991). *Motivational interviewing: preparing people for change.* New York: Guilford Press.

Okifuji, A. (2003). Interdisciplinary pain management with pain patients: Evidence for its effectiveness. *Sem Pain Med, 1*(2), 110–119.

Prochaska, J., & DiClemente, C. (1984). *The transtheoretical approach: towards a systematic eclectic framework.* Homewood, IL: Dow Jones Irwin.

Prochaska, J., Velicer, W., DiClemente, C., Guadagnoli, E., & Rossi, J. (1991). Patterns of change: dynamic typology applied to smoking cessation. *Multivariate Behav Res, 26*, 83–107.

Smith, D. E., Heckemeyer, C. M., Kratt, P. P., & Mason, D. A. (1997). Motivational interviewing to improve adherence to a behavioral weight-control program for older obese women with NIDDM. A pilot study. *Diabetes Care, 20*(1), 52–54.

Song, R., & Lee, H. (2001). Managing health habits for myocardial infarction (MI) patients. *Int J Nurs Stud, 38*(4), 375–380.

Steptoe, A., Kerry, S., Rink, E., & Hilton, S. (2001). The impact of behavioral counseling on stage of change in fat intake, physical activity, and cigarette smoking in adults at increased risk of coronary heart disease. *Am J Public Health, 91*(2), 265–269.

Town, G. I., Fraser, P., Graham, S., McSweeney, W., Brockway, K., & Kirk, R. (2000). Establishment of a smoking cessation programme in primary and secondary care in Canterbury. *N Z Med J, 113*(1107), 117–119.

Turk, D. C. (2002). Clinical effectiveness and cost effectiveness of treatments for patients with chronic pain. *Clin J Pain, 18*(6), 355–365.

Turk, D. C., & Rudy, T. E. (1991). Neglected topics in the treatment of chronic pain patients—relapse, noncompliance, and adherence enhancement. *Pain, 44*(1), 5–28.

U.S. Department of Health and Human Services. (1996). *Physical activity and health: a report of the Surgeon General.* Atlanta, GA: Centers for Disease Control and Prevention, National Center for Chronic Disease Prevention.

Velasquez, M. M., Hecht, J., Quinn, V. P., Emmons, K. M., DiClemente, C. C., & Dolan-Mullen, P. (2000). Application of motivational interviewing to prenatal smoking cessation: training and implementation issues. *Tob Control, 9*(Suppl 3), III36–40.

Von Korff, M., Crane, P., Lane, M., Miglioretti, D. L., Simon, G., Saunders, K., et al. (2005). Chronic spinal pain and physical-mental comorbidity in the United States: results from the national comorbidity survey replication. *Pain, 113*(3), 331–339.

Zweben, A., & Zuckoff, A. (2002). Motivational interviewing and treatment adherence. In W. Miller & S. Rollnick (Eds.), *Motivational interviewing: preparing people for change.* New York: Guilford.

27

Physical Medicine Approaches to Assessing and Treating Pain

Steven Stanos

Lynn R. Rader

A physical medicine and rehabilitation or "physiatric" approach to acute and chronic pain syndromes includes a wide scope of clinical focus. Acute pain syndromes may be easily managed by a focused, directed pharmacologic and active physical therapy approach based on a biomedical model of injury. This model proposes underlying tissue injury correlates with outward manifestations of pain in which treatment is based on removing or decreasing nociceptive input (i.e., treating lumbar nerve root irritation related to disc protrusion treated with steroid epidural injections and oral anti-inflammatory medications). On the other end of the spectrum, assessment and treatment of chronic pain conditions, a more comprehensive biopsychosocial approach, focuses not only on the underlying tissue injury complex but also on related psychological factors (i.e., a patient's pain related depression, anxiety, and maladaptive coping responses) and social issues (i.e., solicitousness of family members, and financial and vocational rewards related to chronic pain condition). The clinician must also differentiate from physical *impairment*, defined as an objective structural or physiological limitation, and *disability*, the resulting loss of function (Mooney, 1987). Individualized treatment goals generally emphasize achieving analgesia, improving psychosocial functioning, and reintegration of recreational or leisure pursuits (i.e., community activities and sports). Additionally, clinicians may participate in the ongoing care of patients with diagnoses related to chronic disabilities (i.e., stroke, spinal cord injury, and cerebral palsy), many of which may have fixed impairments. Minimizing symptom burden may be additionally emphasized.

This chapter will focus on a physiatric musculoskeletal assessment, treatment approaches including active and passive therapies, therapeutic exercise, aquatic therapies, mind-body treatments, and more comprehensive collaborative approaches including multidisciplinary and more integrative interdisciplinary treatment programs. The spectrum of assessment and treatment approaches will be discussed in the context of common acute and chronic pain conditions (i.e., osteoarthritis, myofascial pain, and spine-related disorders). The physiatric approach to chronic pain conditions must also include an understanding of the wide array of important psychological (affective and cognitive) factors that impact the multidimensional experience of pain. Psychological factors may serve to decrease or increase subjective perception of pain and adjustment to ongoing pain-related disability. Affective factors usually include more negative emotions, such as depression, pain-related anxiety, and anger. Cognitive factors include catastrophizing, fear, helplessness, decreased self-efficacy, pain coping, readiness to change, and acceptance. (Please see Chapter 26, "Behavioral Medicine Approaches to Pain Management," for further discussion on psychological issues related to pain.)

Comprehensive Physical Assessment

See Box 27.1 for an outline that covers a comprehensive physical assessment of low back pain.

Physical Exam

Performing a proficient physical exam is a fundamental part of diagnosing and identifying potential areas of dysfunction as a means of narrowing the clinical differential diagnosis and estab-

---

Box 27.1. Comprehensive Assessment: Low Back Pain

I. Global assessment
   a. Gait
   b. Standing posture
      i. Head
      ii. Shoulders
      iii. Pelvis/iliac crests (tilt/rotation)
      iv. Knee (flexed, valgus or varus deformity, rotation)
      v. Feet (rotation, pes planus [high arch], pes cavus [flat foot])
   c. Balance and stability
      i. One- and two-legged testing, eyes open/closed
II. Musculoskeletal
   a. Soft tissue assessment palpation: tenderness, trigger points
   b. Muscle stretch reflexes
   c. Dural tension (straight leg raise [SLR], seated SLR, or slump seated)
   d. Motor strength
   e. Sensory testing (light touch, pin sensation, proprioception)
   f. Range of motion (hip, knee, foot, and ankle)
III. Psychological/illness behavior
   a. Mood, affect
   b. Pain behavior
   c. Equipment (i.e., cervical soft collar, braces, TENS unit)

lishing a rational treatment plan. The physical exam assesses structures that may serve as potential pain generators as well as contribute to loss of function and mobility. A complete musculoskeletal exam includes that of the bony structures, cartilage, joints, ligaments, tendons, bursa, nerves, and skin. Before one performs specialized evaluations of specific areas, the examiner should first assess more global areas related to mobility and function including posture, balance, stability, and gait.

Posture

(Magee, 2002) Posture, the position of the body at one point in time, is made up of the combination of different joints. Proper posture is achieved when the joints line up in such a way as to create the least amount of stress and muscle activation as possible. Theoretically, one should be able to maintain upright posture with active stresses and forces of gravity primarily acting on the iliofemoral ligaments and gastrocsoleus complex. When faulty posture is maintained, abnormal stresses are created on joints leading to potential tissue trauma and eventually sources of pain. Abnormalities in posture may be positional or structural. Positional factors include weak or tight muscles, generalized weakness, excessive weight, muscle spasm, and loss of position sense, whereas structural factors include congenital anomalies, bony abnormalities, and leg length discrepancy.

The patient's posture is assessed in the coronal and sagittal planes, and should also be assessed standing and lying. Even though studies have shown that the reliability for detecting cervical and lumbar lordosis on visual assessment is poor (Fedorak, Ashworth, Marshall, & Paull, 2003), visual inspection and observation remain an important part of the physiatric examination. To begin, one assesses the patient posteriorly, and has the patient stand comfortably with the heels lined up, 4–6 inches apart (the width of the examiner's shoe). The alignment of the head, acromion, angles and distance of the scapulae from the spine (dominant side may be lower), iliac crests, posterior superior iliac spines (PSIS), gluteal folds, and knee and ankle joints should be assessed and any asymmetries noted. In addition, the presence of any rotation about the hip, knee, or ankle joints should be commented on as well as the presence of any pes planus or pes cavus deformities. The entire cervical, thoracic, and lumbar spine should be observed and palpated for scoliotic, rotational, and/or step-off deformities. The examiner should then have the patient flex forward, noting any paravertebral asymmetries, kyphosis or scoliosis, flattening of the lumbar spine, or restrictions. The examiner should then have the patient extend, rotate, and lateral side bend while keeping the pelvis locked, looking for any restrictions or asymmetries at the lumbosacral area or pelvis. From the side of the patient, the examiner should see that the earlobe aligns with the acromion process and iliac crest. Head position, rounding of the shoulders, excessive or loss of lumbar lordosis, and excessive or loss of thoracic kyphosis should be noted. In one study, forward flexed posture (standing occiput-to-wall distance) was found to correlate with amount of vertebral pain, muscular impairments, motor function, and disability in elderly females (Balzini et al., 2003). On lateral inspection and palpation, one should also assess for any anterior or posterior pelvic tilt. This is done by comparing the levels of the ASIS and posterior superior iliac spin (PSIS), a bony landmark located in the dimple area of the pelvis adjacent to the superior lateral border of the sacrum. A normal pelvic angle is 30 degrees, with the PSIS positioned higher than the ASIS.

In the supine lying position, the examiner assesses for rounding or elevation of the shoulders from the table (indicating either tight pectoralis muscles or weak scapular stabilizers), any chest wall deformities, and level of the anterior superior iliac spine (ASIS) to assess for pelvic obliquity. If there is extension of the lumbar spine from the examination table, tight hip flexors may be present. Leg length discrepancy should be assessed by measuring from the ASIS to the ipsilateral medial malleoli. A difference of 1.0–1.5 cm is within the normal limits. Asymmetric rotation of the pelvis more proximally may also lead to a "relative" leg length discrepancy.

Balance and Stability

Balance and stability may be deficient in those with chronic musculoskeletal pain. A study of patients with low back pain found them to demonstrate less balance and postural stability than those without low back pain (Bergmark, 1989). Assessment includes bony structures, ligaments, muscles, and coordinated muscular activity (Panjabi, 1992). Thus, one notes decreased stability and balance when there is tissue damage, muscle weakness, or poor muscular control. Balance may be assessed simply by having the patient stand on one leg. The patient may be unsteady, sway, have a pelvic drop (Trendelenburg sign), or may be unable to lift one leg up safely without losing balance. A Trendelenburg sign, when the pelvis drops on the side opposite of the stance leg, may indicate weak hip abductors. If the patient is able perform a single leg stance without difficulty, the exercise can be made more challenging by having the patient stand on one leg with the eyes closed, or stand on one leg and perform a single leg squat extending the unsupported leg out into the frontal, sagittal, and transverse planes. This stresses the lumbar stabilizers dynamically in multiple planes.

Core stability and balance may also be assessed having the patient perform a bridge with the patient supine, knees and hips flexed and feet on the table. The patient lifts the pelvis from the table, the examiner looks for unsteadiness, pelvic tilting, and/or hamstring cramping. The main muscular stabilizers of the spine, also referred to as "the core," include the multifidi, transversus abdominis, abdominal muscles (internal and external obliques, rectus abdominus), latissimus dorsi, paraspinal muscles, pelvic floor, the diaphragm, and the iliopsoas muscle. The "core" has been likened to a box with the abdominal muscles in the front, the diaphragm as the roof, and pelvic floor and hip muscles as the bottom, and includes more than 20 pairs of muscle groups that stabilize spinal structures, the pelvis, and coordination of movements during functional tasks (i.e., bending, lifting, and squatting; Richardson, Jull, Hodges, & Hides, 1999). Efficient functioning of the "core" helps to distribute, absorb, and limit translational and shearing forces. The core muscle groups include both slow-twitch and fast-twitch muscles fibers. Slow-twitch muscles include the deeper abdominals, which lay closer to the spine which control segmental motion and help to maintain mechanical stiffness of the spine (i.e., transverse abdominus, multifidi, obliques, deep transversospinalis, and pelvic floor muscles. Fast-twitch fibers, on the other hand, include the longer outer and superficial muscles capable of producing large torque forces, possessing greater speed and arcs of motion (i.e., erector spinae, external obliques) and include muscles more commonly strengthened by traditional abdominal exercises (Hreljac, 2005). Decrease in balance and stability is commonly associated with poor core strength. In one study, operative patients with unilateral low back pain had evidence of ipsilateral multifidi atrophy (10%–30%) as compared to contralateral side (Laasonen, 1984). The lumbar stabilizers provide strength, protect the spine, and stabilize the trunk, allowing one to have functional mobility of the limbs and maintain efficient posture and balance.

Gait

Posture and balance alone with support of the upright body and forward motion combine to form a complex activity known as gait. Although gait in of itself is complex, the analysis is likewise. Furthermore, studies have shown that practitioners analyze gait differently according to their profession, using a wide variety of gait indicators (Watelain et al., 2003). Nevertheless, the gait cycle's function is to move the body's center of mass forward, load and unload weight, clear the foot, and advance the limb in a safe, controlled manner. In addition, the gait pattern may be categorized into phases, parameters, and determinants (see Table 27.1)

When there are muscle imbalances, weaknesses, contractures, limb length discrepancies, or valgus or varus abnormalities at the knee, any one of the determinants of gait may be affected and result in deviations and compensations, increase energy expenditure, increase stresses and loads, and increase risk for tissue breakdown and subsequent pain. By examining and describing the phases, parameters, and determinants of gait, one can systematically assess a very complex activity. This knowledge, combined with the information collected previously, including muscle strength, sensation, ROM, and posture, will help the examiner form a systematic assessment of the patient's gait and more appropriately guide patient's rehabilitation therapy.

Range of Motion and Muscle Imbalances

Range of motion, muscle strength, and balance should be assessed as they are important for one to perform the activities of daily living and provide efficient functional mobility. The range of motion about a joint is determined by the shape of the bone, cartilage, muscle strength, tone, and muscle bulk, surrounding tissues and overlying skin. First the examiner assesses the patient's active range of motion, followed by active assistive range of motion, and finally passive range of motion for each joint. The examiner should note differences from side to side, effects on pain and any hyper- or hypomobility. The findings on range of motion testing combined with the results of manual muscle testing may lead to objective findings of muscle imbalances about a joint. This concept has been well described by Janda as the upper crossed and pelvic crossed syndromes. An upper crossed syndrome is characterized by contracted and hypertonic postural muscles (pectoralis major and upper trapezius) and lengthened phasic muscles (rhomboids, serratus anterior, middle and lower trapezius), which may present with related neck and shoulder pain and headaches. Pelvic crossed syndrome is characterized by contracted hip flexors and lumbar extensors, and weak, lengthened phasic muscles (abdominals and gluteus maximus) and may present with chronic low back and buttock pain (Janda, 1994; Jull & Janda, 1987).

Illness Behavior

Before, during, and after the physical examination, one should assess the patient's behavior. Waddell and Main described illness behavior as "what people say and do to express and communicate they are ill" (Waddell & Main, 1998). This behavior is often normal, simply reflecting a physical problem, and may include the way one's individual pain is described in a pain drawing or by signs and symptoms observed by the clinician. In addition, Waddell classically described seven nonanatomic or behavioral symptoms in patients with low back pain. A standardized group of four nonorganic signs, commonly referred to as "Waddell signs," or behavioral responses to the examinations, has been a source of ongoing research (see Box 27.2).

Patients displaying at least three signs were more likely to have evidence of psychosocial distress (Waddell & Main, 1998). Pain

Table 27.1. Phases, Parameters, and Determinants of Gait

Phases of Gait

Stance	Swing
60% of the walking cycle	40% of the walking cycle
Shortened on the painful side	Lengthened on the painful side

Parameters of Gait: Determine the *Quality* of the Gait Cycle

1. Width of support	• Distance between feet • Normally 2–4 inches • Larger when pathology of the dorsal columns or an ataxic gait is present
2. Step length	• Distance between sequential corresponding points of contact by opposite feet • Normally 14–16 inches
3. Step length	• Shortened on the pain-free side
4. Stride length	• Distance between sequential corresponding points of contact by the same foot • Normally 30 inches
5. Pelvic and trunk shift and rotation	
6. Cadence	• Number of steps per minute • Normally 100 steps/minute
7. Center of gravity	• 2 inches anterior to the second sacral vertebrae

Determinants of Gait

1. Pelvic rotation in the horizontal plane
2. Pelvic tilt in the frontal plane
3. Early/late knee flexion
4. Weight transfer and motion at the foot
5. Lateral displacement of the pelvis

Box 27.2. Waddell Symptoms and Signs

Waddell Symptoms

1. Pain at the tip of the tailbone
2. Whole leg pain
3. Whole leg numbness
4. Whole leg giving way
5. Complete absence of any spells with very little pain in the last year
6. Intolerance of, or reactions to, many treatments
7. Emergency admission to hospital with simple backache

Waddell Signs

1. Tenderness: superficial or nonanatomic
2. Simulation tests: axial loading or simulated rotation
3. Distraction tests: physical exam finding is retested with the patient distracted, in other words, straight leg raise (seated and supine)
4. Regional changes: weakness or sensory change

Source: Turk, Wack, & Kerns, 1985.

behaviors, including guarding, bracing, rubbing the painful area, facial grimacing and sighing (F. J. Keefe, Block, Williams, & Surwit, 1981), and others such as distortion of ambulation or posture, negative affect, facial/audible expressions of distress, and avoidance of activity comprise a valid and reliable part of the examination (Turk, Wack, & Kerns, 1985). Furthermore, pain behaviors have been found to correlate with self-report measures of pain intensity, pain disability, and self-efficacy (McCahon, Strong, Sharry, & Cramond, 2005) and may serve as targets for cognitive and behavioral treatment.

Kinetic Chain

In order to have functional movement in space, each joint and part, or link, of the body must move in a coordinated manner. The sequence of the links and the interrelationship of muscle activation and translation of forces within the body is referred to as the kinetic chain (Kibler, 1998). Each link of this system creates force and energy that is transferred from the proximal core stabilizing link ultimately to the distal peripheral link. When one link is weak or injured, other links compensate. Distal links will typically compensate for proximal links, and the added stress and loads result in further injury. For instance, if a person has a tight iliotibial band, a weak gluteus medius with overall poor control of hip rotation, and excessive pronation at the foot, this produces poor biomechanics, abnormal patella tracking, excessive patellofemoral joint pressures, and results in patellofemoral pain. Hence, proper rehabilitation of the patellofemoral joint pain must address factors up and down the kinetic chain, in other words, iliotibial band stretching, strengthening of the gluteus muscle groups and hip external rotators, and correcting pronation (Brukner & Kahn, 2001).

In the lower limb, the kinetic chain is comprised of the hip, knee, and ankle joints. In the upper limb, the kinetic chain is comprised of the shoulder, elbow, and wrist joints. The upper and lower limbs can perform activities in either a closed or open manner. In open chain activities, the distal extremity is free to move in space by contraction of the agonist muscle (for example, the swing phase of gait). In closed chain activities, the distal part of the extremity is immobile and motion is produced at the joints of the chain by muscle cocontraction (the stance phase of gait). Classically, closed kinetic chain exercises are performed in the lower extremities, as in standing squats, and open kinetic chain exercises are typically performed in the upper limbs, as in throwing a ball (DeLee et al., 2003). Although closed chain exercises are more functional in nature, resistance may need to be added to increase strength—such as performing squats while holding dumbbells.

Treatment Approaches

Therapy Professionals

Physiatric management may include incorporating a number of active therapies delivered by a wide range of health-care providers such as physical, occupational, and recreational therapists with individual areas of focus.

Physical therapy focuses on improving range of motion, strength, balance, and aerobic training. Occupational therapy focuses on educating patients regarding proper posture and ergonomics related to functional activities and at the workplace. Physical and occupational therapists employ the use of passive and active therapeutic exercises and passive modalities in guiding patients through the process of tissue recovery and rehabilitation.

Targeted therapeutic exercises are utilized to address specific deficits in posture, flexibility, strength, balance, neuromuscular coordination, and endurance. Passive modalities such as cryotherapy, heat, and electrical stimulation are commonly used to address pain, alter tissue distensibility, and control inflammation.

Pain psychology assessment and intervention focuses on both cognitive and behavioral factors related to pain. One's cognitions may impact mood, behavior, and function. Psychological interventions are focused on unlearning maladaptive responses and reactions to pain while fostering wellness, improving coping and perceived control, and decreasing catastrophizing.

Therapeutic recreation specialists are important members of the rehabilitation team. They evaluate and plan leisure activities that serve to promote mental and physical health. Recreational therapists help patients to establish and incorporate strategies learned from various disciplines of treatment into social and community functions. Application of these techniques (i.e., correct biomechanics, pacing, relaxation techniques) leads to the reduction of stress, fear of movement, and depression while fostering a feeling of self-efficacy and confidence. In addition, therapeutic recreation specialists facilitate the recovery of motor function and reasoning skills, increase social awareness, and promote integration of individuals with disabilities back into the community.

Passive Modalities

A modality describes any physical agent utilized to produce a physiologic response in a targeted tissue. Commonly prescribed passive physical modalities for the treatment of acute and chronic pain include cryotherapy, heat, and electrical stimulation. Modalities are initially incorporated into therapy sessions by physical or occupational therapists, with a goal of educating the patient on appropriate application and use at home. Depending upon the specific pain complaint, modalities may be incorporated in acute conditions, early in treatment as a means of decreasing local swelling, analgesia, and help progression and tolerance of therapies (see Tables 27.2 and 27.3). They are also used as part of a daily treatment regimen (cryotherapy to osteoarthritic knee after exercise, electrical stimulation to low back region during prolonged upright postures), or as a "rescue" treatment for "flare-ups."

Conduction: Transfer of heat between two bodies in direct contact
Convection: Transfer of heat by one body flowing past another
Conversion: Transformation of energy into heat
Evaporation: Liquid vaporizes into a gas, requiring thermal heat

Electrical Stimulation

Transcutaneous electric nerve stimulation (TENS) and interferential current therapy (ICT) involve the transmission of electrical energy to the peripheral nervous system via an external stimulator and conductive gel pads on the skin. TENS is based theoretically on the "gate control theory" proposed by Melzack (Melzack & Wall, 1965). TENS stimulates nonnociceptive, large afferent α-β fibers "closing" the "gate" of facilitated sensory input, normally "opened" by small-diameter nociceptive C-fibers. Electrical stimulation releases endogenous opioids and activates peripherally located alpha-2A adrenergic receptors (King et al., 2005). TENS has been shown to be beneficial in acute pain states, reducing the amount of analgesic medication consumed after surgical procedures, and in chronic pain conditions, in which it helps to relieve pain and foster patient independence (see Table 27.3.).

Table 27.2 Modalities

Cryotherapy

Indication	Effect	Mode	Example	Contraindication
• Acute injury	• Analgesia	Conduction	• Ice	• More than 30 minutes
• Muscle spasticity	• Vasoconstriction	Convection	• Cold pack	• Ischemia/arterial insufficiency
• Osteoarthritis	• Decreases muscle Spindle	Evaporation	• Cryotherapy compression unit	• Raynaud's syndrome
• Minor burns	• Decreases nerve conduction			• Impaired sensation
• Arthritis	• Decreases metabolism		Whirlpool bath	• Burns
• Bursitis	• Decreases enzymatic activity		Vapocoolant spray	• Cryoglobulinemia
• Acute/chronic pain	• Increases tissue stiffness			• Paroxysmal cold hemoglobinuria
• Myofascial pain	• Increase viscosity			• Cold allergy or hypersensitivity
• Contusion				
• Inflammation				

Heat

Indication	Effect	Contraindication
• Chronic inflammation	• Analgesia	• Acute trauma, inflammation
• Arthritis	• Vasodilation, increases blood flow	• Bleeding disorders
• Myofascial pain	• Increases oxygen and leukocytes	• Edema, scars, impaired sensation
• Collagen vascular disease	• Muscle relaxation	• Malignancy
• Strains	• Increases metabolism	• Multiple sclerosis
• Sprains	• Increases capillary permeability	
• Contracture	• Increases collage extensibility	
• Thrombophlebitis		

Superficial Heat (depth 0.5–2.0 cm; amount of heating depends on amount of adipose tissue present)

Example	Mode	Composition	Effect
Hydrocollator packs	Conduction	• Bags of silicone dioxide heated in stainless steel containers in water 65–90 deg. C • Applied to body part over towels	• Increases temperature 3.3 deg. C at 1 cm • Increases temperature 1.3 deg. C at 2 cm (Lehmann, Silverman, Baum, Kirk, & Johnston, 1966)
Paraffin	Conduction	• Paraffin wax and mineral oil in 7:1 ratio heated to 52 deg. C • Body part dipped in bath, wax hardens, repeated 7–12 times, then wrapped in plastic and covered by towel	• Increases temperature 5.5 deg C in forearm subcutaneous tissue • Increases temperature 2.4 deg. C in brachioradialis muscle
Hydrotherapy • Whirlpool • Hubbard tank	Convection	• Water heated to 40 deg. C (body submersion) • Water heated to 43 deg. C (limb submersion) • Heats, massages, debrides • Can elevate core temperature depending on surface area	
Fluidotherapy	Convection	• Hot air blown through medium of dry powder or glass beads • Temperature 46–49 deg. C.	• Produces temperature of 42 deg. C in hand and joint capsule • Produces temperature of 39.5 deg. C in foot and joint capsule (Borrell, Parker, Henley, Masley, & Repinecz, 1980)

Deep Heat (depth 0.5 to 2.0 cm; amount of heating depends on amount of adipose tissue present; heating is by conversion)

Example	Composition and Effect	Intensity	Frequency	Contraindication
Ultrasound (US)	• Electrical current applied to quartz crystal or ceramic produces acoustic vibration above the audible range • Heat greatest at areas of impedance: bones, tendon, skin, muscle	0.8–3.0 W/cm^2	0.8–1.0 MHz	• Heat contraindications • Near brain or spine • Near heart • Near reproductive organs • Near pacemakers • Near tumors

(*continued*)

Table 27.2. (continued)

Deep Heat (depth 0.5 to 2.0 cm; amount of heating depends on amount of adipose tissue present; heating is by conversion)

Example	Composition and Effect	Intensity	Frequency	Contraindication
				• Gravida or menstruating uterus • Eyes • Immature epiphysis • Arthroplasty
	Nonthermal effect • Gaseous cavitation (gaseous bubbles produced by turbulence) • Acoustic streaming (movement of material produced by pressure difference of US waves) • Standing waves (fixed areas of increased pressure produced by superimposition of US waves)	Duration: 5–10 min	Depth: 45 deg. C at 8 cm	

ICT is a variant of TENS that involves the mixing of two unmodulated sine waves with different frequencies (one at 4 kHz, and a second within a variable range) to generate frequencies between 4 and 250 Hz. This allows for the stimulation of deeper tissues with decreased discomfort. The proposed mechanism of action involves the direct stimulation of muscle fibers, as opposed to nerve fibers, to achieve improved muscle blood flow and promotion of the healing process. Variable frequency helps to prevent adaptation. There is less scientific evidence for the use of ICT when compared to TENS.

Manual Techniques

Manual techniques may include a number of different approaches for the treatment of acute and chronic pain and in general include massage, mobilization, and manipulation. Massage therapy for acute and chronic pain has demonstrated mixed results with regard to long-term efficacy (Ernst, 1999; Furlan, Brosseau, Imamura, & Irvin, 2003). Massage techniques, such as stroking or effleurage, involve light movements of the hands over the skin or deeper tissues, in a slow, rhythmic fashion to mobilize tissue. Kneading involves more aggressive grasping, pushing, and squeezing of tissue. Friction massage may help to loosen scar or adhesions between the skin and fascial tissues (ligaments, tendons, and muscles; Haldeman, 1989). Percussive techniques include clapping, cupping, and tapping in a rhythmic manner and may be used for postural drainage of organs or to activate muscle contraction and/or increase circulation.

Various studies have demonstrated the magnitude of pain reduction as modest (Cherkin et al., 2001) and transient between sessions (Hernandez-Reif, Field, Krasnegor, & Theakston, 2001). Diagnostic technique and treatment methods may vary among professional groups (i.e., manual therapist, chiropractors, and osteopathic physicians) leading to difference in treatment outcomes and results of clinical trials (van de Veen et al., 2005).

Mobilization

Mobilization involves passive movement of tissue within the limit of joint range. Manipulation may include similar soft tissue techniques in addition to high-velocity techniques in which forces are generated at a particular joint level beyond the physiological barrier of joint restriction and is more commonly practiced by chiropractic practitioners and osteopathic physicians (Greenman, 1996). Geisser et al. found manual therapy with specific adjuvant exercise to be beneficial in treating chronic low back pain with no significant change in function (M. Geisser, Wiggert, Haig, & Colwell, 2005). Others have demonstrated efficacy of spinal manipulation in short-term studies, although the effect size was small when compared to active therapies (Assendelft, Morton, Yu, Suttorp, & Shekelle, 2003) and placebo (Ferreira, Ferreira, Latimer, Herbert, & Maher, 2002). Osteopathic manipulation in a study of subacute low back pain patients demonstrated similar results as compared to standard medical care but also used less physical therapy and medications (Andersson et al., 1999).

Exercise

Daily exercise is important in maintaining physical health and has been associated with 25% less self-reported musculoskeletal pain as compared to more sedentary controls (Bruce, Fries, &

Table 27.3. Modalities, Continued

TENS Type	Amplitude Frequency	Indication	Duration	Setting Changes
• "Conventional" • Low-intensity • High frequency	1–2 mA/50–100 Hz	Acute pain state	• 1–20 minutes for rapid relief • 30 minutes to 2 hours for short duration of analgesia • Repeat as needed	Increase amplitude or pulse width to avoid adaptation and maintain analgesia
• "Dense-disperse"/"Acupuncturelike" • High-intensity • Low frequency	15–20 mA/1–5 Hz	Chronic pain state	• 30 minutes for short duration • 2–6 hours for long duration • Once daily	Minimal adaptation

Lubeck, 2005). Additionally, inactivity has been shown to be a predictor of future pain with injury (Taimela, Diederich, Hubsch, & Heinricy, 2000). Daily stretching and strengthening exercises may be an effective treatment option for chronic pain conditions. Disuse effects of chronic pain (i.e., deconditioning, loss of flexibility, and maladaptive thoughts and movement patterns) may also be reversed through exercise. A brief overview of physiologic changes of stretching and exercise strengthening will be reviewed.

Stretching

Stretching is used to lengthen tissue, including skin, fascia, muscle, and ligaments, and increase overall range of motion. Increased range of motion will decrease contracture, improve functional mobility, and allow the muscles and joints to function properly. Range of motion exercises vary from passive, in which there is no voluntary muscle contraction and total external force, to active assisted, in which there is partial contraction and external force, and active, in which there is complete contraction and no external force. In general, most range of motion exercises increase blood flow and prevent contracture, whereas active exercise prevents atrophy and increases strength and endurance.

Muscle Conditioning

Once range of motion is normalized, muscle conditioning is addressed, as muscles around a joint impact stability, function, and pain. Muscle conditioning is comprised of strength, endurance, and reeducation.

Muscle strength is increased through isometric, isotonic, or isokinetic exercises. Isometric strengthening is characterized by contraction of the muscle without change in length or movement. Isometric exercises are typically used in acute pain states such as with active inflammation or induced immobilization. Isotonic exercises are those in which muscles contract and the length and movement change, but the load remains the same, such as doing a bicep curl with a dumbbell. On the other hand, with isokinetic exercise, muscle contracts at a constant angular velocity, such as with a Cybex or muscle pulley machine. Muscle strengthening depends on vascularization, energy metabolism, increase in number of myofibrils, and motor unit recruitment. Strengthening may be achieved by isometric, isotonic, and isokinetic exercise. Strengthening muscle tissue results from increasing the load, speed, number, frequency, form, or range of motion of the exercise. Muscle endurance, the ability to sustain and perform repeated contractions, is increased through aerobic activity.

Aerobic activity is defined by low intensity, high-repetition exercise that increases the number of mitochondria and local metabolism. Aerobic exercise may increase the levels of endogenous endorphins (Farrell, Gates, Maksud, & Morgan, 1982) and enkephalins (Grossman & Sutton, 1985) and may be responsible for an additional antinociceptive effect.

Motor Reeducation

Motor reeducation may also be simulated with exercise and is often coordinated by the therapist as the patient progresses in treatment. Motor reeducation involves breaking down a motion into individual chronological movements. The therapist assists the patient in identifying and then unlearning potentially abnormal movement patterns. Proper posture and retraining of movements are practiced and incorporated into the general strengthening, endurance, and flexibility program (Brukner & Kahn, 2001).

Aquatic Therapy

Pool exercise is a common therapeutic modality. The physiologic advantages of water as a therapeutic medium include thermal conductive properties and high specific heat. The viscosity of water provides resistance—for aerobic and strengthening exercises, compressive forces—helping to decrease edema, and buoyancy helps decrease weight bearing (Suomi & Collier, 2003). This may help in decreasing muscle and joint stiffness and pain. Hydrostatic forces with immersion in water leads to cardiopulmonary benefits secondary to centralization of blood flow resulting in increased venous return, stroke volume, and cardiac output and subsequent reflex bradycardia (Anstey & Roskell, 2000; Choukroun, Kays, & Varene, 1989). Patients participating in an aquatic therapy program more than 2 days per week as part of a long-term maintenance treatment program demonstrated reduction in pain and improved function (Ariyoshi et al., 1999).

Mind-Body Therapy (MBT)

MBT is defined by the National Institutes of Health (NIH) as an intervention that may "use a variety of techniques designed to facilitate the mind's capacity to affect bodily function and symptoms." Various mind-body treatments may help to improve coordination, decrease abnormal movement patterns, and improve psychological well-being and include tai chi, body awareness therapy (BAT), and Feldenkrais.

Tai chi, a traditional Chinese mind-body relaxation exercise, consists of approximately 108 intricate exercise sequences performed in a slow, relaxed manner. Tai chi has been found to increase physical and mental health, including physical, social, and emotional function, decrease anxiety, decrease pain perception, and increase flexibility and balance (Audette, Wang, & Smith, 2004; Ross, Bohannon, Davis, & Gurchiek, 1999; Song, Lee, Lam, & Bae, 2003). In addition, MBTs combine the mind with movement to reprogram the nervous system, improve coordination, reduce abnormal motor patterns, and improve physical and emotional health.

Body awareness therapy (BAT) and Feldenkrais (FK) are therapies that use patterns of movement to improve flexibility, posture, breathing, and overall function. Feldenkrais and BAT have been shown to increase body awareness and decrease pain (Gard, 2005). In addition, BAT and FK improve health-related quality of life and self-efficacy of pain to a higher degree than conventional physiotherapy (Malmgren-Olsson & Branholm, 2002).

Clinical Conditions

This section will review theoretical issues related to underlying mechanisms of common pain conditions (osteoarthritis, low back pain, myofascial pain, and fibromyalgia) and principles guiding active physical medicine approaches. These same principles can be applied to other acute and chronic pain conditions.

Osteoarthritis (OA) and Rheumatoid Arthritis (RA)

OA and RA are characterized by an ongoing pathophysiologic cycle. Here, compensatory guarding and pain lead to a loss of range of motion (ROM), decreased strength and endurance, increasing joint contracture and subsequent development of abnormal posture and motor patterns, joint overload, further joint destruction, and pain. Active therapy is aimed at unloading the joint, improving local muscle condition, and increasing joint and muscle flexibility. Because muscles provide the "dynamic" joint stability during movement, signs of OA, such as osteophytes and capsular thickening, may form to increase stability when there is muscle dysfunction and dynamic instability. For example, although controversial, it has been proposed that quadriceps dysfunction and weakness may be a risk factor for progression of knee OA (Slemenda et al., 1997). It was found that independent of body weight, knee extensor strength was 18% lower at baseline in women who developed knee OA compared with controls (Slemenda et al., 1998). Studies have shown that exercise programs resulted in increased quadriceps strength and joint position sense, reduced pain, and improved function. In addition, improvements in quadriceps sensorimotor function resulted in decreased disability of patients with knee osteoarthritis who followed a standard daily exercise regime.

In addition to strength, alignment is equally important for dynamic stability and proper functioning. Sharma et al. (2001) found that quadriceps weakness was not related to progression of knee OA except in lax and malaligned knees.

When malalignment, decrease in function, or instability is present, an orthosis may be indicated. An orthosis is any externally applied device used to modify structural and functional characteristics of the neuromuscular system (Redford, Basmajian, & Trautman, 1995). With the knee often the source of chronic pain in those with OA, braces, neoprene sleeves, and foot orthotics have been found to be helpful to increase stability and decrease pain. Both braces and neoprene sleeves have been found to be better than medical treatment alone. Furthermore, braces are more effective than neoprene sleeves in improving stiffness, pain, and function (Brouwer, Jakma, Verhagen, Verhaar, & Bierma-Zeinstra, 2005). In OA, often described as a "bone on bone" condition, fluoroscopy has shown that braces create distraction between the tibial and femoral condyles (Komistek et al., 1999). Additionally, proprioception, which is reduced in those with knee OA, is increased with the use of braces (Birmingham et al., 2001). In addition to braces, heel wedges can improve abnormal biomechanics that are present in knee OA. For instance, lateral-wedge insoles decreased lateral thrust and reduced pain in 27 of 50 subjects with medial compartment OA (Ogata, Yasunaga, & Nomiyama, 1997), and medial-wedge insoles decrease medial thrust and reduced pain in 10 of 10 knees with lateral compartment OA.

In addition to foot orthotics, walking aids such as canes, forearm crutches, and walkers are used in those with rheumatoid or osteoarthritis. They help to unload the joint, improve body mechanics, and decrease pain. In one study, 49% of the RA patients and 44% of the OA patients owned a walking aid. It was found that in those with RA, age, education, frequency of pain, and disability were associated with possessing a walking aid. In the OA group, however, only age and disability were associated with possessing a walking aid. Only 30% actually used the walking aid; use was in those who were older, who had higher pain intensity and disability, and who experienced a decrease in morning stiffness with the aid (Van der Esch, Heijmans, & Dekker, 2003). It should be noted that for a painful knee, the cane can be held in either hand, whereas for the painful hip, the cane should be held in the contralateral hand.

Strengthening and endurance exercise relieves symptoms in patients with mild or moderate OA (Ettinger et al., 1997). Studies have shown that aerobic walking and home-based quadriceps strengthening exercise reduce pain and disability from knee osteoarthritis (Roddy, Zhang, & Doherty, 2005). Aerobic exercise only, not strengthening, was found to significantly lower depressive symptoms in both high and low depressive symptomatology subgroups. Intensity of the aerobic exercise was not a factor. Aerobic cycling at both high and low intensities was found to be equally effective in improving functional status, gait, pain, and aerobic capacity with OA of the knee (Mangione et al., 1999). Thus, exercise appears to moderately decrease pain, and increase quadriceps strength and physical function (van Baar et al., 1998). Exercise has been shown to increase self-efficacy. Self-efficacy is the belief that one has the capabilities to execute the courses of actions required to manage prospective situations (Baron, 2002). In one study, when persons stopped exercising, self-efficacy beliefs declined. Self-efficacy beliefs increased, however, after resuming exercising (McAuley, Lox, & Duncan, 1993).

Although exercise is beneficial, it must be actively maintained. Long-term follow-up and compliance of patients who participated in a randomized 3-month intervention showed that the beneficial effects declined with time and disappeared during the 6-month follow-up period (van Baar et al., 2001) versus another study (Ettinger et al., 1997) in which significant differences were found in measures of disability, physical performance, and pain after 18 months of exercise in patients with knee OA. Exercise is also beneficial when combined with manual therapy, or passive movements the therapist uses to increase ROM. A randomized trial (Deyle et al., 2000) compared manual therapy to the knee, hip, foot and ankle, and/or lumbar spine combined with exercises for lower-extremity strengthening, range of motion, and endurance to placebo ultrasound treatment. Significant improvements in pain relief, the 6-minute walk test, and self-reported function scores were found in the manual therapy plus exercise group compared to controls. Treatment effects remained at 1-year follow-up.

TENS use and aquatic therapy are also beneficial. TENS use had a positive effect, greatest with high-intensity burst modes, repeated treatments, and when used for at least 4 weeks (Osiri et al., 2000). Aquatic therapy has been found to improve aerobic capacity, walk time, physical activity level, and depression in those with OA (Bunning & Materson, 1991). In addition, those with OA and RA have been able to reduce the amount of postural sway by 18%–30%, a risk factor for fall, with a 6-week aquatic exercise program (Suomi & Koceja, 2000).

Low Back Pain

Physical Therapy Approaches for Spine-Related Disorders

A number of active physical therapy treatments for spine-related conditions have demonstrated efficacy in decreasing pain and improving function (Malmivaara et al., 1995). The heterogeneous nature of underlying spinal conditions possess a challenge for determining the specific or multiple pain generators involved (i.e., disc degeneration, herniation, nerve root compression, facet arthropathy, or sacroiliac dysfunction), thereby directing therapy. One must also be cognizant of related psychosocial factors (pain-related cognitions, fear-avoidance beliefs, depression, anxiety, and anger; Linton, 2000), which may perpetuate the experience of pain and related disability. From a purely mechanical view of low back pain, several subgroups of low back pain exist, and may benefit from different exercise treatments. Treatment approaches include cervical and lumbar range of motion, stabilization exercises (O'Sullivan, Phyty, Twomey, & Allison, 1997), flexion-based exercises (Williams, 2003), specific directional preference exercises (McKenzie, 1981), and neurodynamic techniques. These techniques and underlying theories are reviewed briefly below with the understanding of significant overlap and variability between deliveries by various therapists.

Stabilization Exercises: Core Strengthening and Stabilization

The concept of lumbar stability has been an area of extensive research for over 30 years. Initial theory was based on an understanding pain in the spine was the result of gradual degeneration of joints and related soft tissue as a result of microtrauma and poor control of spinal structures, a dynamic process involving static positions and controlled movements (Barr, Griggs, & Cadby, 2005). Biomechanical changes of spine stability include postural and motor control, which help to reduce tissue strain and provide efficient muscle action (Sahrmann, 2002). Panjabi (1992) classically describes a three-component interdependent system comprising of bone and ligamentous structures, muscles, and neural control system. An important focus of spine stability for low back pain includes assessment and strengthening of core muscle groups, controlling intersegmental stability, and restoring motion, and will be reviewed below (Cholewicki & McGill, 1992).

A basic individualized physical therapy approach includes stretching tight or contracted muscles, activating inhibited muscles, and improving core strength. Exercises are commonly targeted on retraining multifidus (back muscle) and transverses abdominus (a deep abdominal muscle) along with supplemented exercises for the pelvic floor and breathing control (Richardson, Jull, Hodges, & Hides, 1999). Therapists help to train patients to contract these muscles independently from more superficial muscles. As the patient progresses through core strengthening, balance and conditioning are incorporated into their exercise program. These exercises can be facilitated with the use of an exercise or medicine ball, balance boards, Thera-Band elastic strips, and a Dyna Disc, an air-filled plastic disc with adjustable inflations (Akuthota & Nadler, 2004). Research has suggested stability exercises may prevent recurrence of pain and improve function compared to control groups (Hides, 2004; O'Sullivan, Phyty, Twomey, & Allison, 1997).

Directional Preference

The concept of centralization, recognized and popularized by McKenzie, is based on the concept by which pain radiating from the cervical, thoracic, or lumbar spine is sequentially abolished (McKenzie, 1981), neurologic symptoms are decreased (Fritz, Delitto, Vignovic, & Busse, 2000), symptoms are reduced (Delitto, Cibulka, Erhard, Bowling, & Tenhula, 1993; Erhard, Delitto, & Cibulka, 1994) distally to proximally in the affected limb or body region in response to spinal positions or maneuvers (i.e., extension, flexion, side bending). Centralization phenomena can be reliably assessed, and because of its association with more favorable clinical outcomes (physical therapy and lumbar surgery), used to guide treatment in selected patients (Aina, May, & Clare, 2004; Werneke & Hart, 2001; Wetzel & Donelson, 2003).

Peripheralization, the opposite response, involves the distal spread of pain into the limb with similar positioning. Noncentralization has been shown to be a more reliable predictor of poorer outcomes in physical therapy and surgery. In the one trial involving subacute pain (Lindstrom et al., 1992), those who underwent a graded activity program returned to work more quickly, had fewer absences during the next 2 years, and had improved back mobility and fitness.

Neurodynamic Therapy

Neurodynamic therapy is based on the concept of altered mechanosensitivity of the damaged neurogenic tissue. It is based on a more comprehensive functional understanding of peripheral and central nervous system plasticity. Classically, this is represented clinically by a positive straight leg raise (SLR), identifying possible presence of perineuritis. Maitland more formally described as the slump test (or seated SLR), which incorporates cervical flexion and ankle dorsiflexion as a means of assessing mechanosensitivity of neural structures within the spinal vertebral canal (Maitland, 1985). Peripheral nerves may become pain generators due to related innervated connective tissue or injury processes along the nerve myelin sheath. Butler describes abnormal impulse-generating sites (AIGS) as areas of injury along the central nervous system where ion channels accumulate leading to abnormal firing. Therapy is focused peripherally at decreasing AIGS firing by improving mobility of the nerve by decreasing tension or pressure along the perineural structures (Butler, 2000).

Exercise

Exercise benefits in low back pain treatment have been demonstrated with regard to improved muscle performance, strength, and endurance (Liddle, Baxter, & Gracey, 2004; Mannion et al., 2001). General exercise guidelines may be useful in developing an individual treatment program for acute and chronic pain conditions. The American College of Sports Medicine (ACSM; 2000) proposed three areas of focus, including (1) muscle strengthening, (2) flexibility training, and (3) cardiovascular endurance. Exercise-based treatments may help to promote wellness rather than illness behavior (Cohen & Rainville, 2002) and empower patients to take a more active role in their progress toward improved function (Mannion et al., 2001; Rainville, Ahern, & Phalen, 1993). Meta-analysis and reviews have shown exercise-based treatment to be more effective at decreasing pain and improving function with chronic low back pain (Hayden, van Tulder, Malmivaara, & Koes, 2005) as compared to reviews of acute low back pain (van Tulder, Malmivaara, Esmail, & Koes, 2000). Interestingly, a systematic review of exercise therapy concluded that specific back exercises should not be recommended for acute or chronic pain but that exercise in general may be beneficial as part of an active rehabilitation program (van Tulder, Malmivaara, Esmail, & Koes, 2000). Keller et al. examined lumbar paraspinal muscle density, an indication of muscle strength, in patients who underwent lumbar fusion as compared to a nonsurgical group. The nonsurgical group participated in a low-intensity exercise and cognitive behavioral interventional program. The exercise and cognitive intervention group demonstrated significant improvement in lumbar strength (increase by 30%) at 1 year as compared to their surgical counterparts. Lumbar fusion patients demonstrated 10% reduction in muscle density, whereas the exercise group muscle density remained unchanged (Keller et al., 2003). Other studies have also suggested activity in general may itself be therapeutic in reducing pain and improving psychosocial functioning (Abenhaim et al., 2000; Hurwitz, Morgenstern, & Chiao, 2005).

Myofascial Pain Syndrome (MPS)

Myofascial pain is characterized by tenderness in the muscle, characteristic pain referral patterns, and restriction of motion (Simons & Travell, 1999). MPS may be a primary source of pain or present as part of a more complicated multifactorial pain condition. Trigger points are discrete, focal, hyperirritable spots located in a taut band of skeletal muscle, painful on compression, may produce referred pain, referred tenderness, motor and or autonomic dysfunction, and autonomic dysfunction. Myofascial trigger points (MTrP) may be classified as active or latent. Latent trigger points are tender to palpation and may be associated with restricted ROM and stiffness, but are not associated with *spontaneous* complaints of pain. MTrPs are commonly found in postural muscles including the neck, shoulders, and pelvic girdle, upper trapezius, scalene, levator scapulae, quadratus lumborum, and lumbosacral

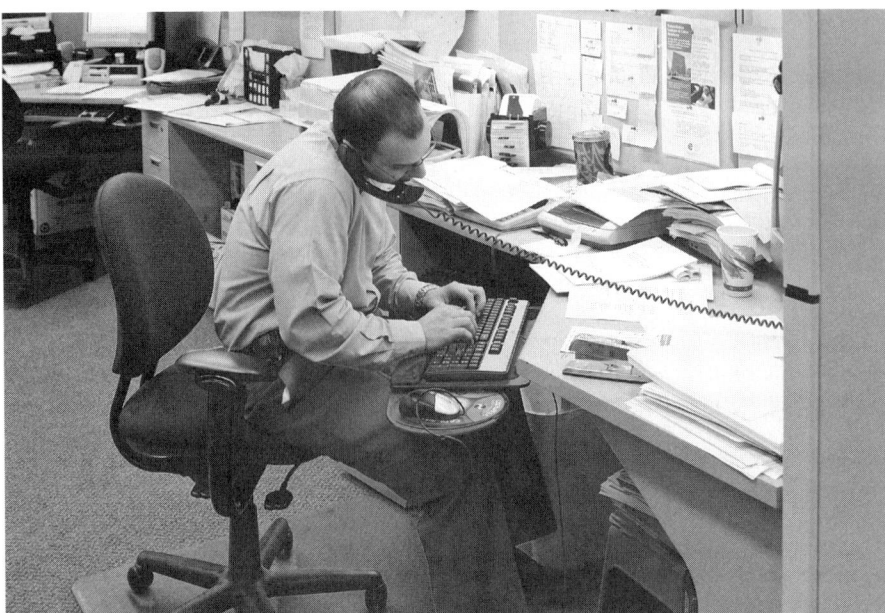

Figure 27.1. Workplace posture: prolonged head forward posture with increased thoracic kyphosis, shoulders rounded anteriorly, and head tilted cradling phone.

muscles. MTrP may develop or be aggravated by acute tissue trauma, repetitive microtrauma, muscle deconditioning, postural abnormalities, poor sleep, and/or metabolic abnormalities (i.e., vitamin deficiencies and hypothyroidism [Han & Harrison, 1997]). Occupational and recreational activities often precipitate or aggravate MPS. Common workplace activities such as holding a telephone receiver between the ear and shoulder, prolonged bending over a table, sitting in chairs with poor back support, improper height of arm rests and computer workstations, and moving boxes using improper body mechanics (Rachlin, 1994) may lead to musculoskeletal dysfunction and MPS (see Figures 27.1 and 27.2).

Diagnosis of MPS is primarily based on clinical findings. Clinically, confirmation of MPS is not related to any specific laboratory tests (e.g., imaging studies, electromyography, or muscle biopsy). Assessment of posture, body mechanics, dynamic joint function, and palpation of MTrP may help to confirm the diagnosis. In assessing active MTrP, one palpates across muscle fibers and feels for a "ropelike" nodularity of tight muscle. These discrete areas may reproduce characteristic pain referral patterns usually traveling in a proximal-to-distal direction. There may be a local "twitch response," characterized by a palpable and visible reflex contraction of involved muscle. A "jump sign" is a pain-related withdrawal reflex secondary to applied pressure to a painful MTrP.

Although the physical exam is sensitive and specific in diagnosing MPS, research has demonstrated fine needle electromyographic findings characteristic of the disorder and may help to develop mechanistic strategies for pharmacologic and nonpharmacologic treatment. Abnormal acetylcholine (Ach) release at the motor endplate and endplate noise is more frequent in MTrP than at endplates outside of the zone or MTrP. Endplate noise is characteristic but not diagnostic of MTrP, and may be increased in any situation in which there is a mechanical, chemical, or other noxious stimuli. With sustained Ach release, sarcomeres shorten, which produces a "contraction knot." This increase in sarcomere activity results in an increase in energy consumption and a relative reduction in circulation, potentially creating localized hypoxia and ischemia. Pronociceptive substances such as bradykinin, serotonin, and histamine are in turn released, sensitizing afferents and producing local tenderness. Central convergence and facilitation at the level of the dorsal horn leads to referred pain in adjacent myotomes and expansion of receptive fields. Increased neuronal excitability at the level of the dorsal horn leads to the release of substance P and glutamate, key players in the development and maintenance of central sensitization.

The autonomic nervous system (ANS) may also be activated by neurovasoreactive substances (i.e., bradykinin, substance P, serotonin, and histamine). With ANS activation, more Ach is released. Audette et al., in a study of dry needle treatment of MTrPs, found bilateral motor unit activation was produced with unilateral needle stimulation of the symptomatic MTrP. Contralateral or mirror-image electromyographic activity may support the concept of abnormal central nervous system processing of sensory input at the level of the spinal cord as a key perpetuator of pain and muscle dysfunction (Audette, Wang, & Smith, 2004). Clinically, ongoing psychological stress, maladaptive posture, and elevated muscle tension may also contribute to the muscle-pain dysfunction cycle (McNulty, Gevirtz, Hubbard, & Berkoff, 1994).

Effective treatment of MPS focuses on pharmacologic and nonpharmacologic treatments including PT, OT, exercise, ergonomic assessment, relaxation, and stress reduction training. PT and OT treatment goals include reducing pain, restoring range of motion, and improving function. Muscles with one or more MTrPs fatigue more rapidly and recover more slowly. Therapies involve a graded stabilization and strengthening program. If strengthening is done too early, there is the risk for overload and subsequent compensation attempts by other muscles that may then develop MTrP. Also, PT and OT are important in helping to reduce fear of movement and are incorporated in a gradually progressive submaximal exercise program, helping the patient to gain confidence in independent movements. Muscle release techniques and other self-management approaches are commonly included. Overall, was the most effective for easing MTrP pain and increasing cervical ROM (Hou, Tsai, Cheng, Chung, & Hong, 2002), over hot pack and active ROM plus stretch and spray plus TENS, which was more effective than hot pack plus active range of motion and stretch and spray.

Interventional treatments, such as trigger-point injections and acupuncture, have been found to be effective in treating MTrP. In comparative studies, dry needling was found to be as effective as injecting an anesthetic solution such as procaine (Novocain) or lidocaine (Xylocaine). Postinjection soreness, however, was more intense and of longer duration than the soreness with lidocaine. In one study, 58% of patients reported verbal rating scores (VRS) 0 on a 0–10 scale immediately after trigger-point injection and 42% had minimal pain scores (1 to 2 on a 10-point VRS; Hong, 1994); however, overall pain relief did not differ, supporting the theory that mechanical disruption of the muscle fibers and the increase in blood flow is important in relieving pain. Porta, in a single-center, randomized study, reported greater reduction pain in patients with chronic MPS injected with botulinum toxin type A (BTX-A) as compared to steroid. Pain reduction gains continued at 60 days in the BTX-A group but decreased in the steroid-treated patients (Porta, 2000). BTX-A has been studied in other MPS-related disorders showing efficacy in cervicogenic pain (Wheeler, Goolkasian, & Gretz, 1998) and mixed outcomes with headache disorders (Blumenfeld, 2003; Padberg, de Haan, & Tavy, 2004; Sundaraj, Ponciano, Johnstone et al., 2004) BTX-A has been compared to dry needling and lidocaine trigger-point injections and has not been found to be cost effective (Kamanli et al., 2005).

Fibromyalgia

Fibromyalgia syndrome (FMS), another common musculoskeletal pain disorder, may share some common characteristics with MPS, and may coexist in patients; however, they remain distinct disorders although there may be significant sign and symptom overlap (see Table 27.4). FMS is characterized by widespread musculoskeletal pain (at least 3 months) and stiffness, with symmetrically distributed tender points, and associated symptoms (i.e., irritable bowel/bladder syndrome, dysautonomia, cognitive and endocrine dysfunction, dizziness, cold intolerance, and/ or mood disorder; Larsen, 1999).

Recent studies support evidence of central changes in brain processing (Bradely, Sotolongo, Alberts, et al., 1999) and neurochemical abnormalities (elevated excitatory neurotransmitter substance P; Russell, Orr, Littman, et al., 1994), nitric oxide (Bradley, Weigent, Sotolongo, et al., 2000), and amino acids (Larson, Giovengo, Russell, et al., 2000) as possible mediators of peripheral and central sensitization.

Tender points (TPs), distinguished from MTrPs associated with MPS, are characterized by eliciting pain with at least 4 kg of pressure to at least 11 of 18 muscle tendon sites, based on common research criteria (Wolfe, Smythe, Yunus, et al., 1990). Reported prevalence rates of FM are approximately 2% in the United States, including 3.4% of women and 0.5% of men (Wolfe, Smythe, Yunus, et al., 1990). FMS patients may have lowered mechanical and thermal pain thresholds and psychological factors including increased levels of catastrophizing (M. E. Geisser et al., 2003).

Treatment involves first giving the patient a diagnosis, which does not have an adverse affect on clinical outcome (White & Pape, 1992), and then behavioral management and education, both of which equally decrease depression, self-reported pain behaviors, observed pain behaviors, and myalgia scores (Nicassio et al., 1997).

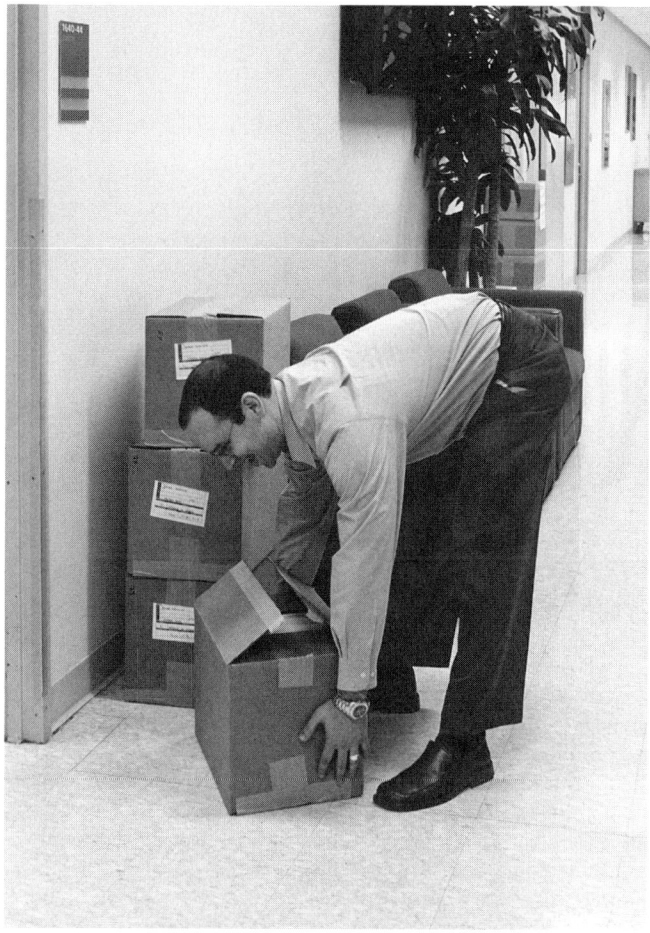

Figure 27.2. Improper lifting mechanics: poor mechanics with excessive flexion of the lumbosacral spine with knees extended. Proper mechanics would include placing the load closer to the body and lifting with the lower extremities by flexing the knees and hips while keeping the spine in a safer, more neutral position.

stretching is the basis of all exercise programs for MPS, as it is vital to reset the muscle fiber length. Aerobic exercises have been found to increase endogenous pain control, improve mood, have additive effects with PT, and prevent recurrence of MPS.

Modalities such as spray and stretch technique involves the therapist passively stretching the target muscle while simultaneously applying a local soft tissue coolant. Chemicals such as dichlorodifluoromethane-trichloromonofluoromethane (Fluori-Methane) or ethyl chloride spray produce a drop in skin temperature, temporary anesthesia, theoretically blocking the spinal stretch reflex, and sensation of pain centrally. The muscle may then be passively stretched toward its normal length, inactivating trigger points, relieving spasm, and reducing referred pain.

Another commonly used modality, TENS, may be used for acute or chronic MFP. See "Electrical Stimulation" above. High-frequency, high-intensity TENS has been shown to reduce pain in MPS. High-power ultrasound applied to the trigger points before stretching was found to be more effective than conventional ultrasound and significantly decrease the length of therapy (Majlesi & Unalan, 2004). One study looked at the immediate effects of various physical therapeutic modalities on cervical myofascial pain and trigger-point sensitivity and found that hot pack plus active ROM plus interferential current plus myofascial release technique

Table 27.4. Myofascial Pain Syndrome Versus Fibromyalgia

Soft Tissue Pain Disorder	Myofascial Pain Syndrome (MPS)	Fibromyalgia (FM)
Points/Lesions Clinical sign	Myofascial Trigger Point (MTrP) • Local tenderness • Referred pain pattern • Trigger points • Pain in taut band of muscle • Local twitch response • "Jump sign" Male = Female	Tender Point (TP) • Local tenderness or • Diffuse pain for 3 months • Tender points • 11 of 18 symmetrical tender points are positive Female>Male
Gender Location	• Occur in any muscle • Asymmetric	• Specific locations: ○ Fat pad, epicondyle, joint, muscle insertion site, muscle • Symmetric
Associated Factors	• Acute tissue trauma • Repetitive microtrauma • Muscle deconditioning • Postural abnormalities • Sensitized nerve foci	• Insidious cause of pain • Increase in pain sensitivity • Sleep disturbance • Increase in catastrophizing • Decreased serotonin production

Fibromyalgia was once considered a "nonrestorative sleep syndrome," and evidence exists that those with FM do not obtain adequate amounts of restorative NREM sleep (Moldofsky, Scarisbrick, England, & Smythe, 1975), which may result from disorders of serotonin metabolism. Thus encouraging proper sleep hygiene and restoring proper levels of serotonin and NREM sleep is important in reducing pain and fatigue.

Physical medicine approaches to managing FMS include a comprehensive program incorporating a range of pharmacologic and nonpharmacologic strategies including active physical therapy, exercise, cognitive and behavioral treatments, and patient education (Goldenberg, Burckhardt, & Crofford, 2004; see Box 27.3). A recent study identified clusters of patients based on severity of TP tenderness, affective distress (depression and anxiety), and psychological traits (sense of self efficacy and catastrophizing) and may help classify individually the level of clinical intervention needed (Giesecke, Williams, Harris, et al., 2003).

Box 27.3. Stepwise Fibromyalgia Management

Step 1

• Confirm diagnosis.
• Explain the condition.
• Evaluate and treat comorbid illness, such as mood disturbance and primary sleep disturbances.

Step 2

• Start a trial of low-dose tricyclic antidepressant or cyclobenzaprine.
• Begin cardiovascular fitness exercise program.
• Refer for cognitive behavioral therapy or combine with exercise.

Step 3

• Provide a specialty referral (e.g., rheumatologist, physiatrist, psychiatrist, pain management).
• Begin trials with selective serotonin reuptake inhibitor, serotonin and norepinephrine reuptake inhibitor, or tramadol.
• Consider combination medication trial or anticonvulsant.

Source: Goldenberg, Burckhardt, & Crofford, 2004.

Pharmacological treatment is the mainstay of treatment of fibromyalgia focusing on achieving analgesia and improved mood and restorative sleep. Medicines are focused at modulating levels of serotonin, norepinephrine, and substance P. Tricyclic antidepressants amitriptyline and cyclobenzaprine, taken at night (Carette et al., 1994), as well as tramadol (Biasi, Manca, Manganelli, & Marcolongo, 1998) have been found to be effective. Serotonin reuptake inhibitors (SSRIs) are helpful, and fluoxetine has been found to decrease fatigue, depression, and pain (Arnold et al., 2002). Newer pharmacologic agents include serotonin norepinephrine dual-reuptake inhibitors (SNRIs), including venlafaxine and duloxetine, and pregabalin, an anticonvulsant and calcium channel modulator, may help to decrease central sensitization and have demonstrated efficacy in decreasing pain and improving sleep (Arnold et al., 2004; Goldenberg, Burckhardt, & Crofford, 2004; Sayar, Aksu, Ak, et al., 2003)

The pain and fatigue reported by individuals with fibromyalgia results in a relatively sedentary lifestyle, hence also a decrease in the fitness level of skeletal muscles. Low-intensity aerobic exercise regimens may be effective in reducing the number of tender points, total myalgic scores, reducing TP tenderness, as well as improving aerobic capacity, physical function, subjective well-being, and self-efficacy. Aerobic exercise also has been found to be better than stretching in decreasing depression, pain, and the emotional aspects and mental health domains of SF-36 (Valim et al., 2003).

FMS patients may have difficulty tolerating general exercise programs due to fatigue and muscle sensitivity. Gowans and deHueck (2004) recommend the following: (1) exercise should be initiated below patient's capacity and increased gradually, (2) patients should be aware of tolerable short-term increase in pain and fatigue after initiating exercise, and (3) capacity to exercise should be increased over time, with similar or lower levels of pain.

Pool therapy has been found to improve cardiovascular capacity, walking time, and number of days of feeling good, and reduce self-reported physical impairment, pain, anxiety, depression, and daytime fatigue in those with FM (Jentoft, Kvalvik, & Mengshoel, 2001).

Cognitive behavioral therapy (CBT) has been found to reduce pain and fatigue, and to improve mood and function in FMS (Rossy et al., 1999). In general, CBT includes three treatment components (educational phase, skills training, and application phase) focusing on changes in negative perceptions of pain, improved coping and relaxation strategy training, and relapse prevention (F. Keefe, 1996). Greater benefits of CBT may be found when used adjunctively with exercise and other active treatments (Williams, 2003).

Multidisciplinary, tertiary, center-based outpatient programs have also been found to be beneficial in patients with FM incorporating structured multimodal treatment (pharmacologic management, physical therapy and exercise, psychological treatment, and education; Buckelew et al., 1998). A recent review found multidisciplinary approaches effective for decreasing pain, decreasing impact of FMS, and increasing self-efficacy and walk time (Burckhardt, 2006). Pfeiffer et al. examined a 1.5-day multidisciplinary treatment program incorporating educational and self-management sessions, physical and occupational therapy, and medical management demonstrating a positive effect on impact of illness in FMS patients with and without concomitant depression (Pfeiffer, Thompson, Nelson, et al., 2003).

In general, when compared to pharmacological treatment, nonpharmacological treatment appears to be more efficacious in improving self-report of FMS symptoms than pharmacological treatment alone (Rossy et al., 1999).

Conclusion

A physical medicine and rehabilitation approach to acute and chronic pain syndromes includes a wide spectrum of treatment focus. Whether assessing or treating acute or chronic pain syndromes, management should include a biopsychosocial approach. Assessment may include a focused joint and functional exam including more global areas of impairment (i.e., gait, balance, and endurance) and disability. More complicated multidimensional chronic pain conditions may require the use of a more collaborative interdisciplinary approach. Treatment options may include active physical therapy, rational polypharmacy, cognitive behavioral therapy, and the use of passive modalities. Treatment goals generally emphasize achieving analgesia, improving psychosocial functioning, and reintegration of recreational or leisure pursuits (i.e., community activities and sports). Progress in all therapies necessitates close monitoring by the health-care provider and necessitates ongoing communication among members of the treatment team. Although this chapter focused on diagnoses related to acute and chronic low back pain, osteoarthritis, and musculoskeletal disorders (myofascial pain and fibromyalgia), assessment and treatment recommendations may be generalized to most other pain conditions.

References

Abenhaim, L., Rossignol, M., Valat, J. P., Nordin, M., Avouac, B., Blotman, F., et al. (2000). The role of activity in the therapeutic management of back pain. Report of the International Paris Task Force on Back Pain. *Spine, 25*(4 Suppl), 1S–33S.

Aina, A., May, S., & Clare, H. (2004). The centralization phenomenon of spinal symptoms—a systematic review. *Man Ther, 9*(3), 134–143.

Akuthota, V., & Nadler, S. F. (2004). Core strengthening. *Arch Phys Med Rehabil, 85*(3 Suppl 1), S86–92.

American College of Sports Medicine. (2002). *American College of Sports Medicine (ACSM) guidelines for exercise testing and prescription.* (6th ed.). Philadelphia, PA: Lippincott Williams and Wilkins.

Andersson, G. B., Lucente, T., Davis, A. M., Kappler, R. E., Lipton, J. A., & Leurgans, S. (1999). A comparison of osteopathic spinal manipulation with standard care for patients with low back pain. *N Engl J Med, 341*(19), 1426–1431.

Anstey, K., & Roskell, C. (2000). Hydrotherapy: Detrimental or beneficial to the respiratory system? *Physiotherapy 86,* 5–12.

Ariyoshi, M., Sonoda, K., Nagata, K., Mashima, T., Zenmyo, M., Paku, C., et al. (1999). Efficacy of aquatic exercises for patients with low-back pain. *Kurume Med J, 46*(2), 91–96.

Arnold, L. M., Hess, E. V., Hudson, J. I., Welge, J. A., Berno, S. E., & Keck, P. E., Jr. (2002). A randomized, placebo-controlled, double-blind, flexible-dose study of fluoxetine in the treatment of women with fibromyalgia. *Am J Med, 112*(3), 191–197.

Arnold, L. M., Lu, Y., Crofford, L. J., Wohlreich, M., Detke, M. J., Iyengar, S., et al. (2004). A double-blind, multicenter trial comparing duloxetine with placebo in the treatment of fibromyalgia patients with or without major depressive disorder. *Arthritis Rheum, 50*(9), 2974–2984.

Assendelft, W. J., Morton, S. C., Yu, E. I., Suttorp, M. J., & Shekelle, P. G. (2003). Spinal manipulative therapy for low back pain. A meta-analysis of effectiveness relative to other therapies. *Ann Intern Med, 138*(11), 871–881.

Audette, J., Wang, F., & Smith H. (2004). Bilateral activation of motor unit potentials with unilateral needle stimulation of active myofascial trigger points. *Am J Phys Med Rehabil 83,* 368–374.

Balzini, L., Vannucchi, L., Benvenuti, F., Benucci, M., Monni, M., Cappozzo, A., et al. (2003). Clinical characteristics of flexed posture in elderly women. *Journal of the American Geriatrics Society, 51*(10), 1419–1426.

Baron, R. A. (2002). *Social psychology* (10th ed.). Boston: Allyn and Bacon.

Barr, K. P., Griggs, M., & Cadby, T. (2005). Lumbar stabilization: Core concepts and current literature, Part 1. *Am J Phys Med Rehabil, 84*(6), 473–480.

Bergmark, A. (1989). Stability of the lumbar spine. A study in mechanical engineering. *Acta Orthopaedica Scandinavica Supplementum, 230,* 1–54.

Biasi, G., Manca, S., Manganelli, S., & Marcolongo, R. (1998). Tramadol in the fibromyalgia syndrome: A controlled clinical trial versus placebo. *Int J Clin Pharmacol Res, 18*(1), 13–19.

Birmingham, T. B., Kramer, J. F., Kirkley, A., Inglis, J. T., Spaulding, S. J., & Vandervoort, A. A. (2001). Knee bracing after ACL reconstruction: Effects on postural control and proprioception. *Med Sci Sports Exerc, 33*(8), 1253–1258.

Blumenfeld, A. (2003). Botulinum toxin type A as an effective prophylactic treatment in primary headache disorders. *Headache 43*(8), 853–860.

Borrell, R. M., Parker, R., Henley, E. J., Masley, D., & Repinecz, M. (1980). Comparison of in vivo temperatures produced by hydrotherapy, paraffin wax treatment, and Fluidotherapy. *Phys Ther, 60*(10), 1273–1276.

Bradely, L., Sotolongo, A., Alberts, K., et al. (1999). Abnormal regional cerebral blood flow in the caudate nucleus among fibromyalgia patients and non-patients is associated with insidious symptom onset. *J Musculoskeletal Pain 7,* 285–292.

Bradley, L., Weigent, D., Sotolongo, A., et al. (2000). Blood serum levels of nitric oxide (NO) are elevated in women with fibromyalgia (FM): Possible contributions to central and peripheral sensitization. *Arthritis Rheum, 43,* S173.

Brouwer, R. W., Jakma, T. S., Verhagen, A. P., Verhaar, J. A., & Bierma-Zeinstra, S. M. (2005). Braces and orthoses for treating osteoarthritis of the knee. *Cochrane Database Syst Rev*(1), CD004020.

Bruce, B., Fries, J. F., & Lubeck, D. P. (2005). Aerobic exercise and its impact on musculoskeletal pain in older adults: A 14 year prospective, longitudinal study. *Arthritis Res Ther, 7*(6), R1263–1270.

Brukner, P., & Kahn, K. (2001). *Clinical sports medicine* (2nd ed.). New York: McGraw Hill.

Buckelew, S. P., Conway, R., Parker, J., Deuser, W. E., Read, J., Witty, T. E., et al. (1998). Biofeedback/relaxation training and exercise interventions for fibromyalgia: A prospective trial. *Arthritis Care Res, 11*(3), 196–209.

Bunning, R. D., & Materson, R. S. (1991). A rational program of exercise for patients with osteoarthritis. *Semin Arthritis Rheum, 21*(3 Suppl 2), 33–43.

Burckhardt, C. (2006). Multidisciplinary approaches for management of fibromyalgia. *Current Pharmaceutical Design, 12,* 59–66

Butler, D. (2000). *The sensitive nervous system.* Australia: Noigroup Publications.

Carette, S., Bell, M. J., Reynolds, W. J., Haraoui, B., McCain, G. A., Bykerk, V. P., et al. (1994). Comparison of amitriptyline, cyclobenzaprine, and placebo in the treatment of fibromyalgia. A randomized, double-blind clinical trial. *Arthritis Rheum, 37*(1), 32–40.

Cherkin, D. C., Eisenberg, D., Sherman, K. J., Barlow, W., Kaptchuk, T. J., Street, J., et al. (2001). Randomized trial comparing traditional Chinese medical acupuncture, therapeutic massage, and self-care education for chronic low back pain. *Arch Intern Med, 161*(8), 1081–1088.

Cholewicki, J., & McGill, S. M. (1992). Lumbar posterior ligament involvement during extremely heavy lifts estimated from fluoroscopic measurements. *J Biomech, 25*(1), 17–28.

Choukroun, M., Kays, C., & Varene, P. (1989). Effects of water temperature on pulmonary volumes in immersed human subjects. *Respir Physiol 75*, 255–266.

Cohen, I., & Rainville, J. (2002). Aggressive exercise as treatment for chronic low back pain. *Sports Med, 32*(1), 75–82.

DeLee, J. C., Drez, D., Jr., & Miller, M. D. (2003). *DeLee and Drez's orthopaedic sports medicine* (2nd ed.). Philadelphia: Saunders.

Delitto, A., Cibulka, M. T., Erhard, R. E., Bowling, R. W., & Tenhula, J. A. (1993). Evidence for use of an extension-mobilization category in acute low back syndrome: A prescriptive validation pilot study. *Phys Ther, 73*(4), 216–222; discussion 213–218.

Deyle, G. D., Henderson, N. E., Matekel, R. L., Ryder, M. G., Garber, M. B., & Allison, S. C. (2000). Effectiveness of manual physical therapy and exercise in osteoarthritis of the knee. A randomized, controlled trial. *Ann Intern Med, 132*(3), 173–181.

Erhard, R. E., Delitto, A., & Cibulka, M. T. (1994). Relative effectiveness of an extension program and a combined program of manipulation and flexion and extension exercises in patients with acute low back syndrome. *Phys Ther, 74*(12), 1093–1100.

Ernst, E. (1999). Massage therapy for low back pain. *Journal of Pain and Symptom Management, 17*.

Ettinger, W. H., Jr., Burns, R., Messier, S. P., Applegate, W., Rejeski, W. J., Morgan, T., et al. (1997). A randomized trial comparing aerobic exercise and resistance exercise with a health education program in older adults with knee osteoarthritis. The Fitness Arthritis and Seniors Trial (FAST). *JAMA, 277*(1), 25–31.

Farrell, P. A., Gates, W. K., Maksud, M. G., & Morgan, W. P. (1982). Increases in plasma beta-endorphin/beta-lipotropin immunoreactivity after treadmill running in humans. *J Appl Physiol, 52*(5), 1245–1249.

Fedorak, C., Ashworth, N., Marshall, J., & Paull, H. (2003). Reliability of the visual assessment of cervical and lumbar lordosis: How good are we? *Spine, 28*(16), 1857–1859.

Ferreira, M. L., Ferreira, P. H., Latimer, J., Herbert, R., & Maher, C. G. (2002). Does spinal manipulative therapy help people with chronic low back pain? *Aust J Physiother, 48*(4), 277–284.

Fritz, J. M., Delitto, A., Vignovic, M., & Busse, R. G. (2000). Interrater reliability of judgments of the centralization phenomenon and status change during movement testing in patients with low back pain. *Arch Phys Med Rehabil, 81*(1), 57–61.

Furlan, A., Brosseau, L., Imamura, M., & Irvin, E. (2003). Massage for low back pain: A systematic review. Cochrane Review, *J Pain Symptom Manage:* Update Software.

Gard, G. (2005). Body awareness therapy for patients with fibromyalgia and chronic pain. *Disabil Rehabil, 27*(12), 725–728.

Geisser, M., Wiggert, E., Haig, A., & Colwell, M. (2005). A randomized, controlled trial of manual therapy and specific adjuvant exercise for chronic low back pain. *Clin J Pain, 21*, 463–470.

Geisser, M. E., Casey, K. L., Brucksch, C. B., Ribbens, C. M., Appleton, B. B., & Crofford, L. J. (2003). Perception of noxious and innocuous heat stimulation among healthy women and women with fibromyalgia: Association with mood, somatic focus, and catastrophizing. *Pain, 102*(3), 243–250.

Giesecke, T., Williams, D., Harris, R., et al. (2003). Subgrouping of fibromyalgia patients on the basis of pressure-pain thresholds and psychological factors. *Arthritis Rheum, 48*, 2916–2922.

Goldenberg, D., Burckhardt, C., & Crofford, L. (2004). Management of fibromyalgia syndrome. *JAMA, 292*, 2388–2395.

Gowans, S., & deHueck, A. (2004). Effectiveness of exercise in management of fibromyalgia. *Curr Opin Rheumatol 16*, 138–142.

Greenman, P. (1996). *Principles of manual medicine* (2nd ed.). Baltimore, MD: Williams and Wilkins.

Grossman, A., & Sutton, J. R. (1985). Endorphins: What are they? How are they measured? What is their role in exercise? *Med Sci Sports Exerc, 17*(1), 74–81.

Haldeman, S. (1989). *Manipulation and message for the relief of pain.* New York: Churchill Livingstone.

Han, S. C., & Harrison, P. (1997). Myofascial pain syndrome and trigger-point management. *Reg Anesth, 22*(1), 89–101.

Hayden, J. A., van Tulder, M. W., Malmivaara, A., & Koes, B. W. (2005). Exercise therapy for treatment of non-specific low back pain. *Cochrane Database Syst Rev*(3), CD000335.

Hernandez-Reif, M., Field, T., Krasnegor, J., & Theakston, H. (2001). Lower back pain is reduced and range of motion increased after massage therapy. *Int J Neurosci, 106*, 131–145.

Hides, J. (2004). *Paraspinal mechanism and support of the lumbar spine.* Edinburgh, Scotland: Churchill Livingstone.

Hong, C. (1994). Lidocaine injection versus dry needling to myofascial trigger point. The importance of the local twitch response. *Am J Phys Med Rehabil, 73*, 256–263.

Hou, C. R., Tsai, L. C., Cheng, K. F., Chung, K. C., & Hong, C. Z. (2002). Immediate effects of various physical therapeutic modalities on cervical myofascial pain and trigger-point sensitivity. *Arch Phys Med Rehabil, 83*(10), 1406–1414.

Hreljac, A. (2005). Etiology, prevention, and early intervention of overuse injuries in runners: A biomechanical perspective. *Phys Med Rehabil Clin N Am, 16*(3), 651–667, vi.

Hurwitz, E. L., Morgenstern, H., & Chiao, C. (2005). Effects of recreational physical activity and back exercises on low back pain and psychological distress: Findings from the UCLA low back pain study. *Am J Public Health, 95*(10), 1817–1824.

Janda, V. (1994). *Muscles and motor control in cervicogenic disorders: Assessment and management.* New York: Churchill Livingstone.

Jentoft, E. S., Kvalvik, A. G., & Mengshoel, A. M. (2001). Effects of pool-based and land-based aerobic exercise on women with fibromyalgia/chronic widespread muscle pain. *Arthritis Rheum, 45*(1), 42–47.

Jull, G. A., & Janda, V. (1987). *Muscles and motor control in low back pain: Assessment and management.* New York: Churchill Livingstone

Kamanli, A., Kaya, A., Ardicoglu, O., Ozgocmen, S., Zengin, F. O., & Bayik, Y. (2005). Comparison of lidocaine injection, botulinum toxin injection, and dry needling to trigger points in myofascial pain syndrome. *Rheumatol Int, 25*(8), 604–611.

Keefe, F. (1996). Cognitive behavioral therapy for managing pain. *Clin Psychologist, 49*, 4–5.

Keefe, F. J., Block, A. R., Williams, R. B., Jr., & Surwit, R. S. (1981). Behavioral treatment of chronic low back pain: Clinical outcome and individual differences in pain relief. *Pain, 11*(2), 221–231.

Keller, A., Brox J. I., Gunderson, R., Holm, I., Friis, A., & Reikeras, O. (2003). Trunk muscle strength, cross-sectional area, and density in patients with chronic low back pain randomized to lumbar fusion or cognitive intervention and exercises. *Spine J, 29*, 3–8.

Kibler, W. B. (1998). *Determining the extent of the functional deficit.* Gaithersburg, MD: Aspen Publishers.

King, E. W., Audette, K., Athman, G. A., Nguyen, H. O., Sluka, K. A., & Fairbanks, C. A. (2005). Transcutaneous electrical nerve stimulation activates peripherally located alpha-2A adrenergic receptors. *Pain, 115*(3), 364–373.

Komistek, R. D., Dennis, D. A., Northcut, E. J., Wood, A., Parker, A. W., & Traina, S. M. (1999). An in vivo analysis of the effectiveness of the osteoarthritic knee brace during heel-strike of gait. *J Arthroplasty, 14*(6), 738–742.

Laasonen, E. M. (1984). Atrophy of sacrospinal muscle groups in patients with chronic, diffusely radiating lumbar back pain. *Neuroradiology, 26*(1), 9–13.

Larsen, J. (1999). Current considerations in pain management for the patient with fibromyalgia syndrome. *Pharm Times, 66*, 2HPT–6HPT.

Larson, A., Giovengo, S., Russell, I., et al. (2000). Changes in the concentrations of amino acids in the cerebrospinal fluid that correlate with pain in patients with fibromyalgia: Implications for nitric oxide pathways. *Pain and Headache, 87*, 201–211.

Lehmann, J. F., Silverman, D. R., Baum, B. A., Kirk, N. L., & Johnston, V. C. (1966). Temperature distributions in the human thigh, produced by infrared, hot pack and microwave applications. *Arch Phys Med Rehabil, 47*(5), 291–299.

Liddle, S. D., Baxter, G. D., & Gracey, J. H. (2004). Exercise and chronic low back pain: What works? *Pain, 107*(1–2), 176–190.

Lindstrom, I., Ohlund, C., Eek, C., Wallin, L., Peterson, L. E., & Nachemson, A. (1992). Mobility, strength, and fitness after a graded activity program for patients with subacute low back pain. A randomized prospective clinical study with a behavioral therapy approach. *Spine, 17*(6), 641–652.

Linton, S. J. (2000). A review of psychological risk factors in back and neck pain. *Spine, 25*(9), 1148–1156.

Magee, D. J. (2002). *Orthopedic physical assessment* (4th ed.). Philadelphia: W. B. Saunders.

Maitland, G. (1985). The slump test: Examination and treatment. *The Australian Journal of Physiotherapy, 31*, 215–219.

Majlesi, J., & Unalan, H. (2004). High-power pain threshold ultrasound technique in the treatment of active myofascial trigger points: A randomized, double-blind, case-control study. *Arch Phys Med Rehabil, 85*(5), 833–836.

Malmgren-Olsson, E. B., & Branholm, I. B. (2002). A comparison between three physiotherapy approaches with regard to health-related factors in patients with non-specific musculoskeletal disorders. *Disabil Rehabil, 24*(6), 308–317.

Malmivaara, A., Hakkinen, U., Aro, T., Heinrichs, M. L., Koskenniemi, L., Kuosma, E., et al. (1995). The treatment of acute low back pain—bed rest, exercises, or ordinary activity? *N Engl J Med, 332*(6), 351–355.

Mangione, K. K., McCully, K., Gloviak, A., Lefebvre, I., Hofmann, M., & Craik, R. (1999). The effects of high-intensity and low-intensity cycle ergometry in older adults with knee osteoarthritis. *J Gerontol A Biol Sci Med Sci, 54*(4), M184–190.

Mannion, A. F., Junge, A., Taimela, S., Muntener, M., Lorenzo, K., & Dvorak, J. (2001). Active therapy for chronic low back pain: Part 3. Factors influencing self-rated disability and its change following therapy. *Spine, 26*(8), 920–929.

McAuley, E., Lox, C., & Duncan, T. E. (1993). Long-term maintenance of exercise, self-efficacy, and physiological change in older adults. *J Gerontol, 48*(4), P218–224.

McCahon, S., Strong, J., Sharry, R., & Cramond, T. (2005). Self-report and pain behavior among patients with chronic pain. *Clin J Pain, 21*(3), 223–231.

McKenzie, R. (1981). *The lumbar spine. Mechanical diagnosis and therapy.* Waikanae, New Zealand: Spinal Publications.

McNulty, W. H., Gevirtz, R. N., Hubbard, D. R., & Berkoff, G. M. (1994). Needle electromyographic evaluation of trigger point response to a psychological stressor. *Psychophysiology, 31*(3), 313–316.

Melzack, R., & Wall, P. (1965). Pain Mechanisms: A new theory. *Science and Justice, 150*, 971–979.

Moldofsky, H., Scarisbrick, P., England, R., & Smythe, H. (1975). Musculoskeletal symptoms and non-REM sleep disturbance in patients with "fibrositis syndrome" and healthy subjects. *Psychosom Med, 37*(4), 341–351.

Mooney, V. (1987). Impairment, disability, and handicap. *Clinical Orthopaedics & Related Research, 221*, 14–25.

Nicassio, P. M., Radojevic, V., Weisman, M. H., Schuman, C., Kim, J., Schoenfeld-Smith, K., et al. (1997). A comparison of behavioral and educational interventions for fibromyalgia. *J Rheumatol, 24*(10), 2000–2007.

Ogata, K., Yasunaga, M., & Nomiyama, H. (1997). The effect of wedged insoles on the thrust of osteoarthritic knees. *Int Orthop, 21*(5), 308–312.

Osiri, M., Welch, V., Brosseau, L., Shea, B., McGowan, J., Tugwell, P., et al. (2000). Transcutaneous electrical nerve stimulation for knee osteoarthritis. *Cochrane Database Syst Rev*(4), CD002823.

O'Sullivan, P. B., Phyty, G. D., Twomey, L. T., & Allison, G. T. (1997). Evaluation of specific stabilizing exercise in the treatment of chronic low back pain with radiologic diagnosis of spondylolysis or spondylolisthesis. *Spine, 22*(24), 2959–2967.

Padberg, M., de Bruijn, S. F., de Haan, R. J., Tavy, D. L. (2004). Treatment of chronic tension-type headache with botulinum toxin: A double-blind, placebo-controlled clinical trial. *Cephalalgia, 24*(8), 675–680.

Padberg, M., de Haan, R., & Tavy, D. (2004). Treatment of chronic tension-type headache with botulinum toxin: A double-blind, placebo-controlled clinical trial. *Cephalgia, 24,* 675.

Panjabi, M. M. (1992). The stabilizing system of the spine. Part I. Function, dysfunction, adaptation, and enhancement. *Journal of Spinal Disorders, 5*(4), 383–389; discussion 397.

Pfeiffer, A., Thompson, J., Nelson, A., et al. (2003). Effects of a 1.5-day multidisciplinary outpatient treatment program for fibromyalgia: A pilot study. *Am J Phys Med Rehabil 82*, 186–191.

Porta, M. (2000). A comparative trial of botulinum toxin type A and methylprednisolone for the treatment of myofascial pain syndrome and pain from chronic muscle spasm *Pain, 85,* 101–105.

Rachlin, E. (1994). Trigger points. In E. Rachlin (Ed.), *Myofascial pain and fibromyalgia: Trigger point management* (pp. 145–157). St. Louis, MO: Mosby.

Rainville, J., Ahern, D. K., & Phalen, L. (1993). Altering beliefs about pain and impairment in a functionally oriented treatment program for chronic low back pain. *Clin J Pain, 9*(3), 196–201.

Redford, J., Basmajian, J., & Trautman, P. (1995). *Orthotics: Clinical practice and rehabilitation technology.* New York: Churchill Livingstone, Inc.

Richardson C, Jull, G. A., Hodges, P., & Hides, J. (1999). *Therapeutic exercises for spinal stabilization and low back pain: Scientific bases and clinical approach.* Edinburgh, Scotland: Churchill Livingstone.

Roddy, E., Zhang, W., & Doherty, M. (2005). Aerobic walking or strengthening exercise for osteoarthritis of the knee? A systematic review. *Ann Rheum Dis, 64*(4), 544–548.

Ross, M. C., Bohannon, A. S., Davis, D. C., & Gurchiek, L. (1999). The effects of a short-term exercise program on movement, pain, and mood in the elderly. Results of a pilot study. *J Holist Nurs, 17*(2), 139–147.

Rossy, L. A., Buckelew, S. P., Dorr, N., Hagglund, K. J., Thayer, J. F., McIntosh, M. J., et al. (1999). A meta-analysis of fibromyalgia treatment interventions. *Ann Behav Med, 21*(2), 180–191.

Russell, I., Orr, M. D., Littman, B., et al. (1994). Elevated cerebrospinal fluid levels of substance P in patients with the fibromyalgia syndrome. *G Bacteriol Virol Immunol [Microbiol], 37,* 1593–1601.

Sahrmann, S. A. (2002). Does postural assessment contribute to patient care? [Comment]. *Journal of Orthopaedic & Sports Physical Therapy, 32*(8), 376–379.

Sayar, K., Aksu, G., Ak, I., et al. (2003). Venlafaxine treatment of fibromyalgia. *Ann of Pharmacother, 37,* 1561–1565

Sharma, L., Song, J., Felson, D. T., Cahue, S., Shamiyeh, E., & Dunlop, D. D. (2001). The role of knee alignment in disease progression and functional decline in knee osteoarthritis. *JAMA, 286*(2), 188–195.

Simons, D., & Travell, J. (1999). *Myofascial pain and dysfunction: The trigger point manual* (2nd ed.). Baltimore: Williams & Wilkins.

Slemenda, C., Brandt, K. D., Heilman, D. K., Mazzuca, S., Braunstein, E. M., Katz, B. P., et al. (1997). Quadriceps weakness and osteoarthritis of the knee. *Ann Intern Med, 127*(2), 97–104.

Slemenda, C., Heilman, D. K., Brandt, K. D., Katz, B. P., Mazzuca, S. A., Braunstein, E. M., et al. (1998). Reduced quadriceps strength relative to body weight: A risk factor for knee osteoarthritis in women? *Arthritis Rheum, 41*(11), 1951–1959.

Song, R., Lee, E. O., Lam, P., & Bae, S. C. (2003). Effects of tai chi exercise on pain, balance, muscle strength, and perceived difficulties in physical functioning in older women with osteoarthritis: A randomized clinical trial. *J Rheumatol, 30*(9), 2039–2044.

Sundaraj, R., Ponciano, P., Johnstone, C., et al. (2004). Treatment of chronic refractory intractable headache with botulinum toxin type A: A retrospective study. *Pain Practice, 4,* 229.

Suomi, R., & Collier, D. (2003). Effects of arthritis exercise programs on functional fitness and perceived activities of daily living measures in older adults with arthritis. *Arch Phys Med Rehabil, 84*(11), 1589–1594.

Suomi, R., & Koceja, D. M. (2000). Postural sway characteristics in women with lower extremity arthritis before and after an aquatic exercise intervention. *Arch Phys Med Rehabil, 81*(6), 780–785.

Taimela, S., Diederich, C., Hubsch, M., & Heinricy, M. (2000). The role of physical exercise and inactivity in pain recurrence and absenteeism from work after active outpatient rehabilitation for recurrent or chronic low back pain: A follow-up study. *Spine, 25*(14), 1809–1816.

Turk, D. C., Wack, J. T., & Kerns, R. D. (1985). An empirical examination of the "pain-behavior" construct. *J Behav Med., 8,* 119–130.

Valim, V., Oliveira, L., Suda, A., Silva, L., de Assis, M., Barros Neto, T., et al. (2003). Aerobic fitness effects in fibromyalgia. *J Rheumatol, 30*(5), 1060–1069.

van Baar, M. E., Dekker, J., Oostendorp, R. A., Bijl, D., Voorn, T. B., & Bijlsma, J. W. (2001). Effectiveness of exercise in patients with osteoarthritis of hip or knee: Nine months' follow up. *Ann Rheum Dis, 60*(12), 1123–1130.

van Baar, M. E., Dekker, J., Oostendorp, R. A., Bijl, D., Voorn, T. B., Lemmens, J. A., et al. (1998). The effectiveness of exercise therapy in patients with osteoarthritis of the hip or knee: A randomized clinical trial. *J Rheumatol, 25*(12), 2432–2439.

Van der Esch, M., Heijmans, M., & Dekker, J. (2003). Factors contributing to possession and use of walking aids among persons with rheumatoid arthritis and osteoarthritis. *Arthritis Rheum, 49*(6), 838–842.

van de Veen, E., de Vet, H., Pool, J., Schuller, W., de Zoete, A., & Bouter, L. (2005). Variance in manual treatment of nonspecific low back pain between orthomanual physicians, manual therapists, and chiropractors. *J Manipulative Physiol Ther, 28,* 108–116.

van Tulder, M., Malmivaara, A., Esmail, R., & Koes, B. (2000). Exercise therapy for low back pain: A systematic review within the framework of the Cochrane collaboration back review group. *Spine, 25*(21), 2784–2796.

Waddell, G., & Main, C. J. (1998). *Illness behavior.* Edinburgh, Scotland: Churchill Livingstone.

Watelain, E., Froger, J., Barbier, F., Lensel, G., Rousseaux, M., Lepoutre, F.-X., et al. (2003). Comparison of clinical gait analysis strategies by French neurologists, physiatrists and physiotherapists. *Journal of Rehabilitation Medicine, 35*(1), 8–14.

Werneke, M., & Hart, D. L. (2001). Centralization phenomenon as a prognostic factor for chronic low back pain and disability. *Spine, 26*(7), 758–764; discussion 765.

Wetzel, F. T., & Donelson, R. (2003). The role of repeated end-range/pain response assessment in the management of symptomatic lumbar discs. *Spine J, 3*(2), 146–154.

Wheeler, A., Goolkasian, P., & Gretz, S. (1998). A randomized, double-blind, prospective pilot study of botulinum toxin injection for refractory, unilateral, cervicothoracic, paraspinal, myofascial pain syndrome. *Spine, 23,* 1662–1666.

White, M. A., & Pape, K. E. (1992). The slump test. *Am J Occup Ther, 46*(3), 271–274.

Williams, D. (2003). Psychological and behavioral therapies in fibromyalgia and related syndromes. *Best Pract Res Clin Rheum 17,* 649–665.

Wolfe, F., Smythe, H., Yunus, M., et al. (1990). The American College of Rheumatology 1990 criteria for the classification of fibromyalgia: Report of the Multicenter Criteria Committee. *Arthritis Rheum., 33,* 160–172.

28

Interventional Pain Medicine

Michel Y. Dubois

Roshni Patel

Interventional pain medicine is an important part of pain management. Although there are many interventional approaches available for treating pain (Box 28.1), the expression "interventional pain medicine" is usually reserved for all procedures done with the use of a needle. Nerve blocks, a prime example, have been used for more than a century for both diagnostic and therapeutic purposes. Many minimally invasive interventions may be effective in diagnosing or managing chronic pain from a variety of sources. Performing these procedures requires an understanding of the relevant anatomy, physiology, and pharmacology, as well as the ability to interpret the results. Most of these techniques should be practiced only after special advanced training.

The efficacy of interventional pain techniques is related to the chemical or physical interruption of the nociceptive afferent, but such intervention also usually affects the afferent limb of the abnormal pathophysiology mechanism, which is a source of chronic pain. The intervention may, therefore, provide long-lasting relief. Although diagnostic regional anesthesia procedures can be applied to every peripheral and central nervous structure, interventional pain techniques can be particularly useful for common conditions, such as neck and back pain, complex regional pain syndrome, and cancer and acute pain. Injection of a variety of substances (local anesthetics, opioids, alpha-2 adrenergic, GABA-agonists, etc.) or the use of physical modalities (heat, neurolytic chemicals, electrostimulation, cold, etc.) are some of the techniques utilized in pain management.

The use of interventional pain medicine in the chemically dependent patient carries some specific caveats. If the patient is actively drug seeking, he/she will not readily accept the prospect of an intervention to take care of the pain problem. This resistance can become a major obstacle to a comprehensive treatment. To avoid exacerbating the problem, one should explain to the patient that interventional pain medicine is one of the modalities of multidisciplinary pain management and may help the patient's overall functioning. Associated and significant psychopathology, examined in the other part of the book, is not rare in the chemically dependent patient. One should be particularly cautious in the use of interventional pain medicine in a patient with psychiatric co-morbidity, such as somatization disorder, untreated depression, or borderline personality disorders. The decision as to the timing and the type of intervention should be the result of a consensus decision made within an interdisciplinary pain management group.

Neural Blockade in Chronic Spinal Pain

Chronic spinal pain, especially low back pain, affects approximately 90% of the adult population in the United States and is usually experienced as a time-limited acute episode, which, in 90% of the cases, will resolve spontaneously, regardless of therapy. The remaining 10%, however, represents one of the greatest challenges in pain medicine. The primary difficulty is that back pain may arise from multiple origins. In addition, in most patients with chronic spinal pain, the source of the pain generator cannot, most often, be precisely identified. Any or all the spinal structures that can contribute to spinal pain (intervertebral disc, facet joint, posterior longitudinal ligament, nerve root, dura, ligamentum flavum, ligaments and muscles) can be (individually, or often in combination) the origin of spinal pain. Generally, patients with spinal pain who have not improved in the first month of conservative therapy, those using medication and physical therapy, patients who have a significant functional impact from their pain, and patients who cannot tolerate medications or effective physical rehabilitation all are potential candidates for neurospinal blockade.

The *pro and cons for neural blockade* are listed in Box 28.2. An important argument for the use of neural blockade is its function as a *diagnostic tool*. It helps to substantiate the suspected etiology and precise location of the pain. It completes an array of diagnostic tests used in the workup of chronic back pain patients, such as electrodiagnostic and imaging studies (MRI, CT, EMG, plain films, etc.). It is usually essential for the diagnosis, when perfor-

> **Box 28.1. "Interventions" for Treating Pain**
>
> - Pharmacotherapy
> - Rehabilitative approaches
> - Psychological approaches
> - Interventional pain techniques
> - Surgical approaches
> - Neurostimulatory approaches
> - Complementary and alternative approaches
> - Lifestyle changes

> **Box 28.2. Neural Blockade: Pros and Cons**
>
> - Is a lesser invasive pain management technique
> - Can be used as a diagnostic tool
> - Provides pain relief
> - Allows other treatment modalities
> - Requires special expertise and facilities
> - May not provide prolonged relief
> - Has the potential for abuse

ming most spinal diagnostic injections, to use a fluoroscopically guided technique, which allows anatomic precision. If local anesthetics are used to help in diagnosis, the use of a limited volume of injectate is essential in order to maintain the specificity of the test (i.e., if too large of a volume is given, the whole region, not just a single nerve, becomes anesthetized). In some cases, such as a discogram procedure, the provocative component while injecting and the analgesia following local anesthetic injection are both helpful diagnostic aids.

The *therapeutic value* of interventions can be explained by several mechanisms. One is the antiinflammatory effect of steroids, which also have a direct inhibitory effect on unmyelinated C-fibers. Another mechanism is the irrigative effect of an injection around the site, for instance, a ruptured disc that was releasing highly irritating chemicals. Another mechanism is the central modulation of the afferent nociceptive signals through either spinal cord stimulation or medications applied directly around the neuraxis itself.

Peripheral Blocks

Peripheral nerves, tendons, joints, and muscles can be readily injected, usually safely, using aseptic techniques, and sometimes under control of fluoroscope. One of the most common interventions is the *trigger-point injection* in myofascial pain, a soft tissue disorder that creates pain in tender areas within muscle groups. The diagnosis is made upon determining a clinical trigger point on examination. These trigger points are usually in a taut band of muscle that may produce referred pain and be extremely painful and disabling. Dry needling or injections with 1% lidocaine at the location of the trigger point may relieve this condition, temporarily or more permanently. In some select cases and in limited quantity, botulinum toxin injections have also been successful. Following pain relief, physical therapy is essential as part of the treatment to avoid recurrence of the condition. Muscle trigger points can frequently be misdiagnosed as common orthopedic conditions (Rachlin, 1994). Trigger points in a neck muscle may simulate pain from a cervical disc, or bicipital tendonitis can create an arm pain which may appear to arise from a radiculitis. Temporal, masseter, and occipital trigger points can be mistaken for cervical arthritis. It is therefore extremely important to examine patients having one of these complaints carefully and to find out whether simple trigger point muscle injections may solve complex clinical complaints.

Spinal Joints

Zygapophysial Joints

Anatomy

The facet joint (zygapophysial articulation) is formed by the superior articular facet of the vertebrae below and the inferior articular facet of the above adjacent vertebrae. The joint is lined by synovium and covered by hyaline cartilage. The joint capsule has a superior and inferior recess.

The facet joint is innervated by the dorsal ramus, which sends branches to its corresponding level and one level below. So each facet joint is innervated by two dorsal rami.

The anatomy of the cervical region is different from the thoracic region, and both differ from the lumbar region. In the cervical region, the facets extend laterally from the lamina and pedicle. In the thoracic region, the facet joint extends superior inferior from the lamina and pedicle. In the lumbar region, the facets extend concave posteriorly, and convex anteriorly.

Facet Joint Syndrome

Facet joint syndrome may result from occupational injury, trauma, whiplash, and degenerative changes related to aging. Pain of the thoracolumbar region facet joint may present with spasms of ipsilateral paraspinal muscles, pain on axial rotation, and hyperextension. Pain of the cervical facet joints may present with pain upon flexion, hyperextension, or lateral rotation of the head, with pain radiating into the cervical muscles and shoulders (Clemans & Benzon, 2005). The pain is usually described as an aching. The most common region associated with the facet joint is the lumbar region, with the pain being described as an aching pain in the lower back, with or without radiation into the buttock, hip, and posterior thigh down to the knee, with or without spasms. Diagnosis is difficult via imaging; CT and MRI, as well as plain radiographs, may not demonstrate any pathology of the facet joint. Also, imaging may reveal multilevel abnormalities of the facet joint that may confuse the picture.

Diagnosis is made by history and physical examination: tenderness on palpation of the facet joint and pain elicited by spine rotation and hyperextension.

Once the diagnosis of facet arthropathy is made, the decision must be made whether to inject one level or multiple levels. The results can be difficult to interpret in this case; it is not as straightforward as a nerve root block. A partial or negative response does not mean that facet disease is not the cause of the axial lower back pain, but rather that multiple level disease may be the cause of the axial back pain.

Treatment involves medication management, physical therapy, and interventional therapeutic techniques including facet intraarticular joint injection, medial branch blocks, or radiofrequency lesioning of one or multiple affected facet joints.

Indications for Facet Joint Injections

- focal tenderness over facet joint with or without radiographic support
- chronic lower back pain with or without radiation (limited to lower back, buttock, hip, into the thigh and knee—but not below the knee)
- facet arthritis on imaging
- postlaminectomy/failed back syndrome
- pain with axial loading, twisting, and hyperextension (Clemans & Benzon, 2005)

Technique for Facet Joint Injection

Radiographic localization with fluoroscopy of the facet joint is performed first. Localization with fluoroscopy eliminates missed needle insertion into the joint as well as false interpretation of the response to the injection. The lumbar facets, because they are the most commonly affected, will be discussed here. The lumbar facet joint is optimally visualized at a 10- to 15-degree oblique view. The skin is prepped with antiseptic, and local anesthetic is applied to the skin. The inferior or superior recess is visualized and localized, and the spinal needle is advanced to the joint. An arthrogram may be

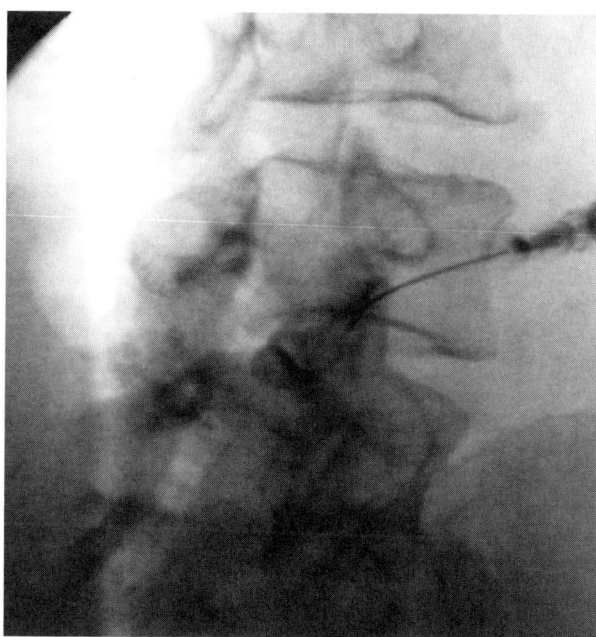

Figure 28.1. Intraarticular lumbar facet joint injection.

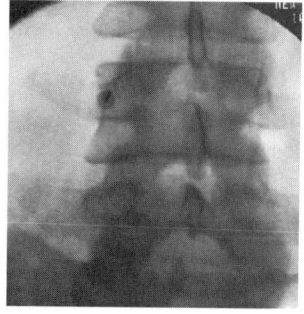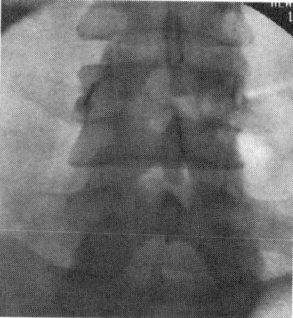

Figure 28.2. Lumbar facet medial branch nerve block (*left*) and radiofrequency lesioning (*right*).

performed with radio-opaque dye, but the physician must be aware of the limited joint space. Special attention must also be given to the pressure during the delivery of the dye and medication injectate, as a complication of the procedure may be destruction of the joint capsule. Once the joint space is confirmed, the injectate is given, usually not more than 2 cc. The solution is composed of a local anesthetic, Bupivacaine 0.25%, for example, and corticosteroid (Figure 28.1).

Medial Branch Block

If an intraarticular facet joint injection is not beneficial, and/or the facet proved too difficult for needle insertion due to degenerative changes of the joint, radiofrequency lesioning of the dorsal ramus may be considered. First, a medial branch block is performed as a diagnostic procedure to predict response to a radiofrequency procedure. Radiofrequency lesioning is a therapeutic procedure performed using an electrode with an active tip in which the electrical current is applied and concentrated around the tip. The target area is the dorsal ramus medial branch that comes around the body of the vertebrae and supplies the facet and one below. The ideal position of the radiofrequency needle (as well as a medial branch block) is caudal to the transverse process and lateral to the medial border of the superior articular process. The needle is advanced until contact is made with the junction of the transverse process and the superior articular process, and then the tip is walked off in 1–2 mm increments, until the needle slips off the superior border of the transverse process. At this point, the needle is in proximity to the medial branch nerve. An AP view is obtained to ensure the needle tip has not entered the intervertebral foramen (Figure 28.2, *left*).

Radiofrequency Lesioning

If the patient responds to the medial branch block, which is a temporary measure to identify whether the facet joint is indeed the cause of the lower back pain, the next step is a more permanent resolution of the pain with radiofrequency lesioning of the affected facet joint.

A radiofrequency lesioning protocol is followed, which involves both motor and sensory stimulation to confirm needle positioning at the medial branch nerve. The lesion settings are for 90 seconds at 80 degrees Celsius, with either thermal or pulsed lesioning (Clemans & Benzon, 2005).

Technique

The patient is placed in a prone position, and the overlying facet joint skin is antiseptically prepped. Fluoroscopy guidance is used to identify the superior medial aspect of the transverse process. Usually a 10- to 15-degree lateral angulation of the C-arm is sufficient to bring the anatomy into view. The skin is then anesthetized with 1% lidocaine. A disposable radiofrequency cannula is then advanced to where it touches the target point (the superior medial aspect of the transverse process). The cannula is then walked off the transverse process edge until it slips off and then the tip is advanced another 2–3 mm. The next step involves electrical sensory and motor stimulation to confirm correct cannula positioning, therefore avoiding complications of the procedure such as permanent weakness or numbness. Motor fasciculations should be absent with stimulation. After the position is confirmed, 2% lidocaine, 1 ml, is injected. Then thermal or pulse lesioning is performed at a temperature of 80 degrees Celsius for 60 seconds (Figure 28.2, *right*).

Complications

- infection
- bleeding
- thecal sac puncture
- permanent damage to the spinal nerve with numbness and weakness
- dysesthesias (Clemans, 2005)

Sacroiliac Joint (SIJ)

The sacroiliac joint is a synovial joint that decreases in mobility with age due to fibrosis. Within the joint articulation, friction is created with the various ligament and muscle attachments within the groove. Prolonged activities such as standing, running, and sitting with stress to one side causes joint loading of the hypomobile joint creating stress leading to lower pelvic, hip, and back pain (Benzon, 2005a).

Sacroiliac joint pain may be caused by multiple etiologies, including but not limited to trauma, antalgic gait, lifting, bending forward, inadequate pelvis stabilization, and prolonged sitting with a sustained stretch on muscle insertions (Simon, 2001). The most common complaint involving the sacroiliac joint is that of aching, which is localized and radiates to the ipsilateral hip and greater trochanter. SIJ pain may produce symptoms similar to degenerative disc disease pain because the joint is innervated by the L3–S1 spinal nerves, resulting in referred pain. For example, pain may be referred to the hip, ischial area, groin, and testicle area.

Many maneuvers during physical examination can produce positive provocation, verification that the SIJ is the etiology of the presenting pain complaint. These include the compression test, in which the patient lies in a lateral position and pressure is applied to the pelvic brim eliciting pain in the SIJ. The distraction test can also be performed in which the patient lies supine and the anterior superior iliac spine is pressed in a posterior lateral direction producing positive pain. Also, the Patrick Test can be performed to diagnose the pain syndrome. This test requires the patient to be supine; a heel is then placed on the opposite knee, and the crossed leg is pushed into the table, causing pain posteriorly in the SIJ.

Treatment

First conservative therapy of deep heat, massage, TENS, physical therapy, and medication is given an adequate trial. If this fails, SIJ injection is the next step.

Procedure

Under fluoroscopic guidance, the posterior superior iliac spine is identified, and the overlying skin is antiseptically prepped. The area is first injected with 1% lidocaine. Then a 22-gauge, 3-inch needle is advanced toward the SIJ at a 45-degree angle. The needle should enter the lower third of the joint. When the needle is correctly positioned in the space, contrast may be given to confirm location. The injectate, which includes methylprednisolone and 0.25% bupivacaine solution, is then given (Figure 28.3).

Complications
- joint rupture
- ligament injection
- avascular necrosis
- bleeding
- infection (Simon, 2001)

Epidural Steroid Injections

Degenerative disc disease, disc extrusion, annular tears, and central protrusion lead to mechanical nociceptor activation. Pain may be associated with chronic inflammation due to chemical irritation, continuous leakage of nucleus pulposus–induced injury, and the inflammation cascade. The inflammation cascade includes release of substances such as nitric oxide, prostaglandins, interleukins, and phospholipase 2 (Molloy, 2005). Steroids interfere with this cascade, and therefore with pain generation. They suppress cytokine and leukocyte production (which play a part in the development of intraneural congestion, edema, and conduction abnormalities). They inhibit platelet adhesion formation, stabilize membrane excitation and coupling, including that of the unmyelinated small C fiber, and reduce central sensitization. The epidural application of steroids is aimed at reducing pain and inflammation.

Anatomy

The spine can be divided into two compartments, which are separated by a frontal plane through the dorsal wall of the intervertebral foramen. The dorsal compartment is composed of facet joints, dorsal dura, and intrinsic back muscles. The ventral compartment is composed of vertebral bodies, vertebral discs, anterior and posterior spinal ligaments, ventral dura, nerve roots, and prevertebral muscles. Pain-sensitive structures in the ventral compartment include the posterior longitudinal ligament, disc, nerve root, and dorsal root ganglion. Back pain is one of the most common pain complaints. Most of the cases resolve spontaneously; however, 10% of these cases have unremitting lower back pain despite medication and physical therapy (Sitzman, 2003). Those patients with persistent back pain are usually referred to pain management physicians for further evaluation and possible interventional therapy. Epidural steroid injections have traditionally been the first intervention tried by pain interventional physicians.

Indications
- back pain with radiculopathy
- nerve root irritation due to mechanical pressure, inflammation, and ischemia (Molloy, 2005)

Technique: Interlaminar Epidural Injection

The epidural space is approached by several regions including cervical, thoracic, lumbar, or caudal. The patient is placed in a prone position, with the lumbar spine slightly flexed to optimize access to the epidural space. The back is cleaned with antiseptic and draped. Fluoroscopy is used to identify the correct interspace. The skin is anesthetized with 1% lidocaine, then the epidural needle is introduced (commonly an 18- or 20-gauge Tuohy needle). The epidural needle is inserted slowly through supraspinous and interspinous ligaments and ligamentum flavum. A glass syringe is attached to the needle during the advancement, and the loss of resistance technique is used until the epidural space is reached. With the loss-of-resistance technique, continuous or intermittent pressure is applied to the plunger while advancing slowly until a sudden loss of resistance to pressure is achieved, signifying that the needle tip has reached the epidural space. Next, usually an epidurogram is performed by injecting radio-opaque contrast into the space to confirm the localization of the epidural space. Before injecting anything into the presumed epidural space, aspiration is done to rule out vascular entry or dural puncture with CSF appearing. After the epidurogram is performed, the medication is injected. The medication injected can be a variety of solutions, based on physician preference. Solutions usually include a depo-steroid, saline, and/or local anesthetic.

Several studies have been done to justify the use of fluoroscopy (Molloy, 2005). Blind needle placement is not advised due to the variation in surface and the epidural space anatomy, especially in the older population and following back surgery (Figure 28.4).

Figure 28.3. Sacroiliac joint injection.

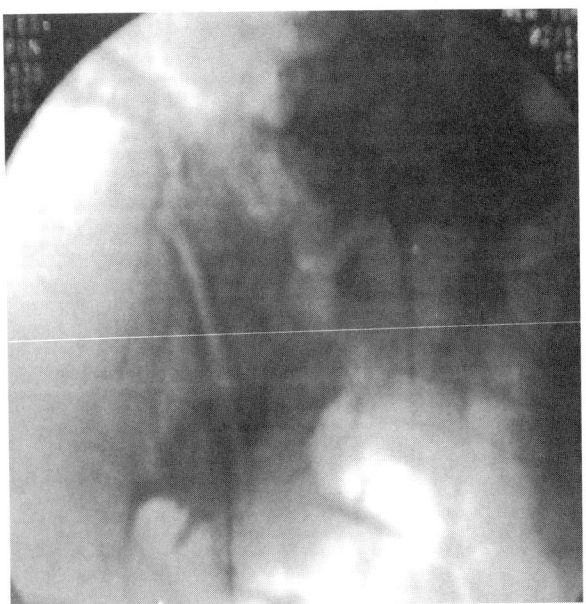

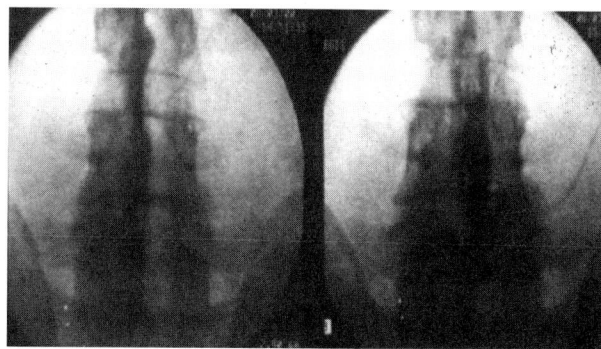

Figure 28.4. Interlaminar lumbar epidural injection: In this case, the epidural space has a midline partition that requires two injections, left and right.

Efficacy

The current standard of practice is based on studies and their results. Efficacy is found to be anywhere from 25% to 89% (Simon, 2001). It was found to be better in the earlier stages of inflammatory back pain (less than 3 months). Repeated injections were found to be beneficial, but evidence also revealed that there was little benefit to do more than three injections (Molloy, 2005). Although millions of epidural steroid injections have been administered, the evidence to support the intervention is mixed.

Complications
- direct damage to spinal nerve root
- intrinsic spinal cord damage
- puncture of dura (1%–5%)
- subarachnoid injection of corticosteroid
- adhesive arachnoiditis
- aseptic meningitis
- transient to permanent paralysis
- durocutaneous fistula
- epidural abscess and hematoma (Molloy, 2005)

Systemic Effects
- iatrogenic Cushing's syndrome
- adrenal suppression
- increase in glucose serum concentrations

Lumbar Transforaminal Epidural Steroid Injections

Transforaminal epidural steroid injections (Fenton, 2003) have both a therapeutic and diagnostic indication. However, the procedure is often bypassed as a potential temporary measure of pain relief and as a diagnostic tool for possible neurosurgical intervention. The most appropriate indication is radiculopathic pain syndromes. Radicular symptoms may or may not be supported by a neurologic exam and imaging, including MRI and CT.

Patients most often first receive an epidural steroid injection, which may give little, if any, relief and which provides no diagnostic information regarding the origin of the pain. A transforaminal epidural steroid injection may be beneficial in that it delivers a small concentrated volume of injectate to the targeted level. This has great diagnostic, as well as a therapeutic, potential.

During the procedure, the patient usually complains of concordant pain that may confirm the correct localization of the cause. This information may help to guide the surgeon in a patient who has multilevel disease. A positive response to a transforaminal injection relates to a positive surgical outcome in studies.

Most of the time, a single level transforaminal epidural steroid injection is performed, for both therapeutic reasons and, primarily, as a diagnostic test. However, sometimes a two-level selective nerve root transforaminal injection is performed. The indications for a two-level block include posterior lateral disc herniation or osteophyte compression of the exiting nerve root and the traversing nerve root. Transforaminal epidural steroid injection is a therapeutic procedure to deliver medication to the affected spinal nerve via the intervertebral foramen. The procedure is used for radicular pain syndromes. This procedure offers the advantage of delivering medication in maximum concentration at the site of inflammation, which an interlaminar epidural steroid injection may not achieve.

Efficacy

An outcome study of fluoroscopy-guided transforaminal lumbar epidural steroid injection (TFESI) found that 75% of patients achieved a greater than 50% benefit in pain reduction (Benzon, 2005b). The study identifies key points when transforaminal ESI may be an option for both therapeutic and diagnostic reasons before a surgical intervention is considered.

Another study compared outcomes of TFESI of corticosteroids versus saline as injectate. The study found 84% reported greater than 50% reduction in pain compared to only 48% in the control group. Also there was a statistically significant drop in the disability scale when compared to the control group (Benzon, 2005b).

Indications
- pain with radiculopathy
- failed medication management
- inflammatory basis of pain
- patient not a surgical candidate
- multilevel disease to define etiology of pain
- minimal imaging findings and normal neurological exam with radicular pain (Benzon, 2005b)

Complications
- abscess formation
- hematoma formation leading to nerve damage
- puncture of dura
- nerve damage by direct invasion
- motor weakness/paralysis by deposition of insoluble injectate inside radicular artery or artery of Adamkewitz (most commonly enters between T9–L2, which supplies the anterior two-thirds of the lower thoracolumbar spine; Rathmell et al., 2004).

Technique

A transforaminal epidural steroid injection can be performed with little or no sedation in an outpatient setting with the assistance of fluoroscopy imaging. Proper positioning of the fluoroscopic image is key. The fluoroscopy image is rotated obliquely until the superior articular process of the targeted nerve root level is visualized in the center of the picture. The needle is targeted inferior lateral to the pedicle and advanced in 1- to 2-mm increments until the needle tip enters the intervertebral foramen. An AP view is obtained to confirm needle positioning into the foramen, but not past the half mark of the pedicle. After aspiration, to rule out vascular or thecal puncture, the injectate is given (Figure 28.5).

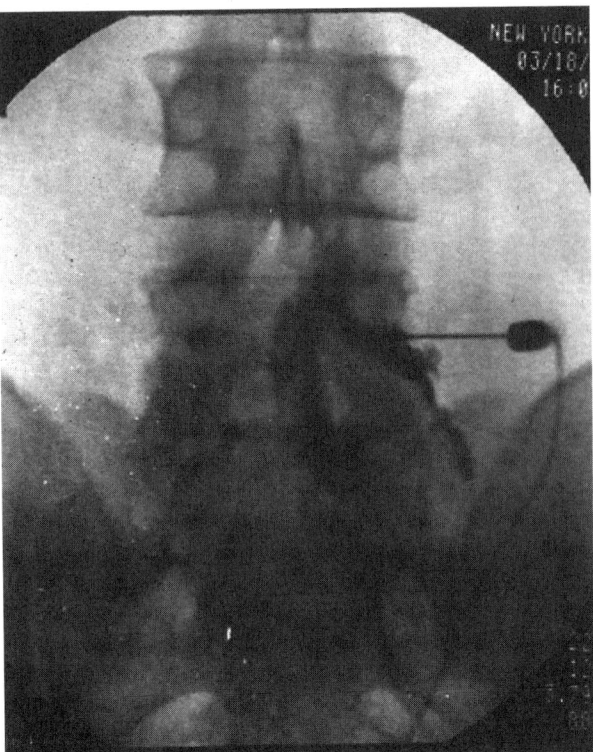

Figure 28.5. Transforaminal lumbar epidural injection at right L5 root; contrast agent injected at this level is seen going to the S1 root.

Cervical Transforaminal Epidural Steroid Injections

Cervical transforaminal steroid injections deserve special mention due to the reported cases of complications, including paraplegia due to spinal cord infarction and death, though extremely rare. Due to the catastrophic, rare complications, cervical transforaminal injections are not recommended. The complication is thought to be related to the deposition of steroid into the radicular artery found in the foramen leading to thrombosis and/or embolus formation and, therefore, spinal cord infarction (Rathmell et al., 2004).

Cadaveric studies have shown great variation in the location and number of radicular arteries in the foramen feeding the anterior and posterior spinal arteries, explaining the unpredictability of complications from needle placement and steroid deposition (Hoeft et al., 2006).

Vertebral Disc

Discography is a provocative test used to diagnose discogenic pain. After 3 decades of use, the test is still controversial. Although some practitioners will rely entirely on this procedure, others may deny even the existence of pain from the disc. This diagnostic test has been used, and abused, to justify major spinal surgery (e.g., spinal fusion). Both the test and the surgery that follows have led to mixed results in patients with chronic back pain, explaining the skepticism of many clinicians. Discography is, however, recognized to be useful in the evaluation of unremitting spinal pain that has lasted for at least 4 months and has failed conservative management (Bogduk, 2004). It is also useful to determine the anatomic abnormalities of a diseased disc and the exact location of the painful disc for future intervention.

Discography has had a recent revival of popularity due to the introduction of new techniques such as IDET and disc decompression, which rely heavily on information coming from the discogram. Discography should be done under strict, sterile conditions using fluoroscope imaging for proper needle placement. It is performed to evaluate the intrinsic disc anatomy and also to evaluate the reproduction of the "usual" pain. After careful positioning of the needle in the disc, a solution, which contains contrast product and allows the morphological study of disc, is injected (Figure 28.6). This fluoroscopic study may be completed with a CAT scan of the injected disc for a more precise evaluation. It is also the purpose of the discogram to get feedback from the patient about the character of any pain that may be felt during the procedure. Both the volume of the injectate and the pressure obtained during the injection are important variables to consider. The injected contrast can cause pain, which usually improves after the follow-up injection of local anesthetic. The specificity of discography is extraordinarily affected by the characteristics of the patient being examined. In a chronic pain patient with psychopathology, the specificity may be at most 20%, whereas in the healthy patient with no chronic pain condition and a normal psychiatric profile, the specificity may be as high as 90%. There are no data on the sensitivity of the test, and its validity is still very much debated, which leads most clinicians to interpret its result with caution.

Disc Decompression

Usually disc removal is a surgical operation, which can be done with a classical back incision or, more often these days, through a small incision using endoscopic microscopy. However, a new technique using needles and minimally invasive methods using "through needle" or "through trocar" instrumentation has recently become available. This technique is referred to as "percutaneous decompression" through a needle. Typically the candidate is a patient with pain coming from a small contained disc herniation causing clinical radicular symptoms. Chemonucleolysis was the first such technique introduced but is now rarely performed

Figure 28.6. Lumbar discograms.

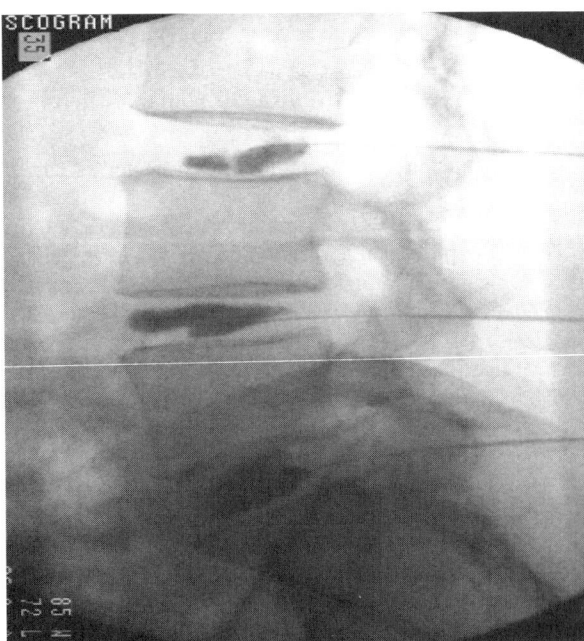

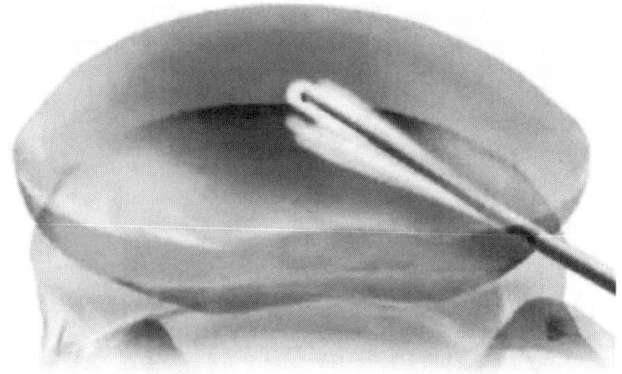

Figure 28.7. Drawing showing the intradiscal action of the nucleoplasty probe.

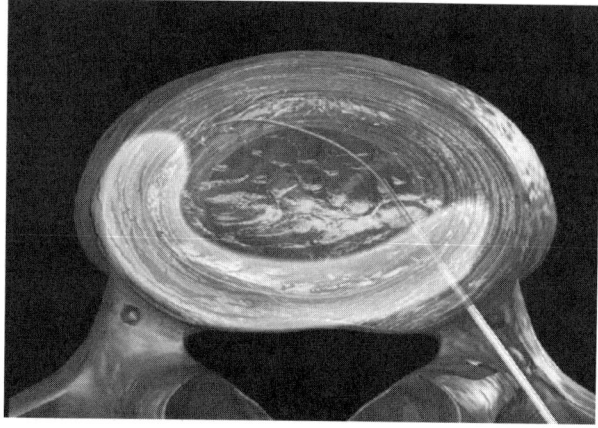

Figure 28.8. The IDET probe in proper position.

due to the frequency of allergic reaction to the substance injected, chemopapain. More recently, laser-assisted percutaneous discectomy relieves the nerve root compression by removing a portion of the central nucleus pulposus. Nucleoplasty, also called "coablation," is now a widely accepted treatment for patients with small contained herniations. Nucleoplasty is achieved using a micro device threaded through a needle and creates a pressure reduction, which is highly dependent on the degree of spine degeneration, in the disc (Figure 28.7). The procedure has, in fact, negligible effect on highly degenerative discs, whereas the intradiscal pressure may be markedly reduced by the procedure in a non- or minimally degenerative disc (Chen et al., 2002). Some preliminary outcome studies seem to suggest that the technique highly beneficial in a selected amount of patients.

IDET: IntraDiscal Electrothermal Therapy

Introduced almost 10 years ago, IDET is a treatment for discogenic low back pain. Discogenic pain has been defined as back pain that has lasted for more than 6 months, is more severe with prolonged sitting or standing, and is commonly nonradicular although it usually projects into the proximal lower extremities above the knees. A number of studies assessing the technique have been published. Its use is still controversial because the diagnosis of "discogenic pain" itself is controversial. IDET discoplasty basically heats the peripheral annular structure of the disc by means of an electrode introduced through an intradiscal needle (Figure 28.8). It has been used on patients with back pain resulting from internal disc disruption who nonetheless have adequate maintenance of at least of 50% disc height. The reported benefits of IDET are related to denervation of the annulus. In early prospective human trials, the technique seemed to provide significant benefits with little risk in carefully selected patients with discogenic back pain. Although a prospective randomized controlled study has shown that there is statistically significant reduction in pain in the treatment group compared with patients who did not have the procedure, another similar study showed no difference (Freeman et al., 2005; Pauza et al., 2004).

Vertebroplasty

Initially used for the treatment of vertebral hemangioma, the percutaneous vertebroplasty is a radiologically guided technique of percutaneous injection of polymethylacrylate via a trocar cannula, which passes through the pedicles into the vertebral body (Figure 28.9). The indication of this technique for spinal pain primarily involves malignant vertebral tumor and painful osteoporotic vertebral body compression fracture (Heini et al., 2000). The advantage of this technique is the stabilization of the vertebral body. In osteoporosis, however, in which fragilization of the entire spine is usually present, it may arguably cause additional fracture above and below the site of the vertebroplasty. In preliminary studies, good results have been reported for both treatment of painful osteoporotic and metastatic vertebral fracture. However, the long-term outcomes are still unclear. Further work is needed to assess this technique and to justify its place among the standard treatments offered to patients with spinal pain.

Central Modulation Techniques

CNS Electrostimulation

Transcutaneous Electrical Nerve Stimulation (TENS)
This common technique is used in the treatment of chronic back pain. It appears to activate peripheral A-beta fibers which

Figure 28.9. Fluoroscopic image of vertebroplasty of a lumbar vertebra.

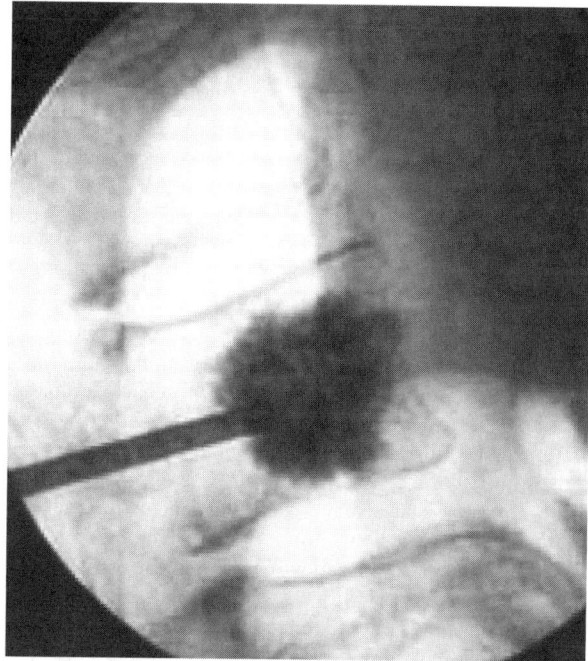

themselves modulate A-delta and C fibers at the level of the spinal cord, therefore producing central inhibitory effects. It is indicated in all types of musculoskeletal pain, but its long-term efficacy has been questioned. It is mainly used today because of its low incidence of side effects and its potential action as a "diversion therapy."

Spinal Epidural Cord Stimulation

Dorsal cord stimulation was first introduced in 1967 by Shealy et al. (1967). It is used, very selectively, in patients with intractable pain for whom conservative treatments have failed. Patients who are most likely to respond to this modality are those with failed back surgery syndrome sometimes complicated by arachnoiditis, radiculopathy, or sympathetic pain. Selection criteria follow a standard protocol that includes factors such as the origin of pain, the response to previous treatments, and psychological profile. Spinal cord stimulation uses pulse electrical energy near the spinal cord and adjunct structures to control pain.

In most common procedures, it involves implantation of a lead in the epidural space to transmit pulse energy across the spinal cord near the desired nerve root. Following initial selection, the patient undergoes a temporary stimulation trial when one or two leads are entered within the epidural space above the area of pain (Figure 28.10) and connected to an external stimulator. If this trial produces significant sustained relief over the painful area, the patient is a candidate for a totally implantable system. A variety of leads and generators are available; some leads can be implanted through a special spinal needle, whereas others require a small surgical implantation. The permanent system includes leads attached to an internal generator implanted under the skin, which may be rechargeable. Some systems also use internal receivers that communicate by radio waves through the skin with an external battery. The patient can activate and deactivate the device at will, whenever required. Results of this technique over the last 30 years have been successful in well-chosen patients. In fact, the latest published series of outcome studies plead in favor of a wider use of the technique (Oakley, 2003). Spinal cord stimulation is not only effective in selected patients, but it is a nondestructive technique that can be used for the control of intractable pain when no other treatments are available. To ensure its success, however, the technique requires special training for the operator, careful selection of the patient, attention to detail, as well as the ability to follow up—long term and on a regular basis—with the implanted patient.

Spinal Drug Delivery Systems

In the last 20 years, neuraxial drug therapy has increased in popularity. Intrathecally administered local anesthetic was the first example of spinal analgesia used clinically without excessive systemic side effects. Today a variety of drugs can be given spinally. Not all drugs are approved by the FDA for intrathecal administration. It is now common to see patients given intrathecal bupivacaine, morphine, fentanyl, clonidine, baclofen, or hydromorphone (Deer et al., 2002). Each drug has its specific indications (clonidine for neuropathic pain, opioids for visceral pain, and baclofen for spasticity), and the patient may receive a mixture of them. Chronic spinal analgesic infusions are primarily for patients who have failed all other, more conservative, treatments. Use of this technique in chronic noncancer pain may be lifelong, and patient selection should therefore be cautious. Administering an opioid chronically in a chemically dependent patient or in a patient with secondary gain may become exclusionary criteria. It is unusual, however, for patients to develop an addiction from chronic intrathecally administered opioids. Side effects follow the pharmacology of the

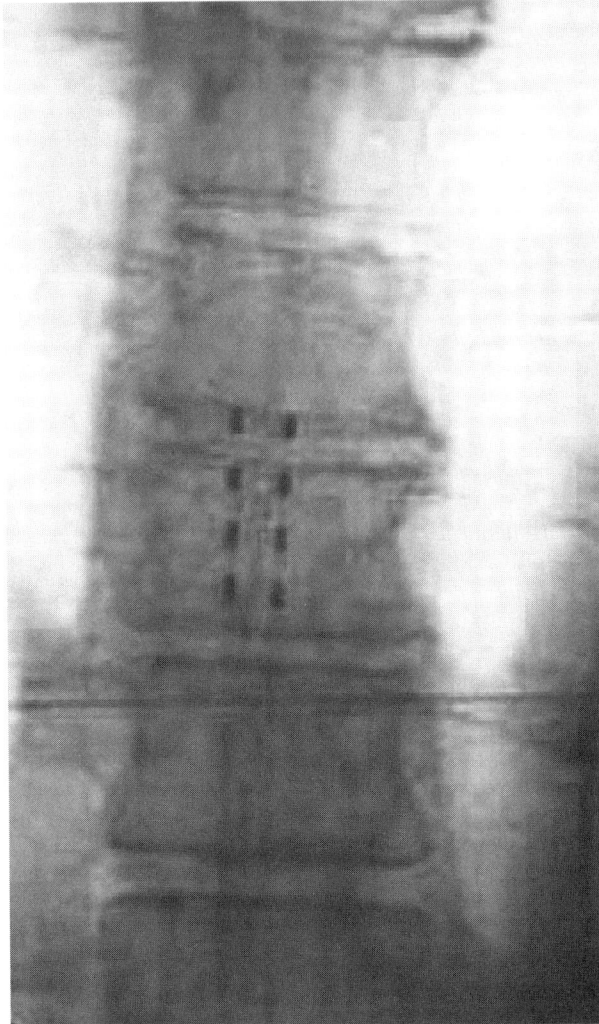

Figure 28.10. Two epidural SCS leads in position in a patient with back pain after multiple lumbar spinal surgeries.

drugs given, such as tolerance for opioids or low blood pressure for clonidine.

Medications can be administered intrathecally by single injection (usually used for diagnostic purposes) or through a catheter, either temporarily or permanently implanted (Figure 28.11). The intrathecal catheter extension is usually tunneled under the skin and is connected rarely to an external pump, more frequently to an implanted pump. Implanted pumps are usually programmable, communicating with an external electronic device that programs the pump through telemetry. A newer feature allows the patient to interact directly with the pump within safe preprogrammed criteria (as with an IV PCA pump). Clinical studies in chronic noncancer pain showed a significant success rate in highly selected patients, especially in patients with failed back surgery syndrome (Deer et al., 2002). Although use of the appropriate drug combination can provide optimal and sustained pain relief (Hassenbusch et al., 2004), reliance on such a device should be limited, not only to highly selected patients but also to facilities that are fully prepared to screen patients properly and provide personnel for the implant and the maintenance of such systems. Once implanted, these patients require close observation for the duration of the entire treatment.

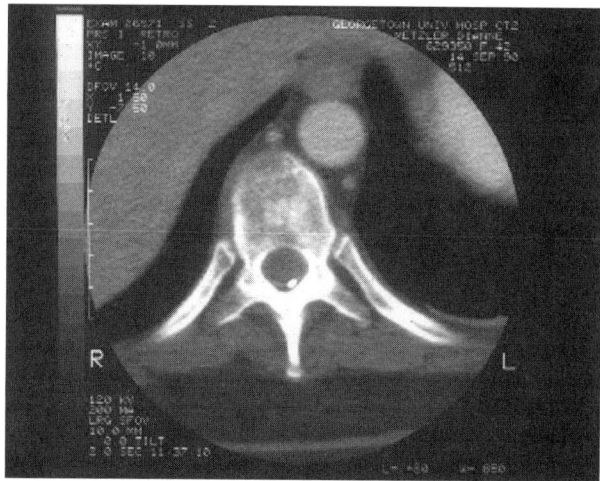

Figure 28.11. Intrathecal catheter of a totally implanted drug delivery system.

Complex Regional Pain Syndrome (CRPS)

Although it can affect other parts of the body, CRPS usually involves the upper or the lower extremities. It is a form of neuropathic pain for which treatment can become very difficult. Usually the patient presents persistent pain following an injury (often modest) that has apparently healed. Pain has all the typical neuropathic characteristics: allodynia, dysesthesias, or hyperalgesia. Also trophic changes are frequently recorded (temperature and color changes, edema) and have been attributed to dysregulation of the autonomic nervous system. "Sympathetic nerve blocks" are done for both diagnostic and therapeutic reasons. *Blockade of the stellate ganglion* is commonly used to treat CRPS I or II of the upper extremity. The stellate ganglion, which lies anterior to the C7 transverse process, is formed by the union of the inferior cervical ganglion and the first thoracic ganglion. An anterior neck approach is used, at the level of the cricoid cartilage (C6 vertebral body). The finger palpation of the Chassaignac tubercle (transverse process of C6) allows precise determination for the location of the nerve block. The carotid artery being retracted laterally, the bone of the transverse process is contacted with the tip of the needle, which is then slightly retracted from the periosteum. Local anesthetic is injected and creates a chemical sympathectomy of the upper extremity and part of the face (Stanton-Hicks et al., 1996). Response to this sympathectomy of the upper extremity ranges from short-term to prolonged relief of symptoms. The diagnostic value and the specificity of this nerve block for CRPS have been questioned, however. Although it is commonly practiced on patients with CRPS as one of the treatment modalities, it may bring only limited pain relief.

The interruption of the *lumbar sympathetic* plexus is frequently used for CRPS of the lower extremity, as well as for stump pain or inoperable ischemic foot pain. The preferred technique today is a single needle technique performed at the level of L2–L3 under fluoroscopic guidance. Confirmation of the location of the needle is offered by the injection of the contrast (Figure 28.12). Sympathectomy is primarily evaluated by an increase in local temperature of the leg and disappearance of the pain. Again, many patients may obtain only short-term benefits from this sympathetic block.

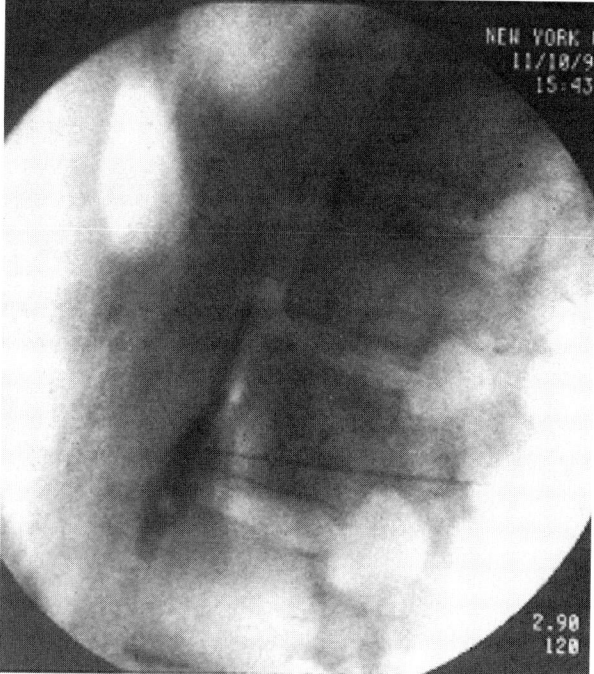

Figure 28.12. Lumbar sympathetic block.

In rare cases of intractable CRPS, *spinal cord stimulation* can also be used; it has been shown to be efficient in well-selected patients (Stanton-Hicks, 2006). A major advantage of this treatment is to provide a window of opportunity best utilized by rehabilitative measures associated with medications and psychological treatment. Effective pain management allows intensive physical therapy, which is essential to obtain functional improvement in a patient who may be otherwise very difficult to treat.

Interventions for Cancer Pain

In addition to peripheral or plexus nerve blocks, neuraxial therapy, using *spinal drug delivery systems*, can be advantageous for the treatment of chronic intractable cancer pain at an advanced stage. Recently, outcomes studies have shown these techniques to not only significantly improve the comfort of patient, but also to have an impact on survival. Neurolytic ablative techniques using destructive modalities can also be used in the context of cancer pain. Any visceral pain due to cancer of the pancreas, liver, or gallbladder, stomach and small intestine can benefit from a *celiac plexus block* (Eisenberg et al., 1995).

It is usually performed with the patient in prone position, and the needle is aimed at the celiac plexus, in front of the junction of the T12–L1 vertebral bodies (Figure 28.13). The neurolytic block is usually done using either alcohol or phenol. It is done only on patients with intractable, usually with well-localized, pain that has been unresponsive to less invasive and reversible techniques, after administering a diagnostic block with local anesthetic. Life expectancy is also a criterion of choice: The block is normally reserved for patients who are not expected to live more than 6–12 months. In most cases, the neurolytic celiac plexus block is done with the help of a precise imaging technique such as CAT scan, which allows the total visualization of the anatomic location of tip of the needle, confirmed by the injection of the contrast agent and local

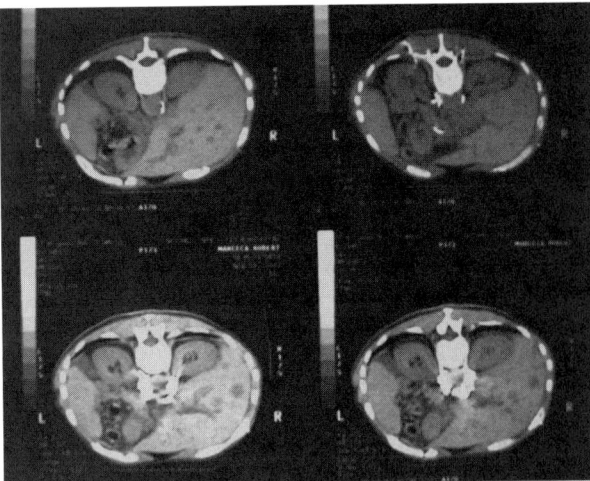

Figure 28.13. Sequential injection of contrast agent seen in CT scan prior to a neurolytic celiac plexus block.

anesthetic, prior to the injection of a neurolytic substance (alcohol, 50%–100%, or phenol, 6%–10% 25–50 cc). If properly performed, this block has minimal side effects and provides sustained pain relief with minimal "maintenance," because this is a one-time shot. The same kind of block can be applied to the superior hypogastric plexus in case of malignant pelvic pain (Plancarte et al., 1997) or to the ganglion impar in case of perineal chronic intractable pain.

Another possible approach for neurolytic blockade is subarachnoid. This block attempts to achieve a dorsal rhizotomy and, ideally, allows sensory block without motor block. This is most useful in intractable cancer pain of the extremities, when a neural structure can be anatomically isolated, and in cancer of the pelvis and perineum. It is also a one-shot treatment applied to patients who, again, are unresponsive to more conventional pain management techniques. It requires a meticulous technique in which the operator identifies which nerve needs to be blocked and at what vertebral level the injection should be done.

The fact that a hyperbaric (phenol) or hypobaric (alcohol) solution may be used has an impact on the patient's position during the block. If properly done, the success rate of this block in advanced cancer patients can be close to 75%. Complications may include bladder and bowel dysfunction and motor weakness. They are, however, transient, and only 20% of patients demonstrate this complication 3 months after the subarachnoid block. Because of the development of continuous spinal infusion techniques such as epidural, intrathecal, long-term infusions of opioids and local anesthetics, this neurolytic central block is not practiced very often, but there are still limited useful indications for the right patients.

Interventions for Acute Pain

Nerve blocks can be extremely useful in the chemically dependent patient for management of acute pain conditions. One of the most common situations occurs after surgery, when pain management with traditional opioid medications presents a major challenge in a patient with a past (or present) history of drug abuse or high tolerance medication.

Single or continuous blocks of nerve plexus are being increasingly used especially after surgery of extremities. Many single nerves (femoral, popliteal, obturator, and sciatic) or plexuses (cervical, lumbar, and brachial) can be blocked, not only by single injection but also by inserting a catheter in the vicinity of the nerve or plexus. The infusion of usually local anesthetics through the catheter provides a continuous block that will provide pain relief for up to 2 or 3 days. The solution of local anesthetic is titrated in such a way that the patient will have diminished sensation of the pain but at the same time will be able to mobilize his/her limb. In some institutions, patients are sent home with a continuous infusion block and a disposable pump, which they retain until the pain is bearable. Diagnostic ultrasound is sometimes used to identify large nerves or plexus trunks in the body and may provide help for a more precise insertion of both the needle and/or the catheter that deliver the continuous infusion.

Another routine pain intervention uses *epidural controlled analgesia* usually following major surgery. Generally a mixture of local anesthetic and opioid is delivered to provide analgesia without creating a motor and sensory blockage. This technique is particularly of value after major thoracic, abdominal, or lower extremity surgery. It has been repeatedly shown to have an impact on patient's outcomes after those surgeries (Liu et al., 1995). The positive effects of postoperative epidural analgesia, which have been demonstrated in several meta-analyses, are summarized in Box 28.3.

Box 28.3 Postoperative Epidural PCA and Patient Outcomes

- Facilitates ambulation
- Decreases respiratory dysfunction
- Decreases thromboembolic disease
- Improves gastrointestinal motility (and splanchnic blood flow)
- Permits earlier hospital discharge
- Decreases morbidity in high-risk patients
- Has economic consequences

Conclusion

Interventional pain medicine is an important component of the diagnosis and treatment of the pain patient. A pain diagnosis is based on history, physical examination, imaging, and electrodiagnostic studies. Nerve blocks should be used whenever necessary to confirm the source of pain. Furthermore, they may provide long-term treatment solutions through, for instance, RF lesioning or permanent spinal neuromodulation. It is essential, however, to know what makes them successful: technical excellence associated with thorough knowledge of anatomy and correct interpretation of indications. Only physicians with appropriate training and experience can provide such a service. Care providers must be aware that patients with chemical dependency who have pain are usually difficult to manage. Properly applied interventions may be tremendously helpful in defining and treating pain in these complex patients.

References

Benzon HT. Pain originating from the buttock: sacro-iliac joint dysfunction and piriformis syndrome. In: Benzon, HT, *Essentials of Pain Medicine and Regional Anesthesia*. Philadelphia, PA: Elsevier Publishing; 2005a: 356–365.

Benzon HT. Selective nerve root blocks and transforaminal epidural steroid injections for back pain and sciatica. In: Benzon HT, *Essentials of Pain Medicine and Regional Anesthesia*. Philadelphia, PA: Elsevier Publishing; 2005b: 341–346.

Bogduk N. Lumbar disc stimulation—provocation discography. In: *ISIS Practice Guidelines for Spinal Diagnostic and Treatment Procedures*. San Francisco: ISIS Press; 2004:20–46.

Chen YC, Lee SH, Chen D. Intradiscal pressure study of percutaneous disc decompression with nucleoplasty in human cadavers. *Spine.* 2002;27:966–973.

Clemans RR, Benzon HT. Facet syndrome: facet joint injections and facet nerve blocks. In: Benzon, H.T., *Essentials of Pain Medicine and Regional Anesthesia.* Philadelphia, PA: Elsevier Publishing; 2005:348–355.

Deer TR, Caraway DL, Kim CK, et al. Clinical experience with intrathecal bupivacaine with opioid for the treatment of chronic pain related to failed back syndrome and metastatic cancer to the spine. *The Spine J.* 2002;2:274–278.

Eisenberg E, Carr DB, Chalmers TC. Neurolytic celiac plexus block for the treatment of cancer pain: a meta-analysis. *Anesth. Analg.* 1995;80:290–295.

Fenton D. Selective nerve root block. In: Fenton D, *Image Guided Spine Interventions.* Philadelphia, PA: Saunders Publishing; 2003:73–74.

Freeman BJ, Fraser RD, Cain CM, et al. A randomized double blind controlled trial of intradiscal electrothermal therapy versus placebo for the treatment chronic discogenic low back pain. *Spine.* 2005;30(21):2369–2377.

Hassenbusch ST, Portenoy RK, Cousins M, et al. Polyanalgesic consensus conference 2003: an update of the management of pain by intraspinal drug delivery—report of expert panel. *J. Pain Symptom Manage.* 2004;27(6):540–563.

Heini PF, Walchli B, Berlemann U. Percutaneous transpedicular vertebroplasty with PMMA: operative technique and early results. A prospective study for the treatment osteoporotic compression fractures. *Eur. Spine J.* 2000;9:445–450.

Hoeft MA, Rathmell JP, Monsey RD, Fonda BJ. Cervical transforaminal injection and the radicular artery: variation in anatomical location within the cervical intervertebral foramen. *Reg. Anesth. Pain Med.* 2006;31:270–274.

Liu S, Carpenter RL, Neal JM. Epidural anesthesia and analgesia: their role in postoperative outcome. *Anesthesiology.* 1995;82:1474–1506.

Molloy R, Interlaminar Epidural steroid injections for lumbosacral radiculopathy. In: Benzon HT, *Essentials of Pain Medicine and Regional Anesthesia.* Philadelphia, PA: Elsevier Publishing; 2005:332–339.

Oakley JC. Spinal cord stimulation: patient selection, technique and outcomes. *Neurosurg. Clin. N. Am.* 2003;14(3):365–380.

Pauza KJ, Howell S, Dreyfuss P, et al. A randomized, placebo controlled trial of intradiscal electrothermal therapy (IDET) for discogenic low back pain. *The Spine J.* 2004;4(1):27–35.

Plancarte R, de Leon Casasola OA, El-Helealy M, et al. Neurolytic superior hypogastric plexus block for chronic pelvic pain associated with cancer. *Reg. Anesth.* 1997;22:562–568.

Rachlin ES. History and physical examination for regional myofascial pain syndrome. In *Myofascial Pain and Fibromyalgia.* St Louis, MO: Mosby; 1994:166.

Rathmell JP, Aprill C, Bogduk N. Cervical transforaminal injection of steroids. *Anesthesiology.* 2004;100:1595–1600.

Shealy CN, Mortimer JT, Reswick J. Electrical inhibition of pain by stimulation of the dorsal column: preliminary clinical report. *Anesth. Analg.* 1967;46:489–491.

Simon S. Sacro-iliac joint injection and lower back pain. In: Waldman SD, *Interventional Pain Management.* Philadelphia, PA: Saunders Publishing; 2001:535–539.

Sitzman T. Epidural injections. In: Fenton D, *Image Guided Spine Interventions.* Philadelphia, PA: Saunders Publishing; 2003:99–110.

Stanton-Hicks M, Raj PP, Racz GB. Use of regional anesthetics for diagnosis of reflex sympathetic dystrophy and sympathetically maintained pain: a critical evaluation. In: *Progress in Pain Research and Management* (vol. 6). Seattle, WA: IASP Press; 1996:217–237.

Stanton-Hicks M. Complex regional pain syndrome: manifestations and role of neurostimulation in its management. *J. Pain Symptom Manage.* 2006;31:S20–S24.

Part IV

Current Approaches to Management of the Chemically Dependent Patient

29

Pharmacologic Approaches to Opioid Dependence and Withdrawal

Eric D. Collins

Opioid Detoxification in Pain Management

In the clinical management of patients with pain (PWPs), the questions of whether, when, and how to stop chronic opioid therapy will inevitably arise. This chapter provides guidelines for medical detoxification from opioids for PWPs maintained on them. The detoxification process is essentially the same for malignant pain syndromes and for chronic nonmalignant pain (CNMP) syndromes. Some decisions about the need for opioid detoxification may be affected by the presence of malignancy, but such differences are beyond the scope of this chapter.

Definitions and Applicability to Opioids

Detoxification is any process by which an individual is taken off a drug that has produced physical dependence. Medical detoxification, or medically supervised withdrawal, describes the process when supervised by a physician, either on an inpatient or outpatient basis. Physical dependence refers to the presence of tolerance and/or withdrawal (defined below), which are usually present together and frequently lead to a need for medically supervised withdrawal. Patients maintained on opioids typically develop tolerance and/or withdrawal symptoms upon opioid discontinuation after only a few weeks of chronic administration (Jaffe & Martin, 1975). Longer durations of treatment virtually always produce physical dependence, the severity of which is roughly correlated with average daily opioid dosage consumed.

Tolerance occurs in the setting of chronic, regular medication administration and refers to the phenomenon in which either the amount of drug required to produce a given effect increases and/or the effects produced by a fixed dose decrease. It is not unique to opioids or even to drugs with abuse potential. With opioids, tolerance can be profound, such that there is no known maximal opioid dosage that an individual can take, as long as the dosage is arrived at sufficiently gradually for tolerance to develop. If tolerance has not developed, large doses of opioids produce fatal respiratory depression. Caution, therefore, must be taken when dosing opioids in any new patient whose level of opioid tolerance is not known.

Withdrawal refers to a syndrome of signs and symptoms that characteristically emerge upon cessation or a sudden dosage reduction of a substance or class of substance that has been taken regularly. Chronic administration of some medications, including opioids, produces nervous system adaptations, which generally offset the acute drug effects. Withdrawal syndromes represent the physical manifestations of these underlying nervous system adaptations. Withdrawal syndromes differ in signs/symptoms, severity, risk, and contribution to resumed use of the drug for different substances and classes of substances. For opioids, the withdrawal syndrome is often sufficiently uncomfortable that patients cannot successfully wean themselves from opioids without medical supervision.

Opioid Withdrawal

The classic signs and symptoms of opioid withdrawal include the following: anxiety, insomnia, irritability, diaphoresis, yawning, lacrimation, rhinorrhea, nausea, vomiting, diarrhea, myalgias, arthralgias, bone pain, abdominal cramping, restlessness, piloerection (goose bumps, giving rise to the term "cold turkey"), myoclonic jerks of large skeletal muscles (giving rise to the term "kick the habit"), mild tremor, altered temperature sense (hot and/or cold flashes), and weight loss (usually from fluid loss and limited food intake during acute withdrawal). There are usually not significant vital sign abnormalities, although blood pressure and heart rate may be elevated, and a few patients will have very slightly elevated body temperature (though they virtually always remain afebrile, if uninfected). Unlike withdrawal from alcohol or sedative-hypnotic medications, withdrawal from opioids is not generally life threatening, except perhaps in the most medically compromised patients, who cannot tolerate marked fluid shifts associated with the symptoms described above (diarrhea, vomiting, sweating, etc.).

The time course of withdrawal varies principally as a function of the half-life of the opioid analgesic on which a patient is maintained. The shorter the half-life, the more acute and severe are the withdrawal symptoms. Generally, opioid analgesics (with the exceptions of long-acting methadone and very short-acting fentanyl) have relatively short half-lives (on the order of 3.5 to 5 hours), and withdrawal from them will begin to manifest approximately 8 to 12 hours after the last administered dose. Initial symptoms are typically slight anxiety, irritability, restlessness, fatigue or lethargy, and increased pain sensitivity. Untreated, symptoms progress over the next 2 to 3 days (to diarrhea, vomiting, severe restlessness, arthralgias, myalgias, rebound pain, and severe opioid craving), with peak withdrawal occurring between 36 and 72 hours after the last dose of opioid ingested. The most severe phase of withdrawal would abate after 5 to 7 days, although few PWPs would ever have to go through such severe withdrawal, barring a manmade or natural disaster precluding access to opioids.

Withdrawal from slow-release oral opioids (e.g., OxyContin, MS Contin) follows a similar time course, though it is delayed by a few hours by the slow release matrix in the medication. Withdrawal from transdermal fentanyl patches will typically begin with later onset following patch removal, because the half-life of elimination of transdermal fentanyl is between 16 hours (Lehmann & Zech, 1992) and 21 to 30 hours perioperatively, depending on age (Thompson, Bower, Liddle, & Rowbotham, 1998). This unusually long half-life of elimination for fentanyl occurs only in the first 24 hours following patch removal; it is due to continued absorption of fentanyl from subcutaneous fat stores for 8 to 16 hours after the patch has been removed.

Because of its long half-life (on the order of 15 to 24 hours), withdrawal from methadone will not begin for 24 to 48 hours. Withdrawal symptoms following discontinuation of methadone peak approximately 4 to 6 days following cessation of the drug, and acute phase symptoms (flulike symptoms, arthralgias, anxiety, restless, and insomnia) could last up to 2 weeks, though they usually subside sooner. And though withdrawal symptoms from methadone will last longer than withdrawal from short-acting opioids, the peak severity of withdrawal from methadone is not as great as from short-acting opioids, other things being equal. Methadone withdrawal as a result of sudden cessation of opioids will not be a common problem in clinical practice, except perhaps in settings in which patients cannot communicate that they were on opioids or are restricted to a setting in which methadone or another opioid is absolutely unavailable.

In all patients, following the acute, more severe withdrawal symptoms, there are residual, low-grade withdrawal symptoms, principally fatigue, disrupted sleep, muscle aches, and anxiety. Such symptoms typically last for weeks, possibly months following maintenance on long-acting opioids such as methadone. The aches and pains may sometimes be mistaken for recurrence of underlying pain symptoms. The residual withdrawal symptoms frequently contribute to patients' inclinations to resume opioids, though they often do not recognize their discomfort as residual withdrawal. And if opioids are resumed, patients will feel relief, not only of pain, but of low-grade withdrawal. This phenomenon contributes to the conviction some patients have that they cannot function without opioids, even in some instances in which the opioids are no longer necessary for analgesia.

Reasons for Opioid Detoxification in Patients With Pain

Although many PWPs do well with chronic opioid therapy, some need to be taken off opioids. There are several common reasons to stop opioids: failure of opioids to produce adequate analgesia, despite increasing doses and opioid rotation; development of worsening pain sensitivity to opioids, unimproved with opioid rotation; development of intolerable and unmitigated side effects due to opioid therapy; and the development, recurrence, or exacerbation of addiction illness, either to opioids or other drugs. For these and sometimes other, less compelling reasons, PWPs and/or their treatment providers may wish to begin a medically supervised withdrawal from opioids. The next section addresses the specifics of how to take patients off opioids safely and reasonably.

Medical Detoxification of Opioid Dependence

Regardless of the reasons for medically supervised opioid withdrawal, the process of detoxification is usually straightforward. The most common method, particularly for PWPs, involves a gradual taper off opioids, either utilizing the current opioid they take for pain (at the time of the planned detoxification) or another, usually long-acting, opioid. It is possible to manage opioid withdrawal symptomatically by use only of nonopioid medications, but the approach is much less acceptable to patients, despite some advantages for the physician, at least from an institutional and regulatory standpoint. For patients who have developed addiction to opioids (i.e., they display the behavioral syndrome of opioid addiction, commonly with compulsive use, loss of control of use, continued use of opioids despite harm, and/or opioid craving [AAPM, APS, & ASAM, 2001]), particularly when the pain syndrome has resolved, the use of buprenorphine will be preferred, because maintenance treatment of patients with opioid addiction using DEA schedule II opioids for more than 3 days requires a special license. Buprenorphine, a schedule III opioid, is specifically singled out as an acceptable agent for maintenance treatment of opioid dependence.

The next several subsections describe the common approaches to medically supervised opioid withdrawal. The first three approaches are usually preferred by patients because they are considerably less unpleasant, at least in terms of the emergence of opioid withdrawal symptoms.

Use of Current Opioid Analgesic

Some PWPs may be tapered off opioids gradually by using the opioid they currently take for analgesia. The main advantage of this approach is that both the patient and physician are already familiar with the medication, making it easier for them to dose the medication appropriately. An advantage with most short-acting opioids also is that they are nearly universally available in small tablet sizes, allowing for gradual dosage reductions and greater patient comfort. Gradual reductions in dosing are not very easy for patients utilizing the transdermal fentanyl patch because the fixed-size delivery system makes fine dosage adjustments very difficult. Most patients maintained on fentanyl transdermal patches will need to be switched to another opioid, as discussed below. Some PWPs maintained on opioids, including transdermal fentanyl, may prefer to switch to a different short-acting opioid, rather than utilize any of the approaches discussed in these sections. The approach for any short-acting opioid follows that described here for patients who will use their current opioid for supervised withdrawal. A common reason to switch to a different short-acting opioid from the current analgesic opioid is to make use of liquid preparations (e.g., hydromorphone 1 mg/mL oral solutions) that allow for much more finely tuned dosage reductions.

Sudden cessation of opioids produces the most severe and uncomfortable withdrawal symptoms, as described earlier in this chapter. Therefore, to minimize patient discomfort, medically supervised opioid withdrawal using opioids involves an opioid taper. The longer the taper schedule, the less severe the withdrawal symptoms, though after several weeks tapering off a short-acting opioid, at least from low to moderate doses, there may not be additional benefit with a longer taper. Many patients will be quite comfortable with dosage reductions of approximately 10% of the starting daily dosage over the first week (down to about 30% of the original dosage) and then daily dosage reductions of about 5% of the original dosage over the second week. Of course, the taper may be made more gradual if patients develop significant withdrawal symptoms or rebound pain. If this happens, it would be unusual that the taper should take longer than a month. As doses get very low, it will eventually become impossible to maintain frequent dosing throughout the day, and the emergence of pain between doses may become clinically significant. For this reason, and because some patients find it more difficult to reduce the doses of the same medication they took for analgesia, the use of a long-acting opioid, as described in the next two sections, may be preferable.

Methadone

Methadone has been well established for over 40 years in the treatment of opioid dependence (Dole & Nyswander, 1965). Its use for pain is also well established and, in some patients, it may be superior to slow release morphine (Fredheim et al., 2006) for analgesia. When used in the management of pain, methadone should be dosed every 6 to 8 hours to provide continuous pain relief. This is the dosing frequency that should also be used when PWPs undergo medically supervised opioid withdrawal (in the absence of an underlying pain syndrome, daily dosing is the norm for detoxification with methadone). There are several advantages to methadone (compared to short-acting opioids) in the management of opioid withdrawal. First, its long half-life allows for a degree of self-taper, so that withdrawal symptoms do not emerge as quickly and are less severe at their peak. Second, methadone has antagonist effects at NMDA receptors (Gorman, Elliott, & Inturrisi, 1997), which, independent of its opioid receptor agonism, may help attenuate both pain (Sang, 2000) and opioid tolerance (Elliott, Kest, Man, Kao, & Inturrisi, 1995) and thus facilitate opioid withdrawal. Third, methadone is available as a liquid, which, as noted previously, allows for very small dosage adjustments and a very gradual withdrawal. Finally, methadone is inexpensive.

When methadone used for opioid withdrawal, care must be taken with the initial dosing, so as to prevent accidental overdose and possible death. As noted above, methadone should be dosed four times daily in PWPs, but blood levels of methadone rise over several days, such that an initially safe dose may produce evidence of opioid toxicity (drowsiness, depressed respiration, miosis, motor impairment, nausea, vomiting, and mild hypothermia) after a few days of dosing and rising blood levels (Dart, Woody, & Kleber, 2005). Table 29.1 provides suggested dosing equivalents for withdrawal for a variety of commonly prescribed opioid analgesics (note that these equivalences are not necessarily the same as equianalgesic dosing of various opioids). It can be difficult to be certain of a patient's actual daily opioid dose because some patients, especially those with addiction, may overestimate their opioid intake in order to reduce the risk that their physician will undermedicate them (and allow withdrawal to develop). For this reason, initial dosing of methadone, in particular, must be observed very closely, with special attention to possible signs of either withdrawal or opioid intoxication. The physician should be particularly watchful during the first week of the methadone induction, especially if there is a methadone dosage increase during that week. A pulse oximeter to monitor hemoglobin oxygen saturation is a useful tool to assess the degree of respiratory depression. Although it should be an extremely rare occurrence, if the oxygen saturation falls 4 points or more below baseline or below 90%, regardless of baseline, the methadone dose utilized is too large. Oxygen saturation below 90% likely represents a medical emergency, the responses to which could include asking the patient to breathe deeply and rapidly for several breaths, repeatedly whenever oxygen saturation falls, and administration of supplemental oxygen and/or a low-dose of naloxone or other opioid antagonist. Administration of an antagonist should be reserved for individuals who are somnolent and appear in danger of persistent hypoxemia, because the antagonist will precipitate a moderate to severe withdrawal syndrome, depending on the dosage utilized. If naloxone is used, it may need to be readministered periodically, because its half-life is much shorter than that of methadone.

Buprenorphine

Buprenorphine, a partial agonist at μ-opioid receptors and an antagonist at κ-opioid receptors, was initially marketed in the United States as a parenteral analgesic (Buprenex) in an ethanol-based solution. The FDA subsequently approved two sublingual tablet formulations of buprenorphine in 2002 (Subutex and Suboxone) for the treatment of opioid dependence. The discussion in this chapter will be restricted to the use of the sublingual products for purposes of medically supervised opioid withdrawal and will not address the use of the parenteral solution (Buprenex). The comparative dosing for these has not been well described, and most of the withdrawal literature involves studies of buprenorphine administered sublingually. Subutex contains buprenorphine only, whereas Suboxone includes naloxone in a buprenorphine to naloxone ratio of 4:1 (e.g., 2 mg buprenorphine:0.5 mg naloxone). The naloxone is intended to reduce the risk of injection buprenorphine abuse because injected naloxone should precipitate some withdrawal in patients dependent on opioids, whereas sublingual naloxone is poorly bioavailable and will not precipitate withdrawal. Intranasal use of crushed Suboxone tablets may also precipitate withdrawal in opioid-dependent individuals.

Table 29.1. Methadone Dosing for Supervised Withdrawal Using Methadone

Methadone 10 mg daily,* given divided or as a single dose, should be considered equivalent to the following medications:

Medication	Oral Dose (mg)	Parenteral Dose (mg)
Codeine	300	180
Morphine	30–40	10–15
Hydrocodone	15	N/A
Oxycodone	15	7.5
Levorphanol	5	N/A
Meperidine[‡]	300	75
Fentanyl	N/A[†]	0.1 (100 mcg)[†]

N/A = not available.

N.B. This table should be considered a rough guide. Physicians may safely calculate the approximate starting dose of methadone using this table and then reduce the dosage by about 25% in order to reduce the risk of respiratory depression.

*Note that these ratios apply for most patients on low to moderate doses of short-acting opioids. With chronic administration of high to very high doses of short-acting opioids, the potency ratios shift, so that methadone becomes at least 10 times as potent as morphine. For example, a patient maintained on oral morphine 1,000 mg daily should be given no more than 100 mg methadone as an initial dose (but see caveat above).

[‡]Note that there should be few conversions from maintenance meperidine because chronic dosing of meperidine leads to accumulation of the metabolite normeperidine, which lowers seizure threshold.

[†]Fentanyl is available as transmucosal lollipops and as transdermal patches. Accurate conversions for these parenteral doses are not available. When considering dosing, note that the fentanyl transdermal patch at 100 mcg/hour is a total daily dose of 2,400 mcg, which is NOT the equivalent of 240 mg methadone. Exercise caution in converting[b] these patients to methadone.

Practitioners who wish to treat opioid dependence using buprenorphine are required to demonstrate that they have acquired special knowledge about the use of buprenorphine and about the management of addiction illness. A common way for physicians who are not addiction specialists to demonstrate their knowledge is to take an approved 8-hour course on utilizing buprenorphine to treat opioid dependence. Although pain practitioners are not required to take the course to utilize sublingual buprenorphine (as an off-label use) in PWPs, it is highly advisable that they do so, in part because they may use it for some of their patients with addiction and in part because of the unique pharmacology of buprenorphine. Like methadone, buprenorphine is long-acting and may be effective in the management of chronic pain (Malinoff, Barkin, & Wilson, 2005). Unlike methadone, its partial agonism at μ-receptors makes induction of buprenorphine potentially challenging because its high receptor affinity means that buprenorphine will displace other opioids from opioid receptors. If buprenorphine is administered too soon after administration of a pure opioid agonist, it will precipitate withdrawal by displacing the pure agonist and substituting its partial agonist effect. Therefore, buprenorphine should be administered only after mild to moderate opioid withdrawal symptoms are present. When this is done, buprenorphine will usually relieve opioid withdrawal (unless too large a dose of buprenorphine is administered).

The usual starting dose of buprenorphine during buprenorphine induction is 2 to 4 mg sublingual (SL). After about an hour, another 2 to 4 mg SL may be administered, if the initial dosage did not precipitate withdrawal. Additional doses may be given later in the day, as needed for opioid withdrawal symptoms and/or pain. The total daily dosage during buprenorphine induction is commonly 12 to 16 mg, but, in some patients maintained on very high doses of opioids, the first day's dosage of buprenorphine may be 24 to 32 mg, and possibly higher, as there are no data available to guide clinical decisions about optimal buprenorphine dosing in PWPs. In rare instances, when patients have been maintained on enormous doses of opioids, buprenorphine alone may initially not sufficiently manage withdrawal symptoms (because its partial agonism produces a ceiling effect), in which case other ancillary medications for withdrawal may be utilized, as discussed in the next section. In the vast majority of patients, buprenorphine alone will be more than adequate for management of opioid withdrawal.

There is quite limited experience with the use of buprenorphine for opioid withdrawal in patients with pain. The information that follows is based on experience in patients with opioid addiction. The use of buprenorphine for opioid withdrawal in PWPs may evolve over time, as practitioners gain more experience with the medication in the pain population. After buprenorphine induction, as described above, most patients may be tapered off buprenorphine over a matter of 1 to 2 weeks, although patients on very high dose opioids will likely have fewer and more manageable withdrawal symptoms if the taper schedule is lengthened to 4 to 6 weeks. A community trial for patients with opioid addiction in both inpatient and outpatient settings utilized a 13-day taper off buprenorphine, with gradual dosage reductions over about 10 days from a maximum of 16 mg on the third day of the procedure (Amass et al., 2004; Ling et al., 2005). The taper was very well tolerated. The withdrawal procedure utilizing buprenorphine for patients being taken off very high doses of opioid analgesics could be structured similarly over about 28 days, with gradual dosage reductions from a starting point of 32 mg of buprenorphine daily. More work is needed in order to refine these currently rough guidelines.

Clonidine and Ancillary Medications

The antihypertensive α_2-adrenergic agonist medication clonidine has been an important nonopioid medication with well-established efficacy in the management of opioid withdrawal in both inpatient and outpatient settings (Charney, Heninger, & Kleber, 1986; M. S. Gold, Redmond, & Kleber, 1978; Kleber et al., 1985). Although clonidine does not have FDA approval for use in opioid withdrawal, its use is well established and should be considered a standard of care in management of opioid withdrawal. Because clonidine has mild analgesic effects (Hidalgo et al., 2005), it may be particularly useful in medically supervised opioid withdrawal of PWPs, particularly when the painful condition remains active. Clonidine is most effective in alleviating the autonomic signs and symptoms of opioid withdrawal and less effective in addressing fatigue, insomnia, restlessness, myalgias, and opioid craving (Charney, Sternberg, Kleber, Heninger, & Redmond, 1981; Jasinski, Johnson, & Kocher, 1985). The usual total daily dose range is 0.6 to 1.8 mg, divided and administered every 4 to 6 hours. Severe withdrawal symptoms may require 0.2 to 0.3 mg every 4 hours, but considerable care must be taken to avoid the marked hypotension, bradycardia, and consequent syncope that may occur with these doses. Prior to each dosage, vital signs should be assessed and clonidine held if the blood pressure (BP) and heart rate (HR) are sufficiently low to make subsequent clonidine administration risky (e.g., "Hold clonidine for BP < 85/55, HR < 50"). Some practitioners favor the use of transdermal clonidine, but the clonidine patch takes a day to reach steady state, and it usually requires supplementation with oral clonidine for breakthrough symptoms. Many practitioners, therefore, use oral clonidine only. Patients who have been taking tricyclic antidepressants will not be likely to benefit from clonidine because tricyclic antidepressants render the alpha-2 receptor hyposensitive to clonidine.

Clonidine may be combined with other medications for opioid withdrawal. In some instances, it may be combined with methadone or buprenorphine, although this is usually necessary only when taper schedules much more aggressive than those suggested above are utilized. Many patients obtain considerable relief from benzodiazepines (preferably long-acting ones to reduce rebound symptoms between doses) for insomnia, anxiety, and restlessness. Myalgias, arthralgias, rebound pain, and abdominal cramping may be treated with non-steroidal anti-inflammatory drugs. Antiemetics, including prochlorperazine and ondansetron, are useful for the nausea and vomiting of opioid withdrawal, and antidiarrheal agents such as octreotide, a powerful antisecretory drug, often help with severe diarrhea, although clonidine itself can reduce withdrawal diarrhea by promoting intestinal absorption (Ippoliti, 1998). A reasonable and more recently available alternative to clonidine is the similar α_2-adrenergic agonist lofexidine, which produces less hypotension than clonidine, with similar clinical benefits on withdrawal (Gowing, Farrell, Ali, & White, 2004). Lofexidine may eventually supplant clonidine as the α_2-agonist of choice for opioid withdrawal, but thus far, because it has only been available in the United States in research settings, there has been less experience with it. Once it is granted FDA approval for use in opioid withdrawal, its use will likely increase considerably.

Anesthesia for Opioid Detoxification From Opioids

Beginning around 1990 and for about 15 years subsequently, there was a lot of interest in the possibility that detoxification from opioids could be improved by the use of general anesthesia. The general approach involved the administration of a high dose of an opioid antagonist (naloxone, naltrexone, and/or nalmefene) to an individual who had been put under general anesthesia to prevent the severe precipitated withdrawal syndrome that emerges when opioid antagonists are administered to individuals physically dependent on opioids. Some suggested that rapid opioid antagonist induction under general anesthesia could be especially useful for opioid detoxification (Breitfeld, Eikermann, Kienbaum, & Peters, 2003), arguing that the process would "reset" opioid receptors and restore sensitivity to opioids. But no randomized controlled trials have demonstrated that the procedure is at all valuable for PWPs. Moreover, the use of general anesthesia and rapid antagonist induction for detoxification from heroin not only lacks efficacy compared to alternative procedures for treatment of heroin dependence, it is considerably more dangerous (Collins, Kleber, Whittington, & Heitler, 2005; Favrat et al., 2005; McGregor, Ali, White, Thomas, & Gowing, 2002). Given the risks attendant to the procedure, including marked increases in corticotropin, cortisol (Elman et al., 2001), catecholamines (Kienbaum et al., 1998, 2000), and sympathetic activity (Hoffman, McDonald, & Berkowitz, 1998) and deaths (C. G. Gold, Cullen, Gonzales, Houtmeyers, & Dwyer, 1999; Hamilton et al., 2002), there appears to be no place for the use of general anesthesia in opioid detoxification for persons with or without chronic pain. Advocates of the procedure will need to demonstrate that the procedure offers benefits peculiar to PWPs and that these benefits offset the risks, most of which appear to be a direct result of the invasive and stressful procedure rather than intrinsic to the opioid withdrawal process.

Summary

Some patients with chronic pain maintained on opioids will require medically supervised opioid withdrawal. This may be accomplished using a gradual taper of one of several opioids, including their maintenance opioid analgesic, methadone, or buprenorphine, or the withdrawal may be accomplished using clonidine and other ancillary medications for opioid withdrawal symptoms. There appears to be no role for anesthesia-assisted methods in accomplishing the withdrawal.

References

AAPM, APS, & ASAM. (2001). *Definitions related to the use of opioids for the treatment of pain*. Retrieved June 26, 2006, from http://www.asam.org/pain/definitions2.pdf

Amass, L., Ling, W., Freese, T. E., Reiber, C., Annon, J. J., Cohen, A. J., et al. (2004). Bringing buprenorphine-naloxone detoxification to community treatment providers: The NIDA Clinical Trials Network field experience. *Am J Addict, 13*(Suppl. 1), S42–66.

Breitfeld, C., Eikermann, M., Kienbaum, P., & Peters, J. (2003). Opioid "holiday" following antagonist supported detoxification during general anesthesia improves opioid agonist response in a cancer patient with opioid addiction. *Anesthesiology, 98*(2), 571–573.

Charney, D. S., Heninger, G. R., & Kleber, H. D. (1986). The combined use of clonidine and naltrexone as a rapid, safe, and effective treatment of abrupt withdrawal from methadone. *Am J Psychiatry, 143*(7), 831–837.

Charney, D. S., Sternberg, D. E., Kleber, H. D., Heninger, G. R., & Redmond, D. E., Jr. (1981). The clinical use of clonidine in abrupt withdrawal from methadone. Effects on blood pressure and specific signs and symptoms. *Arch Gen Psychiatry, 38*(11), 1273–1277.

Collins, E. D., Kleber, H. D., Whittington, R. A., & Heitler, N. E. (2005). Anesthesia-assisted vs. buprenorphine- or clonidine-assisted heroin detoxification and naltrexone induction: A randomized trial. *JAMA, 294*(8), 903–913.

Dart, R. C., Woody, G. E., & Kleber, H. D. (2005). Prescribing methadone as an analgesic. *Ann Intern Med, 143*(8), 620.

Dole, V. P., & Nyswander, M. (1965). A medical treatment for diacetylmorphine (Heroin) addiction: A clinical trial with methadone hydrochloride. *JAMA, 193*, 646–650.

Elliott, K., Kest, B., Man, A., Kao, B., & Inturrisi, C. E. (1995). N-methyl-D-aspartate (NMDA) receptors, mu and kappa opioid tolerance, and perspectives on new analgesic drug development. *Neuropsychopharmacology, 13*(4), 347–356.

Elman, I., D'Ambra, M. N., Krause, S., Breiter, H., Kane, M., Morris, R., et al. (2001). Ultrarapid opioid detoxification: effects on cardiopulmonary physiology, stress hormones and clinical outcomes. *Drug Alcohol Depend, 61*(2), 163–172.

Favrat, B., Zimmermann, G., Zullino, D., Krenz, S., Dorogy, F., Muller, J., et al. (2005). Opioid antagonist detoxification under anaesthesia versus traditional clonidine detoxification combined with an additional week of psychosocial support: A randomised clinical trial. *Drug Alcohol Depend*.

Fredheim, O. M., Kaasa, S., Dale, O., Klepstad, P., Landro, N. I., & Borchgrevink, P. C. (2006). Opioid switching from oral slow release morphine to oral methadone may improve pain control in chronic non-malignant pain: A nine-month follow-up study. *Palliat Med, 20*(1), 35–41.

Gold, C. G., Cullen, D. J., Gonzales, S., Houtmeyers, D., & Dwyer, M. J. (1999). Rapid opioid detoxification during general anesthesia: A review of 20 patients. *Anesthesiology, 91*(6), 1639–1647.

Gold, M. S., Redmond, D. E., Jr., & Kleber, H. D. (1978). Clonidine blocks acute opiate-withdrawal symptoms. *Lancet, 2*(8090), 599–602.

Gorman, A. L., Elliott, K. J., & Inturrisi, C. E. (1997). The d- and l-isomers of methadone bind to the non-competitive site on the N-methyl-D-aspartate (NMDA) receptor in rat forebrain and spinal cord. *Neurosci Lett, 223*(1), 5–8.

Gowing, L., Farrell, M., Ali, R., & White, J. (2004). Alpha2 adrenergic agonists for the management of opioid withdrawal. *Cochrane Database Syst Rev*(4), CD002024.

Hamilton, R. J., Olmedo, R. E., Shah, S., Hung, O. L., Howland, M. A., Perrone, J., et al. (2002). Complications of ultrarapid opioid detoxification with subcutaneous naltrexone pellets. *Acad Emerg Med, 9*(1), 63–68.

Hidalgo, M. P., Auzani, J. A., Rumpel, L. C., Moreira, N. L., Jr., Cursino, A. W., & Caumo, W. (2005). The clinical effect of small oral clonidine doses on perioperative outcomes in patients undergoing abdominal hysterectomy. *Anesth Analg, 100*(3), 795–802, table of contents.

Hoffman, W. E., McDonald, T., & Berkowitz, R. (1998). Simultaneous increases in respiration and sympathetic function during opiate detoxification. *J Neurosurg Anesthesiol, 10*(4), 205–210.

Ippoliti, C. (1998). Antidiarrheal agents for the management of treatment-related diarrhea in cancer patients. *Am J Health Syst Pharm, 55*(15), 1573–1580.

Jaffe, J. H., & Martin, W. R. (1975). Narcotic analgesics and antagonists. In L. S. Goodman & A. Gilman (Eds.), *The Pharmacological Basis of Therapeutics* (5th ed., pp. 245–324). New York: Macmillan.

Jasinski, D. R., Johnson, R. E., & Kocher, T. R. (1985). Clonidine in morphine withdrawal. Differential effects on signs and symptoms. *Arch Gen Psychiatry, 42*(11), 1063–1066.

Kienbaum, P., Scherbaum, N., Thurauf, N., Michel, M. C., Gastpar, M., & Peters, J. (2000). Acute detoxification of opioid-addicted patients with naloxone during propofol or methohexital anesthesia: A comparison of withdrawal symptoms, neuroendocrine, metabolic, and cardiovascular patterns. *Crit Care Med, 28*(4), 969–976.

Kienbaum, P., Thurauf, N., Michel, M. C., Scherbaum, N., Gastpar, M., & Peters, J. (1998). Profound increase in epinephrine concentration in plasma and cardiovascular stimulation after mu-opioid receptor blockade in opioid- addicted patients during barbiturate-induced anesthesia for acute detoxification. *Anesthesiology, 88*(5), 1154–1161.

Kleber, H. D., Riordan, C. E., Rounsaville, B., Kosten, T., Charney, D., Gaspari, J., et al. (1985). Clonidine in outpatient detoxification from methadone maintenance. *Arch Gen Psychiatry, 42*(4), 391–394.

Lehmann, K. A., & Zech, D. (1992). Transdermal fentanyl: clinical pharmacology. *J Pain Symptom Manage, 7*(3 Suppl.), S8–16.

Ling, W., Amass, L., Shoptaw, S., Annon, J. J., Hillhouse, M., Babcock, D., et al. (2005). A multi-center randomized trial of buprenorphine-naloxone versus clonidine for opioid detoxification: findings from the National Institute on Drug Abuse Clinical Trials Network. *Addiction, 100*(8), 1090–1100.

Malinoff, H. L., Barkin, R. L., & Wilson, G. (2005). Sublingual buprenorphine is effective in the treatment of chronic pain syndrome. *Am J Ther, 12*(5), 379–384.

McGregor, C., Ali, R., White, J. M., Thomas, P., & Gowing, L. (2002). A comparison of antagonist-precipitated withdrawal under anesthesia to standard inpatient withdrawal as a precursor to maintenance naltrexone treatment in heroin users: outcomes at 6 and 12 months. *Drug Alcohol Depend, 68*(1), 5–14.

Sang, C. N. (2000). NMDA-receptor antagonists in neuropathic pain: experimental methods to clinical trials [published erratum appears in J Pain Symptom Manage 2000 Mar;19(3):235]. *J Pain Symptom Manage, 19*(1 Suppl.), S21–25.

Thompson, J. P., Bower, S., Liddle, A. M., & Rowbotham, D. J. (1998). Perioperative pharmacokinetics of transdermal fentanyl in elderly and young adult patients. *Br J Anaesth, 81*(2), 152–154.

30

Behavioral Medicine Treatment in the Management of the Chemically Dependent Patient

Joshua Wootton

Where pharmacological approaches to chemical dependency are concerned, addiction is frequently considered essentially a brain disease, but no medication is likely ever to control addiction on its own, without treatment applied to the social and behavioral dimensions of chemical dependency (Leshner, 1997; NIDA, 1999). Even when immediate physiological dependency has been addressed and overcome, there will always remain those environmental and emotional cues that, when encountered, may tend to reawaken the craving and result in relapse (Beck et al., 2001). Visiting a certain neighborhood or location, pursuing activities with a particular group of people, or just being alone and experiencing feelings of boredom, emptiness, or anxiety can all trigger powerful and familiar cravings, even after prolonged periods of abstinence (Franken et al., 2001; Leshner, 1997).

The approach of behavioral medicine is to prepare for this eventuality by encouraging the development of more adaptive coping strategies and supporting the chemically dependent patient through recovery with a tool kit of resources designed to sustain abstinence or, at least, promote harm reduction (Aldridge, 2005). Behavioral medicine is the multidisciplinary field combining behavioral, psychosocial, and biomedical perspectives in the service of understanding the interrelationships among them and developing and applying interventions and techniques directed toward prevention, diagnosis, treatment, and rehabilitation (SBM, 2005). In its broadest definition, it includes the full spectrum of medical, psychotherapeutic, educational, and motivational approaches and interventions through which clinicians seek to address these often complex and difficult-to-parse interrelationships; but the term is usually applied to the psychosocial dimension of the biopsychosocial perspective and, most especially, to the cognitive patterns and learned behaviors that contribute to health or illness (Turk, Meichenbaum, & Genest, 1987).

The Spectrum of Treatments and Treatment Matching

A broad range of approaches to the psychosocial dimension of treatment has been developed for the specialized population of chemical dependency, and almost every theoretical perspective is represented, from the various psychoanalytic schools to person-centered therapy, and existential therapy (Coombs & Howatt, 2005). Treatment may be delivered in a variety of settings—inpatient or outpatient, private or publicly supported—and range from individual to group psychotherapies (Daley, Mercer, & Spotts, 2003; Rounsaville & Carroll, 2003), with or without pharmacological adjuncts, and include vocational rehabilitation and 12-step strategies. For the purposes of this chapter, we will divide the discussion broadly between psychotherapeutic strategies and those interventions and techniques often called mind-body therapies. The latter will include cognitive therapies, behavioral therapies, and the various skills-based therapies designed to elicit deep physiological relaxation.

With such a broad palette of approaches to treatment being applied to chemical dependency, the idea has emerged, not surprisingly, that particular approaches may prove more successful, depending upon the type of patient being treated (NIDA, 1999). Can we, by taking certain variables into account—like personality traits, comorbid psychopathology, and polysubstance versus single substance abuse—match patient with treatment in such a way as to improve the chances of recovery and successful rehabilitation? Despite the widespread acceptance of this notion in behavioral medicine, there is little research to support the efficacy of attempting to match patients with particular approaches to care (Leshner, 1997). Similar rates of efficacy have been found for various treatments of alcoholism, for example, independent of the patient variables investigated (Bower, 1997; NIH/NIAA, 1996). Project MATCH, one of the largest and best designed studies of chemical dependency, failed to show significant differences in outcome among patients assigned to 12-step facilitation therapy, cognitive-behavioral therapy, or motivational enhancement therapy (Project MATCH Research Group, 1997).

There is nevertheless evidence that effective treatment must address the specific needs of the individual, whether vocational, psychological, social, or legal (McLellan et al., 1997; NIDA, 1999). The most effective therapeutic approach can fail if the patient's comorbid psychopathology is ignored or his or her need for medical care, housing, a stable social environment, or family counseling is not addressed (Jones, Knutson, & Haines, 2003; NIDA, 1999; Strain, 2002). The approach of behavioral medicine to treatment for chemical dependency is designed to help patients acquire the perspective and the skills that will return a sense of control to their lives, keeping them free from addiction. Many of the following strategies for treatment may be integrated into a comprehensive approach or philosophy and may be started on an inpatient basis, concurrently with detoxification, or undertaken on a residential basis, in which socialization is a principal focus of rehabilitation, or limited to outpatient care, in the case of higher functioning patients.

Psychotherapeutic Strategies

Psychotherapeutic strategies, like cognitive-behavioral approaches to care, have been adapted for treatment with chemically dependent patients in a variety of modalities, including individual psychotherapy, group psychotherapy, couples therapy, and family therapy. Although most cognitive-behavioral approaches are structured, psychotherapeutic strategies can be brief and focused or long-term and open-ended. In the case of psychoanalytic or psychodynamic treatment, the psychotherapy for chemical dependency may be subsumed into a more comprehensive analysis of the formation of character and defenses, whereas other psychotherapeutic strategies tend to focus on more specific and immediate goals of understanding, interpersonal accommodation, and behavioral change.

The evidence-based psychotherapeutic strategies most frequently applied to chemical dependency include several principal types or models: the supportive-expressive approach, the directive or drug counseling approach, the multidimensional family counseling approach, and motivational enhancement (McGovern & Carroll, 2003; NIDA, 1999). These models represent psychotherapies that have been developed and tested for efficacy through research supported by the National Institute on Drug Abuse (1999), but this list is by no means complete, and, in many cases, psychotherapeutic approaches found in most treatment centers and programs combine elements of these models with mind-body approaches and empirically validated therapies for comorbid disorders in an integrated or comprehensive approach to treatment (Blume, 2005; Coombs & Howatt, 2005; Jarvis, Tebbutt, Mattick, & Shand, 2005; McCrady & Epstein, 1999).

Supportive-Expressive Psychotherapy

Supportive-expressive psychotherapy is an adaptive, psychodynamic model first proposed by Luborsky, more than 20 years ago (1984). It employs supportive psychotherapeutic techniques to encourage patients to explore and discuss their personal experiences, as well as expressive techniques to assist in the identification of interpersonal problems and the dissatisfactions with relationships that may be at the root of the patient's having turned to substance use (McGovern & Carroll, 2003; NIDA, 1999). The focus is on how relationships can be improved and how interpersonal problems can be solved without recourse to substances. This approach has been validated in the treatment of opioid-dependent patients and compares favorably with drug counseling alone in settings in which chemically dependent psychiatric patients are treated with methadone (Woody, McLellan, Luborsky, & O'Brien, 1987, 1995). Luborsky's model of supportive-expressive treatment lends itself well to study in the situation of chemical dependency precisely because it is brief and focused, but it must be noted that a wide variety of psychodynamic and supportive approaches to psychotherapy have been and continue to be applied with good results to the treatment of chemically dependent patients (Coombs & Howatt, 2005; Flores, 2004; Levin, 2002).

Drug Counseling

The general rubric of drug counseling includes a variety of client-centered approaches and techniques, both directive and nondirective, all with the goal of assisting patients in the development of coping strategies and tools for maintaining abstinence by encouraging them with open-ended questions and an empathic therapeutic stance to explore their patterns of substance use (Jarvis, Tebbutt, Mattick, & Shand, 2005; NIDA, 1999). As a psychosocial approach, drug counseling also addresses related areas of impaired functioning, such as problems with work, social adjustment, and family and couples functioning (Egan, 2002).

Individual and group drug counseling have been studied as manual-guided interventions with the goal of mobilizing community resources in the service of identifying triggers to substance use and preventing relapse (McGovern & Carroll, 2003). The role of the drug counselor may include coordinating referrals for medical, psychiatric, vocational, and family services, as well as encouraging the patient's participation in support groups and 12-step programs. The model of drug counseling has been shown to reduce substance use among cocaine addicts and to provide significantly greater improvement than methadone maintenance alone for methadone maintenance patients (Daly & Mercer, 2002; NIDA, 1999).

Multidimensional Family Therapy

Couples and family approaches to treating addiction have become better integrated into comprehensive treatment with the recognition that chemical dependency is not just a problem for the identified patient. The lives of parents, spouses, and children may be intimately involved and affected, and family members are likely to share a role in the development and identification of problems with substance use and can share a role in their prevention and treatment, as well (Mitchell et al., 2001). The therapeutic models typically reflect the various schools of family therapy—strategic, structural, systemic, Bowenian, Ericksonian, contextual—but all tend to uphold the basic principle that family members can support and reward abstinence or moderation and that patients with higher functioning families are typically at lower risk for relapse (Rotunda & O'Farrell, 1997).

The model most frequently studied in chemical dependency is multidimensional family therapy, which was developed as a treatment for adolescent drug users. This approach views adolescent chemical dependency in the context of a network of influences from a variety of sources—parents, peers, community, and culture (NIDA, 1999). Promoting and supporting abstinence and increasing functional behavior, therefore, occurs through different mechanisms, depending on the setting, with different sources of influence sometimes working at cross-purposes. Treatment in the multidimensional model involves both individual and family sessions, with the individual work focusing on developmental tasks, like decision making, negotiation, and problem solving, and the family work focusing on parenting styles and communication (Schmidt, Liddle, & Dakof, 1996). This approach to treating chemical dependency has been shown to have a positive impact on patterns of adolescent substance abuse, behavioral problems, and family functioning (Liddle et al., 2001).

Motivational Enhancement Therapy

Motivational enhancement therapy evolved from the techniques of motivational interviewing, an approach to treatment that begins by recognizing that some patients are ambivalent about treatment and may not be ready to make changes in their lives (Blume, 2005; Miller & Rollnick, 2002). It is based on the stages of change or transtheoretical model developed by Prochaska and DiClemente (1986), which establishes five levels of readiness for change: (1) precontemplation, in which the patient recognizes the dangers of substance use but does not relate them to his or her situation, (2) contemplation, in which the patient begins to consider changing his or her pattern of substance use, (3) preparation, in which he or she engages in an interior dialogue, weighing the pros and cons of changing, (4) action, in which he or she chooses and implements one or more plans or interventions for making change—for example, detoxification or participation in treatment, and (5) maintenance, in which the patient engages in activities designed to maintain abstinence—for example, long-term treatment or participation in a 12-step program.

The paradigm of motivational enhancement therapy consists of an initial assessment of the patient's stage of readiness for treatment, followed by a brief course of individual psychotherapy in which the goal is to educate the patient about the risks of substance abuse and how they may affect his or her life and to strengthen his or her motivation for change (NIDA, 1999). The psychotherapist draws the patient into an exploration of his or her ambivalence to change by focusing attention on the incompatibility of the patient's ideals and goals for life with his or her behavior. The patient emerges with a concrete plan for change, as well as a better understanding of the coping strategies that will be necessary to work toward abstinence and avoid relapse by overcoming situations in which cravings can be reawakened. Several versions of this approach to care have been found to have a positive impact in the treatment of chemically dependent patients (McGovern & Carroll, 2003).

Mind-Body Therapies

Traditional Western medicine has made use of the interconnectedness of mind and body and the influence that each has upon the other, but since the 1960s, both science and clinical practice have grown enormously in their exploration of the mind's capacity to affect the body. The clinical application of this research has developed—or, in some cases, accepted and incorporated—a number of now largely standard and widely practiced therapies, clustered under the general category of mind-body medicine (NIH/NCCAM, 2005). According to one study, nearly 20% of American adults used at least one mind-body practice during a 1-year period between 1997 and 1998, with meditation, guided imagery, and yoga being the most widely used techniques (Wolsko, Eisenberg, Davis, & Phillips, 2004). In a study of active and recovering intravenous drug users, as many as 45% reported regular exposure to at least one complementary and alternative medicine (CAM) approach to treatment (Manheimer, Anderson, & Stein, 2003).

Those mind-body therapies that have undergone rigorous scientific scrutiny and have been shown to be efficacious in clinical practice are generally accepted within the rubric of behavioral medicine. These include cognitive-behavioral therapy, support groups, certain forms of meditation and other techniques designed to elicit the body's natural relaxation response, hypnosis, and biofeedback. Other mind-body therapies that have not, as yet, been so well-studied or their efficacy, empirically established, are often clustered under the category of CAM. These include but are not limited to various forms of dance, music, and art therapy, along with certain movement therapies, including tai chi, qi gong, and yoga. Prayer and spiritual healing are often categorized under CAM, with acupuncture and massage sometimes being included, as well (Deng, Cassileth, & Yeung, 2004; Mamtani & Cimino, 2002).

Much of the efficacy of mind-body therapies is attributed to the physiology of expectancy or placebo response. Placebo effects—here, the ability of the mind to influence healing mechanisms within the body—are believed to be mediated by both cognitive mechanisms and behavioral conditioning. Research demonstrates that the placebo response is mediated by conditioning when unconscious physiological functions, like hormonal secretion, are concerned but by expectation or cognition when conscious physiological processes, like pain and motor functioning, are involved (NIH/NCCAM, 2005). The approach of behavioral medicine to the treatment of chemical dependency employs a number of mind-body therapies in the attempt to influence, both cognitively and behaviorally, those factors that promote dependency. The most frequently applied of these are the cognitive-behavioral and behavioral therapies, along with the broad spectrum of skills-based relaxation techniques, including meditation, guided imagery, hypnosis, and biofeedback. A discussion of support groups, such as 12-step programs, acupuncture, and other CAM therapies not typically subsumed under behavioral medicine is undertaken in other chapters.

Cognitive-Behavioral Therapy

Cognitive-behavioral therapy (CBT) and behavioral therapy are largely synonymous within the clinical community, although there are widely recognized and specialized second- and third-generation forms and hybrids, such as rational-emotive behavior therapy (REBT), dialectical behavior therapy (DBT), integrative behavioral couples therapy, mindfulness-based cognitive therapy, and acceptance and commitment therapy (ACT; Hayes, 2005). There is continued discussion and debate regarding the processes involved in each of these approaches and the mechanisms through which they exert their influence, but the basic model applied to the treatment of chemical dependency is grounded in social learning theory and the principles of operant conditioning. It emphasizes a functional analysis of substance use—how it was acquired in the life of the patient and why it is maintained—along with skills training, through which the patient can come to recognize those situations or states in which he or she is most vulnerable to use and learn to mobilize a range of cognitive and behavioral strategies to avoid or cope successfully with those situations or states (Carroll & Onken, 2005).

CBT begins with the assumption that substance use is functionally related to other problems in the patient's life. Chemical dependency develops as a consequence of an individual's use of substances as a way of coping, albeit a maladaptive one, with distressing affects or overwhelming thoughts. The techniques and interventions of cognitive-behavioral therapists are designed to help the patient identify and challenge the thoughts and behaviors that lead to drinking or drug use and replace them with more adaptive thoughts and behaviors. The emphasis is on the development of coping skills as an effective alternative to relying upon substances as an overgeneralized means of contending with life's difficulties and defending against the distressing emotions that tend to develop in their wake.

The underlying assumption of the therapist's work is that changing certain thoughts—the automatic, practiced, and often uncritical ways in which a patient thinks about substance use—can lead to changes in behavior and that changing certain behaviors can lead to changes in thinking (Aldridge, 2005). In both cases, distressing effects can be ameliorated. If substance misuse is a learned behavior, then the behavior and the cognitive processes supporting it can be modified. A broad spectrum of techniques and interventions have been developed in CBT, and the therapist's job is to select and apply those that are best suited to the individual and likely to be most efficacious in his or her life.

Cognitive techniques applied in CBT to the treatment of the chemically dependent patient are designed to help the patient in the present: What happens if I have the opportunity to use alcohol or drugs now? A change in thinking (I do not need alcohol or drugs in order to feel better) will lead to a change in behavior (I can relax and feel better by talking with my friends or calling my wife or clearing my head with a walk). When thoughts arise that would typically lead to substance misuse, CBT prepares the patient to recognize them and to challenge the distortions behind them. Any intervention that leads the patient to alter his perceptions or beliefs may be considered a cognitive intervention (Reinecke & Freeman, 2003), although a number of useful resources have made the attempt to catalogue those interventions that are most applicable to the situation of chemical dependency or addiction (Beck, Wright, Newman, & Liese, 2001; Blume, 2005; Coombs & Howatt, 2005; Jarvis, Tebbutt, Mattick, & Shand, 2005; McCrady & Epstein, 1999).

Behavioral techniques applied in CBT to the treatment of chemical dependency are designed to disrupt the behavioral patterns that previously supported substance misuse, substituting new, more adaptive behaviors. This can take the form of having the patient attempt to complete the behaviors underlying the sources of anxiety that led to reliance upon alcohol or drugs in the first place. Interventions designed to encourage the patient to confront the source of his or her fears and successfully resolve them can lead to changes in thinking (I can stand up for myself and ask for what I want without using alcohol or drugs). Behavioral techniques can also be designed to encourage the patient to practice and rehearse new strategies for coping. Training in relaxation techniques, for example, can offer patients new ways to soothe themselves, relieving tension and anxiety and, therefore, establishing an alternative pattern of behavior to that of turning to drugs or alcohol. Compendia of the most applicable behavioral techniques in CBT are also provided in the previously mentioned resources. Behavioral interventions can be as simple as contingency management (systematically reinforcing abstinence by offering goods or privileges for a sustained series of substance-free toxicology screens) or as complicated and individualized as in vivo cue exposure (identifying the cues and contexts leading to a particular patient's substance misuse and exposing the patient to them in a controlled and graduated manner designed to foster increased self-control; Coombs & Howatt, 2005).

A number of studies, meta-analyses, and reviews of the literature have established that cognitive-behavioral approaches to the treatment of chemical dependency are strongly validated and empirically supported (Carroll et al., 2004; Carroll & Onken, 2005; Kaminer, Burleson, & Goldberger, 2002; Miller & Wilbourne, 2002; Waldron & Kaminer, 2004). One CBT-based approach to treatment, relapse prevention therapy, has been shown to exhibit efficacy longitudinally, with the skills learned and therapeutic gains made being maintained in the year following treatment (Irvin, Bowers, Dunn, & Wong, 1999; NIDA, 1999). Relapse prevention therapy consists of a number of CBT-based strategies designed to promote abstinence and enhance self-control. Specific techniques typically include helping patients to explore the consequences of continued substance use, developing skills at self-monitoring to recognize the craving for alcohol or drugs while it is still inchoate, and developing strategies for coping with high-risk situations (NIDA, 1999).

Relaxation Techniques

A variety of skills-based techniques fall under the general heading of relaxation training, a therapeutic approach often undertaken in conjunction with CBT. The goals of relaxation training include (1) developing an awareness of the experience of tension, whether somatic or psychological in origin, (2) learning to relax the body, relieving musculoskeletal tension, (3) learning to reduce the subjective or emotional experience of tension or stress through mental imagery or an evoked meditative state, and (4) learning to modulate escalating or sustained tension and stress that might trigger cravings for alcohol or drugs or increase the risk for relapse (Jarvis, Tebbutt, Mattick, & Shand, 2005).

Relaxation techniques are seldom prescribed alone for chemically dependent patients but are instead seen as a component of a more comprehensive approach to care. Their benefit, when integrated into treatment, is that they can effectively modulate the physical and emotional cues frequently associated with craving, relieving musculoskeletal tension and soothing the emotional states—like anxiety, frustration, irritation, anger, and boredom—that may serve as triggers, precipitating the thinking and behaviors associated with patterns of substance misuse. The currently most popular forms of relaxation training include meditation, guided or self-guided imagery, progressive muscle relaxation, and hypnosis (Mamtani & Cimino, 2002; NIH/NCCAM, 2005).

There are numerous forms of meditation, most of which originated in spiritual practice but some of which have been appropriated into the mainstream of behavioral medicine (NIH/NCCAM, 2006). One example of this is relaxation response (RR), a technique derived from Vedic tradition in India, introduced to the West through the more contemporary expression of transcendental meditation (TM) and subsequently adopted by medicine in the treatment of patients with stress-related illnesses (Benson, 2000). Relaxation response is considered one of the most basic forms of meditation, and it offers a template of the four conditions that most meditative forms have in common: (1) a quiet location, reasonably free from distractions, (2) a specific, comfortable posture, (3) a focus of attention—whether a word or phrase, repeated rhythmically like a mantra, or a particular object, or the rhythmic awareness or control of breathing, and (4) an open or passive attitude toward distractions, both interior (like thoughts and mental images) and exterior (like noise and other interruptions; Benson, 2000; NIH/NCCAM, 2006).

Guided or self-guided imagery typically employs the same four conditions as meditation, but the focus is on a mental image or series of images in place of a mantra or object (Wolsko, Eisenberg, Davis, & Phillips, 2004). The images can be evoked either internally, by a memorized script, or guided externally, by another's voice, whether taped or live. Guided imagery is much like hypnosis, in which the hypnotherapist evokes a state of focused concentration and greater susceptibility to suggestion (Mamtani & Cimino, 2002), including suggestions for deeper relaxation. Progressive muscle relaxation (PMR), by contrast, makes use of a movement script in which the patient alternately tenses and then relaxes the major muscle groups, one group at a time. It is often used to elicit relaxation in patients who are resistant to meditation or hypnosis. The goal is to develop the patient's awareness of excess tension by having him or her deliberately and systematically produce and release it (Jarvis, Tebbutt, Mattick, & Shand, 2005).

Biofeedback involves the use of monitoring instruments, usually through a computer program, to provide the patient with information about what is happening physiologically, as he or she responds to different conditions (Mamtani & Cimino, 2002). When employed passively, as a psychoeducational tool, the patient is prompted through a series of conditions, usually from a stressed phase to a relaxed phase, with the instruments monitoring whether deep relaxation is being elicited. Biofeedback may also be used more actively to establish a relay of information back to the patient, such that the patient learns to modify his behavior in response to the direct feedback loop created by the instruments. By observing the information produced by his or her body—heart rate, blood pressure, skin temperature, and muscle tension—the patient learns to monitor and modulate his or her level of autonomic arousal and degree of musculoskeletal tension.

All of the relaxation techniques discussed induce changes in the autonomic nervous system by reducing activity in the sympathetic nervous system and increasing activity in the parasympathetic nervous system (NIH/NCCAM, 2006). Relaxation techniques, by inducing this set of integrated physiological changes, elicit the body's natural relaxation response, modulating the impact of the body's fight-or-flight response. Although the fight-or-flight response is associated with escalating or sustained stress, increased musculoskeletal tension, and heightened affect or affectively laden states, the relaxation response is associated with relief from tension and the evocation of positive emotional states (Davidson et al., 2003; Lazar et al., 2000; NIH/NCCAM, 2005), both of which have direct implications for the management of craving and modulation of cuing in the chemically dependent patient.

Summary

The approach of behavioral medicine in the treatment of chemical dependency is to encourage the development of adaptive coping strategies and to support the patient through recovery with a tool kit of resources designed to promote and sustain abstinence. The range of treatments within behavioral medicine that may be applied to recovery includes the full spectrum of psychotherapies and mind-body therapies through which clinicians seek to address the often complex and difficult-to-parse interrelationships between the biological, psychological, and social factors that influence us. Addressing only the biological factors may result in successful detoxification, but sustaining abstinence and preventing relapse will likely depend on the changes in the psychological and social perspectives that only behavioral medicine can achieve.

References

Aldridge, S. (2005). *Use your brain to beat addiction: The complete guide to understanding and tackling addiction.* London: Cassell Illustrated.

Beck, A. T., Wright, F. D., Newman, C. F., & Liese, B. S. (2001). *Cognitive therapy of substance abuse.* New York: Guilford Press.

Benson, H. (2000). *The relaxation response.* New York: Avon.

Blume, A.W. (2005). *Treating drug problems.* Hoboken, NJ: John Wiley & Sons.

Bower, B. (1997). Alcoholics synonymous: Heavy drinkers of all stripes may get comparable help from a variety of therapies. *Science News, 151,* 62–63.

Carroll, K. M., Fenton, L. R., Ball, S. A., Nich, C., Frankforter, T. L., Shi, J., & Rounsaville, B. J. (2004). Efficacy of disulfiram and cognitive-behavioral therapy in cocaine-dependent outpatients: A randomized placebo controlled trial. *Archives of General Psychiatry, 64,* 264–272.

Carroll, K. M., & Onken, L. S. (2005). Behavioral therapies for drug abuse. *American Journal of Psychiatry, 162,* 1452–1460.

Coombs, R. H., & Howatt, W. A. (2005). *The addiction counselor's desk reference.* Hoboken, NJ: John Wiley & Sons.

Daley, D. C., & Mercer, D. (2002). *Drug counseling for cocaine addiction: The collaborative cocaine treatment study model.* Therapy Manuals for Drug Addiction, Manual 4. Bethesda, MD: National Institute on Drug Abuse.

Daley, D. C., Mercer, D. E., & Spotts, C. E. (2003). Group therapies. In A. W. Graham, T. K. Schultz, M. F. Mayo-Smith, et al. (eds.), *Principles of addiction medicine,* 3rd ed., pp. 839–850. Chevy Chase, MD: American Society of Addiction Medicine.

Davidson, R. J., Kabat-Zinn, J., Schumacher, J., et al. (2003). Alterations in brain and immune function produced by mindfulness meditation. *Psychosomatic Medicine, 65*(4), 564–570.

Deng, G., Cassileth, B. R., & Yeung, K. S. (2004). Complementary therapies for cancer-related symptoms. *Journal of Supportive Oncology, 2,* 419–429.

Egan, G. (2002). *The skilled helper: A problem-management and opportunity-development approach to helping* (7th ed.). Pacific Grove, CA: Brooks/Cole.

Emmelkamp, P. M. G., & Vedel, E. (2006). *Evidence-based treatment for alcohol and drug abuse: A practitioner's guide to theory, methods, and practice.* New York: Routledge.

Flores, P. J. (2004). *Addiction as an attachment disorder.* Lanham, MD: Jason Aronson.

Franken, I. H. A., Hendriks, V. M., Haffmans, P. M. J., & van der Meer, C. W. (2001). Coping style of substance-abuse patients: Effects of anxiety and mood disorders on coping change. *Journal of Clinical Psychology, 57*(3), 299–306.

Hayes, S. C. (2005). Stability and change in cognitive-behavior therapy: Considering the implications of ACT and RFT. *Journal of Rational-Emotive & Cognitive-Behavior Therapy, 23*(2), 131–151.

Irvin, J. E., Bowers, C. A., Dunn, M. E., & Wong, M. C. (1999). Efficacy of relapse prevention: A meta-analytic review. *Journal of Consulting and Clinical Psychology, 67,* 563–570.

Jarvis, J. J., Tebbutt, J., Mattick, R. P., & Shand, F. (2005). *Treatment approaches for alcohol and drug dependence: An introductory guide* (2nd ed.). Chichester, England: John Wiley & Sons.

Jones, E. M., Knutson, D., & Haines, D. (2003). Common problems in patients recovering from chemical dependency. *American Family Physician, 68*(10), 1971–1978.

Kaminer, Y., Burleson, J. A., & Goldberger, R. (2002). Cognitive-behavioral coping skills and psychoeducation therapies for adolescent substance abuse. *Journal of Nervous and Mental Disease, 190,* 737–745.

Lazar, S. W., Bush, G., Gollub, R. L., et al. (2000). Functional brain mapping of the relaxation response and meditation. *Neuroreport, 11*(7), 1581–1585.

Leshner, A. I. (1997). Drug abuse and addiction treatment research: The next generation. *Archives of General Psychiatry, 54*(8), 691–694.

Levin, J. D. (2002). *Treatment of alcoholism and other addictions: A self psychology approach.* Northvale, NJ: Jason Aronson.

Liddle, H. A., Dakof, G. A., Parker, K., Diamond, G. S., Barrett, K. A., & Tejeda, M. (2001). Multidimensional family therapy for adolescent drug abuse: Results of a randomized clinical trial. *American Journal of Drug and Alcohol Dependence, 27,* 651–687.

Luborsky, L. (1984). *Principles of psychoanalytic psychotherapy: A manual for supportive-expressive psychotherapy.* New York: Basic Books.

Mamtani, R., & Cimino, A. (2002). A primer of complementary and alternative medicine and its relevance in the treatment of mental health problems. *Psychiatric Quarterly, 73*(4), 367–381.

Manheimer, E., Anderson, B. J., & Stein, M. D. (2003). Use and assessment of complementary and alternative therapies by intravenous drug users. *American Journal of Drug and Alcohol Abuse, 29*(2), 401–413.

McCrady, B. S., & Epstein, E. E. (1999). *Addictions: A comprehensive handbook.* New York: Oxford University Press.

McGovern, M. P., & Carroll, K. M. (2003). Evidence-based practices for substance use disorders. *Psychiatric Clinics of North America, 26,* 991–1010.

McLellan, A. T., Grissom, G. R., Zanis, D., Randall, M., Brill, P., & O'Brien, C. P. (1997). Problem-service "matching" in addiction treatment: A prospective study in 4 programs. *Archives of General Psychiatry, 54,* 730–735.

Miller, W. R., & Rollnick, S. (2002). *Motivational interviewing: Preparing people for change* (2nd ed.). New York: Guilford Press.

Miller, W. R., & Wilbourne, P. L. (2002). Mesa Grande: A methodological analysis of clinical trials of treatments for alcohol use disorders. *Addiction, 97*, 265–277.

Mitchell, P., Spooner, C., Copeland, J., Vimpani, G., Toumbourou, J., Howard, J., & Sanson, A. (2001). *The role of families in the development, identification, prevention, and treatment of illicit drug problems.* Canberra, ACT, Australia: Commonwealth Government.

NIDA (National Institute on Drug Abuse). (1999). *Principles of drug addiction treatment: A research-based guide.* Bethesda, MD: National Institutes of Health (NIH Publication No. 99-4180).

NIH/NCCAM (National Institutes of Health/National Center for Complementary and Alternative Medicine). (2005). Mind-body medicine: An overview. Retrieved 12/22/2005 from http://nccam.nih.gov/health/backgrounds/mindbody.htm

NIH/NCCAM (National Institutes of Health/National Center for Complementary and Alternative Medicine). (2006). *Meditation for health purposes.* Retrieved 12/22/2005 from http://nccam.nih.gov/health/meditation

NIH/NIAAA (National Institutes of Health/National Institute of Alcohol Abuse and Alcoholism). (1996). NIAAA Reports Project MATCH Main Findings Washington, D.C. Retrieved 12/22/2005 from http://www.niaaa.nih.gov/NewsEvents/NewsReleases/match.htm

Prochaska, J. O., & DiClemente, C. C. (1986). Toward a comprehensive model of change. In W. R. Miller, R. G. Benefield, & N. Heather, (Eds.), *Treating addictive behaviors.* New York: Plenum.

Project MATCH Research Group. (1997). Matching alcoholism treatments to client heterogeneity: Project MATCH posttreatment drinking outcomes. *Journal of Studies on Alcohol, 58,* 7–29.

Reinecke, M. A., & Freeman, A. (2003). Cognitive therapy. In A. S. Gurman & S. B. Messer, (Eds.), *Essential psychotherapies: Theory and practice.* New York: Guilford Press.

Rotunda, R., & O'Farrell, T. J. (1997). Marital and family therapy of alcohol use disorders: Bridging the gap between research and practice. *Professional Psychology: Research and Practice, 26,* 95–104.

Rounsaville, B. J., & Carroll, K. M. (2003). Individual psychotherapy. In A. W. Graham, T. K. Schultz, M. F. Mayo-Smith, R. K. Ries, & B. B. Wilford, (Eds.), *Principles of addiction medicine* (3rd ed., pp. 851–872). Chevy Chase, MD: American Society of Addiction Medicine.

SBM (Society of Behavioral Medicine Web Site Public Information Area). (2005). Definition. Retrieved 12/22/2005 from http://www.sbm.org/about/definition.html/

Schmidt, S. E., Liddle, H. A., & Dakof, G. A. (1996). Effects of multidimensional family therapy: Relationship of changes in parenting practices to symptom reduction in adolescent substance abuse. *Journal of Family Psychology, 10*(1), 1–16.

Strain, E. C. (2002). Assessment and treatment of comorbid psychiatric disorders in opioid-dependent patients. *Clinical Journal of Pain, 18*(4) Supplement, S14–S27.

Turk, D. C., Meichenbaum, D., Genest, M. (1987). *Pain and behavioral medicine: A cognitive-behavioral approach.* New York: Guilford Press.

Waldron, H. B., & Kaminer, Y. (2004). On the learning curve: The emerging evidence supporting cognitive-behavioral therapies for adolescent substance abuse. *Addiction, 99*(s2), 93–105.

Wolsko, P. M., Eisenberg, D. M., Davis, R. B., & Phillips, R. S. (2004). Use of mind-body medical therapies. *Journal of General Internal Medicine, 19,* 43–50.

Woody, G. E., McLellan, A. T., Luborsky, L., & O'Brien, C. P. (1987). Twelve month follow-up of psychotherapy for opiate dependence. *American Journal of Psychiatry, 144,* 590–596.

Woody, G. E., McLellan, A. T., Luborsky, L., & O'Brien, C. P. (1995). Psychotherapy in community methadone programs: A validation study. *American Journal of Psychiatry, 152*(9), 1302–1308.

31

Traditional Chinese Medicine for Pain and Addiction

Gira Patel

David Euler

In 1997, the National Institutes of Health had a consensus conference that concluded acupuncture to be effective in the treatment of tennis elbow, fibromyalgia, low back pain, osteoarthritis, and headaches, just to name a few ailments. This consensus conference opened the door to hundreds of research grants investigating the efficacy and mechanisms of acupuncture. This sparked the public's interest in this procedure.

A growing population of patients are seeking acupuncture and other complementary treatments for pain management; most of them are prescribed a variety of medications including NSAIDs, steroids, neuroleptics, as well as opioids. The most challenging patients, by far, are chronic pain patients addicted to opioids. In this chapter, traditional Chinese medicine[1] is discussed as a CAM modality for the treatment of pain and chemical dependency.

Acupuncture is a medical procedure that involves the insertion of very thin filiform needles into specific areas in the body (called acupuncture points) to achieve clinical results either by modulating the course of a disease or by symptomatically reducing objective and subjective findings. Acupuncture is commonly practiced in conjunction with a technique called moxibustion.[2] The Chinese character for *moxa* forms one half of the two making up the Chinese word that often gets translated as "acupuncture": *zhenjiu*. Practitioners use moxa (artemisia vulgaris or mugwort) to warm regions and acupuncture points with the intention of stimulating circulation through the points and inducing a smoother flow of blood and qi.[3] It is claimed that moxibustion militates against cold and dampness in the body. Medical historians believe that moxibustion predated acupuncture, and needling came to supplement moxa after the 2nd century b.c. Different schools of acupuncture use moxa in varying degrees. For example, Japanese styles of acupuncture may use moxa directly on the skin (direct moxibustion),[4] whereas a TCM-style practitioner will use rolls of moxa and hold them over the point treated (indirect moxibustion). The thermal stimulation of specific areas and acupuncture points with moxa is especially valuable for patients complaining of various types of pain.

Acupuncture has been utilized as a therapeutic modality for thousands of years, but it is only recently that a deeper, more detailed understanding of the underlying mechanisms has developed. The scientific progress understanding the physiology of pain perception paralleled the growth in knowledge of acupuncture analgesia. As with many ancient healing traditions, acupuncture has accumulated a wealth of anecdotal experiences documenting its clinical effectiveness for a large variety of problems. Given the rapid increase of interest within the scientific and clinical medical community in acupuncture, there is a substantial body of evidence to support the efficacy of acupuncture.

History of Acupuncture

Acupuncture originated in China at least 3,000 years ago. Archeological findings of metallic Acupuncture needles date back to the late Shang dynasty (1000 b.c.). Prior to that, bone chips and stone fragments were used to stimulate acupuncture points and meridians. With the development of the Chinese culture and civilization, from the time of the Spring-Autumn period (770–475 b.c.) onward, there appeared different schools of philosophical thought. It was during this period that the theories of yin-yang and five elements (five phases) were applied to medicine. The most important and influential work of this period is the Huangdi Neijing (Yellow Emperor's Internal Classic). Although legend has it that it was written by the legendary Yellow Emperor, it was predominantly the work of a number of scholars and physicians living between the 5th and 1st centuries b.c. A large proportion of the Neijing deals with acupuncture and its related subjects, indicating that acupuncture had by this time developed into a special branch of Chinese med-

---

[1] In this context, acupuncture, moxibustion, and to some degree herbal formulas are discussed.
[2] The Chinese character for *moxa* forms one half of the two making up the Chinese word that often gets translated as "acupuncture": *zhenjiu*.
[3] Theories of traditional Chinese medicine assert that the body has natural patterns of qi associated with it that circulate in channels, called meridians in English. Symptoms of various illnesses are often seen as the product of disrupted or unbalanced qi movement through such channels (including blockages), deficiencies or imbalances of qi, in the various organs. Traditional Chinese medicine seeks to relieve these imbalances by adjusting the flow of qi in the body using a variety of therapeutic techniques. Some of these techniques include herbal medicines, special diets, physical training regimens (qigong), massages to clear blockages, and acupuncture.
[4] Due to modern medical concerns, this type of moxibustion is now commonly done on top of an herbal burn-protecting cream.

icine with its own sphere of learning. From the 3rd century a.d. onward, acupuncture became a more specialized discipline in China with many outstanding practitioners and numerous valuable books devoted exclusively to it.

In the early 17th century, a trend appeared among quite a few scholarly doctors whereby acupuncture, together with surgery, was regarded as an insignificant and petty skill that was inferior to herbal medicine. In 1822, Emperor Dao Guang issued an imperial edict stating that acupuncture and moxibustion were not suitable forms of treatment for a monarch, and should be banned forever from the Imperial Medical Academy. Although the ban was limited to the court, by the second half of the 19th century the general study and practice of acupuncture was at a low ebb. By this stage, however, acupuncture and moxibustion had already arrived in Europe and the West. It was first introduced through reports by Jesuits in the 17th century. In England, James Morris Churchill began to use acupuncture for pain control and Sir William Osler recommended the use of acupuncture in the treatment of lumbago. Over the past 50 years in China, acupuncture, together with the whole system of traditional Chinese medicine, has been designated a national cultural heritage. Since the 1950s, Chinese official policy has been to encourage the study of traditional Chinese medicine and the integration of the two medical systems, traditional Chinese medicine and Western medicine.

Looking back on the long history of Chinese medicine, one can see that the decline of acupuncture was temporary and short-lived. As a well-tried branch of traditional Chinese medicine, acupuncture's roots are deep and vital (Ma, 2000).

Acupuncture as a medical discipline has spread to many countries throughout Asia, Europe, and America. As a result of this pollination, many different forms of acupuncture have evolved. Though all disciplines of acupuncture are based on Chinese classic texts, one may find a great number of different styles including various Japanese styles, Korean hand acupuncture, French Energetics, along with traditional Chinese acupuncture.

Philosophy of Traditional Chinese Medicine

Traditional Chinese medicine has its own internal logic, which is separate from allopathic medicine. The terminology as well as the logical tools are based on the observation of the human as being one organism rather than a sum of organs and tissues. Within that paradigm of thought, a patient complaining of lower back pain, knee pain, osteoporosis, and tinnitus may be diagnosed as suffering from "deficiency of kidney yin" rather than a battery of allopathic diagnoses. According to this logic, Traditional Chinese Medicine creates a multisystem diagnosis, which explains the etiology as well as suggests a treatment strategy. The diagnostic tools of traditional Chinese medicine borrow their names and effects on the human body from nature such as heat, cold, wind, and so forth, as well as philosophical concepts such as yin and yang, qi, and jing. Internal pathogenic factors such as organ disease or external pathogenic factors such as bacteria, viruses, and trauma, may alter the flow of qi and blood and cause disease as well as pain. The degree of pathology, in this system of thought, is a factor of the human body's strength versus the strength of the pathogenic factor. The internal condition of the patient is ever changing, therefore the treatment strategy must be dynamic and flexible to apply to the status quo of the patient. Due to this dynamic tension between the pathogenic factors and the human body, a patient that receives traditional Chinese medicine, whether it is acupuncture or herbal formulas, will be reevaluated before each treatment and the clinical approach adjusted to the current condition.

In order to understand some of the clinical rational behind the treatment strategies, some of the basic concepts should be explained. Qi (pronounced "chee") is a very ancient concept describing movement, nourishment, as well as warmth and life. Some references translate this unique concept as vital energy or life force. It might not be easily translated and should be seen as an emergent property rather than a sum of functions and ideas. Qi is enabling movement. Movement is regarded as a basic condition of life and health. Stagnation, on the other hand, is the basis of disease, pain and death. "The logic underlying Chinese medical theory that assumes that a part can be understood only in its relation to the whole can also be called synthetic or dialectical. In Chinese early Taoist thought this dialectical logic that explains relationships, patterns, and changes is called Yin and Yang theory. This theory is based on the philosophical construct of two polar complements, called Yin and Yang" (Kaptchuk, 1983a). These complementary opposites are neither forces nor material entities; they are ideas describing how things function in relation to each other. In the human body, yin and yang will describe lower and upper body respectively, parasympathetic and sympathetic nervous system, intracellular and extracellular, cold and hot, lubricant and dry, estrogen and testosterone, dull pain and sharp pain, and so forth. The well-known and popular symbol of yin and yang not only describes the two poles but also the ability and dynamic of change (the black dot inside the white field and the white dot inside the black field can be translated as yin within yang and vice versa). "Jing, best translated as Essence, is the substance that underlies all organic life. It is the source of organic change. Jing is supportive and nutritive, and is the basis of reproduction and development" (Kaptchuk, 1983b). Decrease in jing will lead to poor prognosis and eventually death. Shen can be best translated as spirit, the emotional milieu associated with the personality traits and the ability to think in abstract terms, make decisions, and so forth. "If Jing is the source of life, and Qi the ability to activate and move, then Shen is the vitality behind Jing and Qi in the human body. While animate and inanimate movement are indicative of Qi, and instinctual organic processes reflect Jing, human consciousness indicates the presence of Shen" (Kaptchuk, 1983, pp. 7–8). Health is a reflection of the interaction between qi, yin and yang, jing, shen, and the internal organs in the body. These, in turn, are influenced by lifestyle, nutrition, medication, medical procedures, radiation, and so forth.

The stimulation of acupuncture points is geared toward establishing a free flow of qi, jing, and shen within a virtual line or pathway system called meridians; acupuncture points are found along these lines.[5] There are 12 major meridians crossing the body; some start at the face and run down the arm to the fingertips, and some go down the front or back of the head to the toes. Other meridians start at the fingers and toes and terminate at the trunk. In general terms, according to traditional Chinese medicine, if there is a blockage or disturbance in the path of a meridian, it will result in disease and or pain. This blockage can be external, such as an injury or a scar that has not healed completely or formed adhesions and found painful upon palpation or the result of an internal problem. Eleven meridians in the body are associated with a major organ and are referred to in Table 31.1.

When diagnosing and treating a patient according to traditional Chinese medicine (acupuncture, moxibustion, and herbal formulas), the above-mentioned concepts are taken into consideration in attempt to address the underlying cause of the symp-

---

[5]Some acupuncture points can be found outside the meridian system and are called "extra points."

Table 31.1. The Body's Meridians

Upper Extremity Meridians	Lower Extremity Meridians
Lung	Stomach
Large intestine	Bladder
Small intestine	Gall bladder
Heart	Liver
Pericardium	Spleen
Triple warmer	Kidney

tomatic presentation even when the Western diagnosis is not conclusive. Diagnosis of disease using traditional Chinese medicine consists of obtaining a complete medical history including past and present complaints, surgical procedures, traumas, medication (including herbal and food supplements), and other medical modalities (acupuncture, osteopathic, chiropractic, cosmetic, naturopractic, etc.) and incorporating this information with physical findings obtained through palpation. Based on the findings, the practitioner starts to identify patterns that lead to a treatment protocol.

Regardless of the patients' main complaint, it is imperative to treat the root of his or her problem and not just mask the symptomatic presentation. This approach ensures longer lasting treatment effects. For example, a patient complaining of rotator cuff pain but who also has a history of diabetes, would be treated, according to traditional Chinese medicine, for his diabetes first, and then for his shoulder pain (if still necessary). Traditional Chinese medicine is always looking for the underlying cause of a particular disease or symptom. A large population of patients presenting with various pain syndromes respond very well to the allopathic methods found in pain clinics and other medical centers. Unfortunately there is a growing number of patients that do not respond or have side effects associated with these methods. These patients seek alternative and complementary methods to address their complaints. Traditional Chinese medicine allows the practitioner to treat the underlying problems that led to the current complaint as well as the possible reasons that the patient is not healing. Often, combining traditional Chinese medicine with conventional, allopathic, or symptomatic treatments such as steroid injections and NSAIDS can produce phenomenal results. A recent study published in *Pain* (Molsberger et al., 2002) demonstrated that acupuncture with conventional orthopedic treatment (back school, infrared heat therapy, physical exercise, and diclofenac) provided substantially greater pain relief than conventional orthopedic treatment alone. In this case of a combined clinical approach, the constitutional (root) problems are addressed with acupuncture, moxibustion (and sometimes herbs), as well as the symptomatic presentation with a strong local, chemical, or other physical treatment to produce a longer lasting, comprehensive, and tolerable treatment.

Possible Mechanisms of Acupuncture

Acupuncture research is still in its infancy, but there is growing evidence that the stimulation of specific acupuncture points has an effect on the fascia, ascending, descending, segmental, and the autonomic nervous system, as well as on the humeral response to achieve regulatory action (pain reduction and modulation of pathology). The effect of a stimulation at an acupuncture point can be observed systemically with measures such as fMRI mappings of the brain, blood tests for specific hormones, or locally, such as tissue displacement during acupuncture (Langevin et al., 2004; Langevin & Yandow, 2002), the presence of endorphin, norepinephrine, cortisol, serotonin, substance P, and so forth at the loci of stimulation (Shah et al., 2005), or at the target tissue. Outcome studies that examine the effectiveness of acupuncture demonstrate that without any significant side effects, acupuncture does have a positive effect on reducing acute and chronic pain as well as reducing chemical dependency. The following section will review and discuss these findings that examine acupuncture from the perspective of its effect on pain and chemical dependency.

Acupuncture and the Peripheral Nervous System

Traditionally, Chinese acupuncture needle manipulation at specified points is verified to be accurate when the recipient experiences a de qi sensation. It is now believed that this sensation is a result of the activation of group III and IV fibers, in skeletal muscle. An analogy has been drawn in tying the physiologic benefits of sustained physical exercise and the stimulation of the same muscle afferents that are activated with acupuncture stimulation (Kaptchuk, 2002). The distribution of these muscle sensory afferents to the dorsal horn of the spinal cord may play an important role in the observed physiological effect of acupuncture stimulation especially if these afferents are sensitized, as evidenced by elevated substance P found in animal models of acupuncture points.

Also related to the peripheral nervous system, the correlation between acupuncture points and myofascial trigger points has been mapped (Melzack, 1981). Keeping in mind the differences in muscle and skin pain pathways, stimulation of muscle tissue (as in trigger point injections and acupuncture) may have more than a pain-inhibitory effect and can also influence visceral structures and remote somatic structures because of sensory convergence on the same WDR second-order neurons.

Acupuncture and Descending Pain Inhibition

The most well-delineated effect that acupuncture has on pain inhibition is the way it influences the descending inhibitory pain system. In the late seventies and early eighties, a number of studies investigated the relationship between acupuncture and pain inhibition. The studies measured either opioid activity in the brain in relationship to acupuncture analgesia or a reduction in acupuncture analgesia with the administration of opioid antagonists such as naloxone or naltrexone, as well as comparing the analgesic effects of acupuncture with those of morphine. Acupuncture has been shown to influence pain perception by modulating the activity of key subcortical and brainstem sites along the descending pain modulating system pathway (Mayer, 2000).

Acupuncture may produce analgesia effects on the descending pain inhibitory system. According to Chifuyu et al. (1992), the descending pain inhibitory system associated with acupuncture analgesia caused by low-frequency stimulation at an acupuncture point was identified by the results of lesion and stimulation procedures previously determined to differentiate the afferent and efferent paths in rats. Chifuyu et al. (1993) further established that low frequency stimulation of the muscle beneath an acupuncture point with sufficient intensity to cause muscle contraction will produce acupuncture analgesia (AA) in humans as well. Similar stimulation at points other than acupuncture points will not, under normal circumstances, induce analgesia. Although the acupuncture and nonacupuncture points can be differentiated by their interconnected, but different, afferent central pathways, electrophysiological properties of the acupuncture point and the kinds of receptors activated by its stimulation are not yet fully understood. Han and Xie have demonstrated that electroacupuncture can have analgesic effects at the spinal cord level and the CNS level without the need of muscle contraction (Han and Xie, 1984). This finding is much closer to the original type of stimulation achieved before electroacupuncture was invented. Needles were inserted into the acupuncture point and manually rotated at various frequencies to achieve the desired effect.

Given the variety of neurotransmitters involved in the peripheral sensitizing milieu and the windup phenomenon, it is not surprising that there are potentially a number of nonopioid mechanisms of analgesia that may be involved as well. As just one example, low-intensity, high-frequency electrical stimulation has a faster onset of action but doesn't have as a prolonged effect as high-intensity, low-frequency stimulation. The former is thought to be serotonergic mediated and the latter opioid mediated (Debreceni, 1993).

One theory that may help to better explain the long-term effect of electroacupuncture and manual acupuncture is that by stimulating peripheral sensory afferents of the skin and muscle, sustained changes occur in the CNS via central neuromodulation. A fundamental concept that has emerged is that sustained nociceptive input can have profound effects on the CNS causing pathological neuroplastic changes. Interestingly, unlike TENS, manual and electroacupuncture do in fact rely on a more "painful stimulation" of the peripheral nervous system. In effect then, through controlled stimulation of peripheral nociceptors, acupuncture may be causing a reverse neuroplasticity in the CNS.

A clue to the neuroplastic changes that may be occurring in the CNS with electro- and manual acupuncture can be found in the literature looking at c-Fos expression. The expression of the gene c-Fos in CNS occurs in cells felt to be activated after noxious peripheral stimulation. The Fos protein is the nuclear product of the immediate-early gene c-Fos and couples transient intracellular signals to long-term changes in gene expression and is believed to herald neuroplastic changes in the CNS (Morgan, 1991). A body of literature has looked at c-Fos expression in the spinal cord and brain in relation to acupuncture. Acupuncture has been shown to suppress c-Fos expression in the spinal cord and the brain after noxious peripheral stimulation suggesting a possible neuromodulatory mechanism that is independent of endogenous opioid release (Pan et al., 1994).

Balancing the nervous system and regulating the immune response (including the reduction of inflammation) explains some of the positive results in the management of chronic and acute pain as well as the reduction of chemical dependency with acupuncture. But it is yet to be discovered how a specific stimulation[6] of a unique distal acupuncture point[7] affects a specific target organ or tissue (with or without the corresponding activation in the cortex) as well as how the acupuncture stimulation achieves a long-term effect after only a few treatments.

Acupuncture and the Brain

Functional magnetic resonance imaging (fMRI) has made it possible to look into the effect that acupuncture has on brain activation. These studies give some of the strongest evidence for acupuncture point specificity, and help to argue against critics who claim that acupuncture analgesia is due to nonspecific, inhibitory control mechanisms induced by the noxious needle stimulation. Such evidence for point specificity was elegantly demonstrated in a study by Cho et al. An acupuncture point on the lateral aspect of the small toe,[8] which, in some acupuncture systems is believed to be an influential point for vision, was stimulated and observed to cause increased fMRI activity in the occipital lobes in 12 subjects. Stimulation of the eyes directly with light caused a similar activation, whereas stimulation of a sham acupuncture point 2–5 cm away from B67 failed to cause occipital lobe activation (Cho et al., 1998).

Functional magnetic resonance imaging (fMRI) demonstrates some of the CNS pathways for acupuncture stimulation. Acupuncture at specific points[9] has shown to activate structures of descending antinociceptive pathways and deactivate multiple limbic areas subserving pain association. "These findings may shed light on the CNS mechanism of acupuncture analgesia and endogenous pain modulation circuits in the brain" (Wu et al., 1999). Acupuncture at the main points generally produces antistress and antianxiety effects (Mann, 1992). According to fMRI findings and ongoing research by K. K. S. Hui et al. (2000), signal decreases were observed in the amygdala, hippocampus, parahippocampus, hypothalamus, thalamus, ventral tegmental area, nucleus accumbens, septal nucleus, caudate, putamen, cingulated gyrus, anterior insula, temporal pole, and orbitofrontal cortex. Findings in the cortical and subcortical limbic/paralimbic structures in subjects who experienced deqi[10] demonstrate modulation of the cerebrocerebellar and limbic system activity that may constitute an important pathway of acupuncture action. "Acupuncture action involves the interplay between multiple neurotransmitters and modulators. Correlation of the distribution and the known function of these mediators in the cerebrocerebellar and limbic systems with the hemodynamic response to acupuncture suggests that the down-regulation of dopaminergic and norepinephrinergic tone coupled with the up-regulation of serotonergic tone during the procedure may initiate a cascade of reactions that results in the more delayed effects of acupuncture" (Hui, 2005).

Acupuncture and Chemical Dependency

As one of the most recognized alternative medical treatment modalities, acupuncture is increasingly accepted in the medical as well as legal community (U.S. Department of Justice, 1993) as a viable treatment for chemical dependency. The rapidly growing population dependent on habit-forming and addictive medication presents the attending physician with a difficult challenge. On one hand, there is the need to reduce pain, and on the other hand is the increasing dependency of the patient to pain medication as well as the decrease of medication's effect. This, in turn, will increase the dose (or strength) of the medication needed as well as reduce the patient's tolerance to pain. Chronic use of exogenous opiates interferes with opioid receptors and through a negative feedback system results in a decrease of opioid peptides. Hence, when exogenous substances attach to opioid receptor sites, the presynaptic neurons receive the message that endogenous opioid transmission is normal, thus resulting in a reduction in the synthesis of those neurotransmitters (Mackler & Eberwine, 1991).

---

[6]Such as the angle of needle insertion, or type of mechanical or electric stimulation.
[7]Point specificity.
[8]The acupuncture point B67 (Zhiyin) is located at the superior lateral aspect of the fifth toenail.
[9]In this study, acupuncture points St36 (Zusanli) and LI4 (Hegu) were investigated.
[10]A sensation often described as heaviness, fullness, and dull ache at the site of acupuncture.

This vicious cycle can be broken with the use of acupuncture. Acupuncture provides a safe and cost-effective way to reduce chemical dependency and the symptoms associated with detoxification from narcotics and other drugs (whether prescribed medications or "recreational" drugs; Bullock et al., 1987; Lipton et al., 1994) as well as significantly reduce the abundance of side effects resulting from increasing intake of pain medications. Studies have shown that acupuncture relieves withdrawal symptoms by triggering the body to produce more endorphins, thus bringing the body back to a state of equilibrium (Brewington et al., 1994; Jayasuriya, 1987; Sytinsky & Galebskaya, 1979). Normalization of endorphin mechanisms may explain the effectiveness of acupuncture in treating withdrawal symptoms of opiate-related addictions (Kiser et al., 1983; Pert et al., 1981; Pomeranz, 1982). Han et al. have clearly demonstrated that analgesia induced by 100Hz electroacupuncture resulted from accelerating the release of dynorphin from the spinal cord of rats (Chen, 1992; Fei et al., 1987; Han, 2003).

The "reward cascade" theory proposed by Kenneth Blum et al. at the University of Texas Health Center, San Antonio (Blum et al., 1996) may also explain how acupuncture works in nonopiate addictions and how it prevents relapse. This theory involves a deficiency of dopamine in the limbic system of the brain, which causes the patient to believe that the drug is necessary for his or her survival. Reduction of removal of the drug will cause severe withdrawal symptoms. Evidence suggests the importance of serotonin in acupuncture, particularly high frequency (50–2000 Hz) electroacupuncture. Most of this evidence comes from research into the analgesic effects of acupuncture (Han & Terenius, 1982; Lewith & Kenyon, 1984; Sytinsky & Galebskaya, 1979).

Sean Scott and William N. Scott from the Center of Pain Management in Fresno, CA, suggest that acupuncture directly affects the reward cascade by increasing the amount of serotonin in the hypothalamus (Scott & Scott, 1997). When acupuncture stimulation is applied at the correct points, neural impulses are received in the dorsal horn of the spinal cord. These impulses are conveyed to a variety of fibers of the spinoreticular and spinomesencephalic tracts and project to the midbrain, where they directly influence the descending serotonergic pathways (Kendall, 1989). The hypothalamus and midbrain have interconnecting or modulatory neural pathways. Therefore, by stimulating the descending serotonergic pathways with acupuncture, serotonin within the reward cascade is directly affected, leading eventually to an increase of dopamine in the nucleus accumbens and amygdala and a subjective sense of well-being.

Mi Ryeo Kim et al. (2005) demonstrated that the stimulation of a specific acupuncture point (Ht7 Shenmen) significantly decreased both dopamine release in the nucleus accumbens and behavioral hyperactivity induced by a systemic morphine challenge in morphine-pretreated rats. These results suggest that minimizing sensitization may be one mechanism whereby acupuncture reduces morphine craving in addicts.

Acupuncture and General Approaches to Pain

Chronic pain—especially neck, back, hip, shoulder, and knee pain—are common conditions that are often difficult to treat as the origins of the pain can be ambiguous or the patient's lifestyle and posture constantly interfere with the healing process. From a traditional Chinese medical perspective, there are three important considerations: (1) meridian pathway; (2) bilateral structural evaluation of the musculoskeletal system; and (3) internal diseases and other disorders in the patient's medical history (including emotional/psychological problems and events).

Identifying the meridians involved in the patient's symptomatic presentation and main complaint is extremely useful for the treatment strategy. Figure 31.1 (diagram of acupuncture meridians) describes 12 paths crossing the body. In treatment of chronic pain, the first strategy is to identify which meridians are involved in the clinical presentation. For example, in a medial meniscus tear, the inflammation, pain, and swelling as well as the radiology findings will involve the spleen, stomach, and kidney meridians. With this knowledge, the practitioner can then work on points along or associated with those meridians to treat the problem at hand. In addition, pain along a certain meridian can be indicative of a deeper seated problem that needs to be addressed in order to facilitate a complete healing process yielding better clinical results.

Taking the patient with a medial meniscus pain as an example, when looking at Figure 31.1, one can see that the spleen meridian passes through the vastus medialis, crosses the knee at the medial meniscus, and follows the medial aspect of the tibia. It is common that patients with long-standing knee problems also complain of chronic constipation, abdominal pain, bloating, loose stools, craving for sugar,[11] and other gastrointestinal problems. In traditional Chinese medicine, these correlations are commonly made and the treatment of acupuncture points for gastrointestinal problems is essential in the treatment strategy for knee pain.

The second strategy in the treatment of chronic pain conditions is taking a complete assessment of the patient's body alignment. This entails a palpatory and mobility assessment of the ankles, knees, hip joints, ASIS, PSIS, abdomen, chest, neck, and head as well as the entire spine and foot alignment. If the patient presents with palpatory or range of motion findings at any of the above-mentioned areas, it is important that treatment and alignment of the musculoskeletal system be a priority. A structural imbalance distal to the area of pain can either hinder treatment or be the direct cause of the problem the patient complains of.

For example, whiplash injuries are very common and can be challenging to treat. Acupuncture can be a very effective tool in the overall diagnosis and treatment strategy because it takes into consideration the tightness and tenderness at the ASIS region found by palpation and is commonly overlooked by the allopathic medical approach. This finding is an indication of a hip imbalance caused by the forward propulsion of the body mass and abruptly stopped by the seatbelt. This usually goes untreated because the neck is where the patient feels the pain. In treatment of whiplash or any other type of neck pain, if the hip imbalance goes untreated, strain patterns going up from the hip to the shoulder and neck hinder the healing effect and may cause secondary pain blocking the ability of the patient to heal. A good acupuncture treatment strategy will include points along the meridians involved in the strain pattern (also reducing the hip pain) as well as points associated with specific tissues that might be part of the pain pattern (such as fascia, muscles, tendons, and ligaments as well as bones).

The third consideration in the treatment of chronic pain is the evaluation of the patient's complete medical history. Because the purpose of an acupuncture treatment is to modulate the course of a medical condition toward complete recovery and not just to mask

---

[11] In traditional Chinese medicine, certain cravings are indicative of constitutional weaknesses that might lead to various medical problems (called organ syndromes). In the case of a sugar craving, the spleen channel is affected, which might result in medial meniscus weakness (pathway of the spleen channel).

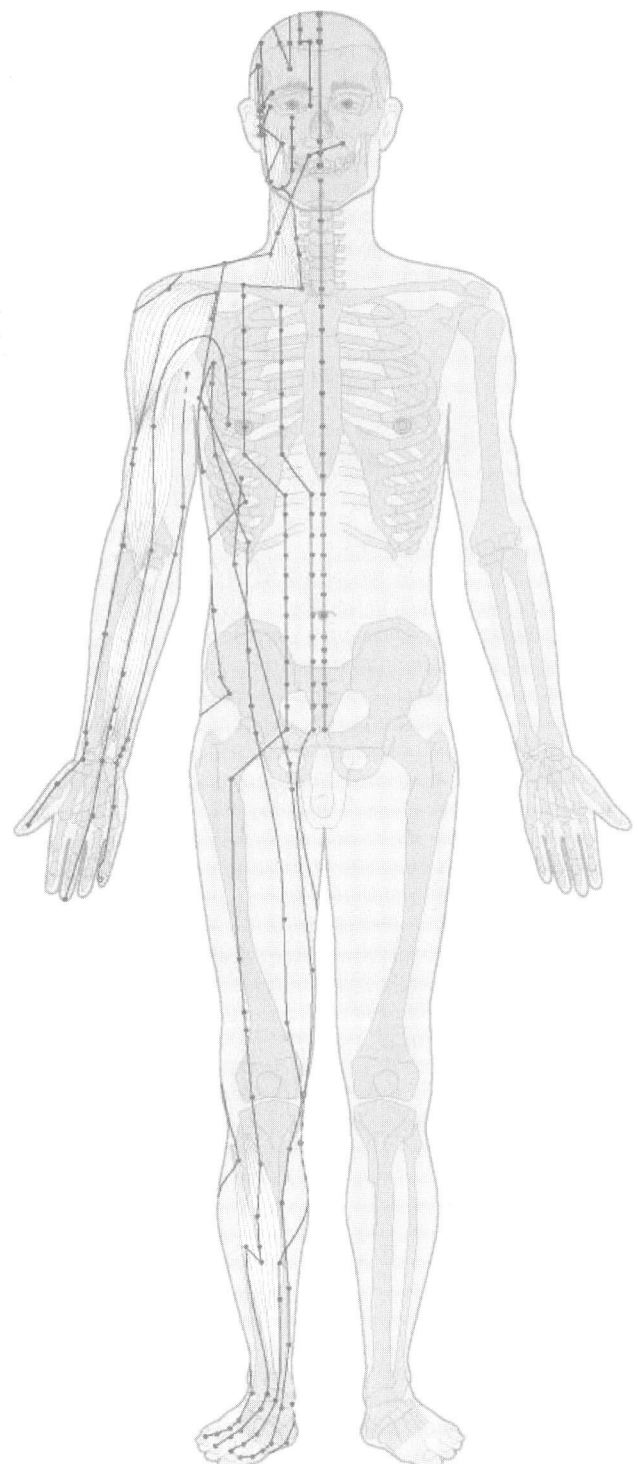

Figure 31.1. Acupuncture chart from www.isrmt.co.uk/images/acupuncture. Contact: info@therapy-school.co.uk.

the symptomatic presentation, the practitioner must evaluate the reasons for the patient's inability to recover. Often the answers can be found through knowledge of past and present medical history. In traditional Chinese medicine, internal/metabolic disturbance such as diabetes, cardiac problems, adrenal gland exhaustion, autoimmune diseases, accumulation of toxin from medications, poor diet and/or genetic predispositions, to name a few, are all part of the treatment strategy that should be addressed in order to treat a current complaint. In addition to the patient's own medical history, traditional Chinese medicine is also interested in family medical history as this also provides clues into the patient's constitutional weaknesses and can help formulate a more effective treatment strategy.

A common example would be a patient who comes to the acupuncture clinic complaining of sciatic pain that did not respond to any allopathic treatment. The patient appears to be in good health with no preexisting medical conditions except for the main complaint of sciatic pain. Yet in the medical history, it is noted that both his father and grandfather had cardiovascular problems. This would lead the acupuncturist to examine reflection zones that correspond to cardiovascular problems, and if these were active, it would be imperative to treat these first, prior to working on the sciatic pain. Often, treating the patient's constitutional weakness will eliminate at least 50% of the pain problem. Previous medical history is also important for the prognosis and determination of length of treatment. For example, a patient with postherpetic nerve pain also suffering from diabetes and thyroid disease will have a longer, more involved treatment course than a patient who is relatively healthy without any other major medical complications.

Utilization of Acupuncture Within a Western Clinical Setting

Acupuncture can be utilized in two ways to treat chronic pain conditions: (1) using acupuncture alone, and (2) using acupuncture plus a combination of allopathic medications and penetrative procedures such as cortisone spinal/paraspinal injections, spinal cord stimulators, radiofrequency ablations, surgical interventions, and so forth. Many patients do not tolerate medications and/or procedures well due to significant side effects and/or ineffectiveness. In addition, many patients simply do not want to start medications for pain conditions as they are fearful of addiction. In these cases, acupuncture (with or without herbal formulas) may be a very effective alternative. Acupuncture may also provide a safe and effective alternative for patients with significant pain who have not improved or deteriorated while taking "conventional" allopathic analgesic medications.

Acupuncture may be very effective when used in combination with allopathic medications. Often, a certain drug may have major side effects that inhibit the patient from taking it; other times medications gives temporary relief of symptoms or they function to "takes the edge off the pain." In these cases, acupuncture can be used in conjunction with the medications to provide optimal function while managing the side effects. Patients taking medications such as Vicodin or Percocet report that the drug helps the pain but doesn't take it away completely. These patients are excellent candidates for acupuncture. In many cases, these patients find that they can spread out their prescribed dosage with less pain once they have started acupuncture.

In addition, a growing number of pain medications take away pain but do not play a role in making the patient more functional. Because acupuncture takes into account the patient's structure and overall health, it can be used with pain medications to help a patient increase functionality while decreasing the pain with medications. This can help patients get out of the pain cycle, thus also helping with possible opioid addiction in the future.

In current practice, patients treated at a pain clinic often get prescribed medication and usually are referred to physical therapy. Many times, though, the patient is not ready for physical therapy as

Table 31.2. The Most Common Problems Treated With Acupuncture

Orthopedic	Neurological	Internal Organs	Miscellaneous
Any injury to bones, ligaments and tendons; joint pain, autoimmune disorders; repetitive strain disorders; phantom pain, herniated/bulging discs, spinal stenosis	Postherpetic neuralgia, diabetic neuropathy, complex regional pain syndrome (CRPS), reflex sympathetic dystrophy (RSD), and other complex pain syndromes, neuromas, sciatic pain, spinal stenosis pain, pinched nerves, Parkinson's syndrome, muscular dystrophy, headache, migraine	Chronic angina pectoris, abdominal pain, pelvic pain syndrome, chronic cystitis, Crohn's disease, and ulcerative colitis pain	Fibromyalgia, myofascial pain

it can aggravate his or her symptoms. A better approach may be to use the medications along with acupuncture to decrease the pain and increase function and resume daily activities. Once this goal is met, it is beneficial for the patient to go to physical therapy in order to strengthen and increase motor function to a greater extent. It is often the case that patients are sent to physical therapy too quickly and end up experiencing more pain and inflammation rendering them fearful of activity, which translates into an increase of dose and/or frequency in the use of their medication. Over time, these patients may become resistant to their medications, forcing the system to try alternatives such as higher dosage, different brands, as well as more toxic drugs. Early intervention with acupuncture can help these patients avoid such outcomes.

Some patients get good relief with medications but suffer from significant side effects such as constipation, diarrhea, nausea, headaches, dry mouth, tinnitus, and so forth. These patients are also excellent candidates for acupuncture. The treatment strategy of the acupuncture, in this case, would be to stimulate the kidney and liver to provide a detoxification in order to reduce (and sometimes eliminate) the side effects. The detox treatment will be provided side by side with the pain-control treatment in an effort to achieve a more "holistic" and long-lasting result.

Acupuncture also may be very useful as a complementary treatment to penetrative procedures. Acupuncture is best utilized in conjunction with these treatments in two ways: (1) Acupuncture may be used to prepare the body to optimally respond to interventions (in terms of structural muscles), and (2) acupuncture may enable interventional treatments to potentially have a longer duration of effect. It is conceivable that a patient who receives a glucocorticoid injection in the vicinity of the spinal cord may obtain suboptimal pain relief due to the muscle spasms surrounding the spine inhibiting the maximum relief a patient should get from the injection. Four or five acupuncture sessions relaxing and realigning the musculoskeletal system may give the injection a better chance to achieve its goal.

Acupuncture has gained popularity due to its efficacy in the management of a very wide range of medical disorders, among them acute and chronic pain syndromes.[12] Table 31.2 shows the most common pain problems treated with acupuncture.

Acupuncture is a cost-effective, low-risk treatment modality for the management and alleviation (sometimes complete) of chronic pain established with a large quantity of randomized control studies. The efficacy of acupuncture has been tested on a large variety of pain disorders ranging from chronic low back pain (Molsberger & Hille, 2002), osteoarthritis of the knees (Witt et al., 2005), and other orthopedic problems to headache disorders including migraine, and so forth. Unfortunately, none of these studies explain the mechanisms by which acupuncture achieves these positive results with no significant side effects.

Osteoarthritis is one of the major causes of pain-related disorders. A trial performed by Berman and colleagues (2005) demonstrated that acupuncture helps decrease pain and increase functionality in patients suffering from osteoarthritis of the knee. Linde et al. (2006) showed that patients with various types of osteoarthritis had a decrease in pain up to 6 months postacupuncture treatments.

Another study by Vas and colleagues compared two groups of patients suffering with osteoarthritis of the knee (Vas et al., 2004). One group received diclofenac and placebo acupuncture and the other group received diclofenac with acupuncture (Vas et al., 2004). The study concluded that diclofenac plus acupuncture was more effective than diclofenac plus placebo acupuncture. The group that received diclofenac plus acupuncture had a decrease in pain and stiffness along with increased physical function. This study demonstrates what has been seen in clinical settings in which acupuncture with allopathic medication can provide greater relief than allopathic medications alone.

Scharf et al. (2006) performed a three-armed randomized trial in 1,007 patients with at least 6 months of pain due to osteoarthritis of the knee (American College of Rheumatology [ARC] criteria and Kellgren-Lawrence score of 2 or 3) in an effort to assess the efficacy and safety of traditional Chinese acupuncture (needling at defined nonacupuncture points) and conservative therapy (physiotherapy and as-needed antiinflammatory drugs). Success rate was defined by at least 36% improvement in Western Ontario and McMaster Universities Osteoarthritis Index (WOMAC) score at 26 weeks. Success rates were 53.1% for TCA, 51.0% for sham acupuncture, and 29.1% for conservative therapy. Acupuncture groups had higher success rates than conservative therapy groups (relative risk for TCA compared with conservative therapy, 1.75 [95% CI, 1.43 to 2.13]; relative risk for sham acupuncture compared with conservative therapy, 1.73 [CI, 1.42 to 2.11]). There was no difference between TCA and sham acupuncture (relative risk, 1.01 [CI, 0.87 to 1.17]; Scharf et al., 2006). There is a high probability that the "sham" acupuncture managed to create a healing effect that is very similar to Japanese styles of acupuncture. In Japanese styles of acupuncture, it is common to use distal points with a little or no stimulation to achieve a healing effect. Unlike the formulaic rigid TCA style, the Japanese style of acupuncture is very generous with point location, meaning that any given acupuncture point can be located within an inch of the TCA point location. There are many credible styles of acupuncture that utilize a variety of different techniques from deep needling with deqi to nonpenetrative techniques, all of which have been shown clinically to decrease the pain levels in any given patient.

Low back pain is another disorder that affects millions of adults in the United States. The medical costs of low back pain are growing at rapid rate. Despite costly treatments, many patients do

---

[12] Acupuncture treatments will not cure genetic disorders, terminal disease, or fix advanced degenerative joint and bone problems, nor will acupuncture repair a broken or torn structure that clearly demands surgery.

not benefit from allopathic treatment. This is in part due to the fact that conventional treatments are too focused on the pain and do not always take into consideration other factors in the patient's medical history. Acupuncture is able to address a wide variety of back pain syndromes regardless of their origins. In a clinical setting, acupuncture has been able to address chronic low back pain associated with bulging discs, arthritis, "failed" back syndrome, and myofascial disease. There have been a number of promising studies that have shown the positive effects of acupuncture. One meta-analysis study showed that acupuncture decreased pain, increased functionality, and decreased the use of analgesic medication in patients suffering from low back pain (Manhelmer et al., 2005). Brinkhaus et al. (2006) showed that patients who received acupuncture over an 8-week period had a greater reduction in pain than those on a waiting list over the same time period. Another study demonstrated that acupuncture coupled with conventional orthopedic treatment (COT) was much more effective than COT alone in relieving chronic low back pain. The results from this study are very encouraging and had the potential to lead to a decrease in consumption of addictive medications.

Other orthopedic problems, such as various types of tendonitis, have been shown to improve with acupuncture. A randomized controlled trial (RCT) recruited 52 athletes with rotator cuff tendonitis. They were treated over a 4-week period and were assessed using the Constant-Murley Score. Patients in the acupuncture group improved significantly over the control group (Kleinhenz et al., 1999). Lateral elbow tendonitis has also been studied with some positive preliminary results (Molsberger & Hille, 1994).

The current available treatments for migraine headache patients are not suitable or effective for all. Many people who receive these medications and/or procedures develop not only a tolerance to them but can also develop "rebound" headaches. In addition, some medications have a wide array of unfavorable side effects. In recent years, there has been a growing body of research that shows that acupuncture is an effective treatment for migraine and chronic daily headaches. A small study was published to see the effect on the change in cerebrovascular blood flow in migraineurs before and after acupuncture stimulation. The results showed that patients who benefited from acupuncture (60%) had less abnormality in cerebrovascular response to visual stimulation. This means that the acupuncture reduced the intensity and/or frequency of migraine headache (Backer et al., 2004).

Another, much larger, RCT measured the effects of acupuncture on patients suffering from chronic headaches, particularly migraines at baseline, 3-month and 12-month follow-up. This study showed that at 12 months, the patients who received acupuncture had a significantly lower headache score than the control group. Furthermore, the study showed that the patients who received acupuncture missed fewer days at work, had a decreased number of visits to the general practitioner, and used less medication than those in the control group (Vickers et al., 2004). Again, this illustrates how acupuncture combined with allopathic medication can have a positive effect on the patient's quality of life.

Chronic pelvic pain in both men and women can be a challenge to treat with allopathic medicine alone as there can be many contributing factors that lead to the pain. Acupuncture can be used as a primary treatment for these conditions. A small study showed that acupuncture significantly reduced pain in men suffering from chronic pelvic pain with intrapelvic venous congestion. The study showed that pain was reduced in these men only 1 week after the fifth session of acupuncture was administered. Magnetic resonance venography (MRV) on these patients also showed that acupuncture decreased the intrapelvic venous congestion (Honjo et al., 2004). Acupuncture may provide safe and effective pain relief during pregnancy. Kvorning et al. (2004) performed an RCT that showed acupuncture to be effective decreasing visual analog scale (VAS) pain scores in pregnant women suffering from low back and pelvic pain. In addition, it also indicated that patients showed a decrease in pain during activity (Kvorning et al., 2004).

Acupuncture and General Approaches to Chemical Dependency

The efficacy of acupuncture in the treatment of substance abuse and drug withdrawal has been amply demonstrated to the scientific community. In fact, acupuncture has become standard procedure in many detoxification programs around the world. In the clinical setting, such as the pain clinic, primary care office, and so forth, the acupuncture treatment may be a very valuable tool for the practitioner and the patient to reduce the amount of medication required as well as eliminate the need for potentially addictive drugs (opiates and opiate derivatives). The use of acupuncture as a method of detoxification may also ensure that the medications needed will not cause internal organ damage so a patient can use these medications for a longer period of time, or as needed.

Chemical dependency in patients is a complex mechanism that includes biochemical cause and effect, psychological needs, cultural factors, as well as socioeconomic considerations. The effects and mechanisms of acupuncture in the detoxification process and reduction of symptoms associated with drug withdrawal have been studied to some degree and found to be effective and useful in the clinical setting. The other aspects of chemical dependency mentioned above are not in the scope of the acupuncture practice.

Many cite acupuncture's most heralded biomechanical action—the stimulation of endorphin production—as the primary physiological basis for its success in the treatment of substance abuse. This might be true for opiates and opiate derivatives, but it does not explain its success in the treatment of nonopiate addiction and how it prevents relapse. The following will be an attempt to explain the successes of the acupuncture treatments in both opiate and nonopiate dependency.

Although the natural painkilling neurotransmitter endorphin is best known for its role in analgesia, it may also be partially responsible for drug craving and physical withdrawal symptoms. Chronic use of exogenous opiates interferes with opioid receptors and through a negative feedback system results in a decrease in opioid peptides. Hence, when exogenous substances attach to opioid receptor sites, the presynaptic neurons receive the message that endogenous opioid transmission is normal, thus resulting in a reduction in the synthesis of those neurotransmitters. When the exogenous opioid is withdrawn, the body must once again begin manufacturing the supplanted endogenous opioids. During this time of replenishment, there is a net reduction of opioids in the body, which results in painful withdrawal symptoms. Acupuncture is thought to relieve withdrawal symptoms by triggering the body to produce more endorphins, thus bringing the body back to equilibrium. Normalization of endorphin systems may explain the effectiveness of acupuncture in treating withdrawal symptoms of opiate-related addictions.

The success that acupuncture treatment has on nonopiate-related addictions has several suggested mechanisms. Evidence suggests the importance of serotonin in acupuncture, particularly high-frequency electroacupuncture (50–2000Hz). Most of this evidence comes from research into analgesic effects of acupuncture. Investigations have shown that acupuncture activates the descending serotonergic pathways via the anterolateral tract. When acupuncture stimulation is applied to the correct points, neural impulses are received in the dorsal horn of the spinal cord. These impulses are conveyed to a variety of fibers of the spinoreticular and spinomesencephalic tracts and project to midbrain where they directly influence the descending serotonergic pathways. The hypothalamus and midbrain have interconnecting feedback or modulatory neuronal pathways. Therefore, by stimulating the descending serotonergic pathways with acupuncture, serotonin within the reward cascade is directly affected, leading eventually to an increase in dopamine in the nucleus accumbens and amygdala, and a subjective sense of well-being. Brain scans using fMRI have shown that acupuncture points, stimulated correctly, do affect these centers as well as other structures, creating a calm response of the brain. This is also evident in the clinic, where patients suffering from withdrawal symptoms fall asleep during treatments and awake not experiencing pain or anxiousness.

The most important feature in diagnosis and devising the treatment strategy, in the Japanese style of acupuncture, is palpation. Pressure pain afflicted by palpation of certain regions in the body is associated with stress and anxiety (especially the sternocleidomastoid muscles and the midline of the sternum). Stress, anxiety, general discomfort, and the inability to rest or relax are among the symptoms presented by patients in the physician's office who are going through withdrawal. Reduction of pressure pain at the areas that represent stress, anxiety, and so forth is an indication of the calming of the sympathetic nervous system and restoration of the balance in the autonomic nervous system. This reduction of pressure pain can be achieved with acupuncture treatments and maintained by inserting small semipermanent needles into the acupuncture points used. A common technique found in many detox clinics is to retain small press tack needles in the ear (utilizing auricular acupuncture) so that the patient can massage them in the case of reoccurring withdrawal symptoms.

Treatment Protocol/Integration With Other Modalities

Treatment protocols can vary from practitioner to practitioner. Generally speaking, patients receive acupuncture 1–2 times a week depending on the severity of the problem. For acute pain problems, it is favorable to see the patient twice a week for 3–4 weeks. After the acute pain subsides, it is beneficial for the patient to come once a week until the pain is gone and he or she is functional again. Chronic pain patients are usually seen once a week for about 7 to 10 sessions. Patients should see a positive change within 7 sessions. If they do not see any change, then it can be deduced that acupuncture alone is not a viable treatment for them. In many cases, internal herbal medicine may need to be combined with the acupuncture.

Acupuncture sessions are generally 1 hour long and consist of treating the front of the body for about 20 minutes and the back of the body for 20 minutes. Session times can vary slightly depending on the severity of the patient's complaints. The number of sessions required can also vary from patient to patient; therefore the above is a guideline. Generally speaking, the effects of the acupuncture sessions build one on the other so that the effect is cumulative. It is important to understand that a patient will go through a healing process, meaning that there will be decreases and increases in symptoms between sessions as the body heals. The net outcome should be favorable. There are two major ways patients may respond to acupuncture treatments. Some patients feel an immediate reduction in pain that may come back in increments over the week, whereas other patients may experience an increase in pain directly after the treatment but will notice a reduction in symptoms the day following treatment. This is important to keep in mind when judging the effectiveness of treatment.

The Role of Herbal Formulas in the Treatment of Pain and Chemical Dependency

Traditional Chinese medicine includes acupuncture moxibustion and the prescription of herbal formulas in combination with nutrition and exercise. As previously mentioned, the acupuncture and moxibustion treatment strategy is individually tailored to the patient (and not the disease); this is also true for the herbal formulas, nutrition, and exercise regime. Herbal medicine, according to traditional Chinese medicine, is not a single herb practice in which one herb at a time is chosen to remedy a particular symptom; rather, it is a combination of herbs, working as a whole, in the attempt to address the entire clinical presentation of the patient. Within this paradigm of thought, a patient presenting with chronic pain and or withdrawal symptoms will be prescribed an herbal formula that considers past medical history, reason for the onset of pain, working diagnosis for the lack of response to medication and other treatments, as well side effects to prescribed medications and the ability of the patient to absorb and assimilate the herbs. Such a formula might include as few as 2–4 herbs or as many as 16–20 herbs.

The formulas in traditional Chinese medicine are not just a random collection of herbs and minerals in which the actions of one herb or mineral are simply added to those of another in a cumulative fashion. They are complex recipes of interrelated substances, each of which affects the actions of the others in the formula. It is this complex interaction that makes the formulas so effective (and difficult to study).[13] An effective formula is one in which the substances are carefully balanced to accentuate the strengths and reduce the side effects. The combination of herbs in a formula creates a new therapeutic agent that can treat much more effectively and completely than can a single substance (Bensky & Barolet, 1990).

The utilization of herbal formulas in the modern, integrated medical practice uses prepared formulas in the form of powders, pills, capsules, and tinctures.[14] This enables the patient to use the herbal formulas with ease and ensures a regular intake over a period of time.[15] Herbal medicine is used for a large variety of medical conditions; pain and withdrawal symptoms are just a small example. Clinical trials and RCTs evaluating the effect of traditional Chinese herbal formulas are not abundant due to the complexity of the differential diagnosis and the large variety of herbal formulas possible to prescribe for any given condition. Nevertheless, there are studies that clearly demonstrate the ability of single herbs as well as herbal formulas to act as analgesics (Li et al., 2000) and to reduce inflammation (Wei et al., 1999; Zhou et al., 2006), and to

---

[13]In the United States, traditional Chinese herbal studies require a minimum of 3 years at an accredited acupuncture school. In most states, a license is required in order to prescribe traditional Chinese herbal formulas.
[14]The formulas are standardized and quality controlled.
[15]Traditional herbal medicine practitioners prescribe herbal packages that the patient has to cook on a daily basis. The cooking process can take a relatively long time and is rather aromatic. From clinical experience, the minority of patients are willing to participate in this form of medicine.

treat angina pectoris (He et al., 2004), osteoarthritis (Winther et al., 2005), and low back pain (Gagnier et al., 2004).

References

Backer M, Hammes M, Sander D, et al. Changes of cerebrovascular response to visual stimulation in migraineurs after repetitive session of somatosensory stimulation (acupuncture): A pilot study. *Headache: The Journal of Head and Face Pain.* Jan 2004; 44(1): 95.

Bensky D, Barolet R. *Formulas & Strategies.* Seattle, WA: Eastland Press, 1990, pp. 14.

Berman BM, Lao L, Langenberg P, et al. Effectiveness of acupuncture as adjunctive therapy in osteoarthritis of the knee. *Ann Intern Med.* Dec 21, 2005; 141(12): 901–10.

Blum K., Cull J., Braverman E., et al. Reward deficiency syndrome. *American Scientist.* March–April 1996; 132–145.

Brewington V., Smith M., Lipton D. Acupuncture as a detoxification treatment: An analysis of controlled research. *J Substance Abuse.* 1994; 2(4): 289–307.

Brinkhaus B, Witt C, Jena S, et al. Acupuncture in patients with chronic low back pain. *Arch Intern Med.* 2006; 166: 450–457.

Bullock M., Umen A., Culliton P., Olander R. Acupuncture treatment of recidivism: A pilot study. *Alcoholism: Clin Exper Res.* 1987; 11(3): 229–295.

Chen XH, Han JS. Analgesia induced by electroacupuncture of different frequencies is mediated by different types of opioid receptors: another cross-tolerance study. *Behav. Brain Res.* 1992b; 47: 1173–1177.

Chifuyu T, Kiyoshi O, Terumichi M, et al. The acupuncture point and its connecting central pathway for producing acupuncture analgesia. *Brain Research Bulletin.* 1993; 30: 53–67.

Chifuyu T, Takao S, Takashi M, et al. Descending pain inhibitory system involved in acupuncture. *Brain Research Bulletin.* 1992; 29: 617–634.

Cho ZH, Chung SC, Jones J P, et al. New findings of the correlation between acupoints and corresponding brain cortices using functional MRI. *Proc. National Acad Sci.* 1998; 95: 2670–2673.

Debreceni L. Chemical releases associated with acupuncture and electric stimulation. *Crit Rev Phys Rehab Med.* 1993; 5(3): 247–275.

Fei H, Xie GX, Han JS. Low and high frequency electroacupuncture stimulations release (Met5) enkephalin and dynorphin A in rat spinal cord. *Chinese Sci. Bull.* 1987; 32: 1496–1509.

Gagnier JJ, Chrubasik S, Manheimer E. Harpgophytum procumbens for osteoarthritis and low back pain: a systematic review. *BMC Complement Altern Med.* Sep 15 2004; 4:13.

Han J, Terenius L. Neurochemical basis of acupuncture analgesia. *Amer Review Pharm Toxicology.* 1982; 22: 193–220.

Han JS. Acupuncture: neuropeptide release produced by electrical stimulation of different frequencies. *Trends Neurosci.* 2003; 6:17–22.

Han JS, Xie GX. Dynorphin: important mediator for electroacupuncture analgesia in the spinal cord of the rabbit. *Pain.* 1984; 18: 367–376.

He J, Huang M, Zhang Q, et al. Treatment of unstable angina pectoris with modified nuan gan jian—a report of 33 cases. *J Tradit Chin Med.* 2004; 24(4):263–5.

Honjo H, Kamoi, K, Naya Y, et al. Effects of acupuncture for chronic pelvic pain syndrome with intrapelvic venous congestion: preliminary results. *Int J Urol.* 2004; 11(8): 607.

Hui KKS et al. The integrated response of the human cerebro-cerebellar and limbic systems to acupuncture stimulation at St36 as evidenced by fMRI. *Neuro Image.* 2005; 27: 479–496.

Hui KKS et al. Acupuncture modulates the limbic system and subcortical gray structures of the human brain: evidence from fMRI. *Human Brain Mapping.* 2000; 9(1): 13–25.

Jayasuriya A. *Scientific basis of acupuncture.* Colombo, Sri Lanka: Chandrakanthi Press (International); 1987: 42–74.

Kaptchuk TJ. *The Web That Has No Weaver.* Chicago: Congdon and Weed; 1983.

Kaptchuk TJ. The placebo effect in alternative medicine: can the performance of a healing ritual have clinical significance? *Ann Intern Med.* 2002; 136(11): 817–25.

Kendall D. A scientific model of acupuncture, parts 1 & 2. *American Journal of Acupuncture.* 1989; 17(3): 251–268; 17(4): 343–360.

Kim MR et al. Effect of acupuncture on behavioral hyperactivity and dopamine release in the nucleus accumbens in rats sensitized to morphine. *Neuroscience Letters.* 2005; 387(1): 17–21.

Kiser R., Khatami M., Gatchel R., et al. Acupuncture relief of chronic pain syndrome correlates with increased plasma met-enkephalin concentrations. *Lancet,* 1983; 2: 1394–1396.

Kleinhenz H, Streitberger K, Windeler J, et al. Randomised clinical trial comparing the effects of acupuncture and a newly designed placebo needle in rotator cuff tendonitis. *Pain.* 1999; 83(2): 235–241.

Kvorning N, Holmberg C, Grennert L, et al. Acpuncture relieves pelvic and low back pain in late pregnancy. *ACTA Obstet Gynecol Scand.* Mar 2004; 83: 246.

Langevin HM, Konofagou EE, Badger GJ, et al. Tissue displacements during acupuncture using ultrasound elastography techniques. *Ultrasound in Medicine and Biology.* 2004; 30: 1173–1183.

Langevin HM, Yandow JA. Relationship of acupuncture points and meridians to connective tissue planes. *Anat Rec.* 2002; 269: 257–265.

Lewith G., Kenyon J. Physiological and psychological explanations for mechanisms of acupuncture as a treatment for chronic pain. *Soc Sci Med.* 1984; 19: 1367–1378.

Li X, Zhang S, Qin L. [Experimental study of analgesic effect of combined Radix Aconiti and Radix Stephaniae Tetrandrae] *Zhongguo Zhong Xi Yi Jie He Za Zhi.* 2000; 20(3):202–4. [Article in Chinese].

Linde K, Weidenhammer W, Streng A, et al. Acupuncture for osteoarthritic pain: an observational study in routine care. *Rheumatology.* 2006; 45: 222–227.

Lipton D, Brewington V, Smith M. Acupuncture for crack-cocaine detoxification. *J Substance Abuse,* 1994; 2(3): 205–215.

Ma K-W. Acupuncture: its place in the history of Chinese medicine, *Acupuncture in Medicine.* 2000; 18(2): 55–99, and in R. Hayhoe (ed.), *East-West Medical Exchange and Their Mutual Influence, Knowledge Across Culture.* Hubei Education Press/OSIE Press; 1993: 154–81.

Mackler S, Eberwine J. The molecular biology of addictive drugs. *Molecular Neurobiology.* 1991; 5: 45–58.

Manhelmer E, White A, Berman B, et al. Meta-analysis: acupuncture for low back pain. *Ann Intern Med.* 2005; 142: 651–663.

Mann F. *Reinventing Acupuncture: A New Concept of Ancient Medicine.* London: Butterworth Heinemann, 1992.

Mayer DJ. Biological mechanisms of acupuncture. *Prog Brain Res.* 2000; 122: 457–77.

Melzack R. Myofascial trigger points: relation to acupuncture and mechanisms of pain. *Arch Phys Med Rehabil.* 1981, 62: 114–117.

Molsberger A, Hille E. The analgesic effect of acupuncture in chronic tennis elbow pain. *Br J Rheumatol.* 1994; 33(12): 1162–5.

Molsberger AF, Mau J, Pawele DB, et al. Does acupuncture improve the orthopedic management of chronic low back pain—a randomized, blinded, controlled trial with 3 months follow up. *Pain.* 2002; 99: 579–587.

Morgan JI, Curran T. Stimulus-transcription coupling in the nervous system: involvement of the inducible proto-oncogenes fos and jun. *Ann Rev Neurosci.* 1991; 14: 421–451.

National Institutes of Health. (1997, November 3–15). Acupuncture. *NIH Consensus Statement Online,* 15(5): 1–34.

Pan B, Castro-Lopes JM, Coimbra A. C-fos expression in the hypothalamo-pituitary system induced by electroacupuncture or noxious stimulation. *NeuroReport.* 1994; 5(13): 1649–1652.

Pert A., Dionne R., Ng L., et al. Alterations in rat central nervous system endorphins following transauricular acupunctur. *Brain Res.* 1981; 224: 83–93.

Pomeranz B. Acupuncture and endorphins. *Ethos.* 1982; 10: 385–393.

Scharf H-P, Mansmann U, Streitberger K, et al. Acupuncture and knee osteoarthritis—a three-armed randomized trial. *Annals.* 2006; 145: 12–20.

Scott S, Scott WN. A biochemical hypothesis for the effectiveness of acupuncture in the treatment of substance abuse: acupuncture and the reward cascade. *American Journal of Acupuncture.* 1997; 25(1): 33–38.

Shah JP, Phillips TM, Danoff JV, et al. An in vivo microanalytical technique for measuring the local biochemical milieu of human skeletal muscle. *Journal of Applied Physiology.* 2005; 99: 1977–1984.

Sytinsky I, Galebskaya L. Physio-biochemical basis of drug dependence treatment by acupuncture. *Addictive Behavior.* 1979; 4: 137–141.

U.S. Department of Justice. *Miami's "Drug Court": A Different Approach.* Washington, DC: Office of Justice Programs; June 1993: 3, 13.

Vas J, Mendez C, Perea-Milla E, et al. Acupuncture as complementary therapy to the pharmacological treatment of osteoarthritis of the knee: randomized controlled trial. *BMJ.* 2004; 329: 1216.

Vickers A, Zollman C, McCarney R, et al. Acupuncture for chronic headache in primary care: large pragmatic, randomized trial. *BMJ.* Mar 2004; 328: 744.

Wei F, Zou S, Young A, et al. Effects of four herbal extracts on adjuvant-induced inflammation and hyperalgesia in rats. *J Altern Complement Med.* 1999; 5(5): 429–36.

Winther K, Apel K, Thamsborg G. A powder made from seeds and shells of a rose-hip subspecies (Rosa canina) reduces symptoms of knee and hip osteoarthritis: a randomized, double-blind, placebo-controlled clinical trial. *Scand J Rheumatol.* 2005; 34(4): 302–8.

Witt C, Brinkhaus B, Jena S, et al. Acupuncture in patients with osteoarthritis of the knee: a randomized trial. *Lancet.* 2005; 366: 136–43.

Wu M-T, Hsieh J-C, Xiong J, et al. Central nervous pathway for acupuncture stimulation: localizing of processing with functional MR imaging of the brain—preliminary experience. *Neuroradiology.* 1999; 212:1; 133–141.

Zhou H, Wong YF, Cai X, et al. Suppressive effects of JCICM-6, the extract of an anti-arthritic herbal formula, on the experimental inflammatory and nociceptive models in rodents. *Biol Pharm Bull.* 2006; 29(2): 253–60.

32

Support Groups and Twelve-Step Programs in the Treatment of the Chronic Pain Patient

Douglas M. Ziedonis

Jeffrey A. Berman

M. Dale Lehn

Stephen Colameco

Chronic pain can cause great emotional and spiritual suffering, including isolation, exaggerated fears, obsession, shame, guilt, irrational thinking, anger, resentment, self-pity, and confusion. Patients often struggle with the question, "Why me?" Medication management, behavioral therapy, and complementary treatment approaches are commonly used and are often effective in helping the individual manage chronic pain; however, some individuals are better able to manage their chronic pain because they receive additional support and anticipatory guidance from peers at chronic pain support and 12-step groups.

Chronic pain can lead to depression, anxiety, obsession and preoccupation with the pain, perceived low self-esteem, and chemical dependence. Peer support groups can help individuals better handle their chronic pain and recover from negativity and self-defeating behaviors in a number of ways. First, they can find hope and strength from the group by hearing similar experiences of others and how they learned to improve the quality of their life. Second, they can overcome feelings of shame through the acceptance of the group. For many, attendance at a support group is often the first time they have heard others describing similar feelings, thoughts, and consequences from chronic pain. They learn that they are not alone! Participation in support groups can also facilitate a calming acceptance of their condition, so participants turn their attention away from suffering and focus on what they can do to improve their emotional and spiritual well-being.

Individuals with substance use disorders often experience chronic pain, and health-care providers usually recommend participation in 12-step recovery groups for the treatment of addiction. However, referring pain patients who are being treated with opiates, benzodiazepines, or muscle relaxants to 12-step programs can be problematic. Unfortunately, many group members do not accept the fact that pain patients receiving any of these medications can be still "working" a program of recovery. For this reason, it is advisable for health-care providers to educate patients about how to share this information with their 12-step group or sponsor in a manner that helps them to maintain their recovery and be "clean and sober." However, there is a reality that prescription drug abuse can occur and can be a complication of chronic pain management. Studies range in their findings on prescription drug abuse amongst patients receiving medication for chronic pain from as few as 2%–5% to as high as 20%–25% (Cicero et al., 2005; Johnston et al., 2005; Sullivan et al., 2005). However, 12-step meetings for prescription drug addiction are available—many attend Narcotics Anonymous (NA). Often, patients who become addicted as a consequence of medical treatment with opiates do not feel comfortable at NA meetings and initially see their situation as being very different from those NA attendees who "chose" on their own to begin drug use that led to addiction and was used to "get high."

This chapter focuses on how chronic pain support groups and newer 12-step programs such as Chronic Pain Anonymous can play an important role in the management of chronic pain. The chapter begins with an overview of the different types of support groups available and factors for the clinician to consider in making recommendations to patients about specific types of support groups or 12-step programs. The next section of the chapter reviews practical information to prepare patients before going to meetings, including helpful strategies that are recommended at support groups and how the 12-step principles have been adapted for chronic pain. Given the book's focus on chemical dependence and chronic pain, this chapter concludes with a section on how to work with the patient who has chronic pain and addiction, including how to monitor addiction recovery status, facilitate 12-step participation, and provide anticipatory guidance regarding the issue of taking pain medication and attending 12-step addiction recovery meetings.

Although more research is needed on evaluating chronic pain support groups, there have been some studies demonstrating that these support groups can be effective in improving an individual's quality of life and ability to live fuller lives even with chronic pain. In addition, some of these studies found that pain symptoms were further reduced with the addition of chronic pain support groups; however, other studies did not (Creamer et al., 2000; Haughli et al., 2001; Hitchcock et al., 1994; Jerome, 1991; Linton et al., 1997; Lorig et al., 2002; Subramaniam et al., 1999; Von Korff et al., 1998; Weis, 2003).

Matching Patient Issues to Types of Support Groups/Twelve-Step Programs

There are a variety of types of chronic pain support groups and 12-step programs that could be of help to patients with chronic pain and the common comorbidities associated with chronic pain such as chemical dependence and mental health problems. Health-care providers have a unique opportunity to provide patients with information about the range of support groups, to encourage patients with particular clinical issues to attend support groups, and to provide anticipatory guidance on how to best make use of the support groups.

Individuals with chronic pain who have become more isolated, irritable, angry, and depressed may benefit from a mental health consultation; however, they also may find a support group to be very helpful. Sometimes just having the experience of knowing others have had similar suffering with chronic pain can be helpful—especially when they learn how others have developed strategies to improve their life. This information and experience can be very empowering and provide new participants with a sense of hope, while, at the same time, teaching what can be controlled and what cannot. At meetings some members may chose to focus on discussing about the difficulties they have encountered as a result of their pain, but for the most part the focus of the support groups is on recovery—providing hope, motivation, and practical solutions to promote wellness.

Support groups aren't for everyone; however, clinicians should be prepared to respond to an initial negative response from the patient in regard to attending a support group. This initial patient resistance may reflect the anxiety of a patient in being labeled as having an emotional problem or as being weak; often it is the patient's anxiety about being in an initially uncomfortable and awkward public setting. Clinicians may get a warmer response from the patient if the clinician encourages group participation and both normalizes support group attendance and provides the individual patient with specific feedback in regard to why a meeting might help their specific situation. A recommendation that conveys positive expectation for attending a support group meeting can make a great difference in the patient's willingness to attend, become active, and also express gratitude to the clinician after participating in the support group meetings.

Support groups vary in their primary goals and the amount of structure they provide. Some support groups tend to focus on providing education and have expert guest speakers, whereas others emphasize peer education. Some meetings are more social and unstructured versus others that are structured and follow a set format. Sometimes individuals benefit from a more structured, didactic program, whereas at other times they may benefit from a less structured program that emphasizes sharing of feelings. There are many choices, and each meeting will be a different experience—so one meeting may be a great match and another a poor match for any given individual. For some patients, participation in meetings that are guided by a "program" of recovery based on progressive "steps" can feel more structured and therefore reduce anxiety thus facilitating a more "upbeat" and "hopeful" atmosphere.

There are several national chronic pain organizations that have a primary activity of organizing support groups and training people with chronic pain to have skills to help guide these groups. Box 32.1 lists several of the major national organizations that have information on local chronic pain support groups, online Internet support groups, and other contact information. Some individuals may want to start with support groups that are on the Internet and later attend face-to-face support group meetings.

Support Groups on the Internet

The Internet has become a resource of information for professionals, patients, and family members interested to learn more about chronic pain, including online support groups. There are interactive Internet sites that allow for discussion amongst individuals with chronic pain. Martelli et al. (2000) provides a good introduction to Internet sites focused on the issue of chronic pain, including information for professionals, patients, and family members. One example, "PainAid" of the American Pain Foundation (http://www.painfoundation.org), provides online "chat rooms" and "conference rooms" that have scheduled live chats on a range of issues, "discussion boards," which are message boards on a broad range of topics, and "ask-the-experts" via online message boards moderated by licensed health-care professionals. Because of the anonymity, ease of access, and no cost, more individuals are reaching out online. One randomized controlled study found that a closed group, moderated, e-mail discussion group was helpful in improving outcomes in the treatment of chronic recurrent back pain (Lorig et al., 2002). This type of e-mail support group may be particularly useful for those who have difficulty with transportation. This study found that individuals who participated in the e-mail discussion group reduced their chronic pain and health distress while also improving their role functioning compared to a control group (Lorig et al., 2002).

Chronic Pain Versus Specific Disorder Focused Support Groups

Another factor to consider is whether a patient might want to attend a general chronic pain support group or one that focuses on a specific cause of chronic pain (such as fibromyalgia or arthritis).

Box 32.1 Chronic Pain Support Groups

American Chronic Pain Association (ASPA), http://www.the acpa.org; address: P.O. Box 850, Rocklin, CA 95677; phone: 1–800–533–3231

National Chronic Pain Society, http://www.ncps-cpr.org/support_groups.php; address: 900 Town & Country St., Suite 310, Houston, TX 77024; phone: 281-357-HOPE (4673); fax: 281-357-4514; e-mail: ncps@houston.rr.com

American Pain Foundation (APF), http://www.painfoundation.org (including PainAid online chat and discussion); address: 201 North Charles Street, Suite 710, Baltimore, MD 21201-4111; phone: 1-888-615-PAIN (7246)

Chronic Pain Anonymous (CPA), http://www.chronicpainanonymous.org; address: P.O. Box 41, Riderwood MD 21139; phone: Dale 410–825–8442 ext. 2

National Chronic Pain Outreach Association—Support Groups listing, http://www.chronicpain.org; address: P.O. Box 274, Millboro, VA 24460; phone: 540-862-9437; fax: 540-862-9485

The American Academy of Pain Medicine (AAPM), http://www.painmed.org; address: 4700 W. Lake, Glenview, IL 60025; phone: 847/375–4731; fax: 877/734–8750; e-mail: aapm@amctec.com

A simple search on the Internet will find support groups of both types. The groups that are devoted to specific medical conditions are more apt to offer educational and resource networking components that helps the attendee learn about new treatment approaches and other condition-specific resources.

Peer-Led Versus Professional-Led Support Groups

Support groups are usually facilitated by people with chronic pain and are not professional therapy groups; however, some institutions have developed support groups that are led by counselors/experts who use the strategies of support groups. Some individuals prefer to have an expert-led support group. The counselor-led group often has three primary goals. The first goal is to make participants aware of the relationship between individuals' body symptoms and their emotions, thoughts, and life situations. The second goal is to help the patient shift the focus away from the pain toward recovery and empowerment. The third goal is to provide education and information on resources in the community. A randomized controlled study of the effectiveness of this type of professional-led support group found that patients who participated in group sessions reported less pain, better pain-coping abilities and less use of health-care resources than the control group (Haugli et al., 2001).

Twelve-Step-Oriented Chronic Pain Support Groups

In recent years, 12-step programs such as Chronic Pain Anonymous have been created with a limited number of meetings. Twelve-step meetings have structured formats that follow the general principles of the Alcoholics Anonymous (AA) 12-step approach. Given the commonalities in the emotional and spiritual suffering caused by these two conditions (alcoholism and chronic pain) it is not surprising that the AA model was adapted for chronic pain. There are different types of 12-step meetings for addictions (e.g., speaker, open/closed, step, discussion, gender-specific), but this range is not available for Chronic Pain Anonymous meetings that incorporate the components of all these traditional meeting types into their meetings. Individuals familiar with Alcoholics Anonymous or other addiction 12-step program approaches may be particularly open to considering how to utilize the 12-step approach to living better with their pain. Most are not aware that there are 12-step Chronic Pain Anonymous meetings. These 12-step meetings create a fellowship of mutual support and opportunity for the chronic pain sufferer to share their experience, strength, and hope.

Co-occurring Substance Use Disorders

Another important factor to consider in recommending a specific type of support group or 12-step meeting is the issue of co-occurring substance use disorder. Many individuals with substance use disorders, active or in stable recovery, also have a chronic pain disorder (Rosenblum et al., 2003). The manner in which health-care providers integrate 12-step programs (for addiction and/or chronic pain) can vary according to the patient's history of substance use, including the five subtypes of individuals with chronic pain and substance use based on their substance use:

1. Active substance abuse or dependence
2. No active substance use and are in recovery or remission
3. Those on agonist therapy with methadone or buprenorphine
4. No prior substance use disorders who for the first time develop a substance use disorder in the context of their chronic pain treatment
5. Those with no past history or current symptoms of a substance use disorder

Patients with an active chemical dependence or mental illness may also benefit from attendance at 12-step meetings or other support groups that target the addiction or mental illness. The 12-step program is a very helpful component of effective treatment and is often integrated into the different levels of addiction treatment programs (outpatient, intensive outpatient, partial hospital, or residential). The chronic pain treatment specialist has the opportunity to both monitor the patient's involvement in 12-step programs and in some situations to actually provide 12-step facilitation. The Recovery Status Exam and 12-step facilitation will be discussed in more detail later in this chapter. For individuals who are in stable recovery, many have already found the value of attending 12-step meetings for substance use disorders; however, they may face negative reactions from peers if they choose to disclose the fact that they are being treated for chronic pain with opiates or other medications. Health-care providers must be prepared to provide anticipatory guidance on how to handle peer pressure that might cause individuals to stop taking pain medication. Such pressures can complicate participation in addiction recovery and may even cause individuals to cease attending addiction recovery meetings, often leading to substance abuse relapse.

Prescription drug dependence is a complicated and more common addiction problem. Clinicians who treat chronic pain must remain vigilant and constantly monitor and assess for the aberrant behaviors that can be indicators of substance use disorders. Prescription drug abuse has increased in the United States in recent years and can either precede chronic pain or be a consequence of chronic pain (Isaacson et al., 2005). In addition to obtaining prescription pills from prescribers and traditional illicit drug dealers, individuals can now purchase prescription medications via the Internet. Many individuals with prescription drug dependence complain that they do not "fit in" with the majority group who attend Narcotics Anonymous. This issue can be managed through 12-step facilitation approaches that emphasize the need for recovery and doing step work rather than focusing on the individual characteristics of those who attend (e.g., intravenous heroin use versus pain pills). Patients are advised to look for similarities amongst the other members (usually the feelings and thoughts that are similar) and to take what is helpful at the meetings and leave the rest behind. Unfortunately, there are limited 12-step meetings that focus just on prescription drugs or the dual problem of chronic pain and addiction. Individuals at highest risk for prescription drug abuse are those with a past or current history of another substance use disorder, a family history of a substance use disorder, or a history of being a trauma victim (Fishbain et al., 1992; Isaacson et al., 2005; Joranson et al., 2000). Balancing substance use disorders and the management of chronic pain can be challenging at times, but can be effective when both issues are addressed simultaneously, including the use of 12-step meetings and support groups.

Another common addiction disorder amongst individuals with chronic pain that often goes untreated is tobacco dependence (see Chapter 21, "Smoking, Pain, and Addiction"). As patients consider ways to live healthier lifestyles, there is a growing interest in quitting smoking to reduce morbidity and mortality. There are support groups and 12-step meetings of Nicotine Anonymous (NicA) that are available for helping tobacco users to quit, and social support during tobacco dependence treatment is very important in addition to medications and psychosocial treatments.

More research is needed on tobacco dependence treatment in the population of patients with chronic pain; however, some studies suggest that tobacco use is associated with more pain symptoms. One study of fibromyalgia and tobacco addiction found that 21.9% were regular tobacco smokers and that after adjustment for age and education there was more pain, global severity, functional disability, and numbness amongst smokers compared to nonsmokers (Yunus et al., 2002). A similar study of chronic spinal disability patients found that smokers had higher posttreatment pain and disability ratings, providing further evidence that ongoing tobacco smoking may negatively affect rehabilitation (McGeary et al., 2004). Treating tobacco dependence is an important public health issue that should be considered by chronic pain specialists, and more research is needed on the use of support groups for this problem.

Co-occurring Mental Illness

Many individuals with chronic pain also have a history of mental illness or may have developed depressive and/or anxiety symptoms or disorders in the context of dealing with their chronic pain (Sullivan et al., 2005). In addition to a consultation from a mental health professional, clinicians might encourage attendance at a chronic pain support group to help them feel less isolated and better able to handle these emotions. Enhancing emotional well-being is an important component of support groups as indicated from a survey of persons with chronic nonmalignant pain who were members of a national self-help organization. In fact, this survey found that depression was one of the worst problems caused by chronic pain, with about 50% of those surveyed reporting that they had contemplated suicide due to feelings of hopelessness associated with their chronic pain (Hitchcock et al., 1994). In addition to support groups for chronic pain, some of these individuals may also benefit from support groups that focus on depression or anxiety disorders. Emotions Anonymous (http://www.emotionsanonymous.org/) is a 12-step organization for recovery from emotional difficulties that utilizes the 12-step philosophy of Alcoholics Anonymous. Other support groups for specific mental health conditions are easily found on a search of the Internet. Research on the patient-led chronic pain support groups have found that these support groups can be effective at helping to reduce anxiety, worries, and sadness and improve self-care and involvement in activities (Subramaniam et al., 1999; Van Korff et al., 1998).

Chronic Pain Support Groups Provide Fellowship, Support, and Helpful Guidance

Chronic pain support groups provide individuals with a connection with others, new information on available resources, a better sense of what they can and cannot control, and specific strategies on how to manage their chronic pain more effectively. Learning how others have dealt with difficult issues can make a big difference in another person's recovery. Many individuals find the most important benefit from the support groups is "the fellowship." Amongst others living with a similar experience they often feel connected, accepted, and understood. This experience can help facilitate the individual's acceptance of their chronic pain condition. Many people with chronic pain will be more open in sharing about their feelings and situation in the context of being with others who understand what they are going through. Through a process of mutual trust, acceptance, and nonjudgmental support, individuals develop a sense of hope.

Box 32.2 Chronic Pain Support Group Do's and Don'ts From the ACPA

DO look to the support groups to help you improve the quality of your life in spite of your pain.
DO continue to seek proper health care while attending support group meetings.
DO feel free to talk about what your pain has done to your life and the changes that have occurred.
DO look to the support group members to listen to what you are saying and give you feedback and support.
DO expect to learn coping skills that can help you to become involved in your recovery. DO expect to have your needs met during group meeting, if you let the group know what you need.
DO let the group contact person know if you are unable to attend a meeting.
DO make your own decisions and accept responsibility for your actions.
DO offer to help with the group. Take responsibility for helping to make the group a success for all members.
DON'T allow prolonged discussion about physical symptoms to take up group time.
DON'T talk about medications in the group. We each experience medication differently and this should be discussed with your personal health care professional.
DON'T compare your progress with that of others. No one is looking for perfection; rather we hope to help you achieve the personal goals you have set for yourself.
DON'T interrupt when someone is talking. Allow him or her to finish before commenting.
DON'T give advice.
DON'T look for a miracle: the ACPA cannot take away your pain. We can help you to live more effectively despite your pain.
DON'T judge other group members.
DON'T discuss personal information about group members outside group. Respect confidentiality.

Reprinted with permission from the American Chronic Pain Association.

The insights learned from members of chronic pain support groups have been put together in useful resources that can serve as a guide to help individuals be prepared and feel more comfortable at the support groups. The American Chronic Pain Association (ACPA; http://www.theacpa.org) has developed some helpful do's and don'ts for people considering attending a support groups (see Box 32.2). The ACPA has also developed a very useful resource for members to help guide individuals on how to manage their chronic pain and groups on important issues to include in support groups (see Box 32.3). This practical and focused 10-step approach is representative of the type of information available at support groups. Groups can help individuals learn ways to relax better and redirect their attention to things that can be controlled versus the chronic pain. Similar to a 12-step perspective, learning to accept the chronic pain condition and to stop fighting or denying the pain is perceived as a big step toward recovery and healing. Many individuals find that staying active, within realistic limits, helps them remain flexible and reduce the sense of suffering.

Some support groups use books from of self-help genre as their main written instructional material to provide information and guide some of the support group discussion. Examples of these books are listed in Box 32.4. This model of using readings to help members of support groups is a core method in Alcoholics Anonymous, which uses *Alcoholics Anonymous* ("the Big Book"; Alcoholics Anonymous, 1955) and *The Twelve Steps and Twelve Traditions* ("Twelve and Twelve"; Alcoholics Anonymous, 1992). Some of the listed chronic pain books are very 12-step–oriented and follow the principles of Alcoholics Anonymous, only adapted

Box 32.3 ACPA's Ten Steps for Moving From Patient to Person

Step 1: Accept the Pain
Learn all you can about your physical condition. Understand that there may be no current cure and accept that you will need to deal with the fact of pain in your life.

Step 2: Get Involved
Take an active role in your own recovery. Follow your doctor's advice and ask what you can do to move from a passive role into one of partnership in your own health care.

Step 3: Learn to Set Priorities
Look beyond your pain to the things that are important in your life. List the things that you would like to do. Setting priorities can help you find a starting point to lead you back into a more active life.

Step 4: Set Realistic Goals
We all walk before we run. Set goals that are within your power to accomplish or break a larger goal down into manageable steps. And take time to enjoy your successes.

Step 5: Know Your Basic Rights
We all have basic rights. Among these are the rights to be treated with respect, to say no without guilt, to do less than humanly possible, to make mistakes, and to not need to justify your decisions, with words or pain.

Step 6: Recognize Emotions
Our bodies and minds are one. Emotions directly affect physical well-being. By acknowledging and dealing with your feelings, you can reduce stress and decrease the pain you feel.

Step 7: Learn to Relax
Pain increases in times of stress. Relaxation exercises are one way of reclaiming control of your body. Deep breathing, visualization, and other relaxation techniques can help you to better manage the pain you live with.

Step 8: Exercise
Most people with chronic pain fear exercise. But unused muscles feel more pain than toned flexible ones. With your doctor, identify a modest exercise program that you can do safely. As you build strength, your pain can decrease. You'll feel better about yourself, too.

Step 9: See the Total Picture
As you learn to set priorities, reach goals, assert your basic rights, deal with your feelings, relax, and regain control of your body, you will see that pain does not need to be the center of your life. You can choose to focus on your abilities, not your disabilities. You will grow stronger in your belief that you can live a normal life in spite of chronic pain.

Step 10: Reach Out
It is estimated that one person in three suffers with some form of chronic pain. Once you have begun to find ways to manage your chronic pain problem, reach out and share what you know. Living with chronic pain is an ongoing learning experience. We all support and learn from each other.

Reprinted with permission from the American Chronic Pain Association.

Box 32.4 Reference Books Used as "Big Books" at Chronic Pain Anonymous Meetings

Chronic Illness and the Twelve Steps: A Practical Approach to Spiritual Resilience, Martha Cleveland, Ph.D.
Living with Pain, A New Approach to the Management of Chronic Pain, Richard L. Reilly, D.O.
12 Steps for Those Afflicted With Chronic Pain, Stephen Colameco, M.D., M.Ed.
Mastering Pain: A Twelve-Step Program for Coping with Chronic Pain, R. Sternbach, M.D.

learning relaxation techniques, and getting involved in hobbies and other activities. The emotional and spiritual suffering of chronic pain is important to acknowledge and perhaps address through interacting with others, attending support groups, and enhancing their spiritual connection with God or a higher power (Cleveland, 1999; Colameco, 2005; Reilly, 1993; Sternbach, 1987).

Typical Format of Chronic Pain Twelve-Step Meetings

There are several forms of Chronic Pain Anonymous' (CPA) 12-step meetings. CPA meetings are open to anyone who wishes to attend. The only agreement is to preserve the anonymity of all those attending and of all stories shared during the meeting. A "typical" CPA meeting uses a standard format that was adapted from Alcoholics Anonymous meetings. The meeting opens with one member of the group (an established regular member) calling the meeting to order and asking someone from the gathering to read the prologue (see Box 32.5), another person to read the 12 steps of CPA (see Box 32.6) and someone else to read the 12 promises (see Box 32.7). These readings set the tone for the meeting. At discussion meetings, group members choose discussion topics. Once topics have been chosen, members raise their hands indicating that they wish to speak to a specific topic already chosen by the group. At speaker meetings, one or more individuals are chosen to be "speakers"; they share their story of how the 12 steps of CPA have affected their lives and helped them to live with chronic pain. Chronic Pain Anonymous does not yet have its own "Big Book," although members are currently writing one following the example of Alcoholics Anonymous. Without a specific CPA Big Book, the CPA has still been able to have some meetings that are modeled after the AA Big Book meetings, but CPA members read from two books—either *Living With Pain* by Richard Reilly or *Chronic Pain and the Twelve Steps* by Martha Cleveland. At meetings that have a Big Book orientation, members take turns reading a section of one of these two books. After the reading, there is an open discussion where any person at the meeting can share their understanding of

for chronic pain. Some books provide helpful steps, like the ACPA's 10-step guide to helping individuals manage their pain and feel like a person again. These books are especially helpful for patients who find that reading is effective in helping them with problems and could be used by the clinicians in the treatment of the patient.

Most of these resources recommend beginning with "acceptance" of the chronic pain and provide some anticipatory guidance on how to manage their preoccupation with their chronic pain in the short term while developing longer term strategies of alternative activities. Some of the short-term strategies include setting realistic goals and keeping busy with other activities to distract them from the chronic pain, such as becoming physically fit,

Box 32.5 Chronic Pain Anonymous: Prologue

CPA is a fellowship of men and women who share their experience, strength, and hope with each other so that they may solve their common problem and help others recover from chronic pain.

The only requirement for membership is a desire to recover from the physical, emotional, and spiritual debilitation of chronic pain. There are no dues or fees for CPA membership. We are self-supporting through our own contributions.

CPA is not allied with any sect, denomination, politics, organization, or institution; does not wish to engage in any controversy, neither endorses nor opposes any causes. Our primary purpose is to live our lives to the fullest by minimizing the effects of chronic pain in our lives and to help others to do the same.

Box 32.6 Chronic Pain Anonymous: The Twelve Steps of Recovering From Pain

1. We admitted we were powerless pain—that our lives had become unmanageable.
2. Came to believe that a Power greater than ourselves could restore us to sanity.
3. Made a decision to turn our will and our lives over to the care of God AS WE UNDERSTOOD HIM.
4. Made a searching and fearless moral inventory of ourselves.
5. Admitted to God, to ourselves, and to another human being the exact nature of our wrongs.
6. Were entirely ready to have God remove all these defects of character.
7. Humbly asked Him to remove our shortcomings.
8. Made a list of all persons we had harmed, and became willing to make amends to them all.
9. Made direct amends to such people wherever possible, except when to do so would injure them or others.
10. Continued to take personal inventory and when we were wrong promptly admitted it.
11. Sought through prayer and meditation to improve our conscious contact with God AS WE UNDERSTOOD HIM, praying only for knowledge of His will for us and the power to carry that out.
12. Having had a spiritual awakening as the result of these steps, we tried to carry this message to those in pain, and to practice these principles in all our affairs.

Disclaimer: The Twelve Steps of Chronic Pain Anonymous, as adapted by Al-Anon with permission of Alcoholics Anonymous World Services, Inc. ("AAWS"), are reprinted with permission of Chronic Pain Anonymous and AAWS. The Twelve Steps of Alcoholics Anonymous, as well as an excerpt from pages 83–84 of the book *Alcoholics Anonymous*, are reprinted with the permission of AAWS. AAWS' permission to reprint the foregoing material does not mean that AAWS has reviewed or approved the contents of this publication, or that AAWS necessarily agrees with the views expressed therein. Alcoholics Anonymous is a program of recovery from alcoholism *only*—use or permissible adaption of A.A.'s Twelve Steps in connection with programs or activities which are patterned after A.A., but which address other problems, or in any other non-A.A. context, does not imply otherwise.

what was read. Chronic Pain Anonymous also offers step meetings. In the tradition of other 12-step programs, CPA has its own steps. At a step meeting, the group reads and discusses the particular step in detail, with emphasis placed on how the step can apply to each person's life. The most important aspect of any CPA meeting is the honest sharing of individual experiences, their expression of strength, and their hope for the future.

Box 32.7 The Twelve Promises (AA)

If we are painstaking about this phase of our development, we will be amazed before we are halfway through.
We are going to know a new freedom and a new happiness.
We will not regret the past nor wish to shut the door on it.
We will comprehend the word *serenity* and we will know peace.
No matter how far down the scale we have gone, we will see how our experience can benefit others.
That feeling of uselessness and self-pity will disappear.
We will lose interest in selfish things and gain interest in our fellows.
Self-seeking will slip away.
Our whole attitude and outlook upon life will change.
Fear of people and of economic insecurity will leave us.
We will intuitively know how to handle situations which used to baffle us.
We will suddenly realize that God is doing for us what we could not do for ourselves.
Are these extravagant promises? We think not.
They are being fulfilled among us—sometimes quickly, sometimes slowly.
They will always materialize if we work for them.

Reprinted with permission from Alcoholics Anonymous World Services, Inc., pp. 83–84.

"Working the Steps" of a Twelve-Step Program

Twelve-step programs like AA and CPA offer many tools for recovery, but the most important is for the individual to actually "work the steps." Other tools such as going to meetings, not isolating, calling peers, getting a sponsor, praying, having an attitude of gratitude, keeping active, using affirmations, and helping others are all useful tools that fit into the process of "working the steps."

To work the steps is a process of methodically learning and applying each of the 12 steps in their order. There are many excellent resources for the professional and the individual who might attend the 12-step programs to learn about how to work the steps. One example is *Twelve-Step Sponsorship: How It Works* (Hamilton, 1996). Box 32.8 lists the 12 steps of Alcoholics Anonymous. Tables 32.9 and 32.6 show two examples of how two different 12-step-based chronic pain support groups have adapted the traditional AA 12 steps for chronic pain. Box 32.9 outlines the 12 steps for those afflicted with chronic pain, and Box 32.6 is Chronic Pain Anonymous' 12 steps of recovering from pain.

Clinicians have two opportunities to help patients in working the steps. One is to administer the Recovery Status Exam (this is described later in this chapter). The other is to engage the patient in 12-step facilitation therapy, which might include reviewing and helping patients to work the steps. Twelve-step facilitation is an evidence-based treatment approach that has been found to be effective in the treatment of addiction (Project MATCH Research Group, 1988).

The first step in all 12-step programs is to accept that life has become unmanageable. Just as alcoholics must admit that they cannot control their drinking (Step 1), chronic pain patients have to accept their powerlessness over their own physiology that is causing the pain symptoms. Their pain is not necessarily taken away, but they are able to live a more meaningful and active life and not be self-absorbed and filled with anger, resentment, self-pity, and other feelings and thoughts that keep them isolated. Members of 12-step programs believe they are powerless to overcome their

Box 32.8 The Twelve Steps of Alcoholics Anonymous

1. We admitted we were powerless over alcohol—that our lives had become unmanageable.
2. Came to believe that a Power greater than ourselves could restore us to sanity.
3. Made a decision to turn our will and our lives over to the care of God as we understood Him.
4. Made a searching and fearless moral inventory of ourselves.
5. Admitted to God, to ourselves, and to another human being the exact nature of our wrongs.
6. Were entirely ready to have God remove all these defects of character.
7. Humbly asked Him to remove our shortcomings.
8. Made a list of all persons we had harmed, and became willing to make amends to them all.
9. Made direct amends to such people wherever possible, except when to do so would injure them or others.
10. Continued to take personal inventory and when we were wrong promptly admitted it.
11. Sought through prayer and meditation to improve our conscious contact with God as we understood Him, praying only for knowledge of His will for us and the power to carry that out.
12. Having had a spiritual awakening as the result of these Steps, we tried to carry this message to alcoholics, and to practice these principles in all our affairs.

The Twelve Steps printed by permission of AA World Services, New York, New York.

Box 32.9 The Twelve Steps for Those Afflicted With Chronic Pain

1. Admitted that we are powerless over our pain, that our lives had become controlled by our suffering, and became willing to try a new way of living.
2. Came to believe that a Power greater than ourselves could help us find strength in our adversity and fulfillment in our lives.
3. Learned to let go of our bitterness and fear by turning our lives and will over to the care of the Higher Power, accepting that even our suffering is part of the Higher Power's plan.
4. Made an honest assessment of our strengths and weaknesses, accepting the fact that our emotions contribute to our suffering.
5. Learned to share the facts of our lives with others, without feeling ashamed, blaming ourselves, or blaming others.
6. Became ready to accept the fact that we are loved by our Higher Power, and are deserving of healing.
7. Humbly asked our Higher Power for the strength to overcome our shortcomings, so that we can carry out the Higher Power's will for us.
8. Made a list of all the persons we had harmed because we were controlled by our pain and our fear, and became willing to make amends to them all.
9. Made direct amends to such people whenever possible, except when to do so would injure them or others.
10. Continued to take a personal inventory of our strengths and our weaknesses, and promptly admitted when we harm others or ourselves.
11. Sought through prayer and meditation to improve our conscious contact with our Higher Power, praying only for knowledge of our Higher Power's will for us and for the power to carry that out.
12. Having had a spiritual awakening as a result of these steps, we sought to carry this message to other sand to practice these principles in all of our affairs.

Source: Colameco, Steven. *Twelve Steps for Those Afflicted With Chronic Pain: A Guide to Recovery from Emotional and Spiritual Suffering.* Reprinted with permission.

---

problem when they are trying to do so alone. They can affect change with the help of their higher power and the program. Prior to taking this first step, their lives had been managed around their experience of pain; this fact had affected their choices in activities, careers, entertainment, or any other actions depending upon the severity level of their chronic pain. Through participation in a 12-step support group, they learn to differentiate between attempts to control over that which they are powerless to change (e.g., chronic pain) versus what they do have the power to control (how they act in response to events, either initially, or in the hours, days, and years afterward). Paradoxically, acceptance of powerlessness gives the individual the courage to attempt to change only the things that they can change. Some patients may have particular difficulties with this concept, and believe it is wrong to admit you are powerless over your pain. This may be due to anger at the condition causing the chronic pain or a fear that if they admit they are powerless they will have surrendered to the pain and "given up" completely. This first step identifies the problem and bridges to the next two steps by taking responsibility for and ownership of their healing from this point forward with the help of their higher power.

In doing this first step, the person must acknowledge the consequences that chronic pain has had on their life and that their lives have become a series of "I cannot do this or that." Group members share how chronic pain leads people to withdraw socially because of the pain and how fear limits their making commitments to others. They often experience a loss of patience with the ones they love. Chronic pain may lead to unemployment, partial employment, financial difficulties, much time and money spent on doctors, physical therapy, or other health practitioners, and limited energy to do the basic chores to support themselves (clean house, do laundry, grocery shop, etc.).

The Serenity Prayer, written by Reinhold Niebuhr, has been used by many people in an effort to accept difficult situations that are out of their control: "God, Grant me the Serenity to accept the things I cannot change, Courage to change the things I can, and Wisdom to know the difference" (Alcoholics Anonymous, 1955). The Serenity Prayer is a pillar of the philosophy espoused Alcoholics Anonymous and other 12-step programs: As with alcohol dependence and other substance use disorders, acceptance of the situation can help many individuals with chronic pain to paradoxically manage their situation better. When patients accept pain as an everyday part of their lives, they are able to achieve a greater sense of inner peace and serenity versus inner turmoil and conflict.

Interestingly, studies of patients' ability to accept chronic pain have found that "acceptance" is an important predictor of better outcomes for those living with chronic pain. These studies were of patients in a self-support group for fibromyalgia and in a pain clinic support group. Patients' acceptance of their pain predicted improved sense of well-being outcomes as measured by the Chronic Pain Acceptance Questionnaire and the Illness Cognitions Questionnaire. In fact, higher levels of acceptance of the chronic pain were associated with better mental well-being outcomes than lower levels of pain severity; however, higher levels of acceptance were not associated with improvements in actual physical functioning. Acceptance of pain was associated with better ability to engage in normal life activities and actually feeling more control over their life. The authors concluded that acceptance of chronic pain is a way to shift one's focus away from pain to nonpain aspects of life. These findings reinforce the value expressed at support group meetings of the importance for individuals to shift away from searching for a cure and total pain relief to a perspective that acknowledges the pain may not change but their life can get better (Lame et al., 2005; Viane et al., 2003).

Step 2 requires 12-step members to believe that God (or a higher power or something greater than and different from themselves) is needed to help them to improve their lives. This process helps the individual to become less self-absorbed and to consider the advantages of connecting with others. Step 3 is about the letting go of compulsive self-reliance, surrendering to the will of a higher power and beginning of placing trust in others. Chronic pain can have a debilitating effect on individuals that challenges their sense of meaning, purpose in life, connection with others and even connection to God. Chronic pain can cause anger and resentment that leads to questions such as, "Why has this happened to me?" Some patients ask themselves, "Why did God do this to me? Why is He punishing me so? What did I do wrong?" Working the third step leads to a growing appreciation of the interconnectedness of our minds, body, and spirit.

The 12-step programs are grounded in the power of spirituality and connecting to a "higher power." Spirituality can be a complicated topic influenced by one's cultural beliefs and other paradigms—including the 12-step view of spirituality (Ellis et al., 1999). In general, spirituality is a way to find meaning, purpose, comfort, inner peace, serenity, and hope. Spirituality may be found in one's religious beliefs, 12-step fellowship, meditation, music, or nature. Spirituality embodies a sense of connection to others and to a higher power and may be found through one's individual values and principles. There is a growing literature of the positive benefits from positive beliefs, religious activities, meditation, and prayer to improving health and a sense of well-being (Marwick, 1995; Matthews et al., 1998). Improving the patient's spiritual health may not cure their chronic pain, but may help them to feel better and to live a fuller and more meaningful life.

Support groups encourage the inclusion of spirituality in the healing process from chronic pain. Spirituality allows participants to think about the things that give them a sense of inner peace, comfort, strength, love, and connection; chronic pain patients learn to set aside a regular daily time to do things that help them spiritually, including community service, volunteer work, prayer, meditation, devotional singing, reading inspirational books, nature walks, quiet time for thinking, yoga, playing a sport, or attending religious services.

Step 4 requires members to undergo honest self-assessment. They must prepare an "inventory" of strengths and weaknesses—the characteristics they want to keep (assets) and those they would like to change (liabilities). In preparing their inventory, members come to see the unhappiness in their lives differently; increased self-awareness helps them understand that how they have reacted to their chronic pain condition contributed to their suffering. This is also a time to look beyond the chronic pain condition and to consider underlying character qualities, secrets, and fears, including "defects of character" such as irresponsibility, grandiosity, resentments, and so forth. AA encourages self-reflection on the seven human deadly sins of pride, greed, lust, anger, gluttony, envy, and laziness and how these apply to their lives (Alcoholics Anonymous, 1992). This inward look can cause feelings of shame, guilt, and grief as they recognize their role in their life situation and how they have affected themselves and others. The fourth step requires members to contemplate their strengths and weaknesses and to accept that there is an emotional component to their physical symptoms. Sometimes taking their own inventory can also lead to reflecting on their life before the chronic pain condition developed.

Step 5 asks pain patients to share their life circumstances with another individual (a sponsor, therapist, or perhaps even the group) and admit to the other person the nature of their responsibility and wrongs that resulted from their character defects. This step can cause much anxiety about sharing with others but usually results in feeling a great relief because this step facilitates the release of the withheld feelings and thoughts. Individuals make an effort to share without feeling ashamed or blaming others. The patient must accept that the pain simply exists; it is not anyone's fault—not the fault of God, nor the physician, nor the driver who may have caused the accident that resulted in chronic pain. According to the AA "Twelve and Twelve," the process of completing Step 5 will allow the "dammed-up emotions of years break out of their confinement, and miraculously vanish as soon as they are exposed. As the pain subsides, a healing tranquility takes its place" (Alcoholics Anonymous, 1992).

Step 6 builds from Step 4 and is the acknowledgment of a "willingness" to address their character defects. This step encourages a clear focusing on the character defects/liabilities they would like to change. Step 7 is linked with Step 6. Step 7 is a step of humility, and it requires asking God (their higher power) for help to remove character defects. In working these steps, the chronic pain patients are encouraged to believe that they are loved and deserving of healing, whereas the AA member is asked to be ready for God to remove character flaws or other shortcomings that have caused a life of unsatisfied demands and a state of continual disturbance and frustration.

Steps 8 and 9 focus on improving interpersonal relationships. In Step 8, the individual makes a list of all the people who have been negatively affected by patient's character defects. The pain patient is instructed to think of all of the individuals he has harmed as a result of his being controlled by pain, or of his fear of never achieving comfort and relief from his pain. For example, he may have screamed at his wife and children over minor household annoyances (i.e., his son spilling tomato soup on the rug), or worse yet, he may have ignored his family altogether, choosing to focus on his relentless pain instead. This patient may also neglect major family responsibilities, such as attending weddings or funerals, for fear of having a pain exacerbation during the event. In Step 9, the individual makes amends to the people they have harmed. The "Twelve and Twelve" text (Alcoholics Anonymous, 1992) gives specific guidance on these and all other steps.

The last three steps are important in how they guide individuals throughout their life. Step 10 is a process of continuing to take a personal inventory of their life and to promptly acknowledge when they have made mistakes. This is a lifelong process of taking their own daily inventory and can be viewed as a quick checkup of Steps 4 through 9 in their current life. Step 11 continues the spiritual growth of members in 12-step programs or connecting with God (their higher power) through prayer and meditation. This is a regular and ongoing part of their life and a time for ongoing self-reflection and connection. Some 12-step members have difficulty with learning how to meditate and will express great interest in recommendations to help them. Strategies that can help facilitate meditation include teaching deep breathing techniques, teaching meditation techniques, using audiotapes that teach meditation (Kornfield, 2001; Weil, 1997), providing music that promotes meditation without guiding the person on a meditation (Ziedonis & Clottey, 2004), and helping the patient to do simple hand drumming or Native American flute playing (Clottey, 2003). The book and CD *Sound Healing: Ease Chronic Pain* (Richman & Nelson, 2005) provides some other helpful suggestions. The final Step 12 is a service step in which individuals are encouraged to help other people who suffer with the same type of problem that they might have (alcoholism or chronic pain, for example) and to continue to live their life using the principles they learned through working the steps.

Twelve Promises

The AA Promises (see Box 32.9) are a very important (although perhaps less well-known) set of virtues that were developed to help AA members learn what to expect if they maintain their sobriety and work the 12 steps of Alcoholics Anonymous. The AA Promises give hope that the individual will find inner peace and freedom in their future. The AA Promises also are important for CPA and other chronic pain 12-step programs to help individuals learn what to expect if they are able to truly accept their pain as a state of being that is a fact of their life beyond their control and if they are able to trust that a "higher power" will help them (Promises 1 and 4). In addition, if the patient is able to recognize the emotional triggers that exacerbates his or her pain (i.e., a fight with one's spouse, missing a deadline, sitting in traffic, etc.), and to learn to mitigate these triggers, he or she would no longer feel useless and dwell in self-pity (Promise 6). Rather than expecting to live in a pain-free state, if patients were to redefine their goal as "keeping pain to a minimum," they are likely to find a "new happiness," which is not a state of complete physical comfort but rather one of serenity and acceptance (Promise 3). The AA Promises provide a sense of realistic hope and expectation that will empower the individual to handle situations (like acute flare-ups, e.g., sickle cell crisis) that they previously could not (Promise 12; Alcoholics Anonymous, 1992).

When Chronic Pain and Addiction Collide: Twelve-Step Facilitation for Addiction

Chronic pain and addiction often collide in the management and treatment of either condition. In treating substance use disorders, 12-step programs are usually considered an important component of the treatment plan. When chronic pain is being treated, an awareness and support for ongoing addiction treatment and involvement in 12-step meetings must be considered whether the person has an active substance abuse problem or is abstinent and doing well in his or her addiction recovery. Health-care providers must know how to monitor their patients' addiction by doing a "recovery status exam" and in some cases by actually doing therapy of 12-step facilitation, including the process of engaging individuals to attend addiction 12-step programs, monitoring individual's involvement and progress in 12-step recovery, and in addressing the issue of prescribing pain medication to individuals active in 12-step meetings. This chapter concludes with a review of these three important issues.

Twelve-Step Recovery Status Examination

Health-care providers who manage patients with chronic pain and chemical dependence have recognized the value of 12-step programs in recovery from addictions. John Chappel (1992) created a helpful Recovery Status Examination that guides clinicians through a series of important assessment questions about their patients' addiction status and involvement in 12-step programs. These items include first assessing about the status of their current use—Are they abstinent? When did they last use? How motivated are they to be abstinent? A second area of assessment is checking the status of their "program of recovery": Are they going to 12-step meetings (which ones, what types)? Do they have a sponsor (how do they work with their sponsor)? Do they have a home group? Do they use a phone list? What step are they working on? Are they sponsoring anyone?

Clinicians can help patients connect to local 12-step meetings or online 12-step meetings, but this requires familiarity with local 12-step programs and ideally having a list of potential contacts whom the patient can call. If the moment is ripe and a patient is "ready" to attend a meeting, the clinician could contact the local AA or NA contact (dial 411 information) or suggest specific meetings/times in the area. AA and NA also have committees whose members are interested in working with clinicians to help get patients to meetings and information to clinicians (Chappel, 1992).

Twelve-Step Facilitation

Specific knowledge of 12-step recovery and facility with the clinical skills needed to successfully refer patients to 12-step recovery programs and support their ongoing participation is referred to as 12 step facilitation (TSF; Nowinski et al., 1995). TSF seeks to help the patient with two primary goals: acceptance of their need for abstinence from alcohol or other drug use and surrender (willingness to participate actively in 12-step fellowship and connect to their higher power) as a way to become and maintain sobriety. These goals are implemented through a series of objectives that consider cognitive, emotional, relationship, behavioral, social, and spiritual issues. This treatment approach is based in the 12 steps and 12 traditions of AA. The primary mechanism of action is active participation and a willingness to accept a higher power as the locus of change in one's life. The clinician must be familiar with the structure, content, and dynamics of 12-step meetings and principles. Knowledge should include the understanding and meaning of specific terminology including meetings, home groups, sponsors, the 12 steps, and 12 traditions. Additionally, the health-care practitioner should be familiar with the literature developed by 12 step groups such as the "Big Book," topic-specific pamphlets (e.g., "AA and Medications"), and slogans used by 12-step recovery groups and individuals ("one day at a time"). The ability to discuss the meanings and applications of these tools for recovery is useful. Clinicians can educate about the 12-step tools and applications that are most suitable for the individual, recognizing that traditional meeting attendance might not be as readily accepted and other options such as reading the 12-step literature or attending online meetings can be encouraged (Chappel, 1992; Nowinski et al., 1995; Ziedonis, Krejci, & Atdjian, 2001).

It is critical that health-care providers know how to help patients overcome resistance to attending a 12-step or mutual-help programs. Patients have many excuses for why they cannot or should not participate in 12-step programs, and 12-step facilitation helps patients overcome their denial and their fear. Sometimes clinicians must remind patients of their painful personal, medical, and social histories associated with their use of alcohol or other drugs to help break through denial, which is a presentation of resistance. Network Therapy, developed by Galanter (Galanter et al., 2002) uses family members and friends in the patient's "network" to enhance motivation, reduce minimization of the consequences of his or her addiction, and to facilitate recovery-oriented behaviors. Patience and persistence by the clinician are necessary in order to develop a strong, therapeutic alliance with the addicted patient, particularly during the first year of recovery. A strong therapeutic alliance allows the clinician to work with low motivation moments that appear as resistance, be it to 12-step meeting participation or making recovery-oriented lifestyle changes to people, places, and things. Clinicians should be prepared to work with patients as long as necessary to promote abstinence and sobriety. Other psychosocial therapies can be blended with 12-step facilitation. Chappel (1992) and Zweben (1995) have suggested ways psychotherapy can help deepen a patient's working of the steps.

Prescribing Prescription Pain Medication to Individuals in Twelve-Step Programs for Addiction

AA as an organization has historically seen medical treatment as necessary to help recovery in certain cases, but clearly it is outside of its purview. AA does not make specific treatment recommendations but does encourage patients to seek medical attention from health-care providers who are knowledgeable about addictions. Patients should not be denied the medical treatment needed to maintain their physical health, even if these medications have an effect on the central nervous system or do have the potential for physical dependence. Individuals with addictions may have complicated comorbid health problems—including Parkinsonism, chronic pain, and depression—that may require the use of medications that affect the brain and may be used in an addictive manner in the community. AA has historically respected the role of physicians in the recovery process (a physician was a cofounder of AA) and even the AA Big Book states: "God has abundantly supplied this world with fine doctors, psychologists, and practitioners of various kinds. Do not hesitate to take your health problems to such persons. Most of them give freely of themselves, that their fellows may enjoy sound minds and bodies. Try to remember that though God has wrought miracles among us, we should never belittle a good doctor or psychiatrist. Their services are often indispensable in treating a newcomer and in following his case afterward" (Alcoholics Anonymous, 1955).

In an official AA publication entitled *The AA Member—Medications and Other Drugs* (1984), alcoholics describe the experience of having been shunned by the group for taking prescription pain or psychiatric medications while in recovery (Dual Recovery Anonymous). Many of them were told that they were weak for continuing these medications, that they were resorting to self-pity and indulgence rather than dealing with their substance abuse issues head-on. In addition, AA leaders and members have told these individuals that taking prescription medications was simply a re-addiction to a new substance. Such members, though well-intended, may not understand the complexities of comorbid medical or psychiatric diagnoses. They take the concept of abstinence from alcohol to the extreme, demanding abstinence from substances that may be vital to health. The concept that a person can take a psychotropic medication for mood stability rather than a "high" may be foreign to them. The reality is that the depressed patient who throws away all of his SSRI at the advice of his well-intentioned AA sponsor may be at risk for committing suicide; the epileptic who does the same with her medications is at risk for a life-threatening seizure. The bias found among some in AA—that taking a psychotropic or pain medication represents a character flaw, that a person must be completely substance-free in order to truly be immersed in the program—is not supported by the AA literature. This point is elegantly stated in the aforementioned publication *The AA Member—Medications and Other Drugs*: "It becomes clear that just as it is wrong to enable or support any alcoholic to become re-addicted to any drug, it's equally wrong to deprive any alcoholic of medication which can alleviate or control other disabling physical and/or emotional problems" (Alcoholics Anonymous, 1984).

Clinicians can help patients by giving them a copy of *The AA Member—Medications and Other Drugs* (available through the AA website) and emphasize that this is official 12-step literature versus peer misinformation and bias. In some cases, actually having a phone meeting or face-to-face meeting with the patient's 12-step sponsor can also help to review any concerns. Patients are encouraged to let the sponsor and others know that the clinicians are also knowledgeable in addictions and 12-step recovery and do not take the decision to use these medications lightly. The clinicians will be monitoring for misuse of substances through a variety of measures.

Conclusion

The management of chronic pain and related comorbidities including psychiatric disorders can be complicated, and there is no single path of recovery that works for everyone. Medications, behavioral therapies, and complementary treatment approaches are often used and can be helpful; however, some individuals will benefit from the support and anticipatory guidance that they receive from peers at chronic pain support groups and 12-step programs. The support groups are particularly helpful in addressing the great emotional and spiritual suffering that patients can experience, including isolation, self-pity, fear, obsession, irrational thinking, anger, resentment, and confusion.

Several national organizations are very helpful in facilitating the development of local support groups and the Internet is a great resource for the specific locations and ways to connect to these support groups in addition to providing online support groups. Some support groups are for chronic pain in general, whereas others are for specific chronic pain disorders; some are led by peers with the common illness, and others by professionals; some are educational in nature, and others provide emotional and spiritual support. Chronic Pain Anonymous is a model example of the development of support groups for people with chronic pain that utilizes the 12-step program principles of recovery beginning with acceptance of the chronic pain and that their life has become unmanageable. Health-care providers must know how to monitor their patient's addiction recovery status and 12-step addiction program involvement. This includes the very important issue of providing anticipatory guidance on taking pain medications while participating in 12-step programs for addiction such as Alcoholics Anonymous or Narcotics Anonymous.

References

Alcoholics Anonymous. *Alcoholics Anonymous* (2nd ed.). New York: AA World Services, Inc.; 1955.

Alcoholics Anonymous. *The AA Member—Medications and Other Drugs*. New York: AA World Services, Inc.; 1984.

Alcoholics Anonymous. *The Twelve Steps and Twelve Traditions*. Center City, MN: Hazelden Press, 1992.

Chappel JN, DuPont RL. Twelve-step and mutual-help programs for addictive disorders. *Psychiatr Clin North Am*. Jun 1999;22(2):425–46.

Cicero TJ, Inciardi JA, Munoz A. Trends in abuse of Oxycontin and other opioid analgesics in the United States: 2002–2004. *J Pain*. Oct 2005;6(10):662–72.

Cleveland M. *Chronic Illness and the Twelve Steps: A Practical Approach to Spiritual Resilience*. Center City, MN: Hazelden Press; 1999.

Clottey K. *Mindful Drumming*. Oakland, CA: Sankofa Publishing; 2003.

Colameco S. *Twelve Steps for Those Afflicted With Chronic Pain: A Guide to Recovery from Emotional and Spiritual Suffering*. Charleston, SC: BookSurge Publishing; 2005.

Creamer P, Singh BB, Hochberg MC, Berman BM. Sustained improvement produced by nonpharmacologic intervention in fibromyalgia: results of a pilot study. *Arthritis Care Res*. Aug 2000;13(4):198–204.

Dual Recovery Anonymous. Dual Recovery Anonymous World Service, Inc. *Medications and Recovery*. http://www.draonline.org/medications.html.

Ellis MR, Vinson DC, Ewigman B. Addressing spiritual concerns of patients: family physicians' attitudes and practices. *J Fam Pract*. 1999;48:105–9.

Fishbain DA, Rosomoff HL, Rosomoff RS. Drug abuse, dependence and addiction in chronic pain patients. *Clin J Pain*. 1992;8(2):77–85.

Galanter MD, Dermatis H, Keller D, Trujillo M. Network therapy for cocaine abuse: use of family and peer supports. *Am J Addict*. 2002;11(2):151–6.

Hamilton B. *Twelve Step Sponsorship: How It Works*. Center City, MN: Hazelden Press; 1996.

Haugli L, Steen E, Laerum E, Nygard R, Finset A. Learning to have less pain—is it possible? A one-year follow-up study of the effects of a personal construct group learning programme on patients with chronic musculoskeletal pain. *Patient Educ Couns*. 2001;45(2):111–8.

Hitchcock LS, Ferrell BR, McCaffery M. The experience of chronic nonmalignant pain. *J Pain Symptom Manage*. 1994;9(5):312–8.

Isaacson JH, Hopper JA, Alford DP, Parran T. Prescription drug use and abuse. Risk factors, red flags, and prevention strategies. *Postgrad Med*. 2005;118(1):19–26.

Jerome JA. Chronic pain support groups. *Clin J Pain*. 1991;7(2):167–8.

Joranson DE, Ryan KM, Gilson AM, Dahl JL. Trends in medical use and abuse of opioid analgesics. *JAMA*. 2000;283(13):1710–4.

Kornfield J. *Meditation for Beginners* [audio CD]. Boulder CO: Sounds True; 2001.

Lame IE, Peters ML, Vlaeyen JW, Kleef M, Patijn J. Quality of life in chronic pain is more associated with beliefs about pain, than with pain intensity. *Eur J Pain.* Feb 2005;9(1):15–24.

Larsen E. *Stage II Recovery: Life Beyond Addiction.* San Francisco: Harper Collins, 1984.

Linton SJ, Hellsing AL, Larsson I. Bridging the gap: support groups do not enhance long-term outcome in chronic back pain. *Clin J Pain.* Sep 1997;13(3):221–8.

Lorig KR, Laurent DD, Deyo RA, Marnell ME, Minor MA, Ritter PL. Can a back pain e-mail discussion group improve health status and lower health care costs?: A randomized study. *Arch Intern Med.* 2002;162(7):792–6.

Martelli MF, Liljedahl EL, Nicholson K, Zasler ND. A brief introductory guide to chronic pain resources on the Internet. *NeuroRehabilitation.* 2000;14(2):105–21.

Marwick C. Should physicians prescribe prayer for health? Spiritual aspects of well-being considered. *JAMA.* 1995;273(20):1561–2.

Matthews DA, McCullough ME, Larson DB, Koenig HG, Swyers JP, Milano MG. Religious commitment and health status: a review of the research and implications for family medicine. *Arch Fam Med.* 1998;7(2):118–24.

McGeary DD, Mayer TG, Gatchel RJ, Anagnostis C. Smoking status and psychosocioeconomic outcomes of functional restoration in patients with chronic spinal disability. *Spine J.* Mar–Apr 2004;4(2):170–5.

Nowinski J, Baker S, Carroll K. *Twelve-Step Facilitation Therapy Manual.* NIH Publication No. 94–3722. Rockville, MD: U.S. Department of Health and Human Services; 1995.

Project MATCH Research Group. Matching alcoholism treatment to client heterogeneity: Project MATCH three-year drinking outcomes. *Alcohol Clin Exp Res.* 1998;22(6)1300–11.

Reilly RL. *Living With Pain: A New Approach to the Management of Chronic Pain.* Minneapolis, MN: Fairview Press, 1993.

Richman H, Nelson J. *Sound Healing: Ease Chronic Pain.* New York: Stewart, Tabori, and Chang; 2005.

Rosenblum A. et al. Prevalence and characteristics of chronic pain among chemically dependent patients in methadone maintenance and residential treatment facilities. *JAMA.* 2003;289:2370–2378.

Sternbach RA. *Mastering Pain: A Twelve-Step Program for Coping With Chronic Pain.* New York: Ballantine Books, 1987.

Subramaniam V, Stewart MW, Smith JF. The development and impact of a chronic pain support group: a qualitative and quantitative study. *J Pain Symptom Manage.* May 1999;17(5):376–83.

Sullivan MD, Edlund MJ, Steffick D, Unutzer J. Regular use of prescribed opioids: association with common psychiatric disorders. *Pain.* 2005;119(1–3):95–103.

Viane I, Crombez G, Eccleston C, Poppe C, Devulder J, Van Houdenhove B, De Corte W. Acceptance of pain is an independent predictor of mental well-being in patients with chronic pain: empirical evidence and reappraisal. *Pain.* 2003;106(1–2):65–72.

Volkow ND. *NIDA Community Drug Alert Bulletin—Prescription Drugs.* NIH Pub. No. 05–5580. http://www.nida.nih.gov/PrescripAlert/index.html. Published September 2005.

Von Korff M, Moore JE, Lorig K, Cherkin DC, Saunders K, Gonzalez VM, Laurent D, Rutter C, Comite F. A randomized trial of a lay person-led self-management group intervention for back pain patients in primary care. *Spine.* 1998;23(23):2608–15.

Weil A. *Meditations for Optimum Health* [audio CD]. New York: Tommy Boy Music; 1997.

Weis J. Support groups for cancer patients. *Support Care Cancer.* 2003;11(12):763–8.

Yunus MB, Arslan S, Aldag JC. Relationship between fibromyalgia features and smoking. *Scand J Rheumatol.* 2002;31(5):301–5.

Ziedonis DM, Clottey K. *The Journey: Mindful Rhythm and Sound to Heal the Soul* [music CD]. Hopewell, NJ: Mindfulness Music; 2004.

Ziedonis DM, Krejci J, Atdjian S. Integrating medications and psychotherapy in the treatment of alcohol, tobacco and other drug addictions. In Kay J (Ed.). *Integrated Treatment of Psychiatric Disorders* (Vol. 20). Washington DC: American Psychiatric Press Inc.; 2001: 79–111.

Zweben JE. Integrating psychotherapy and 12 step approaches. In: Washton AM (Ed.). *Psychotherapy and Substance Abuse: A Practitioner's Handbook.* New York: Guilford; 1995: 124–40.

Part V
Clinical Management of Pain in Chemical Dependency

33

Treatment of Acute Pain in the Opioid-Dependent Patient in the Perioperative Setting

Raymond S. Sinatra

Sukanya Mitra

Patients exhibiting diminished opioid response, whether those presenting with high-grade tolerance or others demonstrating paradoxical treatment induced hyperalgesia, can pose significant and unique challenges to perioperative care providers. This chapter focuses on the clinical implications of opioid tolerance and opioid-induced hyperalgesia, and offers guidelines for patient assessment and acute pain management in the perioperative setting. For opioid tolerant patients in the perioperative setting, higher than standard doses of opioids will often be required. A balanced analgesic approach rather than high-dose opioid monotherapy is preferred. Analgesic regimens should include central or peripheral neural blockade, neuraxial analgesia, and administration of nonopioid adjuvant agents. On the other hand, patients developing opioid-induced hyperalgesia must be recognized and their analgesic plan quickly modified to minimize poor pain control. Opioid rotation, methadone substitution, administration of ketamine, as well as continuous clinical monitoring remain the key cornerstones of perioperative pain management.

Perioperative management of acute pain in opioid dependent patients often presents major clinical challenges. The majority of these individuals may be moderately to profoundly unresponsive to the therapeutic effects of narcotic analgesics (Carroll et al., 2004; Hord, 1992; Jage & Bey, 2000; May et al., 2001), whereas a subset of patients may actually experience increasing discomfort or hyperalgesia following opioid administration (Mao, 2002; Mercadante et al., 2003; Simmonet & Rivat, 2003). In this chapter, treatment options in this challenging situation are discussed, followed by guidelines for patient assessment and perioperative management.

Preoperative Recognition and Assessment of Patients With High Opioid Use

In the perioperative setting, anesthesiologists, surgeons, pharmacists, and nursing staff are increasingly asked to care for chronic pain patients with high baseline opioid requirements (Collett, 2001; Hord, 1992; Jage & Bey, 2000; May et al., 2001; Mitra & Sinatra, 2004; Streitzer, 2001). There may be several factors responsible for the increased acceptance and prescription of opioid analgesics in this population, for example, concerns of analgesic undermedication and inadequate pain control, the favorable side-effect profiles of newer semisynthetic and sustained-release opioids, and morbidity associated with nonsteroidal antiinflammatory drugs (NSAIDS) and COX-2 inhibitors (Collett, 2001; Nissen et al., 2001; Streitzer, 2001).

Another set of patients demonstrating high-grade opioid tolerance includes the opioid abusers or opioid-addicted patients, who may be more problematic both in terms of assessment and management (Hord, 1992; Jage & Bey, 2000; May et al., 2001; Mitra & Sinatra, 2004; Streitzer, 2001). Some of these patients are former addicts enrolled in the methadone maintenance programs. They are exposed to relatively large doses of methadone, 25–100 mg/d, and, as might be expected, exhibit high-grade tolerance to the antinociceptive effects of opioids (Doverty et al., 2001; Savage et al., 1993).

It is critical that surgeons and anesthesiologists identify opioid-dependent patients prior to surgical admission and develop a clear management strategy that employs liberal doses of opioid and nonopioid analgesics to overcome high-grade tolerance (Collett, 2001; Hord, 1992; May et al., 2001; Pasero & Compton, 1997; Streitzer, 2001). In this context, high-grade opioid tolerance has been empirically suggested as the requirement of ≥ 1 mg intravenous or ≥ 3 mg oral morphine equivalent per hour for > 1 month (Mitra & Sinatra, 2004).

Caregivers need be aware of the rapidly changing profile of opioid-based analgesia. It may be worthwhile to recognize both the names of newly developed opioids and method of action of novel delivery systems including oral sustained-release, transmucosal, intranasal, and transdermal preparations. Newly developed and marketed opioids including Actiq, Avinza, Kadian, Combunox, and Palladone are not readily recognizable as opioids yet represent potent or long-acting preparations.

Perioperative Management of Acute Pain in Opioid-Dependent Patients

The perioperative clinical guidelines outlined below (see Box 33.1 for a summary and proposals) may be useful in caring for the patient with high doses and may minimize development of hyperalgesia.

Box 33.1. Guidelines for Perioperative Pain Management in Opioid-Tolerant and/or Opioid-Hyperalgesic Patients

Preoperative

1. *Evaluation.* Evaluation should include early recognition and high index of suspicion, both for opioid tolerance and for opioid hyperalgesia.
2. *Identification.* Identify factors such as previous surgery or trauma resulting in undermedication, inadequate analgesia, or relapse episodes. Distinguish between true opioid tolerance and opioid hyperalgesia.
3. *Consultation.* Meet with addiction specialists and pain specialists in perioperative planning.
4. *Reassurance.* Discuss patient concerns related to pain control, anxiety reduction, and risk of relapse.
5. *Medication.* Calculate opioid dose requirement and modes of administration. Provide anxiolytic or other medications as clinically indicated.

Intraoperative

1. Maintain baseline opioids: oral, transdermal, or intravenous.
2. Increase dose of opioids to compensate for tolerance. In contrast, avoid dose escalation in opioid hyperalgesic patients.
3. Consider use of preemptive and intraoperative ketamine in opioid-induced hyperalgesic patients. Consider additional methadone in patients already receiving it.
4. Provide peripheral neural or plexus blockade; consider neuraxial analgesic technique when clinically indicated.
5. Use nonopioids as analgesic adjuncts.

Postoperative

1. Plan preoperatively for postoperative analgesia; formulate a definite strategy with definite alternatives.
2. Maintain baseline opioids.
3. Use multimodal analgesic techniques.
4. Use patient-controlled analgesia as primary therapy or as supplementation for epidural or regional techniques.
5. Continue with neuraxial opioids: intrathecal or epidural analgesia.
6. Continue continuous neural blockade.

After discharge

1. If surgery provides complete pain relief, opioids should be slowly tapered rather than abruptly discontinued.
2. Develop a pain management plan before hospital discharge. Provide adequate doses of opioids and nonopioid analgesics.
3. Arrange for a timely outpatient pain clinic follow-up or a visit with the patient's addiction specialist.

Modified with permission from Mitra & Sinatra (2004).

The patients should be administered their daily maintenance or baseline opioid dose prior to induction of anesthesia. They may be instructed to take their usual dose of oral opioid on the morning of surgery. Due to the long-lasting analgesic effect of sustained-release opioids, baseline requirements will generally be maintained during preoperative and intraoperative periods. Later, these may be provided orally (e.g., following ambulatory surgery) or parenterally (for those involved in more invasive procedures; May et al., 2001; Pasero & Compton, 1997; Rapp et al., 1995). Those in the opioid maintenance programs with methadone (Kreek, 1976; Rubenstein et al., 1976) or buprenorphine (Johnson et al., 1992) may continue taking these medications on the morning of surgery. Again, redosing is usually not an issue as these are also associated with prolonged duration of activity.

Patients who cannot take or missed their baseline opioids may be given a parenteral equivalent loading dose of hydromorphone or methadone, either at anesthetic induction or during the operative procedure. Patients with transdermal fentanyl patch should maintain it into the operating room. If the preparation was removed, an intravenous fentanyl infusion may be initiated to maintain baseline plasma concentrations. A new patch may then be applied intraoperatively. It may take 6–12 hours to reestablish baseline analgesic effects (Caplan et al., 1989; Sevarino & Ning, 1992); during that time interval, the fentanyl infusion may be gradually decreased in rate and eventually discontinued.

Patients treated with transdermal fentanyl are often highly opioid tolerant. The fentanyl patch should be maintained during the perioperative period and supplemented with higher than normal doses of IV or oral opioids for breakthrough pain. In our practice, we have found greater success with hydromorphone, and fentanyl for PCA use instead of morphine as they provide a more rapid onset are associated with fewer adverse effects and require administration of fewer milligrams of drug.

It may be a safe practice to maintain epidural and intrathecal opioid infusions delivered by internally implanted devices throughout the perioperative period. As an exception, intrathecal infusions of the nonopioid relaxant baclofen (Lioresal) may be discontinued or reduced during the immediate perioperative period due to the risk of hypotension and excessive sedation (Gomar & Carrero, 1994).

Postoperative Pain Management

For those former opioid addicts on buprenorphine maintenance, it may be continued for postoperative pain control, supplemented with methadone or morphine if needed (0.8 mg sublingual buprenorphine is equianalgesic with 20 mg oral methadone; Foley, 1993; Gustin & Akil, 2001). Opioid antagonists such as naloxone and naltrexone, however, should be avoided in opioid-dependent patients (Foley, 1993; Manfredi et al., 1996; Reisine & Pasternak, 1996). Postoperative administration of these drugs, as well as mixed agonist-antagonist opioids that block μ receptors (e.g., nalbuphine, butorphanol, and pentazocine), may all precipitate acute withdrawal symptoms in patients who are dependent on potent opioids (Gustin & Akil, 2001; Manfredi et al., 1996; Reisine & Pasternak, 1996).

Intravenous boluses of fentanyl or sufentanil may initially be used for patients recovering from ambulatory surgery. Oral opioids may be restarted following stabilization in PACU. Depending upon the invasiveness of the procedure, the doses may be higher than baseline requirements (Saberski, 1992).

In most nonambulatory surgeries, following anesthetic induction, oral opioids are discontinued and a parenteral equivalent conversion is needed (Hord, 1992; May et al., 2001; Pasero & Compton, 1997; Saberski, 1992). Although precise dosing guidelines have not been developed, intraoperative and postsurgical analgesic requirements are affected by receptor downregulation and may need to be increased by 30% or higher than amounts typically administered to opioid-naive patients (Collett, 2001; May et al., 2001; Saberski, 1992). The matter is, however, complicated by the fact that parenteral administration bypasses gastrointestinal absorption and first-pass effects; accordingly, most IV or IM doses of opioid can usually be adjusted downward from doses taken orally (Foley, 1993; Pereira et al., 2001). Thus, it is important to appreciate these differences in oral-to-intravenous dose equivalency in order to estimate perioperative baseline and supplemental opioid dose requirements. This is particularly the case with IV morphine and hydromorphone, which have three and two times greater bioavailability and systemic potency than equivalent oral doses, respectively (Foley, 1993; Pereira et al., 2001; Quigley, 2002). In contrast, oxycodone and sustained-release Oxycontin have high oral bioavailability that approaches 83% of an IV dose; hence 1–1.5 mg oral oxycodone becomes equivalent to 1 mg IV morphine (Ginsberg et al., 2003; Poyhia et al., 1993). The baseline requirement of opioids for patients treated with transdermal fentanyl (Duragesic), IV-PCA morphine, or hydromorphone may be fulfilled with an equivalent IV dose of opioid (Foley, 1993).

To provide effective postsurgical analgesia, a continuous parenteral opioid infusion or IV-PCA is a useful option (Macintyre, 2001; Parker et al., 1992). IV-PCA may be started in the PACU as soon as the patient becomes oriented and capable of utilizing the device. It helps to lower the risk of undermedication and breakthrough pain that may occur during patient transport to the surgical care unit. To overcome the opioid tolerance and receptor downregulation, higher than normal doses of morphine or hydromorphone might be considered (Pasero & Compton, 1997; Saberski, 1992), for example, by maintaining a basal infusion equivalent either to the patient's hourly oral dose requirement or 1 to 2 PCA boluses per hour (Parker et al., 1992).

As regards the controversial issue of allowing substance abusers or recovering addicts access to IV-PCA to control postoperative pain, due to the worry regarding excessive self-administration (Hord, 1992; Pasero & Compton, 1997), it is now recognized that, along with oral methadone (Sartain & Mitchell, 2002), IV-PCA may be offered to selected patients provided that pain intensity and opioid consumption are carefully assessed, and that such therapy is supplemented with baseline doses of methadone, neural blockade, and nonopioid analgesics (Boyle, 1991; Fitzgibbon & Ready, 1997; Hord, 1992; Pasero & Compton, 1997).

Clinicians caring for opioid-tolerant patients should recognize that a subset of these individuals might be polydrug dependent, often requiring alcohol, marijuana, or sizable doses of anxiolytics and other psychoactive drugs to help control pain or to provide emotional/psychological support. Despite administration of an adequate opioid dose, individuals codependent upon benzodiazepines, alcohol, muscle relaxants, tricyclic antidepressants, SSRIs, and baclofen may exhibit signs of withdrawal or complain of agitation and inadequate pain control. Polysubstance-dependent individuals often self-medicate with benzodiazepines or other centrally acting agents to help them cope with fear and anxiety associated with chronic pain or other stressful life events (Malcolm, 2003). It is important not to abruptly discontinue or to overlook the powerful psychological effects of a wide variety of centrally acting drugs.

Although relatively few evaluations have been performed in opioid-dependent patients, nonopioid analgesic adjuvant agents may also be employed to reduce opioid-dose requirements and provide multimodal analgesia. There is some evidence for the efficacy of NSAIDs and COX-2 inhibitors (Katz, 2002; Mercadante et al., 1997), low doses of ketamine ($0.5\ mg \cdot kg^{-1}$) or similar agents to antagonize NMDA receptor activation (Clark & Kalan, 1995; Trujullo & Akil, 1991), and clonidine patch $0.1\ mg \cdot h^{-1}$ (Segal et al., 1991).

Neuraxial Analgesia for Postoperative Pain

Through neuraxial administration of opioids, significantly greater levels of analgesia can be delivered to those patients recovering from more extensive procedures in which postsurgical parenteral opioid doses would be expected to be very high; hence, this offers a more efficient method of providing postsurgical analgesia than parenteral or oral opioids (Bromage, 1978; Cousins & Bridenbaugh, 1998; Harrison et al., 1988; Wang et al., 1979).

With both epidural and intrathecal routes of opioid administration in the opioid-dependent patient, upward dose adjustment (1.5–2X opioid-naive patient dose) is required to compensate for tolerance at spinal opioid receptors. Nevertheless, most opioid-dependent patients experience effective pain relief with doses of morphine and hydromorphone that are generally equivalent to a small fraction of their baseline oral requirement. Caution should be used in opioid-dependent patients receiving relatively high opioid doses because unless supplementary oral or parenteral opioids are given, plasma concentrations and supraspinal receptor binding may decline to the point that acute withdrawal may be precipitated (Cousins & Bridenbaugh, 1998; de Leon-Casasola & Lema, 1992).

Although neuraxial analgesia provides effective pain relief, the dose of opioid administered either epidurally or intrathecally may be too low to maintain supraspinal receptor occupancy and prevent systemic opioid withdrawal. For this reason, it is important to maintain baseline opioid requirements either orally or by intravenous PCA in patients who remain "NPO." Monitoring for complications, in particular excessive sedation and respiratory depression, is mandatory when administering opioid drugs in higher than normal concentrations and via different routes of administration.

Other suggested methods to improve neuraxial analgesic efficacy include switching to an opioid that has high intrinsic potency, for example, sufentanil (de Leon-Casasola & Lema, 1992, 1994) and administering opioids such as morphine directly into subarachnoid space (Cousins & Bridenbaugh, 1998; Wang et al., 1979).

Regional Analgesia for Postoperative Pain

Regional anesthesia/analgesia approaches may reduce oral or parenteral opioid requirement and improve distal perfusion. It may be useful in opioid-tolerant patients undergoing procedures on the extremities, especially for most peripheral vascular and reim plantation surgeries and for other procedures requiring graft revision or replacement (Hord, 1992; May et al., 2001; Saberski, 1992). Either tissue infiltration or nerve/plexus blockade with standard doses of bupivacaine or levobupivacaine may be used. Indwelling catheters infused with local anesthetics may be retained up to 48 hours in ambulatory patients.

Management of Opioid-Induced Hyperalgesia

Ketamine may provide useful pain control in opioid-tolerant patients who develop opioid-induced hyperalgesia. The dose of ketamine used may be significantly lower than the dose recommended in a recent review article (Himmelseher & Durieux, 2005), in which the importance of intraoperative ketamine dosing for optimizing perioperative pain relief was highlighted. The authors found evidence to support the efficacy of subanesthetic doses of ketamine as an analgesic adjunct in a variety of surgical procedures and anesthetic techniques (Himmelseher & Durieux, 2005). Findings on opioid-tolerant or hyperalgesic patients are, however, limited. Although more randomized clinical trials are warranted, use of ketamine in this group of patients seems promising.

Other options of managing acute pain in opioid-hyperalgesic patients that have been suggested in recent studies and expert opinions include opioid switching, especially to methadone (Chung et al., 2004; Inturrisi, 2005; Mercadante & Arcuri, 2005), opioid rotation (Fine, 2004), combination of opioids with different receptor selectivity, and adjuvant medication such as intrathecal alpha-2 agonists (De Cock et al., 2005) or NSAIDs (Carroll et al., 2004; Koppert, 2005). Again, these observations are presently based mostly on case reports or expert opinions; controlled studies are needed in this recently recognized and particularly challenging important area.

Conclusion

Perioperative management of opioid tolerant patients presents unique challenges for perioperative care providers. To avoid undermedication and unacceptable discomfort, higher than standard doses of opioids will often be required. In general, it is better to err on the side of slightly overmedicating than significantly undermedicating these patients. At the same time, caregivers should refrain from overreliance on high-dose opioid monotherapy and make every effort to provide a balanced analgesic approach. Analgesic regimens should include central or peripheral neural blockade, neuraxial analgesia, and administration of central and peripheral acting nonopioid adjuvant agents. Nonopioids including NMDA receptor anatagonists, alpha-2 agonists and COX-2 inhibitors may provide effective analgesic potentiation, opioid sparing, and reduction in the rate of tolerance development.

On the other hand, patients developing opioid sensitization or opioid-induced hyperalgesia must be recognized and their analgesic plan quickly modified to minimize poor pain control. In these individuals, opioid dosing should be carefully titrated to diminish pain perception while at the same time avoiding the noxious excitation associated with this class of analgesics. Opioid rotation, methadone substitution, administration of ketamine, as well as continuous clinical monitoring remain the key cornerstones that may be required to optimize perioperative pain management.

References

Boyle RK. Intra- and postoperative anaesthetic management of an opioid addict undergoing caesarean section. *Anaesth Intensive Care* 1991; 19:276–9.

Bromage PR. *Epidural Analgesia.* Philadelphia: WB Saunders, 1978.

Caplan RA, Ready B, Oden RV, et al. Transdermal fentanyl for postoperative pain management. *JAMA* 1989; 261:1036–9.

Carroll IR, Angst MS, Clark JD. Management of perioperative pain in patients chronically consuming opioids. *Reg Anesth Pain Med* 2004; 29:576–91.

Chung KS, Carson S, Glassman D, Vadivelu N. Successful treatment of hydromorphone-induced neurotoxicity and hyperalgesia. *Conn Med* 2004; 68:547–9.

Clark JL, Kalan GE. Effective treatment of severe cancer pain of the head using low-dose ketamine in an opioid-tolerant patient. *J Pain Symp Manage* 1995; 10:310–4.

Collett B-J. Chronic opioid therapy for non-cancer pain. *Br J Anaesth* 2001; 87:133–43.

Cousins MJ, Bridenbaugh PO. *Epidural neural blockade in clinical anesthesia and management.* 3rd ed. Philadelphia: Lippincott Raven, 1998.

De Cock M, Lavand'homme P, Waterloos H. The short-lasting analgesia and long-term antihyperalgesic effect of intrathecal clonidine in patients undergoing colonic surgery. *Anesth Analg* 2005; 101:566–72.

de Leon-Casasola OA, Lema MJ. Epidural sufentanil for acute pain control in a patient with extreme opioid dependency. *Anesthesiology* 1992; 76:853–6.

de Leon-Casasola OA, Lema MJ. Epidural bupivacaine/sufentanil therapy for postoperative pain control in patients tolerant to opioid and unresponsive to epidural bupivacaine/morphine. *Anesthesiology* 1994; 80:303–9.

Doverty M, Somogyi AA, White JM, et al. Methadone maintenance patients are cross-tolerant to the antinociceptive effects of morphine. *Pain* 2001; 93:155–63.

Fitzgibbon DR, Ready JB. Intravenous high dose methadone administered by patient controlled analgesia and continuous infusion for the treatment of pain refractory to high dose morphine. *Pain* 1997; 73(2):59–61.

Foley RM. Opioid analgesics in clinical pain management. In: Herz A, Akil H, Simon EJ, eds. *Handbook of Experimental Pharmacology. Opioids II.* Vol. 104. New York: Springer Verlag, 1993; 697–743.

Ginsberg B, Sinatra RS, Adler LJ, et al. Conversion to oral controlled-release oxycodone from intravenous opioid analgesic in the postoperative setting. *Pain Med* 2003; 4(1):31–8.

Gomar C, Carrero EJ. Delayed arousal after general anesthesia associated with baclofen. *Anesthesiology* 1994; 81:1306–1307.

Gustin HB, Akil H. Opioid analgesics. In: Hardman JG, Limbird LE, eds. *Goodman and Gilman's The Pharmacological Basis of Therapeutics.* 10th ed. New York, McGraw-Hill: 2001; 569–619.

Harrison DH, Sinatra RS, Chung J, et al. Epidural narcotic and patient-controlled analgesia for post-cesarean section pain relief. *Anesthesiology* 1988; 68:454–7.

Himmelseher S, Durieux ME. Ketamine for perioperative pain management. *Anesthesiology* 2005; 102:211–20.

Hord AH. Postoperative analgesia in the opioid-dependent patient. In: Sinatra RS, Hord AH, Ginsberg B, Preble LM, eds. *Acute Pain: Mechanisms and Management.* St Louis, MO: Mosby Yearbook Inc., 1992; 390–8.

Inturrisi CE. Pharmacology of methadone and its isomers. *Minerva Anestesiol* 2005; 71:435–7.

Jage J, Bey T. Postoperative analgesia in patients with substance use disorders: Part I. *Acute Pain* 2000; 3:140–55.

Johnson RE, Jaffe JH, Fudala PJ. A controlled trial of buprenorphine treatment for opioid dependence. *JAMA* 1992; 287:2750–5.

Katz WA. Cyclooxygenase-2-selective inhibitors in the management of acute and perioperative pain. *Cleve Clin J Med* 2002; 69 Suppl 1:SI65–75.

Koppert W. Opioid-induced analgesia and hyperalgesia. *Schmerz* 2005; 19:386–94 [article in German].

Kreek MJ. Long-term pharmacotherapy for opiate (primarily heroin) addiction: opioid agonists. In: Schuster CR, Kuhar MJ, eds. *Handbook of Experimental Pharmacology. Opioids II.* Vol. 118. New York: Springer Verlag, 1996; 487–562.

Macintyre PE. Safety and efficacy of patient-controlled analgesia. *Br J Anaesth* 2001; 87:36–46.

Malcolm RJ. GABA systems, benzodiazepines and substance dependence. *J Clin Psychiatry* 2003; 64 Suppl 3:36–40.

Manfredi PL, Ribeiro S, Cahndler SW, Payne R. Inappropriate use of naloxone in cancer patients with pain. *J Pain Sympt Manage* 1996; 11: 131–4.

Mao J. Opioid-induced abnormal pain sensitivity: implications in clinical opioid therapy. *Pain* 2002; 100:213–7.

May JA, White HC, Leonard-White A, Warltier DC, Pagel PS. The patient recovering from alcohol or drug addiction: special issues for the anesthesiologist. *Anesth Analg* 2001; 92:1601–1608.

Mercadante S, Arcuri E. Hyperalgesia and opioid switching. *Am J Hosp Palliat Care* 2005; 22:291–4.

Mercadante S, Ferrera P, Villari P, Arcuri E. Hyperalgesia: an emerging iatrogenic syndrome. *J Pain Symptom Manage* 2003; 26:769–75.

Mercadante S, Sapio M, Caligara M, et al. Opioid-sparing effect of diclofenac in cancer pain. *J Pain Symptom Manage* 1997; 14(1):15–20.

Mitra S, Sinatra RS. Perioperative management of acute pain in the opioid-dependent patient. *Anesthesiology* 2004; 101:212–27.

Nissen LM, Tett SE, Cranoud T, et al. Opioid analgesic prescribing: use of an audit of analgesic prescribing by general practitioners and the multidisciplinary pain center at Royal Brisbane Hospital. *Br J Clin Pharmacol* 2001; 52:693–8.

Parker RK, Holtman B, White PF. Patient-controlled analgesia—does a concurrent opioid infusion improve pain management after surgery? *JAMA* 1992; 266:1947–52.

Pasero CL, Compton P. Pain management in addicted patients. *Am J Nursing* 1997; 4:17–19.

Pereira J, Lawlor P, Vigano A, et al. Equianalgesic dose ratios for opioids. A critical review and proposals for long-term dosing. *J Pain Symptom Manage* 2001; 22:672–87.

Poyhia R, Vainio A, Kaiko E. A review of oxycodone's clinical pharmacokinetics and pharmacodynamics. *J Pain Symptom Manage* 1993; 8: 63–7.

Quigley C. Hydromorphone for acute and chronic pain. *Cochrane Database Syst Rev* 2002; (1): CD003447.

Rapp SE, Ready LB, Nessly ML. Acute pain management in patients with prior opioid consumption: a case-controlled retrospective review. *Pain* 1995; 61:195–201.

Reisine T, Pasternak G. Opioid analgesics and antagonists. In: Hardman JG, Limbird LE, Molinoff PB, Ruddon RW, Gilman AG, eds. *Goodman and Gilman's The Pharmacological Basis of Therapeutics*, 9th ed. New York: McGraw-Hill, 1996; 521–55.

Rubenstein RB, Spira I, Wolff WI. Management of surgical problems in patients of methadone maintenance. *Am J Surgery* 1976; 131:566–9.

Saberski L. Postoperative pain management for the patient with chronic pain. In: Sinatra RS, Hord AH, Ginsberg B, Preble LM, eds. *Acute Pain: Mechanisms and Management*. St. Louis, MO: Mosby Yearbook Inc., 1992; 422–31.

Sartain JB, Mitchell SJ. Successful use of oral methadone after failure of intravenous morphine and ketamine. *Anaesth Intensive Care* 2002; 30:487–9.

Savage SR. Addiction in the treatment of pain: significance, recognition and treatment. *J Pain Symptom Manage* 1993; 8:265–78.

Segal IS, Jarvis DJ, Duncan SR, et al. Clinical efficacy of oral-transdermal clonidine combinations during the perioperative period. *Anesthesiology* 1991; 74:220–5.

Sevarino FB, Ning T. Transdermal fentanyl for acute pain management. In: Sinatra RS, Hord AH, Ginsberg B, Preble LM, eds. *Acute Pain: Mechanisms and Management*. St. Louis, MO: Mosby Yearbook Inc., 1992; 364–9.

Simmonet G, Rivat C. Opioid-induced hyperalgesia: abnormal or normal pain. *NeuroReport* 2003; 14:1–7.

Streitzer J. Pain management in the opioid-dependent patient. *Curr Psychiatry Rep* 2001; 3:489–96.

Trujillo KA, Akil H. Inhibition of morphine tolerance and dependence by the NMDA receptor antagonist MK-801. *Science* 1991; 251:85–7.

Wang JK, Nauss LA, Thomas JE. Pain relief by intrathecally applied morphine in man. *Anesthesiology* 1979; 50:149–51.

34

Management of Persistent Pain in the Opioid-Treated Patient

Thomas Simopoulos

The opioid-dependent patient (ODP) not uncommonly presents a significant treatment challenge to physicians. Opioids are increasingly being used for managing both malignant and nonmalignant pain. Opioids are a cost-effective, straightforward therapy for some people with persistent pain, and this property fits well into current pain management practice in many settings. However, because long-term opioid therapy may have declining or adverse effects in some patients, alternative modalities are sometimes sought. There exist limitations of long-term opioid therapy alone in some patients, and adopting a multimodal approach to long-term pain management may better address long-term outcomes. This chapter will focus on the use of adjunctive and alternative modalities in the management of chronic nonmalignant pain of patients on chronic opioid therapy with suboptimal outcomes. Of course, many of the management strategies discussed may be employed as well in patients with malignant pain.

Special Considerations in the Opioid-Treated Patient

Not uncommonly, patients with persistent pain on opioid treatment are referred to pain management practices by nonpain specialists who are no longer comfortable prescribing opioids or for declining analgesic effect. There may also be the overly optimistic expectation that they will all wean off their opioids once a successful pain intervention is performed. In addition, the efficacy of pain management strategies is erroneously judged by a reduction or elimination of opioid medications. In clinical practice, however, this task is often not achieved. The reasons for this are that chronic opioid therapy may offer benefits not only for pain control, but also for improving the affective components of chronic pain.

Pain practitioners have come to recognize that opioid therapy alone may be far from simple and may not be sufficient for achieving desired outcomes or pain management. Thus, clinicians continue to seek alternative and/or adjunctive modalities for controlling chronic pain. Satisfying outcomes of opioid therapy are often achieved by the four A's: analgesia, activities of daily living, adverse side effects, and aberrant drug-taking behaviors (Passik & Weinreb, 2000).

A patient with meaningful pain relief, manageable, stable psychosocial function, and minimal or no aberrant drug-taking behavior is unlikely to also require interventional techniques. However, patients with outcomes that are suboptimal in any of these domains may be candidates for interventional techniques to improve pain control, decrease adverse effects, improve adherence and aberrant behavior, and/or improve functional outcomes. The decision to treat chronic pain with opioids is most commonly done outside the context of a multidisciplinary pain center, without a careful biopsychosocial evaluation and clearly defined treatment goals. By the time such patients are seen in the pain center, significant residual pain in the face of long-term, relatively "high-dose" chronic opioid therapy is sometimes present, making further treatment challenging.

In general, chronic effects of opioids on patients may be divided into biological and psychological changes. Opioid tolerance may play a role in propagating physiologic perturbations. Clinically, the distinction between disease progression versus tolerance may not be straightforward, and upward dose adjustments are not uncommon. Opioid tolerance is a pharmacologic process that develops with repeated exposure to opioids and brings about the need for escalating doses in order to maintain equipotent analgesic effects. Prolonged use of relatively moderate to high doses of opioids may conceivably lead to opioid-induced abnormalities in pain sensitivity, hormone levels, and immune function in some patients (Ballantyne & Mao, 2003). Abnormal pain sensitivity or opioid-induced hyperalgesia can limit the ability of patients to tolerate even percutaneous procedures.

A reduction in gonadotropin-releasing hormones may lead to sexual dysfunction that can create significant psychosocial distress (Rajagopal et al., 2004). Adverse effects on the musculoskeletal system in the form of reduced muscle mass, strength, and osteoporosis may ensue as a result of hypogonadism (Ebeling, 1998). Lastly, attenuation in immune function may theoretically predispose patients to infection (Rahim et al., 2002). Table 34.1 summarizes opioid-induced physiologic changes and their potential impact on further pain management and rehabilitation. Persistent treatment of opioid tolerance/opioid induced hyperalgesia with dose escalation may create a vicious cycle and further fuel the adverse effects of prolonged opioid therapy. On the other hand,

Table 34.1. Chronic Potential Adverse Effects of Opioids and Implications on Further Treatment

Adverse Effect Induced by Opioids	Potential Impact on Further Therapy
Abnormal pain sensitivity (opioid hyperalgesia)	Limited ability to tolerate percutaneous procedures and adequate physiologic testing
Immune dysfunction	Increased risk of infection for implantable therapies
Endocrinopathies	Alterations in mood and reduced muscle and bone mass affecting rehabilitation potential

Box 34.1 Essential Components of a Medical Evaluation With a Focus on Pain Management

Detailed history and physical examination
Review of prior diagnostic workups
Review of results of prior treatments for results, side effects, and effectiveness
Reasons for failure of prior therapies
Review of notes from prior caregivers
Impact of pain on activities of daily living and employment
Identification of coexisting psychopathology and its need for further treatment
Identification of significant social issues (e.g., ongoing litigation or divorce)

chronic opioid therapy may be the only medical intervention that has made a significant improvement in the level of pain, and here, clearly, the benefits outweigh the risks.

The opioid-treated patient with persistent pain may not only present with physiologic changes, but also have psychological and social issues whose palliation has come to depend on chronic opioid therapy. Psychopathology such as depressive disorders and anxiety disorders are common in patients with chronic pain; opioids may improve some of the symptoms associated with these conditions (McQuay, 1999).

Evaluation of the Opioid-Treated Patient With Persistent Pain

Taking into account the aforementioned considerations, the opioid-treated patient with persistent pain requires a detailed evaluation in order to determine candidacy for future treatment modalities. The evaluation may be outlined under three categories:

- Obtaining a detailed understanding of the chronic pain condition when possible
- Psychological screening
- Management of present opioids as well as identification of their adverse effects, if any

The formulation of an appropriate treatment plan comes about by integrating the data obtained from each category. A thorough history, physical examination, review of imaging data, and prior treatments is a necessary first step and permits formulation of potential interventions (Box 34.1). In addition, part of the initial evaluation requires the pain practitioner to assess the patient for coexisting psychosocial issues that surround pain complaints. Not uncommonly, the opioid-treated patient with persistent pain presents with complaints that are concerning for psychological and social conditions that may limit further effective pain management and rehabilitation (Jamison, 1996). A psychiatric evaluation may be essential for further diagnosis and management (Box 34.2). Psychopathology that is undertreated or refractory may cause suboptimal outcomes from any future pain management modality (Manchikanti et al., 2002).

The final issue is the ongoing management of opioids. It is critical to identify adverse effects of opioids, if any. Adverse effects can influence treatment options and outcomes (see Table 34.1). Additionally, it may be difficult to accurately ascertain, in the opioid-treated patient with persistent pain who comes to your clinic already on relatively "high-doses" of opioids, the degree of analgesia and functional improvement achieved from opioids. The full treatment plan may take months to develop because of the many complex issues that may surround the opioid-treated patient with persistent pain. Patients on relatively "high-dose" opioids or a strong focus on these medications may derive suboptimal benefit from alternative pain management strategies.

Treatment Principles

In carefully selected opioid-treated dependent patients with suboptimal outcomes, comprehensive and aggressive medical treatment can be employed to achieve functional restoration and reduce the reliance on long-term opioid therapy. The modalities described here are used in patients who may or may not be taking opioids. The approaches to further pain management include pharmacologic, interventional, as well as physical medicine approaches in efforts to foster rehabilitation. The rationale and principles for the use of each modality is described taking into account chronic opioid dependence in the patient with suboptimal outcomes.

Pharmacologic Approaches With Adjuvant Analgesics

Traditionally, the opioid analgesics and the nonsteroidal antiinflammatory drugs (NSAIDS) have been the mainstay for primary analgesia in chronic pain. Exclusive management of chronic pain with chronic opioid therapy has the potential for loss of efficacy. Long-term complications with either NSAIDS or opioids increase the complexity of providing ongoing pain control (Marcus, 2000). Recent data suggests that exposure to chronic opioids may reduce the analgesic effects of NSAIDS (Jakubowski et al., 2005). Fortunately, numerous classes of medications (Box 34.3) have been demonstrated to possess analgesic efficacy especially in chronic nonmalignant pain of neuropathic origin.

The antidepressants have been most commonly employed for the treatment of chronic pain conditions for more than 40 years. Tricyclic antidepressants have been used mostly and proven to be effective in neuropathic pain. Pain that is burning in quality and often associated with a sleep disturbance may be particularly responsive to these agents. Tricyclic antidepressants can potentiate the effects of opioids or even exert an "opioid sparing" effect particularly in cancer-related pain (Ventafridda et al., 1987). Norepinephrine reuptake blockade appears to be a significant predominant mechanism of antidepressant analgesic action, whereas serotonin reuptake inhibition may enhance the effects due to norepinephrine reuptake (Max, 1994). An appreciable analgesic response to tricyclic antidepressants may be seen in painful diabetic neuropathy, postherpetic neuralgia, and headaches (Magni, 1991). An emerging alternative to tricyclics are the atypical antidepressants, particularly the serotonin-norepinephrine reuptake inhibitors venlafaxine and duloxetine. Although duloxetine and venlafaxine have been shown to be effective in the treatment of pain and depression, all other atypical antidepressants and selective

Box 34.3 Adjuvant Pharmacologic Treatments

Tricyclic antidepressants: amitriptyline, nortriptyline, desipramine
Atypical antidepressants: venlafaxine, duloxetine, bupropion
Antiepileptic drugs: gabapentin, pregabalin, topiramate, zonisamide, oxcarbazepine, lamotrigine
Systemic local anesthetics: lidocaine, mexiletine
Corticosteroids: most commonly given as injection depo preparations
Skeletal muscle relaxants: baclofen, tizanidine, cyclobenzaprine
Topical agents: lidocaine, capsaicin
Alpha-2 agonists: clonidine

---

serotonin reuptake inhibitors to date have at best very modest data to support their analgesic efficacy (Goldstein et al., 2005; Sindrup et al., 2003). In summary, antidepressants may exert the following potential benefits in the opioid-treated patient with persistent pain:

- Improvement in overall pain and function
- Enhancement in sleep onset
- Improvement of coexisting mood disorders

The antiepileptic drugs have been used in the treatment of chronic pain for more than 50 years. Pain that is typically characterized as sharp, shooting, or lancinating felt in the area of a sensory deficit may potentially respond to anticonvulsants. This diverse group of drugs has been proven to be effective in trigeminal neuralgia, glossopharyngeal neuralgia, postherpetic neuralgia, and diabetic neuropathy (Calissi & Jaber, 1995; McQuay et al., 1995; Rothrock, 1997). Antiepileptics work through various mechanisms including sodium and calcium channel blockade as well as enhancement of gamma aminobutyric acid (Bajwa & Ho, 2004). The pathophysiology of neuropathic pain, particularly lancinating pain, may involve spontaneous discharges because of exuberant sodium channel upregulation. Blockade of sodium channels analogous to epileptiform discharges may reduce painful shooting sensations (Allen, 1998; Backonja et al., 1998). Similar to antidepressants, anticonvulsants provide partial relief to a variety of neuropathic syndromes that is sustained over time. The potential benefits to the opioid-treated patient with persistent pain are similar to the antidepressants.

Muscle pain is all too common in chronic pain patients and does not consistently respond to opioids. The opioid-treated patient with persistent pain may continue to complain of deep soft tissue pain. Skeletal muscle relaxants are commonly used to relieve muscle spasm without interfering with muscle function. These drugs may exert their action at supraspinal sites and/or possibly at the level of the spinal cord by affecting spinal motor neurons, but the mechanism of analgesia is not fully understood (Cohen et al., 2004). This is not surprising, given that there is a lack of basic science and clinical data to explain deep tissue pain. Numerous clinical trials support the effectiveness of tizanidine in the treatment of muscle spasm of the cervical and lumbar regions (Fryda-Kaurimsky & Muller-Fassbender, 1981).

Systemic administration of local anesthetics, in particular, lidocaine, has been found to be useful in the treatment of some neuropathic conditions such as phantom limb pain, postherpetic neuralgia, diabetic neuropathy, as well as a variety of other peripheral neuropathies (Tremont-Lukats et al., 2005). Systemic lidocaine is equally as effective as intravenous morphine in reducing the pain of postherpetic neuralgia and postamputation stump pain (Rowbotham et al., 1991; Wu et al., 2002). These neuropathic pain conditions are thought to at least partially arise from the cell membranes of injured peripheral nerves, which express an increased sodium channel density that gives rise to spontaneous ectopic discharges (Devor et al., 1993; Kajander et al., 1992). In an analogous fashion to the mechanism of some of the anticonvulsants, lidocaine produces analgesia by blockade of peripheral as well as central sodium ion gate channels, including in the dorsal horn (Mao & Chen, 2000).

Systemic lidocaine in clinical practice can provide relief for some patients for weeks to months, an effect well beyond the half-life of the drug. Indeed, not uncommonly many patients with a significant neuropathic condition report a 50% or greater reduction in pain. But for many patients, the relief is transient and may warrant a trial of oral mexiletine, the most commonly used oral local anesthetic (Hayes, 2006). If mexiletine proves to have intolerable side effects or is ineffective, then antiepileptic drugs with sodium channel blocking features such as oxcarbazepine or zonisamide may be tried.

Fundamentals of Interventional Pain Medicine

Patients may not uncommonly obtain unsatisfactory alleviation of their pain complaints despite rational polypharmacological and cognitive behavioral management strategies. In these situations, physical rehabilitation may not be adequately achieved. Opioid-treated patients with suboptimal outcomes who fall in this category and are well selected may derive benefit from an interventional approach (Table 34.2). The general criteria for the application of these modalities often include:

- Identifiable anatomic cause of the pain
- Reasonable understanding of the mechanism(s) of pain
- Motivation and desire to make a change
- Coping and having an understanding of the painful condition that is usually irreversible
- Commitment to lifestyle modifications
- Willingness to reduce opioid medications (especially in those on "high doses" with little benefit)
- Adequate support to promote these changes
- Long-term future realistic goals and expectations

It should be stressed that the application of these procedures in high-dose opioid-dependent patients often renders less than satisfactory results if the above criteria are not met. The opioid-treated patient with persistent pain has frequently undergone one or more surgical procedures, whether it was spine surgery that did

Table 34.2. Interventional Techniques

Technique	Example
Nerve blockade	Epidural injection
Joint injection	Facet or sacroiliac
Sympathetic block	Stellate, lumbar plexus block
Annuloplasty	Intradiscal electrothermal therapy
Percutaneous disc decompression	Laser discectomy, coblation, mechanical aspiration
Ablative methods	Radiofrequency lesioning, cryoanalgesia, neurolytics
Diagnostic testing	Discography, nerve blockade
Percutaneous injection of polymethymethacrylate	Vertebroplasty
Implantable therapies	Spinal cord stimulators and drug delivery systems

not reverse pain symptoms or a surgery that resulted in inadvertent nerve damage (e.g., postthoracotomy, postmastectomy). The readiness of the patient for additional procedures should be carefully assessed. If a patient is a candidate for intervention, the patient should understand that these techniques have limitations and that little or no long-term pain relief may be derived despite multiple attempts to further elucidate and treat the source of chronic pain.

Nerve blocks represent one of the most common interventions applied in chronic pain. Pain injections may be defined as the use of needle technique intended to reduce inflammation or nociceptive afferent input, around a nerve and/or to reduce myofascial, tendon, or joint pain. Diagnostic regional anesthetic procedures have been applied to almost every peripheral and cranial nerve in order to materially enhance clinical diagnosis and therapy. The systematic blocking of nerves in the axial spine and of the various sympathetic plexuses has been found to be of the greatest utility. The use of neural blockade commonly involves the application of a mixture of local anesthetic and corticosteroid. The deposition of high concentrations of corticosteroid around nerve roots (usually lumbar or cervical) or joints (commonly either lumbar or cervical facet and sacroiliac joints) may reduce or eliminate inflammation or inflammatory/nociceptive mediators. The usual systemic side effects of corticosteroids are largely obviated by direct injection in proximity to the pain generator (e.g., therefore a low dose—"one shot"—administration can occur). Additional potential benefits of corticosteroids include the following (Abram, 1999):

- Inhibition of phospholipase A2, which prevents the formation of prostaglandins that contribute to ongoing inflammation and central sensitization.
- Reduction of the inflammatory edema surrounding nerve roots and dorsal root ganglia and thereby enhanced perfusion.
- Exertion of a membrane stabilizing effect so as to cause a reduction in ectopic discharges.

Epidural application of depocorticosteroids by using the interlaminar or transforaminal approach is the most commonly used procedure in the management of low back pain associated with radicular symptoms, and can be applied to acute and chronic presentations (Dooly et al., 1988). In acute radicular symptoms, epidural steroids may speed the resolution of pain, thereby reducing the dependence on medication and facilitating functional rehabilitation (Narozny et al., 2001). In persistent radicular pain (often postlaminectomy), the relief is usually temporary. A group of these patients are helped by periodic (every 2–3 months) injections (Boswell et al., 2005). This spacing allows for recovery of the hypothalamic-pituitary axis. Long-term corticosteroid complications such as bipedal edema, osteopenia, avascular necrosis of the femoral head, and muscle wasting are exceedingly rare.

Although radiographic guided local anesthetics/corticosteroids have proven an invaluable tool in the management of multiple painful conditions, the duration of relief obtained by a significant number of patients may prove to be too short-lived to be of practical benefit. Ablative interventions defined as procedures designed to more permanently disrupt the nervous system are grouped by agent (e.g., "chemical" phenol or alcohol) or by technique (radiofrequency lesioning [RFL] or cryoanalgesia). Neurolytic agents have found most of their application in cancer-related pain, in situations in which opioid and adjunctive agents prove to be inadequate or produce intolerable side effects. The perineural injection of alcohol or phenol to cause neurolysis of major widespread nerve plexus such as the celiac or hypogastric has been performed to produce relief from painful intraabdominal or pelvic malignancies respectively (Brown, 1988; De Leon-Casasola et al., 1993). The application of these agents in nonmalignant pain is less commonly used, because of unpredictable spread and therefore potential irreversible complications as well as loss of efficacy over time.

On the other hand, application of cryoanalgesia and RFL for nonmalignant pain appears to have a history of benefit with a relatively low risk of complications and reasonably reproducible results over time. Cryoanalgesia is best suited for painful conditions that originate from small, well-localized peripheral nerve lesions such as neuromas or entrapments of sensory nerves that do not respond to injections or other conservative means (Trescot, 2003). A percutaneous cryoprobe with the ability to physiologically stimulate sensory and motor fibers is used to localize the target and exclude the potential for motor damage. The freezing process (-70°C) occurs over several minutes and disrupts the axons and myelin in small focal areas (Evans, 1981). The epineurium and perineurium are left intact so as to allow for regeneration without neuroma formation. The relief may last for several months to years.

RFL has found diverse application of lesioning nerves to painful structures. Because of the ability to physiologically test the needle position analogously to cryoanalgesia and produce very small focal lesions, RFL has proven to be clinically safe and significant complications are rare (Weinbren & Chan, 1999). RFL may exert both thermal and electric field effects on nerves (Van Zundert et al., 2005). In clinical practice, practitioners take advantage of the dual mode of action by using high temperatures for neurolysis and low temperature or pulsed radiofrequency to produce so-called electric field effects on target neural tissue. Box 34.4 summarizes many reported RFL applications.

Although RFL has many potential uses, the majority of clinical data supports its efficacy in facet denervation and trigeminal ganglion lesioning for trigeminal neuralgia (Boswell et al., 2005). Neither cryoanalgesia nor RFL is a cure, and it must be explained to the patient that the relief is temporary. The application of cryoanalgesia or RFL in the opioid-treated patient with persistent pain may prove especially challenging. Opioid-induced hypersensitivity may require the clinician to use more local anesthetic or add a sedative/narcotic to allow the procedure to take place. This may obscure or make physiologic testing less precise, and therefore results may vary markedly.

Internal intervertebral disc disruption in the form of concentric or radial tears within the annulus fibrosis can result in significant axial pain that may lead to a patient on relatively high doses of opioids in efforts to achieve some degree of analgesia. The provocation of the intervertebral disc by injection of contrast (discography) and reproduction of an individual's chronic pain may be used to aid in the diagnosis of "discogenic pain." The usefulness of discography remains controversial especially in

---

Box 34.4 Application of Radiofrequency Lesioning Technology

Medial dorsal rami of lumbar, thoracic, and cervical facet joints
Gasserian ganglion in trigeminal neuralgia
Lateral dorsal rami for sacroiliac syndrome
Rami communicans for painful intervertebral discs
Splanchnic nerve denervation for abdominal pain
Sensory branches of the obturator and femoral nerve for inoperable hip pain
Suprascapular nerve for chronic shoulder pain
Sympathetic chain in sympathetically mediated pain
Dorsal root ganglia at all spinal levels

"high-dose" opioid dependent patients because of the test's subjective nature (Shah et al., 2005). Furthermore, the treatment of discogenic low back pain is even more contentious (Simopoulos et al., 2005). Therapies have ranged from conservative management to spinal fusion with variable results.

Recently developed intradiscal electrothermal therapy (IDET) is a percutaneous procedure for the treatment of painful discs. It involves the placement of a thermal resistive coil into the posterior annulus, followed by subsequent heating (annuloplasty). IDET may cause collagen remodeling and denervation of the intervertebral disc, but the exact mode of action is unknown (Shah et al., 2001). Through both observational studies and controlled trials, IDET appears to benefit a carefully selected subgroup of patients with discogenic low back pain (Bogduk et al., 2005). Of note is that patients on relatively high doses of opioids are often excluded from these studies.

In contrast to IDET, which is used for discogenic low back pain (not associated with disc protrusion), percutaneous disc decompression is used for lumbar radicular pain caused by minor to moderate disc protrusions. Percutaneous disc decompression is used on an outpatient basis similarly to IDET. Various modalities to remove nucleus pulposus cause a reduction in intradiscal pressure and thereby cause the protrusion to recoil to a normal position include the following (Zachary & Fortin, 2003):

- Nucleoplasty (coblation)—molecular dissociation to vaporize nuclear tissue
- Mechanical aspiration of the nucleus (Dekompressor)
- Laser-assisted discectomy—ablation of nuclear material via laser

Annular competence and patient selection are essential for high success rates. Patients who derive the most sustained benefit are those whose complaints are primarily radicular arising from small-contained disc herniations (Alo et al., 2004).

Pathologic vertebral compression fractures are not uncommonly very challenging to treat by conservative means, and extensive surgical procedures are not well tolerated by elderly patients. In addition, opioids are commonly used in the elderly for osteoporotic compression fractures with significant side effects. Opioids may exert hormonal suppression of estrogens, further perpetuating the process of osteoporosis, as does injection of corticosteroids (Ebeling, 1998). Percutaneous vertebroplasty has been demonstrated to be safe and indicated for the treatment of vertebral hemangiomas, malignant tumor, and painful osteoporotic vertebral body compression fractures (Burton & Mendel, 2003). The injection of polymethymethacrylate into the vertebral bodies via cannulas passed through the pedicles provides prompt and long-lasting relief. Patients with acute as well as chronic compression fractures appear to significantly benefit (Brown et al., 2004). Many patients are able to quickly wean off opioids with improvement in quality of life.

Many neuropathic pain conditions may fail to respond to the aforementioned therapies for any significant length of time. Spinal cord stimulation (SCS) is usually applied for intractable neuropathic pain of the extremities and trunk. The primary target of SCS appears to be the dorsal columns of the spinal cord whose activation is thought to cause orthodromic and antidromic inhibition of the dorsal horn (Linderoth & Foreman, 1999). Increased levels of inhibitory neurotransmitters, such as adenosine and gamma aminobutyric acid, may play a role in the mechanism(s) of action. Paresthesias induced by stimulation of the dorsal columns must be felt over the area of chronic pain for the therapy to be effective. The most common applications of SCS are persistent radicular pain following laminectomy and complex regional pain syndromes, although many neuropathic conditions have been reported to benefit (Krames, 1999). Many case series and observational studies report reduction in opioid medication with implementation of SCS.

Before proceeding with the permanent implantation of an SCS device, a stimulation trial is conducted (Stojanovic & Abdi, 2002). The trial involves insertion of epidural leads that allow patients to evaluate the analgesic efficacy in their everyday surroundings. Intraoperative placement of stimulating electrodes and confirmation of adequate coverage of painful areas by paresthesias can be challenging in patients on chronic opioids. The injection of local anesthetic into soft tissues can be very painful, as is the insertion of 14-gauge Tuohy needles. Copious application of local anesthetics, patience, and minimization of strong sedatives are necessary in order to preserve feedback from the patient. Trials are typically conducted for 3 to 7 days, and a permanent implant requires a minimum of 50% pain reduction. Patients treated with relatively "high dose" opioids with persistent pain may not be able to fully evaluate the analgesic benefits of SCS until 2 to 4 days postinsertion of the stimulating electrode because of procedure-related pain. It is therefore prudent to extend trials to 5 to 7 days in order to determine if SCS will offer effective pain relief. Postoperative pain management can be challenging in the opioid-treated patient with persistent pain and at times may require admission into the hospital or the addition of sustained-release opioid medications.

Implantable drug delivery systems in the form of intrathecal pumps may be used to enhance analgesia and/or minimize side effects of systemic medications (usually opioids). An intrathecal pump system consists of an infusion pump placed in the subcutaneous tissue of the abdomen, and a catheter inserted intrathecally and tunneled around the flank into the pump pocket site. Medication is inserted into the pump percutaneously by accessing the septum of the pump and filling the reservoir. Both programmable and nonprogrammable pumps have found widespread use for three general intractable conditions (Krames, 2002):

- *Spasticity*: Usually related to spinal cord injury, multiple sclerosis, or cerebral palsy.
- *Pain related to cancer:* Commonly widespread disease involving the spine or a nerve plexus.
- *Nonmalignant pain:* Most often used for chronic disabling spinal pain, but applied also to a wide range of neuropathic syndromes.

The efficacy for intrathecal devices for severe cancer pain has been established (Smith & Coyne, 2005; Smith et al., 2002, 2005) but still remains underutilized. Intrathecal devices may potentially improve pain control in cancer patients compared to comprehensive medical management as well as lead to a reduction in fatigue, and improvement in appetite, level of consciousness, and survival. In pain due to spasticity, the Food and Drug Administration has approved intrathecal baclofen, which has proven to be effective in even severe cases of spasticity. Because of the level of comorbid illness and severe life-threatening withdrawal symptoms, patients should have close access to centers that provide 24-hour services (Coffey & Ridgely 2001).

The insertion of intrathecal pumps in nonmalignant pain continues to be an option of last resort in many institutions. Patients are generally required to have even more careful psychological and medical evaluation than other therapies. The reasons for this are several: (1) The patient has no control over the infusion. Therefore, patients cannot vary the amount of medicine on a daily basis and as a result, they often continue on oral opioids for break through pain.

Box 34.5 Common Intrathecal Drugs and Admixtures

Morphine (1–20 mg/day)
Hydromorphone (0.5–12 mg/day)
Morphine + clonidine (50–900 mcg/day) + bupivacaine (3–15mg/day)
Hydromorphone + clonidine + bupivacaine
Fentanyl (25–750 mcg/day) + clonidine + bupivacaine
Sufentanil (10–90 mcg/day) + clonidine + bupivacaine
Baclofen (25–600 mcg/day) + opioid
Baclofen + clonidine

They also cannot decrease the infusion on days that the pain level is reduced. (2) The patient must be more proactive in symptom assessment and help distinguish side effects from intrathecal medications versus a potentially new disease. (3) The patient must be prepared for the possibility of serious complications that may take years to manifest, such as an inflammatory intradural mass.

As with SCS, a trial of neuraxial medications is warranted to determine the level of analgesia and functional improvement that would occur if a pump were to be implanted. Trials may be done by continuous catheters either intrathecally or epidurally, or single intrathecal bolus; there is no consensus on which modality is optimal (Anderson et al., 2003). Morphine as monotherapy for many patients is suboptimal; this has resulted in used of admixtures (Taha, 2004; Box 34.5) as well as various recommended approaches (Burton et al., 2004; Hassenbusch et al., 2004). In addition, escalating intrathecal doses of morphine as well as other opioids (especially in high doses) seem to potentially lead to the formation of a catheter tip inflammatory mass (Yaksh et al., 2002). This inflammatory mass, termed granuloma, can have serious neurologic consequences, such as paralysis (Coffey & Burchiel, 2002). Lastly, increasing federal regulations on compounding pharmacies have made preparation of complex admixtures more challenging for pain practitioners to obtain. There has been a lack of formal compatibility and stability data for the various complex mixtures at the various concentrations. Pain physicians utilizing intrathecal therapies may encounter problems with the infusion system that require prompt evaluation to avoid withdrawal or control infection. Given the potential challenges, complications, and long-term labor-intensive commitment, intrathecal therapies for nonmalignant pain are practiced by fewer centers in recent years.

Conclusion

The opioid-treated patient with persistent pain may present with multiple complex issues that involve more than just biologic issues perpetuating the use of opioids. Sorting through the psychosocial issues may take time in order to determine the potential for rehabilitation. Multiple pharmacologic, nonpharmacologic, as well as interventional approaches offer providers other alternatives that when used in conjunction appropriately may be more effective in the long run for chronic pain management than any sole therapy. Ultimately, improved analgesia, in the setting of a multidisciplinary chronic pain rehabilitation program, may lead to enhanced function and return to normal activities.

References

Abram SE. Treatment of lumbar radiculopathy with epidural steroids. *Anesthesiology* 1999; 91:1937–41.

Allen RR. Neuropathic pain: Mechanisms in clinical assessment. In Payne R, Patt RB, Hill CS (eds.). Progress in pain research and management (Vol. 12). Seattle, WA: IASP Press; 1998:159–173.

Alo KM, Wright RE, Sutcliffe J, Brandt SA. Percutaneous lumbar discectomy: Clinical response in an initial cohort of fifty consecutive patients with chronic radicular pain. *Pain Practice* 2004; 4(1):19–29.

Anderson VC, Burchiel KJ, Cooke B. A prospective randomized trial of intrathecal injection vs. epidural infusion in the selection of patients for continuous intrathecal opioid therapy. *Neuromodulation* 2003; 6(3):142–152.

Backonja M, Beydoun A, Edwards KR, Schwartz SL, Fonseca V, Hes M, et al. Gabapentin for the symptomatic treatment of painful neuropathy in patients with diabetes mellitus: A randomized controlled trial. *JAMA* 1998; 280(21):1831–1836.

Bajwa ZH, Ho C. Antiepileptics for pain. In Warfield CA, Bajwa ZH (eds.). *Principles and practice of pain medicine.* McGraw-Hill, 2004:649–654.

Ballantyne JC, Mao J. Opioid therapy for chronic pain. *N Eng J Med* 2003; 349:1943–53.

Bogduk N, Lau P, Govind J, Karasek M. Intradiscal electrothermal therapy. *Tech in Reg Anesth & Pain Med* 2005; 9:25–34.

Boswell MV, Shah RV, Everett CR, Sehgal N, et al. Interventional techniques in the management of chronic spinal pain: Evidence-based practice guidelines. *Pain Physician* 2005; 8:1–47.

Brown D, Moore DC. The use of neurolytics celiac plexus block for pancreatic cancer: Anatomy and Technique. *J of Pain & Symp Mgmt* 1988; 3:206.

Brown DB, Giluta LA, Sehgal M, Shimony JS. Treatment of chronic symptomatic vertebral compression fractures with percutaneous vertebroplasty. *AJR* 2004; 182:319–322.

Burton AW, Mendel E. Vertebroplasty and kyphoplasty: A focused review. *Pain Physician* 2003; 6(3):335–341.

Burton AW, Rajagopal A, Shah HN, et al. Epidural and intrathecal analgesia is effective in treating refractory cancer pain. *Pain Med.* 2004; 5(3): 239–47.

Calissi PT, Jaber LA. Peripheral diabetic neuropathy: current concepts in treatment. *Ann Pharmacother* 1995; 29:769–777.

Coffey RJ, Burchiel K. Inflammatory mass lesions associated with intrathecal drug infusion catheters: Report and observations on 41 patients. *Neurosurgery* 2002; 50:78–87.

Coffey RJ, Ridgely PM. Abrupt intrathecal baclofen withdrawal: Management of potentially life-threatening sequelae. *Neuromodulation* 2001; 4(3):142–146.

Cohen SP, Mullings R, Abdi S. The pharmacologic treatment of muscle pain. *Anesthesiology* 2004; 101(2):495–526.

De Leon-Casasola OA, Kent E, Lema MJ. Neurolytic superior hypogastric plexus block for chronic pelvic pain associated with cancer. *Pain* 1993; 54: 145–51.

Devor M, Govrin-Lippmann R, Angelides K. Na+ channel immunolocalization in peripheral mammalian axons and changes following nerve injury and neuroma formation. *J Neurosci.* 1993; 13(5): 1976–92.

Dooly JF, McBroom RJ, Taduchi T, et al. Nerve root infiltration in the diagnosis of radicular pain. *Spine* 1988; 13:79–83.

Ebling PR Osteoporosis in men. New insights into etiology, pathogenesis, prevention, and management. *Drugs Aging* 1998; 13:421–434.

Evans P. Cryoanalgesia: The application of low temperatures to nerves to produce anesthesia or analgesia. *Anaesthesia* 1981; 36:1003–1013.

Fryda-Kaurimsky Z, Muller-Fassbender H. Tizanidine (DS 103–282) in the treatment of acute paravertebral muscle spasm: A controlled trial comparing tizanidine and diazepam. *J Int Med Res* 1981; 9:501–5.

Goldstein DJ, Lu Y, Derke MJ, Lee TC, Iyengar S. Duloxetine vs. placebo in patients with painful diabetic neuropathy. *Pain* 2005; 116:109–18.

Hassenbusch SJ, Portenoy RK, Cousins M, et al. Polyanalgesic Consensus Conference 2003: An update on the management of pain by intraspinal drug delivery-report of an expert panel. *J Pain Symptom Manage.* 2004; 27(6):540–63.

Hayes K. Adjuvant treatments. In Ballantyne JC (ed.). *The Massachusetts General Hospital handbook of pain management* (3rd ed.). Philadelphia: Lippincott Williams & Wilkins; 2006:127–140.

Jakubowski M, Levy D, Goor-Aryeh I, Collins B, et al. Terminating migraine with allodynia and ongoing central sensitization using parenteral administration of COX 1/COX 2 Inhibitors. *Headache* 2005; 45:850–861.

Jamison R. Psychological factors in chronic pain. *J Back Musculoskeletal Rehab* 1996; 7:79–95.

Kajander KC, Wakisaka S, Bennett GJ. Spontaneous discharge originates in the dorsal root ganglion at the onset of a painful peripheral neuropathy in the rat. *Neurosci. Lett* 1992; 138:225–8.

Krames E. Implantable devices for pain control. Spinal cord stimulation and intrathecal therapies. *Best Pract Res Clin Anaesthesiol* 2002; 16:619–649.

Krames E. Spinal cord stimulation: Indications, mechanism of action and efficacy. *Curr Rev Pain* 1999; 3:419–426.

Linderoth B, Foreman RD. Physiology of spinal cord stimulation: Review and update. *Neuromodulation* 1999; 2(3):150–164.

Magni G. The use of antidepressants in the treatment of chronic pain: A review of the current evidence. *Drugs* 1991; 42:730–748.

Manchikanti L, Fellows B, Singh V. Understanding psychological aspects of chronic pain in interventional pain management. *Pain Physician* 2002; 5(1):57–82.

Mao J, Chen LL. Systemic lidocaine for neuropathic pain relief. *Pain* 2000; 87:7–17.

Marcus D. Treatment of nonmalignant chronic pain. *Am Fam Physician* 2000; 61(5):1331–8.

Max MB. Antidepressants as analgesics. In: Fields HL, Liebeskind JC (eds.). *Pharmacologic approaches to the treatment of chronic pain*. Seattle, WA: IASP Press; 1994:229–246.

McQuay H. Opioids in pain management. *Lancet* 1999; 353:2229–32.

McQuay H, Carroll D, Jadad AR et al. Anticonvulsant drugs for management of pain: a systemic review. *BMJ* 1995; 1311:1047–1052.

Narozny M, Zanetti M, Boos N. Therapeutic efficacy of selective nerve root blocks in the treatment of lumbar radicular pain. *Swiss Med Wkly* 2001; 131:75–80.

Passik SD, Weinreb HJ. Managing chronic nonmalignant pain: Overcoming obstacles to the use of opioids. *Advances in Therapy*. 2000; 17:70–80.

Rahim RT, Adler MW, Meissler JJ Jr., et al. Abrupt or precipitated withdrawal from morphine induces immunosuppression. *J Neuroimmunol* 2002;127:88–95.

Rajagopal A, Vassilopoulou-Sellin R, Palmer JL, et al. Symptomatic hypogonadism in male survivors of cancer with chronic exposure to opioids. *Cancer* 2004; 100:851–858.

Rothrock JF. Clinical studies of valproate for migraine prophylaxis. *Cephalgia* 1997; 17:81–83.

Rowbotham MC, Reisner-Keller LA, Fields HL. Both intravenous lidocaine and morphine reduce the pain of postherpetic neuralgia. *Neurology* 1991; 41:1024–28.

Shah RV, Lutz GE, Lee J, et al. Intradiskal electrothermal therapy: A preliminary histologic study. *Arch Phys Med Rehabil* 2001; 82:1230–1237.

Shah RV, Everett CR, Mckenzie-Brown AM, Sehgal N. Discography as a diagnostic test for spinal pain: A systematic and narrative review. *Pain Physician* 2005; 8:187–209.

Simopoulos TT, Malik AB, Sial KA, et al. Radiofrequency lesioning of the L2 ramus communicans in managing discogenic low back pain. *Pain Physician* 2005; 8:61–65.

Sindrup SH, Bach FW, Masden C, Gram LF, Jensen TS. Venlafaxine versus imipramine in painful neuropathy: a randomized, controlled trial. *Neurology* 2003; 60:1284–9.

Smith TJ, Coyne PJ. Implantable drug delivery systems (IDDS) after failure of comprehensive medical management (CMM) can palliate symptoms in the most refractory cancer pain patients. *J Palliat Med*. 2005; 8(4):736–42.

Smith TJ, Coyne PJ, Staats P, et al. An implantable drug delivery system (IDDS) for refractory cancer pain provides sustained pain control, less drug-related toxicity, and possible better survival compared with comprehensive medical management (CMM). *Ann Oncol*. 2005; 16(5):825–33.

Smith TJ, Staats PS, Deer T, et al. Randomized clinical trial of an implantable drug delivery system compared with comprehensive medical management for refractory cancer pain: Impact on pain, drug-related toxicity, and survival. *J Clin Oncol* 2002; 20:4040–49.

Stojanovic MP, Abdi S. Spinal cord stimulation: A focused review. *Pain Physician* 2002; 5(2):156–166.

Taha J, Favre J, Janszen M, Galarza M, Taha A. Correlation between withdrawal symptoms and medication pump residual volume in patients with implantable SynchroMed pumps. *Neurosurgery* 2004; 55:393–394.

Tremont-Lukats IW, Challapalli V, McNicol ED, Lau J, Carr DB. Systemic administration of local anesthetics to relieve neuropathic pain: A systematic review and meta-analysis. *Anesth Analg* 2005; 101:1738–49.

Trescot AM. Cryoanalgesia in interventional pain management: A focused review. *Pain Physician* 2003; 6:345–360.

Van Zundert J, de Louw AJA, Joosten EAJ, et al. Pulsed and continuous radiofrequency current adjacent to the cervical dorsal root ganglion of the rat induces late cellular activity in the dorsal horn. *Anesthesiology* 2005; 102:125–131.

Ventafridda V, Bonezzi C, Caraceni A, et al. Antidepressants for cancer pain and other painful syndromes with deafferentation component: comparison of amitriptyline and trazodone. *Ital J Neurol Sci* 1987; 8:579–587.

Weinbren J, Chan V. Complications of regional anesthesia in chronic pain therapy. In Finucane BT (ed.). *Complications of regional anesthesia*. Philadelphia: Churchill Livingstone, 1999:139–169.

Wu CL, Tella P, Staats PS, et al. Analgesic effects of intravenous lidocaine and morphine on post-amputation pain: A randomized double blind, active placebo-controlled, crossover trial. *Anesthesiology* 2002; 96:841–8.

Yaksh TL, Hassenbusch S, Burchiel K, et al. Inflammatory masses associated with intrathecal drug infusion: A review of preclinical evidence and human data. *Pain Med* 2002; 3(4):300–12.

Zachary A, Fortin JD. Minimally invasive options to disc surgery. *Pain Physician* 2003; 6:467–471.

35

Chemical Coping
The Clinical Middle Ground

Steven D. Passik

Kenneth L. Kirsh

Pain clinicians recognize that there is a vast middle ground between generally compliant drug-taking behavior on the one hand and frequent/severe aberrant behaviors that are likely to be associated with addiction on the other (see Figure 35.1). Compliant drug-taking behavior is usually associated with opioid therapy that is beneficial to the patient, whereas frequent and severe aberrant behavior is generally associated with opioid exposure that is potentially harmful to the patient. There is a large group of patients in the middle: those who display aberrant behaviors periodically, who may additionally have a mixed response to opioid therapy, the overall results of which are less than satisfying (often in the domain of functionality).

Much of the extant research on the topic of addiction-spectrum issues in pain has focused upon the prediction, assessment, and treatment of substance use disorders (Bottlender & Soyka, 2005; Comfort et al., 2003; Dekel et al., 2004; Schuckit et al., 2005). However, there has been very little work focused on trying to characterize the types of poor outcomes associated with the less severe/less frequent aberrant behaviors. Such behaviors occur more frequently in the middle ground group than in compliant patients though not as frequently as they do in addicted patients. Any harm associated with this level of misuse is subtle. These behaviors are not likely to rise to the level of compulsivity, or be as out of control, nor are they likely to be driven by cravings in a fashion that would make a clinician concerned about frank addiction.

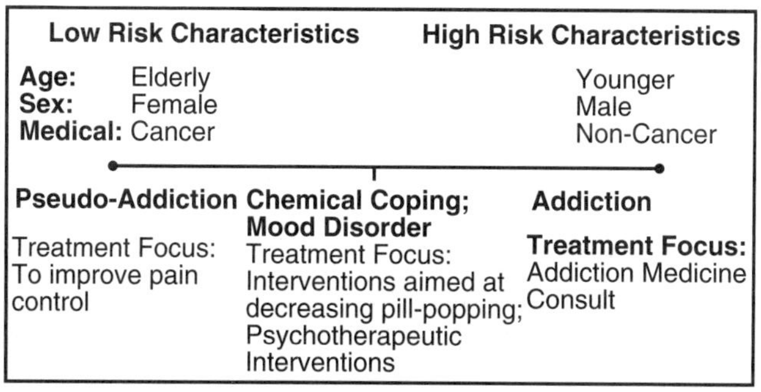

Indications from clinicians are that this poorly described and poorly researched subgroup of chronic patients might outnumber those with substance use disorders by a wide margin. Bruera and colleagues (1995) coined the term *chemical coping* to describe a pattern of maladaptive coping through drug use that they observed in patients struggling with the stress of end-stage cancer. Bruera and colleagues noted that these patients often had histories of alcohol and drug abuse, and that under the onslaught of physical and emotional distress caused by their cancer, they often requested and received large amounts of centrally acting medications. These patients had a proclivity for developing delirium from accidental overmedication. Bruera described these patients as having limited coping repertoires and a tendency to experience distress physically. Others have highlighted the applicability of this concept to a large subset of the population of those with persistent noncancer pain. It is important to have an understanding of chemical coping as a legitimate, understudied phenomenon in chronic pain patients, especially when patients are being considered for long-acting, short-acting, and/or combination opioid therapy.

Definition of a Chemical Coper

As a first step, we must be able to define the concept of chemical coping. In this way, we can then begin to identify these patients in practice and attempt to develop means of treating them. Chemical copers occasionally use their medications in nonprescribed ways to cope with stress. A major hallmark of chemical coping is the overly central place occupied by the procurement of drugs for pain and inflexibility about nondrug components of care. Medication use becomes central to life, whereas other interests become less important. As a result, chemical copers in treatment often fail to move forward toward stated psychosocial goals. They are typically uninterested in treating pain or coping with pain nonpharmacologically. They do not take advantage of other treatment options provided (e.g., they fail to follow up on recommendations to see psychologists or physical therapists). As a manifestation of chemical coping, these patients remain on the fringe of appropriate use of their medication. They occasionally self-escalate their medication dosage in the setting of stress and sometimes need to have prescriptions refilled early. Chemical coping can complicate opioid

Figure 35.1. Spectrum of Problematic Drug Use Behaviors and Risk Characteristics

Low Risk Characteristics		High Risk Characteristics
Age: Elderly		Younger
Sex: Female		Male
Medical: Cancer		Non-Cancer
Pseudo-Addiction	Chemical Coping; Mood Disorder	Addiction
Treatment Focus: To improve pain control	Treatment Focus: Interventions aimed at decreasing pill-popping; Psychotherapeutic Interventions	Treatment Focus: Addiction Medicine Consult

therapy, but many chemical copers are able to comply with their physician's opioid contract enough to avoid being removed from treatment. Theoretically, due to the gender-based differences in substance use, more women than men might be expected to be classified as chemical copers. No attempts have been made in the pain literature to measure, quantify, and study chemical coping and describe this large middle ground (perhaps as many as 35%) of chronic pain patients.

Gender Differences in Chemical Coping

Besides gender-related physical differences in the effects of drugs and in types of drugs prescribed, there are gender-related psychological differences in drug use. Previous research has established that men and women use substances for different reasons (Weiss et al., 2003). Women often use intoxicating substances as an avoidance coping strategy. Some experts believe that drug abuse can be viewed as maladaptive strategy for coping with stress temporarily. Women tend to use emotion-focused and avoidance-based coping strategies more often than men, so women may use drugs to alleviate anxiety, depression, and stress more frequently than men. In addition, women substance abusers have been shown to use drugs in attempts to self-medicate physical or psychological pain more frequently than men (Clayton et al., 1986; Lex et al., 1989, 1994). In other words, women may be more prone to fall into the category of chemical copers than men.

Men, on the other hand, often use drugs and alcohol to avoid boredom and to engage in sensation seeking (Grunberg et al., 1991). Men who are physically ill and/or physically restricted may experience more boredom than men who are physically active. Cancer pain patients and nonmalignant chronic pain patients both experience considerable disability and restriction of daily activities. Therefore, these men may be at higher risk for using drugs to avoid boredom than physically healthy men.

Chemical Coping: Associated Features

Sensation Seeking

Many researchers have found a strong relationship between sensation seeking and substance use and abuse (Andrucci et al., 1989; Jaffe & Archer, 1987; Ratliff & Burkhart, 1984; von Knorring et al., 1987). Sensation seeking has also been linked to opioid dependence specifically (Franques et al., 2003; Kosten et al., 1994; Luthar et al., 1992). *Sensation seeking* is the tendency to seek varied, novel, complex, and intense experiences and sensations and the willingness to take physical, social, legal, and financial risks for the sake of such experiences. Sensation seeking is not an avoidance strategy like chemical coping; instead, it is a desire to experience "altered consciousness." Thus, it may be that sensation seekers are a unique and subtly different subset of those we might label as chemical copers.

Generally, males score much higher on scales of sensation seeking than women. Obviously, individuals who are sensation seekers are at risk for misuse of prescribed drugs. How does sensation seeking correlate with outcomes in men and women with chronic pain on opioid therapy? This, too, has yet to be studied and will add tremendous insight to issues related to pathways of misuse of opioids in pain management that may be gender specific for women (chemical coping) and men (sensation seeking).

Alexithymia and Somatization

Alexithymia, although not a diagnosis, is a useful construct for identifying patients who are not emotionally connected and will likely present with somatic complaints (Sifneos, 1972, 1996). Taken literally, *alexithymia* can be translated from Greek into the terms *a-* (lack), *lexis-* (word), and *thymos* (emotions). Thus, this is an issue wherein the patient is unable to process or understand the emotions he or she is clearly feeling. Given a long enough period of negative affect without the ability to discharge or neutralize these feelings, it is not surprising that bodily systems become involved (Taylor et al., 1991). This effect has been noted in both addict and chronic pain populations (Cook et al., 2004; Kenny & Markou, 2004; Lumley et al., 1994; Thorberg & Lyvers, 2006; Wasan et al., 2005; Zautra et al., 2005).

Somatization is a complex problem in which a person purports to have physical complaints for which there is no known cause. In short, it is seen as a psychological self-protection mechanism or tendency for people to turn psychological distress into bodily complaints. Part of the difficulty in identifying somatization problems lies in the fact that we may be facing genuine physical issues of an unknown pathology or we might be encountering the syndrome as a result of conscious or unconscious psychological processes (Avila, 2006).

Of note, psychodynamic writings about substance abusers have described them as possessing dedifferentiated affect arrays (Krystal & Raskin, 1970). This is an associated feature of alexithymia as well as a tendency toward the notion of drug use as a means of self-medication, which will be discussed next (Khantzian, 1997; Wikler, 1980). There is some question, however, as to whether the tendency for some patients to treat psychiatric distress with medications such as opioids is a means of coping with untreated depression and negative affect or whether the negative affect arises as a result of the drug use (Schuckit & Hesselbrock, 1994; Vaillant & Milofsky, 1982).

Self-Medication

Self-medication is a concept that addresses why patients make attempts to heal themselves or treat their conditions through the use of over-the-counter medications. Taken to an extreme, it also includes attempts to use prescription medications (obtained from family or friends, bought off the street, or obtained for other legitimate reasons), alcohol, or illicit substances in an attempt to medicate a condition or problem. The key additional component is that the drug is being used for purposes counter to their intended use. For example, in the case of prescription drugs being used for reasons other than their prescribed use, we might see patients using opioids as mood stabilizers when they are anxious, depressed, or have had psychosocial issues such as a fight with a spouse. Thus, a core aspect of the chemical coper paradigm is the idea that patients with these behaviors are likely to self-medicate. One idea posed by Richman and colleagues (2001, 2002) suggests that people who have attempted to use active coping techniques that have subsequently failed, in order to escape harassment, are prone to look for escape and self-medication of their problems through the use of alcohol.

The self-medication hypothesis was proposed by Khantzian (1985, 2003) and states that two aspects must be present. First, the patient must be abusing a substance because it in some way relieves a state of distress. Second, the self-medication hypothesis states that there is usually a tendency for pharmacological specificity in the patient's preferred drug class. Opiates are prime candidates for self-medication due to their generally calming and normalizing effects. They tend to assuage feelings of rage as well as the disruption these feelings can have on interpersonal relationships.

Similarly, Markou and colleagues (1998) promoted a self-medication hypothesis specifically tying depression and drug dependence together. They argue that depression has neurobiological effects that are similar to those seen from withdrawal syndromes from alcohol or opiates. As an example, they cite that depression is characterized by changes in dopamine, norepinephrine, and corticotrophin-releasing factors in a similar fashion as that seen from either alcohol or opioid withdrawal. Therefore, patients with an underlying depression might be prone to start using alcohol or opioids in an unconscious attempt to self-correct these dysfunctional systems.

Treatment Options

Drug selection in such patients is often limited to sustained-release delivery to avoid feeding into compulsive pill popping and/or use of opioids in the service of chemical coping (Bruera et al., 1995). The treatment approach might rely mainly on the use of long-acting opioids with a deemphasis on drug taking as a way of managing pain throughout the day. The flare management philosophy (Whitten et al., 2005) is often used in lieu of drug-oriented approaches to breakthrough pain for this group of patients. The emphasis here is for the patient to learn to consider psychological and other forms of dealing with pain spikes as opposed to ad lib drug taking that has a tendency to become hard to manage for such patients. Psychotherapy and rehabilitative approaches are particularly important for this group of patients. They often will not advance in terms of psychosocial functioning unless their coping repertoires are improved. Deconditioning must be overcome and motivation for multiple lifestyle changes must be instilled so that the patient can regain the vitality to live fully with the disease of chronic pain and find a sense of purpose and meaning.

Conclusion

Chemical coping is poorly understood and woefully underresearched. Despite this gap in our knowledge base, it is an often-observed phenomenon. It is generally seen in patients who are amotivated and problematic but not frankly addicted. Although all addicts are chemical copers, not all chemical copers are addicts. Specialized approaches to treatment planning must be put into play to allow these patients to derive some benefit from drug therapies while also providing them the rehabilitative experience they will need to live a full and purposeful life with their chronic pain.

References

Andrucci GL, Archer RP, Pancoast DL, Gordon RA. The relationship of MMPI and Sensation Seeking Scales to adolescent drug use. *J Pers Assess.* 1989 Summer;53(2):253–66.

Avila LA. Somatization or psychosomatic symptoms? *Psychosomatics,* 2006;47:163–166.

Bottlender M, Soyka M. Outpatient alcoholism treatment: predictors of outcome after 3 years. *Drug Alcohol Depend.* 2005 Oct 1;80(1):83–9.

Bruera E, Moyano J, Seifert L, Fainsinger RL, Hanson J, Suarez-Almazor M. The frequency of alcoholism among patients with pain due to terminal cancer. *J Pain Symptom Manage* 1995;10(8):599.

Clayton RR, Voss HL, Robbins C, Skinner WF. Gender differences in drug use: an epidemiological perspective. *NIDA Res Monogr.* 1986;65:80–99.

Comfort M, Sockloff A, Loverro J, Kaltenbach K. Multiple predictors of substance-abusing women's treatment and life outcomes: a prospective longitudinal study. *Addict Behav.* 2003 Mar;28(2):199–224.

Cook JW, Spring B, McChargue D, Hedeker D. Hedonic capacity, cigarette craving, and diminished positive mood. *Nicotine Tob Res.* 2004 Feb;6(1):39–47.

Dekel R, Benbenishty R, Amram Y. Therapeutic communities for drug addicts: prediction of long-term outcomes. *Addict Behav.* 2004 Dec;29(9):1833–7.

Franques P, Auriacombe M, Piquemal E, Verger M, Brisseau-Gimenez S, Grabot D, Tignol J. Sensation seeking as a common factor in opioid dependent subjects and high risk sport practicing subjects. A cross sectional study. *Drug Alcohol Depend.* 2003 Mar 1;69(2):121–6.

Grunberg NE, Winders SE, Wewers ME. Gender differences in tobacco use. *Health Psychol.* 1991;10(2):143–53.

Jaffe LT, Archer RP. The prediction of drug use among college students from MMPI, MCMI, and sensation seeking scales. *J Pers Assess.* 1987 Summer;51(2):243–53.

Kenny PJ, Markou A. The ups and downs of addiction: role of metabotropic glutamate receptors. *Trends Pharmacol Sci.* 2004 May;25(5):265–72.

Khantzian EJ. The self-medication hypothesis of addictive disorders: focus on heroin and cocaine dependence. *Am J Psychiatry.* 1985 Nov;142(11):1259–64.

Khantzian EJ. The self-medication hypothesis of substance use disorders: a reconsideration and recent applications. *Harvard Review of Psychiatry.* 1997;4, 231–244.

Khantzain EJ. The self-medication hypothesis revisited: the dually diagnosed patient. *Primary Psychiatry.* 2003;10(9):47–48, 53–54.

Kosten TA, Ball SA, Rounsaville BJ. A sibling study of sensation seeking and opiate addiction. *J Nerv Ment Dis.* 1994 May;182(5):284–9.

Krystal H, Raskin HA. *Drug Dependence: Aspects of Ego Functions.* Detroit, MI: Wayne State University Press, 1970.

Lex BW, Griffin ML, Mello NK, Mendelson JH. Marijuana and alcohol effects on mood states in young women. *NIDA Res Monogr.* 1989;95:462.

Lex BW, Rhoades EM, Teoh SK, Mendelson JH, Greenwald NE. Divided attention task performance and subjective effects following alcohol and placebo: differences between women with and without a family history of alcoholism. *Drug Alcohol Depend.* 1994 Apr;35(2):95–105.

Lumley MA, Downey K, Stettner L, Wehmer F, Pomerleau OF. Alexithymia and negative affect: relationship to cigarette smoking, nicotine dependence, and smoking cessation. *Psychother Psychosom.* 1994;61(3–4):156–62.

Luthar SS, Anton SF, Merikangas KR, Rounsaville BJ. Vulnerability to drug abuse among opioid addicts' siblings: individual, familial, and peer influences. *Compr Psychiatry.* 1992 May–Jun;33(3):190–6.

Markou A, Kosten TR, Koob GF. Neurobiological similarities in depression and drug dependence: a self medication hypothesis. *Neuropsychopharmacology,* 1998; 18:135–174.

Ratliff KG, Burkhart BR. Sex differences in motivations for and effects of drinking among college students. *J Stud Alcohol.* 1984 Jan;45(1):26–32.

Richman JA, Rospenda KM, Flaherty JA, Freels S. Workplace harassment, active coping, and alcohol-related outcomes. *J Subst Abuse.* 2001;13(3):347–366.

Richman JA, Shinsako SA, Rospenda KM et al. Workplace harassment/abuse and alcohol-related outcomes: the mediating role of psychological distress. *J Stud Alcohol.* 2002; 63(4):412–419.

Schuckit MA, Hesselbrock V. Alcohol dependence and anxiety disorders: what is the relationship? *American Journal of Psychiatry.* 1994;151, 1723–34.

Schuckit MA, Smith TL, Danko GP, Kramer J, Godinez J, Bucholz KK, Nurnberger JI Jr, Hesselbrock V. Prospective evaluation of the four DSM-IV criteria for alcohol abuse in a large population. *Am J Psychiatry.* 2005 Feb;162(2):350–60.

Sifneos PE. Alexithymia: past and present. *Am J Psychiatry.* 1996;153(7 suppl):137–142.

Sifneos PE. *Short-Term Psychotherapy and Emotional Crisis.* Cambridge, Mass: Harvard University Press, 1972.

Taylor GJ, Bagby RM, Parker JD. The alexithymia construct. a potential paradigm for psychosomatic medicine. *Psychosomatics.* 1991;32(2):153–164.

Thorberg FA, Lyvers M. Negative mood regulation (NMR) expectancies, mood, and affect intensity among clients in substance disorder treatment facilities. *Addict Behav.* 2006 May;31(5):811–20.

Vaillant GE, Milofsky ES. The etiology of alcoholism: a prospective viewpoint. *American Psychologist.* 1982;37, 494–503.

von Knorring L, von Knorring AL, Smigan L, Lindberg U, Edholm M. Personality traits in subtypes of alcoholics. *J Stud Alcohol.* 1987 Nov;48(6):523–7.

Wasan AD, Davar G, Jamison R. The association between negative affect and opioid analgesia in patients with discogenic low back pain. *Pain.* 2005 Oct;117(3):450–61.

Weiss SR, Kung HC, Pearson JL. Emerging issues in gender and ethnic differences in substance abuse and treatment. *Curr Womens Health Rep.* 2003 Jun;3(3):245–53.

Whitten CE, Evans CM, Cristobal K. Pain management doesn't have to be a pain: working and communicating effectively with patients who have chronic pain. *The Permanente Journal,* Spring 2005; 9(2):41–48.

Wikler A. *Opioid Dependence: Mechanisms and Treatment.* New York: Plenum Press, 1980.

Zautra AJ, Johnson LM, Davis MC. Positive affect as a source of resilience for women in chronic pain. *J Consult Clin Psychol.* 2005 Apr;73(2):212–20.

36

Buprenorphine in Pain and Addiction

Howard A. Heit

Douglas L. Gourlay

The goal of this chapter is to provide health-care professionals with information regarding the appropriate therapeutic uses of buprenorphine in the context of pain and addiction medicine. Like methadone, buprenorphine can be used both for opioid agonist therapy (OAT) for the disease of opioid addiction as well as the treatment of anticipated or unanticipated acute pain and chronic pain.

Currently available data suggest that 3%–16% of the American population have addictive disorders (Savage 1996). Pain is the most common complaint presenting to the primary care clinician's office (Foley 2000; Glajchen 2001). Approximately 50 to 70 million people are undertreated or not treated for painful conditions (Krames and Olson 1997). Because pain with or without the disease of addiction being present is so common, it is instructive to explore the basic pharmacology and clinical uses of a unique opioid such as buprenorphine.

Pharmacology

Buprenorphine is a semisynthetic highly lipophilic opioid that is a derivative of the morphine alkaloid thebaine (Buprenex [package insert] 2002; Heel, Brogden, et al. 1979). Its primary activity in people appears to be that of a partial agonist at the μ opioid receptor and as an antagonist at the κ receptor (Leander 1988; Martin, Eades, et al. 1976; Reisine and Bell 1993; Richards and Sadeé 1985a, 1985b). The effects of binding at μ opioid receptors include supraspinal analgesia, respiratory depression, and miosis. Buprenorphine, being a partial μ opioid agonist, may have a wider safety profile compared to other full μ agonists, especially with regard to respiratory depression. Further, the slow dissociation of buprenorphine from the receptor may result in fewer signs and symptoms of opioid withdrawal upon termination of buprenorphine therapy than those that occur with full μ opioid agonists, such as morphine, heroin, and methadone (Boas and Villiger 1985). Buprenorphine's antagonist effects at the κ receptor are associated with limited spinal analgesia, dysphoria, and psychotomimetic effects (Sadeé, Rosenbaum, et al. 1982).

Several buprenorphine formulations have been studied. Oral bioavailability of buprenorphine is low because of extensive first-pass hepatic metabolism (Bullingham, McQuay, et al. 1983; Johnson, Fudala, et al. 2005). The administration of buprenorphine by the sublingual route allows for bypassing of the first-pass hepatic metabolism, thus increasing bioavailability.

Buprenorphine is a partial μ agonist and κ antagonist that dissociates very slowly from opioid receptors (Boas and Villiger 1985; Tallarida and Cowan 1982). Buprenorphine has high affinity at the μ opioid receptor that may offer a "blockade effect" to other opioids that typically lasts in excess of 24 hours (Boas and Villiger 1985), making once-daily or even longer dosing possible for the treatment of opioid addiction. Effective analgesia is achieved at relatively low receptor occupancy of 5%–10% (Tyers 1980). The degree of analgesia appears not to be related to plasma concentration of the drug because the dissociation at the receptor site lags behind plasma concentration (Boas and Villiger 1985). Buprenorphine is at least 30–40 times more potent than morphine over its linear range (Cowan, Lewis, et al. 1977; Tigerstedt and Tammisto 1980; Wang, Johnson et al., 1981), with an analgesic effect seen over the 0.1 mg to 10 mg range (Budd 1981). As a partial agonist, the buprenorphine-morphine equivalence at higher doses becomes less certain due to a flattening off of the agonist curve.

As a result of buprenorphine's high receptor site affinity, it may interfere with effectiveness of other full μ analgesics. As with other partial μ agonists, buprenorphine is contraindicated in opioid-dependent patients because it may precipitate severe withdrawal (Clark, Lintzeris, et al. 2002; Sporer 2004).

Buprenorphine use for OAT is based on its pharmacokinetic and pharmacodynamic properties. It has a high affinity for the μ receptor, with slow dissociation resulting in a long duration of action. Because it is a partial agonist, its effects plateau at higher doses, and it begins to behave more like an antagonist (Raisch, Fye, et al. 2002). This antagonist property in higher doses limits the dose-dependent analgesic effect and respiratory depression (Sporer 2004). The high-affinity blockade significantly limits the effect of subsequently administered opioid agonists or antagonists, and the "ceiling effect" confers a high safety profile clinically, a low level of physical dependence, and often mild withdrawal symptoms on cessation after prolonged administration when compared with methadone (Breen, Harris, et al. 2003).

These qualities make it advantageous for the treatment of opioid dependence. The ceiling effect may, however, limit its usefulness in those who would otherwise require higher doses of methadone to achieve stability. Studies involving comparisons between buprenorphine and higher dose methadone are inconclusive and merit further study (O'Connor and Fiellin 2000).

Buprenorphine has been used safely and successfully for many years in France for the treatment of opioid addiction (Bouchez, Beauverie, et al. 1998). More recently, it has been approved for use in the office-based treatment of opioid addiction in the United States under the Drug Addiction Treatment Act of 2000 (DATA 2000). This drug represents the first opioid approved for in-office maintenance treatment of opioid addiction since the implementation of the Harrison Narcotic Control Act of 1914.

Buprenorphine is well absorbed sublingually, with 60%–70% of the bioavailability of intravenous doses (Mendelson, Upton, et al. 1997). Buprenorphine is less well absorbed orally and is quickly metabolized by the liver. The drug is widely distributed, with a peak plasma concentration at approximately 90 minutes and a half-life of 4–5 hours (Ling and Smith 2002). Buprenorphine is lipophilic, and brain tissue levels far exceed serum levels. It is highly bound to plasma protein and is inactivated by enzymatic transformation via N-dealkylation and conjugation (Sadeé, Rosenbaum, et al. 1982). Buprenorphine is mainly metabolized to inactive conjugated metabolites (80%–90%), but nor-buprenorphine, a product of N-dealkylation by the cytochrome P-450 3A4 enzyme, has more potent respiratory depressive effects than the parent drug (Ohtani, Kotaki, et al. 1995, 1997). There are drugs that interfere with the 3A4 system, such as certain antibiotics, antifungals, and HIV protease inhibitors, that could decrease production of nor-buprenorphine. Conversely, there are drugs that induce 3A4 system, such a phenobarbital and certain antiseizure medications, that could increase the levels of nor-buprenorphine (Bridge, Fudala, et al. 2003; Chiang and Hawks 2003). The clinical implications of these interactions are unknown.

Buprenorphine: Opioid Agonist Therapy for the Disease of Addiction

Precise understanding of the definition of addiction is necessary for the health-care professional to evaluate and treat patients with acute or chronic pain with or without this comorbid condition (Heit 2003). Addiction is a primary, chronic, neurobiologic disease, with genetic, psychosocial, and environmental factors influencing its development and manifestations. It is characterized by behaviors that include one or more of the following: impaired control over drug use, compulsive use, continued use despite harm, and craving (American Academy of Pain Medicine, American Pain Society, et al. 2001; Kasser, Geller, et al. 1998; Savage, Joranson, et al. 2003).

Drugs of abuse act at local cellular and membrane sites that are within a neurochemical system that is commonly referred to as the "reward and withdrawal pathway" (Koob and Le Moal 2001). This pathway is in the mesolimbic dopamine system, and it involves, among other structures, the ventral tegmental area, nucleus accumbens, amygdala, and prefrontal cortex of the primitive brain.

Addiction is a neurobiological disease that causes disruption of this pathway. This disruption is mediated via receptor sites and neurotransmitters. Central to this reward and withdrawal pathway is the neurotransmitter dopamine, which has been shown to be relevant not only to drug reward, but also to food, drink, sex, and social reward (Nestler 2001; Nestler and Landsman 2001). Disruption of this neurochemical pathway by drugs of abuse leads to addiction. Drug withdrawal experience tends to build upon itself with repeated drug use and can persist during prolonged periods of drug abstinence, a symptom complex known as the protracted abstinence syndrome (Kasser, Geller, et al. 1998). These processes of neural adaptation related to drug craving or to environmental stimuli associated with drug use, referred to as "cues," lead the genetically susceptible individual to the progressive increase in drug-seeking behavior that often characterizes addiction. This neural process appears to increase the attractiveness of the drug taken and that of the drug-associated stimuli (Nestler, Hyman, et al. 2001).

It is important to remember that addiction is a treatable brain disease that is a distinct medical condition (Leshner 1997; Wise 2000). In the context of opioid addiction, DATA 2000 (Sec. 3501) has allowed for office-based opioid treatment (OBOT) using buprenorphine with or without naloxone. Buprenorphine may be prescribed by certified and specially trained physicians who have received a waiver from the requirement to register as a Narcotic Treatment Program (NTP) from the Center for Substance Abuse Treatment (CSAT) of the Substance Abuse and Mental Health Services Administration (SAMHSA; Sec. 3502. Amendment to Controlled Substance Act. In general—Sec. 303(g) of the Controlled Substance Act [21 U.S.C. 823(g) is amended]).

The buprenorphine-containing products Suboxone and Subutex (Reckitt Benckiser, Berkshire, United Kingdom) are the only two Schedule III drugs currently approved for the treatment of opioid dependence under DATA 2000. The combination product, Suboxone, is available in 2 mg and 8 mg tablets combined with naloxone at 0.5 mg and 2 mg, respectively, whereas the mono product Subutex is available without naloxone. Naloxone is poorly absorbed via the sublingual route but precipitates withdrawal symptoms if administered parenterally to an opioid-dependent person, thereby potentially reducing the risk of parenteral misuse and diversion (Mendelson, Jones, et al. 1997; Sadeé, Rosenbaum, et al. 1982).

Inasmuch as buprenorphine alone as a partial agonist will precipitate opioid withdrawal in active opioid-dependent users, the addition of naloxone to buprenorphine as an abuse deterrent has been questioned on its pharmacological merits (Comer and Collins 2002). However, it is thought by some that the addition of naloxone to buprenorphine might attenuate the "high" derived from the parenteral misuse of the sublingual product, thereby reducing the abuse liability by the parenteral route (Mendelson, Jones, et al. 1999).

Addiction is a chronic disease and should be treated accordingly. Buprenorphine is one of the medications that can be used to treat opioid addiction. Opioids drugs such as fentanyl, heroin, opium, morphine, codeine, oxycodone, hydrocodone, and so forth can all be abused and lead to tolerance and physical dependence. This means that the user's body becomes physically dependent, and, when the drug is stopped, symptoms of withdrawal emerge (American Academy of Pain Medicine, American Pain Society, et al. 2001). Even after the acute withdrawal period, some patients still have cravings and persistent symptoms of withdrawal (post-abstinence syndrome), which, if left untreated, can lead to relapse back to their drug of choice (Kasser, Geller, et al. 1998).

Medical research has shown that in at least some cases, neuroplastic and neuroadaptive changes occur as a result of longtime drug abuse. These brain changes that occur during the development of addiction explain the persistent vulnerability to relapse long after drug taking has ceased. Addiction is a cycle of spiraling dysregulation of the brain reward system that progressively increases, resulting in the compulsive use and loss of control over drug taking. This development of addiction recruits different sources of reinforcement, different neuroadaptive mechanisms, and different neurochemical changes to dysregulate the brain reward system (Koob and Le Moal 2001).

Not all addicted patients who misuse opioids need medications to treat their addiction. Many do very well with counseling, residential therapeutic treatment, or mutual support programs such as Narcotics Anonymous. But in some cases, these approaches alone are not sufficient to maintain functional stability, and maintenance medication is needed. Maintenance medication has a slower onset and is longer acting in its effects on the brain than most other opioid drugs of abuse. Maintenance therapy prevents the "on and off" switch of fluctuating opioid blood levels that lead to euphoria alternating with cravings.

Continuous occupation of the endogenous opioid receptor system allows interacting physiological and behavioral systems to become normalized (Dole 1988). When taken as directed and used in a tightly controlled and structured environment as a maintenance agonist treatment program, a patient on buprenorphine or methadone should no more be considered addicted to the maintenance drug than an insulin-maintained diabetic would be considered "addicted" to insulin.

It some cases, stable methadone maintenance patients will wish to switch to buprenorphine therapy. There are many reasons why this might occur, not the least of which is to avoid the stigma often attached to maintenance treatment with methadone as well as enjoying the more normalized treatment setting of the office-based practice. Unfortunately, because of the partial agonist nature of the medication, buprenorphine is not equivalent in maintenance strength to high-dose methadone. There is a concern that buprenorphine may not be strong enough for some methadone-maintained patients and might lead to dangerous relapses if attempted. With this in mind, it is important for any patient contemplating such a switch to have the option of resuming maintenance treatment with methadone, should they so desire (Johnson, Chutuape, et al. 2000).

Buprenorphine is a partial agonist substitute for the disease of opioid addiction with a μ equivalence of 16 mg sublingual buprenorphine equal to approximately 60 mg equivalents of methadone. Receptor occupancy persists for 24 to 48 hours; therefore, once-daily dosing will be effective for most patients (Borg and Kreek 2003).

In the opioid-dependent patient, buprenorphine is best started when the patient is experiencing the symptoms of withdrawal, which could include sweating, nervousness, abdominal cramps, diarrhea, goose bumps, and/or alterations in one's mood. The dose is adjusted over several days. Complete protocol in doing a buprenorphine induction is beyond the scope of this chapter, and one is encouraged to enroll in a buprenorphine training course presented by the American Society of Addiction Medicine (ASAM) and others. Information for such programs is available from the CSAT website, located at http://www.buprenorphine.samhsa.gov/.

Pain Treatment for a Patient on OAT With Buprenorphine

No data exist on the incidence of either acute or chronic pain in a patient maintained on OAT with buprenorphine. However, chronic pain among chemically dependent patients in methadone maintenance treatment (MMT) and residential treatment facilities (RTF) is quite common and is either undertreated or not treated. Chronic severe pain was reported in 37% of 390 patients in two MMT programs and 24% of 531 patients in 13 RTF, which interfered with physical and psychosocial function. The population used illicit drugs or alcohol to treat their pain and was less likely to be prescribed pain medications (Rosenblum, Joseph, et al. 2003).

The most common triggers for relapse are stress, drug availability, and reexposure to environmental cues (sight, sounds, smells) previously associated with drug taking (Koob and Le Moal 2001). Pain is clearly a stressor and may predispose those in recovery to relapse. It stands to reason that if the patient is in recovery with or without OAT and the pain is undertreated or not treated, he or she may turn to the street for diverted prescription medication or illicit drugs or may use legal drugs such as alcohol to anesthetize him- or herself to their pain (Gourlay, Heit, et al. 2005). For example, older adults with drinking problems are more likely to use alcohol to manage their physical pain (21% versus 56%; Brennan, Schutte, et al. 2005).

Anticipated Pain

Under certain circumstances, patients on OAT with buprenorphine will experience the need for pain management. Painful procedures and events such as elective surgery can be anticipated. This affords both the patient and the treatment team the opportunity to plan and so optimize the management of this acute pain. Communication plays a vital role in ensuring a trouble-free peri- and postoperative course.

Consider the patient on OAT who is going to have an elective procedure/surgery with associated mild to moderate pain. The patient is on a buprenorphine-containing product and is able to take medications by mouth. In most cases, mild to moderately severe pain can be managed simply by temporarily titrating the dose upward while adjusting the dosing schedule of the maintenance drug (in this case, buprenorphine) to a TID or QID dosing regimen.

If breakthrough medication is needed, consider using one with high potency such as oral transmucosal fentanyl lozenge or hydromorphone. Demerol (meperidine) is a particularly poor choice due to its anticholinergic and histaminergic qualities and the accumulation of the potentially toxic metabolite (normeperidine). Normeperidine is a potent CNS irritant that can lead to confusion, disorientation, hallucinations, headaches, and even seizures once individual tolerances are exceeded (Kaiko, Foley, et al. 1983; Mauro, Bonfiglio, et al. 1986). As a result, the American Pain Society has recommended that meperidine should not be used on a chronic basis.

With appropriate preoperative teaching, patient-controlled analgesia (PCA) with fentanyl or hydromorphone can be a very effective tool in the management of postoperative pain, even in those patients who are in recovery from drug or alcohol problems. It is important to note that although the addition of a partial μ agonist to a fully μ dependent patient may precipitate severe withdrawal, the reverse is not true. Although analgesic response may be blunted, full μ agonists can always be added to buprenorphine-maintained patients without fear of precipitating withdrawal. However, care should be exercised during titration due to potentially unpredictable μ sensitivity.

In the case of a patient on OAT who is going to have an elective procedure/surgery with expected moderate to severe pain, buprenorphine may adversely affect the management of acute pain. With effective planning, buprenorphine may be discontinued a few days before surgery. Any full μ agonists can be used to prevent withdrawal, even in the preoperative period and also to treat the resultant acute pain (Heit, Covington, et al. 2004). In this case, the risks of discontinuation of the maintenance drug (i.e., relapse) must be carefully weighed against the potential benefits in order to follow this course. In general, it is wise to avoid, when possible, agents of past misuse or addiction.

Given the current novelty of this drug and the lack of familiarity by health-care providers in the management of acute pain in buprenorphine-maintained patients, preemptive discontinuation may help the acute pain team focus their attention on aggressive pain management rather than simply accepting poor pain control as an inevitable consequence of buprenorphine therapy. Once the acute episode is over, buprenorphine may safely be reintroduced and again titrated to an appropriate maintenance dose in a once-daily fashion.

For the patient on OAT who is going to have an elective procedure/surgery and be NPO, discontinue buprenorphine and start a PCA with full μ agonist. Titrate to effect to prevent withdrawal. Treat the pain with an opioid with high receptor site affinity and potency, such as fentanyl or hydromorphone (second choice), and always avoid meperidine.

Unanticipated Acute Pain

Unlike anticipated pain, when the patient may be optimized prior to the elective procedure, some buprenorphine-maintained patients may experience unanticipated pain such as is seen with trauma or other acute, surgical emergencies. The patient may have mild to moderate pain that may be adequately managed with divided dosing of the maintenance drug. Titration to effect, up to 8 mg TID to QID may adequately manage the acute pain. In this case, breakthrough medicine such as hydromorphone or fentanyl may be used during this acute period. An alternative, if time permits, is to discontinue buprenorphine and switch to a full μ agonist.

If the patient is NPO and has acute moderate to severe pain and treatment with IV opioids is indicated, use PCA analgesic. Titrate to effect to prevent withdrawal and to treat the pain. Fentanyl with its high receptor site affinity and potency may be the IV opioid of choice because it may be easier to titrate. Hydromorphone would be the second choice.

Acute Pain Superimposed on Chronic Pain

One assumes buprenorphine in divided doses controls pain for a patient with mild to moderate chronic pain. If that patient then has acute pain superimposed, an IR/rapid-onset opioid with high receptor site affinity and potency such as hydromorphone or oral transmural fentanyl lozenge can be added. Then one would titrate to effect to treat the acute pain with the IR/rapid-onset opioid. Again, it is wise to avoid previous drugs of misuse. Given the higher risks associated with known substance-use-disordered patients, careful boundary setting, frequent follow-up appointments, and limited prescriptions are strongly recommended.

Off-Label Use of Buprenorphine

The off-label use of the sublingual formulations of buprenorphine (Suboxone/Subutex) for the treatment of pain is not prohibited under DEA requirements. One does not need a wavier from CSAT, only a valid license to prescribe a Schedule III controlled substance (Heit, Covington, et al. 2004).

Buprenorphine "Pearls"

1. Starting buprenorphine when a patient is physically dependent on a full opioid agonist could precipitate acute withdrawal. A full μ agonist, however, may always be given to a buprenorphine-maintained individual without fear of inducing a precipitated withdrawal.
2. As a partial agonist, the effective dose is limited for acute or chronic pain treatment: 6–8 mg in a TID or QID dosing schedule (up to 32 mg/day total) is probably the maximum daily dose.
3. Buprenorphine may not be suitable in a patient requiring a large dose of methadone, in other words, greater than 60 mg of methadone/day. There are, however, patients who do well on buprenorphine even though they struggled with ongoing opioid drug use and even while on high doses of methadone. It is important to remember that not all patients on high doses of methadone, especially those who are relatively unstable, actually *need* high μ agonist effects. Individual patient selection is critical to success.
4. Buprenorphine for chronic pain management has a 6- to 8-hour analgesic duration of action and therefore should be dosed TID or QID for optimum analgesic effect. Once-daily dosing may provide >24 hours of relief in some patients, especially those who are suffering from withdrawal-mediated pain associated with short-acting, immediate-release opioids.
5. Inadequate pain control in buprenorphine-maintained patients should not be attributed to the opioid-blocking effect of this drug. Careful titration to effect of a potent full μ agonist should allow for effective acute pain management in the buprenorphine-maintained patient.

Conclusion

Because of its unique pharmacokinetic and pharmacodynamic properties, buprenorphine has a well-established role in the treatment of the disease of opioid addiction but is regaining popularity in the role of a primary analgesic. Unfortunately, it also poses interesting challenges to the management of both acute and chronic pain. For appropriate prescribing of this medication, the sometimes peculiar pharmacokinetic/pharmacodynamic aspects of buprenorphine must be understood, allowing for proper patient selection and evaluation in order to optimize treatment outcomes. Accepting inadequate pain relief because of the concurrent use of this drug is neither appropriate nor necessary.

References

American Academy of Pain Medicine, American Pain Society, et al. (2001). *Definitions Related to the Use of Opioids for the Treatment of Pain.* Glenview, IL: American Academy of Pain Medicine.

Boas, R. A. and J. W. Villiger (1985). Clinical actions of fentanyl and buprenorphine. The significance of receptor binding. *Br J Anaesth* 57(2): 192–6.

Borg, L. and M. J. Kreek (2003). *Pharmacology of Opioids.* Chevy Chase, MD: American Society of Addiction Medicine.

Bouchez, J., P. Beauverie, et al. (1998). Substitution with buprenorphine in methadone- and morphine sulfate-dependent patients. Preliminary results. *Eur Addict Res* 4 Suppl 1: 8–12.

Breen, C. L., S. J. Harris, et al. (2003). Cessation of methadone maintenance treatment using buprenorphine: transfer from methadone to buprenorphine and subsequent buprenorphine reductions. *Drug Alcohol Depend* 71(1): 49–55.

Brennan, P. L., K. K. Schutte, et al. (2005). Pain and use of alcohol to manage pain: prevalence and 3-year outcomes among older problem and non-problem drinkers. *Addiction* 100(6): 777–86.

Bridge, T. P., P. J. Fudala, et al. (2003). Safety and health policy considerations related to the use of buprenorphine/naloxone as an office-based treatment for opiate dependence. *Drug Alcohol Depend* 70(2 Suppl): S79–85.

Buprenex [package insert] (2002). Richmond, VA: Reckitt Benckiser Pharmaceuticals, Inc.

Budd, K. (1981). High dose buprenorphine for postoperative analgesia. *Anaesthesia* 36(9): 900–3.

Bullingham, R. E., H. J. McQuay, et al. (1983). Clinical pharmacokinetics of narcotic agonist-antagonist drugs. *Clin Pharmacokinet* 8(4): 332–43.

Chiang, C. N. and R. L. Hawks (2003). Pharmacokinetics of the combination tablet of buprenorphine and naloxone. *Drug Alcohol Depend* 70: S39-S47.

Clark, N. C., N. Lintzeris, et al. (2002). Severe opiate withdrawal in a heroin user precipitated by a massive buprenorphine dose. *Med J Aust* 176(4): 166–7.

Comer, S. D. and E. D. Collins (2002). Self-administration of intravenous buprenorphine and the buprenorphine/naloxone combination by recently detoxified heroin abusers. *J Pharmacol Exp Ther* 303(2): 695–703.

Cowan, A., J. Lewis, et al. (1977). Agonist and antagonist properties of buprenorphine, a new antinociceptive agent. *Br J Pharmacol* 60: 537–545.

Dole, V. P. (1988). Implications of methadone maintenance for theories of narcotic addiction. *JAMA* 260(20): 3025–9.

Foley, K. (2000). Dismantling the barriers: providing palliative and pain care. *JAMA* 283(1): 115.

Glajchen, M. (2001). Chronic pain: treatment barriers and strategies for clinical practice. *J Am Board Fam Pract* 14(3): 211–8.

Gourlay, D., H. Heit, et al. (2005). Universal precautions in pain medicine: A rational approach to the treatment of chronic pain. *Pain Medicine* 6(2): 107–12.

Heel, R. C., R. N. Brogden, et al. (1979). Buprenorphine: a review of its pharmacological properties and therapeutic efficacy. *Drugs* 17(2): 81–110.

Heit, H. A. (2003). Addiction, physical dependence, and tolerance: precise definitions to help clinicians evaluate and treat chronic pain patients. *J Pain Palliat Care Pharmacother* 17(1): 15–29.

Heit, H. A., E. Covington, et al. (2004). Dear DEA. *Pain Med* 5(3): 303–8.

Johnson, R. E., M. A. Chutuape, et al. (2000). A comparison of levomethadyl acetate, buprenorphine, and methadone for opioid dependence. *N Engl J Med* 343(18): 1290–7.

Johnson, R. E., P. J. Fudala, et al. (2005). Buprenorphine: considerations for pain management. *J Pain Symptom Manage* 29(3): 297–326.

Kaiko, R. F., K. M. Foley, et al. (1983). Central nervous system excitatory effects of meperidine in cancer patients. *Ann Neurol* 13(2): 180–5.

Kasser, C., A. Geller, et al. (1998). *Principles of Detoxification.* Chevy Chase, MD: American Society of Addiction Medicine.

Koob, G. F. and M. Le Moal (2001). Drug addiction, dysregulation of reward, and allostasis. *Neuropsychopharmacology* 24(2): 97–129.

Krames, E. S. and K. Olson (1997). Clinical realities and economic considerations: patient selection in intrathecal therapy. *J Pain Symptom Manage* 14(3 Suppl): S3–13.

Leander, J. (1988). Buprenorphine is a potent kappa-opioid receptor antagonist in pigeons and mice. *Eur J Pharmacol* 151: 457–461.

Leshner, A. I. (1997). Addiction is a brain disease, and it matters. *Science* 278(5335): 45–7.

Ling, W. and D. Smith (2002). Buprenorphine: blending practice and research. *J Subst Abuse Treat* 23(2): 87–92.

Martin, W., C. Eades, et al. (1976). The effects of morphine and nalorphine-like drugs in the nondependent and morphine-dependent chronic spinal dog. *J Pharmacol Exp Ther* 197: 517–532.

Mauro, V. F., M. F. Bonfiglio, et al. (1986). Meperidine-induced seizure in a patient without renal dysfunction or sickle cell anemia. *Clin Pharm* 5(10): 837–9.

Mendelson, J., R. T. Jones, et al. (1997). Buprenorphine and naloxone interactions in methadone maintenance patients. *Biol Psychiatry* 41(11): 1095–101.

Mendelson, J., R. T. Jones, et al. (1999). Buprenorphine and naloxone combinations: the effects of three dose ratios in morphine-stabilized, opiate-dependent volunteers. *Psychopharmacology (Berl)* 141(1): 37–46.

Mendelson, J., R. A. Upton, et al. (1997). Bioavailability of sublingual buprenorphine. *J Clin Pharmacol* 37(1): 31–7.

Nestler, E. J. (2001). Molecular basis of long-term plasticity underlying addiction. *Nat Rev Neurosci* 2(2): 119–28.

Nestler, E. J., S. E. Hyman, et al. (2001). *Reinforcement and addictive disorders.* New York: McGraw-Hill.

Nestler, E. J. and D. Landsman (2001). Learning about addiction from the genome. *Nature* 409(6822): 834–5.

O'Connor, P. G. and D. A. Fiellin (2000). Pharmacologic treatment of heroin-dependent patients. *Ann Intern Med* 133(1): 40–54.

Ohtani, M., H. Kotaki, et al. (1995). Comparative analysis of buprenorphine- and norbuprenorphine-induced analgesic effects based on pharmacokinetic-pharmacodynamic modeling. *J Pharmacol Exp Ther* 272(2): 505–10.

Ohtani, M., H. Kotaki, et al. (1997). Kinetics of respiratory depression in rats induced by buprenorphine and its metabolite, norbuprenorphine. *J Pharmacol Exp Ther* 281(1): 428–33.

Raisch, D. W., C. L. Fye, et al. (2002). Opioid dependence treatment, including buprenorphine/naloxone. *Ann Pharmacother* 36(2): 312–21.

Reisine, J. and G. Bell (1993). Molecular biology of opioid receptors. *Trends Neurosci* 16: 506–510.

Richards, M. and W. Sadeé (1985a). Burpenorphine is an antagonist at the kappa opioid receptor. *Pharm Res* 2: 178–181.

Richards, M. and W. Sadeé (1985b). In vivo opiate receptor binding of pripavines to mu, delta and kappa sites in the rate brain as determined by an ex vivo labeling method. *Eur J Pharmacol* 114: 343–353.

Rosenblum, A., H. Joseph, et al. (2003). Prevalence and characteristics of chronic pain among chemically dependent patients in methadone maintenance and residential treatment facilities. *JAMA* 289(18): 2370–8.

Sadeé, W., J. Rosenbaum, et al. (1982). Buprenorphine: Differential interaction with opiate receptor subtypes in vivo. *J Pharmacol Exp Ther* 223: 157–162.

Savage, S. R. (1996). Long-term opioid therapy: assessment of consequences and risks. *J Pain Symptom Manage* 11(5): 274–86.

Savage, S. R., D. E. Joranson, et al. (2003). Definitions related to the medical use of opioids: evolution towards universal agreement. *J Pain Symptom Manage* 26(1): 655–67.

Sporer, K. A. (2004). Buprenorphine: a primer for emergency physicians. *Ann Emerg Med* 43(5): 580–4.

Tallarida, R. J. and A. Cowan (1982). The affinity of morphine for its pharmacologic receptor in vivo. *J Pharmacol Exp Ther* 222(1): 198–201.

Tigerstedt, I. and T. Tammisto (1980). Double-blind, multiple-dose comparison of buprenorphine and morphine in postoperative pain. *Acta Anaesthesiol Scand* 24(6): 462–8.

Tyers, M. B. (1980). A classification of opiate receptors that mediate antinociception in animals. *Br J Pharmacol* 69(3): 503–12.

Wang, R. I., R. P. Johnson, et al. (1981). The study of analgesics following single and repeated doses. *J Clin Pharmacol* 21(2): 121–5.

Wise, R. A. (2000). Addiction becomes a brain disease. *Neuron* 26(1): 27–33.

37

Pain and Chemical Dependency in the Emergency Department

Knox H. Todd

Pain is the single most common reason patients seek care in the emergency department (Cordell et al., 2002). Given the prevalence of pain as a presenting complaint, one might expect emergency physicians to assign its treatment a high priority; however, pain is often seemingly invisible to the emergency physician. Multiple research studies have documented that the undertreatment of pain, or oligoanalgesia, is a frequent occurrence (Rupp & Delaney, 2004). Pain that is not acknowledged and managed appropriately causes dissatisfaction with medical care, hostility toward the physician, unscheduled returns to the emergency department, delayed return to full function, and potentially, an increased risk of litigation. Failure to recognize and treat pain may result in anxiety, depression, sleep disturbances, increased oxygen demands with the potential for end-organ ischemia, and decreased movement with an increased risk of venous thrombosis.

Given this state affairs, we should examine the barriers that serve to block the adequate recognition and treatment of pain in emergency departments, as well as other health-care delivery settings. One of these barriers is the physician's fear of being "duped" by patients who fabricate pain symptoms in order to obtain controlled substances for recreational use or diversion. This chapter will focus on the problem of substance abuse and the perceptions of health-care providers regarding substance abuse as they relate to patients who present to the emergency department with complaints of pain.

The Prevalence of Pain

Pain is a near-universal human experience. Acute pain or an acute exacerbation of chronic pain commonly prompts emergency department visits. Acute pain can be defined in terms of duration: characteristically it is of recent onset and lasts no more than a few days to several weeks. It usually occurs in response to tissue injury and disappears when the injury heals. Acute pain serves an adaptive purpose in that it is associated with protective reflexes, such as withdrawal responses to remove a limb from danger, or muscle spasms that serve to immobilize an extremity; however, some responses associated with acute pain may be maladaptive, leading to impaired immune responses, elevated myocardial oxygen demands, hypercoagulation, and atelectasis.

Although less common in the emergency department (ED), chronic pain affects approximately one-third of the U.S. population annually (Portenoy et al., 2004). Domestic and international survey studies have reported chronic pain prevalence rates as high as 40% (Verhaak et al., 1998). Traditionally, chronic pain has been defined as pain lasting at least 3 months; however, it is better considered as pain lasting longer than the usual time period expected for tissue healing, however long this might be. Given our present understanding of pain-related pathology, chronic pain syndromes are often associated with low levels of identified pathology, particularly when only standard diagnostic techniques are employed; however, as we better understand the biological mechanisms underpinning chronic pain, or use more sophisticated diagnostic technologies (e.g., functional magnetic resonance imaging), this may change. Chronic pain serves no adaptive purpose. Recurrent pain is best considered a subset of chronic pain. Most patients with chronic pain experience recurrent, acute exacerbations of their pain syndrome (e.g., low back pain, most patients with sickle cell disease), whereas patients with migraine headaches or inflammatory bowel disease may experience few symptoms between painful episodes.

Of particular importance to the emergency physician's assessment of pain, and as one potential explanation for the phenomenon of oligoanalgesia, acute and chronic pain can be associated with markedly different pain-related behaviors. Although acute pain is usually associated with objective signs of sympathetic nervous system activation and overt signs of physical suffering, patients with chronic pain may not exhibit such typical behaviors and signs of autonomic nervous system overactivity. This disparity between observed patient behaviors and physician expectations of such behaviors in the setting of chronic pain may lead to inaccurate determinations of pain intensity and, ultimately, the undertreatment of pain.

Several studies have attempted to define the prevalence of pain in emergency department settings. Johnston et al. (1998) conducted a prospective study to determine the incidence and severity of pain among patients presenting to noncritical treatment areas within the emergency departments of two urban hospitals in Canada. Fifty-eight percent of adults and 47% of children reported pain on emergency department arrival. For approximately one-half of both groups reporting pain, the intensity of this pain was considered moderate to severe. At the time of discharge, one-third of both groups continued to experience pain of moderate to severe intensity. In fact, 11% of children and adults in this study actually reported clinically important increases in pain intensity during the emergency department stay.

A second prospective study, conducted by Tanabe and Buschmann (1999), found that among adults treated at one Chicago emergency department, fully 78% presented with a chief complaint related to pain. Of these patients, only 58% received analgesics or nonpharmacologic interventions to treat pain. For patients receiving analgesics, an average of 74 minutes elapsed from the time of arrival to the time of treatment. Only 15% of patients were treated with opioids, despite high levels of pain intensity. Interestingly, 16% of patients with pain in this study indicated that they would have refused analgesics had they been offered. The principal reported reason for their refusal was the fear of addiction resulting from opioid exposure, even when opioids were indicated for the treatment of pain.

In 2002, Cordell et al. (2002) reported an analysis of secondary data from an urban, tertiary care emergency department using explicit data abstraction rules to determine the prevalence of pain and to assign painful conditions into standard categories. With inclusion of all age groups, they found evidence of pain in 61% of patients. Pain was the chief complaint for 52% of patient visits. After excluding patients less than 5 years of age for whom chart reviews are obviously less reliable, almost 70% of patient encounters were determined to involve pain complaints.

Although the high prevalence of pain among emergency department patients is well documented, the underlying conditions responsible for pain in this population are less well characterized. In Cordell's retrospective study, 11% of patients presenting to the emergency department were judged to be suffering from pain that was chronic in nature. In a recent prospective multicenter study conducted in the United States and Canada, 44% of ultimately discharged patients presenting to the emergency department with pain reported underlying chronic pain syndromes (Todd et al., 2004). In one-half of these cases, the emergency department visit was prompted by an exacerbation of this chronic pain condition. Importantly, patients with chronic pain reported three to four times the number of annual physician visits when compared to those without chronic pain. Median and mean durations of symptoms for those reporting chronic pain syndromes were 24 and 52 months, respectively. For physicians who view themselves as experts in the management of acute medical and surgical emergencies, chronic pain may represent a less familiar condition with which to contend.

The Prevalence of Substance Abuse

In discussing issues of chemical dependency and aberrant behaviors related to opioid use, a valid system of nomenclature is necessary for clear communication and measurement. The term "substance abuse" is particularly problematic and resistant to precise definition. The American Psychiatric Association (1994) has defined substance abuse as a maladaptive pattern of drug use associated with some manifest harm to the user or others. Other groups using consensus methodology have defined abuse as any use considered to be outside of socially accepted norms (Rinaldi et al. 1988). Determining the bounds of "socially accepted norms" within the broad range of social strata treated within any emergency department is a difficult task. Emergency department physicians may believe that they "know abuse when they see it," and its identification may be influenced by subjective judgments that may, or may not, correspond to socially accepted norms for the index patient's particular social group. Often the term "substance misuse" is applied to behaviors that are not perceived as particularly extreme, for example, taking opioid analgesics to relieve symptoms other than pain such as anxiety or insomnia.

The difficulty in determining whether a given set of behaviors falls within accepted definitions of substance use, misuse, or abuse has important implications outside the clinical realm. Physicians may prescribe controlled substances for the treatment of pain, whereas patients may use these drugs to treat a broad range of symptoms with varying degrees of relatedness to underlying pain syndromes and may, in fact, use drugs in a manner totally unrelated to the physicians' intent, in other words, to obtain euphoric, rather than analgesic, effects. Given the unclear distinctions between use, misuse, and abuse, and a regulatory climate in which practitioners' prescribing patterns are increasingly scrutinized, emergency physicians are understandably reluctant to prescribe controlled substances to patients with whom they expect to have only a transitory relationship.

Using any definition, substance abuse is a highly prevalent problem. The National Survey on Drug Use and Health (formerly the National Household Survey on Drug Abuse) reports that in 2003, an estimated 19.5 million Americans, or 8.2% of the population aged 12 or older, used an illicit drug during the month prior to the survey interview. Illicit drugs included marijuana, cocaine, heroin, hallucinogens, inhalants, and nonmedical use of prescription-type pain relievers, tranquilizers, stimulants, and sedatives (Substance Abuse and Mental Health Services Administration, 2004). Importantly, the survey documents an increase in the lifetime reported nonmedical use of pain relievers between 2002 and 2003, from 29.6 million to 31.2 million persons. To be considered "nonmedical" use, the respondent had to take drugs not prescribed for them or take them only for the "experience or feeling" they caused. Specific analgesics showing statistically significant increases in lifetime use were (in order by magnitude): Vicodin, Lortab, or Lorcet; Percocet, Percodan, or Tylox; hydrocodone; OxyContin; methadone; and Tramadol.

In contrast to the prominence of emergency department-based data collection systems that monitor deleterious outcomes associated with substance abuse, relatively few studies have systematically assessed substance abuse prevalence and treatment needs in the emergency department population. As an example, the Drug Abuse Warning Network (DAWN) is a federally financed, public health surveillance system that monitors drug-related emergency department visits and drug-related deaths investigated by medical examiners and coroners. This reporting system involves hundreds of hospital emergency departments throughout the United States and provides valuable data with which to monitor drug abuse trends. In contrast to this large monitoring research enterprise, relatively little focus has been given to use of the emergency department as a setting in which to intervene in substance abuse problems.

In 1997, Soderstrom et al. assessed the prevalence of psychoactive substance use disorders in a large, unselected group of seriously injured patients treated at a Level I trauma center in Baltimore, using standardized diagnostic interviews and explicit criteria. Psychoactive substance use disorders were diagnosed using the Structured Clinical Interview (SCID), an instrument based on the *Diagnostic and Statistical Manual of Mental Disorders, Revised Third Edition (DSM-IIIR;* Spitzer et al., 1990). Of 1,118 patients consenting to the study, more than half had one or more lifetime abuse or dependence psychoactive substance use disorders, and 18% were currently considered dependent on drugs other than alcohol.

In 1996 and 1997, Rockett et al. used direct interviews to ascertain unmet substance abuse treatment needs in a statewide probability sample survey of adults presenting to seven Tennessee emergency departments (Rockett et al., 2003). Although only 1% of emergency department medical records indicated a diagnosis of alcohol- or drug-related problems, as many as 27% of patients were determined by the researchers to need substance abuse treatment on the basis of explicitly defined case definitions. Less than 10% of patients who were ultimately determined to need substance abuse treatment in this study were actually receiving such care. Thirty-two percent of all patients in this study had a positive saliva or urine assay for psychoactive drugs, and 9% screened positive for opioid use. Unmet substance abuse treatment needs varied directly with the frequency of emergency department visits and inversely with patient age.

A subsequent study by Rockett et al. (2005) examined the association between unmet substance abuse treatment needs in the emergency department and excess utilization of health services in order to estimate the health-care cost savings that might result from effective emergency department–based substance abuse treatment interventions. The researchers estimated that patients with unmet substance abuse treatment needs accounted for an estimated $777 million in extra hospital charges for Tennessee, or $1,568 per emergency department patient when compared to those without substance abuse treatment needs. They suggested that the costs of emergency department–based screening and intervention efforts targeted to substance abuse disorders would be more than offset by savings from decreased health-care utilization and that these programs were likely to be highly cost-effective if implemented.

The Problem of "Drug-Seeking Behavior"

The preceding review makes clear the high prevalence of both pain and substance abuse disorders in the emergency department. Although acute and chronic pain is far more common than substance abuse disorders, it is inevitable that emergency physicians will frequently encounter patients presenting with both pain and substance abuse disorders. Professional discussions of pain treatment in the emergency department frequently center on concerns of being duped by such patients who fabricate painful symptoms in order to obtain opioids, so-called "drug-seeking behavior" (Hansen, 2005). "Drug-seeking behaviors" may represent an entirely appropriate response by those with chronic pain who are routinely undertreated by the medical profession and for whom comprehensive pain treatment centers are in short supply. Although the term "drug seeking behavior" is poorly defined, it is used in the emergency medicine literature and will be used in this chapter with acknowledgment of its imprecision.

Only a limited amount of emergency medicine research has addressed this problematic issue. In 1990, Zechnich and Hedges (1996) attempted to measure community-wide use of emergency department services by patients at high risk for drug-seeking behavior. In this retrospective, observational study, patients were categorized as exhibiting drug-seeking behavior if they sought care at a university hospital in Portland, Oregon, for a specific pain-related diagnosis (i.e., ureteral colic, toothache, back pain, abdominal pain, or headache) and were either independently identified on at least one other local hospital's "patient alert" list or suffered a drug-related death during the year in question. After identifying 33 such patients, they determined the frequency of their emergency department visits at each of seven local hospitals and conducted detailed chart reviews of their visits at three of these hospitals. The patients identified as drug seeking were generally young, and one-half of drug seekers were female. The latter is a surprising finding, given that substance abuse disorders are more than twice as common among males (Substance Abuse and Mental Health Services Administration. 2004). This suggests that drug-seeking behaviors are exhibited (or identified) more commonly among female emergency department patients with substance abuse problems than among males. The 33 patients visited emergency departments, urgent care clinics, or were hospitalized a total of 379 times over the study period, for an average of 12.6 visits per person annually. Interestingly, although chart reviews identified 17 patients who were told that he or she "would receive no further narcotics" at a given facility, these patients subsequently received controlled substances from another hospital in 93% of cases and from even the same facility in 71%. The authors suggested that information sharing between hospitals could help to identify drug-seeking patients and promote more consistent community-wide care and appropriate substance abuse interventions.

The maintenance of lists that include the names and medical information for patients frequently seen in the emergency department is thought to be a common practice. In a mail survey conducted in 1995, Graber et al. described the use of what were referred to as "problem patient files" in the state of Iowa. Fifty-eight percent of emergency department medical directors acknowledged the use of such files and responded that the files were consulted an average of 2.6 times per week. Calls between emergency departments either seeking or responding to requests for information about patients listed in these files were estimated to occur 23 and 20 times per year, respectively. Rarely were explicit policies established for limiting access to these files, and information was added to the records in an informal fashion (Graber et al., 1995).

In 2000, Pope et al. (2000) in Vancouver described a case management program for frequent visitors to their inner-city tertiary care emergency department serving a large number of patients with multiple psychosocial problems, including homelessness and substance abuse. Of 24 patients described in this study, 5 were said to exhibit drug-seeking behavior, and 8 patients suffered from alcohol and drug abuse, personality disorders, and chronic pain. These 24 patients accounted for a staggering 616 visits annually (median 26.5 visits per year). After the implementation of individualized chronic care plans that included social work interventions at the time of the visits, emergency department use by this group of superutilizers dropped to a median of 6.5 visits per person per year.

In 2003, a publication by Geiderman discussed ethical, legal, and regulatory considerations surrounding the use of what were termed "habitual patient files." The article acknowledged the common and informal use of such files, and set forth standards intended to promote the development of formal policies and procedures to govern their use. The author noted that such files have never been demonstrated to be effective in either reducing emergency department use by drug-seeking patients or in altering care patterns and suggested the need for a research program to explore the impact of their use. Finally, the author called for a coordinated and comprehensive program of physician education to promote the identification and treatment of emergency department patients with substance abuse disorders.

Pain and Substance Abuse: A Balanced Perspective

In managing pain, emergency physicians are responsible for beneficence as well as nonmaleficence. We must treat pain and ameliorate suffering while minimizing the extent to which our treatment strategies enable substance abuse by our patients. For the vast majority of patients presenting with acute monophasic pain, whether from trauma, acute medical illness, or procedures performed in the emergency department, there is little danger of enabling substance abuse and a great deal of room for improvement in the quality of analgesic practices. Multiple published studies have documented the continued prevalence of oligoanalgesia among children and adults treated in our emergency departments (Fosnocht et al., 2001; Lewis et al., 1994; Petrack et al., 1997; Selbst & Clark, 1990; Singer & Konia, 1999). For a small subset of emergency department patients, particularly for those presenting with chronic or recurrent pain syndromes, the physician may have legitimate concerns regarding an underlying substance abuse or related disorder. Our task is to balance the often unclear risk of fostering substance abuse, and even diversion, in this subset of patients with the well-known and well-documented risk of undertreating painful conditions.

To the extent we can clarify the nomenclature used to classify patients with pain and substance use disorders, we can begin to identify more effective approaches to both problems. To aid in this effort, we will attempt to clarify various phenomena that have been lumped within the term "drug-seeking behavior."

To begin, it must be said that "drug-seeking behavior" is a term best abandoned by our profession. For the patient in pain, seeking an analgesic of proven effectiveness is the height of rationality. In contrast to the search for controlled substances, it is likely that the most common variety of drug-seeking behavior is the well-documented and relentless quest by patients with self-limited viral upper respiratory infections (or parents of such patients) to obtain antibiotics. The medical profession has a long history of inappropriately prescribing such antibiotics, encouraging antibiotic resistance among common bacterial strains while risking antibiotic side effects without a justifiable expectation of concomitant benefit.

The concern of physicians is that patients may seek controlled substances, particularly opioids and benzodiazepines, for reasons other than those strictly related to pain relief. Such actions are best termed "aberrant drug-related behaviors" as this term suggests that there is a broad range of behaviors that are more acceptable or less acceptable in the context of pain therapy. Although addiction is the most commonly assumed explanation for such aberrant behaviors, there is an extended differential diagnosis for such behaviors that the clinician should consider.

Although confirmatory research is lacking, expert consensus suggests that aberrant drug-related behaviors reflect a broad range of observed activities that are either more, or less, suggestive of an addiction disorder (see Box 37.1). Certainly, the presence of an obvious painful condition (e.g., appendicitis, fracture) should preempt concerns about illegitimate drug-seeking behaviors. At the other extreme, even behaviors that are clearly unacceptable do not necessarily indicate addiction or diversion. Hay and Passik have even reported one case of prescription forgery that was seemingly unrelated to addiction or criminal intent. The forgery occurred when the patient's caregiver was leaving for vacation, prompting excess anxiety and fear of abandonment in this patient with borderline personality disorder (Hay & Passik, 2000). Addiction is but one of many diagnoses that may lead to aberrant drug-related behaviors (see Box 37.2).

Given the high prevalence of chronic pain and the widespread unavailability of chronic pain management resources, particularly for populations served by the emergency department, pseudoaddiction is the most likely cause for a large proportion of drug-related behaviors deemed aberrant. In particular, patient reports of distress associated with unrelieved symptoms, aggressive complaining about the need for higher doses of analgesics, and unilateral dose escalation by the patient are suggestive of pseudoaddiction. Establishing the diagnosis of pseudoaddiction is particularly difficult if the patient has both pain and a comorbid substance use

---

Box 37.1 Spectrum of Aberrant Drug-Related Behaviors That Raise Concern About the Potential for Addiction

Less suggestive of addiction:
- Aggressive complaining about the need for more drug
- Drug hoarding during periods of reduced symptoms
- Requesting specific drugs
- Openly acquiring similar drugs from other medical sources
- Occasional unsanctioned dose escalation or other noncompliance
- Unapproved use of the drug to treat another symptom
- Reporting psychic effects not intended by the clinician
- Resistance to a change in therapy associated with "tolerable" adverse effects with expressions of anxiety related to the return of severe symptoms

More suggestive of addiction:
- Selling prescription drugs
- Prescription forgery
- Stealing or "borrowing" drugs from others
- Injecting oral formulations
- Obtaining prescription drugs from nonmedical sources
- Concurrent abuse of alcohol or illicit drugs
- Repeated dose escalation or similar noncompliance despite multiple warnings
- Repeated visits to other clinicians or emergency rooms without informing prescriber
- Drug-related deterioration in function at work, in the family, or socially
- Repeated resistance to changes in therapy despite evidence of adverse drug effects

From C. L. Shalmi, "Opioids for nonmalignant pain: issues and controversy," in C. A. Warfield, Z. H. Bajwa, eds., *Principles and Practice of Pain Medicine* (2nd ed.). Columbus, OH: The McGraw-Hill Companies Inc., 2004; 607.

Box 37.2 Differential Diagnosis Considerations for Assessing Aberrant Drug-Related Behaviors

Addiction: Out-of-control behavior; compulsive, harmful drug use.
Pseudoaddiction: Undertreated pain leads to desperate acting out; patients may turn to alcohol, street drugs, or doctor-shopping; these behaviors subside once pain is adequately treated.
Organic mental syndrome: Patients often confused and have stereotyped drug-taking behavior.
Personality disorder: Patients impulsive, have sense of entitlement, and may engage in chemical-coping behaviors.
Chemical coping: Patients place excessive emphasis on meaning of their medications and are overly drug focused.
Depression, anxiety, and situational stressors: Patients marked by desire to self-medicate their mood disorder or current life stress.
Criminal intent: Subset of criminal's intent of diverting medications for profit.

From S. D. Passik, K. L. Kirsh, "Addiction in pain management," in B. McCarberg, S. D. Passik, eds., *Expert Guide to Pain Management*. Philadelphia: American College of Physicians, 2005; 293.

disorder; however, the two can obviously coexist. The signature of pseudoaddiction is that aberrant behaviors disappear when adequate analgesics are given to control pain.

The condition that best exemplifies the problem of emergency department-based pseudoaddiction is sickle cell disease. Vasoocclusive pain crises are the most common reason for emergency department visits by patients with sickle cell disease, and the genetics, molecular biology, and pathophysiology of this disease are relatively well understood. Although the management of sickle cell vasoocclusive pain crises is viewed as challenging by emergency physicians, it has been a relatively neglected area of research investigation by the specialty (Linklater et al., 2005). Despite the fact that almost all of the 75,000 annual hospitalizations for pain crises occur after emergency department treatment, the *Annals of Emergency Medicine,* emergency medicine's premier research journal, has published no clinical research on sickle cell pain management within the past 10 years.

Despite our understanding of the sickle cell disease process, many health professionals, largely due to addiction concerns, are reluctant to prescribe adequate doses of opioids for these patients experiencing pain (Yale et al., 2000). In one survey study, 53% of emergency physicians were of the belief that more than 20% of patients with sickle cell disease were addicted to opioids, whereas only 23% of hematologists shared this belief (Shapiro et al., 1997). Also, in this survey, 35% of hematologists reported that they followed pain management protocols when treating painful crises as compared to only 17% of emergency physicians.

Nurses' attitudes regarding the prevalence of addiction among this patient population are even more extreme, with 63% of respondents reporting that addiction was prevalent (Pack-Mabien et al., 2001). Thirty percent of nurses in this survey reported that they were hesitant to administer high-dose opioids for painful vasoocclusive crises. A hesitant approach to emergency department opioid administration in the setting of vasoocclusive pain crises will predictably lead to continued pain, increased anticipation of pain, and increased patient anxiety. This experience may generate pain-avoidance manifestations by patients that are interpreted by physicians as aberrant drug-related behaviors. Eventually, larger doses of opioids may be administered to control pain that is spiraling out of control with resultant excessive sedation. This apparent sedation in the setting of a painful condition may reinforce the physician's disbelief in the reality of his or her patient's initial pain reports.

It has been demonstrated that this cycle of inadequate care can be broken by the institution of pain management protocols that emphasize continuous opioid infusions and sustained courses of orally administered controlled-release opioids. In 1992, Brookoff and Polomano reported the institution of such a structured analgesic regimen on hospital use by patients with sickle cell disease presenting to the emergency department of an inner-city university hospital in Philadelphia with remarkable results. After institution of the pain management protocol, the number of hospital admissions for sickle cell pain decreased by 44%, the number of total inpatient days by 57%, the hospital length of stay by 23%, and the number of emergency department visits by 67%.

The authors asserted that these positive results were seen without a subset of patients being "chased away" from the hospital. Others have reported marked decreases in aberrant drug-related behaviors and the number of emergency department visits by patients with sickle cell disease after instituting long-term management of pain with chronic opioid therapies typically used to treat malignant pain (Shaiova & Wallenstein, 2004).

Aside from considerations of pseudoaddiction, chronic pain is often accompanied by mood disorders and psychiatric comorbidities that complicate the management of these challenging patients (Gureje et al., 1998). The presence of aberrant drug-related behaviors in patients with borderline personality disorders may represent an expression of fear and anger or an attempt to cope with chronic boredom. Patients may use opioids and alcohol in attempts to lessen symptoms of anxiety, panic disorder, depression, or insomnia. Emergency physicians often receive limited training in dealing with such disorders and the specialty's deficiencies in dealing with such problems have been documented (Tse et al., 1999). Psychiatric consultation, if available, may be useful in both suggesting alternative causes for aberrant behaviors and tailoring the physician's therapeutic approach to deal with these complicating factors.

For some patients, aberrant drug-related behaviors represent criminal intent to divert or sell controlled substances. The prevalence of behaviors occasioned by such intent is unknown and it is likely that in many cases, multiple etiologies of aberrant behaviors coexist. Certainly, patients with active or past substance use disorders are at increased risk for injuries and illnesses that can lead to chronic pain (e.g., motor vehicle injury). Thus, the conditions listed in Box 37.2 are not mutually exclusive.

Barriers to Improvement

Barriers to the treatment of pain are discussed by other authors in this volume. There is also a paucity of treatment guidelines and best practice standards for emergency department pain care, in part because of the lack of research in this area by emergency medicine investigators. Although the American College of Emergency Physicians has adopted a statement of general principles regarding pain management (see Box 37.3), the specialty lacks clearly articulated standards to drive pain care and health-care systems do not include adequate mechanisms to ensure accountability for inferior practice (ACEP Board of Directors, 2004).

Given the concentration of patients with substance abuse disorders, the emergency department is an appropriate site for screening and intervention for both alcohol and drug problems; however, emergency physicians receive limited training in recognition and appropriate interventions for such problems, and an air

---

Box 37.3. ACEP Policy Statement, Pain Management in the Emergency Department

The majority of emergency department (ED) patients require treatment for painful medical conditions or injuries. The American College of Emergency Physicians recognizes the importance of effectively managing ED patients who are experiencing pain and supports the following principles.

1. ED patients should receive expeditious pain management, avoiding delays such as those related to diagnostic testing or consultation.
2. Hospitals should develop unique strategies that will optimize ED patient pain management using both narcotic and nonnarcotic medications.
3. ED policies and procedures should support the safe utilization and prescription writing of pain medications in the ED.
4. Effective physician and patient educational strategies should be developed regarding pain management, including the use of pain therapy adjuncts and how to minimize pain after disposition from the ED.
5. Ongoing research in the area of ED patient pain management should be conducted.

of pessimism characterizes physicians' estimation of success for many substance abuse therapies. Translating our knowledge of therapeutic strategies into action against these disorders will require overcoming much clinical inertia.

Although federal regulators and state medical boards do not perceive emergency medicine as a specialty prone to inappropriate prescribing, and investigations of emergency physicians are rare, if not unheard of, many emergency physicians express fears of such scrutiny or sanctions related to prescribing or administering opioids. Although this concern is often voiced, it seems likely that this fear represents concern about other, less obvious physician uncertainties related to pain management and substance abuse disorders. Emergency physicians may be concerned about being overburdened by the inherent difficulties of managing patients with complicated pain syndromes and coexisting substance abuse disorders.

In dealing with complex chronic pain patients, the emergency physician practicing in isolation may exhibit symptoms of despair and direct his or her anger toward the patient with pain, resulting in more alienation of patients who may have already been abandoned by other sectors of the health-care system. This is particularly likely to happen in communities without multidisciplinary treatment centers for either substance abuse disorders or chronic pain and for those with inadequate health-care insurance. Thus the patient with chronic pain joins the larger group of those with unmet health-care needs that currently crowd our emergency departments. The hectic nature of emergency medicine practice often does not allow sufficient time for precisely characterizing patients with complex pain complaints, and clinicians may lump legitimate pain behaviors with the ploys of those seeking opioids inappropriately. Both groups of patients may be ultimately mistrusted and treated with disdain.

Finally, the true prevalence of addiction and aberrant drug-related behaviors is unknown and unstudied. There is little research on risk factors for prescription drug abuse to guide the emergency physician. When the prevalence of such problems is overestimated, oligoanalgesia is the predictable result.

Conclusion

Relieving pain and reducing suffering are primary responsibilities of emergency medicine, and much can be done to improve the care of patients in pain. We have a concurrent duty to limit the personal and societal harm that can result from prescription drug abuse. Our specialty should continue to refine our approach to the problem of pain and substance abuse and reduce the current large amount of variability in our practices. We should continue to more precisely define our own standards for excellence in pain practice and substance abuse interventions while promoting quality improvement initiatives to achieve these goals.

References

ACEP Board of Directors. Policy statement: pain management in the emergency department. *Annals of Emergency Medicine*. 2004;44:198.

American Psychiatric Association. *Diagnostic and Statistical Manual for Mental Disorders—IV*. Washington, DC: American Psychiatric Association, 1994.

Brookoff D, Polomano R. Treating sickle cell pain like cancer pain. *Annals of Internal Medicine*. 1992;116(5):364–8.

Cordell WH, Keene KK, Giles BK, Jones JB, Jones JH, Brizendine EJ. The high prevalence of pain in emergency medical care. *American Journal of Emergency Medicine*. 2002;20(3):165–9.

Fosnocht DE, Swanson ER, Bossart P. Patient expectations for pain medication delivery. *Am J Emerg Med*. 2001;19(5):399–402.

Geiderman JM. Keeping lists and naming names: habitual patient files for suspected nontherapeutic drug-seeking patients. *Annals of Emergency Medicine*. 2003;41(6):873–81.

Graber MA, Gjerde C, Bergus G, Ely J. The use of unofficial "problem patient" files and interinstitutional information transfer in emergency medicine in Iowa. *American Journal of Emergency Medicine*. 1995;13(5):509–11.

Gureje O, Von Korff M, Simon GE, Gater R. Persistent pain and well-being: a World Health Organization study in primary care [Erratum appears in *JAMA* 1998 Oct 7;280(13):1142]. *JAMA*. 1998;280(2):147–51.

Hansen GR. The drug-seeking patient in the emergency room. *Emergency Medicine Clinics of North America*. 2005;23(2):349–65.

Hay JL, Passik SD. The cancer patient with borderline personality disorder: suggestions for symptom-focused management in the medical setting. *Psycho Oncology*. 2000;9(2):91–100.

Johnston CC, Gagnon AJ, Fullerton L, Common C, Ladores M, Forlini S. One-week survey of pain intensity on admission to and discharge from the emergency department: a pilot study. *J Emerg Med*. 1998;16(3):377–82.

Lewis LM, Lasater LC, Brooks CB. Are emergency physicians too stingy with analgesics? *Southern Medical Journal*. 1994;87(1):7–9.

Linklater DR, Pemberton L, Taylor S, Zeger W. Painful dilemmas: an evidence-based look at challenging clinical scenarios. *Emergency Medicine Clinics of North America*. 2005;23(2):367–92.

Pack-Mabien A, Labbe E, Herbert D, Haynes J Jr. Nurses' attitudes and practices in sickle cell pain management. *Applied Nursing Research*. 2001;14(4):187–92.

Petrack EM, Christopher NC, Kriwinsky J. Pain management in the emergency department: patterns of analgesic utilization. *Pediatrics*. 1997;99(5):711–4.

Pope D, Fernandes CM, Bouthillette F, Etherington J. Frequent users of the emergency department: a program to improve care and reduce visits. *CMAJ Canadian Medical Association Journal*. 2000;162(7):1017–20.

Portenoy RK, Ugarte C, Fuller I, Haas G. Population-based survey of pain in the United States: differences among white, African American, and Hispanic subjects. *Journal of Pain*. 2004;5(6):317–28.

Rinaldi RC, Steindler EM, Wilford BB, Goodwin D. Clarification and standardization of substance abuse terminology. *JAMA*. 1988;259:555–557.

Rockett IR, Putnam SL, Jia H, Chang CF, Smith GS. Unmet substance abuse treatment need, health services utilization, and cost: a population-based emergency department study. *Annals of Emergency Medicine*. 2005;45(2):118–27.

Rockett IR, Putnam SL, Jia H, Smith GS. Assessing substance abuse treatment need: a statewide hospital emergency department study. *Annals of Emergency Medicine*. 2003;41(6):802–13.

Rupp T, Delaney KA. Inadequate analgesia in emergency medicine. *Annals of Emergency Medicine*. 2004;43(4):494–503.

Selbst SM, Clark M. Analgesic use in the emergency department. *Ann Emerg Med*. 1990;19(9):1010–3.

Shaiova L, Wallenstein D. Outpatient management of sickle cell pain with chronic opioid pharmacotherapy. *Journal of the National Medical Association*. 2004;96(7):984–6.

Shapiro BS, Benjamin LJ, Payne R, Heidrich G. Sickle cell-related pain: perceptions of medical practitioners. *Journal of Pain & Symptom Management*. 1997;14(3):168–74.

Singer AJ, Konia N. Comparison of topical anesthetics and vasoconstrictors vs. lubricants prior to nasogastric intubation: a randomized, controlled trial. *Academic Emergency Medicine*. 1999;6(3):184–90.

Soderstrom CA, Smith GS, Dischinger PC, et al. Psychoactive substance use disorders among seriously injured trauma center patients. *JAMA*. 1997;277(22):1769–74.

Spitzer RL, Williams JBW, Gibbon M, First MB. *Structured Clinical Interview for DSM-III-R, Patient Edition/Non-patient Edition* (SCID-P/SCID-NP). Washington, DC: American Psychiatric Press, Inc., 1990.

Substance Abuse and Mental Health Services Administration. *Overview of Findings from the 2003 National Survey on Drug Use and Health* (Office of Applied Studies, NSDUH Series H-24, DHHS Publication No. SMA 04-3963, Rockville, MD, 2004).

Tanabe P, Buschmann M. A prospective study of ED pain management practices and the patient's perspective. *Journal of Emergency Nursing.* 1999;25(3):171–7.

Todd KH, Ducharme J, Choiniere M, Johnston C, Crandall C, Puntillo K. Pain and pain-related functional interference among discharged emergency department patients. [abstract]. *Annals of Emergency Medicine.* 2004;44:S86.

Tse SK, Wong TW, Lau CC, Yeung WS, Tang WN. How good are accident and emergency doctors in the evaluation of psychiatric patients? *European Journal of Emergency Medicine.* 1999;6(4):297–300.

Verhaak PF, Kerssens JJ, Dekker J, Sorbi MJ, Bensing JM. Prevalence of chronic benign pain disorder among adults: a review of the literature. *Pain.* 1998;77:231–239.

Yale SH, Nagib N, Guthrie T. Approach to the vaso-occlusive crisis in adults with sickle cell disease. *American Family Physician.* 2000;61(5):1349–56, 1363–4.

Zechnich AD, Hedges JR. Community-wide emergency department visits by patients suspected of drug-seeking behavior. *Academic Emergency Medicine.* 1996;3(4):312–7.

38

Management of Pain in Chemical Dependency in the Primary Care Clinic

Bill H. McCarberg

The management of pain in primary care is a difficult and complex endeavor. Persistent pain management remains an elusive and frustrating goal despite a growing knowledge about the pathophysiology of pain. Primary care physicians struggle with unexplained variability among pain patients. Physical abnormalities are not predictive of pain severity or dysfunction (Flor & Turk, 1988). Large numbers of patients experience pain that may be constant, over long periods of time, and yet their life functioning is not changed in major ways. Conversely, there are other patients with similar structural abnormalities who suffer substantially more and cannot maintain their usual levels of activity (Sanders et al., 1992).

Patients whose lives are significantly disrupted by pain engage in behaviors that are maladaptive, anticipate more distress, amplify sensations associated with pain, spend more time resting, and complain of less ability to control pain (Pinsky, 1993; Reesor & Craig, 1988).

Protocols and guidelines have been established for acute and cancer pain through groups such as the Agency for Health Care Policy and Research and the World Health Organization (Jacox et al., 1992). Yet persistent noncancer pain sufferers lack specific treatment plans. Providers attempt to alleviate pain, often without success. Patients, desperate for pain relief, frequent doctors' offices and are seen as demanding, noncompliant, drug seeking, and difficult. The provider and the patient are found in conflict with each other; however, both doctor and patient want the same outcome: pain control and return to function.

Pain is vastly underrecognized and undertreated. Patients with postoperative pain, end-of-life cancer pain, and HIV-related pain have all been well chronicled as undertreated but represent just a small number compared to the persistent noncancer pain patients. Fewer than half (43%) of Americans with moderate or severe pain feel that they "have a great deal of control" over their pain and 28% "don't believe that there is any real solution" for their pain (Brownlee & Schrof, 1997). Arthritis, low back pain, headache, myofascial pain, fibromyalgia syndrome, chronic pain pelvic, and irritable bowel syndrome are just a few in a list spotlighting this crisis in health care.

The legal community has insinuated itself into our practices with lawsuits for undertreated pain. The Joint Commission on Accreditation of Healthcare Organizations mandated pain criteria for accreditation, and Congress declared this decade (2001–2010) the Decade of Pain Control and Research.

Patients frequently seek care from specialists for their pain: physiatrists for musculoskeletal pain, neurologists for neuropathic pain, oncologists for cancer pain, and an ever-increasing number of other pain care specialists. Despite the plethora of professionals caring for pain problems and the development of specialists in pain management, most patients continue to rely on their primary care clinicians for pain control. And when pain treatment from a specialist fails and the pain becomes part of daily living, patients return to primary care, where they have developed relationships built on trust, experience, and care for their entire family. Most chronic illnesses including chronic pain are managed in primary care (Table 38.1).

It is easy to make an argument that persistent noncancer pain with the complication of substance abuse is so complex that only pain specialists should endeavor to treat these patients. Specialists provide most cancer treatment because the protocols are complex and ever changing. Similarly, it is difficult to keep up with the vast and ever-changing treatments for persistent pain. In the United States, there appears to exist a mismatch of large numbers of patients with persistent noncancer pain (perhaps somewhere between 50 to 80 million) versus pain specialists (perhaps somewhere between 2 to 9 thousand). (As of early 2006, about 2,002 pain specialists have been issued certificates for passing the American

Table 38.1. Chronic Diseases

Condition	Primary Care	Others
Arteriosclerotic cardiovascular disease (ASCVD)	86%	14%
Stroke	91%	9%
Hypertension	92%	8%
Diabetes	90%	10%
Chronic obstructive pulmonary disease (COPD)	89%	11%
Asthma	94%	6%

Data based on 1996 Medical Expenditure Panel Surveys. Annals of Family Medicine, Vol. 2, Suppl. 1, March/April 2004.

Academy of Pain Medicine examination, and the American Board of Anesthesiologists issued about 3, 298 Pain Medicine Certificates.) The immense numbers of patients with persistent pain and the relative lack of specialists, especially in rural areas, make this a primary care problem. In addition, persistent pain is more likely to occur in the chemical-dependent patients because behaviors and lifestyle issues often result in significant injuries and accidents (Heinermann et al., 1988; Honkanen et al., 1983; Reyna et al., 1985; Savage, 2002).

Most persistent noncancer pain starts with an acutely painful event. After appropriate workup and treatment, most of this pain resolves. Even chronic low back pain, which is the most prevalent persistent pain condition, starts with an acute episode and resolves 90% of the time. When specialty referral is initiated and the maximal treatment completed, unresolved pain must be managed. The acute painful event almost always starts at the primary care level, and the chronic unresolved pain returns to primary care.

Texas passed the first Intractable Pain Act in 1989. The Federation of State Medical Boards established model pain guidelines in 1998 in an effort to help physicians practice better pain care. These state medical board guidelines emphasize the importance of opioid therapy for persistent noncancer pain. With improved knowledge from a variety of studies, opioid prescribing has increased dramatically in the last 10 years (Joranson et al., 2000). With legitimate prescribing has also come a tremendous increase in illegitimate use (SAMHSA, 2002a, 2002b, 2004). Addicts with persistent pain may be taking the analgesic drug to treat the addiction. Diversion, which fuels street use and is a growing problem in the adolescent population, is a major concern with the regulatory agencies.

The problem of prescribing opioids to alleviate pain as encouraged by the experts and medical boards has led to an increasing problem of understanding pain treatment in the context of a patient with an addiction history. Just as persistent noncancer pain management resides in primary care, patients with a history of chemical dependency are followed in this same setting.

Primary Care

To understand why pain and chemical dependency is such an issue in primary care, one must also understand what makes the primary care practice unique in the medical environment. Reports of doctors placing signs in their waiting rooms saying "We do not give narcotics here" stem from a variety of practice issues. To improve the crisis of undermanaged pain, we have to address the primary care uniqueness and develop strategies to make pain care automatic, with simple evidence-based choices that fit into our practice style.

It is difficult to generalize about primary care because every practice is different. Patient demographics, panel size, reimbursement rates, practice location, insurance, and midlevel extenders all play roles in making every practice distinct. Some family physicians have developed special interest in persistent pain management and show great skill in managing complex, complicated patients with persistent pain. Despite varying practices, some generalizations can be made for most primary care providers.

1. Time is a precious commodity. There is rarely enough time to completely evaluate any medical condition. Practitioners feel conflicted about following the best, evidence-based standard of care as opposed to simple complaint management in order to get to the next patient. We all would like more time but do not have this luxury. We are constantly making compromises in care because of time. Is the blood pressure of 210/110 more important than the patient's pain complaint? It is not likely that both issues will be addressed thoroughly at an office visit. Returning a patient for follow up is an obvious option, but return visits are limited as well.

2. Long delays in seeing providers often result in patients presenting with lists of medical concerns, each of which must be dealt with during the short office visit. Diabetes, hypertension, and hyperlipidemia would be common chronic problems seen during a visit, not to mention the chronic back pain, insomnia, the spouse who is drinking too much, and the mole that needs evaluation and removal. Once again, this is an issue of time pressure. With an hour visit, each problem could be dealt with, including immunizations and health screening. Because of time, the back pain will not likely be addressed adequately. If a simple solution, such as an opioid, can be given, that option may be chosen. Chemical dependency issues, opioid agreements, and acceptable behavior related to refills will likely not be discussed because of lack of time. The primary care provider may lack sufficient knowledge, but time constraints play a bigger role.

3. In primary care, patient advocacy is preached. Helping patients through the difficult process of sorting out modern medical care depends on someone skillful in the system. This advocacy relies on developing relationships with patients over periods of many years and multiple office visits.

When nothing is helping a patient who suffers in pain, primary care can make the referral process easier, interpret the findings from the specialist, have family meetings to help acceptance and prioritize treatment options. Years of dealing with minor medical problems leads to comfort and trust in the primary provider. Despite having only rudimentary knowledgeable of the specialty-based complex medical problem, patients will seek advice and reassurance from the familiar provider. Trust and respect are the backbone of these interactions. Because this advocacy role is so imbedded in the patient-provider relationship, setting limits can be difficult.

Pain management in a population that has a history of addiction and experimentation places the provider in an unfamiliar and uncomfortable adversarial role. Setting limits on medications, refusing refills, and denying disability claims or requests for handicapped parking abrogates the trust and respect relationship.

Conflict is not uncommon is a primary care office. Patients frequently are resistant to suggestions about weight loss, exercise, smoking cessation, psychosocial referrals, and antidepressant medications. However, this conflict is aimed at the best interest of the patient. Advocacy becomes more difficult when patients demand medications or feel it is their right to be disabled. This uncomfortable conflict leads to an adversarial relationship interfering with patient care. When the next request for a refill of an opioid arrives early again, a busy provider may just refill the prescription rather than discussing the refill with the patient.

Utilizing upfront, clearly defined refill requirements, behavioral goals, and experience with an addiction population, the specialist can more easily control behavior. Specialists often have limited, short-term exposure to patients and not the longitudinal experience of primary care. Even with proper training, limit setting is an uncomfortable conduct for primary care.

4. Tracking patient behavior is a common practice in primary care. We will follow weights, blood pressure, immunization status, hemoglobin A_1C, and mammogram frequency, among many other health-enhancing behaviors. Elaborate methods have been devel-

oped to track these parameters that will become even more automatic with the electronic medical record.

Tracking drug use, however, is often more difficult and not a standardized procedure in most practices. When a patient calls in early for an opioid, alarms are activated; yet we rarely track other drugs. If a patient calls in early for digoxin or insulin, we would not be alerted. Tracking opioid usage is therefore very distinct, and systems are often not in place.

If a patient calls in 5 days early, this may be seen as compliant conduct allowing time for charts to be pulled, agreements to be reviewed, and refills to be initiated. If the patient actually refills the medication 5 days early, then there is the possibility of excess medication being consumed. Are the words "Do not fill until" written on the prescription to ensure appropriate dosing? Only with abusable substances (e.g., opioids, barbiturates, benzodiazepines) is this prescriber behavior warranted yet not practiced by primary care.

Pain specialists who frequently deal with this simple refill procedure will have methods developed, often involving the nursing staff and pharmacists to ensure correct refill intervals. In primary care, in which opioid tracking is not automatic, prescription refills presents a logistical problem without simple solutions.

Cross-coverage for opioid refills also is an issue because differing philosophies about need for medication may exist in a primary care practice. In smaller specialty clinics, coverage is rarely a problem.

5. Primary care deals with many chronic problems. Persistent pain is a chronic problem unlike any other disease process: The diagnosis is uncertain, and the patient's pain behavior often seems out of proportion to known pathology. Guidelines for treatment are lacking. Psychosocial factors appear to play more of a role in complaints than other diseases, and are not adequately addressed when referred for specialty care.

Most primary care providers understand what constitutes advancement to appropriate goals in congestive heart failure, diabetes, and hypertension. When a patient is not improving, we know what steps to take to help patients. On the other hand, what is the goal in persistent pain management? If patients are not making functional and pain-reduction targets, what can we do? Even the referral to experts results in diagnostic uncertainty, differing treatment strategies that add to the confusion.

Given this difficult, complex disease process and unaddressed psychosocial issues, adding a hazardous drug as an opioid may appear to be highly risky. In addition to this, add a history of chemical dependency and most primary care providers feel far beyond their expertise. When behavior around the opioid begins to appear, the inexperienced provider stops prescribing even when improvement can be demonstrated.

6. In the last 15 years and the proliferation of managed care organizations, more providers are aligned with multiple reimbursement arrangements. It is also much more common for patients to have a change in insurance coverage requiring a change of providers. Due to job opportunities and lifestyle choices, our population is much more mobile, which also leads to provider changes. Seeing a single primary care provider from birth to death is not the rule, as it was 2 decades ago. Despite this changing demographic, primary care still often has long histories with patients and is able to identify many characteristic personalities of our patients. We often cannot make an appropriate Axis II diagnosis but know when a patient tends to be anxious or dramatic or exaggerating. We develop this skill not through specialized training but through repeated exposure to multiple patients whom we see daily.

Despite the on-the-job training, it is difficult to identify a patient at risk for abusing a substance and accurately discover when a patient develops addiction. Finding a patient who alters a prescription, borrows a neighbor's opioid, or takes more than prescribed increases our discomfort with using the whole opioid drug class.

Perhaps a more adaptive reaction to a patient's behavior would be setting limits, drafting opioid agreements early in the prescribing process, and implementing pill counts and urine drug screens. It is much more likely that failing to identify the risky opioid user or receiving a call from the substance abuse clinic or the police about our patient will lead us to label the entire persistent pain population as risky. When a patient has a higher risk of addiction due to past substance abuse, comfort with appropriate opioid prescribing in primary care deteriorates. Rather than using reasonable behavior limits, we are more likely to discharge the patient or refuse all problematic medications.

All of the above characteristics of a typical primary care practice make management of persistent pain more difficult than management of other chronic diseases. Deciding not to treat these patients is a very attractive strategy. Yet most in primary care would agree that pain management should and must be our responsibility and indeed, due to our close association with patients, we are the ideal providers to deliver this care.

Pain Management and Chemical Dependency in Primary Care

Primary care is interested and adept at providing longitudinal care for all patients with chronic illnesses and disease states. Chronic pain is not a symptom but a chronic illness amendable to intervention by a dedicated provider with skills in dealing with long-term symptoms and behaviors. Chemical dependency is also a chronic disease requiring a skill set, but particularly important is long-term longitudinal care because relapse is so common. The primary care provider can improve pain management in the chemically dependent patient, but changes have to be made such that this care is appropriate given the pressures of a provider's practice.

The knowledge needed to diagnose, treat, follow, and refer chronic pain patients is needed. Most of the training primary care providers receive involves acute pain or well-understood disease management. Chronic pain must be taught in practical, understandable terms. Diabetes and hypertension have agreed-upon characteristic diagnostic workups that can be recited by any care provider.

Goals of therapy with decision points and treatment algorithms are available and well known in primary care. If a diabetic patient has blood sugars that are not well controlled despite our best efforts or if he or she needs highly technical interventions (insulin pump), referrals are available. The specialist addresses the blood sugar control and also deals with the psychosocial barriers to care. Patients return to primary care when the disease is stable and future treatment has clearly defined outcomes.

Primary care welcomes this type of long-term management because we know exactly what is expected of us and we have the skills to encourage and track desired outcomes. We still may need the endocrinologist to monitor the insulin pump, but we can deal with the depression, diet restrictions, exercise, and other aspects of care.

When long-term management of the chemically dependent patient in pain has clear-cut outcomes and expected behaviors, primary care can manage the chronic illness. Too often patients are returned from specialists without their psychosocial issues adequately addressed. Having completed specialty care, patients are on drug combinations we to do understand with continued high pain levels. Stability of care assured by the specialist often evolves into complaints of inadequate pain treatment, early requests for opioid refills, and disruptive behavior in our offices.

A close association among pain specialists, substance abuse providers, and primary care is a necessity if this treatment is to succeed. Primary care providers can develop the skill set needed to deal with difficult pain problems not by attending lectures on pain management but by having success with their own patients. Having a close relationship with an expert who can help guide us through our own difficult patient decisions makes us pain experts. Interpreting an abnormal urine drug screen is impossibly difficult until done multiple times with the help of the specialist. Interpreting the next abnormal screen and what to do with the results becomes understandable.

The argument can be made for making opioid agreements, required narcotic anonymous attendance, refusing refills, required office behavior and many other characteristics of a pain practice which are foreign to the primary care provider. This will only happen when specialty hand-holding guides us through the process.

Other Suggestions for Pain Management in Primary Care

1. Information is usually gathered from the patient during an office visit and recorded as the history. If a chemically dependent patient is struggling with the control of the use of an opioid, personal reports may be inaccurate or misleading. Just as important is information from spouses or other family members. The Health Information Privacy Policy Act (HIPPA) makes obtaining this information difficult, but opioid agreements allow for this collateral data collection. Every attempt should be made to contact significant others to gather this information.

2. Some patients will be too challenging for the practice style of most primary care providers. Knowing when to refer is of vital importance. Characteristics that suggest referral include repeated relapse, high-dose opioid use without analgesic effect, multiple requests for early refills or lost medications, chaotic social environments, and psychosocial issues including resistant depression, borderline personality disorder, and uncontrolled anxiety. If a patient is making you nervous about prescribing, obtain another opinion.

3. Just as important as when to refer is where to refer. A pain specialist who does injection therapy may perform excellent analgesic blocks yet not address any other concerns. A psychologist unfamiliar with pain or chemical dependency may be equally unhelpful. A pain-trained psychologist as well as an integrated pain clinic with multiple interacting specialties would be more appropriate. Knowing your referral base, just like in other chronic diseases, makes pain management more efficient.

4. At least one small study showed that patients with a history of chemical dependence did better on chronic opioid therapy when there was ongoing attendance at support groups such as Narcotics Anonymous. Attendance at such support groups, including church or psychologically oriented groups, may help control behavior. Part of an opioid agreement could include verified attendance at group meetings, similar to court-ordered attendance at Alcoholics Anonymous.

5. Tighter control over behavior is also essential in a population known for recidivism. This control would include opioid agreements, urine drug screens at each office visit and random collections, more frequent follow-up appointments, shorter dosage intervals, and required cotreatment with an addiction specialist.

It is difficult to generalize about primary care providers because their training, skills, interest, and practice styles are highly variable. Some providers have no interest and will never be able to deal with the persistent pain patients, especially those with chemical dependency. Other providers have become very adept at this type of practice, eager for the knowledge needed, developing relationships with chemically dependent pain patients. Patients and providers cherish these interactions. Some of the most appreciative patients in my practice are the ones in which this patient-provider relationship of trust and understanding has developed.

This is not to imply that persistent pain management in the chemically dependent patient is straightforward and undemanding. The noncompliant diabetic patient is also a challenge in a busy practice. With a coordinated relationship with a few specialists, primary care can take the lead role in pain management, as we have done with every other chronic disease. It is only with the development of this new skill set that our chemically dependent patients will get the pain care they require and deserve.

References

Brownlee S, Schrof JM. The quality of mercy: Effective pain treatments already exist. Why aren't doctors using them? *US News World Rep.* 1997; 122: 54–7.

Flor H, Turk DC. Chronic back pain and rheumatoid arthritis: predicting pain and disability from cognitive variables. *J Behav Med.* 1988; 11: 251–65.

Heinermann AW, Keen M, Donohue R, et al. Alcohol use by persons with recent spinal cord injury. *Arch Phys Med Rehab.* 1988; 69: 619–24.

Honkanen R, Ertama L, Kuosmanen P. The role of alcohol in accidental falls. *J Stud Alcohol.* 1983; 44: 231–45.

Jacox AK, Carr DB, Chapman CR, et al. *Acute Pain Management: Operative or Medical Procedures and Trauma Clinical Practice Guideline No. 1.* Rockville, MD: US Department of Health and Human Services, Agency for Health Care Policy and Research; 1992. AHCPR publication 92–0032.

Joranson DE, Ryan KM, Gilson AM, et al. Trends in medical use and abuse of opioid analgesics. *JAMA.* 2000; 284: 564.

Pinsky J. Chronic pain syndromes and their treatment. In: Brodwin MG, Tellez F, Brodwin SK, eds. *Medical, Psychosocial and Vocational Aspects of Disability.* 1993; Athens, GA: Elliott & Fitzpatrick.

Reesor KA, Craig KD. Medically incongruent chronic back pain physical limitations, suffering, and ineffective coping. *Pain.* 1988; 32: 35–45.

Reyna TM, Hollis H, Hulsebus RC. Alcohol related trauma. *Ann Surg.* 1985; 201: 194–9.

Sanders SH, Brena SF, Spier CJ, et al. Chronic back pain patients around the world: cross-cultural similarities and differences. *Clin J Pain.* 1992; 8:317–323.

Savage SR. Assessment for addiction in pain-treatment settings. *Clin J Pain.* 2002; 18: S28–38.

SAMHSA, Office of Applied Studies. *Emergency Department Trends From the Drug Abuse Warning Network, Final Estimates 1994–2001.* Rockville, MD:SAMHSA; 2002a. DAWN Series D-21, DHHS Publication No. (SMA) 02–3635.

SAMHSA, Office of Applied Studies. *Mortality Data from the Drug Abuse Warning Network, 2001.* Rockville, MD: SAMHSA; 2002b. DAWN Series D-23, DHHS Publication No. (SMA) 03–3781.

SAMHSA, Office of Applied Studies. *Results from the 2003 National Survey on Drug Use and Health: National Findings.* Rockville, MD: SAMHSA; 2004. DHHS Publication No. (SMA) 04–3964.

39

The Palliative Care Patient

Lida Nabati

Janet Abrahm

Dame Cicely Saunders, founder of the modern hospice movement in the 1960s, coined the term "total pain," which embodied the notion that pain, endured by those facing a life-limiting illness, was multifaceted and could include psychological, physical, spiritual, and social elements (Saunders, 1981). From this concept, a new subspecialty, palliative medicine, emerged. In 2007, the American Board of Medical Specialties is expected to recognize palliative medicine as a medical subspecialty.

Among patients with pain and chemical dependence, who is the palliative care patient? The National Consensus Project for Quality Palliative Care (NCPQPC; 2004, p. 1) defines palliative care as "medical care provided by an interdisciplinary team, including the professions of medicine, nursing, social work, chaplaincy, counseling, nursing assistants and other health care professionals, focused on the relief of suffering and support for the best possible quality of life for patients facing serious life-threatening illness, and their families. It aims to identify and address the physical, psychological, spiritual and practical burdens of illness."

This team approach to care is particularly important in the management of the palliative care patient with pain and chemical dependency. As is discussed elsewhere in this volume, it is estimated that one-third of the population has used illicit substances, and the prevalence of substance use disorders in the United States is 6%–15% (Passik et al., 1998a). As these patients develop life-limiting illnesses and become palliative care patients, they are likely to develop new sources of pain and other forms of suffering (Field & Cassel, 1997). Substance use disorders contribute negatively to quality of life even in patients without the added burden of these illnesses, but in palliative care patients, substance abuse complicates the assessment and management of pain and anxiety, and is itself a source of social, spiritual, and existential distress.

Interventions aimed at mitigating the harm of a substance use disorder in a palliative care patient minimize the suffering caused both by the substance use disorder and the terminal illness. Challenges these patients present include the following: (1) using the same guidelines regarding the treatment of their chemical dependency as were used before they developed advanced disease; (2) providing excellent pain management in a setting in which it may be difficult to distinguish pain from anxiety and other causes of distress; and (3) dealing with the guilt and estrangement from family, friends, or even God that these patients may experience. To meet these challenges and serve as effective patient advocates, palliative care teams must work with practitioners caring for patients with chemical dependency and primary caregivers to provide optimal care for them at the end of their lives.

Overview of Palliative Care

The Institute of Medicine's report on end-of-life care confirmed that this type of care in the United States suffers due to inadequate attention in medical school curricula and postgraduate medical training, as well as lack of adequate research funding (Field & Cassel, 1997). Palliative medicine is an emerging specialty that comprises clinical palliative care, education, and research. Hospice care shares a philosophy of care aimed toward relief of suffering, but the current reimbursement system, driven by the Medicare hospice benefit, typically excludes patients who are receiving costly life-prolonging or even palliative therapies from receiving care in hospice programs.

Palliative care services are available to patients at all stages of a life-limiting illness and are often delivered concurrently with disease-modifying therapy. In the United States, this is a growing population, due to aging and increasing rates of chronic illness (Morrison & Meier, 2004). Palliative care and hospice programs serve patients with cancer, congestive heart failure, chronic obstructive pulmonary disease, HIV/AIDS, as well as both advanced renal and liver disease. Palliative care can continue to offer relief of suffering when disease-modifying or life-prolonging therapy can no longer be pursued.

This chapter will discuss the needs of patients with cancer and most noncancer diagnoses. Please see next chapter for special considerations of pain and chemical dependency in the patient with HIV/AIDS.

Prevalence of Pain in the Palliative Care Population

On average, patients with advanced cancer report a median of six symptoms, with pain being the most common (Coyle et al., 1990). It is estimated that 60%–90% of patients with advanced cancer experience pain (Coyle et al., 1990; Curtis et al., 1991; Levy, 1996), and an investigation of prescribing practices in an outpatient palliative care team showed that morphine was the most commonly prescribed medication (Curtis & Walsh, 1993). A qualitative study identified adequate pain and symptom control (comfort) as one of five domains of end-of-life care most valued by patients (Singer et al., 1999). It has been clearly shown, however, that pain is often undertreated in patients with cancer (Cleeland et al., 1994), and the Institute of Medicine report on end-of-life care in the United States, including patients with and without a cancer diagnosis, documented that undertreated pain causes needless suffering (Field & Cassel, 1997).

Chemical Dependency in the Palliative Care Patient

Substance use disorders are not uncommon among patients with terminal cancer, though only 3% of referrals to psychiatry service at Memorial Sloan Kettering Cancer Center in 1990 were for substance abuse issues (Passik et al., 1998b). This may reflect lower rates of patients with substance use disorders presenting for care at a tertiary care cancer center. The prevalence of substance abuse disorders in palliative care populations remains largely unstudied.

Substance abuse can increase patients' risk of several life-limiting illnesses. Alcohol abuse predisposes one, for example, to cancer of the head and neck and esophagus. Intravenous drug use places individuals at risk for viral hepatitis B and C (which can lead to hepatocellular carcinoma) and HIV (which is also associated with increased risk of a variety of cancers). Smoking predisposes patients to several types of cancer (head and neck, lung) and other chronic illnesses (chronic obstructive pulmonary disease and coronary artery disease leading to congestive heart failure).

As reported by CAGE questionnaire screening, rates of alcoholism were as high as 28% in an inpatient palliative care setting in Canada (Bruera et al., 1995). Only one-third of these patients were previously identified as alcoholic. This discrepancy supports the benefit of routine screening for alcoholism in this population.

Aberrant Drug-Related Behaviors

Identifying substance abuse disorders in a medically ill population can be challenging (Kirsh et al., 2002). Many clinicians tend to categorize patients as "addicted" or "not addicted," but this binary classification does not capture adequately the complexity of patients with medical illness, many of whom may have been prescribed controlled substances for legitimate medical purposes. Although *DSM-IV* (American Psychiatric Association, 1994) describes substance dependence and substance addiction, too often these are confused with tolerance or physical dependence, both of which are expected consequences of opioid therapy. Instead, a useful construct describes a spectrum of aberrant drug-related behaviors. At one end of this spectrum are patients with alarming behaviors such as forgery or selling of prescriptions, stealing drugs or obtaining prescription drugs from nonmedical sources, using illicit substances, or repeated noncompliance or unsanctioned dose escalations. Behaviors that are less suggestive of addiction include complaining about needing more drugs, occasional dose escalation, requesting specific drugs, using the opioid to treat symptoms other than pain, and anxiety about recurrent symptoms (Passik et al., 1998a). Further empirical research to identify which aberrant drug-related behaviors are more predictive of a substance use disorder will be important to clinicians caring for this challenging subset of patients with pain. This group may need additional supports in order to safely implement appropriate analgesic therapy (Passik & Kirsh, 2003).

In a palliative care patient with uncontrolled pain, certain behaviors, such as self-escalation of doses or using medications prescribed for others, may mistakenly be interpreted as signs of addictive behavior. Patients requesting specific analgesic medications or routes of administration may similarly be viewed as "addicted." Such patients may be merely advocating for analgesics they have found to be more effective. However, careful consideration of all factors that may cause these behaviors is critical in providing compassionate care.

Differential Diagnosis

In a patient with a life-limiting illness, the differential diagnosis of apparently aberrant drug-related behaviors that accompany a complaint of pain must be thoroughly explored in order to ensure appropriate clinical management. The differential diagnosis includes pseudoaddiction, chemical coping, psychiatric disorders, and other alternatives.

Pseudoaddiction

The iatrogenic phenomenon of pseudoaddiction can easily be mistaken for addiction. First described by Weissman and Haddox, pseudoaddiction results from inadequate management of the patient's pain, not from a patient's desire to "get high." It typically develops in three phases. A patient with inadequately treated pain (for example, someone allowed to take pain medication only every 6 hours when that medication provides pain relief for only 3 hours) may manifest behaviors that may be perceived as aberrant, such as requests for an escalating dose or frequency of analgesics, self-escalation of doses, or hoarding of medication. Regressive behavior (moaning or crying out in pain) or failure to cooperate with the health-care team may develop if the patient's attempts at obtaining more analgesics are unsuccessful. This pattern will continue to escalate until a "crisis of mistrust" arises, leading to feelings of anger and isolation on the part of the patient. Only once a patient trusts that his health-care team "believes" his pain, and that analgesia will be a priority of care, will the aberrant behaviors cease. Pseudoaddiction, therefore, likely arises when the treating clinician has an inadequate understanding of appropriate pain assessment, of the pharmacology of the opioids used for pain management, or excessive fear of addiction in patients managed with opioids (Weisman & Haddox, 1989). Given the fact that pain is typically undertreated in patients at the end of life, pseudoaddiction is an important cause of suffering in this population.

Chemical Coping/Psychiatric Disorders

"Chemical coping" describes a patient who uses pain medicines to alleviate nonpain symptoms, such as anxiety or depression. Careful assessment of psychiatric symptoms and availability of psychiatric consultation are important components of a multidisciplinary comprehensive approach to serving these patients.

Unrecognized and untreated anxiety may explain why a number of cancer patients have used benzodiazepines prescribed for others (Passik et al., 2000a). Patients dependent on nicotine will require replacement in settings in which they are not allowed to smoke or if they become acutely unable to smoke (Quibell & Baker, 2005). The prevalence of anxiety disorders in advanced cancer is 22% (Smith et al., 2003), and though panic disorder at the end of life has not yet been studied, clinical experience has shown this to be a commonly encountered phenomenon (Periyakoil et al., 2005). Depression at the end of life is also quite common. Clinicians must be alert to the presence of depression in the palliative care patient with guilt, hopelessness, or anhedonia, and not rely on somatic or neurovegetative criteria, such as fatigue or anorexia, which are often present in nondepressed patients with advanced medical illnesses (Block, 2000). Counseling, psychotherapy, or psychopharmacologic medication with benzodiazepines, other anxiolytics, or antidepressants may be indicated in these circumstances. If the guilt is associated with spiritual or existential concerns, further questioning and counseling in these areas by the primary or palliative care team or the chaplain should be pursued (Lo et al., 2002).

Alternative Explanations

Delirium is experienced by 28%–83% of patients near the end of life (Casarett & Inouye, 2001; Nowels et al., 2002), and it can explain aberrant drug-related behaviors in patients who are responsible for taking their own medications but are not closely monitored to ensure they are taking the correct amounts at the correct times. Delirium manifests as an alteration of cognition, consciousness, and perception, which may wax and wane. Recognition and treatment of the delirium can eliminate the aberrant drug-taking behavior.

Personality disorders can also cause patients to seem to be taking their medications strangely. If the patient's goal is contact with, or attention from, the health-care team, impulsive or attention-seeking drug-related behaviors may serve this purpose in a patient with a personality disorder.

Spiritual suffering, social isolation and guilt for past behaviors may also manifest as, or intensify, a pain complaint in the palliative care patient with chemical dependence. Spiritual well-being actually protects against despair at the end of life (McClain et al., 2003). But patients with a history of substance abuse or a prior criminal history may be isolated from family and friends and feel guilt about past or ongoing betrayals. They may also fear punishment or be estranged from their religious tradition. They may even resist taking medication so that they can atone before they die ("I'd rather burn here than burn there").

Comprehensive Management

Because substance use disorders in palliative care patients may pose a barrier to optimal treatment for their underlying medical illnesses, identifying and treating the substance use disorder is critical to comprehensive medical management. Additionally, the mission of palliative care is the relief of suffering, and active substance abuse can be viewed as having a negative impact on quality of life and functioning. Therefore, ongoing management of a substance use disorder in the addicted patient, concurrent with other palliative therapies, is important. A collaborative approach, involving the primary treating physician, an addiction or substance abuse specialist, and the resources of a palliative care team is optimal.

Management of pain in any palliative care patient begins with a thorough history and physical, with special attention to assessing coping, psychosocial state, and the patient's goals of care. A thorough assessment of pain includes identifying nullifying or aggravating factors, a detailed description of characteristics of pain, prior workup, and exploration of previous therapeutic modalities used. Skills in communication are a core component of delivering palliative care (NCPQPC, 2004; Tulsky, 2005). Palliative care practitioners use a nonjudgmental stance and "sweeping" or open-ended questions to establish trust, eliminate alienation, and facilitate disclosure when obtaining a history of aberrant drug-related behaviors (Passik & Kirsch, 2005). A substance use history can be similarly obtained, with attention paid to substances used, route of use, and history of substance use treatment.

In a palliative care patient, assessment must be individualized to the patient's goals of care. Burdens of any diagnostic workup or invasive treatment for a pain complaint must be weighed against the potential benefit to the patient. If the burden is too great, starting empiric symptomatic treatment may be more appropriate. Imaging studies, however, should be obtained if possible when they are likely to reveal a specific, reversible etiology for the pain, to provide important prognostic information, or to prevent an outcome that would severely harm the patient's quality of life (e.g., an MRI to evaluate for spinal cord compression in a cancer patient with back pain).

While the etiology is being sought, or if empiric therapy is chosen, the WHO analgesic ladder (Abrahm, 2005a) outlines a basic approach to cancer pain management that includes opioid and nonopioid medications. Patients are also encouraged to use nonpharmacological techniques such as heat, massage, relaxation, and meditation (Abrahm, 2005a). Interventional approaches, such as percutaneous injections of neurolytic substances and continuous infusion of spinal analgesics, can also improve the quality of life for the < 5% of patients with pain refractory to more conventional therapies (Sloan, 2004).

Management of pain in the palliative care patient actively abusing substances, however, can be challenging. A multidisciplinary approach, with close involvement of social work and psychiatry or an addiction specialist, is important to support the palliative care clinician. This work is often labor intensive and exhausting for caregivers, and many oncology clinicians are nihilistic about its chances of succeeding (Passik & Theobald, 2000). Clear guidelines should be set at the initiation of treatment, which should include the following: which providers will prescribe opioids or other controlled substances; the proper use of medications; and how and when new prescriptions are to be obtained. Further, the prescriber should be clear about unacceptable behaviors that would compromise the clinician's continued involvement, such as obtaining prescriptions from other providers. If the practitioner feels it would be useful, a contract or signed statement by the patient can document these expectations and verify that they have been discussed, but one is not required. Patients whose illness prevents them from working at their usual occupations may use drug diversion to support their families (J. Abrahm, personal communication). Urine toxicology can play an important role here, both in monitoring for other illicit substances and in documenting the presence of a prescribed substance when diversion is suspected.

Clinicians should recognize that it is normal to experience frustration and even be at risk for developing negative attitudes toward patients with problematic use of controlled substances or who have a style of interacting with clinicians that arose during their past episodes of substance abuse. Approaching these patients with compassion and a nonjudgmental stance, as one would approach all other patients reporting pain, may facilitate a trusting relationship and decrease the behaviors that cause the patient to seem manipulative or "drug seeking."

In the patient with a history of substance use who is currently abstinent, successful pain management can occur (Dunbar & Katz, 1996; Wesson et al., 1993). Patients with a history of a substance use disorder may need higher doses of analgesics than nonsubstance abusers to achieve acceptable pain control (Kaplan et al., 2000). But patients with a history of alcohol abuse, who maintain abstinence with continued use of a 12-step program, have a low chance of developing problematic use of opioids so long as the patient continues to participate in a 12-step program (Dunbar & Katz, 1996).

Patients on methadone maintenance can also be successfully treated for pain. It is incorrect to assume, however, that the methadone in the maintenance program provides adequate analgesia for those with acute or chronic pain (Alford et al., 2005). Alternative opioids can be used for analgesia, recognizing that patients on methadone likely have significant tolerance to opioids and may need higher doses. And methadone, itself, can be used to treat the patient's pain. For patients on active methadone maintenance, receiving the methadone for maintenance from their program allows them to maintain contact with the additional support and structure that the program offers. Collaboration, therefore, between the team at the facility and the palliative care or primary physician managing the patient's pain would seem ideal.

Both patients with a history of addiction as well as those enrolled in methadone maintenance often need reassurance and support when additional opioids are prescribed for their pain. They and their families fear return of the chemical dependence disorder, and adequate support and careful monitoring can decrease this risk.

Palliative care patients without prior substance abuse disorders should also be monitored for aberrant drug-related behaviors, because this will identify the small minority of cancer or other advanced disease patients who develop a new substance use disorder while taking opioids for pain. Imperfect studies from 20–25 years ago suggest that the actual risk of addiction following opioid therapy for pain appears to be negligible (Macaluso et al., 1988; Porter & Jick, 1980), but there are no recent studies that confirm or refute these findings.

Regulatory Issues and Palliative Care

Regulatory issues now may, but they should not, prevent palliative care patients with or without chemical dependency(ies) from receiving the relief they deserve. The palliative care community works to optimize legal and regulatory issues that affect use of controlled substances and pose barriers to pain relief (NCPQPC, 2004). A number of organizations, including the World Health Organization, the American Medical Association and the Institute of Medicine, call for the removal of policies that affect use of controlled substances and hinder pain management and palliative care (Gilson et al., 2005). Ending practices that serve as hurdles to pain relief, such as limiting numbers of opioid pills per prescription or requiring the use of triplicate forms will benefit all citizens requiring these medications for pain relief.

Incarcerated Patients

Incarcerated men and women have high rates of chronic illness, including HIV/AIDS and hepatitis C (Hammett et al., 2002) and with the aging of the prison population, it is estimated that approximately 3,000 inmates die yearly of natural causes. The incarcerated patient nearing the end of life presents a unique challenge to clinicians. Hospice is emerging as the standard for meeting the needs of terminally ill inmates (Ratcliff & Craig, 2004).

More than half of all inmates are identified as having a substance use disorder at the time of incarceration (Lo & Stephens, 2000; Peters et al., 1998). Substance abuse issues and management of pain, in the setting of regulations of controlled substances in correctional health settings, can be challenging. Experience in the Louisiana State Penitentiary Hospice Program suggests that contrary to what might be expected, inmates may underreport their pain because being able to deal with pain is considered a sign of strength (Tillman, 2000).

Tasks of Patients at the End of Life

Clinicians caring for patients with pain and chemical dependence can help them and their families with spiritual or existential concerns that arise as they end their lives. These concerns include making meaning of their lives, wondering whether they are loved by family and friends, asking for or giving forgiveness, and wondering how to say goodbye or thank you (Byock, 1997). For some patients and families, especially when substance abuse or addiction has colored their relationships, discussing "The Five Things" together will bring healing and closure: "Forgive me; I forgive you; Thank you; I love you, and Goodbye" (Byock, 1997). When patients are unable to speak, or are spending a great deal of time sleeping, clinicians can encourage their families to tell each other what they remember about the patient. For many patients and families, this difficult time can become a time of growth and healing, resolution, remembrance of good times together, and transmission of a legacy (Block, 2001).

When patients are still able to do so, physicians can urge them to talk more about their lives. In the telling, patients prioritize, order, celebrate, and mourn. Clinicians can help patients find solace and closure at the end of life by exploring religious and spiritual beliefs and listening empathetically (Block, 2001; Lev & McCorkle, 1998).

Through these discussions, patients begin to understand that they are cared for as people, not just patients. Some may reveal fears that their clinicians can dispel, such as a fear of dying in uncontrolled pain, of suffocating, or of being abandoned. Some want to reconnect with religious traditions and carry out the rituals that surround dying in their culture or religion (Bigby, 2003). Chaplains, social workers, and psychiatrists best address many of these problems, and the clinician can make these referrals. In our experience, these sources of counseling are particular helpful for the issues of guilt and worthlessness that arise in patients with active or past addiction(s).

Hospice Programs

Hospice programs provide a continuum of care, from home to the inpatient setting. Although by law, 80% of days of patient care must take place in the home, all Medicare-certified hospices are required to provide four levels of care: routine home care, continuous home care, respite care in nursing homes, and inpatient care ("Medicare Hospice Regulations," 2006; Table 39.1).

To be eligible to enroll in a hospice program, both the attending physician and the hospice medical director must simply certify that the patient is terminally ill with a prognosis of 6 months or less, if the disease followed its usual course ("Medicare Hospice Regulations," 2006; Saunders, 1981). There are a number of misconceptions, however, that delay and prevent referrals to hospice (Box 39.1).

The services provided by hospice are listed in Box 39.2. Hospice provides 95% of the cost of prescription drugs related to the terminal diagnosis and necessary for its palliative treatment (and many waive the other 5% if there is no insurance coverage). Hospice programs provide all durable medical equipment, supplies, and oxygen for needs related to the terminal diagnosis; laboratory and diagnostic procedures related to the terminal diagnosis;

Table 39.1. Routine Clinical Care Provided by Hospice Programs

Service	Frequency
"On call"	24 hours/day
Home health aide	≤ 2hr/day
Registered nurse visits	≤ 3/wk + prn
Social workvisits	q 2 wks
Chaplain visits	q 2–4wks
Volunteer	2–4 hrs/wk
Physician	prn
Occupational therapist, physical therapist, and respiratory therapist	prn

Additional mandated services

1. *Continuous home care:* Patients with, for example, refractory cough, dyspnea, pain, or delirium can receive 24 hour/day nursing and home health aide services.

2. *Inpatient care:* Rarely utilized. For refractory symptoms that cannot be controlled at home, even with continuous care. The referring physician admits the patient and may bill for his/her services under Medicare Part B (Medicare hospice regulations, 2006).

3. *Respite care:* The goal of the respite (in a community skilled or intermediate nursing facility) is either to provide a rest for the caregiver or to remove the patient to an adequate facility when the home is temporarily inadequate to meet the patient care needs. Respite care is offered for 5 days for every month the patient is enrolled in hospice.

Box 39.1. Common Misconceptions About Hospice Care

- *Misconception: Patients enrolling in hospice must choose not to be resuscitated.*
- *Misconception: Patients enrolled in hospice lose their primary physicians.* The referring primary care physician or oncologist continues to direct and approve all of the patient's care. If the patient requires either inpatient hospice admission for symptom control or routine admission for a diagnosis unrelated to the terminal illness, the physician may bill Medicare under Part B for any visits.
- *Misconception: Hospice patients cannot be hospitalized and remain enrolled in hospice.*
- *Misconception: Hospice patients cannot participate in research projects while enrolled in hospice.* Yes they can, so long as the project is consistent with the mission of hospice.
- *Misconception: Hospice nursing personnel do not provide sophisticated care.* The palliative care delivered by hospice nurses requires astute assessment and expert intervention tailored to the patient and family goals. Tube feedings, intravenous hydration or nutrition, or intravenous medications to control symptoms may be included in the hospice plan of care.
- *Misconception: Patients can "use up" their hospice eligibility.* Patients who live longer than 6 months will continue to receive services, so long as they continue to meet eligibility criteria for hospice care. And patients who chose to revoke the hospice benefit to seek life-prolonging therapies may choose to reenroll if their goals change.
- *Misconception: Patients must have a live-in caregiver to enroll in hospice.* Hospices that care for "live-alone" patients have special protocols to enhance their safety.

and transportation when medically necessary for changes in the patient's level of care.

Relief of Suffering in the Last Weeks

Patients report that the components of a "good death" include the following: (1) optimizing physical comfort, (2) maintaining a sense of continuity with one's self, (3) maintaining and enhancing relationships, (4) making meaning of one's life and death, (5) achieving a sense of control, and (6) confronting and preparing for death (Block, 2001). Control of physical and psychological suffering is a prerequisite to allowing both patients and caregivers to address these social and spiritual/existential dimensions of their lives and to minimize the suffering of bereaved survivors.

Even in patients on stable drug regimens, physiologic changes in patients at the end of life make it necessary to monitor them carefully for the appearance of opioid-related side effects such as myoclonus or delirium. With decreasing renal function, for example, patients taking sustained-release preparations of morphine or oxycodone may develop these side effects from decreased clearance of the drugs and their metabolites. If the respiratory rate declines to < 6 and opioids are thought to be the cause, opioid doses should be decreased 25% and the patient should be monitored carefully for increasing discomfort. Naloxone is almost never indicated. If a sedated patient has a dangerous reduction of the respiratory rate, thought to be caused by opioids, naloxone can be diluted in 10 ml and given 1 ml at a time until the respiratory rate recovers to > 6. If the naloxone is given undiluted, the patient is likely to experience severe opioid withdrawal.

If the patient becomes unable to take pills, liquid opioid concentrates, transmucosal (Payne et al., 2001), rectal (Davis et al., 2002; Kaiko et al., 1992), transdermal, or pelleted opioids can be used. Kadian and Avinza are morphine sustained-release pellets packaged into capsules that can be opened. The pellets can be sprinkled on food or suspended in liquid and either swallowed or placed into feeding tubes every 12–24 hours. Patients whose opioid dose is too large to be delivered by sublingual, transdermal, or rectal routes will need subcutaneous or intravenous continuous opioid infusions. Parenteral opioid administration is also needed for patients who would benefit from the patient-controlled analgesia option.

The xerostomia that is common in this population is usually due to opioids, not to dehydration (Ellershaw et al., 1995). There is no correlation between reports of thirst or dry mouth and hydration status (Ellershaw et al., 1995), and no controlled studies have shown that rehydration is effective. Moistening the mouth with swabs, or offering sips of water, ice chips, or fruit-flavored ice usually ameliorates the xerostomia.

Box 39.2. Hospice Services

Personnel

Medical director, nurses, social workers, home health aides, chaplains, volunteers, administrative personnel, medical consultations, occupational therapy, physical therapy, speech therapy, bereavement counseling

Items Needed for Palliation of Terminal Illness

Prescription medications
Durable medical equipment and supplies
Oxygen
Radiation and chemotherapy
Laboratory and diagnostic procedures

Other

Transportation when medically necessary for changes in level of care
When needed, continuous care at home or in a skilled nursing facility or inpatient setting
Respite care (care in a nursing facility that provides a "respite" for the caregivers)

Not all patients who exhibit distress are in pain. Delirium may mimic pain. Patients who moan without any apparent provocation, or in response to nonpainful stimuli such as having their lips moistened, may be delirious. Delirium is especially likely in patients with these behaviors who have not reported pain before they became nonverbal. Therapy to prevent and treat constipation in dying patients should be continued because constipation can cause delirium in this population. Delirious patients may appear agitated or hypoactive, or vacillate between these states (Abrahm, 2005a). Symptoms of delirium include insomnia and daytime somnolence, nightmares, restlessness or agitation (which mimics uncontrolled pain), irritability, distractibility, hypersensitivity to light and sound, anxiety, difficulty in concentrating or marshaling thoughts, and fleeting illusions. Table 39.2 lists effective treatments for delirium.

Anxiety

Anxiety in this population is often situational, involving concerns related to the terminal illness. Fear of death, impairment, or pain and concerns about the past all contribute (Stark et al., 2002). Hospitalization can add a sense of isolation, loneliness, a sense of uselessness, and concerns about lack of information or misinformation about what is happening (Storey et al., 2003). Other causes include drugs (corticosteroids, metoclopramide, opioid neurotoxicity, withdrawal from benzodiazepines or alcohol), uncontrolled pain or other symptoms, hypoxia, dyspnea, metabolic abnormalities (sepsis, hypoglycemia), insomnia, and preexisting psychiatric disorders (Storey et al., 2003).

The Final Days

If the patient is not enrolled in hospice, the treatment team needs to explain to the family what to expect as the patient dies and how to recognize when the patient's last days are approaching. Many have limited support from someone who will care for their own family while they support the dying patient, or limited vacation, sick, and family leave days. Signs that the patient is entering the last 10–14 days include the following (Pitorak, 2003):

Table 39.2 Common Disorders at the End of Life

Source	Medication(s)	Dose and Route (PO/SL/IV/SC/PR)*	Source	Medication(s)	Dose and Route (PO/SL/IV/SC/PR)*
Fatigue	Methylphenidate	2.5–5 mg PO 8 a.m./noon; can increase as needed	Cough	Opioid	Nebulized with dexamethasone, e.g., morphine 5–10 mg PO, IV or by nebulizer q2h
Insomnia	Temazepam	7.5–30 PO hs (lower dose in elderly)			
	Zolpidem	5–10 mg PO hs		Lidocaine	2 ml of 2% lidocaine in 1 ml of NL saline for 10"
	Trazodone	25–100 mg PO hs			
Pain (continuous)	Opioid (morphine, oxycodone)	Oral concentrates or IV or SQ infusion		Albuterol/terbutaline	Nebulized
			Hiccups	Baclofen	10–20 mg PO tid
	Fentanyl	Transdermal		Metoclopramide	10–20 mg PO/IV/SC/PR qid
Pain (intermittent)	Morphine, oxycodone	SL oral concentrates		Nifedipine	10–20 mg PO tid
	Hydromorphone	PR		Haloperidol	1–4 mg PO/SC/PR tid
Depression	Methylphenidate	2.5–5 mg PO qam or qam and noon		Chlorpromazine	25–50 mg PO/IV qd–qid
Anxiety	Lorazepam	0.5–2 mg SL q2h	"Death rattle"	Scopolamine	Transderm Scop patch 1–3 q3d
	Clonazepam	0.5–2 mg PO bid		Hyoscyamine	0.125—0.25 SL tid–qid
Delirium	Haloperidol	1–5 mg PO, SQ, IV, PR q2–12h		Glycopyrrolate	0.2–0.6 mg PO/SC/IV tid
	Chlorpromazine	12.5–50 mg PO, IV, PR q4–8h	Nausea	Olanzapine	2.5 to 5 mg SL hs to bid
	Olanzapine wafer	5 mg SL qhs or bid; 5 mg SL prn q4h		Lorazepam, metoclopramide, dexamethasone, or haloperidol	IV or compounded suppositories with desired agents (depending on presumed cause of nausea) q6 PR
Agitated delirium	Midazolam	1–2.5 mg IV/SC load; 0.5–1.5 mg/hr IV/SC or 25% of loading dose; increase as needed	Palliative sedation for refractory symptoms	Midazolam	1–2.5 mg IV/SC load; 0.4 mg/hr IV/SC drip; increase as needed
Dyspnea (anxiety)	Lorazepam	1 mg PO, SL q2h		Pentobarbital	2–3 mg/kg IV load; 1–2 mg/kg/hr IV drip
Dyspnea (other)	Opioid	For example, morphine 5–10 mg PO, IV or by nebulizer q2h		Lorazepam	0.5–1 mg/hour IV
	Chlorpromazine	25–50 mg PO, PR q4–12h		Propofol	2.5–5 ug/kg/minute IV

*PO = oral; SL = sublingual; IV = intravenous; SC = subcutaneous; PR = per rectum
Source: Abrahm, 2005b.

- Dehydration, tachycardia, followed by decrease in heart rate and blood pressure
- Perspiration, clammy skin, cool extremities; just before death, mottling
- Diminished breath sounds, irregular breathing pattern with periods of apnea or full Cheyne-Stokes respiration; grunting or moan with exhale
- Mouth droop; difficulty swallowing; loss of gag reflex with pooling of secretions causing "death rattle"
- Incontinence of bladder or rectum
- Agitation ± hallucinations; stillness, difficult to arouse

For patients in a hospital or nursing home, discussions should begin with the family to learn whether their religious or cultural tradition has any specific requirements for the days immediately preceding or immediately following the death. The family can then begin to assemble the group who will perform the rituals and begin to explain to the unit staff what they will need.

Table 39.2 lists the common causes of disorders in the last days of life and medications that can ease these problems.

Summary

The approach to palliative care patients with substance use disorders and pain is not unique; it comprises careful communication, compassionate delivery of care, and multidisciplinary management. Clinicians should be aware of the complex spectrum of aberrant drug-related behaviors and avoid binary categorization of patients as "addicted" or "not addicted." Coordinated efforts of palliative care teams, primary treating physicians, and addiction specialist should focus care on mitigating the harm and suffering caused by a substance use disorder in patients at the end of life. This can allow for personal and spiritual growth, legacy leaving, and closure.

References

Abrahm JL. 2005a. *A physician's guide to pain and symptom management in cancer patients.* Baltimore, MD: Johns Hopkins University Press.

Abrahm JL. 2005b. Specialized care of the terminally ill. In: DeVita VT, Hellman S, Rosenberg SA, eds. *Cancer principles and practice of oncology*, 2702–2718. Philadelphia, PA: Lippincott Williams & Wilkins.

Alford DP, Compton P, Samet JH. 2005. Acute pain management for patients receiving maintenance methadone or buprenorphine therapy. *Ann Intern Med* 144:127–134.

American Psychiatric Association. 1994. *Diagnostic and statistical manual for mental disorders* (4th ed.). Washington, DC: American Psychiatric Association.

Bigby JA, ed. 2003. *Cross-cultural medicine.* Philadelphia, PA: American College of Physicians.

Block, SD. 2000. Assessing and managing depression in the terminally ill patient. *Ann Intern Med* 132:209–218.

Block, SD. 2001. Psychological considerations, growth, and transcendence at the end of life. *JAMA* 285:2898–2905.

Bruera E, Moyano J, Seifert L, Fainsinger RL, Hanson J, Suarez-Almazor M. 1995. The frequency of alcoholism among patients with pain due to cancer. *J Pain Symptom Manage* 10:599–603.

Byock, I. 1997. *Dying well: the prospect of growth at the end of life.* New York: Riverhead Books.

Casarett DJ, Inouye SK. 2001. Diagnosis and management of delirium near the end of life. *Ann Intern Med* 135:32–40.

Cleeland CS, Gonin R, Hatfield AK, Edmonson JH, Blum RH, Stewart JA, Pandya KJ. 1994. Pain and its treatment in outpatients with metastatic cancer. *N Engl J Med* 330:592–596.

Coyle N, Adelhardt J, Folay KM, Portenoy RK. 1990. Character of terminal illness in the advanced cancer patient: Pain and other symptoms during the last four weeks of life. *J Pain and Symptom Manage* 5:83–93.

Curtis EB, Krech R, Walsh TD. 1991. Common symptoms in patients with advanced cancer. *J Palliat Care* 7:25–29.

Curtis EB, Walsh TD. 1993. Prescribing practices of a palliative care service. *J Pain Symptom Manage* 8:312–316.

Davis MP, Walsh D, LeGrand SB, Naughton M. 2002. Symptom control in cancer patients: the clinical pharmacology and therapeutic role of suppositories and rectal suspensions. *Support Care Cancer* 10:117–138.

Dunbar SA, Katz NP. 1996. Chronic opioid therapy for nonmalignant pain in patients with a history of substance abuse: report of 20 cases. *J Pain Symptom Manage* 11:163–171.

Ellershaw JE, Sutcliffe JM, Saunders CM. 1995. Dehydration and the dying patient. *J Pain Symptom Manage* 10:192–197.

Field MJ, Cassel CK, eds. 1997. *Approaching death: improving care at the end of life.* Washington, DC: National Academy Press.

Gilson AM, Joranson DE, Maurer MA, Ryan KM, Garthwaite JP. 2005. Progress to achieve balanced state policy relevant to pain management and palliative care: 2000–2003. *J Pain Palliat Care Pharmacother* 19:13–26.

Hammett TM, Harmon MP, Rhodes W. 2002. The burden of infectious disease among inmates of and releasees from U.S. correctional facilities, 1997. *Am J Public Health* 92:1789–1794.

Kaiko RF, Fitzmartin RD, Thomas GB et al. 1992. The bioavailabilty of morphine in controlled-release 30 mg tablets. *Pharmacotherapy* 12:107–134.

Kaplan R, Slywka J, Slagle S, Ries K. 2000. A titrated morphine analgesic regimen comparing substance users and non-users with AIDS-related pain. *J Pain Symptom Manage* 19:265–271.

Kirsh KL, Whitcomb LA, Donaghy K, Passik SD. 2002. Abuse and addiction issues in medically ill patients with pain: attempts at clarification of terms and empirical study. *Clin J Pain* 18:S52-S60.

Lev EL, McCorkle R. 1998. Loss, grief, and bereavement in family members of cancer patients. *Sem Oncol Nurs* 14:145–151.

Levy MH. 1996. Pharmacological treatment of cancer pain. *N Engl J Med* 335:1124–1132.

Lo B, Ruston D, Kates LW, et al. 2002. Discussing religious and spiritual issues at the end of life; a practical guide for physicians. *JAMA* 287:749–754.

Lo CC, Stephens RC. 2000. Drugs and prisoners: treatment needs on entering prison. *Am J Drug Alcohol Abuse* 26:229–45.

Macaluso C, Weinberg D, Foley KM. 1988. Opioid abuse and misuse in a cancer pain population. *J Pain Symptom Manage* 3:S24.

McClain CS, Rosenfeld B, Breitbart W. 2003. Effect of spiritual well-being on end-of-life despair in terminally-ill cancer patients. *Lancet* 361:1603–1607.

Medicare hospice regulations. 2006. Title 42 *Code of Federal Regulations*, Part 418.

Morrison RS, Meier DE. 2004. Palliative care. *N Engl J Med* 350:2582–2590.

National Consensus Project for Quality Palliative Care. 2004. *National Consensus Project for Palliative Care: Clinical practice guidelines for quality palliative care.* Pittsburgh, PA: National Consensus Project.

Nowels DE, Bublitz C, Kassner CT, Kutner JS. 2002. Estimation of confusion prevalence in hospice patients. *J Palliat Med* 5:687–695.

Passik SD, Kirsh KL. 2003. The need to identify predictors of aberrant drug-related behavior and addiction in patients being treated with opioids for pain. *Pain Med* 4:186–189.

Passik SD, Kirsh KL. 2005. Managing pain in patients with aberrant drug-taking behaviors. *J Support Oncol* 3:83–86.

Passik SD, Kirsh KL, McDonald MV et al. 2000a. A Pilot survey of aberrant drug-taking behaviors in samples of cancer and AIDS patients. *J Pain Symptom Manage* 19:274–286.

Passik SD, Kirsh KL, Portenoy RK. 1998a. Substance abuse issues in palliative care. In: Berger AM, Portenoy RK, Weissman DE, eds. *Principles and practice of palliative care and supportive oncology* (2nd ed.). Philadelphia, PA: Lippincott Williams & Wilkins.

Passik SD, Portenoy RK, Ricketts PL. 1998b. Substance abuse issues in cancer patients. Part 1: prevalence and diagnosis. *Oncology (Williston Park)* 12:517–21, 524.

Passik SD, Theobald D. 2000. Managing addiction in advanced cancer patients: why bother? *J Pain Symptom Manage.* 19:229–234.

Payne R, Coluzzi P, Hart L, et al. 2001. Long-term safety of oral transmucosal fentanyl citrate for breakthrough cancer pain. *J Pain Symptom Manage* 22:575–583.

Periyakoil VS, Skultety K, Sheikh J. 2005. Pain, anxiety, and chronic dyspnea. *J Palliat Med* 8:453–459.

Peters RH, Greenbaum PE, Edens JF, Carter CR, Ortiz MM. 1998. Prevalence of *DSM-IV* substance abuse and dependence disorders among prison inmates. *Am J Drug Alcohol Abuse* 24:573–587.

Pitorak EF. 2003. Care at the time of death: how nurses can make the last hours of life a richer, more comfortable experience. *Am J Nurs* 103:42–52.

Porter J, Jick H. 1980. Addiction rare in patients treated with narcotics. *N Engl J Med* 302:123.

Quibell R, Baker L. 2005. Nicotine withdrawal and nicotine replacement in the palliative care setting. *J Pain Symptom Manage* 30:205–207.

Ratcliff M, Craig E. 2004. The GRACE Project: guiding end-of-life care in corrections 1998–2001. *J Palliat Med* 7:373–379.

Saunders, C. 1981. The founding philosophy. In: Saunders C, Summers DH, Teller N, eds. *Hospice: the living idea.* Philadelphia, PA: Saunders.

Singer PA, Martin DK, Kelner M. 1999. Quality end-of-life care: patients' perspectives. *JAMA* 281:163–168.

Sloan PA. 2004. The evolving role of interventional pain management in oncology. *J Support Oncol* 2:491–500.

Smith EM, Gomm SA, Dickens CM. 2003. Assessing the independent contribution to quality of life from anxiety and depression in patients with advanced cancer. *Palliat Med* 17509–513.

Stark D, Kiely M, Smith A, Velikova G, House A, Selby P. 2002. Anxiety disorders in cancer patients: their nature, associations, and relation to quality of life. *J Clin Oncol* 20:3137–3148.

Storey P, Knight CF, Schonwetter RS. 2003. *Pocket guide to hospice /palliative medicine.* Glenview, IL: American Academy of Hospice and Palliative Medicine.

Tillman T. 2000. Hospice in prison: the Louisiana State Penitentiary Hospice Program. *J Palliat Med* 3:513–524.

Tulsky, JA. 2005. Beyond advance directives: importance of communication skills at the end of life. *JAMA* 294:359–365.

Weissman DE, Haddox JD. 1989. Opioid pseudoaddiction—an iatrogenic syndrome. *Pain* 36:363–366.

Wesson Dr, Ling W, Smith DE. 1993. Prescription of opioids for treatment of pain in patients with addictive disease. *J Pain Symptom Manage* 8:289–296.

40

Managing Pain and Substance Abuse in the Patient With HIV/AIDS

William Breitbart

Lara K. Dhingra

In the past decade, adults in the United States diagnosed with human immunodeficiency virus (HIV) or acquired immune deficiency syndrome (AIDS) have benefited from profound advances in treatment and access to care. However, despite these improvements in survival and care, pain in HIV/AIDS patients continues to be a major problem affecting quality of life outcomes for the majority of patients diagnosed. Pain rates in HIV/AIDS patients are high (30% to 93%), with patients who have a history of substance abuse particularly underserved in pain management. HIV/AIDS patients with a history of substance abuse are more likely to have their pain underassessed and undertreated than patients without a history of substance abuse. It is well-documented that current or past substance abuse is a formidable barrier to adequate pain management in HIV/AIDS care.

Multiple provider, patient, and system-based factors lead to the undertreatment of pain in HIV/AIDS patients with substance abuse problems. Providers may be unlikely to differentiate risk potential for analgesic abuse based on past or ongoing drug-rehabilitation status and recovery. Providers may be especially reluctant to consider opioids as a therapeutic option for HIV/AIDS patients with drug abuse histories due to concerns about triggering drug relapse. Additionally, HIV/AIDS patients with substance abuse histories may be more nonadherent with pain treatment recommendations, have problems with consistent access to care, and report heightened fears of physiologic dependency or addiction. Notably, more than 40% of HIV/AIDS patients in the United States have a history of substance abuse and 12% have a comorbid substance abuse disorder (Bing et al., 2001; Lucas et al., 2006).

Thus, as the AIDS pandemic grows worldwide, the assessment and treatment of pain in HIV/AIDS patients with a history of substance abuse is critical to improving public health. With the development of new retroviral therapies, survival rates for HIV/AIDS patients able to tolerate these drugs are increasing and the psychosocial needs of the population are changing. Further, the prevalence and diversity of pain syndromes associated with HIV/AIDS are increasing. These challenges present opportunities for clinicians and researchers to enhance the quality of care and quality of life for HIV/AIDS patients, especially patients with substance abuse problems. Improvements in pain therapies, access to care, and health-care provider readiness and capacity to deliver pain interventions in HIV/AIDS patients with a history of substance abuse are essential to achieving our public health goals. Thus, this chapter describes the prevalence and types of pain syndromes encountered in adults with HIV/AIDS, reviews the best practices for pain management in adults with HIV/AIDS and a history of substance abuse, and highlights barriers to adequate pain control in this underserved population.

Prevalence of Pain in HIV/AIDS

Approximately 2 million adults are currently diagnosed with HIV or AIDS in the United States (Centers for Disease Control [CDC], 2004), and more than 40 million adults are diagnosed worldwide (World Health Organization [WHO], 2005). Pain is known to be a major cause of suffering and disability in adults diagnosed with HIV/AIDS. Estimates of pain prevalence in HIV patients range from 30% to 90%, with the occurrence of pain increasing as the disease progresses, particularly in the latest stages of illness (Breitbart et al., 1991, 1996a; 1996b; Dobalin et al., 2004; Hewitt et al., 1997; Kimball & McCormick 1996; Larue et al., 1997; Lebovits et al., 1989; Schofferman & Brody 1990; Singer et al., 1993). Approximately 30% of ambulatory HIV patients with early stage HIV disease (e.g., pre-AIDS; Category A or B disease) experience clinically significant levels of pain, and as many as 56% have episodic painful symptoms with unknown significance (Breitbart et al., 1996a; Larue et al., 1997; Singer et al., 1993). Findings from a cross-sectional survey of 438 ambulatory AIDS patients in New York City showed that 63% reported frequent or persistent pain of at least 2 weeks' duration (Breitbart et al., 1996a). The prevalence of pain increased significantly as HIV disease progressed, with 45% of AIDS patients with Category A3 disease reporting pain, 55% of those with Category B3 and 67% of those with Category C1, 2, or 3 disease reporting pain. In this sample, AIDS patients also were more likely to report pain if they had other concomitant symptoms related to HIV (e.g., fatigue or wasting), had received treatment for an AIDS-related opportunistic infection, or if they were not using antiretroviral medications (e.g., AZT, ddI, ddC, d4t).

The authors thank Lauren Levy, Jennifer Stillman, and Theresa Carpenter for their assistance with preparing this chapter.

Among inpatient populations, estimates of pain prevalence rates in AIDS range between 30% and 93% depending on disease severity (Kimball & McCormick 1996; Larue et al., 1997; Lebovits et al., 1989; Schofferman & Brody, 1990). Approximately 50% of AIDS inpatients in a public hospital in New York City were treated for pain, the most prevalent symptom reported in this sample (e.g., 30%; Lebovits et al., 1989). Further, a French multicenter study also showed that 62% of HIV inpatients had significant pain (Larue et al., 1997). A study assessing hospice patients also showed that more than 50% with advanced AIDS reported pain (Schofferman & Brody 1990), whereas up to 93% reported at least one 48-hour period of unremitting pain during the last 2 weeks of life (Kimball & McCormick, 1996). In this sample, approximately 88% of hospice patients were treated with opioids, with the majority experiencing some pain relief (Kimball & McCormick, 1996). When compared to cancer patients, AIDS patients in hospice or home care settings have similar, or higher, pain prevalence and intensity rates (Larue et al., 1994). AIDS patients with pain typically describe an average of 2.5 to 3 concurrent sites of pain (Breitbart et al., 1996b; Hewitt et al., 1997). (For a further review of pain prevalence and characteristics in AIDS populations, as well as a description of pain presentation in special populations and impact on quality of life, interested readers are referred to Breitbart, 2003.)

Pain Types and Syndromes in HIV/AIDS

Pain syndromes encountered in HIV/AIDS patients are diverse in nature and etiology. Pain syndromes seen in HIV disease can be classified into three types (Box 40.1): (1) those directly related to HIV infection or consequences of immunosuppression; (2) those due to AIDS therapies, and (3) those unrelated to AIDS or AIDS therapies (Breitbart, 1997; Breitbart et al., 1997; Hewitt et al., 1997). Approximately 45% of pain syndromes encountered are directly related to HIV infection or consequences of immunosuppression; 15%–30% are due to therapies for HIV/AIDS-related conditions and diagnostic procedures; and the remaining 25%–40% are unrelated to HIV or its therapies (Hewitt et al., 1997).

To date, the most common pain syndromes reported by HIV/AIDS patients include painful sensory peripheral neuropathy, pain due to extensive Kaposi's sarcoma, headache, oral and pharyngeal pain, abdominal pain, chest pain, arthralgias and myalgias, and painful dermatologic conditions (Breitbart et al., 1991, 1996a; Hewitt et al., 1997; Larue et al; 1994; Lebovits et al., 1989; O'Neill & Sherrard, 1993; Penfold & Clark 1992; Schofferman & Brody, 1990; Singer et al., 1993). Based on a study with 151 ambulatory AIDS patients, the most common pain diagnoses include the following: headaches (46%), joint pain (arthritis and arthralgias, 31%), painful polyneuropathy (distal symmetrical polyneuropathy, 28%), muscle pain (myalgia and myositis, 27%), skin pain (Kaposi's sarcoma and infections, 25%), bone pain (20%), abdominal pain (17%), chest pain (13%), and painful radiculopathy (12%; Hewitt et al., 1997). Further, neuropathic pains (e.g., polyneuropathies or radiculopathies) comprise the largest proportion of pain syndromes in AIDS patients (Box 40.2), with pains of a somatic and/or visceral nature also common (Hewitt et al., 1997). Given the diversity and complexity of pain syndromes encountered by the health-care provider involved in HIV/AIDS care, the next section reviews the best practices for pain management in this population.

An Overview of Pain Management in HIV/AIDS Patients

Pain Assessment

Consistent with any pain problem, the initial step in the delivery of best practices for pain management is conducting a comprehensive assessment of pain symptoms. Further, the health-care provider working with the AIDS population must have a working knowledge of the etiology and treatment of pain in AIDS. This would include an understanding of the different types of AIDS pain syndromes discussed in the section above, and familiarity with the parameters of appropriate pharmacologic treatment. Collaboration and collateral information from the entire health-care team regarding medical and psychosocial status is optimal when attempting to adequately manage pain in the AIDS patient. As such, a careful

---

Box 40.1. Pain Syndromes in AIDS Patients

I. Pain related to HIV/AIDS
 a. HIV neuropathy
 b. HIV myelopathy
 c. Kaposi's sarcoma
 d. Secondary infections (intestines, skin)
 e. Organomegaly
 f. Arthritis/vasculitis
 g. Myopathy/myositis

II. Pain related to HIV/AIDS therapy
 a. Antiretrovirals, antivirals
 b. Antimycobacterials, PCP prophylaxis
 c. Chemotherapy (vincristine)
 d. Radiation
 e. Surgery
 f. Procedures (bronchoscopy, biopsies)

III. Pain unrelated to AIDS
 a. Disc disease
 b. Diabetic neuropathy

Box 40.2. Neuropathies Encountered in HIV/AIDS Patients

I. Predominantly sensory neuropathy (PSN) of AIDS

II. Immune-mediated
 a. Inflammatory demyelinating polyneuropathies (IDPs)
  1. Acute (Guillain-Barre syndrome)
  2. Chronic (CIDP)

III. Infectious
 a. Cytomegalovirus polyradiculopathy
 b. Cytomegalovirus multiple mononeuropathy
 c. Herpes zoster
 d. Mycobacterial (MAI)

IV. Toxic-nutritional
 a. Alcohol, vitamin deficiencies (B6, B12)
 b. Antiretrovirals: ddI (didanosine), ddC (zalcitabine), D4T (stavudine)
 c. Antivirals: foscarnet
 d. PCP prophylaxis: dapsone
 e. Antibacterial: metronidazole
 f. Antimycobacterials: INH (isoniazid), rifampin, ethionamide,
 g. Antineoplastics: vincristine, vinblastine

V. Other medical conditions
 a. Diabetic neuropathy
 b. Postherpetic neuralgia

history and physical examination may disclose an identifiable syndrome (e.g., herpes zoster, bacterial infection, or neuropathy) that can be treated in a standard fashion (Kishore-Kumar et al., 1990; Watson et al., 1992). A routine pain history (Foley, 1985; Portenoy & Foley, 1989) may provide diagnostic clues to the nature of the underlying pain mechanisms and indeed may disclose other treatable disorders.

Consistent with any pain evaluation, it is key that the provider obtain a description of the qualitative features of the pain, its duration, and any behaviors that increase or decrease pain intensity. The provider should assess multidimensional indices of pain intensity (e.g., current, average, at best, at worst) to determine the need for weak *versus* potent analgesics and in order to serially evaluate the effectiveness of treatment. Pain descriptors (e.g., burning, shooting, dull, or sharp) can assist in identifying the mechanisms of pain (somatic, nociceptive, visceral nociceptive, or neuropathic) and may indicate the likelihood of response to various classes of traditional and adjuvant analgesics (e.g., nonsteroidal antiinflammatory drugs, opioids, antidepressants, anticonvulsants, oral local anesthetics, or corticosteroids; Jacox et al., 1994; Portenoy, 1990; WHO, 1986). Such clinical information, when integrated with results from medical, neurological, and psychological assessments (including a history of substance use or abuse), is the cornerstone of effective pain management.

Pharmacotherapies for HIV/AIDS Pain

The World Health Organization (WHO, 1986) has developed practice guidelines for the analgesic management of cancer pain that the Agency for Health Care Practice and Research (AHCPR) recommends for the management of pain related to cancer or AIDS (Jacox et al., 1994). These guidelines, also widely known as the WHO analgesic ladder, have been well validated in cancer populations (Ventafridda et al., 1990b). Although the WHO approach has not yet been validated in AIDS care, it has been recommended by the AHCPR, professional organizations including the American Pain Society (APS, 1992), and empirical studies (Jacox et al., 1994; Lebovits et al., 1989; Lefkowitz & Breitbart, 1992; O'Neill & Sherrard, 1993; Singer et al., 1993). Empirical research supports the successful application of the WHO principles to the management of pain in AIDS, particularly with opioids (Anand et al., 1994; Kimball & McCormick, 1996; Lefkowitz & Newshan, 1997; McCormack et al., 1993; Newshan & Wainapel, 1993; Patt & Reddy, 1993; Schofferman & Brody, 1990).

The WHO approach recommends selecting analgesics guided by the severity of pain (e.g., moderate or severe) and the type of pain (e.g., neuropathic or nonneuropathic). For pain of mild to moderate severity, nonopioid analgesics such as NSAIDS (nonsteroidal antiinflammatory drugs) and acetaminophen are the standard of care. For pain that is persistent and moderate to severe in intensity, opioid analgesics of increasing potency (such as morphine) should be used. Adjuvant agents, such as laxatives and psychostimulants, are useful in preventing and treating opioid adverse effects such as constipation or sedation respectively. Adjuvant analgesic drugs, such as the antidepressant analgesics, may be considered for use concurrently with opioids and NSAIDs in all stages of the analgesic ladder (mild, moderate, or severe pain) but have the most utility in the management of neuropathic pain.

Nonopioid Analgesics

The nonopioid analgesics (Table 40.1) are therapeutic options for mild to moderate pain intensity and for augmenting the effects of opioid analgesics in the treatment of severe pain. The use of NSAIDs in patients with AIDS must be accompanied by heightened awareness of toxicity and adverse effects. Patients with AIDS are at increased risk for renal toxicity related to NSAIDs, as these patients are frequently hypovolemic, on concurrent nephrotoxic drugs, and experiencing HIV nephropathy. The antipyretic effects of the NSAIDs may also interfere with early detection of infection in patients with AIDS. For more detailed information related to adverse events and potential contraindications to the use of NSAIDS in AIDS patients, the reader is referred to Murray and Brater (1990) and Radeck and Deck (1987).

Opioid Analgesics

Opioid analgesics are the cornerstone of pharmacologic treatment for moderate to severe pain intensity in the patient with HIV (Table 40.2). Further, opioid therapy may be safely and effectively used in the management of moderate to severe pain in patients with HIV, including patients with a history of injection drug use (IDU) as their HIV transmission factor (Anand et al., 1994; Kaplan et al., 1996; Kimball & McCormick, 1996; Lefkowitz & Newshan, 1997; Newshan & Lefkowitz, 2001; Newshan & Wainapel, 1993; Patt & Reddy, 1993). Of particular relevance to providers are findings indicating that transdermal fentanyl is effective for chronic pain in chemically dependent and nonchemically dependent AIDS patients (Newshan & Lefkowitz, 2001). (For a description of adverse effect management and other issues related to opioid therapy for pain, the reader is referred to Breitbart, 1989, 1992; Breitbart & Mermelstein, 1992; Bruera et al., 1987; Kaiko et al., 1983; Portenoy & Payne, 1990.)

Table 40.1. Oral Analgesics for Mild to Moderate Pain in AIDS

Analgesic (by class)	Dose (mg)	Duration (hours)	Plasma Half-Life (hours)	Comments
Nonsteroidal				
Aspirin	650	4–6	4–6	The standard for comparison among nonopioid analgesics
Ibuprofen	400–600			Like aspirin, can inhibit platelet function
Choline magnesium	700–1,500			Essentially no hematologic or gastrointestinal side effects; trisalicylate
Weaker Opioids				
Codeine	32–65	3–4		Metabolized to morphine, often used to suppress cough in patients at risk of pulmonary bleed
Oxycodone	5–10	3–4		Available as a single agent and acetaminophen
Propoxyphene	65–13	4–6		Toxic metabolite norpropoxy accumulates with repeated dosing

Table 40.2. Opioid Analgesics for Moderate to Severe Pain in AIDS

Analgesic	Equianalgesic Dose (mg)	Oral Morphine Equivalents (mg)	Duration (hours)	Plasma Half-Life (hours)	Comments
Morphine	30–60*(O) 10 (P)	30–60	4–6	2–3	Standard of comparison for the narcotic analgesics. *30 mg for repeat around-the-clock dosing; 60 mg for single dose or intermittent dosing.
Morphine (sustained release)	90–120 (O)	90–120	8–12	—	Now available in long acting, sustained-release forms.
Oxycodone	20–30 (O)	30–45	3–6	2–3	In combination with aspirin or acetaminophen, it is considered a weaker opioid; as a single agent, it is comparable to the strong opioids, like morphine. Available in immediate release and sustained-release preparation.
Oxycodone (sustained release)	20–40 (O)	30–60	8–12	2–3	
Hydromorphone	7.5 (O) 1.5 (P)	30–40 15–20	3–4 3–4	2–3 2–3	Short half-life; ideal for elderly patients. Comes in suppository and injectable forms.
Methadone	Variable	80	4–8	15–30	Long half-life; tends to accumulate with initial dosing; requires careful titration. Good oral potency.
Levorphanol	4 (O) (P)	30–60 30–60	3–6	12–16 12–16	Long half-life; requires careful dose titration in first week. Note that analgesic duration is only 4 hours.
Meperidine	300 (O) 75 (P)	30–60 30–60	3–6 3–4	3–4 3–4	Active toxic metabolite, or meperidine, tends to accumulate, especially with renal impairment and in elderly patients.
Fentanyl	0.1	24–30	48–72	20–22	Transdermal patch is convenient, bypassing GI analgesia until depot is formed. Unsuitable for rapid titration.

(O) = oral; (P) = parenteral.

** Oral morphine equivalents are estimated ranges calculated based on Pereira J, Lawlor P, Vigano A, Dorgan M, Bruera E. Equianalgesic dose ratios for opioids: a critical review and proposals for long-term dosing. *J Pain Symptom Manage*, 22:672–87, 2001.

Adjuvant Analgesics

Adjuvant analgesics are the third class of medications frequently prescribed for the treatment of chronic pain and have important applications in the management of AIDS pain (Table 40.3). Commonly used adjuvant drugs include: antidepressants, neuroleptics, psychostimulants, anticonvulsants, corticosteroids and oral and topical local anesthetics (Breitbart, 1992; Breitbart & Mermelstein, 1992; Jacox et al., 1994; Portenoy, 1998). Adjuvant analgesic drugs are used to enhance the analgesic effects of opioids, treat concurrent symptoms that exacerbate pain, and provide independent analgesia. They may be used across all stages of the WHO analgesic ladder.

Antidepressants

The analgesic efficacy of antidepressants has been demonstrated across a spectrum of clinical pain syndromes, with the use of antidepressants indicated in the treatment of virtually every type of chronic pain disorder (Portenoy, 1998). For populations with high rates of neuropathic pain (Max et al., 1987; Sindrup et al., 1990), such as AIDS patients, antidepressants may be particularly useful (Portenoy, 1998). Although the efficacy of antidepressants in treating HIV-related painful neuropathies has not yet been conclusively demonstrated, they are widely used to manage diabetic and postherpetic neuropathies. In particular, Duloxetine, an antidepressant with potent dual reuptake inhibition of serotonin and norepinephrine, is a potent analgesic shown to be effective in treating fibromyalgia and diabetic neuropathy (Goldstein et al., 2005) prompting its widespread use in AIDS-related neuropathies.

Neuroleptics and Benzodiazepines

Neuroleptic drugs, including methotrimeprazine, fluphenazine, haloperidol, pimozide, and olanzapine may be effective adjuvant analgesics (Goldstein et al., 2005; Gomez-Perez et al., 1985; Khojainova et al., 2002; Lechin et al., 1989; Maltbie et al., 1979) in AIDS patients with pain. However, their benefits must be weighed against an increased sensitivity to the extrapyramidal effects in AIDS patients with neurological complications (Breitbart et al., 1988). Anxiolytics, such as alprazolam and clonazepam, may also be useful as adjuvant analgesics, particularly in the management of neuropathic pain (Caccia, 1975; Swerdlow & Cundhill, 1981).

Psychostimulants

Psychostimulants, including dextroamphetamine, methylphenidate, pemoline, and modafinil, also augment the analgesic effects of opioids (Bruera et al., 1989), counter sedation (Bruera et al., 1987), and produce antidepressant effects (Breitbart et al., 1988; Bruera et al., 1987). Further, providers may consider pemoline as a therapeutic option for the patient with a substance abuse history. Advantages of pemoline in AIDS pain patients with a substance abuse history include the lack of abuse potential, the lack of federal regulation through special triplicate prescriptions, the mild sympathomimetic effects, and the fact that it comes in a chewable tablet form that can be absorbed through the buccal mucosa. Relatedly, modafinil does not cause tolerance or dependence, has a low abuse potential, and does not require a special triplicate prescription.

Table 40.3. Psychotropic Adjuvant Analgesic Drugs for AIDS Pain

Generic Name	Dose (mg)	Generic Name	Dose (mg)
Tricyclic Antidepressants		**Butyrophenones**	
Amitriptyline	10–150	Haloperidol	1–3
Nortriptyline	10–150	Pimozide	2–6 bid
Imipramine	15.5–150		
Desipramine	10–150	**Atypical Antipsychotics**	
Clomipramine	10–150	Olanzapine	2.5–20
Doxepin	12–150		
Heterocyclic and Noncyclic Antidepressants		**Antihistamines**	
Trazodone	125–300	Hydroxyzine	50 q4h–q6h
Maprotiline	50–300	**Anticonvulsants**	
Serotonin Reuptake Inhibitors		Carbamazepine	200 tid–400 tid
Fluoxetine	20–80	Phenytoin	300–400
Paroxetine	10–60	Valproate	500 tid–1,000 tid
Sertraline	50–200	Gabapentin	300 tid–1,000 tid
Newer Agents		Pregabalin	150–600
Nefazodone	100–500	**Oral Local Anesthetics**	
Venlafaxine	75–300	Mexiletine	600–900
Mirtazapine	15–60	**Topical Local Anesthetics**	
Duloxetine	60–120	Lidocaine	5% (patch)
Psychostimulants		**Corticosteroids**	
Methylphenidate	2.5–20 bid	Dexamethasone	4–16
Dextroamphetamine	2.5–20 bid		
Pemoline	13.75–75 bid	**Benzodiazepines**	
Modafinil	100–400	Alprazolam	0.25–2.0 tid
Phenothiazines		Clonazepam	0.5–4 bid
Fluphenazine	1–3		
Methotrimeprazine	10–20 q6h		

q4h = every 4 hours; q6h = every 6 hours; bid = twice a day; tid = three times a day; qid = four times a day.

Anticonvulsant Drugs

Specific anticonvulsant drugs may have analgesic effects, particularly for neuropathic pain characterized by lancinating dysesthesias (Portenoy, 1998). In addition, anticonvulsant drugs potentially useful for managing neuropathic pain in AIDS patients include carbamazepine, phenytoin, clonazepam, valproate and gabapentin (Portenoy, 1998), pregabalin (Freynhagen et al., 2005), and baclofen.

Corticosteroids

Corticosteroid drugs have analgesic potential for a variety of chronic pain syndromes, including neuropathic pain and pain syndromes resulting from inflammatory processes (Portenoy, 1998). Like other adjuvant analgesics, corticosteroids are usually added to an opioid regimen. In patients with advanced disease, these drugs may also improve appetite, nausea, malaise and overall quality of life, benefits that must be balanced with their adverse effects.

Oral and Topical Local Anesthetics

Local anesthetic drugs, including oral tocainide (Lyndstrom & Lindbloom, 1987), mexiletine (Portenoy, 1998), flecainide (Dunlop et al., 1989), and subcutaneous lidocaine (Brose & Cousins, 1991), have shown efficacy in the management of neuropathic pain (Devers & Galer, 2000) characterized by either continuous or lancinating dysesthesias (Paice et al., 2000). Specific findings indicate that capsaicin is ineffective in relieving pain with HIV-associated distal symmetrical peripheral neuropathy (DSPN), but *is* effective in relieving pain associated with other neuropathic pain syndromes (Paice et al., 2000). Presently, no controlled trials have yet been published in HIV-related neuropathies.

Nonpharmacologic Therapies for AIDS Pain

Physical and behavioral therapies may also prove useful in the management of HIV-related pain. Physical interventions range from bed rest and simple exercise programs to the application of cold packs or heat to affected sites. Other nonpharmacologic interventions include whirlpool baths, massage, the application of ultrasound, and transcutaneous electrical nerve stimulation (TENS). Increasing numbers of AIDS patients are using acupuncture to relieve their pain, with anecdotal reports of efficacy. Several behavioral interventions have demonstrated efficacy in alleviating HIV-related pain, including cognitive-behavioral therapy, hypnosis, progressive muscle relaxation therapy, and distraction techniques such as biofeedback and imagery. When nonpharmacologic and standard pharmacologic treatments fail, anesthetic and even neurosurgical procedures (such as nerve block, cordotomy, and epidural delivery of analgesics) are additional options available to the patient who appreciates the risks and limitations of these procedures.

Barriers to Pain Management in HIV/AIDS Care

The undertreatment of pain in AIDS patients is widely documented (e.g., Lebovits et al., 1989; McCormack et al., 1993). Current findings indicate that all classes of analgesics, particularly opioids, are underutilized in the treatment of pain in AIDS (Breitbart et al., 1996a, 1996b; Larue et al., 1997). Based on the WHO guidelines, analgesic therapy may be adequate for only a minority (15%) of patients treated (Breitbart et al., 1996b).

Multiple patient-, provider-, and system-related barriers are related to the undertreatment of pain in AIDS (Breitbart et al., 1998, 1999; Breitbart et al., 1996b). With regard to patient-related factors, women, patients with less education, and patients with a substance abuse history are more likely to have their pain inadequately managed (Breitbart et al., 1996b). Further, patient reluctance to report pain or take opioid analgesics is associated with the undertreatment of pain, including fears about the addiction potential of opioids, adverse effects, and fears and misconceptions about tolerance (Breitbart et al., 1998). AIDS patients also report limiting their intake of medications (e.g., pills) and relying on nonpharmacologic interventions for pain (Breitbart et al., 1998). Economic and social barriers, including an inability to afford prescription medication, lack of access to pain specialists, and fears that family, friends, and physicians will assume they are misusing or abusing these drugs are also significant barriers associated with undertreatment of pain (Breitbart et al., 1998). Several of these barriers to adequate pain management are reiterated by providers, with many who perceive pain management to be the most important aspect of care of AIDS patients (Breitbart et al., 1999). Provider-related barriers include perceived lack of knowledge, reluctance to prescribe opioids, lack of access to pain specialists, fears regarding drug addiction and/or abuse, and lack of psychological support/drug treatment services (Breitbart et al., 1999).

Prevalence of Current or Past Substance Abuse Problems in HIV/AIDS Patients

Perhaps most relevant to the clinical problem of pain management in HIV/AIDS patients is the growing segment of patients who have a history of substance abuse or who are actively abusing drugs. Approximately 40% of HIV/AIDS patients in the United States have a history of substance abuse, and 12% have a comorbid substance abuse disorder (Bing et al., 2001; Lucas et al., 2006). Further, about 36% of all HIV cases in the United States are caused by injection drug use (IDU) (CDC, 2002; UNAIDS/WHO, 2004). According to the CDC, IDU is the second most common form of AIDS exposure among adults in the United States, and has shown the highest rate of increase compared to other forms of AIDS exposure for the past 5 years, particularly in large urban areas.

Adequacy of Pain Management in Patients With Substance Abuse Problems

Current evidence indicates that HIV/AIDS patients with a history of substance abuse are more likely to have their pain inadequately managed than HIV/AIDS patients without a history of substance abuse (e.g., Breitbart, 1997; Breitbart et al., 1997). In a large cross-sectional study of 516 ambulatory AIDS patients, pain and the adequacy of pain management was compared in current and past substance abusers (Breitbart et al., 1997). No significant differences in the report of pain experience (i.e., pain prevalence, pain intensity, and pain-related functional interference) were observed among patients who acknowledged current substance abuse, those in methadone maintenance, and those in drug-free recovery (Breitbart et al., 1997). Furthermore, there were no differences in pain experience among those who reported IDU as their HIV-transmission factor and those who reported other transmission factors (non-IDU; Breitbart et al., 1997). Hence, the description of HIV-related pain was comparable among IDU and non-IDU groups.

What was different was the treatment received by these two groups. Patients in the IDU group were significantly more undermedicated for pain compared to the non-IDU group (Breitbart, 1997; Breitbart et al., 1997). In a study of 211 HIV patients, pain was compared in HIV patients with and without a current history of IDU (Martin et al., 1999). In the non-IDU group, there was a strong positive association among pain and disease stage, CD4 levels, and mortality rates (Martin et al., 1999). However, pain in the IDU group was significantly higher than in the non-IDU group; further, pain was not significantly associated with disease severity (Martin et al., 1999). As such, there may be a need to differentiate and address pain in patients with different HIV transmission risk factors and psychosocial characteristics (Martin et al., 1999).

Barriers to Pain Management in Patients With Substance Abuse Problems

Multiple patient-, provider-, and system-based factors may *lead* to barriers in the delivery of pain interventions for HIV/AIDS patients with substance abuse histories and the uptake of treatment recommendations. Substance abusers with HIV/AIDS are less likely to have consistent access to health care, yet they are most likely to suffer the greatest burden of disease, including advanced clinical stage and the presence of wasting syndrome (Tsao et al., 2005). In addition to barriers to treatment seeking among this underserved population, there may also be a reluctance or bias on the part of the provider to assume care for patients with substance abuse problems (Gerbert et al., 1999; Weinberger et al., 1992). Indeed, attitudes and perceptions about substance-abusing HIV/AIDS patients held by the public may play a role in treatment-seeking. Studies show that injection drug users are more vulnerable to HIV-related stigma by the general population when they are compared to patients who contracted HIV through blood transfusions or "benign" transmission modalities (Herek, 1990). HIV-related stigma has been shown to affect patients' decision making to seek treatment and adherence with health care (Chesney & Smith, 1999). Additional barriers to pain management include patient- and provider-related fears that narcotic analgesics will trigger the relapse of an addictive disorder or drug abuse problem and will further exacerbate a substance abuse problem. These fears may lead to the undermedication of HIV patients with pain. For many of these reasons, substance abusers with HIV/AIDS are a vulnerable and underserved subpopulation of pain patients.

Pain management in the substance-abusing HIV/AIDS patient is perhaps the most challenging of clinical goals. Perhaps the greatest barrier to providers is their perceived ability to develop trust and foster an alliance with the substance-abusing patient.

Concerns are often raised regarding the credibility of AIDS patients' report of pain, particularly when there is a history of IDU (Breitbart et al., 1997). On one hand, providers must address the possibility that they are being manipulated by a substance-abusing patient complaining of pain. On the other hand, providers must rely on a patient's subjective report, which is often the best or only indication of the presence and intensity of pain, and the degree of analgesia provided by an intervention. Providers who believe they are being manipulated by drug-seeking patients often hesitate to use appropriately high doses of narcotic analgesics to control pain. The fear is that the provider is being "conned" into prescribing narcotic analgesics that will then be abused or diverted. Clearly, providers do not want to contribute to or sustain addiction. However, we believe that this concern often leads to a "knee-jerk defensiveness" on the part of the provider, and a tendency to avoid prescribing opioids and even a full assessment of the pain complaint.

Unfortunately, the presence or severity of pain cannot be objectively proven. Our stance is that the provider should accept and respect the report of pain despite the possibility of manipulation by the patient and proceed in the evaluation, assessment, and management of pain. Additionally, pain in the substance-abusing HIV/AIDS patient is complex. However, empirical findings from the cancer pain literature suggests that it is possible to effectively manage pain in substance abusers with life-threatening illness and to safely and responsibly prescribe opioid analgesics based on several sound principles of pain management outlined in the sections below and Box 40.3 (Macaluso et al., 1988; McCaffery & Vourakis, 1992; Portenoy & Payne, 1992). Furthermore, experience has shown that known addicts can benefit from the carefully supervised, judicious use of opioids for the treatment of pain due to cancer, surgery, or recurrent painful illnesses such as sickle cell disease.

Effective Strategies for Managing Pain in HIV/AIDS Patients With Substance Abuse Problems

The use of opioids for pain control in patients with HIV/AIDS and a history of substance abuse raises several difficult pain treatment questions, including the following: how to treat pain in HIV/AIDS

Box 40.3 An Approach to Pain Management in Substance Abusers With HIV/AIDS

- Substance abusers with HIV/AIDS deserve pain control; we have an obligation to treat pain and suffering in all of our patients.
- Accept and respect the report of pain.
- Be careful when labeling substance abuse; distinguish between tolerance, physical dependence, and addictions (psychological dependence or drug abuse).
- Not all substance abusers are the same; distinguish between active users, individuals in methadone maintenance, and those in recovery.
- Tailor pain treatment based on medical and psychosocial characteristics.
- Utilize the principles of pain management outlined for all patients with HIV/AIDS and pain (e.g., WHO ladder).
- Set clear goals and conditions for opioid therapy: Set behavioral limits, recognize drug abuse behaviors, make consequences clear, use written contracts, and establish a single prescriber.
- Use a multidimensional approach incorporating appropriate pharmacologic and nonpharmacologic interventions; address psychosocial problems using multidisciplinary health-care providers.

patients who have a high tolerance to narcotic analgesics, how to mitigate possible drug seeking or potentially manipulative behavior, how to deal with patients who may offer unreliable medical histories or who may not adhere with treatment recommendations, and how to counter the risk of patients spreading HIV while high and disinhibited.

How to Mitigate Possible Drug-Seeking or Potentially Manipulative behavior

Managing pain in patients with substance abuse problems is best achieved by setting clear expectations, directives, and behavioral limits. Although this is an important aspect of the care of intravenous drug-using patients with HIV/AIDS, it is not entirely sufficient. As much as possible, providers should also attempt to eliminate or reduce drug abuse as an obstacle to pain management by dealing directly with the problems of opiate withdrawal and drug treatment. Providers should err on the side of believing patients when they complain of pain, and should use knowledge of specific HIV-related pain syndromes to corroborate the report of a patient perceived as being unreliable.

As such, setting realistic goals for pain management in patients with a current or recent history of substance abuse problems is helpful. This includes anticipating problems related to prescriptions (i.e., requests for more medication or dose escalations prior to the next scheduled visit) and planning for subsequent interactions between the patient and staff. Other providers involved in the patient's care may benefit from education and awareness highlighting that patients with difficult and stigmatized behaviors often elicit feelings from others that could interfere with providing good care. A focus on the development of clear behavioral limits is helpful for both the patient and staff. Written rules and contracts about what behaviors are expected, and what behaviors are not tolerated and the consequence, should be provided to patients and members of the pain team. For example, the use of urine toxicology monitoring, unannounced pill counts, and strict limits on the amount of drug per prescription can all be very useful strategies, as discussed in Chapter 38, "Management of Pain in Chemical Dependency in the Primary Care Clinic," and Chapter 42, "Urine Drug Testing in Pain and Addiction Medicine," in this book. Consistent monitoring and documenting of the efficacy of pain interventions can be useful in forming diagnostic impressions and corroborating pain recommendations. In particular, the provider should assess patient understanding with changes in opioid regimes and monitor adherence when changing routes of opioid administration or tapering opioids. It must be made clear to patients what drugs and/or regimen would be introduced to control pain when opioids are tapered or withdrawn, and what options are available if that nonopioid regimen is ineffective. If an acute medical condition or crisis should be present, once the crisis has resolved, rehabilitation or detoxification from opioids is appropriate.

How to Treat Pain in HIV/AIDS Patients Who Have a High Tolerance to Narcotic Analgesics

When managing pain in HIV/AIDS patients with current or past substance abuse problems, the provider must understand the current terminology relevant to substance abuse and addiction. It is important to distinguish among the phenomena of *tolerance*, *physical dependence*, and *addiction* or *abuse* (psychological dependence). By definition, tolerance is a pharmacologic property of opioid drugs observed by the need for increasing doses to maintain an (analgesic) effect. Next, physical dependence is characterized by the onset of signs and symptoms of withdrawal if narcotic analgesics are abruptly stopped or if a narcotic antagonist is administered. Tolerance usually occurs in association with physical dependence. Further, addiction is a "primary, chronic, neurobiological disease, with genetic, psychosocial, and environmental factors influencing its development and manifestations. It is characterized by behaviors that include one or more of the following: impaired control over drug use, compulsive use, continued use despite harm, and craving" (American Academy of Pain Medicine, 2001). One of the primary criteria for diagnosing addiction includes the presence of aberrant drug-taking behaviors (see Chapter 48, "Aberrant Drug-Taking: Empirical Studies and Clinical Application"). Finally, in contrast to substance use disorders, pseudoaddiction describes pain patients who appear to be drug seeking and who try to increase their medication use due to inadequate pain relief. Although patients with pseudoaddiction display behaviors perceived as aberrant, these behaviors are motivated by the undertreatment of pain. Importantly, these aberrant behaviors cease when adequate analgesia is achieved (Weissman & Haddox, 1989).

Based on these concepts, it is not surprising that studies show that AIDS patients with previous drug use histories experience opioid analgesia but require substantially more morphine than patients without drug use histories (Kaplan et al., 2000). Providers can apply specific strategies for managing patients with substance abuse histories. We first recommend that providers differentiate risk potential for analgesic abuse based on current or past or drug use and their status in ongoing drug rehabilitation and recovery. Specifically, the provider must distinguish between the "former" addict who has been drug-free for years, the recovering addict in a methadone maintenance program, and the addict who is actively abusing illicit and/or prescription drugs. Actively using addicts and those on methadone maintenance with pain must be assumed to have some physiologic tolerance to opioids and may require higher starting and maintenance doses of opioids.

As stated above, preventing withdrawal is an essential first step in managing pain in this population. Further, "active" addicts with HIV/AIDS will require psychosocial support, including intervention with an addictions medicine specialist to adequately treat substance abuse problems and possible pain-related distress using pharmacologic therapy and/or individual or group psychotherapy. Because patients with a history of drug addiction may have concerns about the use of opioids for pain related to fears of relapse, we recommend that patients be assured of the safety and efficacy of opioids for pain. Opioids, when prescribed and monitored responsibly, can be an essential and safe part of pain management. Further, it is important to provide psychoeducation highlighting differences in the use of the drug for pain *versus* the use of the drug for psychological effects in the absence of pain. Patients should be reassured that the physician will offer consistent monitoring of their progress on opioids and assess their adherence with opioid therapy.

Further, the assessment of pain symptoms and potential etiology is essential in AIDS care, particularly in the substance abuser. Thus, AIDS pain specialists have emphasized the importance of conducting and documenting a comprehensive pain assessment to identify the pain syndrome. As reviewed in the previous section "Pharmacotherapies for HIV/AIDS Pain," certain pain syndromes often respond best to specific interventions (i.e., neuropathic pains respond well to antidepressants or anticonvulsants). It is critical that adequate analgesia be provided while diagnostic studies are underway. If the pain is secondary to a medical condition, pain treatments targeted at the condition may be effective. For example, headache from CNS toxoplasmosis responds well to primary treatments and steroids.

Selection of an appropriate pharmacotherapy for pain management should be guided by the WHO analgesic ladder. This approach is guided by the severity (e.g., moderate or severe) and type of pain syndrome (e.g., neuropathic or nonneuropathic) in selecting analgesics. For mild to moderate pain, NSAIDs are recommended. The NSAIDs are continued with adjuvant analgesics (antidepressants, anticonvulsants, neuroleptics, steroids) if a specific indication exists. Patients with moderate to severe pain, or those who do not achieve relief from NSAIDs, are treated with a "weak" opioid, often in combination with NSAIDs and adjuvant drugs, if indicated. However, the guidelines also suggest that based on the type of pain experienced and the severity, opioids are not to be thought of as a treatment of "last resort." Because findings suggest that AIDS patients with prior drug use histories experience opioid analgesia but require substantially more morphine than patients without drug use histories (Kaplan et al., 2000), agonist-antagonist opioid drugs should be avoided. Although providers must evaluate the risks and benefits of individual therapeutic options and ultimately decide on a specific drug therapy, every effort should be made to give patients more of a sense of control and a sense of collaboration with the provider. However, the use of PRN dosing may be trigger for frequent patient and provider interactions that are a burden on time and staff productivity. As always, a patient's report of beneficial or adverse effects of a specific agent is useful to the provider.

How to Counter the Risk of Patients' Spreading HIV While High and Disinhibited

A multidisciplinary approach is indicated when managing pain in substance abusing HIV/AIDS patients. Collaboration among pain specialists, mental health care providers, and addictions medicine specialists is essential to achieving the best pain outcomes.

Substance abusers with HIV/AIDS have high rates of comorbid psychiatric disorders and multiple physical symptoms that can complicate pain and psychosocial outcomes. The management of psychological distress and other comorbid disorders requires ongoing assessment and treatment, including referral to a mental health care professional.

Conclusion

The rates and duration of survival for the majority of persons diagnosed with HIV in the United States have increased remarkably in the past decade and will continue to rise. Pain rates among the rising population of HIV/AIDS patients are high. Furthermore, HIV/AIDS patients have high rates of current or past substance. Thus, pain management in the growing subgroup of HIV/AIDS patients with current of past substance abuse problems is important to public health. However, substance abusers in this population are a vulnerable and undertreated subgroup of pain patients. HIV/AIDS patients with a history of substance abuse are more likely to have their pain inadequately managed compared to HIV/AIDS patients without a history of substance abuse. Further, patients with substance abuse problems suffer the greatest burden of disease, including advanced clinical stage and the presence of wasting syndrome.

Managing pain in HIV/AIDS patients is a challenging clinical problem that health-care providers will be facing with increasing frequency. Pain syndromes in AIDS/HIV patients with substance abuse histories can be adequately treated with efficacious behavioral and supportive strategies that address barriers to pain care. Interventions that focus on tailoring treatments to this heterogeneous group can be effective with providers' use of serial assessments to monitor narcotic medication use and efficacy suggested. Strategies to promote patients' adherence with pain recommendations and alliance with the entire health-care team can effectively enhance the quality of pain care for HIV/AIDS pain patients with substance abuse problems.

References

American Academy of Pain Medicine, American Pain Society, and the American Society of Addiction Medicine. *Definitions related to the use of opioids for the treatment of pain: A consensus document.* (2001). Retrieved February 21, 2006, from http:#x002F;/www.ampainsoc.org/advocacy/opioids2.

American Pain Society. *Principles of Analgesic Use in the Treatment of Acute Pain and Cancer Pain* (3rd ed.). Skokie, IL: American Pain Society, 1992.

Anand A, Carmosino L, Glatt A. Evaluation of recalcitrant pain in HIV-infected hospitalized patients. *J Acquired Immune Deficiency Syndromes,* 7:52–56, 1994.

Bing E, Burnam A, Longshore D, Fleishman J, Sherbourne C, London A, Turner B, Eggan F, Beckman R, Vitiello B, Morton S, Orlando M, Bozzette S, Ortiz-Barron L, Shapiro M. Psychiatric disorders and drug use among human immunodeficiency virus-infected adults in the United States. *Archives of General Psychiatry,* 58(8): 721–728, Aug 2001.

Breitbart W. Pain in AIDS. In J Jensen, J Turner, Z Wiesenfeld-Hallin (eds.), *Proceedings of the 8th World Congress on Pain, Progress in Pain Research and Management,* Vol. 8. Seattle, WA: IASP Press, 63–100, 1997.

Breitbart W. Pain in HIV disease. In O'Neil J (ed.), *A Clinical Guide to Supportive & Palliative Care for HIV/AIDS.* Rockville, MD: U.S. Dept. of Health and Human Services, Health Resources and Services Administration (HRSA) HIV/AIDS Bureau, pp. 85–122, 2003.

Breitbart W. Psychiatric management of cancer pain. *Cancer,* 63:2336–2342, 1989.

Breitbart W. Psychotropic adjuvant analgesics for cancer pain. *Psycho-Oncology,* 7:133–145, 1992.

Breitbart W, Kaim M, Rosenfeld B. Clinician's perceptions of barriers to pain management in AIDS. *J Pain Symptom Manage,* 18:203–212, 1999.

Breitbart W, Marotta R, Call P. AIDS and neuroleptic malignant syndrome. *Lancet,* 2:1488, 1988.

Breitbart W, McDonald M, Rosenfeld B, Passik S, Hewitt D, Thaler H, Portenoy R. Pain in ambulatory AIDS patients—I: Pain characteristics and medical correlates. *Pain,* 68: 315–321, 1996a.

Breitbart W, Mermelstein H. Pemoline: an alternative psychostimulant in the management of depressive disorder in cancer patients. *Psychosomatics,* 33: 352–356, 1992.

Breitbart W, Passik S, McDonald M, Rosenfeld B, Smith M, Kaim M, Funesti-Esch J. Patient-related barriers to pain management in ambulatory AIDS patients. *Pain,* 76:9–16, 1998.

Breitbart W, Rosenfeld B, Passik S, Kaim M, Funesti-Esch J, Stein K. A comparison of pain report and adequacy of analgesic therapy in ambulatory AIDS patients with and without a history of substance abuse. *Pain,* 72:235–243, 1997.

Breitbart W, Rosenfeld B, Passik S, McDonald M, Thaler H, Portenoy R. The undertreatment of pain in ambulatory AIDS patients. *Pain,* 65:239–245, 1996b.

Brose WG, Cousins MJ. Subcutaneous lidocaine for treatment of neuropathic cancer pain. *Pain,* 45(2):145–148, 1991.

Bruera E, Breuneis C, Patterson AH, MacDonald RN. Use of methylphenidate as an adjuvant to narcotic analgesics in patients with advanced cancer. *Journal of Pain and Symptom Management,* 4:3–6, 1989.

Bruera E, Chadwick S, Brennels C, Hanson J, MacDonald RN. Methylphenidate associated with narcotics for the treatment of cancer pain. *Cancer Treat Rep.,* 71:67–70, 1987.

Caccia M. Clonazepam in facial neuralgia and cluster headache: clinical and electrophysiological study. *Eur Neurol,* 13:560–563, 1975.

Centers for Disease Control and Prevention. *Drug-Associated HIV Transmission Continues in the United States.* Atlanta, GA: National Center for HIV, STD and TB Prevention Divisions of HIV/AIDS Prevention, 2002.

Centers for Disease Control and Prevention. *HIV/AIDS Surveillance Report, 2004.* Vol. 16. Atlanta, GA: U.S. Department of Health and Human Services, Centers for Disease Control and Prevention, 2005. Also available at: http://www.cdc.gov/hiv/stats/hasrlink.htm.

Chesney M, Smith A. Critical delays in HIV testing and care: the potential role of stigma. *Am Behav Scientist,* 42(7):1162–1174, 1999.

Devers A, Galer B. Topical lidocaine patch relieves a variety of neuropathic pain conditions: an open label study. *Clinical Journal of Pain,* 16:205–208, 2000.

Dobalian A, Tsao J, Duncan R. Pain and the use of outpatient services among persons with HIV: results from a nationally representative survey. *Med Care,* 422:129–138, 2004.

Dunlop R, Davies R, Hockley J, Turner P. Letter to the editor. *Lancet,* 1:420–421, 1989.

Foley KM. The treatment of cancer pain. *N Engl J Med,* 313:84–95, 1985.

Freynhagen R, Strojek K, Griesing T, Whalen E, Balkenohl M. Efficacy of pregabalin in neuropathic pain evaluated in a 12 week, randomized, double-blind, multicentre, placebo-controlled trial of flexible- and fixed-dose regimens. *Pain,* 115: 254–263, 2005.

Gerbert B, Maguire BT, Bleeker T, Coates TJ, McPhee SJ. Primary care physicians and AIDS: attitudinal and structural barriers to care. *JAMA,* 266:2837–2842, 1999.

Goldstein D, Lu Y, Detke M, Lee T, Iyengar S. Duloxetine vs. placebo in patients with diabetic neuropathy. *Pain,* 116: 109–118, 2005.

Gomez-Perez F, Rull J, Dies H, et al. Nortriptyline and fluphenazine in the symptomatic treatment of diabetic neuropathy: A double-blind cross-over study. *Pain,* 23:395–400, 1985.

Herek G. Illness, stigma and AIDS. In VandenBos GR (ed.), *Psychological Aspects of Serious Illness.* Washington, DC: American Psychological Association, 1990.

Hewitt D, McDonald M, Portenoy R, Rosenfeld B, Passik S, Breitbart W. Pain syndromes and etiologies in ambulatory AIDS patients. *Pain,* 70:117–123, 1997.

Jacox A, Carr D, Payne R, Berde CB, Breitbart W, et al. *Clinical Practice Guideline Number 9: Management of Cancer Pain.* Rockville, MD: U.S. Department of Health and Human Services, Public Health Service, Agency for Health Care Policy and Research, AHCPR Publication No. 94–0592:139–41, 1994.

Kaiko R, Foley K, Grabinski P, et al. Central nervous system excitation effects of meperidine in cancer patients. *Ann Neurol,* 13:180–183, 1983.

Kaplan R, Conant M, Cundiff D, Maciewicz R, Ries K, Slagle S, Slywka J, Buckley B. Sustained-release morphine sulfate in the management of pain associated with acquired immune deficiency syndrome. *J Pain Symptom Manage,* 12:150–160, 1996.

Kaplan R, Slywka J, Slagle S, Ries K. A titrated morphine analgesic regimen comparing substance users and non-users with AIDS-related pain. *J Pain Symptom Manage,* 19:265–273, 2000.

Khojainova N, Santiago-Palma J, Kornick C, Breitbart W, Gonzales GR. Olanzapine in the management of cancer pain. *Journal of Pain and Symptom Management,* 23:346–350, 2002.

Kimball L, McCormick WC. The pharmacologic management of pain and discomfort in persons with AIDS near the end of life: use of opioid analgesia in the hospice setting. *J Pain Symptom Manage,* 11:88–94, 1996.

Kishore-Kumar R, Max M, Scafer SC, et al. Desipramine relieves post-herpetic neuralgia. *Clinical Pharmacological Therapy,* 47:305–312, 1990.

Larue F, Brasseur L, Musseault P, Demeulemeester R, Bonifassi L, Bez G. Pain and HIV infection: A French national survey [Abstract]. *Journal of Palliative Care,* 10:95, 1994.

Larue F, Fontaine A, Colleau S. Underestimation and undertreatment of pain in HIV disease: multicentre study. *British Medical Journal,* 314:23–28, 1997.

Lebovits A, Lefkowitz M, McCarthy D, et al. The prevalence and management of pain in patients with AIDS. A review of 134 cases. *The Clinical Journal of Pain,* 5:245–248, 1989.

Lechin F, Vander Dijs B, Lechin M, et al. Pimozide therapy for trigeminal neuralgia. *Arch Neurol,* 9:960–964, 1989.

Lefkowitz M, Breitbart W. Chronic pain and AIDS. In RH Wiener (ed.), *Innovations in Pain Medicine,* 36:2–3, 18, 1992.

Lefkowitz M, Newshan G. An evaluation of the use of Duragesic for chronic pain in patients with AIDS [Abstract]. *Proceedings of the 16th Annual Scientific Meeting of the American Pain Society* (Oct. 23–26, 1997, New Orleans, LA), p. 68.

Lucas GM, Griswold M, Gebo KA, Keruly J, Chaisson RE, and Moore RD. Illicit drug use and HIV-1 disease progression: a longitudinal study in the era of highly active antiretroviral therapy. *American Journal of Epidemiology,* 163(5):412–420, 2006.

Lyndstrom P, Lindbloom T. The analgesic tocainide for trigeminal neuralgia. *Pain,* 28:45–50, 1987.

Macaluso C, Weinberg D, Foley K. Opioid abuse and misuse in a cancer pain population. *J Pain and Sympt Manag,* 3:54, 1988.

Maltbie A, Cavenar S, Sullivan J, et al. Analgesia and haloperidol: a hypothesis. *Journal Can Psychiat,* 40:323–326, 1979.

Martin C, Pehrsson P, Osterberg A, et al. Pain in ambulatory HIV-infected patients with and without intravenous drug use. *Euro J Pain,* 3:157–164, 1999.

Max M, Culnane M, Schafer S, Gracely R, et al. Amitriptyline relieves diabetic neuropathy pain in patients with normal and depressed mood. *Neurology,* 37:589–596, 1987.

McCaffery M, Vourakis C. Assessment and relief of pain in chemically dependent patients. *Orthopedic Nursing,* 11:13–27, 1992.

McCormack JP, Li R, Zarowny D., Singer J. Inadequate treatment of pain in ambulatory HIV patients. *Clinical Journal of Pain,* 9:247–283, 1993.

Murray MD, Brater DC. Adverse effects of nonsteroidal anti-inflammatory drugs on renal function. *Annals of Internal Medicine,* 112:559–560, 1990.

Newshan G, Lefkowitz M. Transdermal fentanyl for chronic pain in AIDS: a pilot study. *J Pain Symptom Manage,* 21: 69–77, 2001.

Newshan G, Wainapel S. Pain characteristics and their management in persons with AIDS. *JANAC,* 53–59, 1993.

O'Neill WM, Sherrard JS. Pain in human immunodeficiency virus disease: a review. *Pain,* 54:3–14, 1993.

Paice J, Ferrans CE, Lahley FR, et al. Topical capsaicin in the management of HIV-associated peripheral neuropathy. *J Pain Symptom Manage,* 19:45–52, 2000.

Patt RB, Reddy SR: Pain and the opioid analgesics: alternate routes of administration. *PAACNOTES,* Nov:453–458, 1993.

Penfold R, Clark AJM. Pain syndromes in HIV infection. *Can J Anaesth,* 39:724–730, 1992.

Portenoy RK. Adjuvant analgesics in pain management. In D Doyle, GWC Hanks, N MacDonald (eds.), *Oxford Textbook of Palliative Medicine* (2nd ed.) New York: Oxford University Press, pp. 361–390, 1998.

Portenoy RK. Pharmacologic approaches to the control of cancer pain. *J Psychosocial Oncology,* 8:75–107, 1990.

Portenoy R, Foley KM. Management of cancer pain. In JC Holland, JH Rowland (eds.), *Handbook of Psychooncology.* New York: Oxford University Press, pp. 369–382, 1989.

Portenoy RK, Payne R. Acute and chronic pain. In JH Lowinson, P Ruiz, RB Millman (eds.), *Comprehensive Textbook of Substance Abuse.* Baltimore, MD: Williams and Wilkins, pp. 691–721, 1992.

Radeck K, Deck C. Do nonsteroidal anti-inflammatory drugs interfere with blood pressure control in hypertensive patients? *J Gen Int Med,* 2:108–112, 1987.

Schofferman J, Brody R. Pain in far advanced AIDS. In KM Foley et al. (eds.), *Advances in Pain Research and Therapy,* Vol. 16. New York: Raven Press, Ltd., pp. 379–386, 1990.

Sindrup SH, Gram LF, Brosen K, Eshoj O, Mogenson EF. The selective serotonin reuptake inhibitor paroxetine is effective in the treatment of diabetic neuropathy symptoms. *Pain,* 42:135–144, 1990.

Singer EJ, Zorilla C, Fahy-Chandon B, et al. Painful symptoms reported for ambulatory HIV-infected men in a longitudinal study. *Pain,* 54:15–19, 1993.

Swerdlow M, Cundhill JG. Anticonvulsant drugs used in the treatment of lacerating pains: a comparison. *Anesthesia,* 36:1129–1134, 1981.

Tsao JCI, Dobalian A, Stein JA. Illness burden mediates the relationship between pain and illicit drug use in persons living with HIV. *Pain,* 119: 124–132, 2005.

UNAIDS/WHO—Joint United Nations Programme on HIV/AIDS. *UNAIDS/WHO Epidemiological Fact Sheet on HIV/AIDS and Sexually Transmitted Infections.* Geneva, Switzerland: World Health Organization, 2004.

Ventafridda V, Branchi M, Ripamonti C, et al. Studies on the effects of antidepressant drugs on the antinociceptive action of morphine and on plasma morphine in rat and man. *Pain,* 43:155–162, 1990a.

Ventafridda V, Caraceni A, Gamba A. Field testing of the WHO Guidelines for Cancer Pain Relief: Summary report of demonstration projects. In KM Foley, JJ Bonica, V Ventrafridda (eds.), *Proceedings of the Second International Congress on Pain: Vol. 16. Advances in pain research and therapy.* New York: Raven Press, Ltd., pp. 155–165, 1990b.

Watson CP, Chipman M, Reed K, Evans RJ, Birkett N. Amitriptyline versus maprotiline in post herpetic neuralgia: a randomized double-blind, cross-over trial. *Pain,* 48:29–36, 1992.

Weinberger M, Conover CJ, Samsa GP, Greenberg SM. Physicians' attitudes and practices regarding treatment of HIV-infected patients. *South Med J.* 85:683–686, 1992.

Weissman DE, Haddox JD. Opioid pseudoaddiction and iatrogenic syndrome. *Pain,* 36:363–366, 1989.

World Health Organization. *AIDS Epidemic Update: December 2005.* Geneva, Switzerland: World Health Organization, 2005.

World Health Organization. *Cancer pain relief.* Geneva, Switzerland: World Health Organization, 1986.

41

Sickle Cell

A Disease of Molecules and a Disease of Race

Lauren Shaiova

Craig Blinderman

Daniel Brookoff

It is a sad and shameful fact that...this disease has been largely neglected throughout our history. We can't re-write this record of neglect but we can reverse it.
—President Richard M. Nixon, 1971, discussing sickle cell disease in a televised speech to the nation. Many credit this speech with triggering a burst of interest in sickle cell disease across the nation and prompting congressional passage of the National Sickle Cell Control Act, which greatly increased funding for research, community service and education about sickle cell disease (Scott, 1983).

Sickle cell disease provides a compelling example of how the course and treatment of illness is dependent not only upon the biology of the disease but also upon the social position of the patient. Linus Pauling called sickle cell anemia the "first molecular disease" (Pauling & Itano, 1949) and, to date, four Nobel prizes have been awarded for its study (Strasser, 2002). Unfortunately, this extensive research has done little to ease the suffering of its victims, many of whom are still faced with suspicion and animosity when they come seeking care for painful crises.

The discovery of sickle cell disease is certainly a major landmark in the history of molecular medicine. But it is also a landmark in the history of racial oppression in the United States where, for many years, tests for sickling (Emmel, 1917) were used to determine the presence of "Negro blood" and to justify the passage of laws prohibiting miscegenation (Wailoo, 1997).

By the time of its discovery by Western physicians, sickle cell disease has been recognized in West Africa for over a thousand years. In parts of West Africa, it was given the onomatopoeic names *chwecheechwe, nuidudui,* and *nwiiwii* in reference to the severe pain it caused (Konotey-Ahulu, 1968). Written descriptions of sickle cell disease were published by American plantation owners who described autopsies on slaves with small stature, skin ulcerations, and other signs of chronic hemolytic anemia in the mid-1840s (Lebby, 1846), and similar references can be found in diaries dating back to the late 1600s.

The "official" discovery of sickle cell disease was announced in a presentation by Dr. James Herrick at the 25th annual meeting of the Association of American Physicians on the morning of May 5, 1910, and published soon thereafter in the November issue of *Annals of Internal Medicine* (Herrick, 1910). Apparently, none of Dr. Herrick's colleagues recognized this disorder, characterized by "peculiar elongated forms of red corpuscles," and little notice was taken of his presentation.

The story of Herrick's discovery actually began in 1904, when Walter Clement Noel, a young dental student from Grenada, sought help for joint pains and skin ulcers at Rush Medical School Hospital in Chicago. Clement was born to a family of well-to-do sugar planters but was shorter and less robust than his brothers who worked on the family farm. Being frail and more "bookish" than his siblings, he was sent to the Chicago College of Dental Medicine to study, where the cold weather apparently made his symptoms worse. He was initially evaluated by Dr. Ernest E. Irons, an intern at Rush, who drew blood for several tests including measurement of hemoglobin concentration and a "blood culture," a test that, in those days, involved observing the blood under the microscope at several points over the course of hours to detect bloodborne parasites. Dr. Irons presented his findings of abnormal elongated erythrocytes to Dr. Herrick, who examined Walter Clement Noel and went on to care for him over the following 3 years. In 1907, Dr. Noel returned home to Grenada, where he practiced dentistry until his death at age 32 due to pneumonia.

Herrick was the first to posit that Noel's disease was somehow linked to the cellular abnormalities he had observed under the microscope. He wrote that "some change in the composition of the corpuscle itself may be the determining factor" of this illness (Herrick, 1910). Herrick thus became the first person to link a cellular abnormality to a clinical illness. Herrick remains a role model for physician-researchers to this day. Although he understood the growing importance of technology, he never let that distract him from his clinical focus, exemplifying the principle that "caring for the patient is based on caring about the patient" (James, 2000).

Herrick, who was 43 at the time of his presentation about Walter Clement Noel, went on to practice and teach for many more years. After 1910, he never returned to the study of sickle cell disease. In his autobiography, written in 1949, Herrick barely made mention of sickle cell disease (Herrick, 1949). The Herrick Award, however, continues to be awarded to and coveted by physicians. It is awarded by the American College Cardiology in honor of the

With a special section, "Psychosocial Aspects of Sickle Cell Disease," by Marc Goloff physician who cemented the link between coronary occlusion and myocardial infarction (Herrick, 1912).

Herrick's discovery of sickle cell disease may have been predated by reports of a 25-year-old African American woman who was admitted to the medical ward of the UVA Hospital for several occasions beginning in 1907 for joint pain, leg ulcers, gallstones, and anemia. Her blood films, done in 1909, were noted to show "poikilocytes in a variety of shapes, the most common being of a crescent shape." Russell Haden, then a medical student took blood samples from this woman to Johns Hopkins Hospital, where professors made the diagnosis of pernicious anemia (Washburn, 1911).

Few patients with sickle cell disease were seen at American hospitals over the next 10 years. One such patient presented to the hospital at Washington University in St. Louis in 1915, where her illness was brought to the attention to a wide variety of clinicians and scientists. One of these was the young anatomist Dr. Victor Emmel. Dr. Emmel was interested in "blood cultures," a technique in which a drop of blood was sealed between a slide and a cover slip using petrolatum. Emmel noted that sickling sometimes occurred in red cells that had previously appeared to be normal. After studying the blood cells from this patient, Emmel obtained blood from her nonanemic father. He noted that the father's cells appeared normal on a blood smear on the initial observation of the culture but would later become sickled (Kampmeier, 1929). Emmel's test was the standard laboratory method used to detect sickling in red cells for the next 30 years, after which it was improved by the addition of chemical reducing agents that accelerated the sickling of cells containing hemoglobin-S, giving us the "sickle prep" test that is used to this day (Castle & Daland, 1948).

Using Emmel's test, Guthrie and Huck from Johns Hopkins performed the first study of the genetics of sickle cell disease in 1923. They studied the family of newly diagnosed patient with sickle cell disease and found that the red cells of both the parents and the majority of other relatives would sickle in culture. Using Mendelian principles, the investigators came to the conclusion that this indicated that sickle cell was inherited as a single dominant factor, which they reported in the *Bulletin of the Johns Hopkins Hospital* (Huck, 1923). Of note, Guthrie and Huck did not differentiate between subjects who had anemia and healthy subjects whose cells sickled in culture, people we would now understand to have "sickle cell trait." In the highly race-conscious United States of the 1920s, this was interpreted to mean that interracial marriage threatened to spread this terrible illness from the black population into the white population. Our modern understanding of the inheritance of sickle cell disease tells us that intermarriage would actually *reduce* the incidence of disease.

Because of the misunderstanding of the pattern of inheritance of sickle cell disease, Emmel's test came to be regarded not as an indicator of abnormal hemoglobin but rather as a test for the presence of "Negro blood." Based on Emmel's findings, some American physicians felt that persons with sickle cell disease represented biological liabilities (Bauer & Fisher, 1943) and posed a grave health danger to the white race and called for federal laws prohibiting interracial marriage (Bauer, 1943). A 1947 editorial in the *Journal of the American Medical Association* about sickle cell anemia said, "its occurrence depends entirely on the presence of Negro blood; even in extremely small amounts it appears that the *sine qua non* for the occurrence of sickle cell disease is the presence of a strain, even remote, of Negro blood. The disease is regularly found in countries where there is frank interbreeding with African people.... Race is thus a strong etiological factor" ("Sickle Cell Anemia," 1947).

In 1923, Dr. Virgil Sydenstricker of the University of Georgia studied sickling in the red cells of the healthy relatives of a patient with severe anemia. He described the parents as having "latent sickling." Sydenstricker was also the first to use the term "crisis" and the first to suggest that the anemia in sickle cell was due to hemolysis. Sydenstricker also published the first report of an autopsy of a patient with sickle cell disease in which he described a scarred, atrophic spleen. He went on to perform Emmel tests on a population of healthy black and white subjects, noting that all who tested positive for "latent sickling" were black. In one of Sydenstricker's first lectures on this topic, he found that many physicians in his southern medical audience were apparently already familiar with this disease.

One doctor who attended noted that sickle cell disease was "of industrial as well as medical importance. Efficiency is lowered in the adult and total disability is the result of recurrent attacks" (Sydenstricker, 1924). In a chapter published in 1932, he noted that sickle cell anemia had never been reported in a patient over the age of 30, although "latent sickling" had been detected in patents as old as 78 (Sydenstricker, 1932). Sydenstricker later changed this conclusion when he described a patient with sickle cell anemia who had lived to the age of 59 (Sydenstricker et al., 1962).

In the years following its initial discovery, all of the patients with severe sickle cell disease described in the United States were African Americans of sub-Saharan ancestry. The first case report of sickle cell disease reported in Africa described a 10-year-old Arab boy in Omdurman in the Sudan (Archibald, 1925). The first description of the disease in a black African appeared in a report from Ghana published in 1932 (Russell & Taylor, 1932). In 1944 R. Winston Evans, a colonial pathologist, conducted a study of 600 native men throughout West Africa and found that the incidence of "latent sickling" was more than three times that reported in the United States even though sickle cell anemia in that area was vanishingly rare (Evans, 1944). This apparent discrepancy was explained in 1950 in a paper by A. J. Raper, who concluded that "some factor, imported by marriage with white persons is especially liable to bring out the hemolytic aspect of the disease, while the anomaly remains a harmless one in the communities in which it originated" (Raper, 1950).

Information about the real pattern of inheritance of sickle cell disease was beginning to be understood by the 1940s but many physicians continued to hold to the concept of the sickle gene being a Mendelian autosomal dominant factor. As long as they did this, they would be unable to differentiate between heterozygotes whose "sickle cell trait" was a protective adaption against malarial infection and homozygotes that had a painful and lethal illness. The numbers seemed support these physicians. For example, a 1955 study in the Belgian Congo reported only 2 cases of sickle cell anemia in the entire colony where the rate of positive Emmel tests was greater than 25% (Lambotte-Legrand & Lambotte-Legrand, 1955). It was also noted that people with positive Emmel tests were generally healthier than subjects who tested negative.

The early deaths of Africans with sickle cell disease would explain why sickle cell disease was so rare in Africa at the time. As researchers began to understand the true mechanism of sickle cell disease inheritance, many physicians remained resistant. In a 1952 paper describing his research in central Africa, Lehmann wrote, "I do not believe that in Uganda we could have overlooked sickle cell anemia present in "homozygous" carriers of the trait. Even if they had died early in infancy, it would have been such a 'slaughter of the innocents' that it could not have escaped our attention" (Lehmann, 1952). In fact, it had.

As recently as 1970, more than half of all the children with sickle cell anemia in Zambia died before age 3 (Barclay et al., 1970). In that year, the average lifespan of a person with sickle cell anemia in the United States was less than 18 years (Buchanan et al., 2004). This explains why many physicians in the United States came to consider sickle cell anemia to be a pediatric illness and why most of the specialized centers for the care of people with sickle cell disease are found in children's hospitals. It also explains the paucity of specialists who care for adults with this disease and why the medical care of adults with sickle cell disease is generally so poor.

Today we understand that sickle cell disease is not restricted to people who originated in sub-Saharan Africa but that large concentrations of people with sickle cell can be found in a broad belt of land that extends from southern India through adjacent areas of Arabia, Turkey, Greece, southern Italy, and Sicily. These regions with high concentrations of sickle cell are also endemic areas for the malarial parasite *plasmodium falciparum*. The "balanced polymorphism" of being heterozygous for hemoglobin-S confers resistance to infection with malaria, though it also serves to maintain the disease sickle cell anemia within the population (Allison, 1954).

Sickle cell disease remains the most common hereditary hematological disorder in the United States. The disease is characterized by hemolytic anemia, susceptibility to infections, and painful vasoocclusive crises leading to ischemic tissue injury and organ dysfunction. Painful episodes or "crises" can vary widely in frequency, intensity, and duration. About a third of patients with sickle cell disease rarely seek treatment for painful crisis, whereas another third require frequent visits to the physician or the emergency department for the treatment of pain. These differences may be explained by the presence of genes that code for sustained production of hemoglobin F or other traits (Bonds, 2005).

Sickle cell anemia was the first disease to be defined on the basis of molecular characteristics. The specific defect is the substitution of a valine molecule for the glutamic acid molecule that normally occupies the sixth position on the beta chain of hemoglobin. When the resulting molecule—a molecule of hemoglobin S—is deoxygenated, the valine molecule can bind to leucine and phenylalanine molecules on neighboring hemoglobin molecules, causing aggregation and the formation of long chains of hemoglobin, called hemoglobin polymers. These hemoglobin polymers are poorly soluble within the intracellular matrix of the red blood cell and can gel or precipitate, increasing the viscosity of the erythrocyte.

Polymerized hemoglobin-S can also alter the characteristics of the protein matrix underlying the erythrocyte cell membrane. A normal erythrocyte can withstand an enormous amount of shear stress and stretching because the protein cytoskeleton underlying its membrane contains the unique protein spectrin. Spectrin endows the erythrocyte with the distinctive properties of strength coupled with deformability. Polymerized hemoglobin-S can attach to spectrin and alter its structure, decreasing its deformability and also giving rise to the "sickle" shape (Lux et al., 1976).

When sickled erythrocytes in a test tube are "ghosted"—a chemical procedure that involves lysing the cells and removing their contents—the membrane-coated cytoskeletons that remain retain the sickled shape. When these "ghosts" are treated with detergents to remove the lipid membranes, the remaining cytoskeletons retain their sickled shape, suggesting that the interaction with hemoglobin-S has caused irreversible changes in these proteins (Lux et al., 1976). This also explains why sickling is not seen in reticulocytes, which have incomplete membrane cytoskeletons when they are first released from the marrow. In laboratory experiments, some sickled red cells can be "unsickled." So far, no one has shown that sickling is reversible in the bloodstream. In any case, the change of shape from biconcave disk to sickled cell is not the basis of sickle cell disease.

To appreciate how the changes caused by the polymerization of hemoglobin-S translate into disease, we have to consider how the normal properties of the red blood cell are essential to its unique function. Red blood cells are responsible for transporting oxygen to cells in the tissues. To do this efficiently, these cells must contain very high concentrations of the oxygen-carrying protein hemoglobin and still be able to flow through narrow capillaries. Hemoglobin is a very special protein, not only because it can transport oxygen but also because it can stay in solution at very high concentrations. This allows the erythrocyte to have the flow characteristics of water. This fluidity is crucial to a cell that is 8 microns in diameter and has to deliver oxygen in capillaries that average 3–4 microns in width. The normal concentration of hemoglobin in a red cell is 36gm/dl, which is astoundingly high compared to other cells that have high concentrations of protein. If we were to substitute a protein similar to hemoglobin but without its unique solubility characteristics into the red cell, such as myoglobin, the red cell would change from having the fluidity of water to having the flow characteristics of brick (Brookoff, 1992).

One way we conceptualize the molecular basis of sickle cell disease for our patients is to compare normal hemoglobin-A to Teflon-coated beads that easily roll over each other as the red cell flows in the bloodstream. We can then think of hemoglobin-S as beads in which two bits of the Teflon are removed and replaced with Velcro. The Velcro is only exposed on the bead's surface after the hemoglobin releases its load of oxygen—an event which generally occurs in small capillaries. The deoxygenated hemoglobin-S molecule can form a bond to any other hemoglobin molecule. If that second molecule happens to also be a molecule of deoxygenated hemoglobin-S, this can trigger the formation of a chain of hemoglobin molecules (a hemoglobin polymer), which can precipitate, interact with the red cell cytoskeleton, and make the cell less fluid. When a red blood cell of a person with sickle cell disease is exposed to low oxygen levels, it can go from having the consistency of a drop of water to having the consistency of petroleum jelly.

This change in red cell viscosity is the essence of sickle cell disease. Liquid blood becomes a viscous gel that clogs capillaries, depriving the cells that depend upon that capillary of oxygen and nutrition. Much of the bone pain in sickle cell disease has been shown to be generated by infarction of the marrow and endosteum that are invested with a rich supply of afferent nerve cells. This process of tissue infarction is the cause of most of the pain in vasoocclussive crisis, and it is not reversible. As Dr. Samuel Charache has written, "a sickle cell crisis is an event that has already happened" (Charache, 1986).

In the 1950s and 60s, the growing understanding of the molecular mechanisms underlying sickle cell disease led to the development of an extraordinary series of "rational" therapies aimed at preventing or reversing sickling. These treatments worked in the test tube, but few have yet been proven to help the patients. These mechanistic treatments included maneuvers aimed at keeping hemoglobin-S "locked" into its oxygenated configuration using inhaled carbon monoxide (Sirs, 1963) or infused cyanates (Peterson et al., 1974), which turned out to cause significant peripheral neuropathies. Other investigators tried to inhibit sickling by increasing the volume of red cells and thus the distance between hemoglobin-S molecules. This was done by infusing solutes or water-loading patients. In trials of these therapies, subjects had their blood urea nitrogen levels raised above 150 mg/dl (Cooperative Urea Trials Group, 1974) or sodium levels lowered to less than 105 mEq/L. Another series of treatments aimed at preventing hemoglobin polymerization included intravenous infusions of glyceraldehyde, which turned out to be highly immunogenic, or ethacrynic acid, which caused severe dehydration (Benesch et al., 1974). Although these treatments may have made sense on a molecular level, their toxicities often caused clinical catastrophes, many of which could have been anticipated.

Some of the current molecular treatments for sickle cell disease are based on the finding that cancer patients undergoing chemotherapy developed increased levels of fetal hemoglobin (hemoglobin F). This, coupled with the observation that patients with sickle cell disease who also had the concurrent persistence of hemoglobin F (which is the most common of the hemoglobinopathies) had an improved clinical course, led to the use of cytotoxic cancer chemotherapy drugs in these patients. The first trials were conducted with 5-azacytidine, which did elevate hemoglobin F levels but turned out to be too toxic (Steinberg, 1999). Hydroxyurea eventually became the cytotoxic drug of choice, and it is currently in use for sickle cell disease (Rodgers, 1991). Studies have shown that hydroxyurea can decrease the frequency of painful crises in adults (Steinberg et al., 2003), though the greatest success has come when the drug is started early in childhood (Zimmerman et al., 2004).

At first it was thought that cytotoxic drugs worked by causing "hemoglobin switching" in erythrocyte precursors, but this did not turn out to be true. Instead, the cytotoxic drugs apparently work by destroying normal erythrocyte precursor cells, forcing the marrow to recruit immature stem cells that give rise to red cells with high concentrations of hemoglobin F (Cokic et al., 2003). The long-term effects of these drugs, which are ideally started in childhood, are unknown and currently under study. Other rational treatments for sickle cell disease include regular exchange transfusion (Buchanan et al., 2004) and hematopoietic stem cell transplantation (Walters, 2005), which is the only treatment that has been shown to be curative. Of note, none of the treatments for sickle cell disease was ever found to reverse the damage due to recurrent tissue infarction or chronic iron overload.

The genetic basis of sickle cell disease lies in the inheritance of a single point mutation of the gene coding for the beta chain of hemoglobin. To have the disease, a person must inherit two copies of the mutated gene, one from each parent. The mutation, a single base change (GAT ⇒ GTT) in the sixth codon of exon 1 of the β-globin gene, results in the replacement of the normal glutamic acid with valine at position 6 of the β-globin chain (Ingram, 1956, 1975). Inheritance of one normal gene and one mutated gene results in sickle cell trait, the heterozygous carrier state seen in approximately 1 in 10 African Americans and in up to 30% of sub-Saharan Africans. Sickle cell trait is generally asymptomatic, though it as been linked to hematuria due to papillary necrosis caused by sickling in hypertonic areas of the kidney (Ataga & Orringer, 2000) and rare cases of sudden death related to exertion (Holmes et al., 1998).

Fetuses and young infants with sickle cell disease are usually protected by their high circulating levels of hemoglobin F. Sickle cell disease generally becomes clinically manifest after 6 months of age and usually presents as painful vasoocclussive crisis. Throughout the lifespan of a patient with sickle cell disease, pain is the most common reason for presentation to a health-care provider (Galloway & Harwood-Nuss, 1988). Sickle cell disease also leads to significant morbidity from recurrent bacterial infections, cerebrovascular events, acute chest syndrome, leg ulcers, avascular necrosis, hepatobiliary disease, and complications due to iron overload (often due to a combination of continuous hemolysis and repeated transfusions).

The most important medical intervention that has increased the lifespan of people with sickle cell disease has been the management of bacterial infection through the use of prophylactic penicillin in childhood, the use of pneumococcal vaccine, and careful monitoring. As people with sickle cell disease grow into adulthood, they develop severe microvascular disease similar to that seen in diabetics, which can result in renal failure and blindness.

Sickle cell disease affects 1 in 375 African Americans in the United States and is also present, although less common, in Americans of Hispanic, Native American, East Indian, Greek, Italian, and Eastern Asian origin (Charache et al., 1989; Embury et al., 1996; Rodgers, 1997). The disease is especially devastating in low-income, urban populations with large numbers of African Americans and Hispanics whose burden of disease is amplified by economic disadvantage. The impact of sickle cell disease extends to all aspects of the patient's life, including social interactions, family relations, peer interactions, employment, and spirituality (Ballas, 2002). Patients typically have numerous encounters with healthcare providers as a result of the recurrent nature of the painful crises. This leads to a significant financial burden on patients and their families, as well as the health-care system. The management of the majority of patients with sickle cell anemia is primarily palliative—consisting of general supportive care and targeted symptomatic management of the complications of sickle cell anemia, with the goal of achieving the best quality of life for the patients and their families.

Pathophysiology of Painful Crises in Sickle Cell Disease

The occlusion of microvasculature and the resulting tissue infarction does not completely explain the complex pathophysiology of sickle cell disease. A larger view of sickle cell disease encompasses other pathophysiological processes involving inflammatory mechanisms. The damaged tissue releases several inflammatory mediators, including interleukins, bradykinin, $K+$, $H+$, histamine, substance P, and calcitonin gene-related peptide (Wall & Melzack, 2006). Interleukin-1, for example, leads to the synthesis of prostaglandins via the upregulation of the cyclooxygenase gene, which sensitizes peripheral nerve endings and facilitates pain transmission. These inflammatory mediators may directly activate nociceptive afferent fibers or sensitize such fibers, ultimately resulting in a painful stimulus transmitted via A-δ and C peripheral nerve fibers to the dorsal root ganglion (DRG) in the spinal cord. The nerves synapse in the DRG and ascend contralaterally via the spinothalamic tracts to the thalamus and then to the cerebral cortex, where the stimulus is perceived as painful (Wall & Melzack, 2006). Endogenous inhibitors of the painful stimuli (serotonin, enkephalin, β-endorphin, and dynorphin) may play a role in explaining, in part, the variation in the frequency and severity of painful crises in patients with sickle cell disease (Ballas, 2005).

Damaged red cells can also interact with and stimulate vascular endothelial cells and other tissues kindling chronic inflammatory reactions (Platt, 2000). Reperfusion injury, resulting in the formation of oxygen radicals in ischemic tissue, may explain some of the progressive tissue damage in sickle cell disease, such as that which commonly occurs in the spleen, kidneys, and lungs. This may account for the persistent leukocytosis that is commonly seen in patients with sickle cell disease (Kaul & Hebbel, 2000)

A greater understanding of the role of cells other than erythrocytes in the pathophysiology of sickle cell disease promises to yield more targets for therapy. For example, adhesion of sickle cells to vascular endothelium is mediated, in part, by the endothelial protein P-selectin. Animal studies have shown that blocking the expression of P-selectin or inactivating it with a neutralizing antibody can diminish vasoocclusion by sickle cells (Embury et al., 2004). Persistent leukocytosis also appears to be a generator of disease in sickle cell anemia. In a 10-year study of children with sickle cell disease, three predictors of adverse outcomes (e.g., death, stroke, recurrent chest syndrome, frequent painful crises) were leukocytosis in the absence of infection, episode of dactylitis before age 1, and blood hemoglobin levels of less than 7 g/dl (Miller et al., 2000).

Clinical Manifestations of Sickle Cell Disease

The acute painful episode is the hallmark of sickle cell disease. The painful episode is variable, unpredictable, and can be precipitated by a variety of factors. Some common triggers include physical stress, trauma, dehydration, and infection. The severity, location, and duration of the pain may vary among patients and in the same individual over time (Jacob et al., 2002; Walco & Dampier, 1990). Typically, the pain involves the long bones and joints, with pain in the lower back region being the most often reported site. Pain may occur in other regions of the body, including the scalp, face, jaw, abdomen, and pelvis (Ballas, 2005; Ballas & Delengowski, 1993). The accepted definition of *painful crisis* is one that requires treatment in a medical facility with parenteral opioids for 4 or more hours (Charache et al., 1995; Platt et al., 1991). Severe sickle cell disease is defined as the occurrence of three or more crises per year. Patients with sickle cell disease typically use a variety of terms to describe their pain including "throbbing," "sharp," "dull," "stabbing," and "shooting" (Ballas & Delengowski, 1993). Objective signs (fever, leukocytosis, joint effusions, and tenderness) occur in about 50% of patients at presentation (Ballas et al., 1988). The absence of objective signs during the sickle cell crisis, especially during the first few days, may lead to problems when patients initially seek care from health-care providers (Ballas, et al., 1988).

Phases of the Vasoocclusive Crisis

Studies in both children and adults have characterized the vasoocclusive crisis as having four phases, with the typical painful episode lasting an average of 10 days (Ballas, 1995; Ballas & Smith, 1992; Beyer et al., 1999b; Jacob et al., 2005). Phase 1 is the "prodromal" or "precrisis" phase and typically lasts approximately 3 days. It is associated with a low-intensity, aching pain. The patient may report numbness and paresthesias. This may be related to a decrease in RBC deformability and an increase in RBC density as more red cells clog vascular channels. Phase 2 has been termed the "initial, evolving, infarctive" phase. During this phase, the patient experiences a gradual increase from aches to maximum pain with associated fear, anxiety, and anorexia. This is often accompanied by a decrease in hemoglobin, an increase in the percent of dense RBCs, increased red blood cell distribution width (RDW), and increased hemoglobin concentration distribution width (HDW).

Phase 3 is called the "established" or "postinfarctive/inflammatory" phase and typically lasts for approximately 4–5 days. The patients report severe, constant pain with muscle tenderness on exam. The patient may develop fevers, swelling, joint stiffness, and effusions. Hematologic changes include anemia, reticulocytosis, leucocytosis, and an increase in acute-phase reactants (e.g. C-reactive protein, fibrinogen), LDH (indicating tissue damage/bone marrow infarct), CPK (indicating skeletal muscle damage), RDW, and HDW. Phase 4, or the "resolving/healing/recovery/postcrisis" phase, typically lasts for 1–2 days and heralds the end of the vasoocclusive crisis. This phase is associated with a gradual decrease in pain intensity. Laboratory tests can show thrombocytosis, increased fibrinogen levels and a return to baseline hemoglobin levels with decreased sickle cells, percent of dense red cells, RDW, and HDW. Recent reports appear to support the validity of these phases of vasoocclusive crisis (Jacob et al., 2005).

Other Painful Syndromes in Sickle Cell Disease

Patients with sickle cell disease may suffer from painful syndromes other than acute painful vasoocclusive crisis. Other common pain syndromes in patients with sickle cell disease are listed in Box 41.1.

Acute chest syndrome is characterized by acute episodes of fever, chest pain, leucocytosis, and pulmonary infiltrates. Common triggers of acute chest syndrome include infection (especially community-acquired pneumonia), pulmonary infarction secondary to sickling, or bone marrow-fat embolism (Ballas, 2002). This syndrome can sometimes be very difficult to distinguish from pulmonary thrombosis. The possibility of thrombotic or embolic disease must always be considered in the patient presenting with acute chest syndrome. Acute chest syndrome is the second most common cause of hospitalization for patients with sickle cell disease. It is associated with significant morbidity and mortality in both children and adults. Serum levels of "secretory phospholipase

---

Box 41.1 Classification of Painful Episodes in Sickle Cell Disease

I. Pain secondary to the disease itself
   a. Acute pain syndromes
      1. Recurrent acute painful episodes
      2. Acute chest syndrome
      3. Hepatic crisis
      4. Priapism
      5. Calculus cholecystitis (pigment stones)
      6. Hand-foot syndrome (in children)
      7. Splenic sequestration (in children)
   b. Chronic pain syndromes
      1. Avascular necrosis
      2. Arthropathies
      3. Leg ulcers
      4. Chronic osteomyelitis
      5. Intractable chronic pain
   c. Neuropathic pain
II. Pain secondary to therapy
   a. Withdrawal
   b. Loose prosthesis
   c. Postoperative pain
III. Pain due to comorbid conditions
   a. Trauma
   b. Arthritis
   c. Peptic ulcer disease
   d. Other conditions

Source: Adapted from Ballas SK. Pain management of sickle cell disease. *Hematol Oncol Clin N Am* 2005;19:785–802.

A$_2$," an enzyme that cleaves fatty acids from triglycerides, may be a biomarker for impending chest syndrome (Styles et al., 2000).

Most episodes of acute chest syndrome are initially treated as pneumonia. Because of the possibility of infection with unusual organisms, such as *chlamydia pneumoniae,* broad-spectrum antibiotics are recommended. Clinical signs such as dyspnea, oxygen saturation, and chest radiographs must be carefully monitored because acute deterioration can lead to acute life-threatening emergencies. In cases in which there is increasing dyspnea associated with progressive, widespread radio-opacities and PaO$_2$ of less than 75mmHg, exchange transfusion should be considered. This often results in improvement within 48 hours.

Avascular necrosis (or ischemic necrosis) is the most commonly observed complication of sickle cell disease in adults. The limited terminal artery supply and poor collateral circulation in the femoral and humeral heads and the vertebral bodies make these areas vulnerable to bone infarction, joint damage, and chronic pain. These patients often have findings related to infarction on plain radiographs (e.g., "Lincoln log" appearance of the vertebrae). Pain and disability can be quite severe, requiring total joint replacement in advanced forms of the disease. Because of their compromised microvasculature, patients with sickle cell disease have difficulties recovering from joint replacement surgery. Many orthopedists are understandably reluctant to operate on patients with sickle cell disease. As a result, many of these patients end up suffering with chronic pain in degenerating shoulders or hips for years. Patients with sickle disease who report persistent shoulder, hip, or knee pain and have nondiagnostic radiographs should undergo bone scans to look for necrosis.

Dactylitis (hand-foot syndrome) involves acute, painful non-pitting swelling of one or more extremities. It is usually accompanied by fever and is also referred to as "acute osteopathy." Dactylitis usually occurs in children between the ages of 6 months to 2 years, though there have been cases reported up to age 7. The attacks usually resolve spontaneously within a week but predict future attacks. Recurrent episodes of dactylitis are a risk factor for early death due to sickle cell disease.

Leg ulceration occurs in 5%–10% of adult patients and can be a painful and disabling complication of sickle cell anemia (Ballas, 2005; Koshy et al., 1989). These ulcers are probably due vasoocclusion in blood vessels in the skin and underlying muscle. Although formal studies of venous function in sickle cell disease have reached conflicting conclusions (Billett et al 1991; Chalchal et al., 2001; Mohan et al., 2000), a case-controlled study in Jamaica demonstrated an association of venous incompetence with chronic leg ulceration (Clare, et al., 2002). The cause of venous incompetence is unknown but may be related to turbidity and impaired linear flow at venous valves, hypoxia-induced sickling, the rheological effects of high white cell counts, or the abnormal activation of the coagulation system (Clare, et al., 2002).

Priapism—painful and prolonged penile erection—affects up to half of all males with sickle cell disease (Chinegwundoh & Anie, 2004) and can occur as early as age 4. When first described, it was thought to represent a psychiatric "castration fear complex" (Obendorf, 1934), though it was soon understood to be due to sequestration of sickling cells in the corpora cavernosa (Diggs & Ching, 1934). Risk factors include low hemoglobin F levels and high platelet counts. Though most attacks have no obvious cause, priapism can be triggered by sexual intercourse and alcohol ingestion. Suggested treatments include exchange transfusion, stilbestrol, and direct aspiration of the corpora using a wide-bore needle. No studies have shown evidence of benefit for any of these treatments.

Acute headache in a patient with sickle cell disease may herald a neurologic catastrophe. As an increasing number of children with sickle cell disease and silent cerebral infarcts survive into adulthood, the number presenting with aneurysmal bleeds is expected to increase. Recent studies show that both past thrombotic infarcts and the existence of telangiectasias at the basal ganglia ("moyamoya" vasculopathy) are risk factors for hemorrhagic stroke in adulthood (Buchanan et al., 2004; Diggs & Brookoff 1993).

Neuropathic pain syndromes have been described in sickle cell patients (Asher, 1980; Ballas & Reyes, 1997; Kirson & Tomaro, 1979; Konotey-Ahulu, 1972; Shields et al., 1991). For example, the mental nerve may be compressed as a result of mandibular bone infarction, leading to numbness of the chin and mental nerve neuropathy (Konotey-Ahulu, 1972; Kirson & Tomaro, 1979). Other neuropathic pain syndromes that have been described in sickle cell patients include trigeminal neuralgia (Asher, 1980), acute proximal median mononeuropathy (Shields et al., 1991), entrapment neuropathy, and acute demyelinating polyneuropathy (Ballas & Reyes, 1997).

Anemia and Its Sequelae

Many patients with sickle cell disease will require intermittent transfusions and all will require folic acid at a minimum dose of 1 mg per day. Some patients with severe and chronic hemolysis with concomitant poor dietary habits may require replacement doses of folic acid of 5mg per day (Ballas, 2001). Folic acid needs to be constantly replaced because it becomes depleted with increased erythropoietic activity due to chronic hemolysis. Nonadherence to folic acid replacement regimens is associated with increased frequency of painful crisis. This may be related to the development of hyperhomocysteinemia, a condition linked to folic acid deficiency and associated with peripheral vascular disease, and cerebrovascular and coronary thrombotic events. High homocysteine levels may be a risk factor for the development of cerebrovascular accidents in patients with sickle cell disease.

Although acute painful crisis is the most common type of pain described in the literature on sickle cell disease, most of the pain many adults with sickle cell suffer is chronic bone and joint pain whose exacerbations are often framed in terms of acute crisis. Undertreatment of this chronic pain can lead to unnecessary suffering and even fatal complications. Repeated hospital admissions for pain are strongly associated with a higher mortality rate (Platt et al., 1994).

Pharmacological Management of Painful Syndromes

Acute painful crisis accounts for most of the emergency department visits by people with sickle cell disease. Treating sickle cell pain is complex, and it requires understanding that much of the pain in adults with this illness may be chronic. The frequency of painful crises may increase as the patient ages and is subject to progressive damage of bones, joints, and tissues. "Palliative medicine" is often a reasonable model of care for these patients with progressive complex medical problems ranging from recurrent infection, CNS events, leg ulcers, severe bone pain, avascular necrosis of multiple joints, acute chest syndrome, cardiovascular compromise, renal failure, end organ damage, and eventually untimely death.

The term "palliative" should not be interpreted to mean "nihilistic." The clinician faced with a patient with sickle cell disease should always be aware that a painful crisis may be triggered by a dangerous but reversible cause. When faced with a patient in painful crisis, consideration must be given to the possibility of concurrent infection or thrombosis. The patient's assessment and treatment must also take into consideration the possibility of chronic organ dysfunction due to pulmonary hypertension, cardiomyopathy, renal dysfunction or hepatopathy.

The general approach to the patient with acute painful crisis should always include a thorough history and exam, including a patient self-report of the pain, which can be facilitated using one of the numerous validated pain scales available. Crisis pain can be alleviated only by analgesic medications. Analgesics should be started promptly and titrated to the patient's report of pain, which should always be documented.

The usual strategies for treating sustained, severe pain with opioid analgesics all too often call for intermittent dosing on an "as needed" basis. In this approach, pain medications are given only when the pain recurs. The analgesics used are often short-acting and given with insufficient frequency. This discontinuous provision of analgesia subjects patients with sustained pain to periods of pain, anticipation, and anxiety and can generate the pain-avoidance behaviors that physicians often characterize as "manipulative" and "drug seeking" (Brookoff & Polomano, 1992). To avoid this, intravenous analgesics can be started as continuous infusions or via patient-controlled pumps.

After adequate analgesia is obtained, an oral sustained-release opioid may be started with a provision made for intermittent bolus or "rescue" medication. Uncontrolled pain accounts for more that 90% of hospital admissions in adults with sickle cell disease (Platt et al., 1991). In adult patients with frequent episodes of painful crisis, the use of long-acting opioid medications reduced visits to the emergency department and hospitalizations and shortened the lengths of stay in hospital (Brookoff & Polomano 1992; Shaiova & Wallenstein, 2004).

A precipitating cause for the painful crisis should always be considered. Prompt attention to infection in particular can mean the difference between life and death for a patient with sickle cell disease. Serious infections are usually signaled by fevers, and no patient with a temperature greater than 101°F should be discharged before the source of infection is identified and treated. But radiographs, urinalyses, and antibiotics don't relieve pain. Although laboratory tests and radiographs should be ordered when indicated, they should not be considered to be "routine" treatment of painful crisis.

One institution recently reported success with a dedicated outpatient facility for the treatment of uncomplicated sickle cell pain crisis. Use of this special unit reduced the time spent to pain relief, increased the number of patients discharged to home, decreased hospital admission rates, and reduced the use of the emergency department by patients with sickle cell disease. Over the 5 years studied, savings amounted to more than $1.7 million as a result of fewer hospital admissions and a shorter length of stay (Ballas, 1998). Until recently, treatment of sickle cell–related pain was limited to short-acting opioids administered in emergency departments. The most commonly used opioid has been meperidine, which is relatively contraindicated in these patients who often have significant renal insufficiency.

Patients with sickle cell disease who use the emergency department primarily to manage their disease often end up with substandard care, lacking in continuity and in physicians with the specialized knowledge needed to help mange this illness. Unfortunately, in the United States, many of these patients are left with no alternative.

Selection of Opioid Analgesics

Most opiates have comparable efficacy and safety profiles, with analgesia and side effects being dose dependant. In patients with sickle cell disease we have to consider coexistent organ dysfunction that can alter the metabolism of certain medications. It should also be noted that the "baseline" level of renal or hepatic dysfunction may be worsened during an acute crisis. In most cases of acute crisis, most sickle cell centers and pain specialists that treat sickle cell disease favor the intravenous route of opioid administration. One study that evaluated intravenous versus oral morphine in children with vasoocclusive episodes found equal efficacy and safety in both groups (Jacobson, Kopecky, Joshi, Babul, 1997). In another study, oral morphine was used in conjunction with a nonsteroidal antiinflammatory agent for the treatment of acute painful crisis. This regimen reduced admissions to the hospital when compared to historical controls (Conti, Tso, & Browne, 1996). As mentioned above, meperidine has been the most commonly used opioid for the treatment of painful crisis. The increased risk of seizure and the skin and muscle injury due to its use by intramuscular injection make it relatively contraindicated for repeated use in patients with sickle cell disease (Robieux, Kellner, & Coppes, 1992).

Though opioid medications can usually control the pain of sickle cell disease, many physicians will not prescribe these medications or will prescribe them in inadequate dosages because of undue concerns about addiction or side effects such as respiratory depression (Yale, Nagib, Guthrie, 2000). In a study that examined the effectiveness of analgesia in 21 children with vasoocclusive crisis, 71% did not achieve adequate pain control during the study period (Beyer, 2000). Factors undermining effective treatment included lack of pain assessment, improper choice of medication or inadequate dosing, and misconceptions about the nature of painful crisis among physicians and nurses.

Morphine has long been considered a drug of choice for the treatment of painful crisis, but physicians must be aware that the pharmacokinetics of morphine can vary among patients (Yale, Nagib, & Guthrie, 2000). One study of patients with sickle cell disease reported an eightfold variation in morphine clearance among different individuals (Dampier et al., 1995). Patients with sickle cell disease typically have a more rapid plasma clearance for morphine than other patients, such as those with cancer or postoperative pain. Additionally, patients with severe symptoms have significantly faster clearances than those with moderate pain (Dampier, et al., 1995). This rapid clearance may result in less analgesia in response to commonly administered dosages (Abbuhl, Jacobson, & Murphy, 1986; Dampier et al., 1995). It should be noted that the clearance of morphine and some of its active metabolites can be significantly reduced in cases of hepatopathy and renal failure, both of which are becoming more frequent among people with sickle cell disease as improved disease management (most notably prevention and treatment of infections) results in an aging of this population.

Hydromorphone has been useful in the treatment sickle cell pain. It usually has fewer side effects than morphine due to the lack of the hydroxyl group that is responsible for much morphine-induced nausea. The sustained-release preparation of hydromorphone is currently unavailable in the United States. Other oral opioids such as methadone, oxycodone, and levorphanol have been successfully used to treat chronic pain in patients with sickle cell disease, as has transdermal fentanyl.

Adjuvant Therapy for Acute Pain

Nonsteroidal antiinflammatory medications have been used in combination with opioids or alone for acute episodes of sickle cell pain. These include ketorolac, piroxicam, and ibuprofen, which have been evaluated for monotherapy and in combination with opiates for vasoocclusive crisis. Ketorolac is a successful primary treatment for patients unable to tolerate opiates (Beyer et al., 1999a; Beyer, 2000; Goodman, 1991; Richardson & Steingart, 1993). In single-dose studies, ketorolac did not reduce the opioid requirements of patients with sickle cell pain (Hardwick et al., 1999). However, continued ketorolac administration may provide increased benefit. In a blinded, crossover trial with 20 children, ketorolac provided superior pain control and with fewer side effects than meperidine (Beyer et al., 1999b; Goodman, 1991; Richardson & Steingart, 1993). A more recent study of 70 patients with episodes of pain measuring "7 out of 10" found that ketorolac provided relief in fewer than half the subjects (Beiter et al., 2001).

Steroids have also been shown to reduce sickle cell crisis pain. In a randomized, double-blinded trial of 56 pain episodes in children and adolescents, methylprednisolone in doses of 15 mg/kg (to a maximum dose of 1,000 mg) significantly reduced opioid requirements compared to a placebo-controlled group (Griffin et al., 1994). Stimulants have been used as adjuvant therapy to enhance the effects of opioids, usually for patients who experience oversedation with their pain medications.

The antidepressants and anticonvulsant medications, which are typically used for neuropathic pain, have not been studied for sickle cell pain. One antidepressant to be avoided in males with sickle cell disease would be trazodone, whose erection-potentiating effects could lead to the development of priapism, which (as noted earlier) is another common complication of sickle cell disease.

Sickle Cell Disease and Opioid Addiction

One of the most important barriers to care for patients with sickle cell disease is the exaggerated fear among caregivers of promoting addiction. Studies show that the prevalence of addiction in patients with sickle cells disease is lower than that of the surrounding populations and may be as low as 1% (Portenoy & Hagen, 1990). Nonetheless, a survey of caregivers who frequently see patients with sickle cell disease found that 63% of nurses, 53% of emergency department physicians, and 23% of hematologists believed that drug addiction is prevalent in patients with sickle cell disease (Shapiro et al., 1997).

Exaggerated concerns about addiction and physical dependence among patients with sickle cell disease have compromised the treatment of these patients for a long time.

Studies examining incidence of addiction among patients with sickle cell disease have repeatedly shown that it is not greater than that of the general population and is often significantly lower. A study of 610 patients in London found that none were drug addicts (Brozovic et al., 1986). A study of 198 children and adolescents treated with intravenous opiates for sickle cell pain found only 1 patient who showed signs of addiction (Morrison, 1991). Another study of 160 patients found that 14 "made excessive use of hospital services," tampered with drug delivery systems in the hospital, had a history of illicit drug behavior, or been involved with the police or courts because of drug-related activities (Payne, 1989). Despite

Box 41.2 *DSM-IV* Definitions

The Symptoms of Substance Dependence

A need for markedly increased amounts of the substance to achieve intoxication or desired effects, or markedly diminished effect with continued use of the same amount of substance (tolerance).

The characteristic withdrawal syndrome for substance, nausea, yawning, runny nose, sweating, aching muscles, diarrhea, fever, and insomnia.

The substance is often taken in larger amounts or over a longer period of time than intended.

Persistent desire or unsuccessful attempts to cut down or control substance use.

A great deal of time spent obtaining, using, or recovering from the effects of a substance.

Important social, occupational, or recreational activities given up or reduced because of substance use.

Substance use continued despite knowledge of a persistent or recurrent physical or psychological problem likely to have been caused or exacerbated by the substance.

The Symptoms of Substance Abuse

Recurrent substance use resulting in failures to fulfill major role obligations at work, school, or home.

Recurrent substance use in physically hazardous situations (operating machinery while impaired by a substance).

Recurrent substance-related legal problems.

Continued substance use despite persistent or recurrent social or interpersonal problems caused or exacerbated by the effects of the subjects.

---

this, many of the physicians associated with comprehensive sickle cell centers in the United States continue to find that physicians' attitudes about addiction and toward patients in crisis result in undertreatment of pain (Labbe et al., 2005).

Elander et al. (2003) assessed the extent to which sickle cell patients' use of prescribed analgesics corresponded to symptoms of substance dependence and abuse. The assessment differentiated between behaviors that corresponded to the *DSM-IV* symptoms (see Box 41.2) but involved analgesics used to control pain (pain related symptoms) and those involving analgesic use beyond pain control (nonpain-related symptoms). The objectives were to examine interrater reliability, to determine the frequency of pain-related symptoms and nonpain-related symptoms using *DSM-IV* criteria, and to obtain patients' insights into pain-related and nonpain-related symptoms. The investigators conducted individual interviews about the patients' pain management in inpatient and outpatient settings. Pain-related symptoms accounted for 88% of all symptoms reported. This study also showed that many of the patients had coping strategies that were misinterpreted by their physicians and perceived as aberrant behavior.

The most common manifestation of this problem occurs when an adult patient with sickle cell disease seeks care in a hospital emergency room. The interaction between patient and caregiver can quickly deteriorate into disagreements over how aggressively to treat the pain and kindle suspicions of substance abuse (Barbarin & Christian, 1999). Because severe episodes are so regular, patients with sickle cell disease often manifest high degrees of concern, anxiety, and distress regarding their pain medications, and these translate into behaviors that are often misinterpreted by health professionals as drug-seeking behaviors (Elander et al., 2004).

The problematic behaviors that are driven by fear and desperation related to unrelieved pain or lack of access to adequate pain medication can best be characterized as "pseudoaddiction" (Weissman & Haddox, 1989). Assessment and management of this very complex set of behaviors requires considerable clinical sophistication. Inattention to these issues only worsens the burden and stigma of sickle cell disease.

Psychosocial Aspects of Sickle Cell Disease

Sickle cell disease is associated with a number of severe psychosocial challenges to the sufferer and the family (Holbrook & Phillips, 1994; Thomas & Taylor, 2002). Children and adolescents have demonstrated difficulties in the areas of psychological adjustment, school performance, cognitive functioning, and social adjustment. Adults, in addition to facing ongoing psychological and cognitive issues, must often cope with significant employment and financial stress. An additional harsh reality of sickle disease in the United States is that it is predominantly an African American disease. Due to this fact, the psychosocial impact of sickle cell is unavoidably confounded by factors of ethnicity, racism, economic inequality, and environment (Barbarin & Christian, 1999). Historically, research and intervention efforts have focused more heavily on medical than psychosocial aspects of sickle cell disease (Collins et al., 1998). A number of writers make the case for increasing attention to psychosocial factors.

Psychological Adjustment

A review by Barbarin et al. (1999) found that earlier studies reported high rates of depression and anxiety (Barbarin, Whitten, & Bonds, 1994) and "internal behavior problems" (Thompson et al., 1999) among children with sickle cell disease. Neither of these studies included a control group. Cepeda et al. (1997) found a high proportion of children with sickle cell disease also screened positive for such problems as separation anxiety, oppositional defiance, attention deficit hyperactivity disorder, and enuresis. These investigators did study a comparison group consisting of same-race children being seen for other acute medical disorders. There was no significant difference between groups, suggesting that children with sickle cell disease were not at greater risk for psychological disorder than ill outpatient controls.

Collins et al. (1998) also criticized earlier studies for lack of controls and small sample size. When more carefully matched demographically to nondiseased peers, children and adolescents with sickle cell disease did not differ significantly from controls in the incidence of psychological disorder. Even though psychological problems affected many children with sickle cell disease, a majority were well-adjusted (Treadwell & Gill, 1994).

School Performance and Cognitive Functioning

The literature on sickle cell disease and school performance has been inconsistent (Barbarin & Christian, 1999). Sickle cell disease was associated with poor school performance in some studies. Problems included poor teacher evaluations, below-grade-level performance, and grade retention (Barbarin et al., 1994). One group hypothesized that cerebrovascular accidents among children with sickle cell disease affected cognitive functioning and higher order learning, resulting in diminished learning and academic achievement (Brown, Armstrong, & Eckman, 1993). These findings were contradicted by other writers. Hurtig et al. (1989) found no relationship between illness severity and academic achievement, and Midence et al. (1996) did not find a significant difference in IQ between children with sickle cell disease and healthy controls.

Even when efforts are made to include adequate comparison groups, results have been inconsistent in the area of school performance. Nettles (1994) compared 32 African American children with sickle cell disease with 34 demographically similar healthy controls. Subjects with sickle cell disease were lower on math and reading standardized achievement test scores and higher in school absences. Richard and Berlew (1997) also made a noteworthy effort to use an adequate comparison group, with opposite results. They studied 68 African American adolescents, 42 attending a sickle cell clinic and 26 healthy controls in a general medical clinic. Both groups were similar demographically. No differences were found in mathematics or reading grades, standardized tests, or grade retention. Both groups had high absenteeism and were below the national average in math and reading scores. Similar to the literature on psychological disorders, Barbarin and Christian (1999) emphasize the importance of appropriate comparison groups and looking to other factors in addition to sickle cell disease to explain psychosocial problems.

Social Adjustment

Collins et al. (1998) cited a number of problems in social adjustment among children and adolescents with sickle cell disease. These include impaired social competence, problematic peer and family relations, low self-esteem, poor body image, and a passive versus active coping style. Passive coping style was associated by Gil et al. (1991) with increased emergency room visits and reduced home, school, and social activity. Resnick (1984) asserted that for adult survivors of childhood chronic illness, social adjustment difficulties continued in the form of identity crisis and difficulty in achieving personal goals. Adults with sickle cell disease were found to be significantly distressed in the areas of employment and finances, sleeping and eating, performance of daily activities, and fear of body deterioration (Barrett et al., 1988). These writers further found that employment and financial distress, in particular, were even more severe among adults with sickle cell disease than other chronic illnesses.

Robinson (1999) speculated that children with sickle cell disease who had frequent hospital visits may grow to be impaired in social development due to reduced time with their peers: "Children with chronic illness conditions develop social role skills and social competence within the context of an extended family system, which includes the medical care providers who are instrumental in the 'sick care' of the maturing child" (p. 342). Holbrook and Phillips (1994) suggest that sickle cell crises and medication side effects can interfere with school, work, parenting, and socializing in young adult life, creating increasing strain as adult work and family demands multiply.

Barbarin et al. (1999) proposed an integrative model for predicting social, academic, and psychological adjustment of children with sickle cell disease. Psychological outcomes were most commonly associated with parents' psychological status, quality of relations between parents and siblings, and maturity demands of the child with sickle cell disease. Academic outcomes were significantly predicted by parental academic expectations and the child's rejection of the sick role. Social functioning was also associated with degree to which the child rejected the sick role.

A Disease of African Americans

Sickle cell is overwhelmingly a disease of African Americans. Although found among many ethnic groups throughout the world, sickle cell disease is rarely found in the United States among non-African Americans (Barbarin & Christian, 1999). This fact has significant social and cultural implications for the interaction between patients with sickle cell disease and the medical care system, which can influence patient adjustment and how patients are assessed and responded to by medical providers (Barbarin & Christian, 1999). Barbarin and Christian further assert that funding agencies for sickle cell research have typically leaned toward viewing the illness in medical, versus social or psychological, terms. Research therefore rarely looks at the "potentially independent or compounding influences of ethnicity, racism, and economic inequality" (p. 288).

Barbarin and Christian point to a body of writings beyond those on sickle cell disease on how potential racism and cultural competence among care providers affects the quality of health and human services (e.g., Crawford, 1991; Ewalt et al., 1996). Pinderhughes (1989) examined ways in which unrecognized or unacknowledged social class and ethnic differences can cause misperceptions and miscommunication between health-care providers and chronically ill patients. A common example of this can be found in hospital emergency rooms. An adult with sickle cell disease presents with a painful crisis that can precipitate disagreements on how to treat the pain and arouses suspicions of substance abuse on the part of staff without sufficient experience with sickle cell disease (Barbarin & Christian, 1999): "Ethnicity, class, and the social denigration associated with being in a lower status group clearly intersect with and influence medical staff decision making and, in turn, influence the nature of care provided" (p. 289).

Psychosocial Research and Intervention

The conclusion shared by numerous investigators cited above is that research and intervention into psychosocial factors associated with SCD will result in improved care and outcomes (e.g., Barbarin & Christian, 1999; Collins et al., 1998; Robinson, 1999). Trzepacz et al. (2004) and Thompson et al. (2003) utilized the Child Behavior Checklist wherein caregivers rated emotional, social, and behavioral functioning of children with sickle cell disease. These two groups found that 43% and 30%, respectively, of children with sickle cell disease scored in the clinical range on this instrument. Trzepacz cited these findings to justify further psychosocial research, especially in the area of routine screening of children with sickle cell disease in the course of their medical care, followed by randomized trials of targeted interventions.

The multisite Cooperative Study of Sickle Cell Disease compared measures of psychosocial status and psychological adaptation to health status among 90 African American adolescents. Psychosocial factors predicted adaptation better than biomedical risk factors did (Burlew et al., 2000). Collins et al. (1998) present an excellent overview of psychosocial interventions with patients with sickle cell disease and relative empirical support.

Nonpharmacological Pain Management

The centrality of pain to the course of sickle cell disease makes it an obvious target for the growing field of nonpharmacological pain management. Collins et al. (1998) review the limited literature in this area. Biofeedback utilizes electrophysiological instrumentation to "feed back" internal, nonobservable psychophysiological processes to the patient such as motor neuron activity or measures of sympathetic arousal. This helps teach the patient to modify stress or pain due to muscle tension through the use of relaxation, imagery, and the like. Early studies supported biofeedback for adults with sickle cell disease, although they were limited by small sample size, mixed interventions, and lack of comparison groups (Cozzi, Tryon, & Sedlacek, 1987; Thomas et al., 1984; Zeltzer et al., 1979). Biofeedback is strongly supported for use with children, as well, but no studies have been specific to sickle cell disease (e.g., Attanasio et al., 1985; McGrath, 1990). Progressive muscle relaxation training has been utilized successfully with young chronic pain patients (Walco, Varni, & Ilowite, 1992). Collins et al. (1998) advocate employing this widespread approach with patients with sickle cell disease to reduce tension and pain.

Self-hypnosis is a further extension of relaxation, involving self-suggestion to alter one's subjective experience of pain or tension. This has been successfully utilized to reduce children's pain from medical problems (McGrath, 1990) and in two studies of adults with sickle cell pain (Erickson, 1991; Zeltzer et al., 1979). These findings are suggestive of self-hypnosis' efficacy, but small sample size and lack of adequate controls limit the conclusiveness of results (Collins et al., 1998).

Behavioral Contracting and Coping Skills Training

Behavioral contracts consist of spelling out in writing specific behavioral expectations and goals between provider and patient that are aimed at increasing the patient's well behaviors and self-reliance. They were utilized with success in two early case reports involving adolescents with sickle cell disease (Burghardt-Fitzgerald, 1989; Walco & Dampier, 1987). Examples of gains included reduced reliance on the medical system compared with matched norms, reduced hospitalizations, increased adherence, and decreased pain. Generalization of these results is limited by the case report methodology.

Coping skills training goes beyond behavioral contracting by actively imparting specific cognitive and/or behavioral skills germane to improving the patients' ability to manage their disease and optimize functioning and adaptation in spite of it. Gil et al. (1996) randomly assigned adults with sickle cell disease to training in cognitive coping skills versus a disease education control group. The coping skills group reported increased coping attempts and reduced negative thinking, both of which have been linked with positive adaptation to disease. Reduced experimental pain was reported, as well, but this finding has uncertain generalizability to sickle cell pain (Collins et al., 1998).

Educational Programs

Patient and family education in the treatment of chronic illness, and sickle cell disease in particular, are strongly advocated and supported by a number of writers as "essential for adaptive coping and improved disease management" (Collins et al., 1998, p. 443). Topics can include etiology, mode of transmission, community resources, handling, psychosocial stressors, complications, and strategies for managing pain episodes and complications.

A study of a five-group education program for adults with sickle cell disease found that participation resulted in improved patient–physician relationships, greater ability to express disease-related concerns, and increased seeking of appropriate assistance (Butler & Beltran, 1993). A second investigation of an education program for parents of 200 infants diagnosed with sickle cell disease found excellent compliance with penicillin administration, reduced incidence of pneumococcal sepsis, and enhanced parental knowledge (Day, Brunson, & Wang, 1992).

Self-Help and Support Groups

Support groups are widely offered to sickle cell patients (Collins et al., 1998). These authors believe this modality can be particularly helpful for adolescents with sickle cell disease in self-esteem, social and moral development, and age-appropriate separation-individuation. Empirical support for the efficacy of support groups exists, but is limited by methodological issues such as lack of controls and limited data from participants as opposed to facilitators.

Nash and Kramer (1993) conducted a 5-year study of support groups and found that longer membership was associated with fewer psychosocial stressors and psychological symptoms. Support groups were found to empower patients in advocating for their care and for changes in health delivery (Shelley et al., 1994). Comer (2004) reported decreased depressive symptoms among participants in a support group for adult patients with both sickle cell disease and depression.

Family Counseling and Therapy

Families have been identified as a fundamental unit of care in the management of sickle cell disease (Barbarin, 1994; Barbarin et. al, 1999). Collins et al. (1998) cite a large body of literature underlining the lifelong strains that sickle cell disease and other chronic illnesses place upon the family system. Examples include stress-coping resources, disruption of family routines, financial pressures, relative neglect of healthy siblings, and marital stress.

There is very little published empirical research on family treatment and sickle cell disease. Two groups investigated a manualized control group intervention for families of children and adolescents with sickle cell disease (Collins et al., 1997; Kaslow et al., 1997). Upon completion of the intervention sequence, families with sickle cell were found to be more knowledgeable about the disease, more flexible in their functioning as a family, and less depressed compared with the nontreatment control group with sickle cell disease.

To conclude, children, adolescents, adults, and their families must contend with a number of psychosocial problems associated with sickle cell disease. Barbarin and Christian (1999) assert that ethnic, racial, and socioeconomic factors may cause further difficulties and have a negative impact upon the response of the healthcare system and patient access to care. There is growing recognition of the important roles that assessment and intervention for psychosocial problems can play in improving the care and outcomes for patents with sickle cell disease.

References

Abbuhl S, Jacobson S, Murphy J. (1986) Serum concentrations of meperidine in patients with sickle cell disease. *Emergency Medicine* 15:433–8.
Allison AC. (1954) Protection afforded by sickle-cell trait against subtertian malarial infection. *Br Med J.* 1:290–294.
Archibald RG. (1925) A case of sickle cell anemia in the Sudan. *Trans R Soc Trop Med Hyg.* 19:389–393.
Asher SW. (1980) Multiple cranial neuropathies, trigeminal neuralgia, and vascular headaches in sickle cell disease: a possible common mechanism. *Neurology* 30:210–1.
Ataga KI, Orringer EP. (2000) Renal abnormalities in sickle cell disease. *Am J Hematol.* 64:205–211.
Attanasio V, Andrasik P, Burke EJ, Blake DD, Kabela E, McCarran MS. (1985) Clinical issues in utilizing biofeedback with children. *Clinical Biofeedback and Health* 8:134–141.
Ballas SK. (1995)The sickle cell painful crisis in adults: Phases and objective signs. *Hemoglobin* 19:323–333.
Ballas SK. (1998) *Sickle Cell Pain Progress in Pain Research and Management* (Vol. 11). Seatle, WA: IASP Press.
Ballas SK. (2001) Sickle cell disease: current clinical management. *Seminars in Hematology* 38:307–314.
Ballas SK. (2002) Sickle cell anemia. *Drugs* 62:1143–1172.
Ballas SK. (2005) Pain management of sickle cell disease. *Hematol Oncol Clin N Am* 19:785–802.
Ballas SK, Delengowski A. (1993) Pain measurement in hospitalized adults with sickle cell painful episodes. *Ann Clin Lab Sci* 23:358–61.
Ballas SK, Larner J, Smith ED, et al. (1988) Rheologic predictors of the severity of the painful sickle cell crisis. *Blood* 72:1216–23.
Ballas SK, Reyes PE. (1997) Peripheral neuropathy in adults with sickle cell disease. *Am J Pain Med* 71:53–8.
Ballas SK, Smith ED. (1992) Red blood cell changes during the evolution of the sickle cell painful crisis. *Blood* 79:2154–2163.
Barbarin O, Whitten C, Bonds S. (1994). Estimating rates of psychosocial problems in urban and poor children with sickle cell anemia. *Health and Social Work* 19:112–119.
Barbarin OA (1994) Risk and resilience in adjustment to sickle cell disease: integrating focus groups, case reviews, and quantitative methods. *Journal of Health & Social Policy* [Special Issue: Psychosocial aspects of sickle cell disease: past, present, and future directions of research] 5(3–4):97–121.
Barbarin OA, Christian M. (1999) The social and cultural context of coping with sickle cell disease: I. A review of biomedical and psychosocial issues. *Journal of Black Psychology* 25: 277–293.
Barbarin OA, Whitten CF, Bond S, Conner-Warren R. (1999) The social and cultural context of coping with sickle cell disease: III. stress, coping tasks, family functioning, and children's adjustment. *Journal of Black Psychology* 25(3):356–377.
Barclay GPT, Huntsman RG, Robb A. (1970) Population screening of young children for sickle cell anemia in Zambia. *Trans R Soc Trop Med Hyg.* 64:733–739.
Barrett D, Wisotzek IE, Abel GG, Rouleau JL, Plat AF, Pollard WE, Eckman JR. (1988) Assessment of psychosocial functioning of patients with sickle cell disease. *Southern Medical Journal*, 81:745–750.
Bauer J. (1943) Sickle cell disease. *Arch Surg.* 47:553–63.
Bauer J, Fisher LJ. (1943) Sickle cell disease: with special regard to its nonanemic variety. *Arch Surg.* 47:553–563.
Beiter J, Simon H, Chambliss C, Adankiewicz T, Sullivan K. (2001) Intravenous ketorolac in the emergency department management of sickle cell pain and predictors of its effectiveness. *Arch. Pediatr Adolescent Med* 155:496–500.
Benesch R, Benesch RE, Yung S. (1974) Chemical modifications that inhibit gelation of sickle hemoglobin. *Proc Nat Acad Sci USA* 71:1504–1505.
Beyer J. (2000) Judging the effectiveness of analgesia for children and adolescents during vaso-occlusive events of sickle cell disease. *J Pain Symptom Manage* 19:63–72.
Beyer J, Platt A, Kinney T, Treadwell M.(1999a) Practice guidelines for the assessment of children with sickle cell pain. *J Soc Pediatrics Nurses* 4: 61–73.
Beyer J, Simmons L, Woods G, Woods P. (1999b) A chronology of pain and comfort in children with sickle cell disease. *Pediatrics* 153:913–920.
Billett HH, Patel Y, Rivers SP. (1991) Venous insufficiency is not the cause of leg ulcers in sickle cell disease. *Am J Hematol.* 37:133–134.
Bonds DR. (2005) Three decades of innovation in the management of sickle cell disease: the road to understanding the sickle cell disease clinical phenotype. *Blood Rev.* 19:99–110.
Brookoff D. (1992) A protocol for defusing sickle cell crisis. *Emergency Med.* 7:131–140.
Brookoff D, Polomano R. (1992) Treating sickle cell like cancer pain. *Ann of Int Med.* 116: 364–368.
Brown RT, Armstrong FD, Eckman JR. (1993) Neurocognitive aspects of paediatric sickle cell disease. *Journal of Learning Disabilities,* 25:33–45.
Brozovic, M, Davies S, Brownell A. (1987) Acute admissions of patients with sickle cell disease who live in Britain. *British Medical Journal*, 294:1206–1208.
Buchanan GR, DeBaun MR, Quinn CT, Steinberg MH. (2004) Sickle cell disease. *Hematology* 1:35–55.
Burghardt-Fitzgerald DC. (1989) Pain-behavior contracts: effective management of the adolescent in sickle-cell crisis. *J Pediatr Nurs.* 4:320–324.
Burlew K, Telfair J, Colangelo L, Wright EC. (2000) Factors that influence adolescent adaptation to sickle cell disease. *Journal of Pediatric Psychology* 25(5):287–299.
Butler DJ, Beltran LR. (1993) Functions of an adult sickle cell group: education, task orientation, and support. *Health and Social Work* 18:49–56.
Castle WB, Daland GA. (1948) A simple and rapid method for demonstrating sickling of the red blood cells: the use of reducing agents. *J Lab Clin Med.* 33:1082–1088.

Cepeda ML, Yang Y, Price C, Shah A. (1997) Mental disorders in children and adolescents with sickle cell disease. *Southern Medical Journal* 90:284–287.

Chalchal H, Rodino W, Hussain S, et al. (2001) Impaired venous hemodynamics in a minority of patients with chronic leg ulcers due to sickle cell anemia. *Vasa* 30:277–279.

Charache S. (1986) Advances in the understanding of sickle cell anemia. *Hosp Pract.* 15:173–90.

Charache S, Lubin B, Reid C. (1989) Management and therapy of sickle cell disease (NIH Publication No. 89–2117, Department of Health and Human Services. Public Health Services). Washington, DC: U.S. Government Printing Office.

Charache S, Scott JC, Charache P. (1979) Acute chest syndrome in adults with sickle cell anemia. *Arch Intern Med* 139:67–9.

Charache S, Terrin ML, Moore RD, et al. (1995) Effect of hydroxyurea on the frequency of painful crises in sickle cell anemia. *N Engl J Med* 332:1317–22.

Chinegwundoh F, Anie KA. (2004) Treatments for priapism in boys and men with sickle cell disease. *Cochrane Database Syst Rev.* 4:CD004198.

Clare A, FitzHenley M, Harris J, et al. (2002) Chronic leg ulceration in homozygous sickle cell disease: the role of venous incompetence. *Br J Haematol* 119(2):567–71.

Cokic VP, Smith RD, Beleslin-Cokic BB et al. (2003) Hydroxyurea induces fetal hemoglobin by the nitric oxide-dependent activation of soluble guanylyl cyclase. *J Clin Invest.* 111: 231–239.

Collins M, Kaslow N, Doepke K, Eckman J, Johnson M. (1998) Psychosocial interventions for children and adolescents with sickle cell disease (SCD). *Journal of Black Psychology* 24(4):432–454.

Collins MH, Loundy MR, Brown FL, et al. (1997) Applicability of criteria for empirically validated treatments to family interventions for pediatric sickle cell disease. *Journal of Developmental and Physical Disabilities* 9(4):293–309.

Comer EW. (2004) Integrating the health and mental health needs of the chronically ill: a group for individuals with depression and sickle cell disease. *Social Work in Health Care* 38(4):57–76.

Conti C, Tso E, Browne B. (1996) Oral morphine protocol for sickle cell crisis pain. *Maryland Med. J* 45:33–5.

Cooperative Urea Trials Group. (1974) Treatment of sickle cell disease crisis with urea in invert sugar: a controlled trial. *JAMA* 228:1125–8.

Cozzi L, Tryon WW, Sedlacek K. (1987) The effectiveness of biofeedback-assisted relaxation in modifying sickle cell crises. *Biofeedback and Self-Regulation* 12:51–61.

Crawford M. (1991) The multicultural society: sickle cell disease in children. *Nursing* 4(31):23–25.

Dampier C, Setty B Logan J Loli J, Dean R. (1995) Intravenous morphine pharmacokinetics in pediatric patients with sickle cell disease. *J Pediatrics* 126: 461–7.

Day S, Brunson G, Wang W. (1992) A successful education program for parents of infants with newly diagnosed sickle cell disease. *J Pediatr Nurs.* 7:52–57.

Diggs LW, Brookoff D. (1993) Multiple cerebral aneurysms in patients with sickle cell disease. *Southern Med J.* 86:377–379.

Diggs LW, Ching RE. (1934) Pathology of sickle cell anemia. *Southern Med J.* 27:839–845.

Elander J, Lusher J, Bevan D, Telfer P. (2003) Pain management and symptoms of substance dependence among patients with sickle cell disease. *Soc Sci Med.* 57:1683–96.

Elander J, Lusher J, Bevan D, Telfer P, Burton B. (2004) Understanding the causes of problematic pain management in sickle cell disease: evidence that pseudoaddiction plays a more important role than genuine analgesic dependence. *J Pain Symptom Manage* 27:156–69.

Embury SH et al. (2004) The contribution of endothelial P-selection to the microvascular flow of mouse sickle erythrocytes in vivo. *Blood* 104:3378–3385.

Embury S, Hebbel R, Mohandas N, Steinberg M (1996) *Sickle Cell Disease: Basic Principles and Clinical Practice*. Philadelphia: Lippincott-Raven.

Emmel VE. (1917) A study of the erythrocytes in a case of severe anemia with elongated and sickle-shaped ed blood corpuscles. *Arch Int Med.* 20:586–98.

Erickson CJ. (1991) Hypnoanalgesia in sickle cell anemia [Abstract]. *Pediatric Research* 29:9.

Evans RW. (1944) The sickling phenomenon in the blood of West African natives. *Trans R Soc Trop Med Hyg.* 37:281–286.

Ewalt PL, Freeman EM, Kirk SA, Poole DL. (1996). *Multicultural Issues in Social Work*. Washington, DC: NASW Press.

Galloway S, Harwood-Nuss AL. (1988) Sickle cell anemia: a review. *J Emerg Med* 6:213–226.

Gil KM, Williams DA, Thompson, RJ, Kinney TR. (1991) Sickle cell disease in children and adolescents: the relation of child and parent pain coping strategies to adjustment. *Journal of Pediatric Psychology* 16:643–663.

Gil KM., Wilson JJ, Edens JL, et al. (1996) Effects of cognitive coping skills training on coping strategies and experimental pain sensitivity in African American adults with sickle cell disease. *Health Psychology* 15:3–10.

Goodman E. (1991) Use of ketorolac in sickle cell disease and vasoocclusive crisis. *Lancet* 338:641–2.

Griffin T, McIntire D, Buchanan G. (1994) High dose intravenous methylprednisolone therapy for pain in children and adolescents with sickle cell disease. *N Engl J Med.* 330:733–7.

Hardwick W, Givens T, Monroe K, King W, Lawley D. (1999) Effect of ketorolac in pediatric sickle cell vasoocclusive pain crisis. *Ped Emerg Care* 15:179–82.

Herrick JB. (1910) Peculiar elongated and sickle-shaped red blood corpuscles in a case of severe anemia. *Arch. Int. Med.* 6:517–521.

Herrick JB. (1912) Clinical features of sudden obstruction of coronary arteries. *JAMA* 59:2015–2020.

Herrick JB. (1949) *Memories of Eighty Years* (pp. 270). Chicago: University of Chicago Press

Holbrook CT, Phillips G. (1994) Natural history of sickle cell disease and the effects on biopsychosocial development. *Journal of Health & Social Policy* [Special Issue: Psychosocial aspects of sickle cell disease: past, present, and future directions of research] 5(3–4):7–18.

Holms PS, Kerle KK, Seto CK. (1998) Sickle cell trait and sudden death in athletes. *Am Fam Physician* 58:1760–1.

Huck JG. (1923) Sickle cell anemia. *Bull Johns Hopkins Hosp* 34:335–344.

Hurtig AL, Koepke D, Park KP. (1989) Relation between severity of chronic illness and adjustment in children and adolescents with sickle cell disease. *Journal of Pediatric Psychology*, 19, 117–132.

Ingram, VM. (1956) A specific chemical difference between the globins of normal human and sickle-cell anemia hemoglobin. *Nature* 178: 792–4.

Ingram, VM. (1975) Gene mutations in human hemoglobin. The chemical difference between normal and sickle cell hemoglobin. *Nature* 180:325–8.

Jacob E, Beyer JE, Miaskowski C, et al. (2005) Are there phases to the vasoocclusive painful episode in sickle cell disease? *J Pain Symptom Manage* 29:392–400.

Jacob E, Miaskowski C, Savedra M, et al. (2002) Changes in intensity, location, and quality of vaso-occlusive pain in children with sickle cell disease. *Pain* 102:187–193.

Jacobson S, Kopecky E, Joshi P, Babul N. (1997) Randomized trial of oral morphine for painful episodes of sickle cell disease in children. *Lancet* 350:1358–61.

James TN. (2000) Homage to James B. Herrick: a contemporary look at myocardial infarction and at sickle-cell heart disease. *Circulation* 101:1874–1897.

Kampmeier OF. (1929) Victor Emmanuel Emmel. *Anat Rec.* 42:75–89.

Kaslow NJ, Collins MH, Loundy MR, Brown F, Hollins LD, Eckman J. (1997) Empirically validated family interventions for pediatric psychology: sickle cell disease as an exemplar. *Journal of Pediatric Psychology* 22(2), 213–227.

Kaul DK, Hebbel RP. (2000) Hypoxia/reoxygenation causes inflammatory response in transgenic sickle mice but not in normal mice. *J Clin Invest.* 106:411–420.

Kirson LE, Tomaro AJ. (1979) Mental nerve paresthesias secondary to sickle cell crisis. *Oral Surg* 48:509–12.

Konotey-Ahulu FID. (1968) Hereditary qualitative and quantitative erythrocyte defects in Ghana: an historical and geographical survey. *Ghana Med J.* 7:118–119.

Konotey-Ahulu FID. (1972) Mental nerve neuropathy: a complication of sickle cell crisis. *Lancet* 2:388.

Koshy M, Entsuah R, Koranda A, et al. (1989) Leg ulcers in patients with sickle cell disease. *Blood* 75:1403–8.

Labbe E, Herbert D, Haynes J. (2005) Physicians' attitude and practices in sickle cell disease pain management. *J Palliat Care* 21:246–51.

Lambotte-Legrand J, Lambotte-Legrand C. (1955) Le prognostic de l'anémie drepanocytaire au Congo Belge (à propos de cas de 150 décès). *Ann Soc Belg Med Trop*. 35:53–57.

Lebby R. (1846) Case of absence of the spleen. *Southern J Med. Pharm.* 1:481–3.

Lehmann H. (1952) Discussion of Jelliffe DB: the African child. *Trans R Soc Trop Med Hyg.* 46:42–43.

Lux SE, John KM, Karnovsky MJ (1976). Irreversible deformation of the spectrin-actin lattice in irreversibly sickled cells. *J Clin Invest.* 58:955–63.

McGrath PA (1990). *Pain in Children: Nature, Assessment, and Treatment.* New York: Guilford.

Midence K, McManus C, Fuggle P, Davies S. (1996). Psychological adjustment and family functioning in a group of British children with sickle cell disease: preliminary empirical findings and a meta-analysis. *British Journal of Clinical Psychology* 35:439–450.

Miller ST et al. (2000) Prediction of adverse outcomes in children with sickle cell disease. *New Eng J Med.* 342:83–89.

Mohan, JS, Vigilance, JE, Marshall, JM, Hambleton, IR, Reid, HL, Serjeant, GR. (2000) Abnormal venous function in patients with homozygous sickle cell (SS) disease and chronic leg ulcers. *Clinical Science* 98:667–672.

Morrison RA. (1991) Update on addiction and choice of an opioid in pain management. *Pediatric Nursing* 17:503–6.

Nash NB, Kramer KD. (1993) Self-help for sickle cell disease in African American communities. *Journal of Applied Behavioral Science* 29:202–215.

Nettles AL. (1994) Scholastic performance of children with sickle cell disease. *Journal of Health & Social Policy* [Special issue: Psychosocial aspects of sickle cell disease: past, present, and future directions of research] 5(3–4):123–140.

Obendorf CP. (1934) Priapism of psychogenic origin. *Arch Neurol Psychiatr.* 31:1292–6.

Pauling L, Itano HA. (1949) Sickle cell anemia is a molecular disease. *Science* 110:543–8.

Payne, R (1989) Pain management in sickle cell disease: rationale and techniques. *Ann NY Acad Sci* 565: 189–206.

Pegelow C. (1992) Survey of pain management therapy provided for children with sickle cell disease. *Clinical Pediatrics* 31:211–14.

Peterson CM, Tsairis P, Onishi A, Lu YS, Grady R. (1974) Sodium cyanate induced polyneuropathy in patients with sickle cell disease. *Ann Intern Med.* 81:152–8.

Pinderhughes, E. (1989) *Understanding Race, Ethnicity, and Power: The Key to Efficacy in Clinical Practice.* New York: Free Press.

Platt OS. (2000) Sickle cell anemia as an inflammatory disease. *J Clin Invest.* 106:337–338.

Platt OS, Brambilla D, Rosse W, Millner P, Castro O, Steinberg M, Klug, P. (1994) Mortality in sickle cell disease: life expectancy and risk factors for early death. *New Eng J Med* 330:1639–1644

Platt OS, Thorington DB, Brambilla DJ, et al. (1991) Pain in sickle cell disease: rates and risk factors. *N Engl J Med* 325:11–6.

Portenoy RK, Hagen NA. (1990) Breakthrough pain: definition, prevalence and characteristics. *Pain* 41:273–282.

Raper AB. (1950) Sickle cell disease in Africa and America—a comparison. *J Trop Med.* 53:489–53.

Resnick M. (1984) In R Blun (Ed.). *Chronic illness and disabilities in childhood and adolescence*, pp. 229–326. New York: Grune & Stratton.

Richard HW, Burlew AK. (1997) Academic performance among children with sickle cell disease: setting minimum standards for comparison groups. *Psychological Reports* 81:27–34.

Richardson P, Steingart R. (1993) Meperidine and ketorolac in the treatment of painful sickle cell crisis. *Ann of Emerg Med* 22:1639–40.

Robieux IC, Kellner JD, Coppes MJ, et al. (1992) Analgesia in children with sickle cell crisis: comparison of intermittent opioids vs. continuous infusion morphine and placebo controlled study of oxygen inhalation. *Pediatr Hematol Oncol* 9:317–26.

Robinson MR. (1999) There is no shame in pain: coping and functional ability in adolescents with sickle cell disease. *Journal of Black Psychology* 25(3):336–355.

Rodgers GP. (1991) Recent approaches to the treatment of sickle cell anemia. *JAMA* 256:2097–2100.

Rodgers, GP. (1997) Overview of pathophysiology and rationale for treatment of sickle cell anemia. *Seminars in Hematology* 34(3):2–7.

Russell H, Taylor CJSO. (1932) A case of sickle cell anemia. *West Afr Med J.* 5:68–69.

Schulman E, Natara M. (1995) Pathophysiology and management of sickle cell pain crisis: report of meeting of physicians and scientists. *Lancet* 346:1048–12.

Scott RB. (1983) Historical review of legislative and national initiatives for sickle cell disease. *Am J Pediatr Hematol Oncol.* 5:346–51.

Shaiova L, Wallenstein, D. (2004) Outpatient management of sickle cell pain with chronic opioid pharmacotherapy. *J Natl Med Assoc* 96:984–6.

Shapiro BS, Benjamin LJ, Payne R, Heidrich G. (1997) Sickle cell-related pain: perceptions of medical practitioners. *J Pain Symptom Manage.* 14: 168–174.

Shelley B, Kramer KD, Nash KB. (1994) Sickle cell mutual help assistance groups and the health services delivery system. *Journal of Health & Social Policy* 5:243–259.

Shields RW Jr., Harris JW, Clark M. (1991) Mononeuropathy in sickle cell anemia: anatomical and pathophysiological basis for its rarity. *Muscle Nerve* 14:370–4.

Sickle cell anemia: a race-specific disease [Editorial]. (1947) *JAMA* 133:33–34.

Sirs JA. (1963) The use of carbon monoxide to prevent sickle cell formation. *Lancet* 1:971–2.

Steinberg MH. (1999) Drug therapy: management of sickle cell disease. *N Eng J Med* 340:1021–30.

Steinberg MH, Barton F, Castro O, et al. (2003) Effect of hydroxyurea on mortality and morbidity in adult sickle cell: risks and benefits up to 9 years of treatment. *JAMA* 289:1645–1651.

Strasser BJ. (2002) Linus Pauling's molecular diseases: between history and memory. *Am J Med Genet.*115:83–93.

Styles LA, Aarsman AJ, Vichinsky EP, Kuypers FA. (2000) Secretory phospholipase A(2) predicts impending acute chest syndrome in sickle cell disease. *Blood* 96:3276–3278.

Sydenstricker VP. (1924) Sickle cell anemia. *South Med J.* 17:177–183.

Sydenstricker VP. (1932) Sickle cell anemia (Herrick's syndrome). In Christian HA (ed.), *Oxford Medicine* (Vol. II, pp. 849–860). New York: Oxford University Press.

Sydenstricker VP, Kemp JA, Metts JC. (1962) Prolonged survival in sickle cell disease. *Am Practitioner* 13:584–590.

Thomas JE, Koshy M, Patterson L, Dorn L, Thomas K. (1984) Management of pain in sickle cell disease using biofeedback therapy: a preliminary study. *Biofeedback and Self-Regulation* 9:413–420.

Thomas VJ, Taylor LM. (2002) The psychosocial experience of people with sickle cell disease and its impact on quality of life: qualitative findings from focus groups. *British Journal of Health Psychology*, 7(Part 4):345–363.

Thompson RJ, Armstrong FD, Kronenberger WG, et al. (1999) Family functioning, neurocognitive functioning, and behavior problems in children with sickle cell disease. *Journal of Pediatric Psychology* 24:491–498.

Thompson RJ Jr, Armstrong FD, Link CL, Pegelow CH, Moser F, Wang WC. (2003) A prospective study of the relationship over time of behavior problems, intellectual functioning, and family functioning in children with sickle cell disease: a report from the Cooperative Study of Sickle Cell Disease. *J Pediatr Psychol.* 28: 59–65.

Treadwell JJ, Gill KM. (1994) Psychosocial aspects. In Embury SH, Hebbel RP, Mohandas N, Steinberg MH. (eds.), *Sickle Cell Disease: Basic Principles and Clinical Practice* (pp. 517–529). New York: Raven Press.

Trzepacz AM, Vannatta K, Gerhardt CA, Ramey C, Nol RB. (2004) Emotional, social, and behavioral functioning of children with sickle cell disease and comparison peers. *Journal of Pediatric Hematology/Oncology* 26(10): 642–648.

Urban MO, Gebhart GF. (1998) The glutamate synapse: a target in the pharmacological management of hyperalgesic pain states. *Prog Brain Res* 116:407–420.

Wailoo K. (1997) *Drawing Blood* (pp. 163–187). Baltimore, MD: Johns Hopkins University Press.

Walco GA, Dampier CD. (1987) Chronic pain in adolescent patients. *J Pediatr Psychol.* 12:215–225.

Walco GA, Dampier CD. (1990) Pain in children and adolescents with sickle cell disease: a descriptive study. *J Pediatr Psychol* 15:643–658.

Walco GA, Varni JW, Ilowite NT. (1992) Cognitive-behavioral pain management in children with juvenile rheumatoid arthritis. *Pediatrics* 89:1075–1079.

Wall PD, Melzack R, eds. (1999) *Textbook of Pain* (4th ed.). New York: Churchill Livingston.

Walters MC. (2005) Stem cell therapy for sickle cell disease: transplantation and gene therapy. *Hematology* 2:66–73.

Washburn RE. (1911) Peculiar elongated and sickle-shaped red blood corpuscles in a case of severe anemia. *Va. Med. Semimonthly* 15:490–493.

Weissman DE, Haddox JD. (1989) Opioid pseudoaddiction—an iatrogenic syndrome. *Pain* 36: 363–6.

Yale S, Nagib N, Guthrie T. (2000) Approach to the vaso-occlusive crisis in adults with sickle cell disease. *Am Fam Physician* 61:1349–56.

Zeltzer LK, Kellerman J, Dash J, Holland JP. (1979) Hypnotically induced pain control in sickle cell anemia. *Pediatrics* 64:533–536.

Zimmerman SA, Schultz WH, Davis JS, et al. (2004) Sustained long-term hematologic efficacy of hydroxyurea at maximum tolerated dose in children with sickle cell disease. *Blood* 103:2039–2045.

42

Urine Drug Testing in Pain and Addiction Medicine

Douglas L. Gourlay

Howard A. Heit

The use of urine drug testing (UDT) in clinical medicine has increased over recent years. UDT results have traditionally been used in legal proceedings under supervision of a medical review officer (MRO). In this context, testing has been required by statute or regulation and so is typically not in the "donor's" interest. Health-care professionals, however, can use UDT in a variety of ways. When used initially, they are particularly helpful in assessing risk and so aid in the development of a rational treatment plan. Over time, they can be used to motivate healthy behavioral change, assist in maintenance of changes already made, and assist in monitoring patients' compliance with a mutually agreed-upon treatment plan. By using UDT in a patient-centered fashion, both patient and health-care professional interests are maintained.

The MRO-based model of testing when used in the clinical setting can lead to mistrust and a deterioration of the doctor-patient relationship. Clinical testing can enhance the doctor-patient relationship when the results are used to improve communication. A patient-centered model of UDT should be used to improve quality of care. This chapter will discuss why urine is the biological specimen of choice for drug testing; who, when, and why to test; testing methods; and most importantly, interpretation of results.

UDT is a useful diagnostic tool in a number of medical disciplines, including pain management and addiction medicine as well as the primary care setting. When used in a therapeutic model of patient-centered care, UDT provides valuable information to assist the practitioner in diagnostic and therapeutic decision making around a number of issues.

A study that audited medical records to asses the management of chronic pain patients in family practices found that only 8% of physicians utilized UDTs (Adams et al., 2001). UDTs are used infrequently in the tertiary care oncology center (Passik, 2000a). In the authors' experience, the use of UDTs in a noncancer pain practice is more common but sometimes is utilized in a punitive manner to "catch" the patient with an inappropriate positive or negative UDT. Unfortunately, this often results in dismissal of the patient from the practice. Although drug testing can be used in a variety of ways, it is most commonly used for two quite different purposes: to identify substances that should not be present in the urine (i.e., forensic testing) and to detect the presence of prescribed medications (compliance testing).

In the forensic setting, the system is designed to detect a relatively small number of drug users, in a test population consisting largely of drug-free donors. The ultimate goal of forensic testing is to produce results that can be used, if necessary, in a court of law. When this paradigm is applied to the clinical setting, an adversarial environment invariably results that often harms the doctor-patient relationship.

In the case of treatment compliance testing in a pain practice, the doctor is looking for the presence of prescribed medications as evidence of their use. Positive results are reassuring to both the patient and health-care professional, indicating compliance with the agreed-upon treatment plan. In compliance testing, not finding the prescribed drug or finding unprescribed or illicit drugs is disconcerting and certainly merits further discussion with the patient and, in some cases, with guidance from the testing laboratory. For example, laboratory error and test insensitivity can result in the lab reporting absence of a prescribed drug. Even bingeing by the patient can result in unexpected negative urine reports if the patient runs out of medication prior to sample collection. Therefore, these results by themselves cannot be relied upon to prove drug diversion and are also consistent with addiction, pseudoaddiction, or the use of an opioid for nonpain purposes—so called "chemical coping"(Passik & Weinreb, 2000).

Self report of unprescribed or illicit drug use including alcohol is, however, fraught with problems (Akinci et al., 2001; Lapham et al., 2002; Staines et al., 2001). Pain patients may be hesitant to reveal a past or current history of drug misuse or addiction, feeling that this might disqualify them from treatment of their chronic pain. Although health-care professionals are those most often cited by patients and their families as the "most appropriate" source of advice and guidance about issues related to the use of alcohol, tobacco, and other drugs, they are also reported to be the "least helpful" in actually addressing these issues (Conigliaro, 2003). It takes time to establish effective communication, mutual trust, and honesty in the therapeutic relationship. Substance misuse issues must be identified and managed for effective management of medical problems (Kirsh et al., 2002).

The U.S. Supreme Court (*Board of Education v. Earls*, No. 01–332) has ruled that widespread UDT could be performed in public schools. Substance misuse in adolescent and young adults contributes to the three leading causes of mortality due to injury, homicide, and suicide (Kaul, 2002). Even though a positive result on a UDT cannot measure functional impairment, in part because it does not represent drug concentration in the brain, the association between drug misuse and trauma is well-established (Casavant, 2002; Kaul & Coupey, 2002). The importance of appropriate drug testing and interpretation of results by primary care practitioners is only likely to increase in years to come.

The purpose of the UDT should be explained to the patient at the initial evaluation. Nonemergent use of urine drug testing should never be done without the patient's knowledge and consent. Although every patient has the right to refuse such testing, it is our experience that those pain patients who are "philosophically opposed" to drug testing have problems with drugs. Both prescriber and patient must carefully interpret this position in the context of a possible comorbid substance use disorder such as misuse or addiction and not as evidence of the minor nature of the complaint of pain. The decision to prescribe controlled substances under these circumstances can be problematic and may be difficult to defend in the context of a poor outcome. The UDT must be used, like all other diagnostic tests, to improve patient care (California Academy of Family Physicians and PharmaCom Group, Inc., 2004). The UDT can enhance the relationship between the health-care professional and patient by providing documentation of adherence to mutually agreed-upon treatment plans. This allows the doctor to be a more effective advocate on behalf of the patient with his or her family, workplace, and other third-party interests. The UDT is an objective diagnostic test that is part of the medical record for the treatment of the subjective complaint of pain.

In cases in which the urine sample is inappropriately positive for unprescribed or illicit substances, this will aid in the assessment and diagnosis of drug misuse or addiction. UDT results can be used to encourage change to more functional behavior while supporting positive changes previously made. Thus, the appropriate use of a UDT result requires documentation in the medical record and an understanding of how the results are to be used (Passik et al., 2000).

In the pain management setting, the presence of an illicit or unprescribed drug must not diminish the patient's complaints of pain, but may suggest a concurrent disorder such as addiction that will frustrate the effective management of an underlying pain condition. Although acute pain can be treated in a patient with an active, untreated addictive disorder, it is impossible to successfully treat a complaint of chronic pain in the face of an untreated addiction. To satisfactorily treat either condition, the patient must be willing to accept assessment and treatment of both. Thus, the diagnosis of a concurrent addictive disorder, when it exists, is vital to the successful treatment of chronic pain.

Specimen Choice

Since the 1970s, urine is the preferred biologic specimen for determining the presence or absence of most drugs (Caplan & Goldberger, 2001). This is in part due to the increased window of detection (1–3 days for most drugs or their metabolites; Conigliaro et al., 2003) when compared to serum samples, the relatively noninvasive nature of sample collection, ease of storage, and low cost of testing.

Whom to Test

Although the prevalence of addictive disorders in the pain population is unknown, it is unlikely to be less than that seen in the general population, which is often quoted as 10% (Savage, 1996). It should not be surprising that when UDT is reserved for those patients suspected of having drug-related problems, a significant number appear offended by the request. In fact, when uniformly applied, it is the exception rather than the rule that the pain patient is offended by a request for urine drug testing. Reliance on a history of addiction or aberrant behavior to trigger a UDT (i.e., reports of lost or stolen prescriptions, multiple unsanctioned dose increases) may miss a significant number of those individuals using unprescribed/illicit drugs (Katz & Fanciullo, 2002). The diagnosis of the disease of addiction is often best made prospectively, over time. By continued evaluation of the patient over time, that diagnosis can be made.

The question of whom to test is made easier by having a uniform practice policy (Heit, 2003). By adopting a uniform policy of testing, stigma is reduced while ensuring that those persons dually diagnosed with pain and substance use disorders may receive optimal care. With careful explanation of the purpose of testing, any patient concerns can be easily addressed (California Academy of Family Physicians and PharmaCom Group, Inc., 2004).

Testing Strategies

The health-care professional must know which drugs to test for and by what methods, as well as the expected use of the results. If the purpose of testing is to find unprescribed or illicit drug use, combination techniques such as gas chromatography/mass spectroscopy (GC/MS) or high-performance liquid chromatography (HPLC) are the most specific for identifying individual drugs or their metabolites (Vandevenne et al., 2000).

Caution must be exercised when interpreting UDT results in a pain practice. True negative urine results for prescribed medication may indicate a pattern of bingeing rather than drug diversion. Time of last use of the drug(s) can be helpful in interpreting UDT results.

A basic routine UDT panel should screen for the following drugs/drug classes:

- Cocaine (benzoylecgonine)
- Amphetamines/methamphetamine (including Ecstasy)
- Opiates
- Methadone
- Marijuana
- Benzodiazepines

Urinary creatinine, pH, and temperature should also be ordered and recorded to assist with results interpretation and to increase specimen reliability. The temperature of a urine sample within 4 minutes of voiding should fall within the range of 90°F to 100°F (Heit, 2003). Urinary pH undergoes physiologic fluctuations throughout the day, but should remain within the range of 4.5 to 8.0 (Cook et al., 2000). Urinary creatinine varies with time of day due to variable degrees of hydration (Cook et al., 2000). A specimen consistent with normal human urine has a creatinine concentration greater than 20 mg/dL; less than 20 mg/dL is considered dilute and less than 5 mg/dL is not consistent with human urine (Cook et al., 2000). Test results outside of these ranges should be discussed with the patient and/or the laboratory, as necessary.

Drug class–specific windows of detection are dependent on a number of factors. The detection time of a drug in urine represents how long after administration of a drug a person continues to excrete that drug and/or metabolite at a concentration above a specific test cutoff level. Although influenced by several factors

Table 42.1. Drug Retention Times

Drug	Retention Time
Amphetamines	48 hours
Barbiturates	Short-acting (e.g., secobarbital) 24 hours; long-acting (e.g., phenobarbital) 2–3 weeks
Benzodiazepines	3 days if therapeutic dose ingested; up to 4–6 weeks after extended use (or abuse quantities)
Cocaine metabolite (benzoylecgonine)	2–4 days
Cocaine parent	Few hours
Methadone	Approximately 3 days
Opiates	2–3 days (morphine/codeine) 6-acetyl morphine (metabolite of heroin) < 12 hours opioids (semisynthetic/synthetic) 2–3 days*
Propoxyphene	6–48 hours
Cannabinoids	Light smoker (1 joint) 2–3 days; moderate smoker (4 times/week) 5 days; heavy smoker (smokes daily) 10 days; retention time for chronic smokers may be 20–28 days
Phencyclidine (including ketamine)	Approximately 8 days; up to 30 days in chronic users (mean value = 14 days)

Note: Interpretation of retention time must take into account variability of urine specimens, drug metabolism and half-life, patient's physical condition, fluid intake, and method and frequency of ingestion. *Detected by GC/MS or other high-sensitivity method. These are general guidelines only.

including dose, route of administration, metabolism, urine concentration, and pH, the detection time of most drugs or their metabolites in urine is usually 1–3 days (Casavant, 2002; Vandevenne et al., 2000). Chronic use of a lipid-soluble drug such as marijuana may extend the window of detection to a week or more (Huestis et al., 1995; Vandevenne et al., 2000). Benzodiazepines and their metabolites differ widely in their elimination half-lives, which affect their clinical effect, excretion, and detection (Simpson et al., 1997). The window of detection for commonly tested drugs is presented in Table 42.1.

The method chosen to detect a particular drug will depend on the reason for undertaking the test. Immunoassay drug tests are most commonly used. They are designed to classify substances as either present or absent and are generally highly sensitive but often lack specificity. In pain management, specific drug identification using more sophisticated chromatographic tests is needed. Combined techniques such as GC/MS make accurate identification of a specific drug and/or its metabolites possible. When the patient is being prescribed drugs from several different classes of compounds, which is the case with many pain patients, specific identification is recommended. When properly used, these tests can help reduce cost, ensure accuracy, and improve efficiency.

Immunoassay is subject to cross-reactivity; in other words, substances with similar, and sometimes dissimilar, chemical composition may yield a false positive for the target drug. For this reason, specific identification of positive results (i.e., with GC/MS) is recommended. For example, immunoassay test for cocaine reacts principally with cocaine's primary metabolite, benzoylecgonine, and to a lesser extent cocaine itself (Braithwaite et al., 1995). The immunoassay test reliably identifies cocaine use. In contrast, tests for amphetamine and its derivatives are highly cross-reactive due to structural similarities to many prescription and over-the-counter (OTC) products. These include diet agents, decongestants such as ephedrine and pseudoephedrine, and certain drugs used in the treatment of Parkinson's disease.

The case of amphetamine testing merits further examination. Amphetamines and their derivatives exist in two mirror-image forms called isomers. Although both the d- and l-isomers are biologically active, it is primarily the d-isomer that accounts for this class of drug's central effects and misuse potential. For example, l-methamphetamine is used in OTC medications such as Vicks Nasal Inhalers. A test that is positive by immunoassay screen for methamphetamine must be confirmed by chiral GC/MS, which has the ability to differentiate between isomeric forms of analytes with a level of greater than 200 ng/mL of amphetamine to be a positive test for use of this illicit drug (Shults & St. Clair, 1999). This situation can be avoided by the patient always informing the doctor of any OTC medication that is taken.

Immunoassay tests for natural opiates are very responsive to morphine and codeine, but do not distinguish between the two. Further, UDT by opiate immunoassay also shows a low sensitivity for semisynthetic opioids such as oxycodone and hydrocodone, and shows virtually no cross-reactivity with fentanyl or methadone (Shults & St. Clair, 1999; Simpson et al., 1997). A negative opiate screen does not exclude their use. Laboratory medicine is constantly adding new immunoassay tests for specific agents such as methadone or oxycodone; however, these tests must be specifically requested in the appropriate clinical context (California Academy of Family Physicians and PharmaCom Group, Inc., 2004).

The presence of a prescribed drug in the urine sample makes monitoring of that class of drugs impossible by immunoassay technique alone. Specific drug identification by advanced testing (i.e., HPLC or GC/MS) is necessary to identify which member of the detected class is responsible for the positive screen. For example, a positive opiate screen cannot be explained on the basis of prescribed transdermal or transmucosal fentanyl; there must be another reason (either true or false positive) for the positive result.

Even though an immunoassay test may be negative for oxycodone, it should be positive on HPLC or GC/MS if the drug was used within the window of detection and the test is performed without threshold (limit of detection testing). The clinical importance of this fact with urine drug testing cannot be overstated because compliant patients may have been dismissed from pain management practices secondary to false-negative immunoassay testing when looking specifically for prescribed oxycodone using nonspecific immunoassay opiate testing.

Specimen Reliability

The purpose of UDT, in the context of pain management, is to enhance patient care and to help manage risk. Certain simple measures can be taken to improve the reliability of the results obtained from the donor's urine, including careful labeling of the sample container and the use of temperature-sensing collection bottles. An unusually hot or cold specimen, small sample volume, or unusual color should raise concerns and lead to discussion with the patient. Samples collected in the early morning are usually more reliable due to increased concentration of the specimen.

Ideally, specimen collection should be done randomly. Unobserved urine collection is usually acceptable in the context of a pain and addiction management practice. Consult with the laboratory regarding any unexpected results.

A false-negative result is technically defined as a negative finding in a sample known to contain the drug of interest. This may occur through laboratory or clerical error or, less likely, due to tampering with the urine sample. Methods employed by a minority of patients who may attempt to influence UDT results include adulteration and substitution of urine. Adulteration and substitution should be suspected if the characteristics of the urine sample are inconsistent with normal human urine.

A less ominous reason for an unexpected negative urine drug test is that the patient has been running out of drug early due either to inadequate dosing or problematic use (i.e., bingeing). Regardless of the reason, the results must never be ignored. Schedule an appointment to discuss abnormal/unexpected results with the patient. Discuss results in a positive and supportive fashion. Use results to strengthen the clinician-patient relationship and support positive behavioral change. Always chart the results and interpretation of the UDT. There must be a clear relationship between test results and subsequent actions taken by the treating practitioner. In some cases, patient behavior may be such that it is unwise to continue prescribing controlled substances. It is important for the practitioner and patient alike to remember that a decision to terminate the use of any pharmacotherapeutic regimen, including controlled substances, does not mean termination of care. In some cases, a practitioner's decision to stop prescribing a certain drug or drugs may cause the patient to elect to seek care elsewhere.

Caveats to Interpretation

Clinical urine drug testing, like any other medical test, has various strengths and weaknesses. Inappropriate interpretation of results may adversely affect clinical decisions: for example, discharge of patients from care when prescribed drugs are not detected (compliance testing) and over- or underdiagnosis of addiction/misuse. Health-care professionals should use UDT results in conjunction with other clinical information when deciding to continue with or adjust the established boundaries of the treatment plan.

The following examples illustrate some common urine test scenarios that may mislead the clinician.

Opiates

A patient may be unexpectedly positive for morphine due to the metabolism of prescribed codeine or, in certain situations, opium alkaloids such a morphine and codeine found in foodstuffs (e.g., poppy seeds in some bread/confections; Braithwaite et al., 1995; Casavant, 2002; Shults & St. Clair, 1999). In general, it is unwise to chronically use any specific medication that the patient has previously misused. In specific, codeine or morphine should not be the opioids of choice for chronic pain management in patients with a history of heroin addiction because both heroin and codeine share a common metabolic pathway to morphine (Braithwaite et al., 1995). Results of random urine drug tests, which should be part of the treatment plan, will be positive for morphine. The clinician will not know if the positive result was because of the prescribed opiate or a relapse to the use of heroin. It is only by detecting the presence of 6-monoacetylmorphine (6-MAM), a heroin metabolite, that definitive proof of heroin use is demonstrated. However, because of its very short half-life, this metabolite is seldom found in the urine drug test (Inturrisi et al., 1984). Basic opioid metabolism is presented in Figure 42.1.

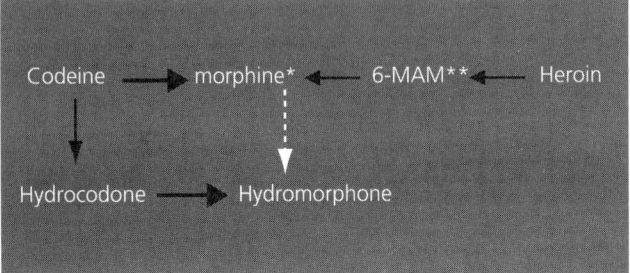

Figure 42.1. Metabolism of opioids: not comprehensive pathways, but may explain the presence of apparently unprescribed drugs (Source: Gourlay D, Heit HA, Caplan Y. California Academy of Family Practice [CAFP], August 2004). *Cone EJ, Heit HA, Caplan YH, Gourlay D. Evidence of morphine metabolism to hydromorphone in pain patients chronically treated with morphine. *J. Anal. Toxicol.* 2006;30(1):1–5. **6-MAM: 6-monoacetylmorphine; an intermediate metabolite.

In certain cases, a UDT may detect traces of unexplained opioids secondary to drug metabolism. For example, a patient taking codeine may show trace quantities of hydrocodone (up to 11%) that is unrelated to hydrocodone use (Oyler et al., 2000). Detection of minor amounts of hydrocodone in urine containing a high concentration of codeine should not be interpreted as evidence of hydrocodone misuse. In the case of a patient who is prescribed hydrocodone, quantities of hydromorphone may also be detected due to hydrocodone metabolism (California Academy of Family Physicians and PharmaCom Group, Inc., 2004). Morphine may be metabolized to produce small amounts of hydromorphone (up to 10%), through a minor metabolic pathway (Cone et al., 2006). Figure 42.1 shows the basic metabolism of opioids and metabolites.

Cocaine

In general, immunoassay results for the presence of the major metabolite of cocaine, benzoylecgonine, are highly reliable. There is little that cross-reacts with this test to give a false-positive result.

In some cases, a patient may be positive for cocaine following certain medical procedures when used as a topical anesthetic. Local anesthetics, however, that end in "caine," such as lidocaine or Novocain, do not result in a false positive for cocaine (Shults & St. Clair, 1999).

Benzodiazepines

Benzodiazepines can pose many challenges in monitoring. Due to a variety of factors, including differences in cross-reactivity, potency, and dose, the detection of benzodiazepines is highly variable (Gronholm & Lillsunde, 2001). For this reason, false-negative results are not uncommon, even in those persons using benzodiazepines as prescribed. This is particularly true of clonazepam, which makes this an attractive choice when selecting a therapeutic agent for either maintenance or substitution treatment because the finding of a positive benzodiazepine screen should alert the clinician to possible relapse back to another benzodiazepine such as diazepam, which is more easily detected. In this case, a negative benzodiazepine immunoassay is reassuring of compliance with treatment goals.

Unexpected Negative Urine

A negative urine test for a prescribed medication may be a result of various factors, including the patient running out of his or her medication early (bingeing). There is no reliable relationship between urine drug concentration and amount of drug ingested. It is also important to ensure that the threshold for reporting has been removed when trying to interpret the apparent absence of any prescribed medication. Communication between the testing laboratory and clinician will help ensure that the urine drug test results accurately reflect the clinical picture.

In all cases, clinical judgment should play the dominant role in interpretation of any UDT result. When UDT is used in a patient-centered fashion, it complements rather than detracts from optimum management of this often complex patient population.

Myths About UDTs

Passive cannabis smoke inhalation rarely explains positive marijuana results with commonly used testing thresholds, therefore, a positive UDT should be considered consistent with deliberate use of marijuana (Katz & Fanciullo, 2002). On the other hand, the prescription medications such as dronabinol (Marinol), which is synthetic δ-9-tetrahydrocannabinol, or Sativex, which is a naturally occurring plant extract containing both δ-9-tetrahydrocannabinol and cannabidiol, will yield a confirmable positive for THC, regardless of the route of administration.

Legally obtained hemp food products are increasingly available in retail stores. However, multiple studies have found that the THC concentrations typical in hemp seed products are insufficient to produce a positive immunoassay result (Bosy & Cole, 2000; Leson et al., 2001).

There have been documented cases of cocaine ingestion by drinking tea made from coca leaves (Shults & St. Clair, 1999). Although such tea may be available for purchase by unknowing consumers, the product—containing cocaine and/or related compounds—is illegal under U.S. Drug Enforcement Administration and Food and Drug Administration regulations. Therefore, in the absence of a legitimate medical explanation, a positive cocaine test indicates illicit use.

Emerging Technologies for Drug Testing

In the past few years, several new techniques have been developed in the field of drug testing. Each has strengths and limitations that will be discussed briefly.

Saliva and sweat testing are being developed primarily for use in the forensic setting. Advantages in using saliva as a test sample include the ease of collection, minimal personal invasiveness, and limited preanalytical manipulation. However, because drugs and/or metabolites in saliva are generally proportional to those in plasma, they may be retained for a shorter period and at lower concentrations compared with urine (Braithwaite et al., 1995; Kintz & Samyn, 2002; Yacoubian et al., 2001).

Sweat collection using a sweat patch is a noninvasive, cumulative measure of drug use up to 1 week, which is most appropriately used to monitor drug use in chemical dependency or probation programs (Wolff et al., 1999). Problems with patch adherence and sensitivity compared to UDT may limit its effectiveness (Huestis et al., 2000).

Hair analysis provides a retrospective, long-term measure of drug use that is directly related to the length of hair tested (Braithwaite et al., 1995; Crouch et al., 2002). However, darkly pigmented hair appears to have a greater capacity to bind certain drugs than hair that is fair or gray, leading to the claim that hair analysis might have a racial bias (Colon et al., 2002; Wolff et al., 1999; Yacoubian et al., 2001). Other disadvantages of hair analysis include irregular growth (approximately ½ inch/month), inability to reliably incorporate certain drugs (i.e., THC), and labor-intensive sample preparation leading to increased cost (Kintz & Samyn, 2002; Yacoubian et al., 2001).

Blood testing (more correctly, serum testing) can give an accurate assessment of drug level at the blood-brain barrier. Although this is useful in the forensic context of assessment of impairment, blood samples are not amenable to rapid screening procedures. They also are expensive, have low-drug concentrations and thus relatively limited windows of detection, and require invasive collection (Braithwaite et al., 1995; Wolff et al., 1999). It is not recommended for routine testing.

Point of care (POC) testing is becoming more readily available for routine use in the primary care setting. The basic principle usually relies on an immunoassay technology to identify specific drugs or classes of drugs. It should be pointed out that these tests are designed primarily to detect drug use in a population of donors who are largely drug free and so are intended to offer preliminary screening with relatively high cutoff thresholds. This limitation becomes more significant when applied to a pain patient population, the vast majority of who are appropriately using prescription drugs that are members of common classes of drugs abuse. This makes POC testing of limited value in the context of monitoring opioid use in pain medicine. In most cases, positive results for general classes of drugs need to be specifically identified by a secondary technique such as GC/MS in order to use UDT to its best advantage. POC testing alone for cocaine use is, however, both reliable and effective in identifying use of this particular drug.

The cost of urine drug testing varies tremendously across the country. In this context, drug testing does not usually require rapid results. The ordering practitioner is encouraged to negotiate the best price for drug testing from several laboratories. As an example, one author's negotiated cost for drugs of abuse urine drug test using immunoassay screening with GC/MS identification is less than $20/sample (Howard A. Heit, personal communication, 2003).

Conclusion

Urine drug testing is an effective tool for the health-care professional in the assessment and ongoing management of patients, especially those who will be or are being treated chronically with controlled substances. A working relationship with a testing laboratory may be very helpful in accurately interpreting urine test results. Most importantly, a health-care professional should have a relationship of mutual trust and honesty with the patient when using urine drug testing in his or her clinical practice. With a carefully thought-out testing strategy and accurate interpretation of results, the interests of both the patient and practitioner are well-served. Refusal to participate in urine drug testing due to philosophical opposition should be considered a relative contraindication to chronic pharmacologic management of chronic pain, especially with controlled substances.

References

Adams NJ, Plane MB, Fleming MF, Mundt MP, Saunders LA, Stauffacher EA. Opioids and the treatment of chronic pain in a primary care sample. *J Pain Symptom Manage* 2001;22(3):791–6.

Akinci IH, Tarter RE, Kirisci L. Concordance between verbal report and urine screen of recent marijuana use in adolescents. *Addict Behav* 2001;26(4):613–9.

Bosy TZ, Cole KA. Consumption and quantitation of delta9-tetrahydrocannabinol in commercially available hemp seed oil products. *J Anal Toxicol* 2000;24(7):562–6.

Braithwaite RA, Jarvie DR, Minty PS, Simpson D, Widdop B. Screening for drugs of abuse. I: Opiates, amphetamines and cocaine. *Ann Clin Biochem* 1995;32 (Pt 2):123–53.

California Academy of Family Physicians and PharmaCom Group, Inc. Urine drug testing in primary care: dispelling the myths & designing strategies. http://www.familydocs.org/assets/Professional_Development/CME/UDT.pdf. Published 2004. Accessed March 7, 2006.

Caplan YH, Goldberger BA. Alternative specimens for workplace drug testing. *J Anal Toxicol* 2001;25(5):396–9.

Casavant MJ. Urine drug screening in adolescents. *Pediatr Clin North Am* 2002;49(2):317–27.

Colon HM, Robles RR, Sahai H. The validity of drug use self-reports among hard core drug users in a household survey in Puerto Rico: comparison of survey responses of cocaine and heroin use with hair tests. *Drug Alcohol Depend* 2002;67(3):269–79.

Cone EJ, Heit HA, Caplan YH, Gourlay DL. Evidence of morphine metabolism to hydromorphone in pain patients chronically treated with morphine. *J Anal Toxicol* 2006;30(1):1–5.

Conigliaro C, Reyes C, Schultz J. *Principles of Screening and Early Intervention* (3rd ed.). Chevy Chase, MD: American Society of Addiction Medicine; 2003.

Cook JD, Caplan YH, LoDico CP, Bush DM. The characterization of human urine for specimen validity determination in workplace drug testing: a review. *J Anal Toxicol* 2000;24(7):579–88.

Crouch DJ, Hersch RK, Cook RF, Frank JF, Walsh JM. A field evaluation of five on-site drug-testing devices. *J Anal Toxicol* 2002;26(7):493–9.

Gronholm M, Lillsunde P. A comparison between on-site immunoassay drug-testing devices and laboratory results. *Forensic Sci Int* 2001;121(1–2):37–46.

Heit HA. *Use of Urine Toxicology Tests in a Chronic Pain Practice* (3rd ed.). Chevy Chase, MD: American Society of Addiction Medicine; 2003.

Huestis MA, Cone EJ, Wong CJ, Umbricht A, Preston KL. Monitoring opiate use in substance abuse treatment patients with sweat and urine drug testing. *J Anal Toxicol* 2000;24(7):509–21.

Huestis MA, Mitchell JM, Cone EJ. Detection times of marijuana metabolites in urine by immunoassay and GC-MS. *J Anal Toxicol* 1995;19(6):443–9.

Inturrisi CE, Max MB, Foley KM, Schultz M, Shin SU, Houde RW. The pharmacokinetics of heroin in patients with chronic pain. *N Engl J Med* 1984;310(19):1213–7.

Katz N, Fanciullo GJ. Role of urine toxicology testing in the management of chronic opioid therapy. *Clin J Pain* 2002;18(4 Suppl):S76–82.

Kaul P, Coupey SM. Clinical evaluation of substance abuse. *Pediatr Rev* 2002;23(3):85–94.

Kintz P, Samyn N. Use of alternative specimens: drugs of abuse in saliva and doping agents in hair. *Ther Drug Monit* 2002;24(2):239–46.

Kirsh KL, Whitcomb LA, Donaghy K, Passik SD. Abuse and addiction issues in medically ill patients with pain: attempts at clarification of terms and empirical study. *Clin J Pain* 2002;18(4 Suppl):S52–60.

Lapham SC, C'De Baca J, Chang I, Hunt WC, Berger LR. Are drunk-driving offenders referred for screening accurately reporting their drug use? *Drug Alcohol Depend* 2002;66(3):243–53.

Leson G, Pless P, Grotenhermen F, Kalant H, ElSohly MA. Evaluating the impact of hemp food consumption on workplace drug tests. *J Anal Toxicol* 2001;25(8):691–8.

Oyler JM, Cone EJ, Joseph RE, Jr., Huestis MA. Identification of hydrocodone in human urine following controlled codeine administration. *J Anal Toxicol* 2000;24(7):530–5.

Passik SD, Schreiber J, Kirsh KL, Portenoy RK. A chart review of the ordering and documentation of urine toxicology screens in a cancer center: do they influence patient management? *J Pain Symptom Manage* 2000;19(1):40–4.

Passik SD, Weinreb HJ. Managing chronic nonmalignant pain: overcoming obstacles to the use of opioids. *Adv Ther* 2000;17(2):70–83.

Savage SR. Long-term opioid therapy: assessment of consequences and risks. *J Pain Symptom Manage* 1996;11(5):274–86.

Shults T, St. Clair S. *The Medical Review Officer Handbook*. Triangle Park, NC: Quadrangle Research; 1999.

Simpson D, Braithwaite RA, Jarvie DR, et al. Screening for drugs of abuse (II): Cannabinoids, lysergic acid diethylamide, buprenorphine, methadone, barbiturates, benzodiazepines and other drugs. *Ann Clin Biochem* 1997;34(Pt 5):460–510.

Staines GL, Magura S, Foote J, Deluca A, Kosanke N. Polysubstance use among alcoholics. *J Addict Dis* 2001;20(4):53–69.

Vandevenne M, Vandenbussche H, Verstraete A. Detection time of drugs of abuse in urine. *Acta Clin Belg* 2000;55(6):323–33.

Wolff K, Farrell M, Marsden J, et al. A review of biological indicators of illicit drug use, practical considerations and clinical usefulness. *Addiction* 1999;94(9):1279–98.

Yacoubian GS, Jr., Wish ED, Perez DM. A comparison of saliva testing to urinalysis in an arrestee population. *J Psychoactive Drugs* 2001;33(3):289–94.

43

The Opioid Contract

Felix A. Chen
Scott M. Fishman
Paul G. Kreis

The medication contract is an instrument commonly used in the treatment of patients placed on long-term opioid therapy. Although these contracts are widely used in the chronic administration of opioids, their efficacy in practice remains to be proven. A *contract* is defined by the *Oxford English Dictionary* as an "explicit bilateral commitment to a well-defined course of action." As such, the physician-patient contract implies several basic assumptions (Quill, 1983): (1) The terms and consequences for breaching the contract are explicitly stated; (2) the doctor and patient each have unique responsibilities; (3) the doctor-patient relationship is consensual, not obligatory; and (4) both physician and patient are willing and able to negotiate. Both parties in the contract are typically required to have a clearly stated understanding of their individual obligations. The term *contract* may not be required to fulfill the spirit or purpose of a contract. In such cases, formation of a documented bilateral agreement may be sufficient to serve as a contract, regardless of whether it is labeled as a contract, agreement, informed consent, or any other term. The contract does not have to be written as verbal contracts can be binding in courts of law.

Despite the relative lack of controlled study regarding the efficacy of opioid contracts, the practice of formal agreements between patient and physician is an appealing tool for overcoming some of the problems that are too often associated with chronic opioid therapy, particularly in situations in which abuse or diversion may be of concern (Kirkpatrick, Derasari, et al., 1998). Thus, physicians and clinical programs involved in dispensing chronic opioid analgesics are adopting the practice of opioid contracts or other formal agreements in their practice. The American Academy of Pain Medicine (2001) has released a sample patient-physician agreement form for long-term controlled substances therapy for chronic pain on their website (Figure 43.1). It is notable that this sample agreement is offered with the warning, "Sample for Adaptation... Please Consult With Your Attorney." This suggests several cautionary messages, including that there is no one standard approach to an opioid contract or agreement and that there may be legal considerations. Although use of opioid contracts or agreements may be second nature for some practices that prescribe chronic opioid therapy, at present it remains unclear how they are best used, or if they may place clinicians at risk for liability or subject patients to reduced autonomy.

Contracts have been best described in cases of managing patients with suicidal ideation (Kernberg, 1993; Smith & Bope 1986; Stanford, Goetz, et al., 1994) or character pathology (Miller, 1990). They are widely used in psychiatric practices, associated with patients with severe personality disorder, suicidal tendencies, or substance abuse (Saxon, Calsyn, et al., 1993). As such, a therapeutic contract (or agreement) may enable a patient to attain an active role in treatment and possibly curb the potential for rebellion against what may be perceived as all-powerful and controlling caregivers (Miller, 1990). Because opioid contracts often target adherence issues, it is ironic that their effectiveness in mitigating adherence to treatment, particularly with drugs such as opioids for chronic pain, is not well-established. Although not exactly related to chronic opioid therapy for analgesia, studies reviewing use of contracts largely from methadone maintenance programs indicate transient efficacy, with improved adherence seen only early in treatment (Maruta, Swanson, et al., 1979; Nolimal & Crowley, 1990). When used in the setting of opioid abuse, contracts were most effective when they placed increased responsibility on the patient and included specific descriptions of these responsibilities (Saxon, Calsyn, et al., 1993). Although convincing data on contract use is limited, there is no direct evidence suggesting that use of contracts is significantly detrimental to treatment.

Treating the patient with a history of substance abuse with comorbid chronic pain presents a particularly difficult dilemma for the prescribing clinician (Wesson, Ling, et al., 1993). The rate of drug and alcohol addiction in the general population can approach 10%–16% (Kissen, 1997), while simultaneously, the prevalence of chronic pain in methadone maintenance treatment program patients can be as high as 37% (Rosenblum, Joseph, et al., 2003). Patients with addiction issues can successfully receive appropriate pain treatment (Dunbar & Katz, 1996); thus a patient's history of previous addiction should not be considered absolute grounds for exclusion from opioid pain medication treatment, although a history of legal problems related to drug use may indicate higher risk of aberrant behavior (Michna, Ross, et al., 2004).

Previous studies have evaluated physicians' views on aberrant behavior (Passik, Kirsh, et al., 2002). Behaviors involving illegal activity such as forging prescriptions or selling prescription drugs as well as altering the route of administration were ranked as most severe. Although several researchers have attempted to develop

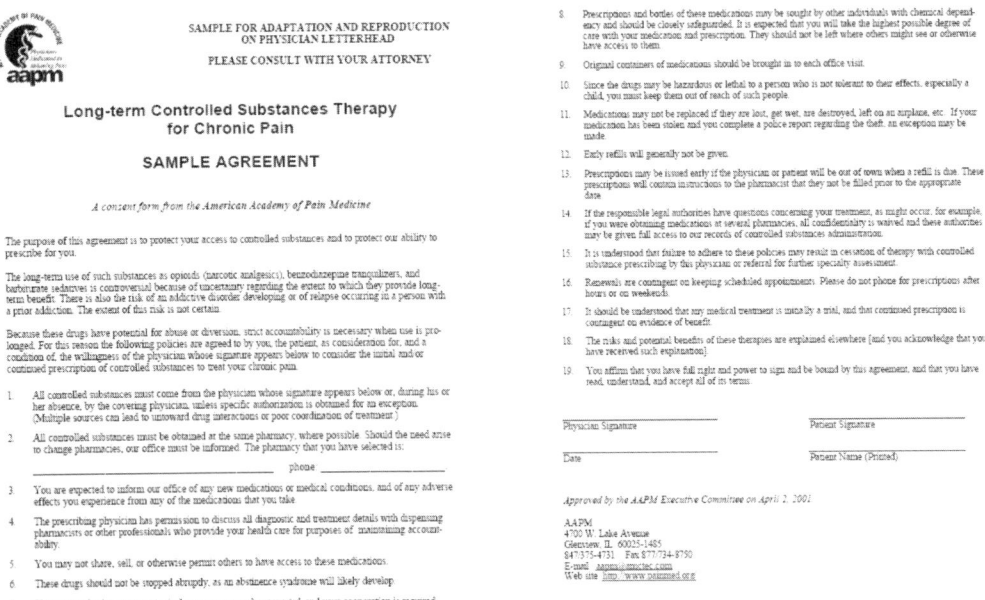

Figure 43.1. Sample opioid agreement provided by the American Academy of Pain Medicine (AAPM; 2001).

screening tools to predict aberrant behaviors (Butler, Budman, et al., 2004; Compton, Darakjian, et al., 1998; Friedman, Li, et al., 2003), unfortunately, there are no validated predictors of aberrant drug-related behavior available to physicians who treat pain (Passik & Kirsh, 2003). Weaver and Schnoll (2002) as well as Passik and Kirsh (2005) describe strategies for the opioid treatment of chronic pain in patients with addiction, including implementation of a medication agreement. The agreement is suggested as a tool for reinforcing the patient's responsibility for his or her prescriptions and medications, while simultaneously providing reassurance to the patient that he or she, in turn, will continue to receive appropriate amounts of pain medication.

Pseudoaddiction is a potentially complicating situation with regard to opioid contracts. Pseudoaddiction is described as undertreatment of pain masquerading as drug-seeking behavior (Weissman & Haddox, 1989), whereby a patient may manifest behaviors classically associated with addiction, including unapproved dose escalations and seeking medications from multiple sources. Although pseudoaddiction may be difficult to distinguish from true addictive behavior, once the patient's pain is adequately treated, the aberrant behavior disappears. In order to avoid mistaking pseudoaddiction for true addiction, the clinician must maintain the possibility that the patient's complaints are genuine, while still monitoring for warning signs of addiction or abuse, keeping in mind that the failure rate of addicted patients on methadone contracts can be significant (Calsyn, Wells, et al., 1996). Although violations of the terms of a typical opioid contract might result in a taper off of opioid analgesics, one may be doing the patient a disservice if this occurs in the context of pseudoaddiction with possible legal ramifications (Fishbain, 2002). Fortunately, the contract can serve to guide all parties, such as for patients with a remote history of addiction with clear terms for documented participation in programs that support sobriety as well as increased function such as Alcoholics or Narcotics Anonymous or psychological or physical rehabilitation activities as part of the pain therapy regimen.

Implementing chronic opioid therapy for chronic pain often requires a clear course of action that is agreed on by all of the involved parties. Although the opioid contract is an appealing tool for serving this purpose, there is presently no standard for what should comprise an effective opioid contract. The medical literature on this topic is not robust in its examination of, or its guidance in, the use of this instrument. Patient-physician interactions around the acceptance of a contract are also not well-described (Burchman & Pagel, 1995).

Burchman and Pagel (1995) have described their successful experience with using an opioid agreement in their pain management center. Their report included the description of using a "medical alert" card identifying the patient who signed the "agreement" as a participant in their program. A previous survey analysis of opioid contracts (Fishman, Bandman, et al., 1999) from 39 academically based pain programs found great variability in contract form and content. Nonetheless, they found consistency among all of the contracts in their overall goals of dealing with patient responsibilities, education, and termination criteria. The purpose of most of these contracts appeared to be to improve adherence to treatment through education, establish clear limit setting, and disseminate administrative information. This report suggested that the contract or agreement usually includes standard information about medication use and abuse, the consequences for violating the contract, and the procedure for opioid discontinuation should it become necessary (Table 43.1). An additional feature included terms for routine, random substance testing as part of the treatment plan or restrictions to a single prescriber or pharmacy. Most of these contracts included statements about how and when changes in medications would be made, including limitations on scheduled prescriptions and appointments. Other notable inclusions reflected the need to involve outside caregivers or agencies, such as the primary care physician, or requirements that the patient agree to tenets of treatment, such as informing the opioid prescriber of relevant information and adherence to medication changes or tapering schedules.

Table 43.1. Specific Statement Groups in Order of Frequency: Subgroups of the General Statement Categories

Rank	Statement Category	# of Contracts	Percent
1.	Avoid improper use of controlled substances (includes overdosing, seeking medication elsewhere, selling medication, stopping medication abruptly).	37	95%
2.	Terms for disciplinary termination (abusing medication, missed appointments, violating contract, inappropriate behavior).	36	92%
3.	Limitations for replacing medication or changing prescriptions.	33	85%
4.	Inform physician of relevant information (i.e., side effects, medications, changes in condition).	29	74%
5.	Submit to random drug screens.	27	69%
6.	Terms regarding appointments (missed appointments, follow-up, appearing without appointment).	24	62%
7.	Include additional health care providers involved in care (primary care physician [PCP], PT, psychologist, etc.).	23	59%
8.	Limits on drug refills (phone allowances, only in person, call in advance, normal office hours).	22	56%
9.	Side effects education (including withdrawal).	22	56%
10.	Terms of nondisciplinary termination (no improvement, pregnancy, tolerance, toxicity, etc.).	20	51%
11.	Education on addiction risks and behaviors.	19	49%
12.	Education on opioids and chronic pain.	19	49%
13.	Health care providers informed of prescription (may include PCP, pharmacist, etc.).	18	46%
14.	Pharmacy issues included (one pharmacy, in-state pharmacy).	17	44%
15.	Goals outlined.	15	38%
16.	Additional risks discussed (other drugs, masking conditions, misusing, pregnancy).	15	36%
17.	Necessity of contract discussed (reasons why necessary, including federal guidelines and abuse).	14	33%
18.	Legal considerations discussed.	13	33%
19.	Single prescriber for all opioid prescriptions.	13	31%
20.	Dosing limitation (how much, interval Rx made, rescue dosing, PRN, dose escalation).	12	31%
21.	Disclaimer for emergency situations (i.e., makes exceptions).	12	31%
22.	Operation of motor vehicle, heavy machinery, or firearms discouraged.	12	31%
23.	Substance abuse exclusion (current or history, including selling drugs).	12	28%
24.	Terms regarding specific medication (type prescribed: long-acting, generic brands, etc.).	11	23%
25.	Time course/trial period is outlined.	9	21%
26.	Agree to medication changes and tapers.	8	18%
27.	Contract issues (includes who receives contract, where contract is kept, violations, and how opioids are maintained).	7	18%
28.	Pregnancy listed as exclusionary.	7	15%
29.	Alcohol use discouraged.	6	15%
30.	Alcohol use prohibited.	6	13%
31.	Agree to take responsibility for medications (e.g., safeguard medication).	5	10%
32.	Family involved in care.	4	10%
33.	Leftover medication brought to clinic.	4	10%
34.	Physician will offer detoxification if necessary.	4	5%
35.	Agree to maintain good health.	2	5%
36.	Benefits of long-term opioids discussed.	2	5%
37.	Patient will inform ER physician of contract.	2	5%
38.	Operation of motor vehicle, heavy machinery, or firearms prohibited.	2	5%
39.	Opioid therapy described as dual responsibility of doctor and patient.	2	5%
40.	Employer may be informed of prescription.	1	3%
41.	Patient will not receive opioids in emergency room.	1	3%
42.	Physician must also agree to a contract.	1	3%
43.	Physician provides treatment information.	1	3%

1. Summary of 39 statement categories among surveyed contracts.

Source: Fishman, Bandman, et al. 1999.

Many of the specific statement groups from the 39 academic centers surveyed are listed in Table 43.1, in order of their frequency within the samples reviewed (Fishman, Bandman, et al., 1999). In general, there are several broad commonalities between most of the surveyed contracts. Most commonly, the contracts involved terms of treatment including treatment parameters and contingency plans for term breaches. Most often these involved expectations of medication use including dosing compliance, secure medication storage, limitations on medication replacements and refills, and submitting to random drug screens. Also commonly found were guidelines for points of termination of treatment, both disciplinary (violation of contract terms) as well as nondisciplinary (treatment failure) via drug taper. Moderately common topics included patient responsibilities, educational information (intent of treatment, opioid medications, addiction risks and behaviors, risks of treatment) and involvement of ancillary health-care providers (addictionologists, psychologists). Less commonly addressed were emergency issues, goals of treatment, legal considerations, and staff responsibilities. It is notable that few contracts discussed the possibility that the patient might be referred back to his or her primary care physician (PCP) for continued opioid prescriptions once the pain stabilized, or the need for the patient to have a PCP during opioid treatment.

The concept of a trilateral opioid agreement has recently emerged as a tool to engage the PCP in chronic opioid prescribing (Fishman, Mahajan, et al., 2002). This trilateral agreement involves signatures from the patient, pain specialist, and the PCP. Prescribing would not begin until all parties signed the agreement assuring that all were in agreement and that once stabilized, the PCP would assume opioid prescribing on a chronic basis. A previous study suggested that almost half of patients surveyed described their primary physician as skeptical or suspicious toward opioid therapy, whereas one-third claimed that the primary physician refused to continue a stable opioid regimen (Donner, Raber, et al., 1998). In studying the trilateral contract, although only 72% of the patients actually obtained their PCP's signature; surprisingly, the number of unsigned contracts was due to patient issues and not reluctance on the part of the patient's PCP. The findings of this study suggest that primary care physicians are not as reluctant to prescribe opioids as previously thought and are willing to collaborate with specialists in managing opioid treatment regimens. Of the patients who did obtain their primary physician's signature, all were transitioned back to their primary without difficulty in obtaining opioids. The trilateral opioid agreement appears to be a potentially useful tool for networking specialty and primary care providers in managing a patient's pain care. A sample of the trilateral opioid agreement is shown in Figure 43.2.

Use of patient-physician contracts poses some potential complications. Contracts have the potential to stigmatize patients, particularly those with histories of substance abuse (Lert & Marne, 1992). For instance, having been given an opioid contract, a patient may believe that the opioids are considered a special problem by his or her clinician because other forms of chronic medication therapy have not required such a contract. Dispelling such understandable conclusions about the patient-physician contract process requires education. To avoid being perceived by the patient as a punishment or manipulation, the contract should be carefully constructed for effective presentation, supported through collaboration with all health-care providers and the patient, and maintained with constancy and balanced, coherent implementation (Miller, 1990). A potentially problematic outcome of a contract is the conclusion by the clinician that the patient is adherent by virtue of signing an agreement. Completion of an opioid contract is in no way tantamount to adherence to the contract, and such reassurance may be nothing more than a rescue fantasy. Thus, a signed opioid agreement should not be used to relax vigilance on monitoring adherence throughout the course of treatment.

The binding nature of the "opioid contract" is also unclear. Because the contract is a bilateral agreement, however, it is possible that there could be legal ramifications if the clinician breaks the

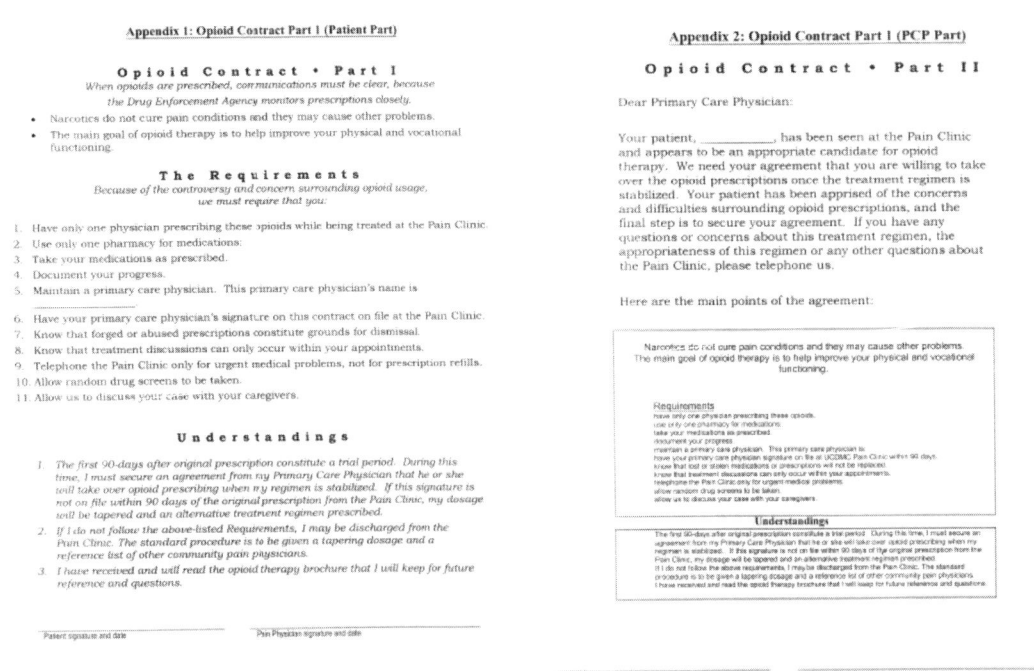

Figure 43.2. Sample trilateral opioid agreement involving the patient, specialist, and primary care physician (Fishman, Mahajan, et al., 2002).

terms of the agreement. Kirkpatrick et al. (1998) have described some of the common regulatory provisions that have an impact on risk-management issues related to opioid contracts, including the defense of a civil medical malpractice case. This report supports the use of a written protocol contract to document the opioid treatment plan and for informed consent.

Because at present there are not clear guidelines for opioid contracts, specific inclusions may require careful consideration. In particular, extreme limitations on personal liberties such as driving are not clearly supported. A recent report (Galski, Williams, et al., 2000) compared cerebrally compromised patients who had passed drivers' tests with patients on chronic opioid therapy. The study found that patients on chronic opioid therapy generally outperformed the cerebrally compromised patients on predriver evaluations and simulated driving evaluations. Nonetheless, driving under the influence of any sedating medication is obviously a risk.

In the study by Fishman et al. (1999), 36% of the reviewed contracts included statements warning patients of the potential dangers of driving a motor vehicle while taking opioids, and two of the contracts clearly prohibited driving altogether. It may be difficult for state and federal authorities to distinguish between acute and chronic use of prescribed opioids, and accident reports or laboratory data can easily be misinterpreted. It is conceivable that, at some point, issue may be taken with patients who use chronic opioids and drive. Although it may be prudent to prohibit driving during periods of initial opioid dosing or after dose escalations, complete prohibition of driving while using opioids is not clearly supported by the medical literature (Fishman, Bandman, et al., 1999; Galski, Williams, et al., 2000). As with any potentially sedating drug such as alcohol or antihistamines, it seems reasonable to always educate and remind our patients that it is each individual's responsibility to monitor themselves and make judgments on a moment-by-moment basis about their capacity to safely operate a motor vehicle or any potentially hazardous machinery or participate in any potentially dangerous activity.

Pregnancy while using prescribed opioids for chronic pain raises similar concerns about the appropriate nature of strict limitations in the opioid contract or agreement. Just as in the case of driving limitations, Fishman et al. (1999) found 36% of the reviewed contracts to include statements reflecting concern regarding potential pregnancy. Half of these contracts clearly prohibited pregnancy, citing it as an exclusion criterion for chronic opioid therapy. The medical literature on pregnancy and therapeutic use of chronic opioids is not conclusive, and such limitations within a formal contract may therefore require careful consideration. There seems to be only one case report on the effect of opioids on the fetus when prescribed for pain in the mother (Wen, Hou, et al., 1996). Because most studies on this topic are limited to the effects of illicit drug abuse (Alroomi, Davidson, et al., 1988; Chiriboga, 1993; Dattel, 1990; Finnegan, 1989; Jacobson, Jacobson, et al., 1994; Kaltenbach & Thornton, Clune, et al., 1990; Ostrea, Ostrea, et al., 1997; Schneider & Hans, 1996; Suess, Newlin, et al., 1997), the effects of opioids on pregnancy in methadone maintenance programs (Finnegan, 1991; Jarvis & Schnoll, 1994) on the fetus of illicit opioids, or prescribed methadone use in a maintenance program (Maas, Kattner, et al., 1990; Stimmel, Goldberg, et al., 1982), drawing firm conclusions about therapeutic opioids in pregnancy is difficult. Overall, there does not appear to be conclusive evidence of detrimental effects from prescribed chronic opioid therapy in pregnancy. Additionally, the long-term effects of pain on the fetus remain to be determined. Thus, the risk-to-benefit analysis in such cases is not clear and it is conceivable that strict contraindications within a formalized contract may raise concerns of unjustifiable limitations. Nonetheless, an opioid contract may be helpful in clarifying the prescriber's concerns about opioids in a pregnancy and establishing a clear agreement for immediate notification should pregnancy occur or be anticipated.

Because the patient-physician contract is a bilateral agreement, there may be legal consequences should the contract be broken by the clinician. This is exemplified by a case in Massachusetts in which a tort was brought against a physician who, being compassionately lenient with the terms of a verbal opioid agreement, refilled an opioid prescription early. The clinician refilled the prescription in a patient who had a history of abuse, but the clinician felt that a second chance was warranted despite knowing that doing so would be contrary to of the terms of the verbal opioid contract. The patient subsequently abused the prescribed opioid and died from overdose. The family sued the physician, who was found liable. The reverse situation may also potentially exist: A well-written contract could provide protection to a clinician in a situation in which a patient demonstrates clear violations of the terms of the contract yet still files suit (Doleys & Rickman, 2003).

Conclusions

The opioid contract is a commonly used instrument for managing chronic opioid medications. Unfortunately, despite its widespread use, the efficacy of the opioid contract in long-term opioid treatment for pain has not been proven, with few studies addressing this topic. Contracts in the use of methadone for heroin addiction treatment have been studied and have demonstrated improved patient compliance only when more responsibility is placed on the patient (Saxon, Calsyn, et al., 1993). Opioid contracts or agreements appear to be widely used for clarifying descriptions and expectations of medication use and abuse, consequences of violating the contract, the procedure for opioid discontinuation should this become necessary, other educational or administrative issues, and terms for adherence monitoring including random drug testing.

The opioid contract may prove most beneficial in the case of the patient with a known addiction history. Previous study of addicted patients on methadone maintenance therapy suggests the medication contract may improve treatment compliance (Calsyn, Wells, et al., 1996; Nolimal & Crowley, 1990; Saxon, Calsyn, et al., 1993). Some patients with addiction problems have demonstrated difficulty with impulsivity, lability, and risk-taking behavior prior to as well as after onset of addiction (Bechara, Dolan, et al., 2002; Giancola, Mezzich, et al., 1998; Simons, Carey, et al., 2004). Subtle brain dysfunction with impaired judgment may also be associated with drug addiction (Bechara, 2001; Clark & Robbins, 2002; Fishbein, Eldreth, et al., 2005). In these cases, the opioid contract could serve as an enduring treatment guideline in the potentially impaired patient, whether due to illicit or iatrogenic etiology.

Although the opioid contract may be helpful, it may not be entirely benign for either the clinician or patient. For instance, it is not clear whether such contracts place clinicians at increased risk of liability should the clinician violate their terms or place patients at risk for reduced autonomy. Careful consideration should be given to restrictions the contract may place on a patient. There may be potential for the opioid contract to appear stigmatizing or punitive. It may also have the potential to inappropriately reassure clinicians of adherence, possibly leading to relaxation of vigilance in monitoring adherence and treatment efficacy.

The contract seems to be of time-tested utility as an educational document for clarifying rationale and expectations of treatment as well as acquiring informed consent. However, the amount of information required to produce an exhaustive document may not be practical in the clinical setting. For the sake of expediency, contracts often include only the most important and relevant points. In our program, we use a double-page contract that clearly but briefly describes the terms of ongoing treatment. The patient acknowledges having reviewed a more comprehensive handout that accompanies the contract, and which details the salient educational and administrative issues involved in treatment. Moreover, we have required that our patients have a primary care physician who must sign the second part of the opioid contract. The primary care physician's signature indicates that the specialist has a partner at the primary care level, which fortifies the treatment network.

Those considering developing or revising an opioid contract or agreement are advised to consider the consistent core themes that have been reported in surveyed contracts as well as many that were not as frequently included but which may be of importance to individual practices (Fishman, Bandman, et al., 1999).

References

Alroomi, L. G., J. Davidson, et al. (1988). Maternal narcotic abuse and the newborn. *Arch Dis Child* 63(1): 81–3.

American Academy of Pain Medicine. (2001). Long-term controlled substances therapy for chronic pain: sample agreement. http://www.painmed.org/productpub/statements/pdfs/controlled_substances_sample_agrmt.pdf. Accessed May 24, 2007.

Bechara, A. (2001). Neurobiology of decision-making: risk and reward. *Semin Clin Neuropsychiatry* 6(3): 205–16.

Bechara, A., S. Dolan, et al. (2002). Decision-making and addiction (part II): myopia for the future or hypersensitivity to reward? *Neuropsychologia* 40(10): 1690–705.

Burchman, S. L., & P. S. Pagel (1995). Implementation of a formal treatment agreement for outpatient management of chronic nonmalignant pain with opioid analgesics. *J Pain Symptom Manage* 10(7): 556–63.

Butler, S. F., S. H. Budman, et al. (2004). Validation of a screener and opioid assessment measure for patients with chronic pain. *Pain* 112(1–2): 65–75.

Calsyn, D. A., E. A. Wells, et al. (1996). Outcome of a second episode of methadone maintenance. *Drug Alcohol Depend* 43(3): 163–8.

Chiriboga, C. A. (1993). Fetal effects. *Neurol Clin* 11(3): 707–28.

Clark, L., & T. Robbins (2002). Decision-making deficits in drug addiction. *Trends Cogn Sci* 6(9): 361.

Compton, P., J. Darakjian, et al. (1998). Screening for addiction in patients with chronic pain and "problematic" substance use: evaluation of a pilot assessment tool. *J Pain Symptom Manage* 16(6): 355–63.

Dattel, B. J. (1990). Substance abuse in pregnancy. *Semin Perinatol* 14(2): 179–87.

Doleys, D. M., & L. Rickman (2003). Other benefits of an opioid "agreement." *J Pain Symptom Manage* 25(5): 402–3; author replay 403–4.

Donner, B., M. Raber, et al. (1998). Experiences with the prescription of opioids: a patient questionnaire. *J Pain Symptom Manage* 15(4): 231–4.

Dunbar, S. A., & N. P. Katz (1996). Chronic opioid therapy for nonmalignant pain in patients with a history of substance abuse: report of 20 cases. *J Pain Symptom Manage* 11(3): 163–71.

Finnegan, L. P. (1991). Treatment issues for opioid-dependent women during the perinatal period. *J Psychoactive Drugs* 23(2): 191–201.

Fishbain, D. A. (2002). Medico-legal rounds: medico-legal issues and breaches of "standards of medical care" in opioid tapering for alleged opioid addiction. *Pain Med* 3(2): 135–42; discussion 143–6.

Fishbein, D. H., D. L. Eldreth, et al. (2005). Risky decision making and the anterior cingulate cortex in abstinent drug abusers and nonusers. *Brain Res Cogn Brain Res* 23(1): 119–36.

Fishman, S. M., T. B. Bandman, et al. (1999). The opioid contract in the management of chronic pain. *J Pain Symptom Manage* 18(1): 27–37.

Fishman, S. M., G. Mahajan, et al. (2002). The trilateral opioid contract. Bridging the pain clinic and the primary care physician through the opioid contract. *J Pain Symptom Manage* 24(3): 335–44.

Friedman, R., V. Li, et al. (2003). Treating pain patients at risk: evaluation of a screening tool in opioid-treated pain patients with and without addiction. *Pain Med* 4(2): 182–5.

Galski, T., J. B. Williams, et al. (2000). Effects of opioids on driving ability. *J Pain Symptom Manage* 19(3): 200–8.

Giancola, P. R., A. C. Mezzich, et al. (1998). Disruptive, delinquent and aggressive behavior in female adolescents with a psychoactive substance use disorder: relation to executive cognitive functioning. *J Stud Alcohol* 59(5): 560–7.

Jacobson, J. L., S. W. Jacobson, et al. (1994). Effects of alcohol use, smoking, and illicit drug use on fetal growth in black infants. *J Pediatr* 124(5 Pt 1): 757–64.

Jarvis, M. A., & S. H. Schnoll (1994). Methadone treatment during pregnancy. *J Psychoactive Drugs* 26(2): 155–61.

Kaltenbach, K. A., & L. P. Finnegan (1989). Prenatal narcotic exposure: perinatal and developmental effects. *Neurotoxicology* 10(3): 597–604.

Kernberg, O. F. (1993). Suicidal behavior in borderline patients: diagnosis and psychotherapeutic considerations. *Am J Psychother* 47(2): 245–54.

Kirkpatrick, A. F., M. Derasari, et al. (1998). A protocol-contract for opioid use in patients with chronic pain not due to malignancy. *J Clin Anesth* 10(5): 435–43.

Kissen, B. (1997). Medical management of alcoholic patients. In B. Kissen & H. Begleiter (eds.), *Treatment and Rehabilitation of the Chronic Alcoholic*. New York: Plenum Publishing Co.

Lert, F., & M. J. Marne (1992). Hospital care for drug users with AIDS or HIV infection in France. *AIDS Care* 4(3): 333–8.

Maas, U., E. Kattner, et al. (1990). Infrequent neonatal opiate withdrawal following maternal methadone detoxification during pregnancy. *J Perinat Med* 18(2): 111–8.

Maruta, T., D. W. Swanson, et al. (1979). Drug abuse and dependency in patients with chronic pain. *Mayo Clin Proc* 54(4): 241–4.

Michna, E., E. L. Ross, et al. (2004). Predicting aberrant drug behavior in patients treated for chronic pain: importance of abuse history. *J Pain Symptom Manage* 28(3): 250–8.

Miller, L. J. (1990). The formal treatment contract in the inpatient management of borderline personality disorder. *Hosp Community Psychiatry* 41(9): 985–7.

Nolimal, D., & T. J. Crowley (1990). Difficulties in a clinical application of methadone-dose contingency contracting. *J Subst Abuse Treat* 7(4): 219–24.

Ostrea, E. M., Jr., A. R. Ostrea, et al. (1997). Mortality within the first 2 years in infants exposed to cocaine, opiate, or cannabinoid during gestation. *Pediatrics* 100(1): 79–83.

Passik, S. D., & K. L. Kirsh (2003). The need to identify predictors of aberrant drug-related behavior and addiction in patients being treated with opioids for pain. *Pain Med* 4(2): 186–9.

Passik, S. D., & K. L. Kirsh (2005). Managing pain in patients with aberrant drug-taking behaviors. *J Support Oncol* 3(1): 83–6.

Passik, S. D., K. L. Kirsh, et al. (2002). Pain clinicians' rankings of aberrant drug-taking behaviors. *J Pain Palliat Care Pharmacother* 16(4): 39–49.

Quill, T. E. (1983). Partnerships in patient care: a contractual approach. *Ann Intern Med* 98(2): 228–34.

Rosenblum, A., H. Joseph, et al. (2003). Prevalence and characteristics of chronic pain among chemically dependent patients in methadone maintenance and residential treatment facilities. *JAMA* 289(18): 2370–8.

Saxon, A. J., D. A. Calsyn, et al. (1993). Outcome of contingency contracting for illicit drug use in a methadone maintenance program. *Drug Alcohol Depend* 31(3): 205–14.

Schneider, J. W., & S. L. Hans (1996). Effects of prenatal exposure to opioids on focused attention in toddlers during free play. *J Dev Behav Pediatr* 17(4): 240–7.

Simons, J. S., K. B. Carey, et al. (2004). Lability and impulsivity synergistically increase risk for alcohol-related problems. *Am J Drug Alcohol Abuse* 30(3): 685–94.

Smith, C. W., Jr., & E. T. Bope (1986). The suicidal patient. The primary care physician's role in evaluation and treatment. *Postgrad Med* 79(8): 195–202.

Stanford, E. J., R. R. Goetz, et al. (1994). The No Harm Contract in the emergency assessment of suicidal risk. *J Clin Psychiatry* 55(8): 344–8.

Stimmel, B., J. Goldberg, et al. (1982). Fetal outcome in narcotic-dependent women: the importance of the type of maternal narcotic used. *Am J Drug Alcohol Abuse* 9(4): 383–95.

Suess, P. E., D. B. Newlin, et al. (1997). Motivation, sustained attention, and autonomic regulation in school-age boys exposed in utero to opiates and alcohol. *Exp Clin Psychopharmacol* 5(4): 375–87.

Thornton, L., M. Clune, et al. (1990). Narcotic addiction: the expectant mother and her baby. *Ir Med J* 83(4): 139–42.

Weaver, M. F., & S. H. Schnoll (2002). Opioid treatment of chronic pain in patients with addiction. *J Pain Palliat Care Pharmacother* 16(3): 5–26.

Weissman, D. E., & J. D. Haddox (1989). Opioid pseudoaddiction—an iatrogenic syndrome. *Pain* 36(3): 363–6.

Wen, Y. R., W. Y. Hou, et al. (1996). Intrathecal morphine for neuropathic pain in a pregnant cancer patient. *J Formos Med Assoc* 95: 252–4.

Wesson, D. R., W. Ling, et al. (1993). Prescription of opioids for treatment of pain in patients with addictive disease. *J Pain Symptom Manage* 8(5): 289–96.

44

Opioids and the Treatment of Chronic Pain

Daniel S. Bennett

Pamela Squire

Daniel Brookoff

I need my Percocets doc, that's the only medication that works for me. And it has to be brand-name. I've been given the generics before and they really don't seem to work... and, anyway, they tear up my stomach. And it has to be now because I ran out last Tuesday and I plan to be leaving town soon...
—Quoted in Brookoff, 1992

The debate over the use of opioid formulations with different kinetic properties is at the heart of the controversy over whether the long-term prescription of opioids for chronic noncancer pain fosters drug abuse and addiction. Advocates for patients with chronic pain have been loath to see this as a hazard of a treatment that has helped so many of their patients. At the same time, professionals who focus on the treatment of drug abuse and addiction are faced with a rising tide of prescription opioid abuse and understandably may associate this with an increase in the prescription of opioid medications for chronic noncancer pain.

Most practitioners on both sides of the issue would agree that the availability of safe opioid medications is vital to the public health. Scientific studies indicate that over a third of Americans will suffer with chronic pain at some point in their lives (Sternbach, 1986) and that many will require treatment with an opioid analgesic. When properly managed, long-term opioid therapy for chronic pain is safe and effective (Portenoy, 1996a), whereas undertreatment is associated with serious morbidity and even mortality (Hill, 1987). Despite 20 years of growing acceptance, opioid therapy for chronic noncancer pain continues to be associated by some with drug abuse; this is true despite the absence of any prospective study showing this correlation. Specifically, it is the long-term prescription of "immediate"-onset (i.e., short-acting) opioid formulations (or controlled-release formulations that can be easily converted to immediate-release forms [which is true of the majority of these preparations]) that links pain management and prescription opioid abuse.

Many government officials, members of the public, and even some physicians postulate that the prescription of opioid medications by doctors is the driving force behind a growing problem of prescription drug abuse in the United States—the assumption being that most of these drugs are initially obtained with a doctor's prescription. Nearly all of the opioids that are being abused or diverted are either easily convertible controlled-release medications or immediate-acting formulations. Most of the abusers and addicts are not patients being treated for pain but rather adolescents and young adults whose consumption of opioids focuses on "recreational" rather than medical use.

Some pain physicians have defused the concern about opioids within their own practices by choosing not to prescribe short-acting opioids or controlled-release formulations that are easily converted into short-acting drugs, such as the currently available versions of controlled-release oxycodone, believing that controlled-release opioids have been associated with less abuse and diversion than the short-acting formulations. Others have eschewed the prescribing of opioids altogether, denying patients who may benefit from them adequate pain control.

Many other physicians continue the long-term prescription of short-acting opioids. This divergence among physicians raises questions such as, what do short-acting opioids treat that cannot be treated with controlled-release formulations? Do immediate-onset kinetics pose an increased risk for abuse? What is the proper role of immediate-onset opioid formulations in the long-term treatment of chronic pain? Most important, what is the "topography" of pain that rationalizes the use of immediate or ultrarapid formulations over wholly sustained-release preparations?

A Brief Historical Perspective

Until recently, immediate-acting opioids were the only formulations that were available to physicians. The introduction of controlled-released morphine in 1982 revolutionized the treatment of chronic pain (Kaiko et al., 1989). Patients were able to achieve stable serum levels of opioid medication using oral formulations with convenient dosing while avoiding frequent abstinence symptoms associated with the use of immediate-acting preparations alone; many, however, either didn't realize or failed to accept that up to 30% of the formulation was in fact "immediately" released. Regular dosing provided for relatively stable serum levels, compared with prior immediate-release preparations. In addition to controlling pain, controlled-release morphine appeared to have less potential for abuse than short-acting morphine formulations (Brookoff, 1993), *despite* the fact that release of the drug could be accelerated by chewing the tablet. In the 25 years since its introduction, controlled-release morphine has not been subject to widespread abuse or diversion.

With the introduction of transdermal fentanyl in 1991, patients with chronic pain could obtain stable serum levels of opioid comparable to a continuous intravenous infusion with dosing intervals as long as 72 hours; this was the first truly sustained-release preparation (i.e., no immediate release of the agent). Transdermal fentanyl had a delayed onset with peak level sometimes taking 24–48 hours to achieve after first application of the patch (this is a property of the lipophilic drug as it builds a reservoir within the fatty tissue; Duragesic package insert, 2003). Because it left a depot of drug in the skin with a half-life of up to 14 hours (i.e., longer than morphine), repeated regular applications of the patch generally provided for stable serum levels without significant peaks or troughs.

Because fentanyl is such a potent opioid, most formulations of this drug have been assumed to have high potentials for abuse, although data do not bear this out (Joranson et al., 2000; SAMHSA, 2003). This line of thought probably developed as *intravenous* solution of fentanyl has been the drug of choice among physicians who are addicted to opioids since its first appearance in American operating rooms in 1965. This hasn't been the case for transdermal or transmucosal application of the drug in the general population, however.

It is interesting to note that fentanyl that is abused by drug addicts on the street is administered by *injection*, not by the transdermal or transmucosal routes (the sole means by which the drug is used to treat chronic pain). Gilson points out that the introduction and increase in medical utilization of transdermal fentanyl in the United States throughout the 1990s did *not* lead to a significant increase in the "street use" of fentanyl (Gilson et al., 2004). Nearly all of the fentanyl used in this fashion has come from clandestine laboratories that are actually manufacturing an analogue molecule, 3-*methyl*fentanyl, which is also known by its "street names" such as "China White" or "synthetic heroin" (Hibbs et al., 1991), not by a legitimate pharmaceutical route.

Abuse and diversion of the reservoir-patch formulation of transdermal fentanyl and the transmucosal form of fentanyl have been rare. There have been anecdotal reports of drug abusers attempting to apply a fentanyl patch or its contents to a mucous membrane, but these have been self-limited and isolated episodes that have quickly ended in catastrophe for the abusers (Kuhlman et al., 2003; Liappas et al., 2004). Attempts to remove and inject the fentanyl-containing gel, likewise, have been short-lived and disastrous (Reeves & Ginifer, 2002; Tharp et al., 2004). There have also been reports of abusers trying to convert fentanyl patches into "teabags" (Barrueto et al., 2004), but the extremely low bioavailability of orally ingested fentanyl prevented this from becoming a preferred route of administration. There have even been reports that some abusers tried to convert transdermal fentanyl into a "solid state system" by freezing the patch and then cutting it up and "chewing it like Chiclets" (U.S. Department of Justice, 2004). These reports were never substantiated and were rendered rather unlikely by the fact that the freezing point of the contents of a fentanyl reservoir patch is somewhere below negative 50 degrees Celsius. The same remains true of the transmucosal form of fentanyl, which has not been associated with a substantial increase in street use of the drug. It is probably the rapid redistribution of the drug in the body, secondary to the lipophyllic properties of the drug, that have led to this low penetrance in the community of fentanyl abuse over other opioids such as oxycodone.

In 1996, controlled-release oxycodone (OxyContin) was introduced, and it soon became the most commonly used long-acting opioid for the treatment of chronic pain in the United States. Its formulation (similar to morphine) provided for release of 30% of the drug within the first hour after ingestion with steady release of the remainder over the next 8–12 hours (Kaiko et al., 1996). In distinction to morphine (associated with terminal cancer) and fentanyl (whose use had previously been essentially confined to anesthesiologists), oxycodone quickly became a familiar drug to family doctors and primary care practitioners, who had prescribed the short-acting form for acute and postoperative pain; this was in part a direct effect of the marketing of the drug by the manufacturer. Many quickly endorsed its use for their patients with chronic pain.

With the introduction of sustained-release oxycodone into the American market, the use of opioids for the treatment of chronic pain increased markedly. The slow-release mechanism of OxyContin turned out to be easily breached by chewing or crushing the tablet. This converted it into a massive-dose, quick-onset drug; the hydrophilic nature of the drug produced quick and sustained serum concentrations. In addition, it is conceivable that oxycodone may have a unique effect on the reward centers of the brain, a problem with the abuse of the drug (and in weaning patients off of it). By 2000, within 4 years of its introduction, there was a plethora of OxyContin abuse in the United States that has been characterized as "a uniquely horrifying case of a powerful drug wreaking havoc in American communities" (Acker, 2003). Because OxyContin tablets were available in dosage strengths that far exceeded those in the immediate-release formulations of oxycodone such as Percocet or Percodan, this latest outbreak was accompanied by considerably more overdose deaths than any of the previous outbreaks of oxycodone abuse recorded in the United States (Meier, 2002).

Generic formulations of controlled-release morphine, transdermal fentanyl, and controlled-release oxycodone have since come to the American market. Some of the new controlled-release morphine formulations allow for once-per-day dosing (with kinetics that approximate true sustained dosing) and have shown no apparent increase in abuse. The newly released transdermal fentanyl formulations use a solid-matrix delivery system, which should be easier to convert into a quick-release formulation than the "reservoir" design of the original patch; these have also thus far not shown an increase in abuse. The federal Drug Abuse Warning Network has recorded a steady increase in the number of fentanyl-related deaths and medical emergencies in the 2 years since the introduction of generic brands; one of these is known to "dump" drug into the system.

The generic forms of controlled-released oxycodone are as easy to breach and convert to a rapid-onset drug as the original formulation. In 2004, a slow-onset, controlled-release formulation of hydromorphone (Palladone) was approved but was taken off the market within 6 months of its release when it was discovered that the drug could be easily extracted from its methacrylate matrix by dissolving the tablet in alcohol. Another formulation of controlled-release hydromorphone in a once-daily, osmotic-release formulation may be approved soon (Palangio et al., 2002).

A controlled-release formulation of oxymorphone has recently been approved. This drug has been available for over 30 years as an injection and suppository (Numorphan), but the level of use has been negligible. Oxymorphone is a metabolite of oxycodone and apparently may possess much of the pain-relieving properties with less of the CNS stimulation associated with the parent drug

(Sloan et al., 2005). Also in development are controlled-release preparations of oxycodone that will be more difficult to convert to a rapid-release form due to its excipients (Remoxy) or that will contain small amounts of naltrexone to deter abuse (Oxytrex). The problem is that the parent drug oxycodone conceivably may potentiate the reward centers of the brain—it will remain to be seen if these "Antabuse" methods make any difference.

Controlled-release opioids have been shown to provide analgesia and improve quality of life for patients with chronic pain (McCarberg & Barkin, 2001). There has been growing acceptance of their use in chronic noncancer pain (American Pain Society, 2002). As mentioned, immediate-release opioids remain, and it is unclear if they are any different than their "sustained-release" counterparts.

It is still recommend to use other therapies when possible, but in moderate-severe chronic pain, opioids are no longer to be reserved as the "last resort" (Portenoy, 1996b).

What Are We Treating With Immediate-Onset Opioids?

The traditional paradigm for treatment of chronic pain calls for the use of controlled-release opioids for the treatment of "baseline" pain and immediate-release and ultrarapid-onset opioids for episodes of "breakthrough" pain. This thinking comes mostly from studies involving patients with advanced cancer (Walsh, 2000), although these studies were poor in comparing around-the-clock dosing of immediate-release opioids versus sustained-release formulations.

"Breakthrough pain" is now defined as a transient increase in the intensity of moderate to severe pain, occurring in the presence of well-established baseline pain. It is typically rapid in onset (within 3–4 minutes) and of short duration (median 30 minutes). Breakthrough pain may be somatic, visceral, or neuropathic in origin. When due to movement, breakthrough pain is referred to as "incident" pain. Breakthrough pain may be due to inadequate dosing of the long-acting medication (referred to as "end-of-dose failure") or may be idiopathic and unrelated to the dosing schedule or activity (Bennett et al., 2005a; Bennett et al., 2007; Portenoy & Hagen, 1990).

A study of cancer patients in a hospice setting showed that the average number of daily breakthrough pain episodes was four (49% of these episodes occurred suddenly, and 38% were characterized as "severe" or "excruciating"). Seventy-two percent of the breakthrough episodes studied lasted less than 30 minutes (Zepetella et al., 2000). Breakthrough pain was common among these cancer patients, was frequent, short-lasting, often unpredictable, and not necessarily related to the chronic pain making treatment difficult (Zepetella et al., 2000). A survey was recently conducted and showed that the noncancer population had similar types of breakthrough pain episodes (Portenoy, Bennett, et al., 2006).

What Makes an Opioid Abusable?

The molecular identity of a drug is not the only feature of an opioid medication that determines its potential for abuse. There are other factors, including dosage form and combination with excipients that can make a major difference in abuse potential. Formulations that make it difficult to extract the psychoactive ingredient, compounds with a slow onset of effect that cannot easily be converted to "fast-release" forms, formulations that limit bioavailability, and formulations that are difficult to reverse-engineer all have been thought to reduce the potential for abuse (Voth et al., 1991); no prospective study specifically addressing these issue exists, however. Katz and colleagues developed an extractability rating system for prescription opioid analgesic products in preliminary efforts to assess the abuse liability of various prescription opioid products (Katz, 2005).

In order to curtail abuse while adequately treating pain, we need to understand the features that make one opioid formulation more attractive than another to potential abusers. In one recent study assessing the drug preferences of opioid abusers (who were not pain patients), OxyContin, Vicodin, Dilaudid, and Percocet were ranked the highest and Talwin NX and transdermal fentanyl patches were ranked the lowest (Butler et al., 2006). The key indicators of "attractiveness" were the following: the quality of the "high," duration of the "high," availability of a pill form, higher overall availability (e.g., lower scheduling), cost, side effects, withdrawal effects, peer influence, and real or perceived dangers (Butler et al., 2006).

Compared to abusers of other prescription formulations, OxyContin abusers were more likely to show a pattern of serious drug abuse (e.g., multiple drugs, self-injections). Eighty-three percent had used other illicit drugs before they started using OxyContin. Rarely was medical or nonmedical use of OxyContin the initiating factor leading to the abuse of other drugs (Sees et al., 2005). Another study found a similar prevalence of prescription opioid abuse with the abusers ranking brand-name OxyContin highest, followed by hydrocodone, other oxycodone formulations, methadone, morphine, hydromorphone, fentanyl, and buprenorphine (Cicero et al., 2005). Abuse of OxyContin and hydrocodone showed the most pronounced growth over the survey period (Cicero et al., 2005). It should be noted that individual metabolic differences could make certain opioid drugs more attractive to specific groups of people—for example, those who rapidly metabolize hydrocodone to hydromorphone (Cone et al., 2006). It important to note that drug abuse represents complex multifactorial interactions involving the patient (e.g., genetic, environment, culture, peer group), individual experience-dependent brain state (e.g., past history, expectations, learning) and addiction agent(s), and is not strictly due to ingestion of drugs (although agents may vary in different patients in terms of their reinforcing effects). Furthermore, in a particular patient environment, a psychoactive drug may be in vogue one week, whereas a depressant (i.e., opioid) may be in vogue the next.

Figure 44.1. Mark Collen, *CP II*, © 2008 Pain Exhibit. Reproduced by permission

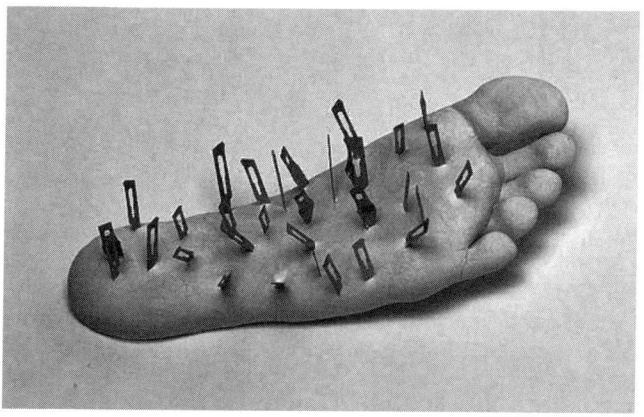

The Significance of Prescription Opioid Abuse

Opiophobia has long been a problem for doctors, patients, regulators, and the general public. (Bennett & Carr, 2002). This phobia has accelerated since the onset of the current enlarging scope of prescription drug abuse, which became apparent in the last decade. In some counties in the United States, deaths from narcotic overdoses have come to outnumber deaths attributed to traffic accidents (e.g., Allegheny County, PA). A growing proportion of these overdose deaths have been related to the diversion and abuse of prescription opioid medications. According to the March 2004 annual report of the Office of National Drug Control Policy, prescription drugs diverted for abuse have increased 163% since 1995 and today constitute a major share of the "street drug" trade, second only to marijuana and far outpacing cocaine and heroin.

A report issued in May 2004 by the Florida State Medical Examiner indicated that for the first time in history, controlled prescription drugs were found to have caused more than half of all the drug-related deaths in the state (Florida Department of Law Enforcement, 2003). A recent study of adolescents in the United States showed that past-year (nonprescribed) use of OxyContin was reported by 1.8% of 8th graders, 3.2% of 10th graders, and 5.5% of 12th graders (Johnston et al., 2006). A study in Canada reported lifetime use by 1.3% students in grades 7–12 (Adlaf et al., 2006). Most of the adolescents who abused OxyContin (70%) used it sporadically, usually *in addition* to the repertoire of other drugs commonly used by adolescents (Adlaf et al., 2006). Although some conclude that the nonmedical use of opioids is predictable based on the potency and extent of prescriptive use (Dasgupta et al., 2006), other studies maintain that the rates of drug abuse and resultant morbidity secondary to the use of opioid analgesics remain low, in spite of the increase in medical use of these substances (Novak et al., 2004).

The Population at Risk for Prescription Drug Abuse: Whom Are We Trying to Protect?

The increase in the abuse of prescription opioids is a growing public health concern and should be addressed by identifying the causes and sources of diversion without interfering with legitimate medical treatment and proper patient care (Gilson et al., 2004). This should be done without adding additional stigma to people burdened with chronic medical illness. *Most* patients with chronic pain do not escalate their dosages or abuse their medications (Cooper et al., 1992; Portenoy, 1990). Many studies indicate that there is little overlap between the population taking prescribed psychotropic medications and the drug-abusing population (Dupont, 1988). Although claims of overutilization of analgesic medications are often made, research suggests that *underutilization occurs much more frequently,* particularly with regard to the use of medications to treat patients with chronic noncancer pain (Morgan, 1986).

At the same time, we have to be aware that increases in prescription opioid abuse reflect, in part, changes in medication prescribing practices and changes in drug formulations (higher doses). Though the short-term use of immediate-onset opioid analgesics for acute or postoperative pain appears to be generally benign, the long-term administration of these medications has been associated with clinically meaningful increases in the overall rates of abuse or addiction (Compton & Volkow, 2006). One recent study of over a hundred prescription drug abusers entering drug rehabilitation found that 84% reported that had been given a prescription for opioids for pain at some point from a physician and 61% reported that they did have chronic pain (Passik et al., 2006b).

One approach to ameliorating this problem would be to design drug formulations that are associated with reduced abuse. This has certainly been successful in the past. For example, the addition of naloxone to rapid-onset formulations of pentazocine in 1978 reduced abuse of this medication by up to 80% (Fudala & Johnson, 2006; Goldstein, 1985). Pharmaceutical companies are currently in the process of developing "abuse resistant" opioid formulations, and organizations have been founded to develop less abusable drugs (Schuster, 2006).

Does the Use of Immediate-Onset Opioids Promote Aberrant Behavior Among Patients With Chronic Pain?

There is little evidence that long-term therapy with immediate-release opioids adversely affects the majority of people being treated for chronic painful conditions. There is some evidence that long-term therapy with short-acting opioids may predispose certain patients with chronic pain to aberrant behaviors or addiction. The patients who may be most at risk are probably those who suffer with concomitant psychiatric illnesses, many of whom have a higher prevalence of substance use than patients with chronic pain, and those with a prior history of substance abuse. A prior history of substance abuse disorder and younger age were associated with abusive behaviors (Reid et al., 2002). Depressive and anxiety disorders are more common and more strongly associated with prescribed opioid use than other drug abuse disorders (Sullivan et al., 2005).

The recurrent "on-off" quality of immediate-acting drugs may produce long-term, perhaps permanent, alterations in affected neuronal systems and may underlie the development of dependence, tolerance, withdrawal, and relapse characteristics of (although distinct from those of) the addictive diseases (Kreek et al., 2005). The clinical picture of failed therapy may be complicated by noncompliance, concealed consumption of psychotropic substances, and diversion of prescribed opioids for various purposes as selling for profit or sharing excess opioids with others (Jage, 2005).

In a large community survey, 3% of respondents were found to be taking prescription opioids regularly. Respondents with common mental disorders (major depression, dysthymia, generalized anxiety disorder, or panic disorder) were more likely to report regular opioid use than people without these disorders; and among these people, respondents reporting "problem drug use" were more likely to have concurrent alcohol or substance abuse problems.

It should be stressed that the majority of patients with chronic noncancer pain show few aberrant medication-related behaviors (Passik et al., 2006a). By regularly assessing the "four A's" (analgesia, activities of daily living, adverse events, and aberrant drug-taking behaviors), the efficacy of treatment and emergence of abusive behaviors can be easily monitored. Routine use of a questionnaire assessing the "four A's" showed that most pain patients on chronic opioids achieved positive outcomes, with the majority exhibiting no aberrant behaviors. Indicators of addiction or diversion turned out to be rare (<5%; Passik & Weinreb, 2000). Many aberrant opioid-related behaviors are due not to addiction *per se* but rather to *misuse* of the medications in a misguided attempt to treat distressing conditions other than physical pain; this behavior is referred to as *chemical coping*. A survey tool that begins to address this includes questions such as, do you take your pain medications to help you sleep? due to stress? because of an argument with a family member? (Passik et al., 2004). A more comprehensive *chemical coping inventory* is currently under development by Bennett and Passik (Kirsh, 2006).

"Ultrarapid"-Onset Opioids

In addition to immediate-acting opioids (which can take 40 minutes to begin working), a new class of "ultrarapid"-onset opioids has been introduced to treat breakthrough pain. The first formulation of this class to be introduced into the market in the United States was oral transmucosal fentanyl citrate (OTFC) lozenge Actiq, which can deliver steady-state levels of medication within 20 minutes of the onset of use (Coluzzi et al., 2001). A large number of studies have demonstrated its efficacy for the treatment of breakthrough pain (Zepetella & Ribeiro, 2006). The newest formulation of ultra-rapid acting fentanyl is Fentora, which has a slightly faster onset and greater bioavailability (48% for Fentora vs. 22% for Actiq) secondary to bicarbonation of the fentanyl citrate, which provides greater absorption of the uncharged particle (Darwish et al.,). Other ultrarapid-onset opioid formulations may soon become available, including opioids delivered as an "oral compressed powder" (Shaiova et al., 2004), in a nasal spray, or via an iontophoretic patch (Sinatra, 2005). At present, the on-label prescription of Actiq and Fentora is restricted to the treatment of breakthrough pain in patients with cancer; in actuality the largest number of prescriptions for these formulations are in patients with noncancer pain, and in those who have pain despite cancer remission.

With a duration of delivery of 15 minutes, a single OTFC device can rapidly deliver up to 800 micrograms of fentanyl into the bloodstream (Egan et al., 2002). OTFC has been found to be better than oral morphine for the treatment of severe episodic pain in cancer patients (Coluzzi et al., 2001) and better or equivalent to intravenous morphine for the treatment of postoperative pain (Lichtor et al., 1999).

In healthy volunteers, OTFC has pharmacokinetics similar to an intravenous injection of fentanyl (Egan et al., 2000); this is a property of the lipophilic class of opioids and is attractive in the treatment of rapid-onset breakthrough pain.

In healthy volunteers, oral OTFC was been shown to produce "subjective pleasant sensations" (e.g., a "high") and at higher doses it also produced sedation and respiratory depression (Stanley et al., 1989). It is important to note that these studies were not undertaken in patients with chronic pain but in healthy volunteers. These healthy volunteers provide a good model for the population most at risk from the introduction of a highly abusable and potent prescription drugs, the so-called "casual" rather than "hardcore" abusers. This group includes many teenagers, for whom prescription analgesics are among the most widely abused drugs, second only to marijuana according to the 2003 National Survey on Drug Use and Health. *Thus, it is not the medical use of the medication that should be at question, but controlling the distribution of these valuable medications to keep them from misuse.*

In summary, despite the concern that these medications are being abused by drug addicts, these formulations do appear to hold significant benefits for selected patients with chronic pain (Furlan et al., 2006). Through careful patient selection, prescription of "lower risk" opioid formulations, and the use of currently available survey tools to monitor patients for signs of abuse or addiction, we should be able to provide adequate relief for our patients with chronic pain without promoting drug abuse (Ives et al., 2006). Long-term therapy with any type of opioid will have to be accompanied by an ongoing assessment of aberrant behaviors (Portenoy, 1996b; Webster & Webster, 2005). A rational approach to the safe prescription of long-term opioids has been framed by Gourlay and colleagues (2005) as the use of "universal precautions in pain medicine." The role of the ultrarapid-onset opioids in the long-term treatment of chronic noncancer pain is still undergoing refinement, but their place adds to the "toolbox" of the pain medicine physician.

Figure 44.2a. Pain diagram, front view.

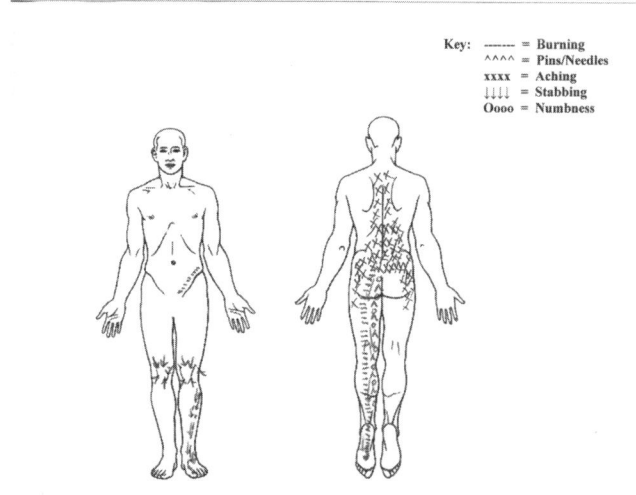

Figure 44.2b. Pain diagram, side view.

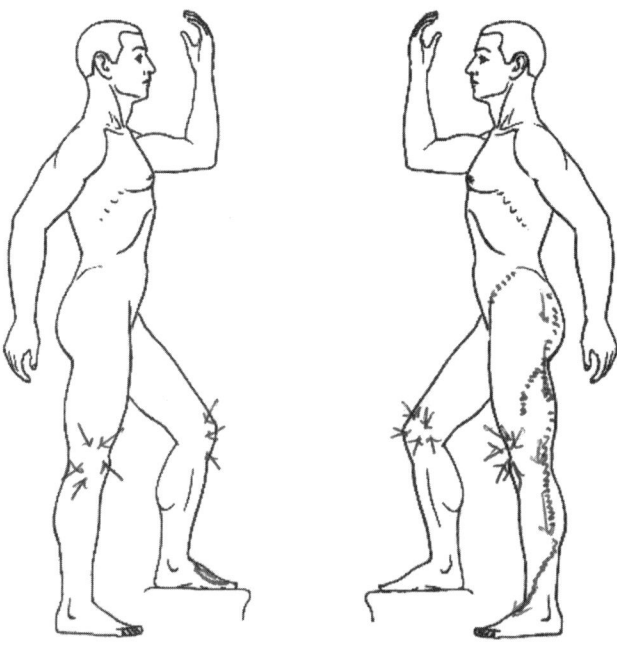

The Real Question: What Is the Best Opioid Preparation to Treat the "Topography" of Pain in the Individual Patient?

There are no prospective studies that show a particular opioid preparation is the "culprit" in abusive behaviors. If the pain medicine physician appropriately screens for known addictive past as well as predictive determinants of abuse behavior (and appropriately comanages these factors), the determinant for the type of opioid preparation should be directly related to the type of pain present in the individual patient; this is referred to as the "topography" of the pain.

This concept is certainly not a novel one; in diabetes, the type of insulin preparation is directly determined by the "topography" of the levels of blood glucose. Similarly, the type of hypertensive medication is determined upon the nature of the blood pressure anomaly; sustained increases in diastolic pressure are treated differently from intermittent increases in diastolic pressure.

As we have no uniform way of measuring an individual person's pain, a detailed pain diary (which is carefully monitored by the prescribing physician) is the only way we can accomplish *a la carte* therapy. Prior to beginning the diary, the practitioner must look for suspect "flags" that would prompt multidisciplinary treatment (i.e., previous addictive disease or flags for abuse/addictive behaviors).

It is the opioid trial that defines who is and who is not a *responder* and to what type of opioid they respond to. Only a *responder* to an opioid should remain on the medication, and thus any further discussions should be focused on defining the opioid *responder* and the potential problems that may occur with aberrant medication use in that group. This process should be ongoing as it is yet unclear as to the exact situations under which *chemical coping* occurs.

The Opioid Trial

The construct of the opioid trial is to provide a framework in which (1) a baseline pain assessment can be visualized, (2) opioid can be given and "effect" can be determined against baseline pain as to (a) diminution in intensity, and (b) sustainability of, or betterment in

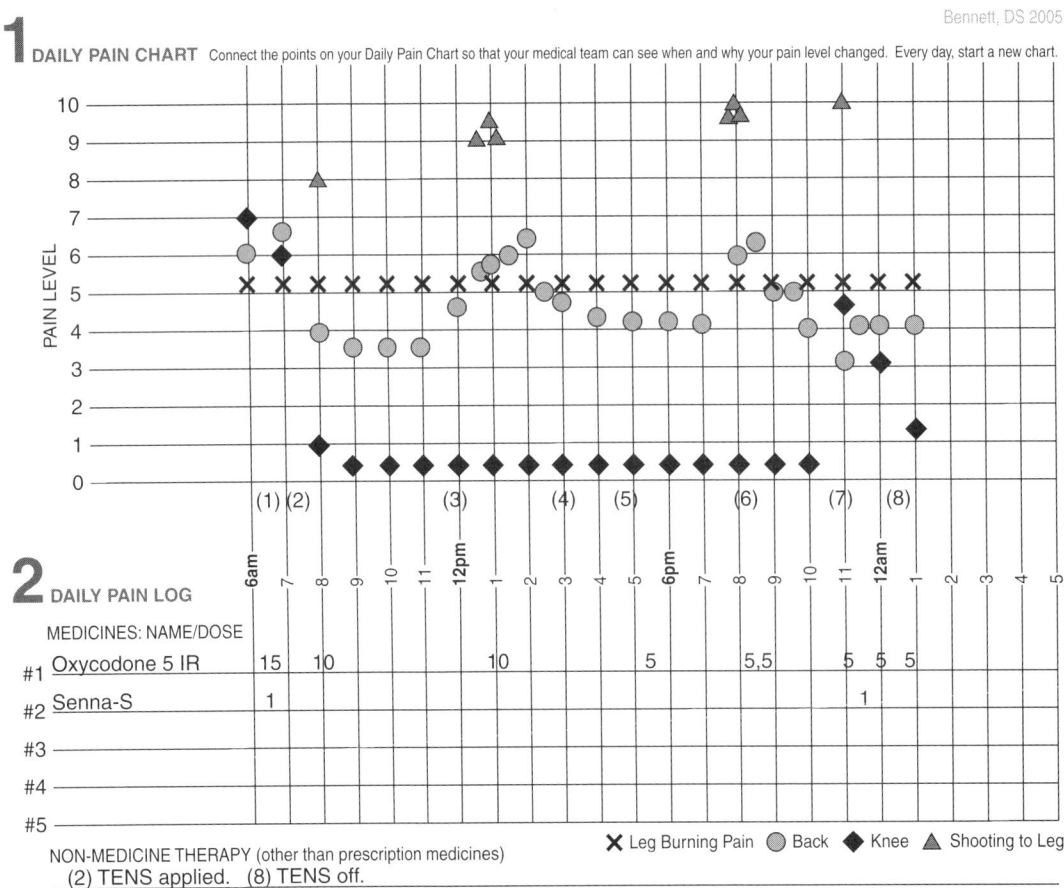

Figure 44.3. Pain journal, initial graph.

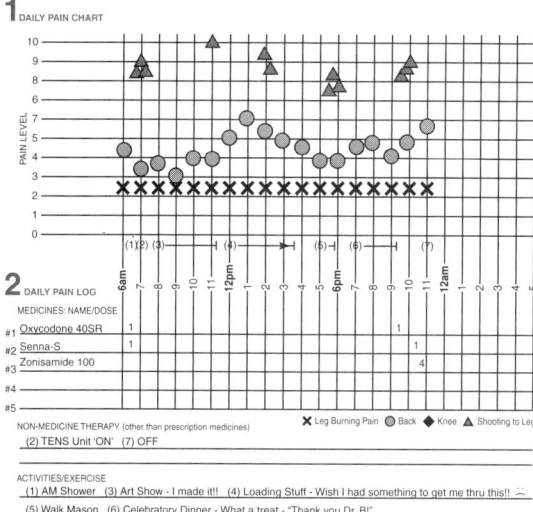

Figure 44.4 Pain journal, weeks 2–4

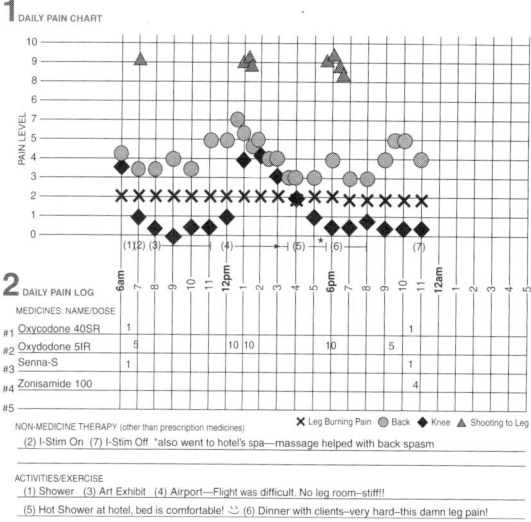

Figure 44.5. Pain journal, weeks 4–6

function as a result of the addition of the medication, and (3) the optimal dose against side effect for the opioid achieves the positive goals of 2(a)(b). If the answer to 2(a)(b) is that there is no response that is positive (i.e., no diminution in pain and/or increase/sustainability of function, or such overt side effects that therapy with an opioid is contraindicated), then the patient is considered a *nonresponder* or *responder but intolerant of therapy* and the specific opioid should be discontinued. It is the responder group that then is monitored for any future aberrant behaviors (i.e., chemical coping or more ominous addictive behaviors).

Last, use of intrathecal opioids cannot be considered a "replacement" of therapy in a nonresponder group. It may be an alternative in patients with ongoing abuse issues (with extreme caution) who are responding to therapy if these same individuals respond positively to an intrathecal opioid trial. However, data to support this claim remain speculative, and one certainly cannot prevent tampering with the medication reservoir.

The following case illustration shows how an opioid/medication trial is accomplished:

Mary, a 34-year-old woman with no history of violence, sexual abuse, aberrant drug behavior, or alcohol abuse, was involved in an auto accident. The result was a crushed left knee requiring full arthrodesis, L4-S1 posterior fusion with autograft, and left SI joint fusion secondary to overt instability. She had a 6-month course of rehabilitation after implantation of a spinal cord stimulator that completely controlled severe neuropathic pain in the lumbosacral region and lower extremities secondary to nerve root injuries at L4-S1 (because of "fear of electricity" spinal cord/nerve root stimulation was discontinued). She presents with left leg persistent pain, left knee pain, worsened with weight bearing and movement (right knee DJD with pain), and left SI joint pain of two types: an "aching" pain that is persistent, asso-

Figure 44.6 Pain journal, weeks 6–8

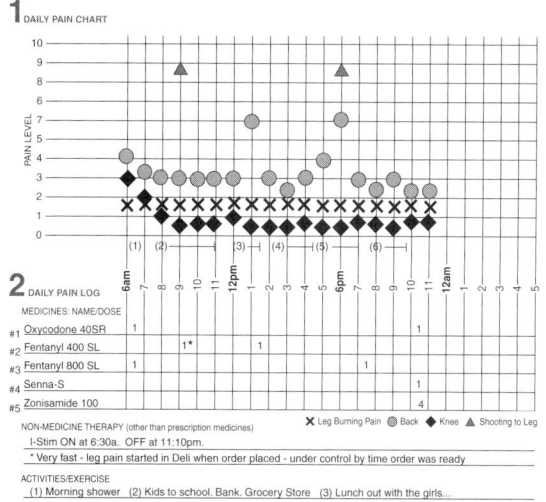

Figure 44.7 Pain journal, weeks 8–12

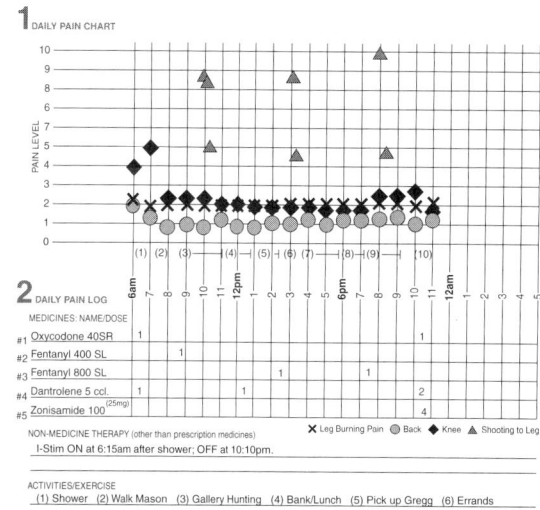

ciated with hardware, and "sharp" pain that is produced with weight bearing and increases in intensity over time (see Figure 44.2).

Mary was given a pain diary and was told to complete this daily for 1 week, taking 1 day and graphing her pain during waking hours; she brought this with her to the follow-up appointment (see Figure 44.3). This diary served as her *baseline pain diary*. Note that her pain is of two distinct types, one is a constant, or baseline, pain, and the others are spontaneous (non-activity-related) or incident (activity-related) pain.

Mary was started on an immediate-release medication, limiting the number of times per day (and therefore the total mg/day). She was again told to complete a pain journal for two weeks, taking 1 day to graph pain during waking hours (see Figure 44.4). *Note that a sustained-release medication was **not** given until a daily dose requirement was established.* Also note that a component of her leg pain is rapid in onset, in which the SI joint pain/back and "burning" leg pain is slower to develop but increases with intensity the longer she is weight bearing. She was placed on a sustained-release preparation (i.e. oxycodone SR) and was allowed to remain on an immediate-release preparation for breakthrough pain episodes. She was told to start an antiseizure mediation after 1 week (i.e. zonisamide). She continued opioid trial for another 2 weeks in a similar fashion (see Figure 44.5).

Figure 44.6, comprising weeks 6–8, shows that the baseline pain is rather well controlled. The gradual-onset SI joint pain responds to proactive ingestion of the immediate-release preparation. What is problematic is the rapid-onset knee pain as well as paroxysms of "shooting" left leg pain. An ultrarapid agent (i.e., OTFC) was added. A muscle relaxant was also added. She again was sent home with a pain journal in a similar fashion.

Figure 44.7 shows the final opioid regimen with comments. You can see that the final regimen comprises a long-acting agent for baseline pain, an intermediate agent for gradual-onset incident pain, and a rapid-onset agent for rapid-onset incident pain. In addition, an antiseizure medication and a direct-acting muscle relaxant were also utilized. Utilizing this combination of balanced analgesia, *side effects were minimized* and *the medication regimen "mimicked" the patient's daily pain topography*, which of course changed with her workweek (i.e., less weight bearing on nonwork days).

Conclusions

Although there are concerns with regard to the long-term use of opioid medications in the treatment of chronic pain (i.e., non-cancer pain and cancer survivors with pain), the use of opioid medications has been found to be effective in individuals whose pain responds to this class of medication. Opioids therefore remain a powerful tool in the therapeutic armamentarium of the pain medicine physician. Factors that predispose to aberrant medication behaviors, such as depression, previous psychological trauma, or a history of previous substance abuse, should be carefully evaluated and comanaged; the degree to which specialized services for substance abuse need to be accessed is dependent upon the individual patient. Although the prevailing dogma has been that immediate- and ultrarapid-release opioids potentiate abuse, there are no data to support this claim. The type of opioid and the preparation that is dispensed should therefore rely on the topography of the pain and not the biases of the prescribing physician.

References

Acker CJ. Take as directed: the dilemmas of regulating addictive analgesics and other psychoactive drugs. In Meldrum ML (ed.), *Opioids and Pain Relief: A Historical Perspective*. Seattle WA: IASP Press; 2003.

Adlaf EM, Paglia-Boak A, Brands B. Use of OxyContin by adolescent students. *CMAJ*. 2006; 174: 9–10.

American Pain Society. *Guidelines for the Management of Pain in Osteoarthritis, Rheumatoid Arthritis and Juvenile Chronic Arthritis* (2nd ed.). Glenview, IL: American Pain Society; 2002.

Barrueto F Jr, Howland MA, Hoffman RS, Nelson LS. The fentanyl teabag. *Vet Hum Toxicol*. 2004; 46:30–1.

Bennett DS, Burton A, Fishman S, et al. Consensus panel recommendations for the assessment and management of breakthrough pain: part I assessment. *Pharmacy & Therapeutics*. 2005a; 30(5):296–301.

Bennett DS, Burton A, Fishman S, et al. Consensus panel recommendations for the assessment and management of breakthrough pain: part II management. *Pharmacy & Therapeutics*. 2005b; 30(6):354–61.

Bennett DS, Carr D. Opiophobia as a barrier to the treatment of pain. *Journal of Pain & Palliative Care Pharmacotherapy*. 2002; 16(1):105–9.

Bennett DS, Rauck R, Simon S. Prevalence and characteristics of breakthrough pain in patients managed in pain specialty clinics who were receiving opioids for chronic back pain. *Journal of Opioid Management*. 2007; 3(2):101–6.

Booth JV et al. Substance abuse among physicians: a survey of academic anesthesiology programs. *Anesth Analg*. 2002; 95:1024–30.

Brookoff D. Abuse potential of various opioid medications. *J Gen Int Med*. 1993; 12:688–90.

Brookoff D. Drug complications—case and comment. *Patient Care*. 1992; 9:206–7.

Butler SF, Benoit C, Budman SH, Fernandez KC, McCormick C, Venuti SW, Katz N. Development and validation of an opioid attractiveness scale: a novel measure of the attractiveness of opioid products to potential abusers. *Harm Reduct J*. 2006; 3:5–17.

Cicero TJ, Inciardi JA, Munoz A. Trends in abuse of OxyContin and other opioid analgesics in the United States: 2002–2004. *J Pain*. 2005; 6:662–72.

Coluzzi PH et al. Breakthrough cancer pain: a randomized trial comparing oral transmucosal fentanyl citrate and morphine sulfate immediate release. *Pain*. 2001; 91:123–30.

Compton WM, Volkow ND. Major increases in opioid analgesic abuse in the United States: concerns and strategies. *Drug Alcohol Depend*. 2006; 81: 103–7.

Cone EJ, Heit HA, Caplan YH, Gourlay D. Evidence of morphine metabolism to hydromorphone in pain patients chronically treated with morphine. *J Anal. Toxicol*. 2006; 30:1–5.

Cooper JR, Czechowicz DJ, Petersen RC, Molinari SP. Prescription drug diversion control and medical practice. *JAMA*. 1992; 268:1306–10.

Darwish M, Kirby M, Robertson Jr P, Tracewell W, Jiang G. Absolute and relative bioavailability of fentanyl buccal tablet and oral transmucosal fentanyl citrate. *J Clin Pharm*. 2007; 47(3):343–50.

Dasgupta N, Kramer ED, Zalman MA, Carino S Jr, Smith MY, Haddox JD, Wright C. Association between non-medical and prescriptive usage of opioids. *Drug Alcohol Depend*. 2006; 82:135–42.

Dupont RL. Abuse of benzodiazepines: the problems and the solutions. *Am J Drug Alcohol Abuse*. 1988; 14(suppl 1):1–69.

Duragesic (fentanyl transdermal system) [package insert]. Titusville, NJ: Janssen Pharmaceutica Products, L.P.; 2003.

Egan TD et al. Multiple dose pharmacokinetics of oral transmucosal fentanyl citrate in healthy volunteers. *Anesthesiology*. 2000; 92:665–73.

Egan T et al. The pharmacokinetics and safety of oral transmucosal fentanyl citrate administered to healthy volunteers as two 400 microgram or as a single 800 microgram dose. *Pain Med*. 2002; 3:187–88.

Fisher MA, Glass S. Butorphanol (Stadol): a study in problems of current drug information and control. *Neurology*. 1997; 48:1156–60.

Florida Department of Law Enforcement. *2003 Report by the Florida Medical Examiners Commission on Drugs Identified in Deceased Persons.* http://www.fdle.state.fl.us/press_releases/20040526_MER_Report.html.

Fudala PJ, Johnson RE. Development of opioid formulations with limited diversion and abuse potential. *Drug Alcohol Depend.* 2006; 83 (suppl 1): S40–7.

Furlan AD, Sandoval JA, Mailis-Gagnon A, Tunks E. Opioids for chronic non-cancer pain: a meta-analysis of effectiveness and side effects. *CMAJ.* 2006; 174:1589–1600.

Gillis JC, Benfield P, Goa KL. Transdermal butorphanol. A review of its pharmacodynamic and pharmacokinetic properties and therapeutic potential in acute pain management. *Drugs.* 1995; 50:157–75.

Gilson AM, Ryan KM, Joranson DE Dahl JE. A reassessment of trends in the medical use and abuse of opioid analgesics and implications for diversion control: 1997–2002. *J Pain Symptom Management.* 2004; 28:176–88.

Goldstein G. Pentazocine. *Drug Alcohol Depend.* 1985; 14:313–24.

Gourlay DL, Heit HA, Almahrezi A. Universal precautions in pain medicine: a rational approach to the treatment of chronic pain. *Pain Medicine.* 2005; 6:107–12.

Greenwald MK, June HL, Stitzer ML, Marco AP. Comparative clinical pharmacology of short-acting mu opioids in drug abusers. *J Pharmacol Exp Ther.* 1996; 277:1228–36.

Hibbs J, Perper J, Winek CL. An outbreak of designer drug-related deaths in Pennsylvania. *JAMA.* 1991; 265(8):1011–3.

Hill CS. Painful prescriptions. *JAMA.* 1987; 257(15):2081.

Ives TJ, Chelminski PR, Hammet-Stabler CA, Malone RM, Perhac JS, Potisek NM, Shilliday BB, Dewalt DA, Pignone MP. Predictors of opioid misuse in patients with chronic pain: a prospective cohort study. *BMC Health Serv Res.* 2006; 6:46–53.

Jage J. Opioid tolerance and dependence—do they matter? *Eur J Pain.* 2005; 9:157–62.

Johnston LD, O'Malley PM, Bachman JG et al. *Monitoring the future national results on adolescent drug use: overview of key findings, 2005.* Bethesda, MD: National Institute on Drug Abuse; 2006.

Joranson, DE, Ryan KM, Gilson AM, Dahl J, Office of Applied Studies, Substance Abuse and Mental Health Services Administration. The DAWN Report: trends in medical use and abuse of opioid analgesics. *JAMA.* 2000; 283(13):1710–14.

Kaiko RF, Benziger DP, Fitzmartin RD, Burke BE, Reder RF, Goldenheim PD. Pharmacokinetic-pharmacodynamic relationships of controlled-release oxycodone. *Clin Pharmacol Ther.* 1996; 59:52–61.

Kaiko RF, Grandy RP, Oshlack B, Pav J, Horodniak J, Thomas G, Ingber E, Goldenheim PD. The United States experience with oral controlled-release morphine: review of nine dose titration studies and clinical pharmacology of 15-mg, 30-mg, 60-mg and 100-mg tablet strengths in normal subjects. *Cancer.* 1989; 63(11 suppl):2348–54.

Katz N. Development of an extractability rating system for prescription opioid analgesic products. Abstract presented at American Pain Society meeting; March 30–April 2, 2005; Boston, MA.

Kirsh KL, Jass C, Bennett DS, Hagen JE, Passik SD. Initial development of a survey tool to detect issues of chemical coping in chronic pain patients. *Palliative and Supportive Care.* 2007; 5:1–8.

Kreek MJ, Bart G, Lilly C, Laforge KS, Nielsen DA. Pharmacogenetics and human molecular genetics of opiate and cocaine addictions and their treatments. *Pharmacologic Reviews.* 2005; 57:1–26.

Kuhlman JJ Jr, McCaulley R, Valouch TJ, Behonick GS. Fentanyl use, misuse and abuse: a summary of 23 postmortem cases. *J Anal Toxicol.* 2003; 27:499–504.

Liappas IA et al. Oral transmucosal abuse of transdermal fentanyl. *J Psychopharmacology.* 2004; 18:277–80.

Lichtor JL, et al. The relative potency of oral transmucosal fentanyl citrate compared with intravenous morphine in the treatment of moderate to severe postoperative pain. *Anesth Analg.* 1999; 89:732–8.

Loder E. Post-marketing experience with an opioid nasal spray for migraine: lessons for the future. *Cephalalgia.* 2006; 26:89–97.

McCarberg BH, Barkin RL. Long-acting opioids for chronic pain: pharmacotherapeutic opportunities to enhance compliance, quality of life and analgesia. *Am J Ther.* 2001; 8:181–6.

Meier B. OxyContin deaths said to be up sharply. *New York Times.* April 15, 2002:A14.

Miller E, Brookoff D, Richey S, Burns C. Use of transdermal fentanyl without rescue opioids in the treatment of chronic nociceptive pain. Poster presentation (#901) at annual meeting of the American Pain Society, 2003.

Morgan JP. American opiophobia: customary underutilization of opioid analgesics. In Stimmel B (ed.), *Advances in Alcohol and Substance Abuse.* New York: Haworth Press; 163–73; 1986.

Novak S, Nemeth WC, Lawson KA. Trends in medical use and abuse of sustained-release opioid analgesics: a revisit. *Pain Med.* 2004; 5:59–65.

Palangio M, Northfelt DW, Portenoy RK, Brookoff D, Doyle RT Jr, Dornseif BE, Damask MC. Dose conversion and titration with a novel, once-daily OROS osmotic technology, extended-release hydromorphone formulation in the treatment of chronic malignant and non-malignant pain. *J Pain Symptom Manage.* 2002; 23:355–68.

Passik SD, Hays L, Eisner N, Kirsh KL. Psychiatric and pain characteristics of prescription drug abusers entering drug rehabilitation. *J Pain Palliat Care Pharmacother.* 2006b; 20:5–13.

Passik SD, Kirsh KL, Donaghy KB, Portenoy RK. Pain and aberrant drug-related behaviors in medically ill patients with and without histories of substance abuse. *Clin J Pain.* 2006a; 22:173–81.

Passik SD, Kirsh KL, Whitcomb LA. A new tool to assess and document pain outcomes in chronic pain patients receiving opioid therapy. *Clin Ther.* 2004; 26:552–61.

Passik SD Weinreb HJ. Managing chronic non-malignant pain: overcoming obstacles to the use of opioids. *Adv Ther.* 2000; 17:70–80.

Poklis A. Fentanyl: a review for clinical and analytical toxicologists. *J Toxicol Clin Toxicol.* 1995; 33(5)4329–47.

Portenoy, RK. Chronic opioid therapy in non-malignant pain. *J Pain Symptom Management.* 1990; 5:546–62.

Portenoy RK. Opioid therapy for chronic nonmalignant pain: a review of the critical issues. *J Pain Symptom Manage.* 1996a; 11:203–17.

Portenoy RK. Opioid therapy for chronic nonmalignant pain: clinicians' perspective. *J Law, Medicine and Ethics.* 1996b; 24:296–309.

Portenoy, RK, Bennett, DS, Rauck, R et al. Prevalence and characteristics of breakthrough pain in patients with chronic noncancer pain. *J of Pain.* 2006; 7(8):583–91.

Portenoy RK, Hagen NA. Breakthrough pain: definition, prevalence and characteristics. *Pain.* 1990; 41:273–81.

Reeves MD, Ginifer CJ. Fatal intravenous misuse of transdermal fentanyl. *Med J Australia.* 2002; 177:552–54.

Reid MC, Engles-Horton LL, Weber MB, Kerns RD, Rogers EL, O'Connor PG. Use of opioid medications for chronic noncancer pain syndromes in primary care. *J Gen Intern Med.* 2002; 17:173–9.

Schuster CR. History and current perspectives on the use of drug formulations to decrease the abuse of prescription drugs. *Drug Alcohol Depend.* 2006; 83(suppl 1):S8–14.

Sees KL, Di Marino ME, Ruediger NK, Sweeney CT, Shiffman S. Nonmedical use of OxyContin tablets in the United States. *J Pain Palliat Care Pharmacother.* 2005; 19:13–23.

Shaiova L, Lapin J, Manco LS, Shasha D, Hu K, Harrison L, Portenoy RK. Tolerability and effects of two formulations of oral transmucosal fentanyl citrate (OTFC, Actiq) in patients with radiation-induced oral mucositis. *Support Care Cancer.* 2004; 12:268–73.

Sinatra R. The fentanyl-HCl patient-controlled transdermal system (PCTS): an alternative to intravenous patient-controlled analgesia in the postoperative setting. *Clin Pharmacokinet.* 2005; 44 (suppl 1): 1–6.

Sloan P, Slatkin N, Ahdieh H. Effectiveness and safety of oral extended-release oxymorphone for the treatment of cancer pain: a pilot study. *Support Care Cancer.* 2005; 13:57–65.

Stanley TH et al. Oral transmucosal fentanyl citrate premedication in human volunteers. *Anesth. Analg.* 1989; 69:21–7.

Sternbach RA. Survey of pain in the United States: the Nuprin pain report. *Clin J Pain.* 1986; 2:49–53.

Substance Abuse and Mental Health Services Administration (SAMHSA) Office of Applied Studies. 2003. *Emergency Department Trends from the Drug Abuse Warning Network, Final Estimates 1995–2002.* DAWN

Series: D-24, DHHS Publication No. (SMA) 03–3780. Rockville, MD: SAMHSA.

Sullivan MD, Edlund MJ, Steffick D, Unutzer J. Regular use of prescribed opioids: associations with common psychiatric disorders. *Pain.* 2005; 119:95–103.

Tharp AM, Winecker RE, Winston DC. Fatal intravenous fentanyl abuse: four cases involving extraction of fentanyl from transdermal patches. *Am J Forensic Med Pathol.* 2004; 25:178–81.

U.S. Department of Justice, Drug Enforcement Administration, Diversion Control Program. Drugs and chemicals of concern: fentanyl. http://www.deadiversion.usdoj.gov/drugs_concern/fentanyl.htm. Published 2006.

Voth EA, et al. Responsible prescribing of controlled substances. *Am Fam Physicians.* 1991; 44:1673–78.

Walsh D. Pharmacologic management of cancer pain. *Sem Oncol.* 2000; 27:45–63.

Ward CF, Ward GC, Saidman LJ. Drug abuse in anesthesia training programs. A survey: 1970 through 1980. *JAMA.* 1983; 250(7):922–5.

Webster, LR, Webster, RM. Predicting aberrant behaviors in opioid-treated patients: preliminary validation of the Opioid Risk Tool. *Pain Medicine.* 2005; 6(6):432–42.

Zepetella G, O'Doherty CA, Collins S. Prevalence and characteristics of breakthrough pain in cancer patients admitted to a hospice. *J Pain Symptom Manage.* 2000; 20:87–92.

Zepetella G, Ribeiro MD. Opioids for the management of breakthrough (episodic) pain in cancer patients. *Cochrane Database Systemic Rev.* 2006; 1:CD004311.

45

Federal and State Policies at the Interface of Pain and Addiction

Martha A. Maurer

Aaron M. Gilson

David E. Joranson

Relief of pain and suffering is an essential part of quality medical practice (Federation of State Medical Boards 2000, 2004). The medical and scientific communities, as well as regulatory agencies, have acknowledged the essential role of opioid analgesics as safe and effective in managing moderate to severe pain when under the supervision of a knowledgeable practitioner (Meldrum 2005; Miaskowski et al. 2005; Portenoy 1996; World Health Organization 1996). However, pain affects many patient populations, including those who need an opioid analgesic as part of a pain management program (Bernabei et al. 1998; Baker, Haffer, & Denniston 2003; Institute of Medicine Committee on Care at the End of Life 1997; SUPPORT Study Principal Investigators 1995). Misinformation about addiction, sensational media coverage of drug abuse, and highly publicized cases against certain prescribers have contributed to the stigmatization of opioid analgesics (Bennett & Carr 2002; Brushwood & Kimberlin 2004; Fishman 2005; Hyman & Brookoff 1998). Despite progress to improve the regulatory environment for pain management in several states (Gilson, Maurer, & Joranson 2005), many health-care professionals continue to fear being investigated and are unwilling to manage pain with opioid analgesics (Gilson & Joranson 2001; Institute of Medicine 1997; Martino 1998).

Patients who experience chronic pain who also abuse drugs, have a diagnosable addictive disease, or have a history of substance abuse are at increased risk for inadequate relief because of an inaccurate understanding about pain and addiction (Gilson & Joranson 2002; Joranson & Gilson 2003; Savage et al. 2003). Persons with addictive disease should not automatically forfeit their access to effective pain management, and legal prescribing for pain must not be mistaken for illegal prescriptions to maintain addiction.

Policy Basis for Prescriptions

Federal law does not prohibit issuing a prescription for the purpose of treating pain in a patient with history of substance abuse or current addiction, including patients being treated for drug dependence in opioid treatment programs (OTPs), as long as it is done in the usual course of professional practice (Food and Drugs 1974). Such prescribing is considered within the scope of legitimate medical practice, although it should be emphasized that prescribing for pain in patients with addictive disease may require special expertise, extra care, and monitoring for functional changes (American Academy of Pain Medicine, American Pain Society, and American Society of Addiction Medicine 2004; Federation of State Medical Boards 2004; Miaskowski et al. 2005). The Drug Enforcement Administration's (DEA) *Pharmacist's Manual* outlines the requirements of the federal Controlled Substances Act (CSA) and DEA regulations, stating that "A practitioner may prescribe methadone or any other narcotic to a narcotic addict for analgesic purposes" (Drug Enforcement Administration 2003, p. 56). Correspondence from the DEA additionally confirms that it is legal to prescribe opioid analgesics for pain relief to patients who are enrolled in OTPs (Good 2000).

Federal and state controlled substances laws do prohibit prescribing controlled substances to maintain addiction (or "drug dependence") without a special authorization.[1] Therefore, it is critically important for patients, prescribers, dispensers, and law enforcement officials to understand what constitutes addiction, to know correct terminology, to use terms correctly, and to know whether the policy in their state defines addiction-related terminology correctly.

For example, the use of decreasing doses in a pain patient to avoid withdrawal from a physical dependence on an opioid analgesic is a clinical procedure known as "tapering," which is different from the separately regulated practice of "detoxification" of a drug dependent person or addict. Without a correct understanding of this crucial distinction, a physician who tapers a pain patient to avoid withdrawal symptoms could mistakenly be viewed by a law enforcement officer as conducting unauthorized detoxification treatment, which could lead to an investigation for illegal distribution of controlled drugs for other than a legitimate medical purpose (i.e., treatment of addiction without a separate registration).

Case

The following case is an example of how the purpose of a physician's prescriptions can be misunderstood and lead to costly law enforcement investigations. In this case, the DEA proposed to deny the registration of an Ohio physician.

---

[1] To be legal, a practitioner must obtain a separate registration to use opioids to treat addiction and can only dispense, but not prescribe, approved opioids such as methadone and buprenorphine.

The Drug Enforcement Administration initiated its investigation of the Respondent in April 1991 after receiving information from the... Sheriff's Department that Respondent was prescribing controlled substances to known drug abusers and drug traffickers.... [t]he patient chart had printed on its face: "Drug addiction to Vicodin."... After reviewing these charts and Respondent's testimony at the hearing, the administrative law judge concluded that Respondent issued controlled substances prescriptions to these individuals for legitimate medical purposes, such as relief of pain, muscle spasms, and anxiety.... [t]he administrative law judge found that no nexus had been established between the volume of controlled substances that the Respondent prescribed... and an illegitimate purpose for such prescribing practices.... [t]he DEA did not meet its burden of proof. (Gillis, Granting of Registration 1993, p. 37507)

The DEA granted the physician's registration.

If legal definitions are accurate and applied correctly, the physical dependence or tolerance that may be experienced by patients being treated with opioids for their pain will not be confused with addiction or drug dependence. Alternatively, if the legal definition of addiction in a particular jurisdiction can be satisfied only by physical dependence or tolerance, the scene is set for costly mistakes and disruption of medical practice when clinicians are charged with unprofessional conduct or criminal misconduct when treating patients appropriately.

Terminology Definitions

Addiction and related terminology have a long history of being misunderstood. Scientists, clinicians, policymakers, regulators, and the public conceptualize and define addiction very differently. This inconsistency has the potential to interfere with appropriate clinical management of both pain and addiction (Savage et al. 2003). Unfortunately, inconsistent terminology also is present in state controlled substances and professional practice statutes and in regulations that govern prescribing and dispensing for pain management.

Inaccurate addiction-related terminology stems in part from past World Health Organization (WHO) Expert Committee documents developed to communicate its understanding of addiction at the time. For example, in 1952, the WHO defined *addiction* as primarily a direct effect of certain drugs such as morphine, stating that "...some drugs, notably morphine and pharmacologically morphine-like substances, whose specific pharmacological action, under individual conditions of time and dose, will always produce compulsive craving, dependence, and addiction in any individual" (World Health Organization 1952, p. 10). In 1964, the WHO introduced the term *drug dependence* to replace addiction, and emphasized that both physical and compulsive drug use were common factors (World Health Organization 1964). A subsequent reconceptualization of *drug dependence* focused on behavioral factors, as well as drug characteristics: "A state, psychic and sometimes also physical, resulting from the interaction between a living organism and a drug, characterized by behavioral and other responses that always include a compulsion to take the drug on a continuous or periodic basis in order to experience its psychic effects, and sometimes to avoid the discomfort of its absence. Tolerance may or may not be present" (World Health Organization 1969, p. 6).

After almost 25 years, this term was replaced by *dependence syndrome,* a more modern medical and scientific conceptualization of addictive disease stressing biological, psychological, social, and drug features (World Health Organization 1993). Neither withdrawal symptoms nor tolerance are sufficient to fulfill the new definition, so that physical dependence resulting from therapeutic opioid use would not be considered pathological. The current *International Classification of Diseases (ICD-10)*, using the WHO terminology, provides clinical criteria for diagnosing dependence syndrome, which emphasizes compulsive behaviors (World Health Organization 1992). The *ICD-10* also clarifies that the necessary characteristic of compulsivity would exclude patients with pain who are taking opioids for therapeutic purposes.

Recognizing the need for accurate and consistent nomenclature, three national professional organizations, representing pain management and addiction medicine, formed a liaison committee in 2001 to develop consensus definitions of addiction-related terms (American Academy of Pain Medicine, American Pain Society, and American Society of Addiction Medicine 2001). A primary goal of this consensus process was to provide an unambiguous conceptual distinction between three phenomena: *physical dependence, tolerance,* and *addiction*. According to this medical and scientific consensus, *addiction* is primarily characterized by compulsive and maladaptive drug use. Neither physical dependence nor tolerance, which are normal adaptations of the body to the long-term presence of particular drugs in the body including withdrawal syndrome, are sufficient to define *addiction* (American Academy of Pain Medicine, American Pain Society, and American Society of Addiction Medicine 2001; Savage et al. 2003). These are the standing definitions of all three parent organizations, and can be used to inform the clinical practice of medicine, pharmacy, and nursing.

A national regulatory organization also has worked to enhance health-care professionals' understanding of addiction-related terminology. In 1998, the Federation of State Medical Boards (the Federation) created "Model Guidelines for the Use of Controlled Substances for Pain Management" (called Model Guidelines) for health-care regulatory boards to adopt to provide guidance for licensees in their state (Federation of State Medical Boards 1998). The Model Guidelines recognize that additional monitoring and expertise are needed for treating pain in patients with addictive disease, and they include definitions that do not confuse addiction with physical dependence or tolerance (Federation of State Medical Boards 1998). Although no changes were made to the relevant provisions when the Federation updated the guidelines in 2004 (now called the "Model Policy for the Use of Controlled Substances for the Treatment of Pain" [Model Policy]), the original definitions relating to pain and addictive disease were replaced with the consensus definitions (see Table 45.1 for changes to the Federation definitions between the Model Guidelines and the Model Policy; Federation of State Medical Boards 2004).

The purpose of this chapter is to examine the extent that federal and state policies, which define addiction or drug dependence, are consistent with current medical and scientific understanding.

Methodology

The Pain & Policy Studies Group (PPSG) has developed a research methodology to evaluate federal and state policies that can affect professional practice and patient access to pain medications

Table 45.1. Definitions of Addiction-Related Terms

Source	Addiction	Physical Dependence	Tolerance
FSMB 1998	Addiction is a neurobehavioral syndrome with genetic and environmental influences that results in psychological dependence on the use of substances for their psychic effects and is characterized by compulsive use despite harm. Addiction may also be referred to by terms such as "drug dependence" and "psychological dependence." Physical dependence and tolerance are normal physiological consequences of extended opioid therapy for pain and should not be considered addiction.	Physical dependence on a controlled substance is a physiologic state of neuroadaptation which is characterized by the emergence of a withdrawal syndrome if drug use is stopped or decreased abruptly, or if an antagonist is administered. Physical dependence is an expected result of opioid use. Physical dependence, by itself, does not equate with addiction.	Tolerance is a physiologic state resulting from regular use of a drug in which an increased dosage is needed to produce the same effect, or a reduced effect is observed with a constant dose.
FSMB 2004 and APS/AAPM/ASAM 2001	Addiction is a primary, chronic, neurobiologic disease, with genetic, psychosocial, and environmental factors influencing its development and manifestations. It is characterized by behaviors that include the following: impaired control over drug use, craving, compulsive use and continued use despite harm. Physical dependence and tolerance are normal physiological consequences of extended opioid therapy for pain and are not the same as addiction.	Physical dependence on a controlled substance is a physiologic state of neuroadaptation which is characterized by the emergence of a withdrawal syndrome if drug use is stopped or decreased abruptly, or if an antagonist is administered. Physical dependence is an expected result of opioid use. Physical dependence, by itself, does not equate with addiction.	Tolerance is a physiologic state resulting from regular use of a drug in which an increased dosage is needed to produce a specific effect or a reduced effect is observed with a constant dose over time.

(Joranson et al. 2000). The methodology is based on the principle of *balance* and uses 16 criteria to identify policy provisions that have the potential to either enhance or impede the use of controlled substances for pain management and can affect treatment of patients for pain. This study examined two criteria relevant to federal and state policies that define addiction-related terms: (1) that physical dependence or analgesic tolerance are *not* confused with "addiction," and (2) that physical dependence or analgesic tolerance are confused with "addiction." Our evaluation identified formal definitions of terms, as well as statements that correctly conceptualize such addiction-related terms.

The PPSG conducted systematic content evaluations of:

- Federal statutes and regulations governing controlled substances,
- State statutes and regulations governing controlled substances and medical and pharmacy practice, and
- Other state health-care regulatory policies such as medical board guidelines and policy statements or joint board policy statements.

Such policies were collected and evaluated at four times; the first evaluation was in 2000, and it was repeated in 2003, 2006, and 2007 to capture new, amended, or repealed policies (Pain & Policy Studies Group 2007a). The policies were evaluated by 3 policy researchers, who applied the criteria to identify policy language that, if implemented into practice, could either enhance or impede the medical use of controlled substances for pain management.

Findings

Both federal law and policies in most states contain numerous instances of addiction-related terminology. Such terminology is either consistent or inconsistent with current medical and scientific conceptualizations of addiction phenomena.

Federal Law

Since 1970, the Federal Controlled Substances Act has defined an *addict* as a person who "habitually uses any narcotic drug so as to endanger the public morals, health, safety, or who is so far addicted to the use of narcotic drugs as to have lost the power of self-control with reference to his addiction" (Controlled Substances Act 1970, p. 836). Despite the archaic language, this definition does not appear to confuse addiction with either physical dependence or tolerance, because the main component of *addict* is loss of control and harm. The definition has little potential to confuse patients using opioids for pain treatment with persons who compulsively use opioids nonmedically due to an addictive disease.

Unfortunately, a separate U.S. federal policy contains an archaic addiction-related definition that stems from a 1969 definition of *drug dependence* from the WHO: "The term 'drug dependent person' means a person who is using a controlled substance... and who is in a state of psychic or physical dependence, or both, arising from the use of that substance on a continuous basis. Drug dependence is characterized by behavioral and other responses which include a strong compulsion to take the substance on a continuous basis in order to experience its psychic effects or to avoid the discomfort caused by its absence" (Public Health and Welfare 1973). Not only does this federal definition not conform to current medical and scientific understanding of addiction, but it clearly has the potential to legally label as an "addict" a patient with pain who is being treated with opioids. In addition, many states adopted this definition when they based their Controlled Substances Acts on this federal model.

State Policies

In 2007, 36 (71%) states had 46 policies containing terminology that did not confuse physical dependence or tolerance with addiction (see Table 45.2). We provide example policy language to show how state regulatory board policies are consistent with the current understanding of addiction issues:

Connecticut Medical Examining Board Policy Statement (2005): "Current practice guidelines accept that tolerance and physical dependence are normal consequences of sustained use of opioid analgesics and are not pathognomonic of addiction" (Connecticut Medical Examining Board 2005).

Kansas State Board of Healing Arts Guideline (1998): "Addiction is a neuro-behavioral syndrome with genetic and environmental influences that results in psychological dependence on the use of substances for their psychic effects and is characterized by compulsive use despite harm. Addiction may also be referred to by terms such as 'drug dependence' and 'psychological dependence.' Physical dependence and tolerance are normal physiological consequences of extended opioid therapy for pain and should not be considered addiction" (Kansas State Board of Healing Arts 1998).

Louisiana State Board of Medical Examiner's Regulation: "The development of controlled substance tolerance or physical dependence does not equate with substance abuse or addiction" (Medical Professions).

Ohio State Medical Board Regulation (1998): "(A) Physical dependence and tolerance by themselves do not indicate addiction. (B) Physical dependence and tolerance are normal physiological consequences of extended opioid therapy, and do not, in the absence of other indicators of drug abuse or addiction, require reduction or cessation of opioid therapy" (Drug Treatment of Intractable Pain 1998).

Sixteen (31%) states had policy language that allowed physical dependence alone to define *addiction* or *drug dependence*. Again, examples are provided:

Arizona Controlled Substances Act: "'Drug dependent person' means a person who is using a controlled substance and who is in a state or psychic or physical dependence, or both, arising from the use of that substance on a continuous basis" (Uniform Controlled Substances Act).

Medical Licensing Board of Indiana Regulations: "'Addict' means a person who is physiologically and/or psychologically dependent upon a drug which is classified as a narcotic, controlled substance or dangerous drug" (Medical Licensing Board of Indiana).

Tennessee Board of Medical Examiners Policy Statement (1995): "Also, remember that with certain conditions, drug holidays are appropriate. This allows you to check to see whether the original symptoms recur when the drug is not given—indicating a continuing legitimate need for the drug or whether withdrawal symptoms occur—indicating drug dependence" (Tennessee Board of Medical Examiners 1995, p. 2).

Interestingly, 12 states (24%) had a policy containing an addiction-related definition that is consistent with current medical and scientific understanding as well as another policy with a definition that conflicts with today's conceptualizations of addiction. In all but 1 state, it was the statutes that contained policy language that conflicts, whereas health-care regulatory board policies contained the language that clearly distinguishes addiction from physical dependence and tolerance. Additionally, all inaccurate statutory definitions were adopted before the correct health-care regulatory board policy language.

Overall, the majority of correct addiction-related terminology was found in health-care regulatory board policies, whereas most of the incorrect policy language was found in statutes (see Table 45.3). Health-care licensing board regulations and guidelines/policy statements contained nearly all (98%) instances of correct addiction-related terminology, whereas 74% of the incorrect definitions were found in statutes.

Figure 45.1 shows the trends in addiction-related terminology found in state policy over the 7-year study period. There was a notable increase in number of correct definitions, while addiction-related definitions that conflicted with the current understanding remained relatively unchanged (Maurer, Gilson, & Joranson 2007).

Discussion

Historically, definitions of addiction-related terminology characterized tolerance and physical dependence as necessary components of addiction. Current scientific knowledge, however, considers these to be separate, although interrelated, conditions; this conceptual distinction must be accurately reflected in laws governing the medical use of controlled drugs. Distinguishing between patients with pain and those with addictive disease can have critical legal implications for physicians and clinically impact patient care. Inappropriate investigations can damage professional careers and have a chilling effect on the entire medical community. Inaccurate legal definitions of addiction and related terms can lead to the following: confusion over whether a prescription is considered

Table 45.2. States With Relevant Policy Language

States With Addiction-Related Terms That Do Not Confuse Physical Dependence With Addiction	States With Addiction-Related Terms That Do Confuse Physical Dependence With Addiction	States With Multiple Definitions That Conflict
AL, AZ, CA, CO, CT, DC, FL, HI, ID, KS, KY, LA, MA, MD, ME, MI, MO, MS, NC, NE, NM, NV, NY, OH, OK, PA, SC, SD, TN, TX, UT, VA, VT, WA, WI, WV (36 total)	AZ, CO, GA, HI, ID, IN, LA, MD, MO, NC, NJ, NV, OK, PA, TN, WY (16 total)	AZ, CO, HI, ID, LA, MD, MO, NC, NV, OK, PA, TN (12 total)

Table 45.3. Correct and Incorrect Addiction-Related Terms by Type of Policy

Provisions	Addiction-Related Terms Consistent With Current Medical and Scientific Understanding	Addiction-Related Terms Inconsistent With Current Medical and Scientific Understanding
Statutes	1	14
Regulations	14	3
Licensing board guidelines/policy statements	31	2

legal, the stigmatization of pain patients as addicts, the placement of such patients at risk for undertreatment, and the erroneous suggestion that mere use of opioids for chronic pain will result in drug addiction.

Some of the addition-related terminology in state laws today still reflects an understanding of addiction phenomenology and biology at a time when early research considered it to be a largely physiological phenomenon; some state laws have not yet adapted to the scientific evolution of knowledge about addiction. In addition, most of the inaccurate definitions were adopted before pain management became a visible health-care priority and before regulatory policies clarified that pain management is a legitimate medical purpose and an expected part of quality clinical practice. It is recognized that the outdated policy language found in drug control policies, such as state controlled substances acts and related regulations, was not intended to limit pain management but rather to prevent addiction as it was understood at the time. In fact, the majority of correct definitions were found in state health-care regulatory board policies because they are based on more recent Federation model policies that define and use these terms accurately.

As an alternative approach, the most recent model for state drug law, entitled the Uniform Controlled Substances Act (USCA) and recommended to states for adoption in 1994, does not define addiction-related terms such as *addict, drug dependent person,* or *habitual user* (National Conference of Commissioners on Uniform State Laws 1994). The USCA further contains a cautionary statement that if state law defines such terms, the state legislature should ensure that the definition "cannot be construed to include a patient using a controlled substance pursuant to the lawful order of a practitioner" (National Conference of Commissioners on Uniform State Laws 1994, p. 13).

Despite the UCSA's caveat, many states' laws contain archaic definitions that are in need of reform. Changes to legislative definitions have been slow to occur, but it is encouraging that one instance of change did occur subsequent to the policy evaluation reported in this chapter. Rhode Island's legislature recently modified an inaccurate definition that created the potential to confuse addiction with physical dependence or tolerance. For more than 30 years, the Rhode Island Legislature had defined *drug dependent person* as someone "who is using a controlled substance and who is in a state of psychic or physical dependence, or both, arising from the use of that controlled substance on a continuous basis..." (Uniform Controlled Substances Act). In 2005, the Legislature revised both the terminology and definition as follows: "'Drug addicted person' means a person who exhibits a maladaptive pattern of behavior resulting from drug use, including one or more of the following: impaired control over drug use; compulsive use; and/or continued use despite harm, and craving" (Uniform Controlled Substances Act 2005). It is clear that the revised definition could not mistake a pain patient being treated with opioid analgesics as an addict. Perhaps the improvement to Rhode Island's definition can serve as a model for other state legislatures to conform their laws more closely to current scientific and clinical understanding by changing or repealing their outdated definitions.

Federal policy changes regarding the use of opioids in addiction treatment programs demonstrate that such policy can be improved. In the past, "narcotic dependence" was the primary criterion for admission to federally regulated narcotic treatment

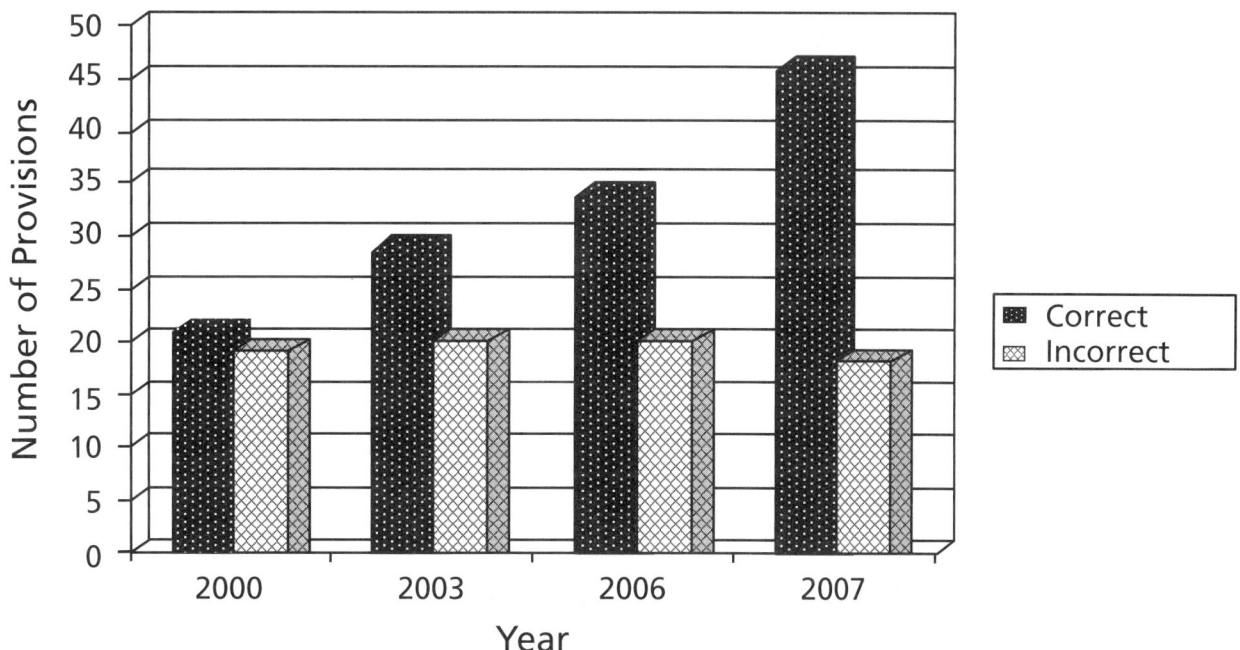

Figure 45.1. Recent trends in the number of correct and incorrect addiction-related provisions in state policy.

programs (now called OTPs). *Narcotic dependent* was defined as "an individual who physiologically needs...a morphine-like drug to prevent the onset of signs of withdrawal" (Food and Drugs 1971, p. 158). As a result, any chronic pain patient who was physically dependent on opioid analgesics for chronic pain could be considered "narcotic dependent" and admitted to a detoxification or maintenance treatment program designed only for addiction treatment (Joranson 1997). In 2001, however, the federal regulations for the treatment of addiction, as well as admissions criteria to OTPs, were modified extensively (Public Health 2003). Physical dependence was no longer the sole condition for admissions, additionally requiring evidence of opioid addiction; in fact, a person can be admitted to an OTP when they are not physically dependent. The new policy also emphasizes the need to differentiate between the disease of opioid addiction and physical dependence as a consequence of prolonged opioid use from pain management (Center for Substance Abuse Treatment 2000). As a result, OTP policy was revised to become more consistent with the current medical and scientific knowledge about chronic addictive disease.

Regulatory definitions of addiction that clearly distinguish it from physical dependence or tolerance are essential for creating rational drug control and health-care policies that can affect both pain management and addiction treatment. Recognizing that this issue has global implications, the WHO published guidelines for national opioid control policies that contain criteria to determine whether there is "terminology in national drug control policy that has the potential to confuse the medical use of opioids for pain with drug dependence" (World Health Organization 2000, p. 26). The WHO guidelines are the first criteria-based policy evaluation tool that addresses the quality of addiction-related terminology, underscoring the importance of medical care of individuals with pain requiring the use of medications that have an abuse and addiction liability.

Conclusions

State policies with incorrect definitions of addiction-related terminology have been identified by a systematic criteria-based policy evaluation. Policymakers, regulators, and professional and patient groups should make use of resources now available to locate the specific provisions in each state that have the potential to confuse pain patients with abusers or persons with addictive disease, as well as those that might prevent patients with cancer, HIV/AIDS, or other chronic diseases from receiving pain relief if they have addictive disease (Pain & Policy Studies Group 2007a, 2007b).

State boards should also consider adopting the Federation's Model Policy as a guideline or policy statement because it contains accurate definitions and recognizes that treatment of pain, including in persons with addictive disease, may require extra care and monitoring. Once a regulatory board adopts precise addiction-related definitions, relevant statutory definitions must be identified and reviewed to assess whether they conform to or are incompatible with the new regulatory terms; if incompatible, efforts must be made to repeal or modify the statutory language to prevent potential licensee confusion and a detrimental impact on clinical practice and patient care. In this way, state policies will be consistent with federal policy, as well as with medical consensus statements and guidelines from national and international authorities, including the Liaison Committee, the WHO, and the International Narcotics Control Board.

Untreated addictive disease and unrelieved pain have devastating effects on the individual, family, friends, and society. The ultimate goal is to address both in a balanced way so that the treatment of one does not interfere in the treatment of the other. Patients with addiction and debilitating pain must not be precluded from the relief that is available to others. We recognize that providing effective pain management to patients with addictive disease is clinically complex and demanding, but patients with pain should not be excluded from access to pain medications when medically indicated. Current medical practice standards acknowledge that addictive disease does not necessarily contraindicate the treatment of pain using opioids. The required task for regulators and legislative policymakers is to create a policy environment that conforms to these current standards.

References

American Academy of Pain Medicine, American Pain Society, and American Society of Addiction Medicine. 2001. *Definitions related to the use of opioids for the treatment of pain.* Glenview, IL: AAPM, APS, ASAM.

American Academy of Pain Medicine, American Pain Society, and American Society of Addiction Medicine. 2004. *Public policy statement on the rights and responsibilities of healthcare professionals in the use of opioids for the treatment of pain.* Glenview, IL: AAPM, APS, ASAM.

Baker, F., S. C. Haffer, & M. Denniston. 2003. Health-related quality of life of cancer and noncancer patients in Medicare managed care. *Cancer* 97, 3:674–681.

Bennett, D. S., & D. B. Carr. 2002. Opiophobia as a barrier to the treatment of pain. *Journal of Pain and Palliative Care Pharmacotherapy* 16, 1:105–109.

Bernabei, R., G. Gambassi, K. Lapane, F. Landi, C. Gatsonis, R. Dunlop, L. Lipsitz, K. Steel, & V. Mor. 1998. Management of pain in elderly patients with cancer. *Journal of the American Medical Association* 279, 23:1877–1882.

Brushwood, D. B., & C. A. Kimberlin. 2004. Media coverage of controlled substance diversion through theft or loss. *Journal of the American Pharmacists Association* 44, 4:439–444.

Center for Substance Abuse Treatment. 2000. *Guidelines for the Accreditation of Opioid Treatment Programs.* Washington, DC: U.S. Department of Health and Human Services.

Connecticut Medical Examining Board. 2005. *Statement of the Connecticut Medical Examining Board on the Use of Controlled Substances for the Treatment of Pain.* Hartford: Connecticut Medical Examining Board.

Controlled Substances Act. Pub L. No. 91–513, 84 Stat 1242 (1970).

Drug Enforcement Administration. 2003. *Pharmacist's manual: An informational outline of the controlled substances act of 1970* (8th ed.). Washington, DC: U.S. Department of Justice.

Drug Treatment of Intractable Pain, Federation of State Medical Boards of the United States Inc. 1998. *Model guidelines for the use of controlled substances for the treatment of pain.* Euless, TX: Federation of State Medical Boards of the United States Inc.

Federation of State Medical Boards of the United States Inc. 2000. *A guide to the essentials of a modern medical practice act* (9th ed.). Dallas, TX: Federation of State Medical Boards.

Federation of State Medical Boards of the United States Inc. 2004. *Model policy for the use of controlled substances for the treatment of pain.* Dallas, TX: Federation of State Medical Boards of the United States Inc.

Fishman, S. M. 2005. From balanced pain care to drug trafficking: The case of Dr. William Hurwitz and the DEA. *Pain Medicine* 6, 2:162–164.

Food and Drugs. 1971. 21 C.F.R. § 1306.04(a).

Food and Drugs. 1974. 21 C.F.R. § 291.505(a)(5).

Gillis, David H., MD. 1993. Granting of Registration. *Fed Reg.* 1993;58(131): 37507.

Gilson, A. M., & D. E. Joranson. 2001. Controlled substances and pain management: Changes in knowledge and attitudes of state medical regulators. *Journal of Pain and Symptom Management* 21, 3:227–237.

Gilson, A. M., & D. E. Joranson. 2002. U.S. policies relevant to the prescribing of opioid analgesics for the treatment of pain in patients with addictive disease. *Clinical Journal of Pain* 18, 4(suppl):S91–S98.

Gilson, A. M., M. A. Maurer, & D. E. Joranson. 2005. State policy affecting pain management: Recent improvements and the positive impact of regulatory health policies. *Health Policy* 74, 2:192–204.

Good, P. M. *Pain management and narcotic addiction treatment.* Letter from Chief of the Liaison and Policy Section, DEA Office of Diversion Control, to Dr. Howard Heit regarding DEA pain management and addiction treatment policy; March 3, 2000.

Hyman, C. S., & D. Brookoff. 1998. State medical boards and pain management. *Journal of Pain and Symptom Management* 15, 6:379–382.

Institute of Medicine Committee on Care at the End of Life. 1997. *Approaching Death: Improving Care at the End of Life.* Washington, DC: National Academy Press.

Joranson, D. E. 1997. Is methadone maintenance the last resort for some chronic pain patients? *American Pain Society Bulletin* 7, 5:1, 4–5.

Joranson, D. E., & A. M. Gilson. 2003. Legal and regulatory issues in the management of pain. In A. W. Graham, T. K. Schultz, M. F. Mayo-Smith, R. K. Ries, & B. B. Wilford (eds.), *Principles of Addiction Medicine* (3rd ed.). Chevy Chase, MD: American Society of Addiction Medicine, Inc.

Joranson, D. E., A. M. Gilson, K. M. Ryan, M. A. Maurer, J. A. Nischik, & J. M. Nelson. 2000. *Achieving balance in federal and state pain policy: A guide to evaluation.* Madison: Pain & Policy Studies Group, University of Wisconsin Comprehensive Cancer Center.

Kansas State Board of Healing Arts. 1998. *Guidelines for the Use of Controlled Substances for the Treatment of Pain.* Topeka: Kansas State Board of Healing Arts.

Martino, A. M. 1998. In search of a new ethic for treating patients with chronic pain: What can medical boards do? *Journal of Law, Medicine & Ethics* 26, 4:332–349.

Maurer, M. A., A. M. Gilson, & D. E. Joranson. 2007. *How do state policies address pain and addiction?* Poster presented at the 7th International Conference on Pain & Chemical Dependency; New York, NY; June 21–24, 2007. Madison: University of Wisconsin Pain & Policy Studies Group/WHO Collaborating Center for Policy and Communications in Cancer Care.

Medical Licensing Board of Indiana, 844 Indiana Administrative Code § 5–1-1(1).

Medical Professions. 46 Louisiana Administrative Code.§ XLV.6917.

Meldrum, M. L. 2005. The ladder and the clock: Cancer pain and public policy at the end of the twentieth century. *Journal of Pain and Symptom Management* 29, 1:41–54.

Miaskowski, C., J. Cleary, R. Burney, P. Coyne, R. Finley, R. Foster, S. Grossman, N. Janjan, J. Ray, K. Syrjala, S. Weisman, & C. Zahrbock. 2005. *Guideline for the Management of Cancer Pain in Adults and Children. APS Clinical Practice Guidelines Series, No. 3.* Glenview, IL: American Pain Society.

National Conference of Commissioners on Uniform State Laws. 1994. *Uniform Controlled Substances Act.* Adopted at its Annual Conference Meeting in its One-Hundred-and-Third-Year; Chicago, IL; July 29–August 5, 1994.

Ohio Administrative Code. 1998. § 4731–21–04.

Pain & Policy Studies Group. 2007a. *Achieving Balance in Federal and State Pain Policy: A Guide to Evaluation* (4th ed.). Madison: University of Wisconsin, Paul P. Carbone Comprehensive Cancer Center.

Pain & Policy Studies Group. 2007b. *Achieving Balance in State Pain Policy: A Progress Report Card* (3d ed.). Madison: University of Wisconsin, Paul P. Carbone Comprehensive Cancer Center.

Portenoy, R. K. 1996. Opioid therapy for chronic nonmalignant pain: A review of the critical issues. *Journal of Pain and Symptom Management* 11, 4:203–217.

Public Health. 2003. 42 C.F.R § 8.12.

Public Health and Welfare. 1973. 42 U.S.C.S § 201.

Savage, S. R., D. E. Joranson, E. C. Covington, S. H. Schnoll, H. A. Heit, & A. M. Gilson. 2003. Definitions related to the medical use of opioids: Evolution towards universal agreement. *Journal of Pain and Symptom Management* 26, 1:655–667.

SUPPORT Study Principal Investigators. 1995. A controlled trial to improve care for seriously ill hospitalized patients: the Study to Understand Prognoses and Preferences for Outcomes and Risks of Treatments (SUPPORT). *Journal of the American Medical Association* 274, 20:1591–1598.

Tennessee Board of Medical Examiners. 1995. Management of prescribing with an emphasis on addictive or dependency-producing drugs. *BME Prescribing Policy*, pp. 1–2. Nashville: Tennessee Board of Medical Examiners.

Uniform Controlled Substances Act. 36 Arizona Revised Statutes § 2501-A-5.

Uniform Controlled Substances Act. 21 General Laws of Rhode Island § 28–1.02(15).

Uniform Controlled Substances Act. 2005. 21 General Laws of Rhode Island § 28–1.02(18).

World Health Organization. 1952. *WHO Expert Committee on Drugs Liable to Produce Addiction: Third Report (Technical Report Series 57).* Geneva, Switzerland: World Health Organization.

World Health Organization. 1964. *World Health Organization Expert Committee on Addiction-Producing Drugs (Technical Report Series 273).* Geneva, Switzerland: World Health Organization.

World Health Organization. 1969. *WHO Expert Committee on Drug Dependence: Sixteenth Report.* Geneva, Switzerland: World Health Organization.

World Health Organization. 1992. *The ICD-10 Classification of Mental and Behavioral Disorders: Clinical Descriptions and Diagnostic Guidelines.* Geneva, Switzerland: World Health Organization.

World Health Organization. 1993. *WHO Expert Committee on Drug Dependence: Twenty-Eighth Report.* Geneva, Switzerland: World Health Organization.

World Health Organization. 1996. *Cancer pain relief: With a guide to opioid availability* (2nd ed.). Geneva, Switzerland: World Health Organization.

World Health Organization. 2000. *Achieving balance in national opioids control policy: Guidelines for assessment.* Geneva, Switzerland: World Health Organization.

46

Documentation and Potential Documentation Tools in Long-Term Opioid Therapy

Kenneth L. Kirsh

Howard S. Smith

The use of long-term opioid therapy (LTOT) to treat chronic nonmalignant pain is growing, based in part on evidence from clinical trials and a growing consensus among pain specialists (Collett, 1998; Portenoy, 1996a, 1996b; Urban et al., 1986; Zenz et al., 1992). The appropriate use of these drugs requires skills in opioid prescribing, knowledge of addiction medicine principles, and a commitment to perform and document a comprehensive assessment repeatedly over time. Inadequate assessment can lead to undertreatment, compromise of the effectiveness of therapy when implemented, and prevention of an appropriate response when problematic drug-related behaviors occur (JCAHO, 1999; Katz, 2002; Max et al., 1999).

Regulatory agencies, state medical boards, and various peer-review groups (among others) not only expect appropriate medical care but also require proper documentation. In cases of LTOT for persistent noncancer pain (PNCP), aside from the usual "SOAP" (subjective/objective/assessment/plan) style medical progress notes, various other issues require documentation. Although there are no explicit requirements spelled out as to what and how to document issues related to LTOT, it is felt by some that the use of specific tools/instruments in the chart on some or all visits may boost adherence to documentation expectations as well as consistency of such documentation (Passik et al., 2005). Assessment tools may also be helpful in the analysis of persistent pain (Wincent et al., 2003).

It must be cautioned that physicians who adequately assess patients before and during opioid therapy may still encounter problems as a result of poor documentation. In a chart review of 300 patients with chronic pain, 61% had no documentation of a treatment plan (Clark, 2002). Similarly, a review of the initial consultation notes of 513 patients with acute musculoskeletal pain revealed that only 43% of historical findings and 28% of physical examination findings were documented (Solomon et al., 2000). In a review of 520 randomly selected visits at an outpatient oncology practice, quantitative assessment of pain scores was virtually absent (<1%), and qualitative assessment of pain occurred in only 60% of cases (Rhodes et al., 2001). Finally, a review of medical records of 111 randomly selected patients who underwent urine toxicology screens in a cancer center found that documentation was infrequent: 37.8% of physicians failed to list a reason for the test, and 89% of the charts did not include discussion of the results of the test (Passik et al., 2000).

Areas of Interest for Documentation

Clearly, strategies are needed to translate these recommendations for patient assessment during long-term opioid therapy to frontline practice. This effort would certainly benefit from the availability of a consistent method of documentation. As one potential framework, it is important to consider four main domains in assessing pain outcomes and to better protect your practice for those patients you maintain on an opioid regimen: (1) pain relief, (2) functional outcomes, (3) side effects, and (4) drug-related behaviors. These domains have been labeled the "four A's" (analgesia, activities of daily living, adverse effects, and aberrant drug-related behaviors) for teaching purposes (Passik & Weinreb, 2000). There are, of course, many different ways to think about these domains, and multiple attempts to capture them will be discussed below.

The PADT

The Pain Assessment and Documentation Tool (PADT), based on the four A's mentioned above, is a simple charting device that is intended to focus on key outcomes and provide a consistent way to document progress in pain management therapy over time. Twenty-seven clinicians completed the preliminary version of the PADT for 388 opioid-treated patients (Passik et al., 2004). Nineteen clinicians (17 physicians, 1 nurse, and 1 psychologist) participated in a debriefing phase. Twelve of the 19 clinicians had participated in the field trial before the debriefing. The debriefing interview for these clinicians used the same standard questions to evaluate both the original and revised PADT. Seven clinicians who participated in the development of the PADT, but not in the field trial, reviewed only the revised PADT.

The result of this work is a brief, two-sided chart note that can be readily included in the patient's medical record. It was designed to be intuitive, pragmatic, and adaptable to clinical situations. In the field trial, it took clinicians between 10 and 20 minutes to complete the tool. The revised PADT is substantially shorter and should require a few minutes to complete.

By addressing the need for documentation, the PADT can assist clinicians in meeting their obligations for ongoing assessment and documentation. Although the PADT is not intended to replace a progress note, it is well-suited to complement existing documentation with a focused evaluation of outcomes that are clinically relevant and address the need for evidence of appropriate monitoring at some regular interval (i.e. quarterly).

The decision to assess the four domains subsumed under the shorthand designation, the "four A's," was based on clinical experience, the positive comments received by the investigators during educational programs on opioid pharmacotherapy for nonmalignant pain, and an evolving national movement that recognizes the need to approach opioid therapy with a "balanced" response. This response recognizes both the legitimate need to provide optimal therapy to appropriate patients and the need to acknowledge the potential for abuse, diversion, and addiction (Passik & Weinreb, 2000). The value of assessing pain relief, side effects, and aspects of functioning has been emphasized repeatedly in the literature (Clark, 2002; Cleeland & Ryan, 1994; Daut et al., 1983; McCarburg & Barkin, 2001; Melzack, 1975). Documentation of drug-related behaviors is a relatively new concept that is being explored for the first time in the PADT.

Assessing LTOT Adverse Effects

Documentation of adverse effects in a majority of charts from many pain clinics tend to be addressed (or in many cases, not addressed) in their chart by a brief note of the presence or absence of one or more adverse effects (e.g., nausea, itching), noted by busy clinicians. Similar to the goal of the PADT, having a standardized form that is used at every visit and filled out by the patients before being seen by health-care providers may offer certain advantages.

Patients with persistent pain on oral opioid therapy have asked to "come off" the opioids because of adverse effects, even if they perceived that opioids were providing reasonable analgesic effects (Kalso et al., 2004). The distress that may be caused by opioid adverse effects may also be seen with acute postoperative pain patients, who may occasionally ask to stop their opioids despite that they are perceived as effective analgesics, because of the significant distress and suffering that they perceive they are experiencing from an opioid adverse effect.

It therefore appears crucial to assess opioid adverse effects, and optimally this should be done in a manner as to be able to follow trends as well as compare the patient's perceived intensity of the adverse effects versus the intensity of pain and/or other symptoms or adverse effects.

An alternative, short and simple, patient-administered quantitative tool that can be rapidly utilized clinically with the patient completing it in the waiting room is the Numerical Opioid Side Effect (NOSE) assessment tool (see Box 46.1; Smith, 2006a). The NOSE instrument is self-administered, can be completed by the patient in minutes, and can be entered into electronic databases or inserted into a hard-copy chart on each patient visit. The NOSE assessment tool is easy to administer, as well as easy to interpret, and may provide clinicians with important clinical information that could potentially impact various therapeutic decisions. Although most clinicians probably routinely assess adverse effects of treatments, it is sometimes difficult to find legible, clear, and concise

Box 46.1. Numerical Opioid Side Effect (NOSE) Assessment Tool

	Not Present										As Bad As You Can Imagine
	0	1	2	3	4	5	6	7	8	9	10
1. Nausea, vomiting, and/or lack of appetite	○	○	○	○	○	○	○	○	○	○	○
2. Fatigue, sleepiness, trouble concentrating, hallucinations, and/or drowsiness/somnolence	○	○	○	○	○	○	○	○	○	○	○
3. Constipation	○	○	○	○	○	○	○	○	○	○	○
4. Itching	○	○	○	○	○	○	○	○	○	○	○
5. Decreased sexual desire/function and/or diminished libido	○	○	○	○	○	○	○	○	○	○	○
6. Dry Mouth	○	○	○	○	○	○	○	○	○	○	○
7. Abdominal pain or discomfort/cramping or bloating	○	○	○	○	○	○	○	○	○	○	○
8. Sweating	○	○	○	○	○	○	○	○	○	○	○
9. Headache and/or dizziness	○	○	○	○	○	○	○	○	○	○	○
10. Urinary retention	○	○	○	○	○	○	○	○	○	○	○

documentation of such information in outpatient records. Furthermore, the documentation that does exist may not always attempt to "quantify" the intensity of treatment-related adverse effects or lend itself to looking at trends.

Assessing LTOT Efficacy

The Initiative on Methods, Measurements, and Pain Assessment in Clinical Trials (IMMPACT) recommended that six core outcome domains—(1) pain, (2) physical functions, (3) emotion, (4) participant rating of improvement and satisfaction with treatment, (5) symptoms and adverse events, and (6) participant disposition—should be considered when designing chronic pain clinical trials (Turk et al., 2003). The authors believe that the use of a unidimensional tool such as the numerical rating scale-11 (NRS-11) provides a suboptimal assessment of persistent noncancer pain as well as LTOT efficacy. Clinicians should attempt to assess multiple domains (preferably with multidimensional tools) in efforts to achieve a global picture of the patient's baseline status as well as the patient's response to LTOT in various domains.

It has been proposed that the use of a collection of various tools may provide adjunct information and help clinicians to create a more complete picture regarding longitudinal trends of overall progress/functioning for their patients with PNCP on LTOT (Smith, 2006b).

Assessing individual outcomes during outpatient multidisciplinary chronic pain treatment is often an extremely challenging task. There are many tools and instruments currently available, but the Treatment Outcomes in Pain Survey (TOPS) tool has been specifically designed to assess and follow outcomes in the chronic pain population (Rogers et al., 2000a, 2000b). TOPS has been described as an augmented SF-36 (Rogers et al., 2000a, 2000b). The Medical Outcomes Study (MOS) Short Form 36-item questionnaire (SF-36) compares the health status of large populations without a preponderance of one single medical condition (Ware & Sherbourne, 1992). The SF-36 assesses eight domains, but it has not been found to be especially useful for following the changes in function and pain in chronic pain populations.

The eight domains of the SF-36 are bodily pain (BP), general health (GH), mental health (MH), physical functioning (PF), role emotional (RE), social functioning (SF), role physical (RP), and vitality (VT). The TOPS scale initially had nine domains, but one (satisfaction with outcomes) was modified in subsequent versions. The nine domains of TOPS are pain symptom, family/social disability, functional limitations, total pain experience, objective work disability, life control, solicitous responses, passive coping, and satisfaction with outcomes. This enhanced SF-36 (TOPS scale) was constructed by obtaining patient data from the SF-36 with 12 additional role functioning questions. These additional questions were taken in part from the 61-item Multidimensional Pain Inventory (MPI; Kerns et al., 1985) and the 10-item Oswestry Disability Questionnaire (Fairbanks et al., 1980), with 4 additional pain-related questions that are similar to those found in the MOS pain-related questions that are similar to those found in the MOS pain-related questions (Tarlor et al., 1989), the Brief Pain Inventory (Daut et al., 1983), and a 6-item coping scale from the MOS (Tarlor et al., 1989). The question adapted from the Oswestry Disability Questionnaire (designed for back pain patients) includes questions that relate to impairment (pain), physical functioning (how long the patient can sit and/or stand) and disability (ability to travel or have sexual relations; Fairbanks et al., 1980).

Although the TOPS instrument is an extremely useful tool, it is time-consuming, is based entirely on the patient's subjective responses, and requires that the clinician has access, whether by a special computer program or by sending forms away, for scoring. As a result, it may not be an ideal instrument to use in every pain clinic and may not provide the clinician with an answer immediately about how the patient is doing relative to previous visits (although it may have that potential given adequate time, scanning equipment, and computer software.) The patient-generated index is an instrument that attempts to individualize a patient's perception of his or her quality of life (Ruta et al., 1994).

Translational Analgesia

A concept that may possess potential utility for clinicians is translational analgesia. Translational analgesia refers to improvements in physical, social, or emotional function that are realized by the patient as a result of improved analgesia, or essentially what the pain relief experienced by the patient "translates" into in terms of perceived improved quality of life (Smith, 2006c). In most cases, a sustained and significant improvement in pain perception that is deemed worthwhile to the patient should "translate" into improvement in quality of life or improved social, emotional, or physical function. Improvements in social, emotional, or physical domains are often spontaneously reported by patients, but in most cases should be able to be ascertained or elicited via "focused" interview techniques with the patient and/or significant others/family and/or "focused" physical exam. Improvements may be subtle and could include the following: going out more with friends, making more contact with family/friends, taking more frequent walks, doing more activities of daily living (laundry), or improved mood/relations with family members. It is important to note that this issue is certainly not exclusive to opioid therapy and is thought to apply to other treatments.

We do not deem it inappropriate or inhumane to taper relatively "high-dose" opioid therapy in a patient with PNCP who notes that his or her numerical rating scale-11 (NRS-11) "pain score" has dropped from 9/10 to 8/10 after escalating to over a gram of long-acting morphine preparation per day but in whom the patient as well as the patient's family/significant other cannot describe (and the clinician cannot elicit) any significant "translational analgesia." A patient with PNCP who remains a "hermit/couch potato" despite equivocal or minimally improved analgesia should not be considered as a therapeutic success.

Rome et al. (2004) has demonstrated that at least a subpopulation of patients seems to do better after tapering off opioids. Furthermore, more evidence regarding the hyperalgesic actions of opioids in certain circumstances is mounting (Holtman & Wala, 2005; Ruscheweyh & Sand Kuhler, 2005).

The periodic assessment of the patient with persistent noncancer pain should be performed in multiple domains (e.g., social domain, analgesia domain, functional domain, emotional domain). We believe the relatively common practice of evaluating patients with persistent noncancer pain by obtaining a NRS-11 pain score at each assessment and basing opioid analgesic treatment solely on this score to be suboptimal. Although multiple tools exist that assess multiple domains used in research, there is no widely accepted and used simple, convenient, and universally acceptable instrument that is utilized in busy clinical pain practices. The SAFE score is a multidomain assessment tool that may have potential utility for rapid, dynamic assessment in the busy clinic setting (Smith et al., 2003, 2005). The SAFE Score is a clinician-generated tool and may best be utilized in conjunction with the Translational Analgesic Score (TAS) as an adjunct.

Box 46.2. Translational Analgesic Score (TAS)

For each of the following questions, respond by comparing your current state over the past month to your baseline status before you started your current treatment regimen by circling a number from 0 to 10, with 0 being no improvement and 10 being maximal improvements:

1. Over the past month, my pain treatment has improved my ability to do usual daily activities—including household work, work, school, and/or social activities.
   0 1 2 3 4 5 6 7 8 9 10

2. Over the past month, my pain treatment has improved my ability to concentrate on work or daily activities.
   0 1 2 3 4 5 6 7 8 9 10

3. Over the past month, my pain treatment has improved the degree to which I feel too tired to do work (feeling that I could not get going and everything I do is an effort) or too tired to perform daily activities and/or socialize because of my pain.
   0 1 2 3 4 5 6 7 8 9 10

4. Over the past month, my pain treatment has improved the degree to which I feel distress, restless, agitated, or could go and lie down and/or be alone because of my pain.
   0 1 2 3 4 5 6 7 8 9 10

5. Over the past month, my pain treatment has improved my mood or feelings of being depressed, frustrated, anxious, irritable, tense, hopeless, annoyed, or just plain fed up because of my pain.
   0 1 2 3 4 5 6 7 8 9 10

6. Over the past month, my pain treatment has improved my ability to sleep.
   0 1 2 3 4 5 6 7 8 9 10

7. Over the past month, my pain treatment has improved my ability to walk, sit, and/or stand for long periods.
   0 1 2 3 4 5 6 7 8 9 10

8. Over the past month, my pain treatment has improved my ability to go up stairs, and/or move or lift objects.
   0 1 2 3 4 5 6 7 8 9 10

9. Over the past month, my pain treatment has improved the extent to which my pain interferes with optimal interpersonal relationships and/or intimacy.
   0 1 2 3 4 5 6 7 8 9 10

10. Over the past month I, my significant other, my family, coworkers, and/or friends noticed improvements in my socializing, recreational activities, physical functioning, concentration, mood, interpersonal relationships, activities of daily living, and/or overall quality of life.
    0 1 2 3 4 5 6 7 8 9 10

Please write below specific examples of things you can now do or currently do frequently that you couldn't do or only did rarely when your pain was not controlled as well as it is now.

_____

_____

TAS = _____

The TAS is expressed as a number between 0 and 10, with a decimal being the average of the responses to the 10 questions (or fewer—if the patient is paraplegic, then he or she would not answer the questions regarding going up stairs, etc.).

As an example, a patient's response to the TAS tool is shown below:

1. Over the past month, my pain treatment has improved my ability to do usual daily activities—including household work, work, school, and/or social activities.
   0 1 2 3 ④ 5 6 7 8 9 10

2. Over the past month, my pain treatment has improved my ability to concentrate on work or daily activities.
   0 1 2 ③ 4 5 6 7 8 9 10

3. Over the past month, my pain treatment has improved the degree to which I feel too tired to do work (feeling that I could not get going and everything I do is an effort) or too tired to perform daily activities and/or socialize because of my pain.
   0 1 2 ③ 4 5 6 7 8 9 10

4. Over the past month, my pain treatment has improved the degree to which I feel distress, restless, agitated, or could go and lie down and/or be alone because of my pain.
   0 1 ② 3 4 5 6 7 8 9 10

5. Over the past month, my pain treatment has improved my mood or feelings of being depressed, frustrated, anxious, irritable, tense, hopeless, annoyed, or just plain fed up because of my pain.
   0 1 2 3 ④ 5 6 7 8 9 10

6. Over the past month, my pain treatment has improved my ability to sleep.
   0 1 2 3 4 ⑤ 6 7 8 9 10

7. Over the past month, my pain treatment has improved my ability to walk, sit, and/or stand for long periods.
   0 1 ② 3 4 5 6 7 8 9 10

8. Over the past month, my pain treatment has improved my ability to go up stairs, and/or move or lift objects.
   1 2 3 4 5 6 7 8 9 10

9. Over the past month, my pain treatment has improved the extent to which my pain interferes with optimal interpersonal relationships and/or intimacy.
   0 ① 2 3 4 5 6 7 8 9 10

10. Over the past month, I, my significant other, my family, my coworkers, and/or my friends have noticed improvements in my socializing, recreational activities, physical functioning, concentration, mood, interpersonal relationships, activities of daily living, and/or overall quality of life.
    0 1 ② 3 4 5 6 7 8 9 10

TAS = 2.6

The Translational Analgesic Score (TAS)

The TAS is a patient-generated tool that attempts to quantify the degree of "translational analgesia" (see Box 46.2; Smith, 2005). It is simple, rapid, and user-friendly, and therefore can be utilized in a busy pain clinic. The patient can be handed the TAS sheet with questions to fill out at each visit while in the waiting room, and the responses are averaged for an overall score that is recorded in the chart. We encourage clinicians to have all patients write down specific examples of things that they can now do or do frequently that they couldn't do or did rarely when their pain was less controlled. Alternatively, the patient's responses can be entered directly or indirectly into a computerized record (with graphs of trends) if the pain clinic's medical records are electronic.

As shown in Box 46.2, the patient answered all 10 questions. Because the average is the sum of all responses (26) divided by 10, the TAS for this patient is 2.6.

A patient who at each visit consistently has a TAS of 10.0 clearly represents a therapeutic success in his or her current treatment.

On the other hand, a patient who at each visit consistently has a TAS of 0.0 would represent a suboptimal therapeutic result (by TAS criteria). We also encourage clinicians to document at least one or two specific examples of translational analgesia (e.g., perhaps various activities that the patient can now perform as a result of pain relief or can now perform frequently as a result of pain relief that the patient could not do or only do infrequently pretherapy) on the bottom or reverse side of the TAS score sheet.

Treatment decisions regarding escalation or tapering of opioids, changing agents, adding agents, and obtaining consultations, as well as instituting physical medicine or behavioral medicine techniques, remain the medical judgment of practitioners and should be based on a careful reevaluation of the patient and not based on a number.

The concept of translational analgesia is not meant to imply that opioids should be tapered, weaned, and/or discontinued. If a patient has a TAS that is very low and essentially unchanged over time (especially in conjunction with a SAFE score in the "red zone"), then this should prompt the clinician to reevaluate the patient and consider a change in therapy. This could mean pursuing various therapeutic options, including perhaps increasing the dose of opioids. However, if a patient has a high TAS and a SAFE score in the green zone, the patient should probably continue LTOT.

The SAFE Score

Another tool that has been advocated to help with this purpose is called the SAFE (social, analgesia, function, and emotional) score (Smith et al., 2003, 2005). Although it has not yet been rigorously validated, it is simple and practical and may possess clinical utility. It is a score generated by the health-care provider that is meant to reflect a multidimensional assessment of outcome to LTOT. It is not meant to replace more elaborate patient-based assessment tools but could possibly serve as an adjunct and possibly in the future shed some light on the difference between patients' perception of how they are doing on opioid treatment versus the physician-based view of outcome.

The SAFE tool is both practical in its ease and clinically useful (Box 46.3). The following are the goals of the SAFE tool:

- Demonstrate that the clinician has routinely evaluated the efficacy of the treatment from multiple perspectives.
- Guide the clinician toward a broader view of treatment options beyond adjusting the medication regimen.
- Document the clinician's rationale for continuation, modification, or cessation of LTOT.

Box 46.3. Sample SAFE Form

	Rating	Criterion				
Social Marital, family, friends, leisure, recreational		1 supportive harmonious socializing engaged	2	3	4	5 conflictual discord isolated bored
Analgesia Intensity, frequency, duration		1 comfortable effective controlled	2	3	4	5 intolerable ineffective uncontrolled
Function Work, activities of daily living, home management, school, training, physical activity		1 independent active productive energetic	2	3	4	5 dependent unmotivated passive deconditioned
Emotional Cognitive, stress, attitude, mood, behavior, neurovegetative signs		1 clear relaxed optimistic upbeat composed	2	3	4	5 confused tense pessimistic depressed distressed
Total Score						

The patient's status in each of the four domains is rated as follows: 1 = Excellent; 2 = Good; 3 = Fair; 4 = Borderline; 5 = Poor.

Table 46.1. Green Zone Cases Using the SAFE Scoring Tool

Example A		Example B	
Social	3	Social	2
Analgesia	2	Analgesia	4
Function	3	Function	3
Emotional	3	Emotional	1
Green Zone "SAFE" score	11	*Green Zone* "SAFE" score	10

Scoring System for the SAFE Tool

At each visit, the clinician rates the patient's functioning and pain relief in four domains: social (social functioning), analgesia (pain relief), function (physical functioning), and emotional (emotional functioning). The ratings in each of the four domains are then combined to yield a "SAFE" score, which can range from 4 to 20.

Interpretation of Scores

The *green zone* is a SAFE score of 4 to 12 and/or decrease of 2 points in total score from baseline. With a score in green zone, the patient is considered to be doing well and the plan would be to continue with the current medication regimen or consider reducing the total dose of the opioids.

The *yellow zone* is a SAFE score of 13 to 16 and/or a rating of 5 in any category and/or an increase of 2 or more from baseline in the total score. With a score in the yellow zone, the patient should be monitored closely and reassessed frequently.

The *red zone* is a SAFE score greater than or equal to 17. With a score in the red zone, a change in the treatment would be warranted.

Treatment options depend on the pattern of scores. If attempts are made to address problems in specific domains and the patient is still not showing an improvement in the SAFE score, then the patient may not be an appropriate candidate for long-term opioid therapy.

Table 46.1 illustrates green zone cases. In example A, there is good analgesic response to opioids, with a fair response in the other domains. No change in treatment would be necessary unless adverse reactions to the medications require an adjustment or discontinuation. In example B, there is borderline analgesic response, but good social and emotional responses and a fair physical functioning response. Some pain specialists may determine that the medication regimen should be optimized. For others, this pattern of ratings may reflect a reasonable improvement in quality of life for the patient. Therefore, continuing the present medication regimen would be a reasonable option.

Table 46.2 illustrates how the SAFE tool can be used to track changes in the status of the same patient on two consecutive visits. In the change in scores from example C to example D, although analgesia deteriorates from fair to borderline, there is significant improvement in the other domains. The clinician may feel this is

Table 46.2. Tracking a Change in Status Using the SAFE Scoring Tool

Example C		Example D	
Social	5	Social	3
Analgesia	3	Analgesia	4
Function	5	Function	3
Emotional	5	Emotional	3
Red Zone "SAFE" score	18	*Green Zone* "SAFE" score	13

Table 46.3. Tracking a Change in Status Using the SAFE Scoring Tool

Example E		Example F	
Social	3	Social	3
Analgesia	2	Analgesia	2
Function	3	Function	4
Emotional	3	Emotional	4
Green Zone "SAFE" score	11	*Yellow Zone* "SAFE" score	13

satisfactory for this particular patient and continue with the current medication regimen. Once again, too narrow a focus on analgesic response may lead to unnecessary dose escalation. This case also illustrates the situation in which even though the total score at visit D is greater than 12 and would be a *yellow zone*, it is assigned as a *green zone* because there was a decrease of more than 2 in the total score. Alternately, the clinician may determine that a borderline analgesic response is not optimal. The choices for intervention may include rotating to another opioid agent, increasing the current opioid dose, adding adjuvant medications, referring for non-pharmacological treatment, or discontinuing high-dose opioids.

Table 46.3 again illustrates again a single patient on two consecutive visits. Here, analgesia has remained good over time, but there has been a negative impact on the domains of function and emotion. Pain specialists who are focused on the pain scores of such a patient may be comfortable with continuing the established treatment plan. However, using SAFE, an expanded view of the patient's overall status will alert the clinician to monitor the patient's physical and emotional functioning in future visits. If the ratings in the psychological and physical domains persist, then the clinician may recommend that the patient pursue psychosocial treatment or physical rehabilitation in addition to maintaining the medication regimen.

Conclusion

Assessment and documentation are cornerstones for both protecting your practice and obtaining optimal outcomes for patients on opioid therapy. There are a growing number of assessment tools for clinicians to guide the evaluation of a group of important outcomes during opioid therapy and provide a simple means of documenting patient care. They all have the capability to prove helpful in clinical management and offer mechanisms for documenting the types of practice standards that those in the regulatory and law enforcement communities seek to ensure.

References

Clark JD. Chronic pain prevalence and analgesic prescribing in a general medical population. *J Pain Symptom Manage.* 2002;23:131–137.

Cleeland CS, Ryan KM. Pain assessment: global use of the Brief Pain Inventory. *Ann Acad Med Singapore.* 1994;23:129–138.

Collett BJ. Opioid tolerance: the clinical perspective. *Br J Anaesth.* 1998; 81:58–68.

Daut R, Cleeland C, Flannery R. Development of the Wisconsin Brief Pain Questionnaire to assess pain in cancer and other diseases. *Pain.* 1983;17: 197–210.

Fairbanks J, Couper J, Davies J et al. The Oswestry Low Back pain Disability Questionnaire. *Physiotherapy.* 1980;66:271–3.

Holtman JR, Wala EP. Characterization of morphine-induced hyperalgesia in male and female rats. *Pain.* 2005;114:62–70.

Joint Commission on the Accreditation of Healthcare Organizations (JCAHO). *Patient Rights and Organization Ethics.* Referenced from the

Comprehensive Accreditation Manual for Hospitals, Update 3, 1999. http://www.jointcommission.org/ Accessed 7/13/2007.

Kalso, E, Edwards JE, Moore, RA, et al. Opioids in chronic non-cancer pain: systematic review of efficacy and safety. *Pain.* 2004;112:372–80.

Katz N. The impact of pain management on quality of life. *J Pain Symptom Manage.* 2002;24(suppl 1):S38–S47.

Kerns R, Turk D, Rudy T. The West Haven-Yale Multidimensional Pain Inventory (WHYMPI). *Pain.* 1985;23:345–6.

Max MB, Payne R, Edwards WT, et al. *Principles of Analgesic Use in the Treatment of Acute Pain and Cancer Pain* (4th ed.). Glenview, IL: American Pain Society; 1999.

McCarberg BH, Barkin RL. Long-acting opioids for chronic pain: pharmacotherapeutic opportunities to enhance compliance, quality of life, and analgesia. *Am J Ther.* 2001;8:181–186.

Melzack R. The McGill Pain Questionnaire: major properties and scoring methods. *Pain.* 1975;1:277–299.

Passik SD, Kirsh KL, Whitcomb L, Schein JR, Kaplan MA, Dodd SL, Kleinman L, Katz NP, Portenoy RK. Monitoring outcomes during long-term opioid therapy for noncancer pain: results with the Pain Assessment and Documentation Tool. *Journal Opioid Management,* 2005;1(5):257–266.

Passik SD, Kirsh KL, Whitcomb LA, Portenoy RK, Katz N, Kleinman L, Dodd S, Schein J. A new tool to assess and document pain outcomes in chronic pain patients receiving opioid therapy. *Clinical Therapeutics,* 2004;26(4):552–561.

Passik SD, Schreiber J, Kirsh KL, Portenoy RK. A chart review of the ordering and documentation of urine toxicology screens in a cancer center: do they influence patient management? *J Pain Symptom Manage.* 2000;19:40–44.

Passik SD, Weinreb HJ. Managing chronic nonmalignant pain: overcoming obstacles to the use of opioids. *Adv Ther.* 2000;17:70–83.

Portenoy RK. Opioid therapy for chronic nonmalignant pain: a review of critical issues. *J Pain Symptom Manage.* 1996a;11:203–217.

Portenoy RK. Opioid therapy for chronic nonmalignant pain. *Pain Res Manage.* 1996b;1:17–28.

Rhodes DJ, Koshy RC, Waterfield WC, Wu AW, Grossman SA. Feasibility of quantitative pain assessment in outpatient oncology practice. *J Clin Oncol.* 2001;19:501–508.

Rogers WH, Wittink H, Wagner A, et al. Assessing individual outcomes during outpatient multidisciplinary chronic pain treatment by means of an augmented SF-36. *Pain Med.* 2000a;1:44–54.

Rogers WH, Wittink H, Ashburn MA, et al. Using the "TOPS," an outcome instrument for multidisciplinary outpatient pain treatment. *Pain Medicine.* 2000b;1:55–67.

Rome JD, Townsend CP, Bruce BK, et al. Chronic noncancer pain rehabilitation with opioid withdrawal: comparison of treatment outcomes based on opioid use status at admission. *Mayo Clin Proc.* 2004;79:759–68.

Ruscheweyh R, Sand Kuhler J. Opioids and central sensitization: II. Induction and reversal of hyperalgesia. *Eur J Pain.* 2005;9:149–52.

Ruta DA, Garratt AM, Leng M, et al. A new approach to quality of life: the patient-generated index. *Medical Care.* 1994;32:1109–26.

Smith HS. The Numerical Opioid Side Effect (NOSE) assessment tool. *Journal of Cancer Pain and Symptom Palliation.* 2006a;1:

Smith HS. Translational analgesic and the translational analgesic score. *Journal of Cancer Pain and Symptom Palliation.* 2006b;1:

Smith HS. Perspectives in persistent noncancer pain. *Journal of Cancer Pain and Symptom Palliation.* 2006c;1:

Smith H, Audette J, Witkower A. Assessing analgesic therapeutic outcomes. In: Smith H. (ed.), *Drugs for Pain.* Philadelphia, PA: Hanley and Belfus; 2003.

Smith HS, Audette J, Witkower A. Playing It "SAFE." *Journal of Cancer Pain and Symptom Palliation.* 2005;1:3–10.

Solomon DH, Schaffer JL, Katz JN, et al. Can history and physical examination be used as markers of quality? An analysis of the initial visit note in musculoskeletal care. *Med Care.* 2000;38:383–391.

Tarlor A, Ware J Jr., Greenfield S., et al. The Medical Outcomes Study: an application of methods for monitoring the results of medical care. *JAMA* 1989;262:925–930.

Turk DC, Dworkin RH, Allen RR, et al. Core outcome domains for chronic pain clinical trials: IMMPACT recommendations. *Pain.* 2003;106:337–45.

Urban BJ, France RD, Steinberger EK, Scott DL, Maltbie AA. Long-term use of narcotic/antidepressant medication in the management of phantom limb pain. *Pain.* 1986;24:191–196.

Ware JE Jr., Sherbourne CD. The MOS 36-item short-form health survey (SF-36). I. Conceptual framework and item selection. *Med. Care (Phila).* 1992;30:473–83.

Wincent A, Linden Y, Arner S. Pain questionnaires in the analysis of long lasting (chronic) pain conditions. *Eur J. Pain.* 2003;7:311–21.

Zenz M, Strumpf M, Tryba M. Long-term oral opioid therapy in patients with chronic nonmalignant pain. *J Pain Symptom Manage.* 1992;7:69–77.

Part VI
Aberrant Drug-Taking Considerations

47

Screening for the Risk of Substance Abuse in Pain Management

Lynn R. Webster

Opioids are a safe, effective treatment for many chronic pain conditions. However, a certain segment of the pain population will end up abusing opioids in defiance of medical direction. Whether due to addiction, uncontrolled pain, a comorbid psychiatric condition, or some other cause, opioid misuse poses a threat to the intended benefits of pain relief and improved function.

Although misuse of medication is, unfortunately, a common clinical occurrence, it is manageable in most cases. The vital first step is the appropriate assessment of the patient prior to the start of opioid therapy. By gaining insight into the patient's individual risk for abuse, the clinician is able to set and maintain the corresponding level of monitoring, thus optimizing chances for a good clinical outcome.

All clinicians who treat pain with opioids should assess patients for potential abuse or addiction, yet this step is often skipped. In one study, health-care practitioners missed more than 80% of substance use disorders (SUD) for lack of a 5-minute assessment (Brown, Hermann, Jones, & Wu, 2004). Research has uncovered a number of reasons physicians shy away from assessing a patient's potential for problematic drug behavior, including the following:

- Lack of confidence in their own addiction-management capabilities
- Perception of time limitations
- Pessimism regarding effectiveness of treatment
- Fears that a patient may be sensitive about substance abuse issues (Friedmann, McCullough, & Saitz, 2001)

These concerns are understandable but surmountable given the proper tools and training. To begin with, clinicians should find it helpful to acquaint themselves with the various factors linked most closely to the risk of abuse.

Risk Factors for Abuse

One frequent myth holds that every patient is equally likely to abuse the opioids prescribed for chronic pain. Opioid prescribing is presumed to be a gamble in which patients may win a better life or lose their well-being to the disease of addiction at the toss of the dice. The evidence refutes this scenario.

In fact, certain patient risk factors are well linked in the scientific literature to an increased likelihood of opioid abuse. Knowing in advance whether a patient possesses these risk factors can give a clinician the edge in monitoring the progress of treatment. Classification categories vary, but patients typically fall into three groups: high, moderate, and low risk. The higher the degree of risk, the more stringent the monitoring measures called for. The purpose of dividing patients into risk categories is never to deny high-risk patients the pain treatment they need but to set the correct level of monitoring and help prevent abuse.

Some of the risk factors for opioid abuse, gleaned from the scientific literature and clinical practice, include the following:

- Personal history of substance abuse (Webster & Webster, 2005)
- Family history of substance abuse (Webster & Webster, 2005)
- Age (young; Webster & Webster, 2005)
- History of preadolescent sexual abuse (Webster & Webster, 2005)
- Mental disease (Webster & Webster, 2005)
- Social patterns of drug use (Savage, 2002)
- Psychological stress (Savage, 2002)
- Lack of a 12-step program (Dunbar & Katz, 1996)
- Polysubstance abuse (Dunbar & Katz, 1996)
- Poor social support (Dunbar & Katz, 1996)
- Cigarette dependency (Friedman, Li, & Mehrotra, 2003)
- History of repeated drug/alcohol rehabilitation (Friedman, Li, & Mehrotra, 2003)
- Focus on opioids (Atluri & Sudarshan, 2002)
- Nonfunctional status due to pain (Atluri & Sudarshan, 2002)
- Exaggeration of pain (Atluri & Sudarshan, 2002)
- Unclear etiology for pain (Atluri & Sudarshan 2002)

No consensus yet exists among clinicians and researchers as to which risk factors are most predictive of abuse, but a preponderance of evidence supports certain factors—such as a personal history of substance abuse—as strong indicators.

Technical writing and manuscript review was provided by Beth Dove of Lifetree Clinical Research and Pain Clinic.

Research aimed at addressing the assessment needs of the opioid-prescribed pain population is "in its infancy" (Robinson et al., 2001, p. 220). The fact is, the available tools to screen for prescription opioid abuse do not yet meet the medical needs. Yet a number of already available screening tools offer some clinical utility, though it is important to be aware of their inadequacies as applied to chronic pain patients.

Limitations of Familiar Screening Tools

Of the currently available tools to screen patients for substance abuse, many share some common problems:

- They are designed to identify patients who already have problems managing substance intake, not to predict who may develop problems.
- They are not designed to screen specifically for opioid abuse.
- They often take a long time to administer and require unique skills to interpret.

Diagnostic Versus Screening Tools

Most screening tools are not designed to diagnose SUDs. If patients demonstrate positive scores on abuse screening tools, they are considered candidates for an additional step to diagnose whether an actual SUD is present. Many of the instruments that are somewhat cumbersome to administer and score are diagnostic tools, not intended for initial screening.

One of these is the Structured Clinical Interview (SCID; Kranzler, Kadden, Babor, Tennen, & Rounsaville, 1996), a thorough assessment widely used by research centers and substance abuse treatment centers, in which staff is specially trained to administer and score it. Another tool that is especially effective for evaluating the need for substance abuse treatment is the Addiction Severity Index (ASI; McLellan, Kushner, Metzger, et al., 1992), a 200-item, hour-long assessment of seven potential problem areas designed to be administered by a trained interviewer. These two assessments are valuable for evaluating many psychiatric, social, and substance problems, but their lengthiness and the special training required to administer them render them impractical for widespread clinical use.

In contrast, brief screening tools are less cumbersome but are usually designed to identify patients who already have problems with substances, not to predict who may develop problems, and are not designed to screen specifically for opioid abuse. Two examples are the widely used, alcohol-specific CAGE (from the key phrases "cut down," "annoyed," "guilty," "eye-opener"; Ewing, 1984) and another tool called TICS (from Two-Item Conjoint Screening tool; Brown, Leonard, Saunders, & Papasouliotis, 2001), a 2-question measure of sensitivity to substance abuse.

Assessment Tool Criteria

Research is beginning to address these concerns. Efforts are underway to design assessments derived from the scientific literature or expert opinions that address the specific needs of opioid-treated pain patients and that are useful in a busy practice. The desired criteria include the following:

- *Predictive:* Assessments that detect current substance abuse are helpful but do not provide for the establishment of a suitable level of monitoring prior to beginning opioid therapy.
- *Brief:* Time limitations on office visits dictate the need for a brief assessment. Longer assessments are impractical for many clinicians and may lead to the assessment process being skipped altogether.
- *Easy to administer and interpret:* The need for special training to score and interpret results does not the meet the requirement for widespread clinical utility.
- *Geared to opioid abuse rather than alcohol or other substances:* Screening all patients for general substance abuse is an advisable part of medical practice. However, patients who are being considered as candidates for long-term opioid therapy present a more specific assessment need given a high opiate-specific, genetic component linked in the scientific literature to opiate abuse (Tsuang et al., 1998).
- *Validated in patients with pain:* The need is for an assessment that is validated for use in chronic pain patients being considered for long-term opioid therapy.
- *Applicable to a variety of clinical settings:* Little is known about the differences between chronic pain patients treated in primary care and chronic pain patients treated in pain clinics. But because patients in pain are treated in a variety of settings, the best type of assessment would apply in a variety of patient pain populations.
- *Self-administered:* A self-administered tool preserves time and clinical resources making it more likely to be used.

Most of the available assessments contain some but not all of these attributes. Each tool has unique advantages and disadvantages.

Features of Available Tools

Some of the available substance abuse screening tools, old and new, are listed in Table 47.1. The table is assembled to determine at a glance whether specific assessments have the following qualities:

- Specific to alcohol, nonalcohol drugs or both
- Predictive of subsequent abuse problems
- Validated in the population of interest, in this case pain patients
- Self-administered
- Brief

Some of the first instruments developed were originally designed to address alcohol abuse and are still widely used. In some cases, these instruments can be modified to assess for opioid abuse. Though useful, clinical tests to determine their efficacy in opioid-treated pain patients are usually lacking. They could, however, have some clinical utility in the field of chronic pain as individuals addicted to alcohol are at increased risk for abusing another substance. One study showed that a majority of individuals admitted for alcohol treatment also abused one or more additional substances in the 3 months leading up to their admission for alcohol treatment (Staines, Magura, Foote, Deluca, & Kosanke, 2001).

Alcohol-Specific Tools

The following assessment tools have been designed to assess for alcohol abuse but are also sometimes used to assess for opioid abuse:

- *CAGE (Ewing, 1984):* A 4-item, verbal test validated in several studies as an effective screen for lifetime alcohol disorders.

Table 47.1. Assessment Characteristics

Tool	Alcohol/ Drugs	Predictive	Pain Patients	Administered	Length
Addiction Severity Index (ASI)	Yes/Yes	No	No	Self/Interview	200 items, 1 hour
Alcohol Use Disorders Identification Test (AUDIT)	Yes/No	No	No	Self/Interview	10 items, 2 minutes
Structured Clinical Interview for *DSM-IV* (SCID; Psychoactive Substance Use Module Only)	Yes/Yes	Yes	No	Interview	30–60 minutes
CAGE (from "cut down, annoyed, guilty, eye-opener")	Yes/No	No	No	Interview	4 items, <1 minute
CAGE-AID	Yes/Yes	No	No	Interview	4 items, <1 minute
TICS (Two-Item Conjoint Screening Tool)	Yes/Yes	No	No	Interview	2 items, <1 minute
Screener and Opioid Assessment for Patients with Pain (SOAPP)	Yes/Yes	Testing ongoing	Yes	Self/Interview	24 items, 10 minutes
Prescription Drug Use Questionnaire (PDUQ)	Yes/Yes	Yes	Yes	Interview	42 items, 20 minutes
RAFFT (from "relax, alone, friends, family, trouble")	Yes/Yes	No	No	Self	5 items, approx. 1 minute
Drug Abuse Screening Test (DAST)	No/Yes	No	No	Self	20 items, 5 minutes
Michigan Alcohol Screening Test (MAST)	Yes/No	No	No	Self/Interview	Long version: 25 items, 15 minutes; Short versions: 9 to 13 items
Screening Instrument for Substance Abuse Potential (SISAP)	Yes/Yes	Yes	No	Interview	5 items
Substance Abuse Subtle Screening Inventory-3 (SASSI-3)	Yes/Yes	No	No	Self	1 page, 15 minutes
Severity of Opiate Dependence Questionnaire (SODQ)	No/Yes	No	No	Self	21 items, approx. 5 minutes
Opioid Risk Tool (ORT)	Yes/Yes	Yes	Yes	Self	5 items, 1 minute

Two affirmative answers are considered a positive screen, although many clinicians consider even one affirmative reply cause for concern.[1] The CAGE was later adapted to include other drug abuse as well as alcohol.

- *Michigan Alcoholism Screening Test (MAST; Storgaard, Nielsen, & Gluud, 1994):* Long and short versions are available. The long version has 25 items, whereas shorter versions contain 10 to 13 items. This is one of the first alcohol screening tests and one of the most widely used. It is particularly useful for assessing lifetime alcohol-related problems. An evaluation is underway to add a screening component for other drugs to the MAST. Its accuracy rates are similar to those of the CAGE, though it takes much longer to administer. A still longer 37-item test called the Self-Administered Alcoholism Screening Test (SAAST; Davis, Hurt, Morse, & O'Brien, 1987) has been derived from the MAST.
- *Alcohol Use Disorders Identification Test (AUDIT; Saunders, Aasland, Babor, de la Fuente, & Grant, 1993):* This is a 10-item written test available through the World Health Organization to identify harmful alcohol consumption in numerous populations, including primary care, psychiatric units and prison populations. Training requirements to administer it make it less popular with clinicians than quick, verbal assessments like the CAGE.

Conjoint Screening Tools

Building on the field of alcohol screening, several instruments have been created or adapted to screen simultaneously for alcohol and other drug abuse. The advantages of a conjoint screening tool are to save time and to encourage a patient to answer more honestly than when answering separate questions. However, a person who abuses alcohol only may answer negatively, wishing to avoid the appearance of illicit or prescription drug use.

Two of the briefer tools that fall into this category are the CAGE-AID (Box 47.1; Brown & Rounds, 1995) and the TICS (Box 47.2). The suffix of the CAGE-AID stands for "adapted to include drugs," and its sensitivity and specificity (shown in the corresponding table) is still high, though the specificity is less than the alcohol-specific CAGE.

The TICS claims to identify 80% of drug and alcohol problems in young and middle-age patients by asking two easily remembered questions. Advantages include being brief and easy to remember and administer. However, these two tools are not opioid specific and are designed to detect current and lifetime substance abuse, not to assess the risk of future abuse.

Box 47.1 The CAGE-AID Questionnaire

In the past have you ever:
1. Tried to cut down or change your pattern of drinking or drug use?
2. Been annoyed or angry by others' concern about your drinking or drug use?
3. Felt guilty about the consequences of your drinking or drug use?
4. Had a drink or used a drug in the morning (eye-opener) to decrease hangover or withdrawal symptoms?

Implications for prescribing:
- One positive response to any question suggests caution.
- Two or more positive responses may have a sensitivity of 60%–95% and specificity of 40%–95% for diagnosing alcohol or drug problems and strongly suggest assessment by an addiction specialist before opioids are prescribed.
- CAGE screen may have less predictive value in the elderly, college students, women, and certain ethnic groups.

Adapted from the CAGE alcohol-screening tool to include drugs.

---

[1] Some practitioners recommend adapting CAGE and other assessment questions to be open-ended rather than inviting a yes/no response. Example: "How often have you..." and so on.

Box 47.2 TICS: A Two-Item Conjoint Screen

1. In the last year, have you ever drunk or used drugs more than you meant to?
2. Have you felt you wanted or needed to cut down on your drinking or drug use in the last year?

In primary care patients, at least one affirmative answer to these two questions yielded nearly 80% sensitivity and specificity.

Drug Abuse Tools

Modeled on the MAST, the self-administered Drug Abuse Screening Test (DAST; Box 47.3; Gavin, Ross, & Skinner, 1989) contains many items to identify problems caused by drug abuse other than alcohol. Some of the problems it assesses include drug-related blackouts, employment difficulties and social and family discord. It also contains an item to screen for prescription drug abuse. The DAST is fairly brief and can be administered without special training. It is valuable for determining which patients should seek substance-abuse treatment but has not been validated for pain patients. Like the MAST, it has been suggested that the DAST's focus on problems with employment, violence, and illegal activities and its lack of questions about home and children make it more applicable to men than women.

Box 47.3 The Drug Abuse Screening Test (DAST)

The following questions concern information about your involvement and abuse of drugs. Drug abuse refers to

1. the use of prescribed or "over-the-counter" drugs in excess of the directions
2. any nonmedical use of drugs

The questions DO NOT include alcoholic beverages. The DAST does not include alcohol use.

The questions refer to the past 12 months. Carefully read each statement and decide whether your answer is yes or no. Please give the best answer or the answer that is right most of the time. Click on the box for Yes or No.

1. Have you used drugs other than those required for medical reasons? Yes / No
2. Have you abused prescription drugs? Yes / No
3. Do you abuse more than one drug at a time? Yes / No
4. Can you get through the week without using drugs? Yes / No
5. Are you always able to stop using drugs when you want to? Yes / No
6. Have you had "blackouts" or "flashbacks" as a result of drug use? Yes / No
7. Do you ever feel bad or guilty about your drug use? Yes / No
8. Does your spouse (or parents) ever complain about your involvement with drugs? Yes / No
9. Has drug abuse created problems between you and your spouse or your parents? Yes / No
10. Have you lost friends because of your use of drugs? Yes / No
11. Have you neglected your family because of your use of drugs? Yes / No
12. Have you been in trouble at work because of your use of drugs? Yes / No
13. Have you lost a job because of drug abuse? Yes / No
14. Have you gotten into fights when under the influence of drugs? Yes / No
15. Have you engaged in illegal activities in order to obtain drugs? Yes / No
16. Have you been arrested for possession of illegal drugs? Yes / No
17. Have you ever experienced withdrawal symptoms (felt sick) when you stopped taking drugs? Yes / No
18. Have you had medical problems as a result of your drug use (e.g., memory loss, hepatitis, convulsions, bleeding, etc.)? Yes / No
19. Have you gone to anyone for help for a drug problem? Yes / No
20. Have you been involved in a treatment program especially related to drug use? Yes / No

The RAFFT (Bastiaens, Riccardi, & Sakhrani, 2002) is a 5-question screening tool for alcohol and drug abuse that has performed well in adolescents. It is brief and easy to score. However, in a study of adult psychiatric patients, it was reported to be less specific than in adolescents.

The Substance Abuse Subtle Screening Inventory (SASSI; Lazowski, Miller, Boye, & Miller, 1998) is a widely used instrument made available through the SASSI Institute located in Bloomington, IN. The one-page questionnaire combines face-valid questions with subtle items that do not address substance abuse directly. The intent is to circumvent a presumed reluctance on the part of subjects to speak frankly about substance abuse. The SASSI's main utility is to plan for treatment in a variety of criminal justice, mental health, vocational, educational, and other settings. The revised SASSI-3 demonstrated a 95% agreement with diagnoses of substance dependence in a range of clinical settings. The SASSI is also available in a format geared to adolescents.

The Severity of Opiate Dependence Questionnaire (SODQ; Sutherland, Edwards, Taylor, Phillips, Gossop, & Brady, 1986), validated in English and Australian heroin users, is intended as a measure of opiate dependence, not as an initial screen for opioid-treated pain patients. The multiple-choice questions encompass five sections addressing patterns of use, degree of withdrawal symptoms, and other signs of physical and psychological dependence. The SODQ helps measure signs of addiction, including whether there is an increased focus on obtaining the substance, an awareness of one's own compulsion, and an inability to stop even after a period of abstinence. Its specificity to opiates is an advantage, though it may not address disparities between users of illegal street drugs and prescription drug abusers. No cutoff score has been established, leaving it to clinical judgment whether or not an individual suffers from opiate dependence based on test answers.

A New Generation of Opioid-Specific Tools

One thing should be clear from the preceding brief overview of the most widely available tools: Though clinically useful, the available tools are not yet tailored to the specific needs of opioid-treated pain patients. That is beginning to change. A number of new tools to screen and assess for the risk of prescription drug abuse have debuted recently. They include items related to mental disorders, past sexual abuse, and lifestyle factors that are aimed at helping clinicians isolate the reasons for medication misuse found in pain populations. These newer tools are demonstrating validity in limited clinical trials, though more research is needed to demonstrate their applicability to broader patient populations.

The Prescription Drug Use Questionnaire (PDUQ)

The new generation of opioid-specific instruments includes the 42-item Prescription Drug Use Questionnaire (PDUQ; Compton, Darakjian, & Miotto, 1998) (Box 47.4). This 42-item interview collects a wealth of data detailing the patient's pain condition, opioid use, social and family factors, and psychiatric history. In a pilot study, scores were recorded from 6 to 15 for nonaddicted subjects, from 11 to 25 for substance-abusing subjects and from 15 to 28 for substance-dependent subjects. All subjects scoring above 15 later satisfied the criteria for SUD; therefore, the questionnaire appears to have some predictive validity. A drawback is that at 42 questions, the PDUQ takes longer to administer than is practical in many clinical situations.

Box 47.4 The Prescription Drug Use Questionnaire (PDUQ)

Evaluation of the Pain Condition

1. Does the patient have more than one painful condition (i.e., chronic back pain complicated by acute migraines or frequent dental work)?
2. Is the patient disabled by pain (i.e., unable to complete social or vocational activities of daily living)?
3. Is the patient receiving disability (i.e., SSI, worker's comp.)?
4. Is the patient involved in litigation around the pain-precipitating incident?
5. Has the patient explored and/or tried nonopioid or nonpharmacological pain management techniques (i.e., physical therapy, TENS unit, relaxation, biofeedback) to manage pain?
6. Does the patient believe that his/her pain has been adequately treated over the past 6 months?
7. Does the patient express anger/mistrust of past health-care providers?
8. Does the patient believe that he/she is addicted to opioid analgesics?
9. Does the referring physician believe that the patient is addicted to opioid analgesics?

Opioid Use Patterns

9a. How long has the patient been on continuous opioids?
10. Does the patient have more than one prescription provider (including dentists, ER physicians)?
11. Is there a pattern of the patient increasing prescribed analgesic does or frequency?
12. Is there a pattern of the patient calling in for early prescription refills?
13. Does the patient report using analgesics for symptoms other than those prescribed for (i.e., insomnia, anxiety, depression)?
14. Does the patient save/hoard unused medication or have partially unused bottles of medication at home?
15. Does the patient report supplementing analgesics with alcohol or other psychoactive drugs (i.e., Soma, benzodiazepines)?
15a. if yes, please list:
16. Has the patient ever forged a prescription?
17. Is there a pattern of the patient reporting losing his/her medication?
18. Does the patient have preferences for specific analgesics and/or routes of administration (i.e., IV, IM routes over oral)?
19. Is there a pattern of the patient making emergency room visits for analgesics?
20. Has the patient ever obtained analgesic from nonmedical (street) sources?
21. Has any M.D./D.D.S. limited care, expressed concern, or refused to prescribe opioid analgesics because of patient's opioid use patterns?

Social/Family Factors

22. Have family members expressed concern that the patient is addicted?
23. Are family members concerned about opioid analgesic side effects or tolerance?
24. Is there a pattern of family interaction that sustains the patient's opioid analgesic use (i.e., family member overly concerned re: pain or withdrawal)?
25. Is there a pattern of family interaction that sustains the patient's illness behavior or pain symptoms (i.e., family member assuming caretaker role)?
26. Does the spouse/significant other have a history of alcoholism/drug abuse/drug misuse?
27. Has a family member or friend ever obtained analgesic for the patient?
28. Has the patient ever taken analgesics prescribed for a friend or family member?
29. Does a family member or friend have access (either legal or illegal) to opioid analgesics (i.e., a family member in the medical profession)?

Family History

30. Is there a positive history of addiction (to any drug including alcohol) in the patient's mother, father, sibling, or blood relative?
31. Is there a positive family history of chronic pain in the patient's mother, father, sibling, or blood relative?

Patient History of Substance Abuse

32. Did intoxication play a role in pain-precipitating incident?
33. Has the patient ever been diagnosed with addiction to any drug or alcohol?
34. Does the patient have a drug or alcohol treatment history?
35. Has opioid analgesic detoxification been previously attempted?

Psychiatric History

36. Has the patient ever been diagnosed with a psychiatric disorder?
37. Did psychiatric symptoms precede onset of pain?
38. Is there a large psychological component to the pain condition, other than those related to addiction (i.e., multiple psychological stressors)?
39. Is there evidence of a somatoform disorder?
40. Does the patient report a history of sexual or physical abuse?
41. Does the patient currently meet *DSM-IV* criteria for any Axis I, II, or III conditions?
41a. if so, please list diagnoses:
42. Please list all pain-producing medical conditions:

The Opioid Risk Tool (ORT)

Two briefer assessments that also have been validated in initial clinical tests are the author's Opioid Risk Tool (ORT; see Table 47.2; Webster & Webster, 2005) and the 24-item Screener and Opioid Assessment for Patients with Pain (SOAPP; Butler, Budman, Fernandez, & Jamison, 2004).

The ORT is a 5-question, self-administered assessment that takes less than 5 minutes to complete. In initial trials, the ORT accurately predicted which patients were at highest and lowest risk for displaying aberrant, drug-related behaviors associated with abuse or addiction. Examples of these behaviors include using more opioids than prescribed, selling prescriptions, losing prescriptions or reporting them stolen, canceling clinic visits, and forging prescriptions.

Designed for a patient's initial visit, the ORT assesses for personal and family history of prescription, alcohol, and illegal drug abuse, age, history of preadolescent sexual abuse and the presence of depression, attention deficit disorder (ADD), obsessive-compulsive disorder (OCD), bipolar disorder, and schizophrenia. A review of the scientific literature showed these risk factors to be predictive of the later development of an SUD.

In the study, 185 new patients being treated with opioids for chronic pain took the ORT on their initial visits. Based on their scores, they were grouped into categories of high, moderate or low risk and then monitored for 12 months. Of the low-risk patients, 17 out of 18 (94.4%) did not display an aberrant behavior. Of the high-risk patients, 40 out of 44 (90.9%) did display an aberrant behavior.

Table 47.2. The Opioid Risk Tool (ORT)

Item	Mark each box that applies	Item score if female	Item score if male
1. Family History of Substance Abuse			
Alcohol	[ ]	1	3
Illegal drugs	[ ]	2	3
Prescription drugs	[ ]	4	4
2. Personal History of Substance Abuse			
Alcohol	[ ]	3	3
Illegal drugs	[ ]	4	4
Prescription drugs	[ ]	5	5
3. Age			
(mark box if 16–45)	[ ]	1	1
4. History of Preadolescent Sexual Abuse			
	[ ]	3	0
5. Psychological Disease			
Attention deficit disorder, obsessive-compulsive disorder, bipolar, schizophrenia	[ ]	2	2
Depression	[ ]	1	1
Total			

Total risk category: low risk: 0 to 3; moderate risk: 4 to 7; high risk: 8 and above.

The Screener and Opioid Assessment for Patients With Pain (SOAPP)

The SOAPP is a 24-item, self-assessment questionnaire that takes about 10 minutes to complete. It is intended for use with any chronic pain patient being considered for long-term opioid therapy. In initial testing, 175 patients who were taking opioids for chronic pain took the SOAPP. Six months later, 95 of the patients were readministered the SOAPP and also were tested for medication misuse using the PDUQ, urine drug tests, and staff observation. Fourteen of the 24 questions were found to predict aberrant behavior in the 6 months that followed the initial assessment (Butler, Budman, Fernandez, & Jamison, 2004). A score of 7 or higher is considered positive for likelihood to abuse.

The SOAPP questions were selected with the input of a panel of pain experts. Like the ORT, it was designed specifically to help clinicians make decisions about the level of monitoring needed for/by their patients on opioids. Information from the website devoted to the development of the SOAPP (http://www.painedu.org/soap-development.asp) proclaims acceptable reliability and reasonable predictive validity but also stresses the ongoing nature of the testing.

Recent tweaking of the SOAPP has produced two additional versions, one containing 14 questions and a short form containing 5 questions (Table 47.3). The short form, which has a cutoff score of 4, loses a bit of accuracy, which the researchers posit as a tradeoff that might be acceptable given the savings in time. The 14-question SOAPP appears to have sensitivity and specificity comparable to the original SOAPP.

The Screening Instrument for Substance Abuse Potential (SISAP)

Another tool that should be mentioned is the Screening Instrument for Substance Abuse Potential (SISAP; see Box 47.5; Coambs & Jarry, 1996). The SISAP is a 5-item screen that is intended to help clinicians assess patients' risk for abusing opioids based on their alcohol consumption, marijuana use, whether they smoke cigarettes, and their age. Tested against a large database of nearly 5,000 telephone survey responses in a Canadian epidemiological survey of alcohol and drug use, the SISAP correctly classified 91% of substance abusers and 78% of nonsubstance abusers. The instrument netted very few false negatives but did have a high false positive rate with 18% of the sample falsely identified as substance abusers. It has not been prospectively validated in a chronic pain population nor has it proven useful, as yet, in clinical settings.

Box 47.5 Screening Instrument for Substance Abuse Potential (SISAP)

1. If you drink alcohol, how many drinks do you have on a typical day?
2. How many drinks do you have in a typical week?
3. Have you used marijuana or hashish in the past year?
4. Have you ever smoked cigarettes?
5. What is your age?

Interpretation of SISAP results.

Use caution when prescribing opioids for the following patients:
1. Men who exceed 4 drinks per day or 16 drinks per week
2. Women who exceed 3 drinks per day or 12 drinks per week
3. A patient who admits to marijuana or hashish use in the past year.
4. A patient under 40 who smokes.

Table 47.3. SOAPP Matrix

The following is an overview of the three SOAPP tools and the questions they contain.

Question #	24 Q	14 Q	5Q
1. How often do you feel that your pain is "out of control"?	X		
2. How often do you have mood swings?	X	X	X
3. How often do you do things that you later regret?	X		
4. How often has your family been supportive and encouraging?	X		
5. How often have others told you that you have a bad temper?	X		
6. Compared with other people, how often have you been in a car accident?	X		
7. How often do you smoke a cigarette within an hour after you wake up?	X	X	X
8. How often have you felt a need for higher doses of medication to treat your pain?	X		
9. How often do you take more medication than you are supposed to?	X		
10. How often have any of your family members, including parents and grandparents, had a problem with alcohol or drugs?	X	X	
11. How often have any of your close friends had a problem with alcohol or drugs?	X	X	
12. How often have others suggested that you have a drug or alcohol problem?	X	X	
13. How often have you attended an AA or NA meeting?	X	X	
14. How often have you had a problem getting along with the doctors who prescribed your medicines?	X		
15. How often have you taken medication other than the way that it was prescribed?	X	X	X
16. How often have you been seen by a psychiatrist or a mental health counselor?	X		
17. How often have you been treated for an alcohol or drug problem?	X	X	
18. How often have your medications been lost or stolen?	X	X	
19. How often have others expressed concern over your use of medication?	X	X	
20. How often have you felt a craving for medication?	X	X	
21. How often has more than one doctor prescribed pain medication for you at the same time?	X		
22. How often have you been asked to give a urine screen for substance abuse?	X	X	
23. How often have you used illegal drugs (for example, marijuana, cocaine, etc.) in the past five years?	X	X	X
24. How often, in your lifetime, have you had legal problems or been arrested?	X	X	X

Source: Butler, Budman, Fernandez, & Jamison, 2004. All versions of the SOAPP, information on validity, and instructions for use can be obtained, free of charge for clinical use, at www.painedu.org.

Accuracy of Assessment Tools

To be useful in a clinical setting, a screening tool should be both reliable and valid based on the cutoff score or scores chosen. A reliable tool yields repeatable, consistent results throughout a variety of administrations. Validity is an indication that the tool actually measures what it is intended to measure. Sensitivity and specificity are two measures that indicate how valid a given assessment is within the population tested.

Sensitivity and Specificity

It is important that clinicians understand the degree to which the tools are able to accurately predict behavior. Measures of sensitivity and specificity are used to determine this accuracy. Sensitivity is the proportion of times a positive score detects a true positive, in other words, the percentage of subjects who test positive and go on to display a measure's criteria for an SUD or aberrant behavior indicating possible abuse. Specificity is the proportion of times a negative score detects a true negative, in other words, the percentage of subjects who go on not to display the measure's criteria for an SUD after testing negative.

A tool with high sensitivity will correctly identify most patients with problems but may also incorrectly identify as high risk some patients who will not demonstrate problems (false positives). Likewise, a tool with high specificity will correctly identify most patients who do not exhibit substance abuse but may also incorrectly identify as negative patients who will demonstrate problems (false negatives).

The meaning of a test's results can be observed in the test's negative and positive predictive values. A positive score on a test with high positive predictive power means the problem tested for will probably be present. A negative score on a test with high

Box 47.6 Selecting the Correct Assessment Tool

Examples of brief tools are the following:

- CAGE-AID
- TICS
- ORT*
- SISAP*
- SOAPP*

*These three are intended specifically for opioid-treated patients.
For patients whose affirmative responses to substance-related items on briefer instruments indicate a need for more in-depth assessment, more detailed assessments include the following:

- ASI (useful for making treatment-related decisions)
- SCID (a thorough assessment)
- PDUQ (particularly useful tool for opioid-treated patients)
- SODQ (to check for presence and severity of opiate dependence)

negative predictive power means the problem tested for will probably be absent.

Tests that are good at identifying patients who are at high risk for opioid abuse often are subject to false positives. Therefore, a test with a high degree of sensitivity is likely to correctly classify as high risk a patient who goes on to exhibit aberrant behaviors but may also classify patients as high risk who do not display problems. The current version of the SOAPP is a good example. The tool's sensitivity is high, correctly identifying about 90% of patients who will display aberrant behaviors. However, its specificity of 69% means that 31% of people who scored high will not display aberrant behaviors.

The ORT effectively predicted the behavior of high- and low-risk patients but is muddier at discerning the significance of the moderate-risk group. Patients whose scores placed them in the ORT's middle category were as likely as not to display aberrant behavior.

In general, the wide net cast by tools sensitive enough to detect high-risk patients may pull in many patients who will not end up abusing. This may be an acceptable tradeoff until tools can be refined. From a clinical perspective, it is better to falsely identify a person as a high-risk opioid consumer than to fail to identify a person who will harm him or herself by abusing substances.

Stigma should not be a factor as the classification is "high-risk patient," not "substance abuser." If, as a result, the individual is more stringently monitored than necessary at first, no harm is done. The monitoring level can be adjusted after an acceptable level of compliance has been established. A person whose monitoring level fails to meet the risk level is more likely to encounter harm while attempting to manage opioid intake. As research grows more sophisticated and specific to the needs of opioid-treated pain patients, more precise assessments will be found.

Honesty in Self-Report

Self report is always subject to inaccuracy or dishonesty from the patient providing the information. It is logical to suspect that a person whose opioid use is out of control could be less than reliable in reporting a history of substance abuse to the person who will be providing opioids. Yet research supports that most patients are surprisingly honest when discussing SUDs with health-care professionals. The ORT, which was administered in an interdisciplinary pain clinic, contains data demonstrating that most patients answered honestly even when asked sensitive questions about prior substance abuse.

An exception concerns individuals intent on criminal diversion, an act that is usually well camouflaged. No tool is designed to detect patients at risk for diversion.

Another complicating factor can be the naïve individuals who feel guilty for using opioids for pain and who inadvertently provide inaccurate information. These individuals sometimes self-report any use of opioids as an abuse or describe themselves as addicted.

It is important to build trust and rapport during the assessment process to encourage and facilitate the honest sharing of information. The validity of the information provided is more likely when the following criteria are met:

- Confidentiality is observed.
- Patients fear no negative consequences from disclosing information.
- The information disclosed has a likelihood of subsequent verification.
- The clinician is nonjudgmental and matter-of-fact.
- The clinician treats substance use questions as an important, routine component of the medical history, no different from data on diet, exercise, and smoking.

Substance abuse counseling experts suggest that confrontational approaches are less effective than empathic ones. A caring, nonjudgmental clinician who is, nonetheless, willing to set and implement treatment boundaries is an indispensable component of providing good medical care.

Little data exist to support or refute the validity of a self-administered test as opposed to an interview format. It is probably true that a certain depth to the investigation is lost when the clinician is unable to gauge a patient's response face to face via verbal cues and facial expressions. However, such interpretations require special training not available in most pain treatment settings. The widespread clinical utility of a self-administered tool make it more practical, and the accompanying savings in time and clinical resources are probably worth the trade-off.

Future Directions

Tools that are geared to opioid-prescribed patients, such as the ORT, the SOAPP, the PDUQ and the SISAP, represent a new direction for researchers. Each of these, except for the PDUQ, could be considered brief. They fulfill many of the needs for opioid-treated patients. However, more testing is needed to confirm their usefulness among chronic pain patients and to assess their validity in a variety of clinical settings.

One revelation that is clear from the research is that a brief assessment may be as valid as or more so than a lengthier one for predicting which patients will exhibit risky behavior. The Holy Grail is to discover which questions elicit answers that reliably predict who is at risk for opioid abuse. As research continues, it will likely take the direction of discovering the briefest, most accurate assessments possible.

Some emphasis in this direction is already apparent. The single question, "Has your use of alcohol or other drugs ever caused a problem for you or those close to you?" (Fine & Portenoy, 2004) has been suggested as having good predictive validity for prior addiction. In theory, if the answer is positive, the question may be valuable in indicating the need for a more detailed assessment and increased monitoring if opioids are prescribed.

Compton et al., the researchers behind the 42-question PDUQ, discovered that 3 of its items were able to correctly classify addicted or nonaddicted subjects in 92% of the cases:

- The tendency to increase analgesic dose or frequency
- To have a preferred route of administration
- To consider oneself addicted

Though the researchers concluded it is much too early to reduce the questionnaire to these 3 questions, they lauded the clinical utility of such a reduction if it could be adequately supported by the data.

Ideally, assessment tools should identify not only those individuals predisposed to abuse but those who may abuse if stressed past a breaking point. Pain is one of the stressful factors that, if uncontrolled, could cause abuse in individuals who otherwise would not be vulnerable to an SUD.

Choosing an Assessment Tool

Pending further research, clinicians should assess patients by using the best available combination of questions found to be associated with the risk of opioid abuse. The choice of which assessment tool to use will depend on the clinician's expertise or access to specialists in the field, the time available, and other aspects of the clinical situation. For new patients, predictive tools can help clinicians assess potential risk before treatment begins. For a current patient, when a pattern of aberrant behavior is suspected, a diagnostic tool would be helpful. (See Box 47.6 for examples).

Deciding which instruments or formats to use is less important than implementing assessment strategies as a routine practice. As opioid therapy progresses, it is important to perform ongoing assessment, not only to screen for drug-related behaviors, but to ensure that pain is adequately controlled, and that goals for improved physical function and quality of life are met. The goal is an environment in which opioids may be safely prescribed and consumed.

Conclusion

No clinician, however skilled and experienced, can predict with certainty whether a person will or will not abuse the opioids prescribed for pain. However, known risk factors may help determine the general probabilities of who may display behavioral cues suggesting abuse or addiction.

All clinicians who prescribe opioids for chronic pain should assess patients for potential abuse. The goal is not to deny pain treatment to any patient but to set and maintain a level of monitoring proportionate to the individual's risk. Higher risk patients will require more careful monitoring and clinical vigilance. The clinician should remain mindful that these patients have the same rights to adequate analgesia as low- or moderate-risk patients.

Clinicians should follow these steps:

1. Become familiar with the individual risk factors for opioid abuse.
2. Screen new patients during their initial clinic visits using clinically validated assessments to evaluate, diagnose and possibly predict abuse or addiction in patients.
3. Set the level of monitoring appropriate to the degree of risk demonstrated by the patient.
4. Monitor for and document any aberrant, drug-related behaviors that may be associated with abuse or addiction.
5. Reassess the patient regularly for improved or impaired function; every visit should include some degree of reassessment. The importance of this step cannot be overemphasized.
6. Never make judgments prior to an appropriate assessment: Do not assume that a high-risk patient will always abuse opioids or that a low-risk patient never will.

By using a clinical instrument to assess the probability of an individual developing aberrant behavior, the clinician can tailor the monitoring of patients according to their risk profiles. More importantly, patients who are at high risk can be identified before beginning opioid therapy and directed to appropriate counseling or treatment of the disorders that make them high risk. The hope is that this awareness will result in better clinical outcomes and less abuse.

References

Atluri S, Sudarshan G. A screening tool to determine the risk of prescription opioid abuse among patients with chronic non-malignant pain. *Pain Physician* 2002; 5(4):447–448.

Bastiaens L, Riccardi K, Sakhrani D. The RAFFT as a screening tool for adult substance use disorders. *Am J Drug Alcohol Abuse* 2002; 28(4): 681–691.

Brown GS, Hermann R, Jones E, Wu J. Using self-report to improve substance abuse risk assessment in behavioral health care. *Jt Comm J Qual Saf* 2004; 30(8):448–454.

Brown RL, Leonard T, Saunders LA, Papasouliotis O. A two-item conjoint screen for alcohol and other drug problems. *J Am Board Fam Pract* 2001; 14(2):95–106.

Brown RL, Rounds LA. Conjoint screening questionnaires for alcohol and other drug abuse: criterion validity in a primary care practice. *Wis Med J* 1995; 94(3):135–40.

Butler SF, Budman SH, Fernandez K, Jamison RN. Validation of a screener and opioid assessment measure for patients with chronic pain. *Pain* 2004; 112(1–2):65–75.

Coambs RB, Jarry JL. The SISAP: a new screening instrument for identifying potential opioid abusers in the management of chronic nonmalignant pain in general medical practice. *Pain Res Manage* 1996;1:155–162.

Compton P, Darakjian J, Miotto K. Screening for addiction in patients with chronic pain and a "problematic" substance use: evaluation of a pilot assessment tool. *J Pain Symptom Manage* 1998; 16(6):355–363.

Davis LJ, Hurt R, Morse RM, O'Brien P. Discriminant analysis of the Self-Administered Alcoholism Screening Test. *Alcoholism Clin Exp Res* 1987; 11(3):269–273.

Dunbar SA, Katz NP. Chronic opioid therapy for nonmalignant pain in patients with a history of substance abuse: report of 20 cases. *J Pain Symptom Manage* 1996; 11(3):163–171.

Ewing JA. Detecting alcoholism: the CAGE questionnaire. *JAMA* 1984; 252(14):1905–1907.

Fine P, Portenoy RK. Opioid misuse, abuse, and addiction. In: *A clinical guide to opioid analgesia.* New York: McGraw Hill; 2004:89.

Friedman R, Li V, Mehrotra D. Treating pain patients at risk: evaluation of a screening tool in opioid-treated pain patients with and without addiction. *Pain Med* 2003; 4(2):182–185.

Friedmann PD, McCullough D, Saitz R. Screening and intervention for illicit drug abuse: a national survey of primary care physicians and psychiatrists. *Arch Intern Med* 2001; 161(2):248–251.

Gavin DR, Ross HE, Skinner HA. Diagnostic validity of the Drug Abuse Screening Test in the assessment of DSM-III drug disorders. *British Journal of Addiction* 1989; 84:301–307.

Kranzler HR, Kadden RM, Babor TF, Tennen H, Rounsaville BJ. Validity of the SCID in substance abuse patients. *Addiction* 1996; 91(6):859–868.

Lazowski LE, Miller FG, Boye MW, Miller GA. Efficacy of the Substance Abuse Subtle Screening Inventory-3 (SASSI-3) in identifying substance dependence disorders in clinical settings. *J Pers Assess* 1998; 71(1):114–28.

McLellan AT, Kushner H, Metzger D, et al. The fifth edition of the Addiction Severity Index. *J Subst Abuse Treat* 1992; 9(3):199–213.

Robinson RC, Gatchel RJ, Polatin P, Deschner M, Noe C, Gajraj N. Screening for problematic prescription opioid use. *Clin J Pain* 2001; 17(3):220–228.

Savage SR. Assessment for addiction in pain-treatment settings. *Clin J Pain* 2002; 18(4 Suppl):S28-S38.

Staines GL, Magura S, Foote J, Deluca A, Kosanke N. Polysubstance use among alcoholics. J Addict Dis 2001; 20(4):53–69.

Storgaard H, Nielsen SD, Gluud C. The validity of the Michigan Alcoholism Screening Test (MAST). *Alcohol Alcohol* 1994; 29(5):493–502.

Saunders JB, Aasland OG, Babor TF, de la Fuente JR, Grant M. Development of the Alcohol Use Disorders Identification Test (AUDIT): WHO Collaborative Project on Early Detection of Persons with Harmful Alcohol Consumption—II. Addiction 1993; 88(6):791–804.

Sutherland G, Edwards G, Taylor C, Phillips G, Gossop M, Brady R. The measurement of opiate dependence. *Br J Addict* 1986; 81(4):485–494.

Tsuang MT, Lyons MJ, Meyer JM, et al. Co-occurrence of abuse of different drugs in men. *Arch Gen Psych* 1998; 55(11):967–972.

Webster LR, Webster RM. Predicting aberrant behaviors in opioid-treated patients: preliminary validation of the Opioid Risk Tool.*Pain Med* 2005; 6(6):432–442.

48

Aberrant Drug Taking
Empirical Studies and Clinical Application

Kenneth L. Kirsh

Steven D. Passik

What exactly do we mean by the term *aberrant drug taking*? Is this a worthwhile term that can aid in the understanding of a complex series of behaviors surrounding medication compliance, or does it simply muddy the waters of already complex terminology around addiction and abuse? Do we even need this additional terminology? These are fundamental questions that must be answered if we are to push the science and understanding of the interface of pain and chemical dependency forward. The purpose of this chapter is to provide an overview of aberrant drug taking and how it can apply to the redefinition of pain patient behaviors. In addition, we discuss the new horizon of attempts to assess and codify the meaning behind these behaviors.

Interpreting Aberrant Behaviors

Aberrant behaviors may be indicative of one of several problems, and a differential diagnosis should be explored if questionable behaviors occur during pain treatment. A true addiction is only one of several possible explanations when aberrant behaviors arise, but is more likely when behaviors such as multiple unsanctioned dose escalations and obtaining opioids from multiple prescribers occur. The diagnosis of pseudoaddiction must be considered if the patient is reporting distress related to unrelieved symptoms (Weissman & Haddox, 1989). Behaviors such as aggressively complaining about the need for higher doses of a medication or occasional unilateral drug escalations may be indications that the patient's pain is undermedicated. Impulsive drug use may also indicate the existence of another psychiatric disorder, the diagnosis of which may have therapeutic implications.

For example, patients with borderline personality disorders may be categorized as exhibiting aberrant drug-taking behaviors when utilizing prescription medications to express fear and anger or to improve chronic boredom. Similarly, patients who use opioids to self-medicate symptoms of anxiety or depression, insomnia, or problems of adjustment may be classified as aberrant drug takers. Occasionally, aberrant drug-related behaviors appear to be causally related to mild encephalopathy, with confusion regarding the appropriate therapeutic regimen.

Problematic behaviors rarely imply criminal intent, such as when patients report pain but intend to sell or divert medications. These diagnoses are not mutually exclusive and a thorough psychiatric assessment is vitally important in an effort to categorize questionable behaviors properly in both the population without a prior history of substance abuse and the population of known substance abusers who have a higher incidence of psychiatric comorbidity (Passik & Portenoy, 1998; Passik, Portenoy, & Ricketts, 1998).

Aberrant Behaviors in Select Medical Populations

Alterations in physical and psychosocial functioning caused by medical illness and its treatment, which may be difficult to differentiate from the morbidity associated with drug abuse, also challenge the main concepts utilized to define addiction. This may particularly complicate the ability to assess a concept that is crucial to the diagnosis of addiction: "use despite harm." For example, it can be difficult to discern problematic behaviors in the patient who develops social withdrawal or cognitive changes after brain irradiation for metastases. Even if impaired cognition is clearly related to medication used in treatment, this effect might only represent a narrow therapeutic window rather than the patient's utilization of analgesic to attain these psychic effects (Passik & Portenoy, 1998; Passik, Portenoy, & Ricketts, 1998). Additionally, in situations where disease and pain have severely limited psychological, social, and vocational functioning, it can be difficult to ascribe harm to particular drug-taking behaviors in the context of so much dysfunction.

It also is important to highlight the types of aberrant drug-taking behaviors that occur on a frequent basis. In part, we must recognize that patients with different disease states and pain sources are likely to be assessed according to different standards and based upon preconceived notions on the part of health-care professionals. We briefly highlight two sample populations of patients with pain and their potentially aberrant drug-taking behaviors. If a large proportion of patients are discovered to engage in a specific behavior, it may be normative and judgments concerning aberrancy should be influenced accordingly (Passik & Portenoy, 1998; Passik, Portenoy, & Ricketts, 1998).

AIDS

Determining rates of drug abuse and addiction is complex in the HIV/AIDS population. These patients tend to be generally younger and characterized by injection drug use as a risk factor in 30%–63% of patients (O'Conner et al., 1994: Siegal et al., 1995; Stark et al., 1995). Specifically, more women than men have injection drug use as a risk factor for HIV/AIDS (Brown et al., 1996; Myers et al., 1995). In addition, clinical observation suggests that the inadequate management of symptoms may be the impetus for aberrant drug-related behaviors. Indeed, there is compelling evidence that pain is undertreated in the HIV/AIDS population (Breitbart et al., 1996).

Treating chronic pain in populations with HIV/AIDS is difficult but can be successfully accomplished. One of the main barriers to effective pain management in this population is the concern and difficulty experienced by clinicians, leading one researcher to note that treatment professionals must recognize and temper their own values and concerns regarding treatment approaches (Faltz, 1998). To highlight this, one study compared a sample of AIDS patients with prior drug use history to a sample of AIDS patients without. All had significant pain issues related either to AIDS or its treatment and were treated with sustained-release morphine. The researchers found that patients with illicit drug use history can be treated successfully for AIDS-related pain. However, the group with a positive history for illicit drug use required significantly higher doses of opioid for an equivalent analgesic effect. This need for higher dosing could easily be misinterpreted as an aberrant behavior in many clinical settings. Interestingly, the two groups did not differ significantly based on quality of life, baseline pain ratings, causes of pain, pain intensity at study end, or demographic variables (Kaplan et al., 2000).

Sickle-Cell Anemia

Nearly 60,000 Americans have sickle-cell anemia, and approximately 2.5 million people have the sickle-cell trait. For persons with the disease, pain is the most commonly experienced symptom (Payne, 1989). The pain is frequently persistent, unpredictable, and intense, creating a unique challenge for management that often results in undertreatment (Jacob, 2001). In addition to the episodic pain, conditions such as bone infarctions, aseptic necrosis, and sickle arthropathy may create a chronic pain problem (Gil, 1989).

Only a small number of patients exhibit behaviors indicative of opioid addiction, but they tend to have frequent contacts with health-care professionals, which can alter the views about both the individual patient as well as others with sickle-cell disease (Marks & Schar, 1973). Perceptions of health-care professionals lean toward the presence of an inordinate amount of drug use problems in this population (Elander et al., 2006). For instance, a survey of nurses serving sickle-cell patients found that 30% were uncomfortable with the notion of administering high doses of opioids and over 60% believed that addiction problems were prevalent in their patients (Pack-Mabien et al., 2001).

Similarly, a study examined the beliefs of emergency room physicians and hematologists regarding addiction in sickle-cell patients, the two groups of physicians that typically come into contact with these patients. The results indicated that emergency room physicians held more negative views, with 53% of those surveyed believing that more than 20% of their sickle-cell patients had addiction problems. In comparison, only 23% of the hematologists felt the same way regarding the prevalence of addiction (Shapiro et al., 1997). It is important to understand these biases while also realizing that this population has been shown to be prone toward problems of pseudoaddiction rather than true addiction (Lusher et al., 2006).

Studies Examining Aberrant Drug-Taking Behaviors

In an effort to further investigate the issues associated with identifying and assessing potentially aberrant drug-taking behaviors in cancer and chronic pain patients, our group has conducted several studies. Various approaches were utilized in examining these issues including chart reviews, structured interviews, and brief surveys.

Chart Reviews

Because urine toxicology screens (UTSs) may be helpful in the diagnosis and monitoring of patients with known or suspected substance abuse, as well as assisting clinicians in managing therapy with controlled prescription drugs in the medically ill, Passik and colleagues (2000a) conducted a study to examine the use of UTSs in a cancer center. In conducting the study, the medical records of 111 randomly selected patients were reviewed utilizing a data collection instrument designed specifically for this study. Although inpatient chart reviews were comprised of only patients who underwent UTSs upon admission, outpatient chart reviews consisted of examining 1 month prior to and after obtaining UTSs. The majority of the patients' diagnoses included cancer, human immunodeficiency virus (HIV), and chronic nonmalignant pain syndromes. Of the 111 patients, 56 (50.5%) had evidence of illicit drug use, a prescription medication that had not been ordered, or alcohol use. The remainder of the sample, 50 (49.5%) patients, had negative screens. Positive UTSs were detected more frequently when the patient had HIV (100% versus 46.6%), or was undergoing treatment for chronic nonmalignant pain (100% versus 43.9%).

Although it was found that documentation of the UTSs in the medical records was infrequent (37.8% of the charts had no reason listed for obtaining the tests, and 29% of the ordering physicians could not be identified), documentation was more likely to exist when the results of the UTSs were positive (14.3% versus 0%). Results also indicated that UTSs are seldom used in the tertiary care oncology center and the documentation concerning the ordering and subsequent use of the test is unsystematic in patient management, with the majority of the records (89%) not containing the results of the UTSs.

Structured Interviews

In a related study, Passik and colleagues (2000b) investigated the issues regarding the assessment of drug-taking behaviors in medically ill populations utilizing a structured interview approach. In conducting this study, a drug-taking behavior and attitudes questionnaire was developed on the basis of clinical experience of specialists in pain management and addiction medicine. This questionnaire explored the self-reports of medication use, past and present drug abuse, patients' beliefs concerning the risk of addiction in pain treatment, and aberrant drug-taking behaviors and attitudes at a major cancer center. In utilizing this instrument, samples of cancer patients ($n = 52$) and women with HIV/AIDS ($n = 111$) were surveyed.

Results indicated that past drug use and abuse were reported more frequently than present drug use and abuse in both groups. Although current aberrant drug-related behaviors were rarely reported, attitude-related items revealed that patients would consider participating in aberrant behaviors or would possibly excuse them in others if pain or symptom management were insufficient. It was also found that aberrant behaviors and attitudes were acknowledged more often by women with HIV/AIDS, and that patients greatly overestimated the risk of addiction in pain treatment. Experience with this questionnaire indicated that both cancer and HIV/AIDS patients respond in a forthcoming manner to drug-taking behavior questions, and describe attitudes and behaviors that may by critically pertinent to the diagnosis and management of substance use disorders in the medically ill population.

Passik and researchers (2006) conducted a related study for the purpose of characterizing the effects of undertreatment of pain in HIV-positive substance abusers in terms of their aberrant drug-taking behaviors, and to examine the correlates of these behaviors. In addition, the frequencies of these behaviors were contrasted to those of cancer patients who have a lower baseline rate of substance abuse and who were either adequately or inadequately managed for pain.

A battery of standardized quality of life instruments was selected to accompany the aberrant drug-taking interview. Data collection involved questionnaires and face-to-face interviews conducted with 100 adult cancer patients and 73 HIV-positive patients. Patients for the HIV sample met *DSM-IV* criteria (based upon a computerized SCID screen) for a current or past substance use disorder (SUD). The cancer patients were recruited for the study only if they did not meet *DSM-IV* criteria for a SUD; thus, the cancer patients were considered a comparison control group.

Analyses revealed a general trend that supported the hypothesis that undertreatment of pain led to an increase in aberrant drug-taking behaviors in addicts, but not in the cancer patients without a history of substance abuse. In the HIV group, 21% reported ongoing substance abuse, whereas 53% were recovered addicts and 24% did not meet SCID criteria for a SUD. Most of the HIV sample used over-the-counter (OTC) medicines to treat their pain, but slightly less than half of the interim sample reported them helpful in alleviating their pain. The majority (88%) reported successful management of their pain with opioid medications, but curiously, 87% reported their pain was uncontrolled.

In an effort to address the issues of poor pain outcomes as they relate to addiction, Passik and colleagues (2004, 2005) conducted a study to examine the relationship between aberrant drug-taking behaviors and pain outcomes during long-term treatment with opioids for nonmalignant pain. In particular, the focus of the study was on providing the nature, frequency, and predictive value of drug-taking behaviors in pain management. This effort could ultimately assist physicians in the assessment and management of these behaviors, whether they resulted from the undertreatment of pain or a substance use disorder.

The main objective of the study was to develop a user-friendly checklist that physicians could utilize to examine the four domains of outcomes in chronic opioid therapy: analgesia (pain relief), activities of daily living (psyhcosocial functioning), adverse effects (side effects), and aberrant drug-taking behaviors (addiction-related outcomes; Passik & Weinreb, 2000). In addition, it was hoped that the checklist could be used to monitor pain and treatment outcomes for patients receiving long-term opioid therapy for chronic pain. Participating physicians throughout the United States evaluated patients who had been receiving opioid therapy for at least 3 months. A structured interview approach and clinical observations were used. Cross-sectional results suggest that the majority of patients with chronic pain achieve relatively positive outcomes in the eyes of their prescribing physicians in all four relevant domains with opioid therapy. Analgesia was modest but meaningful, functionality generally stabilized or improved, and side effects were tolerable. Potentially aberrant behaviors were common but viewed only as an indicator of a problem (i.e., addiction or diversion) in approximately 10% of cases.

Brief Surveys of Physicians

Passik and colleagues (2002) conducted a pilot survey of 100 pain clinicians to rate aberrant drug-taking behaviors on their degree of aberrance in an effort to ascertain the degree to which clinicians perceive the severity of particular aberrant drug-taking behaviors. The survey instrument utilized in this study consisted of 7 items designed to gather physician demographics including specific discipline, number of opioids prescribed per year, and the percentage of patients seen who had a previous substance use disorder. The survey also had a 13-item list of aberrant drug-taking behaviors that physicians were asked to rate from most (1) to least (13) aberrant.

Results revealed that each aberrant behavior listed was rated at each possible position at least once, which indicates a great degree of variability among physicians' perceptions. However, an examination of the mean aberrancy ratings for these behaviors indicated a clustering of behaviors that seemed to be perceived as more problematic. Specifically, illegal behaviors (such as the sale of prescription drugs [mean = 4.00], forging of prescriptions [mean = 4.47], and altering the route or delivery system of a drug [mean = 4.41]) were viewed as more aberrant than seemingly less aberrant behaviors (such as unkempt appearance [mean = 10.95], unsanctioned dose escalation of a drug once or twice [mean = 9.79], and the hoarding of drugs [mean = 8.63]). Overall, though, it became evident that aberrant drug-taking behaviors can represent a host of meanings depending on the individual perceptions and past experiences of the physicians surveyed. In short, we must be cautious of how we interpret these behaviors in our patients and avoid making spurious correlations based on relatively limited personal experience as opposed to empirically derived data.

Assessing Aberrant Behaviors: A New Horizon

In order to avoid personal bias and offhanded judgments of patient behaviors, it is necessary to develop a means to categorize and track various aberrant drug-taking behaviors and what they might signify (i.e., addiction versus pseudoaddiction versus chemical coping, etc.). Although there is a lack of empirical data to truly categorize aberrant behaviors at this time, a groundswell of attempts to at least assess these behaviors has begun to occur. Some of these attempts are discussed, in turn, below.

As mentioned above, Passik and colleagues (2004, 2005) have devised a clinical tool that can be used to assess four relevant domains of behavior in pain patients, including the issue of aberrant drug-taking behaviors. Called the Pain Assessment and Documentation Tool (PADT), it has been designed to be a brief and clinically meaningful way for physicians to assess the behaviors of their patients. For a full discussion, please see Chapter 46, "Documentation and Potential Documentation Tools in Long-Term Opioid Therapy," in this volume.

Compton and colleagues (1998) have also attempted to create an assessment tool for patients already being treated with an opioid regimen. The Prescription Drug Use Questionnaire is a 42-item tool designed to separate patients meeting criteria for addiction from those engaging in other forms of aberrant behaviors. In their study, while assessing a relatively small number of problem patients ($n = 52$), they were able to easily differentiate addicts from nonaddicts according to the items on the questionnaire. Utilizing a "yes/no" format, the questionnaire assesses the patient's pain condition, opioid use patterns, social and family factors, family history, patient history of substance abuse, and psychiatric history.

The Opioid Risk Tool (ORT) is another recent attempt designed to better identify whether patients are likely to engage in aberrant behaviors if placed on opioid therapy (Webster & Webster, 2005). Although the PADT and Prescription Drug Use Questionnaire are useful for assessing patients already on opioids as a means of ongoing monitoring, the ORT was designed to be used as a prescreening instrument. The ORT is a brief tool that measures risk factors associated with substance abuse such as personal and family history of substance abuse, age, history of preadolescent sexual abuse, and certain psychological diseases. Patients are rated on these items and receive scores of 0–3 (low risk), 4–7 (moderate risk), or ≥8 (high risk), indicating the probability of their displaying opioid-related aberrant behaviors. Tested on 185 pain patients, 17 out of 18 in the low-risk category (94.4%) did not display an aberrant behavior, whereas 40 out of 44 (90.9%) in the high-risk category did display an aberrant behavior. The ORT displayed excellent discrimination for both the male ($c = 0.82$) and the female ($c = 0.85$) prognostic models.

Conclusion

Understanding the meaning and context behind aberrant drug-taking behaviors is crucial in determining whether a patient's behavior is a symptom of addiction or one of the many gray areas that lie between addiction and fully compliant behavior. Although previous studies have shed light on the particular diagnostic meanings of various behaviors and have afforded clinicians the opportunity to recognize those behaviors that are true "red flags" in a given population, far too often clinicians are prejudiced in their perceptions of these behaviors due to anecdotal accounts. Certain behaviors are universally judged as aberrant regardless of limited data suggesting this is true, whereas other behaviors found common in nonaddicts that may seem aberrant based on face value may have little predictive value for true addiction.

There are several points that need to be made concerning what we have learned so far. First, it seems apparent that patients are usually forthcoming about illicit drug use and aberrant drug-related behaviors when they are asked about them. Although it may have been thought to be an issue when patients would refrain from divulging risky behaviors for fear of reprisal, this does not appear to be the case. In addition, the undertreatment of pain remains, even in the face of continual enlightenment and improved savvy of physicians concerning pain treatment. Lastly, research has shown that aberrant drug behaviors can be measured systematically, but that the screens and tools still need to be refined.

The future holds several challenges regarding the state of pain management in medically ill patients. Empirical data is needed to understand what aberrant drug-related behaviors are normative in the medically ill. This will ultimately need to be done separately for different types of disease. For instance, common aberrant behaviors that we have uncovered about cancer patients (such as increasing medication dose once or twice) may or may not be similar to those behaviors found in patients with other disorders such as sickle-cell anemia or chronic lower back pain. In essence, what is needed is a formal study of the epidemiology of pain behaviors in multiple illnesses.

References

Breitbart W, Rosenfeld BD, Passik SD, et al. The undertreatment of pain in ambulatory AIDS patients. *Pain,* 1996;65:239–251.

Brown LS, Siddiqui N, Chu AF. Natural history of HIV-1 infection and predictors of survival in a cohort of HIV-1 seropositive injecting drug users. *J Nat Med Assoc,* 1996;88:1–5.

Compton P, Darakjian J, Miotto K. Screening for addiction in patients with chronic pain and "problematic" substance use: evaluation of a pilot assessment tool. *J Pain Symptom Manage.* 1998 Dec;16(6):355–63.

Elander J, Marczewska M, Amos R, Thomas A, Tangayi S. Factors affecting hospital staff judgments about sickle cell disease pain. *J Behav Med.* 2006 Feb 22; [Epub ahead of print]

Faltz B. Counseling substance abuse clients with human immunodeficiency virus. *J Psychoactive Drugs,*1988;20:217–221.

Gil KM. Coping with sickle disease pain. *Ann Beh Med,* 1989;11:49–57.

Jacob E. Pain management in sickle cell disease. *Pain Manage Nurs,* 2001;2:121–131.

Kaplan R, Slywka J, Slagle S, Ries K. A titrated analgesic regimen comparing substance users and non users with AIDS-related pain. *J Pain Symptom Manage,* 2000;19:265–273.

Lusher J, Elander J, Bevan D, Telfer P, Burton B. Analgesic addiction and pseudoaddiction in painful chronic illness. *Clin J Pain.* 2006 Mar–Apr;22(3):316–24.

Marks RM, Schar EJ. Undertreatment of medical inpatients with narcotic analgesics. *Ann Intern Med,* 1973;78:173–181.

Myers K, Metzger D, McLellan H, et al. Will preventative HIV vaccine efficacy trials be possible with female injection drug users? *J Acq Imm Def Synd Hum Retro,* 1995;10:5–11.

O'Conner PG, Selwyn PA, Schottenfeld RS. Medical care for infection-drug users with human immunodeficiency virus infection. *N Engl J Med,* 1994;331:7–10.

Pack-Mabien A, Labbe E, Herbert D, Haynes J. Nurses' attitudes and practices in sickle cell pain management. *Appl Nurs Res,* 2001;14:187–192.

Passik SD, Kirsh KL, Donaghy K, Portenoy RK. Pain and aberrant drug-related behaviors in medically ill patients with and without histories of substance abuse. *Clin J Pain,* 2006 Feb;22(2):173–181.

Passik SD, Kirsh KL, McDonald MV, et al. A pilot survey of aberrant drug-taking attitudes and behaviors in samples of cancer and AIDS patients. *J Pain Symptom Manage,* 2000b:19(4), 274–286.

Passik SD, Kirsh KL, Whitcomb LA, Dickerson P, Theobald DE. Pain clinicians' rankings of aberrant drug-taking behaviors. *Journal of Pain and Palliative Care Pharmacotherapy,* 2002;16(4):39–49.

Passik SD, Kirsh KL, Whitcomb LA, Portenoy RK, Katz N, Kleinman L, Dodd S, Schein J. A new tool to assess and document pain outcomes in chronic pain patients receiving opioid therapy. *Clinical Therapeutics,* 2004;26(4):552–561.

Passik SD, Kirsh KL, Whitcomb LA, Schein JR, Kaplan M, Dodd S, Kleinman L, Katz NP, Portenoy RK. Monitoring outcomes during long-term opioid therapy for non-cancer pain: results with the pain assessment and documentation tool. *J Opioid Management,* 2005 Nov/Dec;1(5):257–266.

Passik SD, Portenoy RK. Substance abuse issues in palliative care. In Berger A, et al., eds. *Principles and practice of supportive oncology.* Philadelphia, PA: Lippincott-Raven Publishers, 1998:513–524.

Passik SD, Portenoy RK, Ricketts PL. Substance abuse issues in cancer patients part 1: prevalence and diagnosis. *Oncology,* 1998;12(4):517–521.

Passik SD, Schreiber J, Kirsh KL, et al. A chart review of the ordering of urine toxicology screens in a cancer center: do they influence pain management? *J Pain Symptom Manage,* 2000a;19(1):40–44.

Passik SD, Weinreb HJ. Managing chronic nonmalignant pain: overcoming obstacles to the use of opioids. *Advances In Therapy,* 2000;17:70–80.

Payne R. Pain management in sickle cell disease: rationale and techniques. *Ann NY Acad Sci*, 1989;565:189–206.

Shapiro B, Lennete B, Payne R, Heidrich G. Sickle-cell related pain: perceptions of medical practitioners. *J Pain Symptom Manage*, 1997;14:168–174.

Siegal HA, Carlson RG, Falck RS, Wang J. Drug abuse treatment experience and HIV risk behaviors among active drug injectors in Ohio. *Am J Pub Health*, 1995;85:1–6.

Stark, K, Sieroslawski, J, Wirth D, et al. HIV risk behavior among injection drug users in Warsaw. *AIDS*, 1995;9:2–8.

Webster LR, Webster RM. Predicting aberrant behaviors in opioid-treated patients: preliminary validation of the opioid risk tool. *Pain Med*, 2005 Nov–Dec;6(6):432–42.

Weissman DE, Haddox JD. Opioid pseudoaddiction: an iatrogenic syndrome. *Pain*, 1989;36:363–366.

49

Abuse Liability Assessment of Prescription Opioids in Chronic Nonmalignant Pain Patients

James P. Zacny

The purpose of this chapter is to introduce the reader to the concept of abuse liability assessment (ALA) of opioids; how ALA of prescription opioids might be done in chronic nonmalignant pain (CNMP) patients; some of the problems that need to be addressed when designing ALA studies in this population and interpreting the results of the studies; and research questions that might be addressed in the conduct of such studies. Given the paucity of studies that have addressed issues of abuse liability of opioids in CNMP patients (Moulin et al. 1996; Tassain et al. 2003), this chapter is meant to serve as a catalyst to stimulate discussion between pain researchers, pain clinicians, addiction medicine specialists, and abuse liability researchers on this topic.

This chapter is timely for two reasons. In the United States, as well as in other countries, there is evidence of increasing use of prescription opioids for the treatment of CNMP (Bell 1997; Coniam 1989; Caudill-Slosberg et al. 2004; Turk & Brody 1992). For example, in a recently published study that examined national trends in office visits and analgesic treatment for chronic musculoskeletal pain, it was established that the use of prescription opioids doubled from 8% in 1980 to 16% in 2000 (Caudill-Slosberg et al. 2004). A more recent phenomenon that has occurred and is presented in another chapter of this volume is the increase in nonmedical use and abuse of prescription opioids in the United States.

One question that has been broached is the prevalence of prescription opioid abuse in the CNMP patient population (Brands et al. 2004; Passik 2001; Savage 1999; Zacny et al. 2003). Several studies have addressed this issue, but small sample sizes, different inclusion/exclusion criteria, and different definitions of what constitutes abuse make it difficult to draw conclusions on the actual prevalence of prescription opioid abuse in this population (Chabal et al. 1997; Cowan et al. 2002, 2003; Fishbain et al. 1992; Mahowald et al. 2005; Michna et al. 2004; Portenoy & Foley 1986; Reid et al. 2002). Against this backdrop of increasing licit use of prescription opioids and unknown prevalence of abuse of prescription opioids in CNMP patients, I will suggest that ALA of prescription opioids in CNMP patients might provide important information that will complement studies that are focused on aberrant behaviors (see other chapters in this volume that address issues surrounding the identification and assessment of these behaviors), as well as studies that examine the epidemiology of abuse/misuse of prescription opioids.

What Is Abuse Liability Assessment?

Abuse liability can be defined as the likelihood that a psychoactive drug will sustain patterns of nonmedical self-administration that result in disruptive or undesirable consequences (Balster & Bigelow 2003). Abuse liability is distinguished from the actual abuse of the drug because the latter can be influenced by such factors as availability, fads, and cost.

Traditionally, human ALA studies have been conducted with drug abusers. One reason is that drug abusers represent a population most at risk for illicit use of drugs (Griffiths et al. 2003). Secondly, they are the most likely to be sensitive to the effects of a drug that would be suggestive of abuse liability (Balster & Bigelow 2003; Griffiths et al. 2003). ALA methodologies and testing instruments were primarily developed at the Addiction Research Center (part of the U.S. Public Health Service) in Lexington, Kentucky, starting in the 1930s. Initially, abuse liability testing of opioids did not involve assessment of how the drug made an abuser feel. The focus was on whether an opioid was capable of producing the same degree of physical dependence as morphine. If so, then that opioid was said to have abuse liability of the morphine type (Himmelsbach 1942, 1943).

In 1961, that changed with the publication of a study (Fraser et al. 1961) in which both subjects and trained observers rated effects of opioids using the Single Dose Questionnaire (SDQ). The SDQ had subjects rate on a numerical scale the extent to which they felt certain effects including relaxed, high, nodding, skin itchy, and sleepy, what they thought the drug was (e.g., a barbiturate, an opiate, etc.), and importantly, how much they liked the drug.

By 1963, Drs. Hill, Haertzen, and colleagues had developed and published the Addiction Research Center Inventory (ARCI) containing several scales that were empirically demonstrated to be sensitive to the effects of a number of abused and nonabused drugs (Hill et al. 1963). The ARCI was shortened in 1971 and consisted of 5 scales, one of them being the Morphine-Benzedrine Group (MBG) scale (Martin et al. 1971). Most researchers consider this scale to tap

---

The preparation of this chapter was funded in part by grant DA08573 from the National Institute on Drug Abuse.

into the euphorigenic effects of a drug. Box 49.1 lists the statements that make up the MBG (Euphoria) scale. Additional measures of abuse liability include drug wanting, how much a person would be willing to pay on the street for a drug, drug identification, visual analog scales (VAS), and reinforcing effects. Reinforcing effects of a drug, although usually positively correlated with some abuse liability-related subjective effects (e.g., euphoria) of a drug, are a separate and distinct measure of actual drug-seeking behavior. For a fuller discussion of the various procedures and measures used in preclinical and human drug ALA, the interested reader is referred to a special volume of the journal *Drug and Alcohol Dependence* that discusses abuse liability assessment of central nervous system drugs (2003, Volume 70, Issue 3 Supplement).

A prototypic opioid ALA study in opioid abusers would employ a placebo-controlled, double-blind, crossover design. Several doses (including those that were supratherapeutic) of an opioid with unknown abuse potential (Drug X), placebo, and typically two doses of a mu agonist opioid such as morphine, known to have abuse liability, would be tested (Jasinski 1977). One would then compare responses to Drug X to see how its subjective effects profile and physiological profile (pupil constriction, or miosis) compared to that of morphine as well as placebo. If Drug X had a profile similar to that of morphine, most notably increased MBG (Euphoria) scores and liking ratings, then this drug would be said to have the same degree of abuse liability as that of morphine. In general, most opioids that have high efficacy at the mu opiate receptor have substantial abuse liability in opioid abusers; abusers report predominantly abuse liability-related effects (e.g., liking and euphoria), and few unpleasant effects (Zacny & Walker 1998).

A number of investigators have also examined subjective and physiological effects of opioids in recreational drug users (people with some history of nonmedical psychotropic drug use that does not meet psychiatric diagnostic criteria for substance abuse) using the same or similar ALA methodology (e.g., Eissenberg et al., 2000; Kaplan et al. 1997; Lasagna et al. 1955; Marsch et al. 2001; Petry et al. 1998; Zacny & Guttierrez 2003). In a majority of these studies, there is more variability in abuse liability-related effects than in opioid abusers, with a significant proportion of subjects reporting varying degrees of unpleasant effects.

One might ask why ALA of prescription opioids needs to be done in CNMP patients if studies are currently being done or have been done in opioid abusers and recreational drug users. The studies may inform to some degree on the abuse liability of prescription opioids in CNMP patients, but there is the concern that CNMP patients differ from the other two populations in significant ways. The first difference is level of pain: presumably absent in opioid abusers and recreational drug users and by definition present in CNMP patients. It has been well established that pain can alter the subjective, reinforcing, and physiological effects of opioids in humans (Borgbjerg et al. 1996; Conley et al. 1997; Hanks et al. 1981; Portenoy & Foley 1986; Wolff et al. 1940; Zacny et al. 1996). Also, in preclinical studies, pain can alter the reinforcing effects of an opioid and the rate at which tolerance to the analgesic effects of opioids occur (Colpaert et al. 2001; Dib & Duclaux 1982; Vaccarino et al. 1993). Thus, results obtained in pain-free subjects may not be indicative of how CNMP patients might react to prescription opioids.

Another difference between opioid abusers and many CNMP patients is history of opioid abuse, and substance abuse in general. All opioid abusers have a history of opioid abuse, and many of them are polydrug abusers (Kassebaum & Chandler 1994; Leri et al. 2003; Oliveto et al. 1999). One cannot make an assumption that all CNMP patients are abusing their prescription opioids and also abusing other substances, and indeed, nothing in the scientific literature suggests this would be the case. A prescription opioid such as hydromorphone has been established as having abuse liability in opioid abusers (Preston et al. 1985), but it would be inappropriate to conclude that the same degree of abuse liability resides in CNMP patients.

Finally, abuse liability researchers are calling for ALA of prescription drugs in the populations that are prescribed them (Kleber 1989). In 2002, the College on Problems of Drug Dependence, a major international society of drug abuse researchers, convened a conference on ALA of central nervous system drugs. One purpose of the conference was to identify research needs to improve the sensitivity and predictive validity of the methodologies used in ALA (Schuster & Henningfield 2003). One of the key research priorities identified by a select panel of abuse liability researchers was "Research should be undertaken on models for predicting abuse liability in the intended patient population in order to determine abuse risk and determinants of iatrogenic addiction" (The Expert Panel, 2003, p. S112).

I have made the case that the abuse liability of prescription opioids in CNMP patients cannot necessarily be inferred from studies with opioid abusers and nondrug-abusing volunteers. Abuse liability researchers are recognizing the need for more ALA drug studies in patient populations that are likely to be prescribed the drugs. In the next section, I will discuss how one might conduct studies examining the abuse liability of prescription opioids in CNMP patients. In the section, I will also discuss potential problems that one might encounter when doing such studies.

Issues Pertinent to Abuse Liability Assessment of Prescription Opioids in Chronic Nonmalignant Pain Patients

There are many challenges that will be encountered when designing an ALA study in this population. CNMP patients are a heterogeneous population, and many decisions will have to be made regarding inclusion and exclusion criteria. Prospective volunteers from the chronic pain community will differ in type of pain, duration of pain, type and dose of opioid, duration of time on opioid

---

Box 49.1 Morphine-Benzedrine Group (Euphoria) Scale

Please indicate "true" or "false" for each statement based on how you feel right now.

1. I would be happy all the time if I felt as I do now.
2. I feel as if I would be more popular with people today.
3. Today I say things in the easiest possible way.
4. I feel more clear-headed than dreamy.
5. Things around me seem more pleasing than usual.
6. I have a pleasant feeling in my stomach.
7. I feel a very pleasant emptiness.
8. I feel that I will lose the contentment I now have.
9. I feel in complete harmony with the world and those about me.
10. I feel less discouraged than usual.
11. I can completely appreciate what others are saying when I am in this mood.
12. I would be happy all the time if I felt as I feel now.
13. I am in the mood to talk about the feelings I have.
14. I feel so good that I know other people can tell it.
15. I feel as if something pleasant had just happened to me.

therapy, adjuvant medications taken, disease state, substance abuse history, and age. These are just examples of many variables that need to be considered in determining the profile of CNMP patients who will be eligible for the ALA study. Design issues include when to conduct the study, for example, when a patient is just starting opioid therapy or when the patient has been taking an opioid for some time. How to include a placebo into the design will raise a challenge, including ethical considerations, in many cases. To a large extent, the research question will inform on inclusion/exclusion criteria and the design of the study.

I will now present a hypothetical prescription opioid ALA study in CNMP patients, and discuss the challenges that will be encountered when interpreting the results of the study. My research question is whether immediate-release (IR) hydromorphone has greater abuse liability than IR oxycodone. Testing relative abuse liability of prescription opioids is important to do, and results could influence clinical practice: If, for example, the two opioids confer the same degree of pain relief, but one has putatively greater abuse liability than the other, a physician might want to consider prescribing the opioid with lesser abuse liability. I will choose a methodology from a study that was recently published in which chronic pain patients who were on controlled-release opioids and had stable pain levels were tested with immediate-release (IR) morphine to determine if IR morphine had memory- and psychomotor-impairing effects (Kamboj et al. 2005). The elegance of this study lay in the fact that because pain was being controlled (or stabilized to an acceptable level) by the controlled-release opioid, a placebo could be ethically included into the design.

My subject population will be patients on controlled-released opioids. Subjects will be taking similar doses (expressed in morphine equivalents) of controlled-release opioids because I want to give the same dose of the IR opioids to all patients. I will allow patients with chronic musculoskeletal or neuropathic pain to enroll in the study. There are many other considerations I will need to take into account when establishing inclusion/exclusion criteria (see above), but for the sake of brevity I will not discuss them. Using a double-blind crossover design with a 1-week washout period between sessions, I will test two therapeutic doses of each opioid that are putatively equianalgesic, and placebo. Dependent measures will include subjective effects questionnaires (e.g., the ARCI, a VAS that includes a measure of drug liking, and a variant of the SDQ) and measures that assess the sensory and affective nature of pain. Measures will be assessed before capsule ingestion (i.e.,

baseline) and at fixed intervals afterward. At each assessment time point, subjects will be instructed to rate how they currently feel and what their level of pain is. Capsule ingestion will occur 4 hours after the patients have taken their controlled-release opioid (presumably when plasma levels of the controlled-release opioid are at steady state). Figure 49.1 presents three hypothetical outcomes at the 90-minute time point after capsule ingestion. Only the high doses of each opioid are included in the figure for ease of comparison. Measures in Figure 49.1 are drug liking ratings and a change score that represents degree of pain relief (level of pain at baseline minus current level of pain). I chose the 90-minute time point because this is when the IR drugs are presumably exerting their peak (or close to peak) effects.

Outcome A shows similar increased liking and pain relief ratings with the two opioids, relative to placebo. Should one conclude from this outcome that the two opioids have abuse liability, per se, because liking is increased relative to placebo? I do not believe such a conclusion would be warranted, because both opioids reduced an aversive, unpleasant state, pain. It would be reasonable to assume that patients might report increased liking of a drug that reduces pain. In this case, liking is not necessarily a predictor of abuse liability. By the same token, MBG (Euphoria) scores might be elevated after administration of the two opioids relative to placebo. Refer back to Box 49.1 and in the majority of the statements, a person answering "true" might be comparing reduced level of pain and perhaps concurrent reduction of aversive emotional states such as anger and irritability to how they used to feel (some level of pain and aversive emotional states). In this case, two key measures of abuse liability would not necessarily inform on the "real" abuse liability of the two opioids.

Outcome B shows that hydromorphone produced higher ratings of liking and pain relief than oxycodone. Would one conclude that hydromorphone has greater abuse liability than oxycodone in a chronic pain population? No, because the basal state of pain has been reduced to different degrees by the two opioids. Again, prototypic measures of abuse liability such as liking ratings and MBG (Euphoria) scores would be of little use in identifying the true abuse potential of these opioids in chronic pain patients if Outcome B occurred.

A more complicated set of results is depicted in Outcome C. The two opioids produce the same degree of pain relief, but hydromorphone engenders a greater degree of liking (and euphoria) than oxycodone. In this case, could one conclude that hydro-

Figure 49.1 Three hypothetical outcomes of a study examining the relative abuse liability of oxycodone to hydromorphone in a placebo-controlled trial. Endpoints shown in the graph are pain relief (open bars) and drug liking (solid bars).

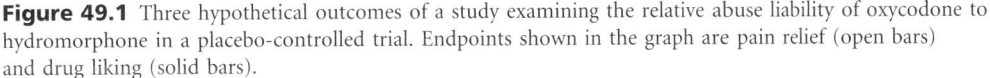
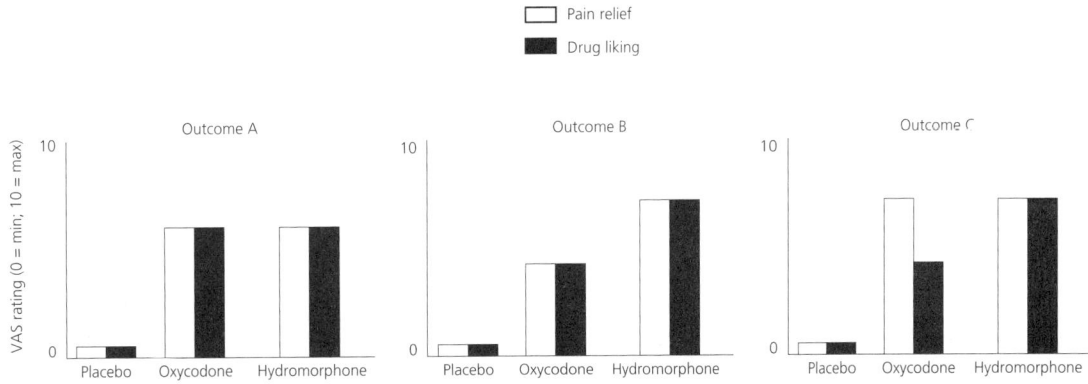

morphone has a greater degree of abuse liability than oxycodone? Perhaps, but other dependent measures would need to be examined to determine if a conclusion regarding relative abuse liability could be drawn. If oxycodone produces a greater number or severity of side effects than hydromorphone, the lower liking ratings and MBG (Euphoria) scores in the oxycodone condition might reflect that. Would this different side effect profile be indicative of a greater likelihood of hydromorphone abuse in chronic pain patients? Perhaps not, if anything the patient on hydromorphone might be more compliant in taking his/her pain reliever than a patient on oxycodone, but that would not necessarily suggest a higher likelihood of abuse. Consider the same question in opioid abusers: would this different side effect profile be indicative of a greater likelihood of hydromorphone abuse than oxycodone abuse? I would suggest that it would, all other things being equal (availability, price, duration of effect). So here again is an example where increased liking and MBG (Euphoria) scores do not necessarily predict abuse liability of the two opioids in CNMP patients.

However, what if the side effect profiles are identical with the two drugs, and that besides conferring an equivalent degree of pain relief the two drugs reduce to a comparable degree unpleasant emotional states such as irritability and anxiety? This might be a situation in which the positive effects reported by subjects under the effects of hydromorphone may not be due solely to an attenuation of dysphoria. One has to look at the entire profile of subjective effects of the two drugs to see what other subjective effects differ between the two drugs. It may be the case that hydromorphone induces a state in which patients report feeling high, carefree, dreamy, and having pleasant thoughts, whereas these effects are *absent* after oxycodone administration. Such a different profile of subjective effects, including increased liking ratings and MBG (Euphoria) scores after hydromorphone administration, would be evidence that hydromorphone may indeed have increased abuse liability relative to oxycodone in chronic pain patients, and that oxycodone should be the first-line opioid prescribed over hydromorphone.

There is a second approach utilizing an ALA methodology that could potentially be used in assessing abuse liability of prescription opioids in CNMP patients. One could allow chronic pain patients to self-administer an opioid and examine usage, and perhaps patterning of self-administration. This approach of studying self-administration of drugs within a therapeutic context is not a new concept and has been used in the study of drugs including opioids for the treatment of pain (Berge 1997; Rowbotham et al. 2003; Winstead et al. 1977), benzodiazepines for the treatment of anxiety and insomnia (Roache et al. 1997; Roehrs et al. 1996, 2001; Winstead et al. 1974), and stimulants for the treatment of obesity and attention deficit hyperactivity disorder (Bigelow et al. 1980; Fredericks & Kollins 2004). I will present a brief description and results of three of these studies as exemplars of the others.

In the first study, Bigelow and colleagues (1980), using a double-blind design, randomly assigned 59 overweight women to have access to *d*-amphetamine (5 mg), fenfluramine (20 mg), or placebo. Patients were told that the usual recommended dosage of their medication was 1 capsule three times per day (before meals), but due to individual variations in sensitivity to effects and side effects they should self-regulate their own intake in the range of 0–6 capsules per day. The study period was 4 weeks. The mean number of medication capsules administered during the 4-week period did not differ across groups. However, *d*-amphetamine was used for a significantly longer time than placebo and fenfluramine. Amphetamine was considered to be a reinforcer in that it engendered a longer duration of use than placebo. Interestingly, fenfluramine was used for a significantly shorter time than placebo, indicating that it functioned as a punisher. Patients lost the most weight in the *d*-amphetamine group. The authors made two interesting comments when discussing the results: (1) "... the reinforcement effect did not result in excessive drug intake; patients were quite conservative in this regard, and no patient self-administered even as much as half of the available medication or showed a trend of progressively increasing medication intake" (p. 1123), and (2) "... [this] is in interesting contrast to the patterns of drug self-administration observed among drug abusers" (p. 1123).

Similar results were obtained in another double-blind study that examined whether alprazolam functioned as a reinforcer in anxious patients (Roache et al. 1997): During the 4-week choice phase, the patient with the greatest usage consumed an average of 4.4 alprazolam capsules per day, although the maximum per day was set at 8. The drug did function as a reinforcer in 11/14 patients (i.e., was chosen more often than placebo, which patients also had access to), and within-subject correlations between amount of alprazolam used and daily fluctuations in anxiety were significant in the majority of patients (69%). This would indicate that although the drug functioned as a reinforcer, the majority of patients were self-medicating, which in this context was appropriate. There was a 2-week sampling phase that preceded the choice phase, and alprazolam generated significantly higher liking ratings than placebo. The authors made a comment in the discussion section that is similar to what I have said earlier: "Whereas such ratings have been used to predict abuse potential in drug abusers.... it is reasonable to suggest that non-drug abusing patients may 'like' a medication perceived as 'helpful' without suggesting that they are abusing it" (p. 153).

The final study I wish to present involved the self-administration of levorphanol in patients with neuropathic pain (Rowbotham et al. 2003). The authors did not have a placebo control group because the patients in this group would have had unrelieved chronic pain. Inclusion of a control group was less of a problem in the studies with stimulants and benzodiazepines described above, but withholding an opioid in the presence of severe pain would be unethical. However, if one does not include a control group, any pain relief noted during a trial could be due to a placebo effect, however unlikely this may seem in neuropathic pain. What the authors did, realizing that opioid-induced analgesia within limits is dose-related, was to use a low dose of the opioid (0.15 mg) in one group and a higher dose (0.75 mg) in the second group. Evidence that levorphanol was responsible for lower pain scores would be shown if the high-dose group reported greater pain relief than the low-dose group, assuming that more levorphanol was consumed in the former group. Maximum number of capsules that could be administered was 7 capsules t.i.d. (i.e., total of 21 capsules per day). After a 4-week titration phase came a 4-week study period in which number of capsules, daily pain ratings, and drug subjective and side effects were assessed.

Pain reduction was significantly greater in the high-dose group, and they did consume more levorphanol, on average, than the low-dose group. Average amount of levorphanol consumed (number of capsules in parentheses) by the low- and high-dose groups were 2.7 mg per day (18.3 capsules) and 8.9 mg per day (11.9 capsules), respectively. Relative to baseline ratings, the following subjective and side effects were increased in both groups:

"dry mouth," "itchy skin," "sweating," "sleepy," "carefree," and "drunken." Patients in the high-dose group reported significantly greater effects than the low-dose group in ratings of "itchy skin," "sweating," and "skin clammy." The increased rating of "carefree" in both groups might be considered an abuse liability-related effect, but the increase was relative to baseline when pain ratings were appreciably higher than in the 4-week study period. Here again, a measure that could be considered abuse liability-related in a nonpain population cannot be interpreted as easily in this study of chronic pain patients. However, the *patterning* of opioid usage could be considered a measure of abuse liability. Abuse liability might be considered if patients reported stable ratings of pain relief throughout the 4-week study period with escalated capsule administration. (However, if patients reported increased levels of pain that preceded increased capsule intake, this could readily be interpreted as a tolerance, or inadequate dosing, issue.)

What was reported by Rowbotham and colleagues was a pattern that I would suggest is evidence of a lack of abuse: "Daily capsule intake and ratings of intensity of pain were stable during the last two weeks of therapy, suggesting that there was no tolerance in the form of a loss of analgesic efficacy that might be reflected in a rapid escalation of doses" (p. 1230). If Rowbotham had used a more comprehensive subjective effects battery, one could have also examined the relationship between subjective effects, pain levels, and capsule intake. If patients reported stable levels of pain relief but increased capsule intake with a concomitant increase in abuse liability-related subjective effects (e.g., liking ratings and MBG scores), I contend this would be evidence of levorphanol abuse in those patients who exhibited increased capsule intake.

The Rowbotham et al. (2003) study had a number of desirable design and methodological features and could serve as a template for future opioid ALA studies in CNMP patients. However, in designing future opioid ALA studies after the Rowbotham et al. (2003) model, a number of procedural modifications might be considered. In the Rowbotham et al. (2003) study, patients kept a daily record to record their intake of study capsules, their use of concomitant medications, and their daily pain on a VAS. Patients were phoned every 7–14 days so that compliance and safety could be monitored. There is still the possibility that patients were not filling out the diary on a daily basis. Compliance might be enhanced in several ways, including paging patients every day and asking them to transmit their information via telephone (or in a diary). Timing of capsule administration could be estimated via bottles equipped with a computer chip to register the date and time of each bottle opening (see Roache et al. 1997). However, even with the use of special bottles that record instances of bottle opening, patients could conceivably be giving the opioid to another person or throwing away the opioid. To determine whether patients are taking their prescribed opioids, testing for opioids in the urine could be done. Rowbotham et al. (2003) did assess presence of opioids in the urine at the end of the 4-week study phase, but results of this assessment were not reported in the paper. More frequent urine testing would also be recommended, not just to assess for presence of the prescribed opioid but also to assess for inappropriate drug usage (e.g., cocaine, nonprescribed opioid medications; Katz & Fanciullo 2002; Katz et al. 2003). It might also be of benefit if a system were developed to prompt patients to rate their pain every time they took their prescribed opioid. In this way, one could do a more molecular analysis of self-administration of opioids in the context of pain. However, with this more molecular analysis, one would have to come up with criteria indicative of prescription opioid abuse or misuse. This could be a challenge as many patients are told to take their prescription opioids on an around-the-clock basis (i.e., timed schedule; Nicholson 2003; Savage 1999). Therefore, a patient taking an opioid when pain levels are low would not necessarily be abusing or misusing the opioid. In the Rowbotham et al. study (2003), patients filled out the variant of the SDQ three times during the 4-week study period. However, more frequent assessments of subjective and side effects could be built into a self-administration study design. Also, perhaps ALA measures should include aberrant behaviors that are described in other chapters in this volume. In the beginning of this section, I listed one research avenue that might be explored in ALA of prescription opioids in CNMP patients, i.e., assessing the relative abuse liability of one opioid versus another (in my example, hydromorphone versus oxycodone). In closing, I would like to present another research avenue for consideration. One axiom of assessing the abuse liability of a drug is that abuse liability is not an inherent property of a drug but can be modulated by a whole host of factors, including organismic and environmental variables (Falk & Feingold 1987; Johanson 1990; Schuster 1989). The simplest example is psychotropic drug use history: Opioid abusers exhibit more and greater abuse liability-related effects when administered an opioid than people with a much lighter history of recreational use of drugs, including opioids. In other words, history of opioid abuse should be considered as a risk factor for subsequent (or continued) abuse.

There are many other potential risk factors that might predispose a CNMP patient to abuse prescription opioids. Some of the risk factors come from studies that retrospectively examine chart reviews of patients on long-term opioid therapy and assess whether there are variables that are related to abuse of the opioid (as evidenced by aberrant behaviors; see Passik et al. 2006). Several risk factors have been identified, including drug or alcohol abuse, mental health disorders, gender, younger age, cigarette use, duration and dose of the prescribed opioids, number of adverse effects from the opioids, and family history of substance abuse (Michna et al. 2004; Reid et al. 2002; Simoni-Wastila & Strickler 2004). A complementary approach is to examine these risk factors in ALA studies. For example, one could investigate whether CNMP patients who are dependent on tobacco and are on long-term prescription opioid therapy show a greater degree of abuse liability-related behaviors than nonsmoking patients. If so, this is evidence from a novel methodology that would bolster and complement the results from the retrospective chart survey studies. One can be more confident that a certain variable functions as a risk factor if the use of different approaches produces the same conclusion.

Future Directions

In this chapter, I have discussed how ALA might be done in CNMP patients, and why ALA should be done in this population. Such studies will be challenging to do because "the devil is in the details" and there are many details to be considered. Designing and conducting ALA studies in CNMP patients would be best served by multidisciplinary collaborations. Abuse liability researchers need to listen to pain researchers, pain clinicians, and to addiction medicine specialists who deal with CNMP patients and issues on an everyday basis to better understand critical research questions that need to be addressed. By the same token, pain researchers, pain clinicians, and addiction medicine specialists need to talk to abuse liability researchers to determine what ALA methodology might provide the most meaningful data when addressing a given research question. These collaborative efforts have the potential to open up a novel area of potentially fruitful research that to a large extent remains untapped today.

References

Balster RL, Bigelow GE (2003) Guidelines and methodological issues concerning drug abuse liability assessment. *Drug Alcohol Depend* 70(3 Suppl):S13–S40.

Bell JR (1997) Australian trends in opioid prescribing for non-cancer pain, 1986–1996. *Med J Aust* 167:26–29.

Berge TI (1997) Pattern of self-administered paracetamol and codeine analgesic consumption after third-molar surgery. *Acta Odontol Scand* 55:270–276.

Bigelow GE, Griffiths RR, Liebson I, Kaliszak JE (1980) Double-blind evaluation of reinforcing and anorectic actions of weight control medications. *Arch Gen Psychiatry* 37:1118–1123.

Borgbjerg FM, Nielsen K, Franks J (1996) Experimental pain stimulates respiration and attenuates morphine-induced respiratory depression: a controlled study in human volunteers. *Pain* 64:123–128.

Brands B, Blake J, Sproule B, Gourlay D, Busto U (2004) Prescription opioid abuse in patients presenting for methadone maintenance treatment. *Drug Alcohol Depend* 73:199–207.

Caudill-Slosberg MA, Schwartz LM, Woloshin S (2004) Office visits and analgesic prescriptions for musculoskeletal pain in US: 1980 vs. 2000. *Pain* 109:514–519.

Chabal C, Erjavec MK, Jacobson L, Mariano A, Chaney E (1997) Prescription opiate abuse in chronic pain patients: clinical criteria, incidence, and predictors. *Clin J Pain* 13:150–155.

Colpaert FC, Tarayre JP, Alliaga M, Bruins Slot LA, Attal N, Koek W (2001) Opiate self-administration as a measure of chronic nociceptive pain in arthritic rats. *Pain* 91:33–45.

Coniam SW (1989) Prescribing opioids for chronic pain in non-malignant disease. In: RG Twycross (ed.), *The Edinburgh Symposium on Pain Control and Medical Education. Royal Society of Medicine International Congress and Symposium Series*. London: Royal Society of Medicine; 149:205–210.

Conley KM, Toledano AY, Apfelbaum JL, Zacny JP (1997) The modulating effects of a cold water stimulus on opioid effects in volunteers. *Psychopharmacology* 131:313–320.

Cowan DT, Allan L, Griffiths P (2002) A pilot study into the problematic use of opioid analgesics in chronic noncancer pain patients. *Int J Nursing Stud* 39:59–69.

Cowan DT, Wilson-Barnett J, Griffiths P, Allan LG (2003) A survey of chronic noncancer pain patients prescribed opioid analgesics. *Pain Med* 4:340–351.

Dib B, Duclaux R (1982) Intracerebroventricular self-injection of morphine in response to pain in the rat. *Pain* 13:395–406.

Eissenberg T, Riggins EC 3rd, Harkins SW, Weaver MF (2000) A clinical laboratory model for direct assessment of medication-induced antihyperalgesia and subjective effects: initial validation study. *Exp Clin Psychopharmacol* 8:47–60.

The Expert Panel (2003) Abuse liability assessment of CNS drugs: conclusions, recommendations, and research priorities. *Drug Alcohol Depend* 70:S107–S114.

Falk JL, Feingold DA (1987) Environmental and cultural factors in the behavioral actions of drugs. In: HY Meltzer (ed.), *Psychopharmacology: The Third Generation of Progress.*New York: Raven Press; 1503–1509.

Fishbain DA, Rosomoff HL, Rosomoff RS (1992) Drug abuse, dependence, and addiction in chronic pain patients. *Clin J Pain* 8:77–85.

Fraser HF, van Horn GD, Martin WR, Wolbach AB, Isbell H (1961) Methods for evaluating addiction liability. (a) "attitude" of opiate addicts toward opiate-like drugs, (b) a short-term "direct" addiction test. *J Pharmacol Exp Ther* 133:371–387.

Fredericks EM, Kollins SH (2004) Assessing methylphenidate preference in ADHD patients using a choice procedure. *Psychopharmacology* 175:391–398.

Griffiths RR, Bigelow GE, Ator NA (2003) Principles of initial experimental drug abuse liability assessment in humans. *Drug Alcohol Depend* 70(3 Suppl):S41–S54.

Hanks GW, Twycross RG, Lloyd JW (1981) Unexpected complication of successful nerve block. Morphine induced respiratory depression precipitated by removal of severe pain. *Anaesthesia* 36:37–39.

Hill JE, Haertzen CA, Wolbach AB, Miner EJ (1963) The Addiction Research Center Inventory: standardization of scales which evaluate subjective effects of morphine, amphetamine, pentobarbital, alcohol, LSD-25, pyrahexyl and chlorpromazine. *Psychopharmacologia* 4:167–183.

Himmelsbach CK (1942) Clinical studies of drug addiction. Physical dependence, withdrawal and recovery. *Arch Int Med* 69:766–772.

Himmelsbach CK (1943) Further studies of the addiction liability of Demerol. *J Pharmacol Exp Ther* 75:5–9.

Jasinski DR (1977) Assessment of the abuse potentiality of morphine-like drugs (methods used in man). In: WR Martin (ed.), H*andbook of Experimental Pharmacology, Volume 45/I. Drug Addiction I: Morphine, Sedative Hypnotic and Alcohol Dependence.* Heidelberg, West Germany: Springer Verlag; 197–258.

Johanson CE (1990) Behavioural pharmacology, drug abuse, and the future. *Behavioural Pharmacology* 1:385–393.

Kamboj SK, Tookman A, Jones L, Curran HV (2005) The effects of immediate-release morphine on cognitive functioning in patients receiving chronic opioid therapy in palliative care. *Pain* 117:388–395.

Kaplan HL, Busto UE, Baylon GJ, Cheung SW, Otton SV, Somer G, Sellers EM (1997) Inhibition of cytochrome P450 2D6 metabolism of hydrocodone to hydromorphone does not importantly affect abuse liability. *J Pharmacol Exp Ther* 281:103–108.

Kassebaum G, Chandler SM (1994) Polydrug use and self control among men and women in prisons. *J Drug Educ* 24:333–350.

Katz N, Fanciullo GJ (2002) Role of urine toxicology testing in the management of chronic opioid therapy. *Clin J Pain* 18(4 Suppl):76–82.

Katz NP, Sherburne S, Beach M, Rose RJ, Vielguth J, Bradley J, Fanciullo GJ (2003) Behavioral monitoring and urine toxicology testing in patients receiving long-term opioid therapy. *Anesth Analg* 97:1097–1102.

Kleber HD (1989) Drug abuse liability testing: human subjects issues. In: MW Fischman, NK Mello (eds.), *Testing for Abuse Liability of Drugs in Humans.* Rockville, MD: NIDA Research Monograph No. 92, DHHS publication number (ADM) 89–1613, pp. 341–356.

Lasagna L, von Felsinger JM, Beecher HK (1955) Drug-induced mood changes in man. *J Amer Med Assoc* 157:1006–1020.

Leri F, Bruneau J, Stewart J (2003) Understanding polydrug use: review of heroin and cocaine co-use. *Addiction* 98:7–22.

Mahowald ML, Singh JA, Majeski O (2005) Opioid use by patients in an orthopedics spine clinic. *Arthritis Rheum* 52:312–321.

Marsch LA, Bickel WK, Badger GJ, Rathmell JP, Swedberg MD, Jonzon B, Norsten-Hoog C (2001) Effects of infusion rate of intravenously administered morphine on physiological, psychomotor, and self-reported measures in humans. *J Pharmacol Exp Ther* 299:1056–1065.

Martin WR, Sloan JW, Sapira JD, Jasinski DR (1971) Physiologic, subjective, and behavioral effects of amphetamine, methamphetamine, ephedrine, phenmetrazine, and methylphenidate in man. *Clin Pharmacol Ther* 12:245–258.

Michna E, Ross EK, Hynes WL, Nedeljkovic SS, Soumekh A, Janfaza D, Palombi D, Jamison RN (2004) Predicting aberrant drug behavior in patients treated for chronic pain: importance of abuse history. *J Pain Symptom Manage* 28:250–258.

Moulin DE, Iezzi A (1996) Randomised trial of oral morphine for chronic non-cancer pain. *Lancet* 347:143–147.

Nicholson B (2003) Responsible prescribing of opioids for the management of chronic pain. *Drugs* 63:17–32.

Oliveto AH, Feingold A, Schottenfeld R, Jatlow P, Kosten TR (1999) Desipramine in opioid-dependent cocaine abusers maintained on buprenorphine vs. methadone. *Arch Gen Psychiatry*56:812–820.

Passik SD (2001) Responding rationally to recent reports of abuse/diversion of OxyContin® [Letter to the editor]. *J Pain Symptom Manage* 21:359–360.

Passik SD, Kirsh KL, Donaghy KB, Portenoy RK (2006) Pain and aberrant drug-related behaviors on medically ill patients with and without histories of substance abuse. *Clin J Pain* 22:173–181.

Petry NM, Bickel WK, Huddleston J, Tzanis E, Badger GJ (1998) A comparison of subjective, psychomotor and physiological effects of a novel muscarinic analgesic, LY297802 tartrate, and oral morphine in occasional drug users. *Drug Alcohol Depend* 50:129–136.

Portenoy RK, Foley KM (1986) Chronic use of opioid analgesics in non-malignant pain: report of 38 cases. *Pain* 25:171–186.

Preston KL, Bigelow GE, Liebson AL (1985) Self-administration of clonidine, oxazepam, and hydromorphone by patients undergoing methadone detoxification. *Clin Pharmacol Ther* 38:219–227.

Reid MC, Engles-Horton LL, Weber MB, Kerns RD, Rogers EL, O'Connor PG (2002) Use of opioid medications for chronic noncancer pain syndromes in primary care. *J Gen Intern Med* 17:173–179.

Roache JD, Stanley MA, Creson DR, Shah NN, Meisch RA (1997) Alprazolam-reinforced medication use in outpatients with anxiety. *Drug Alcohol Depend* 45:143–155.

Roehrs T, Bonahoom A, Pedrosi B, Rosenthal L, Roth T (2001) Treatment regimen and hypnotic self-administration. *Psychopharmacology* 155:11–17.

Roehrs T, Pedrosi B, Rosenthal L, Roth T (1996) Hypnotic self administration and dose escalation. *Psychopharmacology* 127:150–154.

Rowbotham MC, Twilling L, Davies PS, Reisner L, Taylor K, Mohr D (2003) Oral opioid therapy for chronic peripheral and central neuropathic pain. *N Engl J Med* 348:1223–1232.

Savage S (1999) Opioid therapy of chronic pain: assessment of consequences. *Acta Anaesthesiol Scand* 43:909–917.

Schuster CR (1989) Does treatment of cancer pain with narcotics produce junkies? In: CS Hill, WS Fields (eds.), *Advances in Pain Research and Therapy, Vol. 11: Drug Treatment of Cancer Pain in a Drug-Oriented Society*. New York: Raven Press, Ltd.; 1–3.

Schuster CR, Henningfield J (2003) Conference on abuse liability assessment of CNS drugs. *Drug Alcohol Depend* 70:S1–S4.

Simoni-Wastila L, Strickler G (2004) Risk factors associated with problem use of prescription drugs. *Am J Public Health* 94:266–268.

Tassain V, Attal N, Fletcher D, Brasseur L, Degieux P, Chauvin M, Bouhassira D (2003) Long term effects of oral sustained release morphine on neuropsychological performance in patients with chronic non-cancer pain. *Pain* 104:389–400.

Turk DC, Brody MC (1992) What position do APS's physicians take on chronic opioid therapy? *Am Pain Soc Bull* 2:1–5.

Vaccarino AL, Marek P, Kest B, Ben-Eliyahu S, Couret LC Jr, Kao B, Liebeskind JC (1993) Morphine fails to produce tolerance when administered in the presence of formalin pain in rats. *Brain Res* 627:287–290.

Winstead DK, Anderson A, Eilers MK, Blackwell B, Zaremba AL (1974) Diazepam on demand: drug-seeking behavior in psychiatric inpatients. *Arch Gen Psychiatry* 30:349–351.

Winstead DK, Parker M, Willi FJP (1977) Propoxyphene on demand: analgesic-seeking behavior in psychiatric patients. *Arch Gen Psychiatry* 34:1463–1468.

Wolff HG, Hardy JD, Goodell H (1940) Studies on pain: measurement of the effect of morphine, codeine, and other opiates on the pain threshold and an analysis of their relation to the pain experience. *J Clin Invest* 19:659–680.

Zacny J, Bigelow G, Compton P, Foley K, Iguchi M, Sannerud C (2003) College on problems of drug dependence taskforce on prescription opioid non-medical use and abuse: position statement. *Drug Alcohol Depend* 69:215–232.

Zacny JP, Gutierrez S (2003) Characterizing the subjective, psychomotor, and physiological effects of oral oxycodone in non-drug-abusing volunteers. *Psychopharmacology* 170:242–254.

Zacny JP, McKay MA, Toledano AY, Marks S, Young CJ, Klock PA, Apfelbaum JL (1996) The effects of a cold-water immersion stressor on the reinforcing and subjective effects of an opioid in healthy volunteers. *Drug Alcohol Depend* 42:133–142.

Zacny JP, Walker EA (1998) Behavioral pharmacology of opiates. In: RE Tartar, RT Ammerman, PJ Ott (eds.), *Handbook of Substance Abuse: Neurobehavioral Pharmacology*. New York: Plenum Press; 343–362.

50

Aberrant Behavior and Drug Abuse Treatment in Pain Patients

Peggy Compton

Although the safety and efficacy of daily opioid therapy for the treatment of chronic nonmalignant pain (CNMP) is increasingly demonstrated in large clinical trials and across multiple indicators (Finnerup et al., 2005; Kalso et al., 2004; Maier et al., 2002), concerns persist about the provision of this class of drugs with high abuse potential to individuals on a long-term basis (Ballentyne & Mao, 2003; Foley, 2003; McQuay, 2001; Von Korff & Deyo, 2004). Both retrospective reports from known addicts and clinician experience with patients requiring pain medication suggest that addiction is a potential outcome of opioid analgesic therapy and a source of drug-seeking behaviors. The potential for developing opioid tolerance or hyperalgesia (Chu et al., 2004) notwithstanding, concerns about causing or supporting addiction via the provision of chronic ongoing opioids for the treatment of pain are reflected at clinical, legal, and political levels (Gilson & Joranson, 2002; Morgan, 1985–1986).

Unfortunately, empirical data are sparse on the incidence, presentation, and outcome of opioid addiction in the patients on chronic opioid analgesic therapy for the treatment of CNMP. In the extant clinical trial literature, pain patients deemed at high risk for medication abuse tend to be excluded from study participation, or dropped for reasons of "medication noncompliance." In a busy clinical environment and under the scrutiny of state medical boards and the Drug Enforcement Agency, clinicians are motivated to be conservative in their prescription of opioids for chronic pain, and to limit treatment in cases in which medication abuse is perceived to be a problem. Estimates of the prevalence of addiction in this patient population is further complicated because within the context of chronic pain and sanctioned opioid access, known indicators of addiction become less diagnostic (Miotto et al., 1996; Sees & Clark, 1993). Clinicians have tended to rely on the presence of certain aberrant medication use behaviors (i.e., drug seeking, use of multiple providers, escalated use) as evidence of addictive disease, yet the limitations of these to do so are less well-understood.

Yet, it is critical that when present, addictive disease be correctly identified and aggressively managed in the patient with CNMP. Addiction is a disease with high rates of morbidity and mortality, thus recognizing the presence of the disorder is critical in all patient populations. Importantly, identification of the disease allows for the consideration and implementation of addiction treatment strategies in pain treatment, thus improving both pain and addiction outcomes. This chapter will review relationships between aberrant medication use behaviors and the disease of addiction, suggest a clinical algorithm for approaching pain patients with aberrant behaviors, and consider principles of treatment for addictive disease in the patient with CNMP and on ongoing opioid therapy.

Addiction in Chronic Pain Patients on Opioid Therapy

Over the past decade, it has become clear that the standard psychiatric diagnostic criteria used for diagnosing for addiction (or *substance dependence,* as defined in the fourth edition of the *Diagnostic and Statistical Manual* in the general population (*DSM-IV*; American Psychiatric Association, 2004) are inadequate or imprecise for identifying the same in an individual on chronic opioid therapy for the treatment of pain. Firstly, imbedded in these criteria are two commonly used terms that are often confused with and/or considered indicative of addiction, but are not equivalent to true addictive disease. Both *physical dependence,* the development of a drug-specific withdrawal syndrome on the abrupt cessation of the drug effects, and *tolerance,* or a diminution of drug effect over time, are neuroadaptive states resulting from chronic opioid exposure. These are expected physiologic responses in any individual exposed to continuous opioid administration, regardless of addiction status. Accumulating evidence suggests that physical dependence and tolerance to opioids may actually develop to a lesser degree in individuals with pain than those without pain, again making these diagnostic criteria less reliable in the population with chronic pain (Vaccarino & Couret, 1993; Vaccarino et al., 1993).

Strict adherence to the *DSM-IV* criteria (APA, 2004) can result in other diagnostic errors. Not only can the presence of tolerance and/or physical dependence result in false-positive cases, continued opioid use by the patient despite a sincere desire to cut down or stop may also be evident in nonaddicted pain patients (Sees & Clark, 1993). On the other hand, actual cases of addictive disease may be missed secondary to the sanctioned, legal, and relatively unscrutinized access to opioids provided pain patients. Perhaps most importantly, significant clinical overlap exists between the functional deficits of patients who suffer ongoing pain and those who suffer active addiction, making the latter difficult to distinguish from the former in this patient population.

In response to the diagnostic confusion and challenges inherent in determining whether a patient with chronic pain and taking opioid analgesics is, in fact, addicted to the analgesic medications, the American Society of Addiction Medicine, the American Academy of Pain Medicine (AAPM) and the American Pain Society issued a consensus statement in 2001, proposing a definition for addiction specific to assessing the use of opioids in the context of pain treatment:

> *Addiction* in the context of pain treatment with opioids is characterized by a persistent pattern of dysfunctional opioid use that may involve any or all of the following:
>
> - adverse consequences associated with the use of opioids
> - loss of control over use of opioids
> - preoccupation with obtaining opioids, despite the presence of adequate analgesia (AAPM, 2001)

Impressive are how well these criteria capture the critical behavioral elements of addictive disease (inability to control use, use despite harm, preoccupation with use or craving); these are present in all cases of the disease, even those complicated by pain and regular opioid use.

Importance of Addiction Assessment in Chronic Pain Patients on Opioid Therapy

Reported prevalence rates of addictive disease in samples of chronic pain patients vary widely depending on the clinical setting and the measure(s) of addiction utilized, leaving the pain clinician unsure of the frequency with which addiction to pain medications will occur in practice. Best estimates indicate that the rate of addiction in chronic pain patients mirrors the lifetime prevalence of the disease in society in general, and averages around 10% (Clark, 2002; Fishbain, 1996; Fishbain et al., 1992). These data suggest that known risk factors for addiction in the general population should be good predictors for problematic prescription opioid use in patients with CNMP, and include a positive history of early substance use, a personal or family history of substance abuse, and the presence of comorbid psychiatric disorders (DeWitt et al., 2000). Population-based risk estimates for addictive disease in pain patients on chronic opioid therapy are likewise difficult to ascertain as exposure rates to opioid therapy in pain patients are clinically truncated, and inconsistency persists in the measurement or identification of true cases of addiction.

Precision in case identification is critical in the case of addictive disease due to its profound, negative, and wide-reaching effects on patient health outcomes. As with any progressive chronic disease, addiction has a pathological basis, known risk factors, and a predictable course that, if left untreated, results in high rates of morbidity and untimely death. Beyond the direct pathophysiologic and pharmacologic effects of drugs of abuse, active addiction interferes with the successful medical management of all diseases or health problems suffered by the patient, in that its behavioral symptoms preclude active and/or adequate participation in a therapeutic regimen. Active addiction not only complicates, but thwarts, therapy provided for any concurrent health condition, including pain (i.e., Passik & Theobald, 2000; Trafton et al., 2004).

Beyond individual outcomes, addiction is a significant public health problem in this country. In a classic evaluation on the true causes of death in the United States, McGinnis and Foege (1993) named the abuse of alcohol and illicit drugs as among the top 10 causes of death in our country, and the document "Healthy People 2010" listed substance abuse as 4th of 10 U.S. leading public health indicators (U.S. Department of Health and Human Services, 2000). The health consequences of addiction extend beyond direct medical sequelae to include such problems as unintentional injury (especially motor vehicle accidents), the spread of infectious disease (HIV/AIDS, hepatitis); disruptions of family life, household roles/responsibilities; domestic violence, sexual assault, suicide and homicide (Robert Wood Johnson Foundation, 2001). Costs related to substance abuse, including treatment, prevention, health care, lost productivity, crime, and social welfare, were most recently estimated to be $160 billion ($315 billion if alcohol was included), 46% of which is borne by government, and the other 44% borne by patients themselves (Office of Drug Control Policy, 2001).

Thus, addiction is a prevalent, costly, and ultimately lethal disease, and prevents the provision of effective health care, both at the level of the individual and society at large. It is therefore not only incumbent upon the clinician, but imperative, that he or she assess for and diagnose addictive disease in all patients, and especially those at increased risk due to the provision of chronic opioid therapy for the relief of CNMP (see Cohen et al., 2002). Not only do these patients have easy access and repeated exposure to potent and abused medications, but, related to the mixed presentation of untreated addiction and unrelieved chronic pain, are likely to mis- or underdiagnosed as addicted. This is an unique clinical situation, in that opioids are prescribed for a health condition that in and of itself can mask or misrepresent the typical indicators of addiction, while failing to recognize its presence will have devastating consequences for the overall health of the patient.

Aberrant Behaviors in Chronic Pain Patients on Opioid Therapy

As described in Chapter 6, "Basic Science of Addiction," addiction is a disease of behavior, and the *DSM-IV* criteria upon which the diagnosis is made rely almost exclusively on patient behaviors that would otherwise be considered aberrant or dysfunctional (i.e., failure to fulfill major role obligation, recurrent use in hazardous situations, recurrent legal, social or interpersonal problems, large amounts of time spent in activities related to use; APA, 1994). Similarly, in the context of chronic pain treatment, addiction is diagnosed by the presence of certain observable patient behaviors considered aberrant. For example, "behaviors suggestive of addiction" identified in the AAPM consensus statement (2001) include an inability to adhere to the prescription schedule, insistence on certain forms or routes of medication, and resistance to other nonopiate treatments.

Identification of aberrant behaviors as risk factors for predicting the occurrence of addiction in this population has been the subject of much scholarly discourse over the past decade, and expert clinicians are actively engaged in identifying those in chronic pain patients (Adams et al., 2004; Butler et al., 2004; Michna et al., 2004; Passik et al., 2004; Robinson et al., 2001). In an early paper describing the medication use behaviors of addicted pain patients, Wesson and colleagues (1993) advised that patients with a pattern of frequent medication loss, who request for specific opioids drugs, who are unable to bring in available/unused opioids from home, and who continue abuse of alcohol and street drugs should be considered at high risk for having addictive disease. These and others have been subsequently identified in the literature, and consensus is growing about those which can be considered more or less predictive.

The concurrent validity of specific behaviors associated with addiction in chronic pain patients was examined within the assessment framework proposed by Miotto and colleagues (1996), which evaluates the pain patient along five domains to determine if the disease is present. In addition to considering the patient's description of the pain syndrome, the following were evaluated: social and/or family factors sustaining use, family/patient history of substance abuse, psychiatric history, and opiate analgesic use patterns. Preliminary testing of the model in a sample of patients identified as having "problematic" substance use behaviors (i.e., drug seeking, medication hoarding, doctor shopping, frequent ER visits) found that there were significant differences between those behaviors endorsed by nonaddicted pain patients and those diagnosed as addicted by an addiction medicine specialist. Specifically, addicted patients were more likely to report behaviors evidencing *impaired control* over medication their use and to evidence *compulsive patterns* of use (see Table 50.1). Of note is that the addicted pain patients rarely reported engaging in illegal activities (prescription forgery, buying on street) to obtain drug, presumably due to legal opioid access (Compton et al., 1998).

Impaired Control/Compulsive Use

Consistent with these findings and the AAPM consensus statement (2001), behaviors that reflect poorly controlled and/or compulsive medication use are appreciated as indicators of addiction in pain patients. In their Prescription Abuse Checklist, Chabal and colleagues (1997) focused on medication-related behaviors, and suggest that patterns of early refills or escalating drug use in the absence of clinical change and prescription "problems" (e.g., lost, spilled, stolen medications), as well as utilizing supplemental sources of opiates as evidence of addiction in this patient population.

Likewise, behaviors more or less indicative of aberrancy as described by Kirsh et al. (2002)—including drug hoarding during periods of reduced symptoms, acquisition of similar drugs from other medical sources, concurrent abuse of related illicit drugs, multiple unsanctioned dose escalations, stealing or borrowing drugs from others, and obtaining prescription drugs from nonmedical sources—all reflect compulsive and poorly controlled medication use patterns. Savage (2002) identified behaviors indicative of impaired control over use and compulsive use as reports of lost or stolen prescription or medications, frequent early renewal requests, urgent calls or unscheduled visits, abusing other drugs or alcohol, the inability to produce other medications on request, and opioid withdrawal noted on clinic visits. Behaviors common across these analyses that suggest poorly controlled and compulsive medication use are listed in Table 50.2.

Preoccupation With Opioid Use

Another class of behaviors identified as evidence for addiction in patients with chronic pain includes those that reflect a preoccupation with obtaining opioids, a concern which may persist even in the presence of patient-reported adequate analgesia. Such behaviors were of central interest in the analyses of Chabal and colleagues (1997), who considered an overwhelming focus on opiate issues during clinic visits that persisted beyond the third appointment, and/or to the degree that it impeded progress with other treatment issues, as a strong indicator of the disease. Similarly, Kirsh et al. (2002) and Savage (2002) add that the following are reflective of an inappropriate fixation on the abused substance: aggressive complaining about the need for higher doses during office visits, missing appointments unless opioid renewal is expected, unwillingness to try nonopioid treatments, an inability to tolerate nonopioid medications, requests for formulations with high reward, and reporting that only opioids provide pain relief (see Table 50.2).

Challenges to Assessing Addiction in Chronic Pain Patients

Thus, consistent with the AAPM 2001 consensus criteria, aberrant behaviors that reflect (1) an inability to control use, (2) compulsive use, and (3) an overwhelming preoccupation with use, are those that are highly suggestive of addiction. Yet the presence of these "drug-seeking" behaviors is not diagnostic, and must clearly be considered within the context of the pain condition, patient history, psychiatric status, and family and social issues. Pain patients often seek medication for legitimate or appropriate reasons. The distinction between appropriate drug seeking and addiction is clear in the case of drugs without psychoactive effect (e.g., insulin, antibiotics, nonopioid analgesics), but becomes less apparent when an opioid analgesic is sought by the patient, regardless of the apparent validity of the complaint.

Patients in pain may take what appear to be extraordinary steps to ensure adequate medication supply but, rather than indicating addictive disease, may in fact be appropriate responses to

Table 50.1. Aberrant Behaviors Occurring More Frequently in Addicted Versus Nonaddicted Chronic Pain Patients or Opioid Therapy ($p < 0.05$)

Impaired Control	Compulsive Use
Use of multiple prescription providers	Independently and rapidly increasing analgesic dose/frequency
Patterns of early prescription refills	Uses of analgesics for nonpain symptoms
Emergency room visits for analgesics	Saving or hoarding unused medication
	Supplementing with alcohol/psychoactive drugs
	Having a route of administration preference

Source: Compton et al., 1988.

Table 50.2. Aberrant Behaviors Associated With Addiction in Chronic Pain Patients on Opioid Therapy

Impaired Control/Compulsive Use	Preoccupation With Use
Escalation of medication use in absence of increased pathology/clinician sanction	Unwillingness to try nonopioid treatments; reporting that only opioids provide pain relief
Patterns of lost/stolen prescriptions	Missing appointments unless opioid renewal is expected
Use of supplemental sources to obtain medication	Inability to tolerate nonopioid medications
Concurrent use of alcohol or illicit drugs	Overwhelming, ongoing focus on opiate issues during clinic visits

either poorly or well-relieved pain. In the case of inadequate analgesia, drug-seeking behaviors arise when a patient cannot obtain tolerable relief with the prescribed dose of analgesic and seeks alternate sources or increased doses of analgesic, a phenomenon termed *pseudoaddiction* (Weissman & Haddox, 1989). Alternately, patients receiving good pain relief may evidence drug-seeking behaviors because they, understandably, fear not only the reemergence of pain but perhaps also the emergence of withdrawal symptoms. Rather than indicative of addictive disease, such behaviors, termed *therapeutic dependence,* are actually efforts of an anxious patient to maintain a tolerable level of comfort. Similar behavior may be seen in patients with "brittle" diabetes who take insulin or in patients with angina who take nitroglycerin, but because neither medication is addictive, it's accepted or even welcomed as an indication that the patient is concerned about his or her health.

Ultimately, the best behavioral indicator of addiction in the chronic pain patient is a failure to evidence functional improvement despite an otherwise adequate trial of opioid therapy. As noted, addiction is a disease characterized by behaviors that preclude optimal functioning in multiple life domains (i.e., vocational work, family relationships, recreational and leisure activities), and as long as the disease is active and untreated, functional deterioration will continue. In fact, the inability to fulfill expected roles and obligations secondary to drug use is the first of the *DSM-IV* criteria utilized for the diagnosis of substance use disorders.

Similarly, unrelieved chronic pain results in analogous functional deficits or limitations. Rarely does chronic pain treatment result in the patient becoming entirely pain-free; meaningful primary outcome indicators of treatment efficacy focus on the ability of the patient to participate in activities of daily living and carry out his or her role function in social, family, and vocational domains to an acceptable degree. With respect to chronic pain treatment, functional restoration is operationalized as improvements in the patient's physical capabilities, psychological intactness, family and social interactions, and degree of health-care utilization.

Thus, it would be expected that if opioid therapy were effective in treating chronic pain, improvements in functioning would be enjoyed. Yet, as noted above, patients suffering addiction, whether in pain or not, are by definition limited their ability to engage in behaviors consistent with successful role function. In the face of active addiction, opioid analgesic provision will not lead to improved functional outcome, and if allowed to run its natural course, further deterioration will occur. Clinical studies have supported that analgesic abuse in CNMP patients is associated with failure in an improvement of pain symptoms (Ciccone et al., 2000; Dunbar & Katz, 1996).

Diagnostic Approach to Assessment

Suggested is an approach to the patient with chronic pain who evidences behaviors described as aberrant with respect to his or her use of the medication (see Figure 50.1). As noted, these are "drug-seeking" behaviors that can reflect an inability to control drug use, compulsive patterns of drug use, and inordinate concern over drug prescription. The algorithm is designed to assist the clinician in determining whether a chronic pain patient on opioid therapy and exhibiting drug-seeking behavior suffers from addiction or not (Compton & Estepa, 2000).

To rule out pseudoaddiction and therapeutic dependence in patients who appear drug seeking, it is important to consider these behaviors as evidence of unrelieved pain or anxiety until proven otherwise. After investigating new or additive sources of pain, a

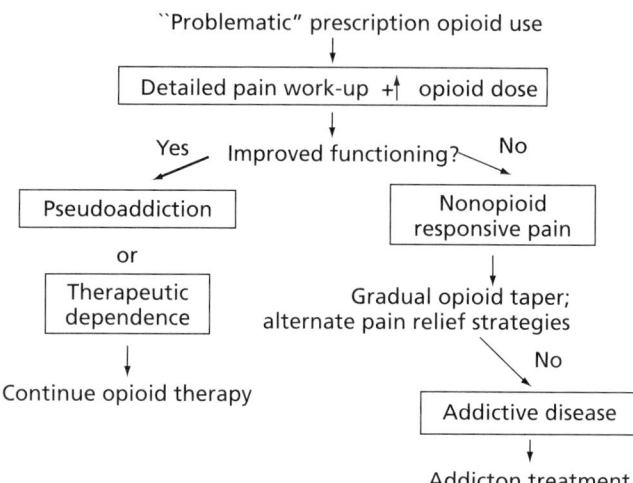

Figure 50.1. Algorithm for the evaluation of drug-seeking behaviors in chronic pain patients on opioid maintenance.

trial of increased opioid dose and/or provision of an extra, "safety," prescription should be initiated. If the drug-seeking behavior ceases and functioning improves with the provision of additional opioid, addiction can be safely ruled out. If, on the other hand, the patient's drug seeking behavior continues and functioning does not improve despite best efforts at provision of opioid analgesia, consultation with a pain specialist is indicated. It may be that the type or nature of the pain suffered by the patient is not opioid responsive, and will require alternate interventional approaches. If properly supported, patients without addiction are unlikely to refuse changes in treatment strategy (including opioid taper) in the hope of experiencing improved pain relief. Worrisome is if the patient strongly resists opioid discontinuation or is noncompliant with nonopioid pain relief strategies; coupled with unimproved functioning, the presence of addictive disease becomes evident.

Reflecting the AAPM consensus criteria (2001), this approach can elicit behaviors that reflect both a loss of control over use of opioids and a preoccupation with obtaining opioids. Provision of supplemental opioids to an addicted pain patient will result in dose escalation and a need for early refills; by definition, the addict cannot control or limit his or her medication use, and increased access will result in increased use. Preoccupation with opioids will be evident in the addict's resistance to try nonopioid therapies, and as mentioned above, his or her concern about maintaining an opioid supply will be greater than that for pain relief. Although the clinician runs the short-term risk of being "duped" by a drug-seeking addict by increasing opioid access, the benefits gained by improving pain relief and/or identifying addictive disease are significant.

Addiction Treatment for the Chronic Pain Patient on Opioid Therapy

Providing effective addiction treatment for the pain patient on opioid therapy is complicated by the relatively institutionalized separation between service delivery for pain and for addiction. Pain specialists typically work from a medical model and focus on neurological contributions to the pain experience, whereas addiction treatment is housed within the domain of psychiatry and is, in fact, often marginalized from the other psychiatric services. In the real world, this separation of the two specialties translates into patients in pain clinics receiving suboptimal addiction services, and those in addiction clinics receiving suboptimal pain treatment, if at all (Jamison et al., 2000; Rosenblum et al., 2003). Few settings are staffed and resourced to provide the integrated care required by these patients.

Optimal treatment for these patients is further limited in that potential interventions remain untested and are only recently becoming the subject of empirical investigation. Too often, patients with chronic pain are discharged from pain treatment when addiction is identified or suspected, thus the efficacy of addiction treatment for these patients becomes a moot issue. Suggested below are several principles upon which to base addiction treatment for the chronic pain patient on opioid therapy.

Firstly, the best treatment for addiction is the *prevention of addiction*. When initiating or formalizing opioid treatment, both the clinician and patient are encouraged to approach addiction as an infrequent but potential adverse effect of opioid therapy. A treatment agreement or contract is recommended, but is best utilized as a vehicle for teaching the patient about appropriate patterns of medication use and how to self-identify behaviors that are associated with addictive medication use. Discussion should move beyond urine toxicology testing (which suggests a punitive approach) to include definitions and concrete empirical indicators of compulsivity and impaired control, so that patients have increased awareness of the role of self-regulation in effective medication use.

It is important to identify aberrant medication use behaviors *early in pain treatment*, as addiction outcomes are significantly better if the disease is caught in its earlier stages. Addicted patients have a tendency to use their medication to treat all their troubling symptoms—insomnia, depression, loneliness—not just their physical pain, and over time drugs or alcohol become their primary coping mechanism. Pain patients should be counseled to use pain medications only for the symptom for which it was prescribed (pain), and alternate sources of dysphoria (depression, stress) or discomfort (insomnia) should be addressed with evidence-based strategies. Addicted drug-seeking pain patients are also likely to use their medication in ways that intensify psychoactive effects, such as taking it on an empty stomach, combining it with alcohol or other drugs, and saving up doses over the course of a day and take them all at once. The use of a pain diary detailing the social and emotional context of opioid use can be extremely helpful in identifying medication use behaviors that may be early signs of addictive disease. Any unusual administration patterns (including medication underuse) should be explored immediately and addressed aggressively.

Controversy exists about the use of *random urine toxicology screens* as a means of making pain treatment decisions (Heit & Gorlay, 2004; Katz & Fanciullo, 2002). In nonpain settings, the only recreational drug use that typically raises clinician concern is that of alcohol and tobacco, as even nonaddictive alcohol/tobacco use brings with it significant pathology. Further, treatment is not terminated if tobacco or alcohol addiction is present, and aggressive interventions for these addictions are instituted. Yet in the case of the pain patients on opioids, any unsanctioned drug use can be grounds for immediate treatment discharge. Unlike the patient without chronic pain, recreational drug use is not tolerated, and addiction, if present, is too often left untreated in these patients.

Yet, as previously noted, the *concurrent abuse of alcohol or drugs* is a correlate of opioid addiction in pain patients, and must not be ignored. Rather than grounds for discharge, it is suggested that urine evidence of unsanctioned drug use be explored as whether or not it constitutes addiction, and to treat accordingly. In that addiction generalizes across drugs of abuse, it is likely that addiction to illicit drugs outside of pain treatment portends addictive opioid use, whereas a patient who is able to maintain recreational, controlled drug use patterns may actually be protected (genetically or otherwise) from developing addictive opioid disease.

Further, it is suggested that *pain treatment not be terminated* if the patient is found to suffer opioid addiction. Consultation with addiction medicine is recommended, as is expansion of the treatment plan to include responses to addiction treatment. In some cases, insight into impaired control and regular 12-step meeting attendance is sufficient to treat early opioid addiction in a pain patient. For others, providing an alternate dispenser of medication (i.e., pharmacist) can help with dosing control. If less intensive interventions fail, addiction is severe, and/or patients are unable to control their addictive opioid use, formalized residential or inpatient drug treatment should be considered. Both are helpful in that access to opioids, alcohol, and other drugs is highly controlled, thus opioid analgesic requirements in the absence of addictive opioid use can be evaluated. Regardless of treatment approach, it should be recognized that opioid withdrawal is a demonstrated precipitant of opioid-induced hyperalgesia (Kaplan & Fields, 1991; Kim et al., 1988); if part of the treatment plan, detoxification should proceed slowly to minimize withdrawal discomfort, and complaints of increased pain should be treated aggressively using nonopioid strategies.

The functional improvements enjoyed via effective drug treatment will do nothing but improve pain outcomes, whereas leaving it untreated will lead to increased morbidity and death. Similarly, if the patient is suffering unrelieved pain, addiction interventions will be ineffective; the significant behavioral changes required of addiction treatment are very difficult to begin or sustain under conditions of painful stress. Optimal patient outcomes rely on directed addiction treatment in the context of well-managed pain.

Conclusions

Addiction is a behavioral disease, thus specific behaviors which are aberrant with respect to patterns of medication use (poorly controlled and compulsive) are always present in cases of the disorder. Yet, because unexpected medication use patterns can occur in pain patients without addiction, aberrant behaviors must be evaluated to rule out other reasons for drug seeking, and to obtain clear evidence of impaired control, compulsive use, and opioid preoccupation. Untreated addiction has devastating consequences for the patient, whereas when the disease is well-treated, patients improve on all health domains. This is particularly true in the case of CNMP, for which functional improvements cannot be appreciated until the functional deficits of addiction are managed. It is suggested that because addiction and CNMP share similar profiles of presentation and desired treatment outcomes, the patient is best served by treating chronic pain and analgesic opioid addiction as integrated phenomena, because unless both are managed, improvements in function will not be appreciated.

References

Adams LL, Gatchel RJ, Robinson RC, Polatin P, Gajraj N, Deschner M, Noe C. (2004). Development of a self-report screening instrument for assessing potential opioid medication misuse in chronic pain patients. *J Pain Symptom Manage* 27:440–459.

The American Academy of Pain Medicine, The American Pain Society, and the American Society of Addiction Medicine. (2001). *Public policy of ASAM: Definitions related to the use of opioids in pain treatment.* http://www.asam.org/ppol/paindef.htm. Accessed 2/28/06.

American Psychiatric Association. (1994). *Diagnostic and Statistical Manual of Mental Disorders* (4th ed.). Washington DC: APA.

Ballentyne JC, Mao, J. (2003). Opioid therapy for chronic pain. *NEJM* 349:1943–53.

Butler SF, Budman SH, Fernandez K, Jamison RN. (2004). Validation of a screener and opioid assessment measure for patients with chronic pain. *Pain* 112:65–72.

Chabal C, Erjavec MK, Jacobsen L, Mariano A, Chaney E. (1997). Prescription opiate abuse in chronic pain patients: Clinical criteria, incidence, and predictors. *Clin J Pain* 13:150–155.

Chu L, Angst M, Clark, D. (2004). Opioids in non-cancer pain: Measurement of opioid-induced tolerance and hyperalgesia in pain patients on chronic opioid therapy. *J Pain* 5:S73.

Ciccone DS, Just N, Bandilla EB, Reimer E, Ilbeigi MS, Wu W. (2000). Psychological correlates of opioid use in patients with chronic nonmalignant pain: A preliminary test of the down hill spiral hypothesis. *JPSM* 20:180–192.

Clark JD. (2002). Chronic pain prevalence and analgesic prescribing in a general medical population. *JPSM* 23:131–137.

Cohen MJM, Jasser S, Herron PD, Margolis CG. (2002). Ethical perspectives: Opioid treatment of chronic pain in the context of addiction. *Clinical Journal of Pain* 18:S99–S107.

Compton P, Darakjian J, Miotto K. (1998). Screening for addiction in patients with chronic pain and "problematic" substance use: evaluation of a pilot assessment tool. *J Pain Symptom Manage* 16:355–363.

Compton P, Estepa C. (2000). Differential diagnosis: Addiction in patients with chronic pain. *Lippincotts Prim. Care Pract.* 4:254–272.

DeWitt DJ, Adlaf EM, Offord DR, Ogborne AC. (2000). Age of first alcohol use: A risk factor for the development of an alcohol diagnosis. *Am J Psychiatry* 157:745–750.

Dunbar SA, Katz NP. (1996). Chronic opioid therapy for nonmalignant pain in patients with a history of substance abuse: Report of 20 cases. *J Pain Symptom Manage* 11:163–71.

Finnerup NB, Otto M, McQuay HJ, Jensen, TS, Sindrup, SH. (2005). Algorithm for neuropathic pain treatment: An evidence based proposal. *Pain* 118:289–305.

Fishbain DA. (1996). Report on the prevalence of drug/alcohol abuse and dependence in chronic pain patients (CPPs). *Subst Use Misuse* 8:945–6.

Fishbain DA, Rosomoff HL, Rosomoff RS. (1992). Drug abuse, dependence, and addiction in chronic pain patients. *Clin J Pain* 8:77–85.

Foley, KM. (2003). Opioids and chronic neuropathic pain. *New England Journal of Medicine* 348:1279–1281.

Gilson AM, Joranson DE. (2002). U.S. policies relevant to the prescribing of opioid analgesics for the treatment of pain in patients with addictive disease. *Clin J Pain* 18:S91–S98.

Heit, HA, Gorlay, DL. (2004). Urine testing in pain medicine. *JPSM* 27:260–267.

Jamison, RN, Kauffman JKatz, NP. (2000). Characteristics of methadone maintenance patients with chronic pain. *JPSM* 19:53–62.

Kalso E, Edwards JE, Moore A, McQuay HJ. (2004). Opioids in chronic non-cancer pain: systematic review of efficacy and safety. *Pain* 112:372–380.

Kaplan H, Fields HL. (1991). Hyperalgesia during acute opioid abstinence: Evidence for a nociceptive facilitating function of the rostral ventromedial medulla. *J Neurosci* 11:1433–1439.

Katz, N, Fanciullo GJ. (2002). The role of urine toxicology testing in the management of chronic opioid therapy. *Clinical Journal of Pain* 18:S76–S82.

Kim DH, Barbaro NM, Fields HL. (1988). Dose response relationship for hyperalgesia following naloxone precipitated withdrawal from morphine. *Soc Neurosci Abstr* 14:174.

Kirsh KL, Whitcomb LA, Donaghy K, Passik SD. (2002). Abuse and addiction issues in medically ill patients with pain: Attempts at clarification of terms and empirical study. *Clinical Journal of Pain* 18:S52–S60.

Maier C, Hildebrandt J, Klinger R, Henrich-Eberl C, Lindena G, MONTAS Study Group. (2002). Morphine responsiveness, efficacy and tolerability in patients with chronic non-tumor associated pain—results of a double-blind placebo-controlled trial (MONTAS). *Pain* 97:223–233.

McGinnis JM, Foege WH. (1993). Actual causes of death in the United States. *JAMA* 270:2207–12.

McQuay, H. (2001). Opioids in chronic non-malignant pain. *BMJ* 322:1134–1135.

Michna E, Ross EL, Hynes WL, Nedeljkovic SS, Soumekh S, Janfaza D, Palombi D, Jamison RN. (2004). Predicting aberrant drug behavior in patients treated for chronic pain: importance of abuse history. *J Pain Symptom Manage* 28:250–258.

Miotto K, Compton P, Ling W, Conolly, M. (1996). Diagnosing addictive Disease in chronic pain patients. *Psychosomatics* 37:223–235.

Morgan JP. (1985–86). American opiophobia: Customary underutilization of opioid analgesics. *Adv Alcohol Subst Abuse* 5:163–73.

Office of Drug Control Policy. (2001). *The Economic Costs of Drug Abuse in the United States, 1992–1998.* Washington DC: Executive Office of the President (Publication No. NCJ-190636).

Passik SD, Kirsh KL, Whitcomb L, Portenoy RK, Katz NP, Kleinman L, Dodd SL, Schein JR. (2004). A new tool to assess and document pain outcomes in chronic pain patients receiving opioid therapy. *Clinical Therapeutics* 26:552–561.

Passik SDS, Theobald DE. (2000). Managing addiction in advanced cancer patients: Why bother? *JPSM* 19:229–234.

Robert Wood Johnson Foundation. (2001). *Substance Abuse: The Nation's Number One Health Problem.* Princeton, NJ: RWJF.

Robinson RC, Gatchel RJ, Polatin P, Deschner M, Noe C, Gajraj N. (2001). Screening for problematic prescription opioid use. *Clin J Pain* 17:220–228.

Rosenblum A, Jospeph H, Fong C, Kipnis S, Cleland C, Portenoy RK. (2003). Prevalence and characteristics of chronic pain among chemically dependent patients in methadone maintenance and residential treatment facilities. *JAMA* 289:2370–2378.

Savage SR. (2002). Assessment for addiction in pain-treatment settings. *Clin J Pain* 18:S28–S38.

Sees KL, Clark HW. (1993). Opioid use in the treatment of chronic pain: assessment of addiction. *J Pain Symptom Manage* 8:257–264.

Trafton JA, Oliva EM, Horst DA, Minkel JD, Humphreys K. (2004). Treatment needs associated with pain in substance use disorder patients: implications for concurrent treatment. *Drug and Alcohol Dependence* 73:23–31.

U.S. Department of Health and Human Services. (2000). *Healthy People 2010: Understanding and Improving Health and Objectives for Improving Health.* (2nd ed., 2 vols.). Washington, DC: U.S. Government Printing Office. http://www.healthypeople.gov/document/.

Vaccarino AL, Couret LC. (1993). Formalin-induced pain antagonizes the development of opiate dependence in the rat. *Neuroscience Letters* 161:195–198.

Vaccarino AL, Marek P, Kest B, Ben-Eliyahu S, Couret LC Jr, Kao B, Liebeskind JC. (1993). Morphine fails to produce tolerance when administered in the presence of formalin pain in rats. *Brain Res* 627(2):287–290.

Von Korff, M & Deyo, RA. (2004). Potent opioids for musculoskeletal pain: Flying blind? *Pain* 109:207–209.

Weissman DE, Haddox JD. (1989). Opioid pseudoaddiction—an iatrogenic syndrome. *Pain* 36:363–366.

Wesson DR, Ling W, Smith DE. (1993). Prescription of opioids for the treatment of pain in patients with addictive disease. *JPSM* 8:289–296.

Part VII
Pain and Chemical Dependency
The Interface

51

Pain Management and the So-Called "Risk" of Addiction
A Neurobiological Perspective

Eliot L. Gardner

Some of the most widely used and most broadly effective medications for the management of pain (e.g., opioids) are also compounds that support self-administration at both the human and animal level, have addictive and abuse liability, and produce physical dependence. Other medications commonly used in pain management (e.g., monoamine reuptake inhibitors, GABA mimetics) do not possess these attributes. But as these other medications are most commonly used in an adjunctive manner in combination with "primary" "strong" analgesics (most often opioids), the question of the so-called "risk of addiction" has permeated pain management for decades—often to the severe detriment of proper compassionate medical care and good patient management. The purpose of the present mini-review is to examine at the neurobiological level the "risk of addiction" posed by such primary analgesics as opioids and to draw conclusions therefrom that may help pain management physicians optimize their patient care.

Terminology: A Long-Standing Confusion

Discussions of the risk of addiction in pain medicine have long been confused by lack of clarity in distinguishing drug dependence from drug addiction. Although this may be forgivable at the lay level, it is unacceptable (and far too common) at the professional level. Indeed, the standard diagnostic manual in the field of psychiatry (American Psychiatric Association, 2000) uses the term *dependence* to describe the compulsive drug-seeking and drug-taking behaviors that are termed *addiction* in much of the medical literature. Because physical dependence occurs quite normally with repeated dosing of many drugs, not all of them abused or addictive, this has led to confusion. It has also led to suboptimal care from clinicians who have been erroneously led to believe that a patient receiving opioids for pain is "addicted" simply because signs of tolerance and withdrawal (physical dependence) are present.

In a recent review article by the directors of the National Institute on Drug Abuse (NIDA) and the National Institute on Alcohol Abuse and Alcoholism (NIAAA), the authors conclude that the use of term *dependence* to describe compulsive drug-seeking and drug-taking behaviors is "confusing" and counterproductive, and that the proper term to describe such behaviors is *addiction* (Volkow and Li 2004). Others have also addressed this problem (e.g., Heit, 2003; O'Brien and Gardner, 2005) and published definitions that appropriately distinguish addiction from dependence.

For present purposes, *addiction* will refer to compulsive drug-seeking and drug-taking behaviors, whereas *dependence* will refer to the normal state of physical dependence that accompanies the repeated use of many medications, the vast majority of which (e.g., antidepressants, cardiac medications, diabetic medications) are nonaddictive. The disease of addiction (and it *is* a disease), then, is a behavioral and mental disorder characterized by (a) impaired control over drug self-administration, (b) compulsive drug self-administration, (c) continued self-administration despite obvious harm to self and others, and (d) drug craving. Addiction medicine specialists often term drug addiction the "disease of the 5 Cs": *chronic* disease with impaired *control, compulsive* use, *continued* use despite harm, and drug *craving*. Pain management experts will readily recognize that these "5 Cs" rarely apply to pain patients under proper management, even under what might otherwise seem heroic opioid dosing. Importantly, addictive behaviors appear to be habit-based (Di Chiara, 1998, 1999; Everitt et al., 2001; Robbins and Everitt, 2002). Thus, drugs with addictive potential may also be termed *habit forming*, a useful term because so many medications that produce physical dependence are nonhabit forming and thus nonaddictive.

Two other important concepts to define at the outset (because their misunderstanding leads to much medical mismanagement and undertreatment) are pseudotolerance and pseudoaddiction. Pseudotolerance refers to the need to increase drug dosage due to disease progression, superimposed new disease, changes in physical activity, and/or lack of compliance with prescribed dose regimen(s) (Pappagallo, 1998). Pseudoaddiction is drug seeking and drug taking (which can sometimes appear compulsive or even obsessional) due to undertreatment of the disease for which the drug provides relief (Weissman and Haddox, 1989). Confusing pseudotolerance with tolerance, or pseudoaddiction with addiction, leads straightforwardly and obviously to poor patient care.

Brain Mechanisms Subserving Pain and Analgesia

The vast majority of physicians are well acquainted with the peripheral and spinal neural pathways and mechanisms that mediate pain and analgesia. For those wishing an update on this still evolving area, reference to any standard medical or neuroscience text (e.g., Kandel et al. 2000) will suffice. Less well-known are the *brain* substrates of pain and analgesia. Pioneering work in this area was carried out more than 30 years ago by Pert and Yaksh (1974, 1975), and remains definitive today (e.g., Manning et al., 1994). In their momentous multiyear research project, Pert and Yaksh (1974, 1975) surgically implanted rhesus monkeys with arrays of microinjection cannulae in their brains, and trained the animals to perform on a footshock pain titration behavioral paradigm. Animals could neither avoid nor escape the painful footshock, but could activate a manipulandum to lower the pain intensity as much as they wished. After baseline levels of voluntary acceptance of pain were established for each animal (pain tolerance), microinjections of morphine were administered to a wide variety of brain sites. Analgesia was defined as voluntary acceptance of higher pain levels than baseline (increased pain tolerance).

Two principal brain regions were found wherein microinjections of morphine resulted in dose-dependent analgesia that was completely reversible by systemic naloxone. The first and most significant analgesia–meditating brain area was found to be within the periventricular–periaqueductal gray matter of the brain stem, extending from the lower portion of the third ventricle up through the subthalamic nucleus and into the intralaminar thalamic nuclear group. This distribution of active sites coincides anatomically with the terminal regions and associated areas of the extralemniscal somatosensory system—long known to mediate the aversive quality of pain (for reviews of this latter point, see Casey and Melzack, 1967, and Pert and Yaksh, 1974). The second analgesia-mediating brain area was found to lie more laterally in the brain stem, running from the lateral reticular nucleus up through the substantia nigra, dorsolateral to the red nucleus, and into the most lateral aspects of the centre median and parafascicular nuclei of the thalamus. This distribution of active sites coincides anatomically with the medial portions of the neospinothalamic somatosensory system—long known to mediate pain sensation, especially its sensory-discriminative aspects (for reviews of this latter point, see Casey and Melzack, 1967, and Pert and Yaksh, 1974).

In a remarkable historical coincidence, while Pert and Yaksh were carrying out their pioneering work on the neuroanatomical location of active analgesic sites in the primate brain, the first reports of the location of opioid receptors in the brain began to emerge (e.g., Hiller et al., 1973; Kuhar et al., 1973)—showing an anatomic overlap with the active analgesic sites. Subsequent work has confirmed these findings. Thus, generally speaking, the present understanding of central brain sites and mechanisms of analgesia is that opioid medications activate central opioid receptors adjacent to and/or within the above-cited neuroanatomic loci (in addition, of course, to activating spinal and peripheral opioid receptors), activating neural substrates that then act to close pain-gating mechanisms (Melzack and Wall, 1965, 1970) at a variety of levels from the dorsal horn of the spinal cord all the way up through brain stem to the thalamus. Subsequent research has confirmed this general picture, up to and including human level (e.g., Hosobuchi, 1981).

For present purposes, the crucial aspect of this corpus of knowledge is that the brain sites and mechanisms mediating pain and analgesia differ from those mediating either opioid-induced physical dependence (as defined above) or opioid-induced addictive behaviors (as defined above). This will become clear as we review the brain substrates of physical dependence and of addiction (see below).

Brain Mechanisms Subserving Physical Dependence

Pioneering work in this area was carried out more than 20 years ago by Bozarth and Wise (1984), and remains definitive. Similar to the approach taken by Pert and Yaksh (1974, 1975), cited above, Bozarth and Wise surgically implanted experimental animals with arrays of microinjection cannulae in their brains, and then determined where in the brain microinjections of opioids produce physical dependence and where in the brain microinjections of opioids support drug-seeking and drug-taking behaviors. They found a complete double-dissociation between brain substrates for physical dependence and those for addiction (Bozarth and Wise, 1984). Thus, microinjections of opioids into brain loci near the locus coeruleus and the dorsal pontine/mesencephalic border produce classic signs of opioid physical dependence (and withdrawal symptoms upon abrupt cessation of opioid administration) but utterly *fail* to support opioid-seeking or opioid-taking behaviors. Conversely, opioids are avidly self-administered when the microinjector tips are in the ventral tegmental area (Bozarth and Wise, 1981, 1982), lateral hypothalamus (Olds, 1979; Stein and Olds, 1977), or nucleus accumbens (Olds, 1982), but such microinjections utterly *fail* to produce opioid physical dependence or withdrawal symptoms upon abrupt cessation of opioid self-administration. Further research has indicated that the central neurotransmitter system activated during physical withdrawal is norepinephrine (NE), probably originating from the locus coeruleus NE nucleus of the brain stem. This would explain why medications that dampen central brain NE activation (e.g., clonidine) are clinically effective for managing physical dependence and withdrawal. Central corticotrophic releasing factor (CRF) circuits may also be activated during physical withdrawal (Koob, 1999). For more comprehensive reviews the reader is referred to Gardner (2000, 2005) and to Wise and Gardner (2002).

For present purposes, the crucial aspect of this work is that the brain sites and mechanisms mediating opioid-induced physical dependence (and physical withdrawal) differ from those mediating pain and analgesia (above) or those mediating addictive opioid-seeking and opioid-taking behaviors (below).

Brain Mechanisms Subserving Addiction

A brief overview of brain mechanisms subserving addiction is complicated by the fact that there are multiple aspects to the disease of addiction, including (a) the highly rewarding acute "high" or "rush" sought by the drug abuser, (b) the transition of addictive drug-seeking and drug-taking behaviors from reward-driven to habit-driven, and (c) the extraordinary vulnerability to relapse to drug seeking and drug taking that characterizes the disease of addiction. We shall deal with these in turn.

Brain Mechanisms Subserving Drug-Induced Reward and Reward-Driven Drug Seeking

The pleasure/reward circuitry of the brain consists of an "in series" sequence of neural circuitry in the ventral limbic mesencephalon, diencephalon, and forebrain (Wise and Bozarth, 1984; for reviews, see Gardner, 2000, 2005). The "first-stage" neural elements of this circuitry originate from a group of ventral limbic forebrain nuclei located rostral to the anterior hypothalamus and loosely termed by neuroanatomists as the "anterior bed nuclei of the medial forebrain bundle." The candally running first-stage axons join together in the medial forebrain bundle (MFB) and project posteriorly to the ventral tegmental area (VTA) of the ventral limbic mesencephalon. These first-stage axons are myelinated and have moderately fast conduction velocities. They are of unknown neurotransmitter type, although Gratton and Wise (1985) have presented convincing evidence that a portion may be acetylcholinergic. It is these first-stage fibers that support the phenomenon of electrical brain-stimulation reward (BSR), in which animals and humans avidly self-administer brief trains of mild electrical stimulation to the MFB. Such BSR is the most intensely rewarding stimulation known, surpassing even that of crack cocaine. The first-stage neurons synapse in the VTA upon the cell bodies/dendrites of the "second-stage" reward neurons.

These second-stage neurons are nonmyelinated and dopaminergic, from which comes the view that dopamine (DA) is the "reward" neurotransmitter of the brain (only partially correct, as there are many DA neural circuits in the central nervous system—from mesencephalon to retina—subserving *many* diverse mental and behavioral functions). It is these second-stage fibers that subserve drug-induced reward, leading to the view that addictive drugs "hijack" the normal reward circuitry of the brain—activating it more intensely than normal biologically essential rewarding stimuli such as food, sex, or even the sight of a friend's face. The second-stage reward neurons ascend rostrally within the MFB to synapse in their target nucleus—the nucleus accumbens (Acb) of the ventral limbic forebrain—upon the cell bodies/dendrites of the "third-stage" reward neurons.

These third-stage reward neurons are GABAergic medium spiny neurons that appear to also co-localize an endogenous opioid neurotransmitter. The third-stage reward neurons project from the Acb to synapse in their target nucleus—the ventral pallidum (VP). It is this "in series" reward circuit that mediates drug-induced reward and reward-driven drug-seeking and drug-taking behaviors. These brain-reward mechanisms are currently believed to constitute the fundamental substrate upon which addictive drugs act to produce their rewarding and incentive motivational effects (Wise, 1996a, 1996b; Wise and Gardner, 2002). For a fuller explication, the reader is referred to Gardner (2005).

For present purposes, the crucial aspect of this extremely large body of knowledge is that the brain sites and mechanisms mediating opioid-induced reward and opioid-induced reward-driven drug-seeking and drug-taking behaviors differ from both those mediating opioid-induced analgesia and those mediating opioid-induced physical dependence (see also, e.g., Ide et al., 2004; Kuzmin et al., 1992; Lattanzi et al., 2001; Semenova et al., 1995; You et al., 2001; Zvartau et al., 1986, for additional evidence that opioid-induced analgesia, physical dependence, and drug reward are mediated by separate neurobiological loci and processes, under different genetic control mechanisms).

Brain Mechanisms Subserving Habit-Driven Drug Seeking

Although reward-driven brain mechanisms (largely DA-mediated) initially subserve the aberrant drug-seeking and drug-taking behaviors that characterize the disease of addiction, tolerance develops rapidly to the initial rewarding effects of opioids. This is clearly observed in laboratory animals by measuring opioid-activated brain-reward substrates directly by electrophysiological means (Gardner and Lowinson, 1993; Nazarro et al., 1981). It is also observed clinically at the human level—after a period of addictive opioid use, people with the disease of addiction frequently report that "I no longer get 'high' from the heroin; now I need to use the heroin to just get 'straight' [i.e., to bring chronically depressed hedonic tone back toward some degree of normality]." This "getting straight" has all the qualities of obsessionality and compulsivity (if not more) than "getting high" initially had when the patient with the disease of addiction started down his or her long and self-damaging road to affliction.

As addictive opioid drug seeking and drug taking becomes less and less reward-driven (by activation of *ventral* neostriatal DA sites and mechanisms—the VTA-Acb DA neural system), it becomes more and more habit-driven (by activation of *dorsal* neostriatal DA sites and mechanisms). Thus, at present levels of understanding, addiction—especially as the disease progresses and develops—is believed to be a disorder of DA-dependent habit formation (Di Chiara, 1999; Everitt et al., 2001; Robbins and Everitt, 2002). The DA dependency is crucial, as DA appears to be essential for the "stamping in" of the stimulus-reward and response-reward associations that underlie the most characteristic signs and symptoms of the disease of addiction—the aberrantly strong motivational and reinforcing control over behavior by drug-associated stimuli at the expense of other sources of reward (Gardner and David, 1999; Wise, 2004).

For present purposes, the crucial aspect of this view of *developed* addiction is that the dorsal neostriatal DA sites and mechanisms mediating opioid-induced habit-driven drug seeking and drug taking differ from both those mediating opioid induced analgesia and those mediating opioid-induced physical dependence.

Brain Mechanisms Subserving Relapse to Drug Seeking

Another highly pathognomonic characteristic of opioid addiction is the extraordinary vulnerability of recovering or recovered opioid abusers to relapse to former patterns of drug seeking and drug taking. Even among those whose lives have been savaged by addiction—losing jobs, livelihoods, homes, possessions, wives, children, and friends—the risk of relapse remains extremely high.

Relapse to drug-seeking and drug-taking behaviors in humans or animals long pharmacologically detoxified and behaviorally extinguished from their prior drug-taking habits is characteristically (and uniquely) triggered by one (or a combination) of three specific relapse triggers: (a) non-contingent exposure to an addictive drug (even secondarily; e.g., entering a room filled with smoke from other cigarette smokers), (b) exposure to environmental cues (sights, sounds, smells) that were previously associated with drug taking, or (c) stress (even mild stress being sufficient to trigger relapse). Through the use of the reinstatement laboratory animal model of relapse (for review, see Shalev et al., 2002; Shaham et al., 2003), a great deal has been learned about the brain loci and underlying mechanisms mediating relapse produced by these three classical triggers.

Drug-Triggered Relapse

Relapse to drug-seeking and drug-taking behaviors triggered by noncontingent reexposure to an addictive drug appears to be mediated by DA neurotransmitter substrates coincident with the second-stage DA reward neurons that originate in the VTA and project to the Acb. This has been established by the fact that microinjections of addictive drugs robustly trigger relapse when given directly into the VTA-Acb mesoaccumbens DA reward circuitry (most especially the VTA or Acb themselves), but not into other brain loci (e.g., Stewart, 1984; Stewart and Vezina, 1988). Provocatively, cross-triggering of relapse (from one class of addictive drug to another) has been shown. Thus, an injection of amphetamine or the DA agonist bromocriptine triggers relapse to opioid self-administration behavior (Stewart and Vezina, 1988; Wise et al., 1990). Such cross-triggering of relapse between different classes of addictive drugs implicates common neurobiological, neurochemical, and neuropharmacological relapse substrates in the brain, common to addictive drugs of different pharmacological classes.

It is the finding that the drugs and doses that trigger relapse are drugs and doses that increase DA function within the mesoaccumbens system (for reviews, see Kalivas and McFarland, 2003; Shaham et al., 2003; Shalev et al., 2002) that has led to the presumption that a mesoaccumbens DA substrate underlies drug-triggered relapse. For example, DA agonists (both direct and indirect) trigger relapse to both cocaine- and heroin-seeking behaviors (e.g., De Vries et al., 1999), as does direct activation of DA neurons in the VTA (Stewart, 1984; Vorel et al., 2001). Direct local intracerebral microinjections of amphetamine, cocaine, or DA itself into mesoaccumbens DA terminal regions (Acb or medial prefrontal cortex) trigger drug seeking (Cornish and Kalivas, 2000; McFarland and Kalivas, 2000; Park et al., 2002; Stewart and Vezina, 1988). Both general DA antagonists and selective DA D_1 or D_2 receptor antagonists attenuate drug-triggered relapse (e.g., Ettenberg et al., 1996; Shaham and Stewart, 1996). Direct local intracerebral microinjections of DA antagonists into the medial prefrontal cortex attenuate cocaine-triggered relapse (Capriles et al., 2003; McFarland and Kalivas, 2000; Park et al., 2002).

However, the situation is not as straightforward as initially believed. The indirect DA agonist GBR-12909 strongly triggers relapse to either cocaine or heroin self-administration, but the direct DA D_1 receptor agonist SKF-82958 fails to trigger relapse to either cocaine or heroin, and the direct DA D_2 receptor agonist quinpirole triggers relapse to cocaine but not to heroin (De Vries et al., 1999). The nonselective direct DA receptor agonist apomorphine inhibits relapse (De Vries et al., 1999). Self and colleagues found that selective DA D_2 receptor agonists trigger relapse to cocaine self-administration, whereas DA D_1 receptor agonists not only fail to trigger relapse but actually protect against cocaine-triggered relapse (Self, 1998; Self et al., 1996). Glutamate mechanisms may well play a role in drug-triggered relapse (e.g., Park et al., 2002), as may endogenous opioid, GABAergic, and endocannabinoid mechanisms, although these may converge on a final substrate (for review, see Shaham et al., 2003). Thus, current best evidence suggests that activation of DA substrates in the Acb (especially involving D_2 receptors) is a crucial underlying neural mechanism for drug-triggered relapse to addictive drug-seeking behaviors (Self and Nestler, 1998).

For present purposes, the crucial import of these findings is that the VTA-MFB-Acb DA sites (including DA projections to medial prefrontal cortex) and mechanisms mediating drug-triggered relapse differ from both those mediating opioid-induced analgesia and those mediating-opioid-induced physical dependence.

Stress-Triggered Relapse

Stress and related negative affective states such as anger, anxiety, or depression also trigger relapse to drug seeking and drug taking at the human (Shiffman, 1982; Shiffman et al., 1996; Sinha et al., 1999) and animal levels (e.g., Erb et al., 1996; Shaham, 1993; Shaham and Stewart, 1995; Shaham et al., 1996; for reviews, see Shaham et al., 2000a, 2003). Importantly, neither the amount nor degree of stress needs to be large. A mild stressor such as mere food deprivation for less than a day (i.e., the same feeding regimen of many household pets) is enough to trigger relapse in animals (e.g., Shalev et al., 2000, 2003).

Mechanistically, it was originally believed that stress-triggered relapse to drug seeking involved the same mesoaccumbens DA brain circuitry and mechanisms as drug-triggered relapse DA. Recent work, however, suggests otherwise, as neither D_1- nor D_2-selective DA receptor antagonists attenuate stress-triggered relapse to opioid self-administration (see, e.g., Shaham and Stewart, 1996). Rather, both (a) brain CRF in the amygdala and (b) brain NE in the brain stem appear to be involved in stress-triggered relapse. Acute intracerebroventricular injections of CRF strongly trigger relapse to drug seeking (Shaham et al., 1997), and the CRF antagonists α-helical-CRF, CO-154526, and D-Phe-CRF$_{12-41}$ potently block stress-triggered relapse to opioid-seeking behaviors (Shaham et al., 1997, 1998). Thus, CRF, a major brain peptide neurotransmitter involved in mediating stressor effects, is importantly involved in subserving stress-provoked relapse to drug seeking and drug taking. Counterintuitively, corticosterone (well implicated in mediating other stress-triggered bodily effects) appears not to play a role (Erb et al., 1998). Rather, it is the central brain CRF circuitry originating in the central nucleus of the amygdala and projecting to the bed nucleus of the stria terminalis that appears to be most critically involved.

As noted, NE (another major brain neurotransmitter involved in response to stress) also appears involved in mediating stress-triggered relapse to drug-seeking behaviors. For example, the α-NE receptor agonists clonidine, lofexidine, and guanabenz (which decrease NE cell firing and neurotransmitter release) block stress-triggered relapse to opioid drug seeking (e.g., Shaham et al., 2000b). Counterintuitively, the locus coeruleus/dorsal NE bundle system (so often implicated in other brain-mediated stress effects) appears not to be involved. Rather, stress-triggered relapse appears to involve the lateral tegmental NE nuclei (Shaham et al., 2000b) and their NE projections through the ventral NE bundle (Moore and Bloom, 1979) to the central nucleus of the amygdala, bed nucleus of stria terminalis, hypothalamus, medial septum, and Acb (for review, see Shaham et al., 2003).

For present purposes, the crucial import of this body of research is that the central amygdaloid/CRF and lateral tegmental/NE sites and mechanisms mediating stress-triggered relapse differ from both those mediating opioid-induced analgesia and those mediating opioid-induced physical dependence.

Cue-Triggered Relapse

Exposure to environmental cues (sights, sounds, and other sensory stimuli) previously associated with drug-taking behaviors is also a strong trigger for relapse to drug seeking and drug taking at both human and animal levels (e.g., Katner et al., 1999; McFarland and Ettenberg, 1997; Meil and See, 1996). Because environmental cues previously paired with drug-taking behaviors significantly enhance DA levels in both the Acb and amygdala (Gerasimov et al., 2001; Katner and Weiss, 1999; Weiss et al., 2000), and because pharmacological blockade of DA D_1 or D_2 receptors attenuated cue-triggered relapse to drug-seeking behaviors in some early experiments, the conclusion was initially drawn that cue-triggered relapse involves the same mesoaccumbens DA brain circuitry and mechanisms as drug-triggered relapse.

However, this turned out to be incorrect, for a number of reasons. First, lesions of the basolateral amygdala eliminate cue-triggered relapse to drug-seeking behaviors in behaviorally extinguished animals, without interfering with drug self-administration per se (Meil and See, 1997). Second, tetrodotoxin (TTX)-induced inactivation of the basolateral amygdala eliminates cue-triggered relapse but has no effect on drug-triggered relapse (Grimm and See, 2000). Third, TTX-induced inactivation of the Acb eliminates drug-triggered relapse but has no effect on cue-triggered relapse (Grimm and See, 2000). These findings demonstrate a clear neuroanatomical dissociation between the neural substrates for drug-triggered and cue-triggered relapse and implicate deep temporal lobe loci involved in the encoding, storage, and retrieval of emotional memories (such as the amygdala) in cue-triggered relapse. Recently, it has been shown that two such deep temporal lobe memory-encoding/retrieval loci—the basolateral amygdala and the ventral subiculum of the hippocampus—are critically involved in cue-triggered relapse (Hayes et al., 2003; Taepavarapruk and Phillips, 2003; Vorel and Gardner, 2001; Vorel et al., 2001). Furthermore, glutamatergic neuronal projections from the basolateral amygdala and hippocampal ventral subiculum to the DA mesoaccumbens reward-related circuitry seem to be crucially involved in mediating such cue-triggered relapse (Hayes et al., 2003; Vorel et al., 2001).

For present purposes, the crucial import of this body of research is that the lateral amygdaloid and hippocampal glutamatergic sites and mechanisms mediating cue-triggered relapse differ from both these mediating opioid-induced analgesia and these mediating opioid-induced physical dependence.

Effect of Chronic Pain on Brain Mechanisms Subserving Addiction and on Addictive Drug Seeking Itself

From the above, it may be well understood that addiction to opioids involves—indeed, is critically dependent upon—a number of underlying brain substrates and mechanisms including the following: (a) activation of the ventral mesolimbic DA VTA-Acb neural axis—which subserves the acute "high" or "rush" produced by opioids, *reward*-driven addictive drug use, and drug-triggered relapse to drug seeking and drug taking; (b) activation of dorsal mesostriatal DA neural substrates located within the dorsal neostriatum—which subserves the "stamping in" of the stimulus-reward and response-reward associations critical to addictive drug seeking and drug taking and which subserves *habit*-driven addictive drug use; (c) activation of amygdaloid central nucleus CRF substrates—which subserves stress-triggered relapse to drug seeking and drug taking; (d) activation of lateral tegmental noradrenergic substrates located within nucleus A2 of the brain stem (Moore and Bloom 1979)—which also subserves stress-triggered relapse to drug seeking and drug taking; and (e) activation of amygdaloid lateral nucleus and hippocampal glutamatergic substrates—which subserves environmental cue-triggered relapse to drug seeking and drug taking.

The important question arises: Does chronic pain activate or inhibit (or neither) these brain loci, mechanisms, and substrates that underlie addictive drug use and whose activation facilitates the development of, maintenance of, and relapse to drug abuse?

Effect of Chronic Pain on DA Substrates Underlying Reward-Driven Addictive Drug Use and Drug-Triggered Relapse to Addictive Drug Use

In laboratory animals, it has been clear for several years that chronic pain robustly *inhibits* opioid-enhanced extracellular DA efflux and opioid-enhanced DA turnover in the VTA-MFB-Acb neural axis mediating reward-driven addictive drug use and drug-triggered relapse to addictive drug use (e.g., Narita et al., 2004, 2005; Ozaki et al., 2002, 2004; Suzuki, 2001). This inhibitory effect of chronic pain on VTA-MFB-Acb addiction substrates may involve several underlying mechanisms, including (a) sustained activation by chronic pain of counteraddictive endogenous kappa opioid systems within the VTA-MFB-Acb reward axis (Narita et al., 2005; Suzuki, 2001; Suzuki et al., 1999); (b) inhibition by chronic pain of mu opioid receptor functions within the VTA-MFB-Acb reward axis (Narita et al., 2004; Ozaki et al., 2002, 2003); (c) suppression by chronic pain of mu-opioid receptor phosphorylation (especially by mitogen-activated protein/kinase [MAPK], and specifically by extracellular signal-regulated kinase [ERK]) within the VTA-MFB-Acb reward axis (Narita et al., 2004); (d) downregulation by chronic pain of mu opioid receptors in the VTA-MFB-Acb reward axis (Narita et al., 2004); and (e) sustained inhibition by chronic pain of ERK-dependent synthesis or activation of the reward neurotransmitter DA itself within the VTA-MFB-Acb reward axis (Narita et al., 2004; Ozaki et al., 2004).

Effect of Chronic Pain on Addictive Drug-Seeking Behaviors

Given the above-cited *suppressive* effects of chronic pain on the brain loci and mechanisms underlying acute drug reward and reward-driven drug-seeking behaviors, it should come as no surprise that an extensive body of preclinical research in animal models of addictive behaviors (e.g., Gardner, 2000; O'Brien and Gardner, 2005; Wise and Gardner, 2004) has repeatedly shown that chronic pain robustly *suppresses* opioid-seeking behaviors (Narita et al., 2004, 2005; Oe et al., 2004; Ozaki et al., 2001, 2002, 2003, 2004; Suzuki et al., 1996, 1999, 2001). Compellingly and importantly, this *loss* by morphine of its addictive potential when used in the presence of (and to control) chronic pain extends to other drugs with addictive potential as well. In the presence of chronic pain, both cocaine and methamphetamine also lose their ability to provoke addictive drug-seeking behaviors (Suzuki et al., 1996).

Thus, an extensive body of preclinical animal behavioral evidence is congruent with the conclusion of the World Health Organization that when opioids are used (even at heroic doses) to control chronic pain, addiction and drug abuse are not a major concern (World Health Organization, 1996).

Effect of Chronic Pain on VTA-MFB-Acb Substrates of Brain Reward as Measured Electrophysiologically

Given the above-cited *suppressive* effects of chronic pain on the brain loci and mechanisms underlying brain reward, it should also come as no surprise that pain *suppresses* brain reward as measured directly using the BSR electrophysiological paradigm in laboratory animals (Kishore and Desiraju, 1990).

Effect of Chronic Pain on the Development of Opioid Physical Dependence

Although evidence cited above strongly argues for a dissociation between opioid-induced physical dependence and opioid-induced addictive drug-seeking behaviors—on neuroanatomical, neurophysiological, and neurotransmitter bases (see also Ator and Griffiths, 1992; Griffiths and Weerts, 1997; and Yanagita, 1987, for additional evidence that mere physical dependence does *not* increase the reward value of addictive drugs)—it is nonetheless of interest to note that chronic pain also robustly inhibits the development of (indeed, often totally abolishes) opioid-induced physical dependence (Vaccarino and Couret, 1993; Vaccarino et al., 1993).

*Under*medication of Chronic Pain *Enhances* Risk of Addiction

Unrelieved or undertreated chronic pain is one of the most highly stress-provoking life events that human beings can be subjected to (especially in a social and political climate that equates drug-seeking behaviors for relief of genuine pain with "addictive" drug-seeking behaviors). As noted above, stress is one of the cardinal triggers for relapse to prior addictive drug-seeking and drug-taking behaviors in pharmacologically detoxified and behaviorally extinguished animals and humans (Shaham et al., 2003; Shalev et al., 2002). It follows logically, then, that undertreated pain can be a stressor that *provokes* and *triggers* relapse to addictive drug use. Thus, even in patients with prior histories of addictive drug use, elimination of the stress produced by undermedication of pain is a medical imperative.

As if concerns regarding stress-triggered relapse were not cautionary enough by themselves, an additional body of evidence speaks strongly to the ability of stress to provoke addictive drug-seeking and drug-taking behaviors via other neurobiological and neurobehavioral mechanisms. First, stress has been long known to *augment* extracellular DA overflow in the VTA-MFB-Acb reward axis (e.g., D'Angio et al., 1987; Louilot et al., 1986; Rougé-Pont et al., 1998), thus mimicking the relapse-provoking effects of noncontingent drug administration. Second, at the behavioral level itself, stress is known to *augment* addictive drug-*seeking* behaviors (e.g., McLaughlin et al., 2006a, 2006b). Third, also at the behavioral level, stress is also known to *augment* addictive drug-*taking* behaviors per se (e.g., Adams, 1995; Piazza et al., 1990; Rougé-Pont et al., 1993). Fourth, stress *augments* the rewarding effects of addictive drugs (Piazza et al., 1990). Fifth, stress *augments* the neurobiological and neurobehavioral *sensitization* induced by addictive drugs (e.g., Deroche et al., 1992a, 1992b; Rougé-Pont et al., 1995). As sensitization of drug-induced reward (e.g., Kim et al., 2004; Vezina et al., 2002; Woolverton et al., 1984) and drug-induced incentive motivation (Bindra, 1968; Bindra and Stewart, 1971; Toates, 1986, 1994) have been posited to underlie the development of addictive drug-seeking and drug-taking behaviors (Berridge and Robinson, 1998; Robinson and Berridge, 1993, 2000, 2001, 2003), such findings would appear to make it all the more imperative to medically quell the stress produced by undertreated pain in order to *prevent* drug addiction and abuse. Sixth, recent evidence suggests that patients with an increased vulnerability to drug addiction/abuse have a heightened sensitivity to pain (e.g., Stewart et al., 1995) and that this may be referable to a common genetic determinant—specific polymorphisms of the catechol-*o*-methyltransferase gene that is crucial to the regulation of the reward neurotransmitter DA within the VTA-MFB-Acb reward axis (e.g., Agarwal et al., 1983; Anokhina et al., 1988; Ishiguro et al., 1999; Tiihonen et al., 1999; Wang et al., 2001). Congruently, the endogenous opioid systems of the brain are more reactive to drugs of abuse (leading to *increased* vulnerability to addictive opioid use) in subjects at high risk for addiction (see, e.g., Gianoulakis, 1996). For *all* these reasons, elimination of the stress produced by undertreatment of pain is a medical imperative; failure to do so *invites* rather that prevents addiction.

Conclusions

A large body of neurobiological evidence has been briefly reviewed that strongly suggests that proper—even aggressive—opioid use during treatment of genuine chronic pain does *not* lead to increased risk of drug addiction, even in former addicts. This is congruent with the findings of the World Health Organization (1996) in human patients, and is congruent with current clinical guidelines in both the fields of addiction medicine and pain medicine (e.g., Schnoll and Weaver, 2003). Furthermore, via a host of neurobiological and neurobehavioral mechanisms and substrates, the stress caused by undertreatment of pain *invites* rather than prevents addiction. For all these neurobiological and neurobehavioral reasons, proper—even aggressive—management of genuine chronic pain is a medical necessity as well as a moral and ethical imperative. Failure to do so is bad medicine, and opens the treating physician to accusations of medical mismanagement.

References

Adams N. Sex differences and the effects of tail pinch on ethanol drinking in Maudsley rats. *Alcohol* 12:463–468, 1995.

Agarwal DP, Phillipu G, Milech U, Ziemsen B, Schrappe O, and Goedde HW. Platelet monoamine oxidase and erythrocyte catechol-*o*-methyltransferase activity in alcoholism and controlled abstinence. *Drug Alcohol Depend* 12:85–91, 1983.

American Psychiatric Association. *Diagnostic and Statistical Manual of Mental Disorders* (4th ed., Text Revision). Washington, DC: American Psychiatric Association, 2000.

Anokhina IP, Kogan BM, and Drozdov AZ. Disturbances in regulation of catecholamine neuromediation in alcoholism. *Alcohol Alcohol* 23:343–350, 1988.

Ator NA and Griffiths RR. Oral self-administration of triazolam, diazepam and ethanol in the baboon: drug reinforcement and benzodiazepine physical dependence. *Psychopharmacology* 108:301–312, 1992.

Berridge KC and Robinson TE. What is the role of dopamine in reward: hedonic impact, reward learning, or incentive salience? *Brain Res Rev* 28:309–369, 1998.

Bindra D. Neuropsychological interpretation of the effects of drive and incentive-motivation on general activity and instrumental behavior. *Psychol Rev* 75:1–22, 1968.

Bindra D and Stewart J (Eds.). *Motivation* (2nd ed.). Baltimore: Penguin, 1971.

Bozarth MA and Wise RA. Intracranial self-administration of morphine into the ventral tegmental area in rats. *Life Sci* 28:5551–5555, 1981.

Bozarth MA and Wise RA. Localization of the reward-relevant opiate receptors. *NIDA Res Monogr* 41:158–164, 1982.

Bozarth MA and Wise RA. Anatomically distinct opiate receptor fields mediate reward and physical dependence. *Science* 224:516–517, 1984.

Capriles N, Rodaros D, Sorge RE, and Stewart J. A role for the prefrontal cortex in stress- and cocaine-induced reinstatement of cocaine seeking in rats. *Psychopharmacology* 168:66–74, 2003.

Casey KL and Melzack R. Neuronal mechanisms of pain: a conceptual model. In Way EL (Ed.), *New Concepts in Pain and Its Clinical Management*. Philadelphia: Davis, pp. 13–31, 1967.

Cornish JL and Kalivas PW. Glutamate transmission in the nucleus accumbens mediates relapse in cocaine addiction. *J Neurosci* 20:RC89, 2000.

D'Angio M, Serrano A, Rivy JP, and Scatton B. Tail-pinch stress increases extracellular DOPAC levels (as measured by in vivo voltammetry) in the rat nucleus accumbens but not frontal cortex: antagonism by diazepam and zolpidem. *Brain Res* 409:169–174, 1987.

Deroche V, Piazza PV, Maccari S, Le Moal M, and Simon H. Repeated corticosterone administration sensitizes the locomotor response to amphetamine. *Brain Res* 584:309–313, 1992a.

Deroche V, Piazza PV, Casolini P, Maccari S, Le Moal M, and Simon H. Stress-induced sensitization to amphetamine and morphine psychomotor effects depend on stress-induced corticosterone secretion. *Brain Res* 598:343–348, 1992b.

De Vries TJ, Schoffelmeer ANM, Binnekade R, and Vanderschuren LJMJ. Dopaminergic mechanisms mediating the incentive to seek cocaine and heroin following long-term withdrawal of IV drug self-administration. *Psychopharmacology* 143:254–260, 1999.

Di Chiara G. A motivational learning hypothesis of the role of mesolimbic dopamine in compulsive drug use. *J Psychopharmacol* 12:54–67, 1998.

Di Chiara G. Drug addiction as dopamine-dependent associative learning disorder. *Eur J Pharmacol* 375:13–30, 1999.

Erb S, Shaham Y, and Stewart J. Stress reinstates cocaine-seeking behavior after prolonged extinction and a drug-free period. *Psychopharmacology* 128:408–412, 1996.

Erb S, Shaham Y, and Stewart J. The role of corticotrophin-releasing factor and corticosterone in stress- and cocaine-induced relapse to cocaine seeking in rats. *J Neurosci* 18:5529–5536, 1998.

Ettenberg A, MacConell LA, and Geist TD. Effects of haloperidol in a response-reinstatement model of heroin relapse. *Psychopharmacology* 124:205–210, 1996.

Everitt BJ, Dickinson A, and Robbins TW. The neuropsychological basis of addictive behaviour. *Brain Res Rev* 36:129–138, 2001.

Gardner EL. What we have learned about addiction from animal models of drug self-administration. *Am J Addict* 9:285–313, 2000.

Gardner EL. Brain-reward mechanisms. In Lowinson JH, Ruiz P, Millman RB, and Langrod JG (Eds.). *Substance Abuse: A Comprehensive Textbook* (4th ed.). Philadelphia: Lippincott Williams and Wilkins, pp. 48–97, 2005.

Gardner EL and David J. The neurobiology of chemical addiction. In Elster J and Skog O-J (Eds.). *Getting Hooked: Rationality and Addiction*. Cambridge, England: Cambridge University Press, pp. 93–136, 1999.

Gardner EL and Lowinson JH. Drug craving and positive/negative hedonic brain substrates activated by addicting drugs. *Semin Neurosci* 5:359–368, 1993.

Gerasimov MR, Schiffer WK, Gardner EL, Marsteller DA, Lennon IC, Taylor SJ, Brodie JD, Ashby CR Jr, and Dewey SL. GABAergic blockade of cocaine-associated cue-induced increases in nucleus accumbens dopamine. *Eur J Pharmacol* 414:205–209, 2001.

Gianoulakis C. Implications of endogenous opioids and dopamine in alcoholism: human and basic science studies. *Alcohol Alcohol* 31(Suppl.1):33–42, 1996.

Gratton A and Wise RA. Hypothalamic reward mechanism: two first-stage fiber populations with a cholinergic component. *Science* 227:545–548, 1985.

Griffiths RR and Weerts EM. Benzodiazepine self-administration in humans and laboratory animals—implications for problems of long-term use and abuse. *Psychopharmacology* 134:1–37, 1997.

Grimm JW and See RE. Dissociation of primary and secondary reward-relevant limbic nuclei in an animal model of ability to relapse. *Neuropsychopharmacology* 22:473–479, 2000.

Hayes RJ, Vorel SR, Spector J, Liu X, and Gardner EL. Electrical and chemical stimulation of the basolateral complex of the amygdala reinstates cocaine-seeking behavior in the rat. *Psychopharmacology* 168:75–83, 2003.

Heit H. Addiction, physical dependence, and tolerance: precise definitions to help clinicians evaluate and treat chronic pain patients. *J Pain Palliat Care Pharmacother* 17:15–29, 2003.

Hiller JM, Pearson J, and Simon EJ. Distribution of stereospecific binding of the potent narcotic analgesic etorphine in the human brain: predominance in the limbic system. *Res Commun Chem Pathol Pharmacol* 6:1052–1062, 1973.

Hosobuchi Y. Periaqueductal gray stimulation in humans produces analgesia accompanied by elevation of beta-endorphin and ACTH in ventricular CSF. *Mod Probl Pharmacopsychiatry* 17:109–122, 1981.

Ide S, Minami M, Satoh M, Uhl GR, Sora I, and Ikeda K. Buprenorphine antinociception is abolished, but naloxone-sensitive reward is retained, in μ-opioid receptor knockout mice. *Neuropsychopharmacology* 29:1656–1663, 2004.

Ishiguro H, Shibuya H, Toru M, Saito T, and Arinami T. Association study between high and low activity polymorphism of catechol-O-methyl-transferase gene and alcoholism. *Psychiatr Genet* 9:135–138, 1999.

Kalivas PW and McFarland K. Brain circuitry and the reinstatement of cocaine-seeking behavior. *Psychopharmacology* 168:44–56, 2003.

Kandel ER, Schwartz JH, and Jessell TM. *Principles of Neural Science* (4th ed.). New York: McGraw-Hill, 2000.

Katner SN, Magalog JG, and Weiss F. Reinstatement of alcohol-seeking behavior by drug-associated discriminative stimuli after prolonged extinction in the rat. *Neuropsychopharmacology* 20:471–479, 1999.

Katner SN and Weiss F. Ethanol-associated olfactory stimuli reinstate ethanol-seeking behavior after extinction and modify extracellular dopamine levels in the nucleus accumbens. *Alcohol Clin Exp Res* 23:751–760, 1999.

Kim JA, Pollak KA, Hjelmstad GO, and Fields HL. A single cocaine exposure enhances both opioid reward and aversion through a ventral tegmental area-dependent mechanism. *Proc Natl Acad Sci USA* 101:5664–5669, 2004.

Kishore KR and Desiraju T. Inhibition of positively rewarding behavior by the heightened aggressive state evoked either by pain-inducing stimulus or septal lesion. *Indian J Physiol Pharmacol* 34:125–129, 1990.

Koob GF. Stress, corticotrophin-releasing factor, and drug addiction. *Ann NY Acad Sci* 897:27–45, 1999.

Kuhar MJ, Pert CB, and Snyder SH. Regional distribution of opiate receptor binding in monkey and human brain. *Nature* 245:447–450, 1973.

Kuzmin A, Patkina N, Pchelintsev M, and Zvartau E. Isradipine is able to separate morphine-induced analgesia and place conditioning. *Brain Res* 593:221–225, 1992.

Lattanzi R, Negri L, Giannini E, Schmidhammer H, Schutz J, and Improta G. HS-599: a novel long acting opioid analgesic does not induce place-preference in rats. *Br J Pharmacol* 134:441–447, 2001.

Louilot A, Le Moal M, and Simon H. Differential reactivity of dopaminergic neurons in the nucleus accumbens in response to different behavioral situations. An in vivo voltammetric study in free moving rats. *Brain Res* 397:395–400, 1986.

Manning BH, Morgan MJ, and Franklin KBJ. Morphine analgesia in the formalin test: evidence for forebrain and midbrain sites of action. *Neuroscience* 63:289–294, 1994.

McFarland K and Ettenberg A. Reinstatement of drug-seeking behavior produced by heroin-predictive environmental stimuli. *Psychopharmacology* 131:86–92, 1997.

McFarland K and Kalivas PW. The circuitry mediating cocaine-induced reinstatement of drug-seeking behavior. *J Neurosci* 21:8655–8663, 2000.

McLaughlin JP, Land BB, Li S, Pintar JE, and Chavkin C. Prior activation of kappa opioid receptors by U50,488 mimics repeated forced swim stress to potentiate cocaine place preference conditioning. *Neuropsychopharmacology* 31:787–794, 2006a.

McLaughlin JP, Li S, Valdez J, Chavkin TA, and Chavkin C. Social defeat stress-induced behavioral responses are mediated by the endogenous kappa opioid system. *Neuropsychopharmacology* 31:1241–1248, 2006b.

Meil WM and See RE. Conditioned cued recovery of responding following prolonged withdrawal from self-administration cocaine in rats: an animal model of relapse. *Behav Pharmacol* 7:754–763, 1996.

Meil WM and See RE. Lesions of the basolateral amygdale abolish the ability of the drug associated cues to reinstate responding during withdrawal from self-administered cocaine. *Behav Brain Res* 87:139–148, 1997.

Melzack R and Wall PD. Pain mechanisms: a new theory. *Science* 150:971–979, 1965.

Melzack R and Wall PD. Evolution of pain theories. *Int Anesthesiol Clin* 8:3–34, 1970.

Moore RY and Bloom FE. Central catecholamine neuron systems: anatomy and physiology of the norepinephrine and epinephrine systems. *Annu Rev Neurosci* 2:113–168, 1979.

Narita M, Suzuki M, Imai S, Narita M, Ozaki S, Kishimoto Y, Oe K, Yajima Y, Yamazaki M, and Suzuki T. Molecular mechanism of changes in the morphine-induced pharmacological actions under chronic pain-like state: suppression of dopaminergic transmission in the brain. *Life Sci* 74:2655–2673, 2004.

Narita M, Kishimoto Y, Ise Y, Yajima Y, Misawa K, and Suzuki T. Direct evidence for the involvement of the mesolimbic κ-opioid system in the morphine-induced rewarding effect under an inflammatory pain-like state. *Neuropsychopharmacology* 30:111–118, 2005.

Nazzaro JM, Seeger TF, and Gardner EL. Morphine differentially affects ventral tegmental and substantia nigra brain reward thresholds. *Pharmacol Biochem Behav* 14:325–331, 1981.

O'Brien CP and Gardner EL. Critical assessment of how to study addiction and its treatment: human and non-human animal models. *Pharmacol Ther* 108:18–58, 2005.

Oe K, Narita M, Imai S, Shibasaki M, Kubota C, Kasukawa A, Hamaguchi M, Yajima Y, Yamazaki M, and Suzuki T. Inhibition of the morphine-induced rewarding effect by direct activation of spinal protein kinase C in mice. *Psychopharmacology* 177:55–60, 2004.

Olds ME. Hypothalamic substrate for the positive reinforcing properties of morphine in the rat. *Brain Res* 168:351–360, 1979.

Olds ME. Reinforcing effects of morphine in the nucleus accumbens. *Brain Res* 237:429–440, 1982.

Ozaki S, Narita M, Narita M, Iino M, Miyoshi K, and Suzuki T. Suppression of the morphine-induced rewarding effect and G-protein activation in the lower midbrain following nerve injury in the mouse: involvement of G-protein-coupled receptor kinase 2. *Neuroscience* 116:89–97, 2003.

Ozaki S, Narita M, Narita M, Iino M, Sugita J, Matsumura Y, and Suzuki T. Suppression of the morphine-induced rewarding effect in the rat with neuropathic pain: implication of the reduction in μ-opioid receptor functions in the ventral tegmental area. *J Neurochem* 82:1192–1198, 2002.

Ozaki S, Narita M, Narita M, Ozaki M, Khotib J, and Suzuki T. Role of extracellular signal-regulated kinase in the ventral tegmental area in the suppression of the morphine-induced rewarding effect in mice with sciatic nerve ligation. *J Neurochem* 88:1389–1397, 2004.

Ozaki S, Narita M, and Suzuki T. Basic research for psychological dependence on morphine under chronic pain. *Nippon Rinsho* 59:1704–1712, 2001.

Pappagallo M. The concept of pseudotolerance. *J Pharm Care Pain Symptom Control* 6:95–98, 1998.

Park WK, Bari AA, Jey AR, Anderson SM, Spealman RD, Rowlett JK, and Pierce RC. Cocaine administered into the medial prefrontal cortex reinstates cocaine-seeking behavior by increasing AMPA receptor-mediated glutamate transmission in the nucleus accumbens. *J Neurosci* 22:2916–2925, 2002.

Pert A and Yaksh T. Sites of morphine induced analgesia in the primate brain: relation to pain pathways. *Brain Res* 80:135–140, 1974.

Pert A and Yaksh T. Localization of the antinociceptive action of morphine in primate brain. *Pharmacol Biochem Behav* 3:133–138, 1975.

Piazza PV, Deminiere JM, Le Moal M, and Simon H. Stress- and pharmacologically-induced behavioral sensitization increases vulnerability to acquisition of amphetamine self-administration. *Brain Res* 514:22–26, 1990.

Robbins TW and Everitt BJ. Limbic-striatal memory systems and drug addiction. *Neurobiol Learn Mem* 78:625–636, 2002.

Robinson TE and Berridge KC. The neural basis of drug craving: an incentive-sensitization theory of addiction. *Brain Res Rev* 18:247–291, 1993.

Robinson TE and Berridge KC. The psychology and neurobiology of addiction: an incentive-sensitization view. *Addiction* 95(Suppl.2):S91-S117, 2000.

Robinson TE and Berridge KC. Incentive-sensitization and addiction. *Addiction* 96:103–114, 2001.

Robinson TE and Berridge KC. Addiction. *Annu Rev Psych* 54:25–53, 2003.

Rougé-Pont F, Piazza PV, Kharouby M, Le Moal M, and Simon H. Higher and longer stress-induced increase in dopamine concentrations in the nucleus accumbens of animals predisposed to amphetamine self-administration. A microdialysis study. *Brain Res* 602:169–174, 1993.

Rougé-Pont F, Marinelli M, Le Moal M, Simon H and Piazza PV. Stress-induced sensitization and glucocorticoids. II. Sensitization of the increase in extracellular dopamine induced by cocaine depends on stress-induced corticosterone secretion. *J Neurosci* 15:7189–7195, 1995.

Rougé-Pont F, Deroche V, Le Moal M and Piazza PV. Individual differences in stress-induced dopamine release in the nucleus accumbens are influenced by corticosterone. *Eur J Neurosci* 10:3903–3907, 1998.

Schnoll SH and Weaver MF. Addiction and pain. *Am J Addict* 12(Suppl.2):S27–S35, 2003.

Self DW. Neural substrates of drug craving and relapse in drug addiction. *Ann Med* 30:379–389, 1998.

Self DW, Barnhart WJ, Lehman DA, and Nestler EJ. Opposite modulation of cocaine-seeking behavior by D1- and D2-like dopamine receptor agonists. *Science* 271:1586–1589, 1996.

Self DW and Nestler EJ. Relapse to drug-seeking: neural and molecular mechanisms. *Drug Alcohol Depend* 51:49–60, 1998.

Semenova S, Kuzmin A, and Zvartau E. Strain differences in the analgesic and reinforcing action of morphine in mice. *Pharmacol Biochem Behav* 50:17–21, 1995.

Shaham Y. Immobilization stress-induced oral opioid self-administration and withdrawal in rats: role of conditioning factors and the effect of stress on "relapse" to opioid drugs. *Psychopharmacology* 111:477–485, 1993.

Shaham Y, Erb S, Leung S, Buczek Y, and Stewart J. CP-154,526, a selective, non-peptide antagonist of the corticotrophin-releasing factor₁ receptor attenuates stress-induced relapse to drug seeking in cocaine- and heroin-trained rats. *Psychopharmacology* 137:184–190, 1998.

Shaham Y, Erb S, and Stewart J. Stress-induced relapse to heroin and cocaine seeking in rats: a review. *Brain Res Rev* 33:13–33, 2000a.

Shaham Y, Funk D, Erb S, Brown TJ, Walker C-D, and Stewart J. Corticotropin-releasing factor, but not corticosterone, is involved in stress-induced relapse to heroin-seeking in rats. *J Neurosci* 17:2605–2614, 1997.

Shaham Y, Highfield D, Delfs J, Leung S, and Stewart J. Clonidine blocks stress-induced reinstatement of heroin seeking in rats: an effect independent of locus coeruleus noradrenergic neurons. *Eur J Neurosci* 12:292–302, 2000b.

Shaham Y, Rajabi H, and Stewart J. Relapse to heroin-seeking under opioid maintenance: the effects of stress, heroin-priming, and withdrawal. *J Neurosci* 16:1957–1963, 1996.

Shaham Y, Shalev U, Lu L, de Wit H, and Stewart J. The reinstatement model of drug relapse: history, methodology and major findings. *Psychopharmacology* 168:3–20, 2003.

Shaham Y and Stewart J. Stress reinstates heroin-seeking in drug-free animals: an effect mimicking heroin, not withdrawal. *Psychopharmacology* 119:334–341, 1995.

Shaham Y and Stewart J. Effects of opioid and dopamine receptor antagonists on relapse induced by stress and re-exposure to heroin in rats. *Psychopharmacology* 125:385–391, 1996.

Shalev U, Grimm JW, and Shaham Y. Neurobiology of relapse to heroin and cocaine seeking: a review. *Pharmacol Rev* 54:1–42, 2002.

Shalev U, Highfield D, Yap J, and Shaham Y. Stress and relapse to drug seeking in rats: studies on the generality of the effect. *Psychopharmacology* 150:337–346, 2000.

Shalev U, Marinelli M, Baumann MH, Piazza P-V, and Shaham Y. The role of corticosterone in food deprivation-induced reinstatement of cocaine seeking in the rat. *Psychopharmacology* 168:170–176, 2003.

Shiffman S. Relapse following smoking cessation: a situational analysis. *J Consult Clin Psychol* 50:71–86, 1982.

Shiffman S, Paty JA, Gnys M, Kassel JA, and Hickcox M. First lapses to smoking: within-subjects analysis of real-time reports. *J Consult Clin Psychol* 64:366–379, 1996.

Sinha R, Catapano D, and O'Mally S. Stress-induced craving and stress responses in cocaine dependent individuals. *Psychopharmacology* 142:343–351, 1999.

Stein EA and Olds J. Direct intracerebral self-administration of opiates in the rat. *Soc Neurosci Abstr* 3:302, 1977.

Stewart J. Reinstatement of heroin and cocaine self-administration behavior in the rat by intracerebral application of morphine in the ventral tegmental area. *Pharmacol Biochem Behav* 20:917–923, 1984.

Stewart J and Vezina P. A comparison of the effects of intra-accumbens injections of amphetamine and morphine on reinstatement of heroin intravenous self-administration behavior. *Brain Res* 457:287–294, 1988.

Stewart SH, Finn PR, and Pihl RO. A dose-response study of the effects of alcohol on the perceptions of pain and discomfort due to electric shock in men at high familial-genetic risk for alcoholism. *Psychopharmacology* 119:261–267, 1995.

Suzuki T. Modification of morphine dependence under chronic pain and its mechanism. *Yajugaku Zasshi* 121:909–914, 2001.

Suzuki T, Kishimoto Y, and Misawa M. Formalin- and carrageenan-induced inflammation attenuates place preferences produced by morphine, methamphetamine and cocaine. *Life Sci* 59:1667–1674, 1996.

Suzuki T, Kishimoto Y, Misawa M, Nagase H, and Takeda F. Role of the kappa-opioid system in the attenuation of the morphine-induced place preference under chronic pain. *Life Sci [Pharmacol Lett]* 64:PL1–PL7, 1999.

Suzuki T, Kishimoto Y, Ozaki S, and Narita M. Mechanism of opioid dependence and interaction between opioid receptors. *Eur J Pain* 5(Suppl. A):63–65, 2001.

Taepavarapruk P and Phillips AG. Neurochemical correlates of relapse to d-amphetamine self-administration by rats induced by stimulation of the ventral subiculum. *Psychopharmacology* 168:99–108, 2003.

Tiihonen J, Hallikainen T, Lachman H, Saito T, Volavka J, Kauhanen J, Salonen JT, Ryynänen O-P, Koulu M, Karvonen MK, Pohjalainen T, Syvälahti E, and Hietala J. Association between the functional variant of the catechol-O-methyltransferase (COMT) gene and Type 1 alcoholism. *Mol Psychiatry* 4:286–289, 1999.

Toates F. *Motivational Systems.* Cambridge, England: Cambridge University Press, 1986.

Toates, FM. Comparing motivational systems—an incentive motivation perspective. In Legg CR and Booth DA (Eds.), *Appetite: Neural and Behavioural Bases.* New York: Oxford University Press, pp. 305–327, 1994.

Vaccarino AL and Couret LC Jr. Formalin-induced pain antagonizes the development of opiate dependence in the rat. *Neurosci Lett* 161:195–198, 1993.

Vaccarino AL, Marek P, Kest B, Ben-Eliyahu S, Couret LC Jr, Kao B, and Liebeskind JC. Morphine fails to produce tolerance when administered in the presence of formalin pain in rats. *Brain Res* 627:287–290, 1993.

Vezina P, Lorrain DS, Arnold GM, Austin JD, and Suto N. Sensitization of midbrain dopamine neuron reactivity promotes the pursuit of amphetamine. *J Neurosci* 22:4654–4662, 2002.

Volkow ND and Li TK. Drug addiction: the neurobiology of behavior gone awry. *Nat Rev Neurosci* 5:963–970, 2004.

Vorel SR and Gardner EL. Drug addiction and the hippocampus. *Science* 294:1235a, 2001.

Vorel SR, Liu X, Hayes RJ, Spector JA, and Gardner EL. Relapse to cocaine-seeking after hippocampal theta burst stimulation. *Science* 292:1175–1178, 2001.

Wang T, Franke P, Neidt H, Cichon S, Knapp M, Lichtermann D, Maier W, Propping P and Nöthen MM. Association study of the low-activity allele of catechol-O-methyltransferase and alcoholism using a family-based approach. *Mol Psychiatry* 6:109–111, 2001.

Weiss F, Maldonado-Vlaar CS, Parsons LH, Kerr TM, Smith DL and Ben-Shahar O. Control of cocaine-seeking behavior by drug-associated stimuli in rats: effects on recovery of extinguished operant-responding and extracellular dopamine levels in amygdala and nucleus accumbens. *Proc Natl Acad Sci USA* 97:4321–4326, 2000.

Weissman DE and Haddox JD. Opioid pseudoaddiction—an iatrogenic syndrome. *Pain* 36:363–366, 1989.

Wise RA. Neurobiology of addiction. *Curr Opin Neurobiol* 6:243–251, 1996a.

Wise RA. Addictive drugs and brain stimulation reward. *Annu Rev Neurosci* 19:319–340, 1996b.

Wise RA. Dopamine, learning and motivation. *Nat Rev Neurosci* 5:483–494, 2004.

Wise RA and Bozarth MA. Brain reward circuitry: four circuit elements "wired" in apparent series. *Brain Res Bull* 12:203–208, 1984.

Wise RA and Gardner EL. Functional anatomy of substance-related disorders. In D'haenen H, den Boer JA, and Willner P (Eds.). *Biological Psychiatry.* New York: Wiley, pp. 509–522, 2002.

Wise RA and Gardner EL. Animal models of addiction. In Charney DS and Nestler EJ (Eds.). *Neurobiology of Mental Illness* (2nd ed.). London: Oxford University Press, pp. 683–697, 2004.

Wise RA, Murray A, and Bozarth MA. Bromocriptine self-administration and bromocriptine-reinstatement of cocaine-trained and heroin-trained lever pressing in rats. *Psychopharmacology* 100:355–360, 1990.

Woolverton WL, Cervo L, and Johanson CE. Effects of repeated methamphetamine administration on methamphetamine self-administration in rhesus monkeys. *Pharmacol Biochem Behav* 21:737–741, 1984.

World Health Organization. *Cancer Pain Relief.* Geneva: World Health Organization, pp. 24–37, 1996.

Yanagita T. Dependence characteristics and risk assessment of agonist-antagonist analgesics. *Drug Alcohol Depend* 20:317–327, 1987.

You ZD, Li JH, Song CY, Lu CL, and He C. Oxytocin mediates the inhibitory action of acute lithium on the morphine dependence in rats. *Neurosci Res* 41:143–150, 2001.

Zvartau EE, Patkina NA, and Morozova AS. Reinforcing, but no analgesic, effect of opioid stimulation of the ventral tegmental area. *Biull Eksp Biol Med* 102:172–174, 1986.

Index

The AA Member—Medications and Other Drugs, 280
abdominal pain in HIV, 330
aberrant drug-taking behaviors, 154–55, 405, 419, 421–22
　See also addiction
abstinence, for cocaine dependency, 146–48
abuse, definition, 9–10, 137
　See also addiction
abuse liability assessments, 411–16
acamprosate, for alcohol abuse, 71, 100–101, 134
Accreditation Council for Graduate Medical Education (ACGME), 26
acetaminophen
　abuse, 21
　for HIV/AIDS-related pain, 331
　prevalence of use, 310
Act and React Test system, 197
ACTH, 53
Actiq, 371
acupuncture, 227, 259–67
　brain activation in, 262
　for chronic pain, 264–66
　descending pain inhibition in, 261–62
　historical overview of, 259–61
　for HIV/AIDS-related pain, 333
　logic and philosophy of, 260–61
　meridians, 260, 261t, 263, 264f
　moxibustion, 259
　for opioid detoxification, 266–67
　in pain management, 263–66
　peripheral nervous system stimulation in, 261
　treatment protocols, 267
acute pain management
　buprenorphine for, 305–6
　in the emergency department, 309–10
　nerve blockade for, 243
　patient-controlled analgesia, 287
　in perioperative settings, 285–88, 305–6

postoperative pain management, 286–87
for sickle-cell disease, 343–46
　See also pain management
addiction, 21
　aberrant drug-taking behaviors, 154–55, 405, 419, 421–22
　behavior of. *See* behavior of addiction
　chemical coping, 299–301, 312f, 322–23
　co-occurrence of tobacco use with, 153–56, 273, 396
　definitions of, 10–11, 12t, 33, 49, 52, 59, 97, 304, 312f, 336, 378–82, 420, 427
　DSM-IV symptoms of, 59
　five Cs, 427
　language and terminology of, 9–13, 137, 378–82, 427
　methadone-maintenance therapy for, 117–18, 249
　morphology, 34–36
　neurobiology of. *See* neurobiology of addiction
　opioid dependence. *See* names of specific substances
　physical dependence. *See* physical dependence
　prescription drug abuse. *See* prescription drug abuse
　prevalence of, 131–32, 310–11, 411–16, 420
　pseudoaddiction. *See* pseudoaddiction
　risk factors for, 396–97, 406, 427–32
　science of. *See* neurobiology of addiction
　undertreatment of pain, vii, 6, 334, 360, 431–32
addiction medicine, vii
addiction memory, 53
Addiction Research Center, 4, 5t
Addiction Research Center Inventory, 411–12

Addiction Severity Index, 397t
addiction spectrum, 299f, 312f
addictive stimuli, 33, 53, 63–64
additivity, 203–4
A-delta fibers, 184
adjuvant treatments, 203–8, 292–93
　α-2 adrenergic agonists, 205
　antidepressants, 204t, 205, 292
　anti-epileptic drugs (AEDs), 204–5
　biphosphonates, 207
　for bone pain, 207
　calcitonin, 207
　cannabinoids, 206, 207
　capsaicin, 205–6
　GABA agonists, 206–7
　for HIV/AIDS-related pain, 331–32, 336
　local anesthetics, 205
　neuroimmunomodulatory agents, 206, 332
　NMDA antagonists, 206
　NSAIDs. *See* nonsteroidal antiinflammatory drugs
　pharmacological mechanisms of, 203, 204t
　for sickle-cell disease, 346
　for visceral pain, 207–8
adolescent prescription drug abuse rates, 20
adverse effects
　of baclofen, 207
　of methadone, 116, 117
　of opioid analgesia, 179–80, 190, 196–98, 291–92, 325
　assessment of, 194, 196, 386t, 387
　on cognitive and psychomotor tasks, 197–98
　documentation of, 385–86
　historical overview, 15–16
　on libido and potency, 198
　of tricyclic antidepressants (TCAs), 205
aerobic exercise, 220, 223
　for arthritis, 224
　for fibromyalgia, 228

for myofascial pain syndrome (MPS), 227
age factors in substance abuse, 19–20, 131–32, 396
　elderly adults, 23, 141
　young adults, 20
Agency for Health Care Policy and Research, 317
Agency for Health Care Practice and Research guidelines, 331
agonist-antagonist analgesics, 176, 177t, 178–79, 194
agonist blockade, 117
AIDS. *See* HIV/AIDS management
Alcoholics Anonymous, 273, 274–75, 276t, 279–80
　See also 12-step programs
Alcoholics Anonymous ("the Big Book"), 274
alcohol use disorders, 131–34
　age and gender factors in, 131–32
　assessment tools, 396–98
　CAGE screening tool, 396, 397
　Cloninger's typology of alcoholics, 132
　co-occurrence of benzodiazepine abuse, 140–41
　co-occurrence of cocaine dependence, 147
　co-occurrence of opioid dependence, 396
　co-occurrence of tobacco use, 155
　diagnosis of, 131
　etiology of, 132
　genetically based susceptibility to, 100, 130, 132
　neurobiology of, 133
　neuroimaging of, 43–44
　prevalence of, 131–32
　in traumatic brain injury, 132–33
　treatment options
　　Alcoholics Anonymous, 273, 274–75, 276t, 279–80
　　pharmacological treatments, 71, 74, 100–101, 133–34
　　psychosocial approaches, 134

437

Alcohol Use Disorders Identification Test, 397
aldehyde dehydrogenase release, 198
alexithymia, 300
alfentanil, reward effects of, 51
allodynia, 164, 183, 184, 241
  mechanical, 169
  in post-laminectomy syndrome, 166–67
  See also chronic pain
α-2 agonists, 110
  for chronic pain, 205, 293
  for postoperative pain, 287, 288
$α_4β_2$ nicotine receptors, 74
alprazolam
  abuse of, 137, 138–39, 140–41
  for HIV/AIDS-related pain, 332, 333t
alvimopan, 196
amantadine
  adjuvant role of, 206
  for cocaine dependency, 149
American Academy of Addiction Psychiatry, 11
American Academy of Pain Medicine
  certification in pain medicine, 317–18
  sample opioid contract, 359, 360f
  standardization of terminology, 9, 11, 12t, 420
American Board of Anesthesiologists, 318
American Board of Medical Specialties, 321
American Chronic Pain Association, 272
  support group do's and don'ts, 274t
  10-step approach, 274–75
American College of Emergency Physicians, policy statement on pain management, 313t
American Medical Association, 9
  Code of Medical Ethics, 26
American Pain Foundation, 272
American Pain Society, 9, 12t
American Psychiatric Association, 9, 11
American Society of Addiction Medicine, 9, 11, 12t, 420
amitriptyline
  adjuvant role of, 188, 204t, 205, 293t
  for fibromyalgia, 228
  for HIV/AIDS-related pain, 333t
ampainsoc.org, 17, 18
amphetamines
  drug-retention times, 355t
  isomers of, 355
  neuroimaging of, 41–42
amygdala, role in learning of, 40, 50f
analgesia. *See* adjuvant treatments; opioid analgesia; pain management
anandamide, 124
anesthesia
  for chronic pain, 293

  for HIV/AIDS-related pain, 333
  for opioid detoxification, 250–51
Anger, Irritability, and Assault Questionnaire, 102
angiotensin-converting enzyme, 164
annuloplasty, 293–96
Anslinger, Harry, 4
anterior cingulate cortex, 40
anticipation, 40
anticonvulsants. *See* anti-epileptic drugs
antidepressants
  adjuvant role of, 204t, 205, 292
  for HIV/AIDS-related pain, 331–32, 333t
  for sickle-cell disease, 346
  for smoking cessation, 100
  See also SNRIs; SSRIs; tricyclic antidepressants
Anti-Drug Abuse Act of 1988, 5t
anti-epileptic drugs, 141
  adjuvant role of, 204–5
  for chronic pain, 293
  for HIV/AIDS-related pain, 333
  for sickle-cell disease, 346
antihistamines, for HIV/AIDS-related pain, 333t
antinociceptive system, 15, 89, 94, 170
  See also opioid receptors
antiretroviral drugs
  drug interactions of, 116
anxiety disorders, 99, 312f, 322–23
  benzodiazepine use, 140–42
  co-occurrence of chronic pain with, 274
  relapse, 430
  self-medication, 300–301
anxiolytics
  for end-of-life anxiety, 326t
  for HIV/AIDS-related pain, 332
  use of, 140–42
  withdrawal from, 140
apparent opioid tolerance, 109
aquatic therapy, 223
arrestins, 92
arthritis
  acupuncture for, 265
  aerobic exercise for, 224
  HIV-associated, 330t
  neurogenic inflammation in, 171
  physical medicine approaches to, 223–24
art therapy, 255
aspiration, mechanical, 293–96
aspirin, for HIV/AIDS-related pain, 331t
assessment, 396–403, 406–8, 419–20
  of abuse liability, 411–16
  of alcohol abuse, 396–98
  choosing a tool, 402–3
  conjoint screening tools, 397–98
  of impulsivity, 101–3
  NRS-11 scale, 192, 389
  Numeral Opioid Side Effect assessment, 194, 196, 386t, 387
  of opioid abuse, 398–403, 407–8

  of outcomes, 387
  Pain Assessment and Documentation Tool, 385–86, 407, 408
  pain journals and graphs, 372f, 373–74
  reliability and validity in, 400–401
  self-report method, 402
  Social, Analgesia, Function, Emotional scale, 194, 389–90
  Structured Clinical Interview, 310–11, 397, 397t, 406–7
  Translational Analgesia Score, 387–89
  Two-Item Conjoint Screening Tool, 396, 397–98
Association for Pain and Chemical Dependency, ix
associative learning. *See* learning
astrocytes, 167–68
avascular necrosis in sickle-cell disease, 343t, 344
aversives, 22
Avinza, 325
axon reflex, 183

baclofen, 73
  adjuvant role of, 204t, 206–7
  adverse effects of, 207
  for alcohol dependency, 133–34
  for chronic pain, 293
  for cocaine dependency, 149
  intrathecal administration of, 240, 296t
  in perioperative settings, 286
balance
  musculoskeletal assessment of, 218
  principle of, 17–18, 23, 189, 379
barbiturates
  drug interactions, 116
  drug-retention times, 355t
Barratt Impulsiveness Scale, Version 11, 102
baseline craving, 147, 149
baseline pain, 369
basic impulse generator, 98f
behavioral approaches to pain management, 211–14
  cognitive-behavioral therapy, 211–12, 228–29, 253, 255–56
  drug counseling, 254
  mind-body therapies, 253, 255–57
  motivation enhancement therapy, 134, 214, 254–55
  multidimensional family therapy, 254
  during opioid detoxification, 253–57
  readiness inventory, 214
  relaxation techniques, 256–57
  for sickle-cell disease, 348–49
  support groups, 255, 271–80, 320
  supportive-expressive psychotherapy, 254
  transtheoretical model of change, 213–14

behavior of addiction
  behavioral switching, 50
  conditioned place preference, 51–52, 60, 65, 72
  conditioned stimuli, 40, 44, 63–64
  cue-exposure. *See* cue-exposure paradigms
  drug-seeking behavior, 311
  habit learning, 61–63
  impulsivity, 97–103
  incentive sensitization, 59–61
  neurobehavioral mechanisms, 59–65
  See also learning; reward and reinforcement
benzodiazepines
  abuse of, 137–42
  for alcohol dependency, 133–34
  anticonvulsant properties of, 141
  in chemical coping, 322
  cognitive impact of, 141
  drug-retention times of, 355t
  for HIV/AIDS-related pain, 332, 333t
  urine tests for, 356
  withdrawal syndrome, 139–40
benzomorphans, 194
β-arrestin, 92, 94, 109
β-endorphin, 53, 75, 164
beta blockers, for benzodiazepine withdrawal, 140
bioethics, 25–29
biofeedback, 257, 333
biology of addiction. *See* neurobiology of addiction
biphosphonates, adjuvant use of, 204t, 207
blood testing, 357
body awareness therapy, 223
body mechanics, 225–27
bone pain
  adjuvants for, 207
  HIV-associated, 330
Bonica, John, 167
Boston Collaborative Drug Surveillance Project, 4–6
botulinum toxin, in interventional pain medicine, 234
bradykinin, 206
  in peripheral nociception, 166
  in somatic pain, 163–64
  in visceral pain, 165
brain-derived neurotrophic factor, 206
brain sites, ix–x
breakthrough pain
  immediate-release formulations for, 369
  ultrafast-release formulations for, 371
Brief Pain Inventory, 387
bupivacaine
  adjuvant role of, 205
  intrathecal administration of, 240, 296t
buprenorphine (Buprenex), 17, 303–6
  dose recommendation for, 306

with methadone, 306
off-label uses of, 306
for opioid detoxification, 249–50, 304–6
in perioperative settings, 286, 305–6
pharmacological properties of, 177t, 178t, 179, 303–4
in postoperative settings, 286
potential adverse effects of, 197
for traumatic pain, 306
bupropion
adjuvant role of, 205
for chronic pain, 293t
for smoking cessation, 100
Burroughs, William S., 71
buspirone, for benzodiazepine withdrawal, 140
Buss-Durkee Hostility Inventory (BDHI), 102
butorphanol
pharmacological properties of, 177t, 178–79
in postoperative settings, 286
butyrophenones, for HIV/AIDS-related pain, 333t

CAGE screening tool, 396, 397
calcitonin, adjuvant use of, 207
calcitonin-gene related peptide (CGRP), 164, 166, 171
cAMP (cyclic adenosine monophosphate)
response element binding protein, 52, 54, 81–85, 89, 98, 175
second messenger pathway, 89, 175
cancer pain, ix
bone metastasis, 207
breakthrough pain, 369, 371
chemical coping in, 299–301
intrathecal pumps for, 295
methadone for, 116–17
opioid analgesia for, 189–94, 192
pain management of, 4–6
spinal drug delivery systems for, 242–43
ultrarapid release formulations for, 371
WHO analgesic ladder for, 17, 323, 331, 336
cannabinoids, 74, 123–26
adjuvant role of, 206, 207
analgesic mechanisms of, 124–25
analgesic synergy of, 126
receptors, 74, 123–125
drug-retention times, 355
interactions with opioids of, 125–26
neuroimaging of, 43–44
role in pain perception of, 123–24
tolerance of, 125–26
urine drug tests for, 355, 357
capsaicin, 22
adjuvant role of, 204t, 205
for chronic pain, 293

carbamazepine
adjuvant role of, 204t, 205
for benzodiazepine withdrawal, 140
for chronic pain, 204
drug interactions of, 116
for HIV/AIDS-related pain, 333t
carbenoxolone, for mirror-image allodynia, 169
caring attitudes, 28–29
categorical imperative, 27
causalgia, 170
CBT. See cognitive-behavioral therapy
C-carfentanil PET, 42
C-DASB PET, 43
C-diprenorphine PET, 40
celiac plexus blockade, 242–43
cellular mechanisms of opioid signaling, 89–94
arrestins in, 92
impulsology model of, 97–99
receptor interacting/scaffolding proteins in, 92–94
regulators of G protein signaling (RGS) in, 81–83, 89–91, 94
See also neurochemistry of addiction
central glucocorticoid receptors, in opioid tolerance, 110
central hypocorticism, 198
centralization, 225
central nervous system. See CNS
central sensitization, 170–71, 184
cerebral blood flow and metabolism, 40–43
cervical transforaminal epidural steroid injections, 238
C-fibers, 166, 184
C-flumazenil PET, 44
c-Fos, 83, 171
change, stages of, 213t
Chaussier, Francois, 167
chemical coping, 156, 299–301, 312f, 322–23
Chemical Coping Inventory, 156
chemokines, 168
chest pain
HIV-associated, 3302
noncardiac, 171
ch'i, 161, 162
Chinese medicine, 161, 162, 259–68
acupuncture, 259–67
herbal formulations, 267–68
logic and philosophy of, 260–61
meridians, 260, 261t, 263, 264f
moxibustion, 259
Chlamydia pneumoniae, in sickle-cell disease, 343t, 344
chlordiazepoxide, abuse of, 138–39
chlorpromazine, for end-of-life disorders, 326t
cholecystokinin (CKK), in opioid tolerance, 110
choline magnesium, for HIV/AIDS-related pain, 331t
cholinergic system, 34
chronic arthritis. See arthritis

Chronic Illness and the Twelve Steps (Cleveland), 275
chronic pain, ix, 4–6, 161–72
benzodiazepan abuse in, 141–42
breakthrough pain, 369
central sensitization and NMDA receptors in, 170–71
demographic factors of, 22–23
dorsal root reflexes in, 171
endogenous pain relief in, 170
historical overview of, 15, 17–18, 161–63
intrathecal pumps for, 295
management of. See pain management
methadone for, 117
mirror-image pain, 169
mononeuritis multiplex in, 167
nerve growth factor in, 166–68
neurobiology of drug-seeking and, 431–32
neurogenic inflammation in, 171
neuropathic pain in, 166–70
neuroplasticity in, 167
opioid analgesia for, 189–94
peripheral nociception in, 166–67
in post-laminectomy syndrome, 166–67
somatic pain and inflammation, 163–65
use of tobacco in, 153–56
visceral pain, 165–66
Chronic Pain Anonymous, 273, 280
meeting formats of, 275–76
prologue of, 275t
12 steps of recovering from pain, 276t
Churchill, James Morris, 260
c-Jun transcription factor, 83
Classification of Mental and Behavioural Disorders (ICD-10), 101
Cleveland, Martha, 275
clodronate, adjuvant use of, 204t, 207
clomipramine, for HIV/AIDS-related pain, 333t
clonazepam
abuse of, 137
for end-of-life anxiety, 326t
for HIV/AIDS-related pain, 332, 333t
withdrawal from, 140
clonidine
adjuvant role of, 204t, 205
for benzodiazepine withdrawal, 140
for chronic pain, 293
intrathecal administration of, 240, 296t
for opioid detoxification, 250
in opioid tolerance, 110
Cloninger's typology of alcoholics, 132
clorazepate, abuse of, 138–39
C-McN56552 PET, 43
CNI-1493, for spinal cord allodynia, 169
CNS
depressants and stimulants, 22

electrostimulation, 239–40
pathways, ix–x
coablation, 239, 293–96
cocaine use, 145–50
abstinence treatment methods for, 146–48
clinical components of addiction to, 145
co-occurrence of alcohol dependence, 147
co-occurrence of benzodiazepine use, 141
craving in, 146–50
drug-retention times in, 355t
evaluation of, 146
hedonic dysregulation in, 149–50
neuroimaging of craving in, 41–42
pharmacological treatment approaches for, 148–50
psychological treatment approaches for, 146–48
relapse prevention in, 148
reward effects of, 52
urine tests for, 356
codeine
drug interactions with, 195
for HIV/AIDS-related pain, 331t
metabolism of, 356
methadone equivalent to, 249t
pharmacological properties of, 177t, 178t
in smokers, 155
urine tests for, 355, 356
cognition
assessments of, 217
impact of opioids on, 197
cognitive-behavioral therapy (CBT)
for alcohol abuse, 134
for chronic pain, 211–12
cognitive restructuring in, 212
for fibromyalgia, 228–29
for HIV/AIDS-related pain, 333
for opioid detoxification, 253
stress responses to pain, 212
College of Problems of Drug Dependence, 9
compartment syndrome, opioid analgesia for, 192
complementary and alternative medicine. See Chinese medicine
conditioned place preference
in incentive sensitization, 60
in reward and reinforcement, 51–52
treatment options for, 65, 72
conditioned stimuli, 33, 53, 63–65, 72
constipation, 180, 196–97
contingency management, for alcohol abuse, 134
Controlled Substances Act
of 1970, 16, 28, 377, 379
of 2002, 12
coping, 103
core strengthening, 225
coronaridine, 105

corticosteroids
    for HIV/AIDS-related pain, 333
    in inflammation treatment, 165
corticotropin-releasing factor, 53
    in inflammation, 165
    in stress-induced craving, 149
cortisol, 53
COX-2 inhibitors, for postoperative pain, 287, 288
C-raclopride PET, 41, 44
craving
    categories of, 147
    neuroimaging of, 40–44
    psychological dependence, 181
    treatment of, in cocaine use, 145, 146–50
CREB transcription factor, 52, 54, 81–85, 89, 98, 175
criminal intent, 312f
Crohn's disease, neurogenic inflammation in, 171
cryotherapy, 221t, 293–96
cue-exposure paradigms, 40, 44, 63–64
    assessments of, 412
    of cocaine craving, 147, 149
    of relapse, 430–31
    in smoking and drug dependency, 154
    treatment options, 65, 147–48
    See also conditioned place preference
cyclic adenosine monophosphate. See cAMP
cyclobenzaprine
    for chronic pain, 293
    for fibromyalgia, 228

dactylitis, in sickle-cell disease, 343t, 344
Dale, William, 188–89
dance therapy, 255
Dao Guang, emperor of China, 260
deafferentation pain, 169
Decade of Pain Control and Research, 317
deep vein thrombosis, opioid analgesia for, 192
dehydration, 325
delirium, 323
delta opioid receptors, 51–52, 81, 89, 93, 175, 186
ΔFosB transcription factor, 52, 54, 81, 84–85, 89, 99
Δ⁹-tetrahydrocannabinol (THC), 123, 206
    See also cannabinoids
De Materia Medica (Dioscorides), 161
dementia, impulsivity in, x
Demerol, pharmacological properties of, 177t. See also meperidine
demographic data
    age factors, 19–20, 23, 131–32, 141, 396
    on drug-related death, 19
    ethnicity factors, 20

gender factors. See gender factors
geographic factors, 20–21, 22
of heroin use, 19, 22
of prescription drug abuse, 19–21
prevalence of addiction, 131–32, 310–11, 411–16, 420
denial, in cocaine use, 145, 150
deontological ethics, 27
dependence, definition, 10–11, 137, 181, 378, 427
    See also addiction
depression, 312f, 322–23
    co-occurrence of chronic pain, 274
    relapse in, 430
    self-medication in, 300–301
descending modulatory systems, 184–85
desensitization, 92
desipramine
    adjuvant use of, 205
    for chronic pain, 293t
    for HIV/AIDS-related pain, 333t
desmethyldiazepam, 138–39
determinants of gait, 219t
detoxification
    acupuncture for, 266–67
    anesthesia for, 250–51
    behavioral approaches to, 253–57
    buprenorphine treatment for, 249–50, 304–6
    Chinese herbal formulations for, 267–68
    definition of, 12, 377
    medical, 181, 247–51
    methadone-maintenance therapy, 117–18, 249
    tapering, 12, 248–49, 377, 387–89
    See also pain management in chemically dependent patients; withdrawal
dexamethasone
    adjuvant role of, 204t
    for HIV/AIDS-related pain, 333t
dextroamphetamine, for HIV/AIDS-related pain, 332, 333t
dextromethorphan, 113
    adjuvant role of, 206
    for opioid tolerance, 110
diabetes, mononeuritis multiplex in, 167
diacetylmorphine, 16
Diagnostic and Statistical Manual
    on alcohol use disorders, 130
    classification of impulsivity, 101
    criteria for addiction, 419–20
    definitions of terms in, 10–11, 137
    symptoms of addiction, 59
diagnostic approaches. See assessment
diaries, 372f, 373–74
diazepam
    abuse of, 138–39, 140–41
    for alcohol dependency, 133–34
didanosine, drug interactions of, 116
Dilaudid
    abuse of, 369

pharmacological properties of, 177t
    See also hydromorphone
Dioscorides, 161
diphenylheptanes, 113, 194
    See also methadone
disability, definition of, 217
disc decompression, 238–39, 293–94
discography, 238–40, 293–96
discontinuance syndrome, 137
discontinuation, 12
disulfiram, 71
    for alcohol abuse, 100, 134
    for cocaine dependency, 149
dizocilpine (MK-801), 73
D-methadone, adjuvant use of, 204t, 206
documentation in long-term opioid analgesia, 385–90
    of adverse effects, 194, 196, 385–86
    of assessments, 385–86
    of outcomes, 387–91
    Social, Analgesia, Function, Emotional scale, 194, 389–90
    translational analgesia, 387–89
    of urine drug tests, 385
Dole, V. P., 17
Dolophine, pharmacological properties of, 177t. See also methadone
dopamine, 39, 97
    in alcohol dependence, 133
    in development of addiction, 33–34, 49–52, 97–99
    receptors, x, 41–42, 72–73, 98, 148–49, 431
    drug action on, 33
    GABAergic release, 33–34
    in mediation of craving, 44
    mesolimbic dopamine system, 49–52
    neurochemistry of, 71–73
    nicotine stimulation of, 155
    in obsessive-compulsive disorder, 99
    release of, 71–72, 81–85
    in reward and reinforcement, 72–73, 97, 429
    in stimulant use, 41–42
    See also neurochemistry of addiction
dorsal root reflexes, 171
dorsolateral prefrontal cortex
    in conflict resolution, 99
    in memory, 40
doxepin
    adjuvant role of, 205
    for HIV/AIDS-related pain, 333t
Dreser, Heinrich, 5t
driving, 363
dronabinol, adjuvant use of, 204t, 207–8
Drug Abuse Screening Test, 397t, 398
Drug Abuse Warning Network, 19, 137, 310

Drug and Alcohol Services Information System (DASIS), 19
    See also Treatment Episode Data Set
drug counseling, 254
drug dependence, definition of, 379–80
    See also addiction
drug-drug interactions, 203–4
drug effect outcome expectancies, 154
Drug Enforcement Administration, 5t, 16–17, 18, 377
drug-related death, demographics of, 19
drug-retention times, 354–55
drug-seeking behavior, 33, 61, 311, 323, 335, 422
    effect of chronic pain on, 431–32
    neurobiology of, 428–30
    See also pseudoaddiction
dry mouth, 325
dry needling, 226, 227, 234
duloxetine
    adjuvant role of, 205
    for chronic pain, 292–93
    for fibromyalgia, 228
    for HIV/AIDS-related pain, 332, 333t
Duragesic, pharmacological properties of, 177t. See also fentanyl
duty, definition of, 27–28
dynorphins, 50f, 84f, 98–99, 170, 175–76
dysesthesias, 241

ecstasy, neuroimaging of, 42–43
educational treatment, for alcohol abuse, 134
efavirenz, drug interactions of, 116
eicosanoids, 163–64
elderly adults
    benzodiazepam abuse among, 141
    prescription drug abuse among, 23
electrical stimulation, 220–22, 227
emergency department management of pain, 309–14
    American College of Emergency Physicians policy statement, 313t
    assessment and treatment, 312–13
    drug-seeking behavior, 311
    prevalence of pain, 309–10
    prevalence of substance abuse, 310–11
    sickle-cell disease care, 346
Emmel, Victor, 341
emotion-focused coping, 103
endocannabinoid system, 123–26
    See also cannabinoids
end-of-life care, 5t
endogenous opioid system. See opioid receptors
endorphins, 164–65, 175–76

enkephalin, 35–36, 50, 72, 74–75, 170, 175–76
environmental cues. See cue-exposure paradigms
epidural-controlled analgesia, 243, 293–94
    for HIV/AIDS-related pain, 333–34
    spinal cord stimulation, 240, 295
    steroid injections, 236–38, 294
ethics of pain management, 25–29
    categorical imperative, 27
    Hippocratic Oath, 28
ethnicity factors, in prescription drug abuse, 20
etidronate, adjuvant use of, 207
euphoria
    in cocaine use, 145, 146
    pharmacological blocks of, 148–49
evaluation and measurement. See assessment
exercise therapy, 222–23, 225
exogenous opioids. See opioid drugs
expectancies, 154
Eysenck Impulsiveness Questionnaire, 102

FAAH inhibitors, analgesic mechanisms of, 125, 126
facet joint pain, 234–35, 293–94
family therapy
    for alcohol abuse, 134
    for cocaine use, 148
    multidimensional family therapy, 254
    for sickle-cell disease, 349
F-cyclofoxy PET, 40
F-desmethoxyfallipride PET, 44
federal policies. See legal and regulatory management
Federation of State Medical Boards' Model Guidelines, 18, 378, 379t, 382
Feldenkrais method, 223
fentanyl, 11, 195
    abuse of, 368, 369
    for acute pain, 306
    adverse effects of, 197–98
    drug interactions with, 195
    for end-of-life disorders, 326t
    for HIV/AIDS-related pain, 331, 332t
    intrathecal administration of, 240, 296t
    methadone equivalent to, 249t
    in perioperative settings, 286
    pharmacological properties of, 177t, 178, 195
    in postoperative settings, 287
    reward effects of, 51
    routes of administration of, 368
    ultrarapid release formulation of, 371
    urine tests for, 355
    withdrawal from, 247–48
Fentora, 371. See also fentanyl
fetal alcohol syndrome, 132

F-FDG PET, 40, 41, 42, 43
fibromyalgia syndrome
    opioid analgesia for, 191
    physical medicine approaches to, 227–29
five Cs, 427
5-HT. See serotonin
The Five Things, 324
flare reaction, 164
6-flourodopa, 41
fluidotherapy, 221t
flunitrazepam, abuse of, 138–39, 141
fluorocitrate, for spinal cord allodynia, 169
fluoxetine
    adjuvant role of, 205
    for fibromyalgia, 228
    for HIV/AIDS-related pain, 333t
fluphenazine, for HIV/AIDS-related pain, 332, 333t
fMRI studies, 42, 44
Foley, K. M., ix
food. See reward and reinforcement
Fos family of transcription factors, 52, 54, 81, 83–85, 89, 99
four As, 370, 385–86

GABA (gamma-aminobutyric acid), 33–34, 35, 39, 72
    in alcohol dependence, 133
    endogenous pain relief, 170
    receptors, 39
    mu-opioid receptor activation, 74–75
    in relapse, 54
    in rewards, 49–52, 50f
    treatments using, 73, 149
gabapentin
    adjuvant role of, 204t
    for alcohol dependency, 134
    for benzodiazepine withdrawal, 140
    for chronic pain, 190, 293
    for HIV/AIDS-related pain, 333t
    for neuropathic pain, 204
    for postoperative pain, 205
gait, 219
Galen, 15, 163
gamma-aminobutyric acid. See GABA
GDTAs. See goal-directed therapy agreements
gender factors
    in alcohol use disorders, 131
    in chemical coping, 300
    in κ-opioid receptors, 178
    in opioid analgesia, 192
    in prescription drug abuse, 20
    in self-reporting of substance abuse, 407
    in sensation-seeking behaviors, 300
    in undertreatment of pain in HIV/AIDS, 334
genetic susceptibility to addiction, 54, 100, 118–19
    A118G mutation, 119

in alcohol use disorders (AUDs), 100, 130, 132
    in tobacco addiction, 155
geographic factors, in prescription drug abuse, 20–21, 22
glial cells, 167–68
glutamate carboxypeptidase II inhibitors, 73–74
glutamate receptor antagonists, for blocking cocaine euphoria, 148–49
glutamate system, 34, 49–50, 72
    metabotropic glutamate receptors, 73, 85
    N-acetylaspartylglutamate, 73–74
    NMDA receptors, 73, 109–10, 113, 149, 170–71, 206, 287, 288
    in opioid tolerance, 109–10
glycine$_B$ receptor antagonists, 73
goal-directed therapy agreements, 193
the Golden Rule, 27
Good, Patricia, 5t
G protein
    coupled receptors, 81, 89, 92, 175, 186
    signaling, 81, 89–91
        in cannabinoid tolerance, 125–26
        endocannabinoid system, 123–24
        in opioid tolerance, 109
gradual discontinuation, definition of, 12
grapefruit juice, drug interactions of, 116
graphs of pain, 372f, 373–74
growth hormone deficiency, 198
guanethidine, for sympathetically maintained pain, 169
guided imagery, 253, 256

habituation, 11, 61–63
hair analysis, 357
halazepam, abuse of, 138–39
haloperidol
    for end-of-life delirium, 326t
    for HIV/AIDS-related pain, 332, 333t
Harrison Narcotics Tax Act of 1914, 4, 5t, 16, 28
Harvey, William, 165
headache
    acupuncture for, 266
    anti-epileptic drugs for, 204
    HIV-associated, 330
    neurogenic inflammation in, 171
    opioid analgesia for, 191
    in sickle-cell disease, 343t, 344
Health Information Privacy Policy Act, 320
heat therapy, 221t
hedonic dysregulation, 145, 149–50
henbane, 161
heptahelical G protein coupled receptors. See G protein, coupled receptors
herbal medicine, Chinese, 267–68

heroin use
    co-occurrence of benzodiazepine use, 141
    classification of, 16
    demographic data, 19, 22
    historical overview of, 3–4, 5t, 16, 21
    reward effects of, 51, 52
    urine tests for, 356
Herrick, James, 339–40
Hippocrates, 3, 161, 163
Hippocratic Oath, 28
histamine, 206
HIV/AIDS management, 329–37, 406–7
    nonpharmacological approaches to, 333–34
    pain assessments, 330–31
    pharmacological approaches to, 331–33
    prevalence of pain in, 329–30
    substance abuse problems in, 334–36
    types of pain in, 330
    undertreatment of pain in, 334
HIV-related polyneuropathy, 205
hospice care, 321, 324–27
    end-of-life care, 325–27
    personnel, 325t
    routine care, 324, 325t
HPA. See hypothalamic-pituitary adrenal axis
5-HT. See serotonin
Hunter, Charles, 4
Hurwitz, William, 5t
hydrocodone, 11
    abuse of, 369
    for chronic pain, 191
    demographics of abuse of, 19, 21, 310
    as metabolite of other opioids, 356
    methadone equivalent to, 249t
    urine tests for, 355
hydromorphone, 369
    for acute pain, 306
    adverse effects of, 197
    controlled-release formulation of, 368
    for end-of-life disorders, 326t
    for HIV/AIDS-related pain, 332t
    intrathecal administration of, 240, 296t
    as metabolite of other opioids, 356
    in perioperative settings, 286–87
    pharmacological properties of, 176, 177t, 178t, 179, 194–95
    postoperative use of, 287
    for sickle-cell disease, 345
hydrotherapy, 221t
hydroxyzine, for HIV/AIDS-related pain, 333t
hyocyamus, 161
hyperalgesia, 7, 183, 184, 241
    opioid-induced, 7, 109–10, 187, 287–88
    in perioperative settings, 287–88
    in somatic pain, 164

hyperalgesia (*continued*)
  in visceral pain, 165–66
  See also chronic pain
hyperglycemia, mononeuritis multiplex in, 167
hypodermic needles, 4, 16
hypogonadotrophic hypogonadism, 198
hypothalamic-pituitary-adrenal axis, 53

iatrogenic opioid abuse, 21
ibandronate, adjuvant use of, 204t, 207
I-β-CIT SPECT, 44
ibogamines, 105–7
  See also 18-methoxycoronaridine
ibudilast, intracellular mechanisms of, 187–88
ibuprofen
  for HIV/AIDS-related pain, 331t
  for sickle-cell disease, 346
ICD-10 Classification of Mental and Behavioural Disorders, 101
I-IBZM SPECT, 41, 43, 44
I-iomazenil SPECT, 44
illness behavior, 219–20
imagery, for HIV/AIDS-related pain, 333
imaging. *See* neuroimaging
imipramine
  adjuvant role of, 205
  for HIV/AIDS-related pain, 333t
immunoassay drug tests, 355
impairment, definition of, 217
implantable therapies, 293, 295–96
impulsivity, x, 97
  basic impulse generator, 98f
  clinical management of, 101
  emotion-focused coping in, 103
  evaluation of, 101–3
  impulsology paradigm, 97–103
  neurochemistry of, 97–99
  pharmacotherapies for, 99–101
  risk-taking behavior, 99
incarcerated patients, 324
incentive sensitization theory of addiction, 59–61
inflammation
  cascade, 236
  neurogenic, 171
  in somatic pain, 163–65
infliximab, adjuvant role of, 206
inhibition, 184–85
Initiative on Methods, Measurements, and Pain Assessment in Clinical Trials, 387
Institute of Medicine Liaison Committee on Pain and Addiction, 9
interferential current therapy, 220–22
interleukins, 164, 169, 206
International Classification of Diseases, ed. 10 (ICD-10), 11, 378

Internet resources
  ampainsoc.org, 17, 18
  fsmb.org, 18
  medsch.wisc.edu/painpolicy, 18
  support groups, 272
interventional pain medicine, 233–42, 293–96
  for acute pain, 243
  for cancer pain, 242–43
  CNS electrostimulation, 239–40
  for complex regional pain syndrome, 241
  for discogenic pain, 238–40
  dry needling, 226, 227, 234
  epidural-controlled analgesia, 236–38, 243
  facet joint injections, 234–35, 293–94
  for HIV/AIDS-related pain, 333–34
  intradiscal electrothermal therapy, 239, 293, 295
  intrathecal routes, 240, 241, 242f, 295–96
  percutaneous disc decompression, 238–39, 293, 295
  radiofrequency lesioning, 235, 293–94
  sacroiliac joint injections, 235–36
  spinal cord stimulation, 240, 242, 293, 295
  spinal drug delivery systems, 240, 242f, 293–96
  subarachnoid blockade, 243
  sympathetic nerve blocks, 242
  vertebroplasty, 239, 293, 295
intradiscal electrothermal therapy, 239, 293, 295
intraliminar epidural injections, 236–37
intrathecal catheters, 240, 241, 242f
intrathecal pumps, 240, 241, 242f, 295–96
intravenous patient-controlled analgesia, 287, 306, 345
ipsilateral allodynia, 169
irritable bowel syndrome, 165–66, 171
ischemic necrosis, in sickle-cell disease, 343t, 344

jing, 260–61
Joint Commission on Accreditation of Healthcare Organizations, 317
joint pain, 234–35, 293–94, 330
journals of pain, 372f, 373–74
Jun family of transcription factors, 83
Junky (Burroughs), 71

Kadian, 325. *See also* morphine
Kant, Immanuel, 25, 27
Kaposi's sarcoma, 330
κ-opioid receptors, 51–52, 54, 81, 89, 175–76
  activation of, 170
  effects of cannabinoid on, 126

gender differences in, 178
genes for, 186
RanBPM interaction with, 93
ketamine, 113
  adjuvant role of, 204t, 206, 207
  drug-retention times for, 355t
  for opioid tolerance, 110
  for postoperative pain, 287–88
ketorlac, for sickle-cell disease, 346
kinetic chains, 220
Kolb, Lawrence, 4

labels of patients, 12–13
Lambert, Alexander, 5t
lamotrigine, 74
  adjuvant role of, 204t, 205
  for chronic pain, 204, 293
language of pain and addiction, 9–13, 137, 378–82, 427
laser discectomy, 239, 293–96
laudanum, vii, 3, 5t, 49, 162
law enforcement. *See* legal and regulatory management
learning
  behavioral switching, 50
  cue-exposure paradigms. *See* cue-exposure paradigms
  dopamine release in, 72, 97–98
  habituation, 11, 61–63
  impulsology paradigm, 97–99
  in reinforcement-mediated behavior, 33, 50
  See also behavior of addiction; reward and reinforcement
legal and regulatory management, 16–17, 22, 379
  Anti-Drug Abuse Act of 1988, 5t
  Controlled Substances Act of 1970, 16, 28, 377, 379
  Controlled Substances Act of 2002, 12–17
  definitions of terms in, 378–82
  of documentation, 385
  by Drug Enforcement Administration, 5t, 16–17
  guidelines of Federation of State Medical Boards, 378, 382
  harm reduction approach, 17, 93–94
  Harrison Narcotics Tax Act of 1914, 4, 5t, 16, 28
  history of, 4, 5t, 16–17
  Marijuana Tax Act of 1937, 16
  of narcotic treatment programs, 381–82
  National Sickle Cell Control Act, 339
  opioid contracts, 362–63
  of pain management, 377–82
  Pain & Policy Studies Group research methodology, 378–82
  in palliative care, 324
  prescription policies, 377–78
  in primary care clinics, 317–18
  Pure Food and Drug Act of 1906, 16
  safe harbor laws, 17

state policies, 380
Uniform Controlled Substances Act, 381
urine drug tests, 353–57
Webb v. United States, 16
See also World Health Organization
leg ulceration, in sickle-cell disease, 343t, 344
leukemia inhibitory factor, 206
leukotriene, 164
levetiracetam, for chronic pain, 204
Levo-Dromoran, pharmacological properties of, 177t
levorphanol
  for chronic pain, 191
  for HIV/AIDS-related pain, 332t
  methadone equivalent to, 249t
  pharmacological properties of, 176, 177t, 178t, 179
  for sickle-cell disease, 345–46
lidocaine
  adjuvant role of, 204t, 205
  for chronic pain, 190, 293
  false-positive test results for cocaine, 356
  for HIV/AIDS-related pain, 333t
  in interventional pain medicine, 234
  in topical patch therapy, x
lifting mechanics, 227f
limbic-hypothalamic-pituitary-adrenal axis, relapse of, 53
limbic "priming" circuit, 34f, 35–36
Living with Pain, A New Approach to the Management of Chronic Pain (Reilly), 275
locus coeruleus, 82–83
lofexidine, for opioid detoxification, 250
long-term memory, 98
long-term opioid therapy, 189, 193–94
  See also opioid analgesia
lorazepam
  abuse of, 137, 138–39, 141
  for chronic pain, 204
  for end-of-life anxiety, 326t
  withdrawal from, 140
Lorcet
  demographics of abuse of, 21
  prevalence of use of, 310
lordosis, 218
Lortab
  demographics of abuse of, 21
  prevalence of use of, 310
low-affinity channel blockers, 73
low back pain
  acupuncture for, 265–66
  nerve blockade approaches for, 233–40
  physical medicine approaches for, 217t, 224–25
  See also spinal pain
Luborsky, L., 254
lumbar discogram, 238f
lumbar plexus blocks, 293–94
lumbar stability, 225

lumbar sympathetic blockade, 242
lumbar transforaminal epidural steroid injections, 237, 238f

maintenance therapy, 71
managed care arrangements, 319
mandrake, 161
manual muscle testing, 219
manual therapies, 222
maprotiline, for HIV/AIDS-related pain, 333t
marijuana. See cannabinoids
Marijuana Tax Act of 1937, 16
massage therapy, 222, 333
Mastering Pain: A Twelve-Step Program for Coping with Chronic Pain (Sternbach), 275t
MDMA. See ecstasy
mechanical allodynia, 169
mechanical aspiration, 293–96
mechanothermal receptors, 184
medial branch blocks, 235
medical detoxification. See detoxification
Medical Outcomes Short Study Short Form, 387
medical review officers, 353
medication contracts, 359–64
　samples, 359, 360f, 362f
　specific statement groups in, 361t, 362
　trilateral agreements, 362
meditation, 255
memantine, 73
　adjuvant role of, 204t, 206
　for cocaine dependency, 149
memory
　disorders of, 99
　dorsolateral prefrontal cortex in, 40
　impact of benzodiazepines on, 141
　long-term, 98
　motor, 34f, 35–36
　working, 99
meperidine, 11, 194
　for HIV/AIDS-related pain, 332t
　methadone equivalent to, 249t
　pharmacological properties of, 177t, 178
　for sickle-cell disease, 345
Merck, Heinrich Emanuel, 16
mesoaccumbens dopamine system, 34, 59–61
　See also dopamine
mesolimbic dopamine system, 33, 49–52
　in conditioned place preference studies, 51–52
　in natural rewards, 50
　in opiate-mediated rewards, 50f, 51–52
　in self-administration studies, 51–52
　See also dopamine
metabotropic glutamate receptors, 73

methadone, vii, 11, 113–19
　adjuvant role of, 206
　adverse effects of, 116, 117, 196
　analgesic benefits of, 116–17, 305
　chemical structure of, 113
　for chronic pain, 22–23
　co-occurence of buprenorphine use, 306
　co-occurrence of benzodiazepine use, 141, 143
　demographics of use, 19, 310
　dosing for supervised withdrawal treatment, 249t
　drug interactions, 116
　drug-retention times, 355t
　genetically based susceptibility to, 118–19
　for hyperalgesia, 287–88
　mechanism of, 113, 117–18
　medical uses of, 17
　methadone-maintenance therapy, 117–18, 249
　for opioid tolerance, 110, 113–14
　in palliative care, 324
　in perioperative settings, 286
　pharmacology, 114–16, 176–78, 179
　in postoperative settings, 286–88
　for sickle-cell disease, 345–46
　synergistic effects, 116
　urine tests for, 355
　withdrawal treatment, 247–48, 249t, 306
methamphetamines, neuroimaging of, 41–42
methotrimeprazine, for HIV/AIDS-related pain, 332, 333t
18-methoxycoronaridine, 74, 105–7
3,4-methylenedioxymethamphetamine. See ecstasy
3-methylfentanyl, 368
methylnaltrexone, 196
methylphenidate
　for end-of-life disorders, 326t
　for HIV/AIDS-related pain, 332, 333t
methylprednisolone
　adjuvant role of, 204t, 206
　for sickle-cell disease, 346
mexiletine
　adjuvant role of, 204t, 205
　for chronic pain, 293
　for HIV/AIDS-related pain, 333t
M_5 muscarinic receptor, 74
MGL inhibitors, analgesic mechanisms of, 125, 126
Michigan Alcohol Screening Test, 397, 398
microglia, 167–68
midazolam, for end-of-life agitation, 326t
migraine headache. See headache
Milner, P., 33, 49
mind-body therapies, 253
　biofeedback, 257
　cognitive-behavioral therapy, 211–12, 228–29, 253, 255–56

complementary and alternative medicine, 255
　guided imagery, 255, 256
　relaxation techniques, 256–57
mirror-image pain, 169
mirtazapine
　for benzodiazepine withdrawal, 140
　for HIV/AIDS-related pain, 333t
misuse, definition of, 9–10, 137
　See also addiction
mixed agonist-antagonist analgesics, 176, 177t, 178–79, 194
MK-801, 73
MMT. See methadone-maintenance therapy
mobilization, 222
modafinil
　for cocaine dependency, 149, 150
　for HIV/AIDS-related pain, 332, 333t
Model Guidelines for the Use of Controlled Substances for Pain Management, 18, 378, 382
moderately opioid responsive pain, 192
modulation, 184–85
Monitoring the Future project, 19, 138
6-monoacetylmorphine, 356
morphine, 113, 194
　adverse effects, 197–98
　analgesic synergy, 116, 126
　for chronic pain, 190–91, 204
　controlled-release formulations of, 367–68
　DEA classification, 17
　drug interactions with, 195
　for end-of-life disorders, 326t
　genetically based susceptibility to, 118–19
　historical overview, 3–4, 5t, 16
　for HIV/AIDS-related pain, 332t
　intracellular mechanisms, 187
　intrathecal administration, 240, 296
　metabolism, 356, 369
　methadone equivalent to, 249t
　pellet forms of, 325
　pharmacological properties, 176, 177t, 178t, 179
　in postoperative settings, 286–87
　reward effects of, 51
　for sickle-cell disease, 345
　urine tests for, 355, 356
　withdrawal from, 248
　See also opioid drugs
Morphine-Benzedrine Group scale, 411–12
morphine glucuronides, 176, 178t, 194
morphine-like agonists, 176–78, 190
morphology of addiction, 34–36
motivation enhancement therapy
　for alcohol abuse, 134
　for opioid withdrawal, 254–55
　for pain management, 214

motive circuit, 34–35
motor "memory" circuit, 34f, 35–36
motor reeducation, 223
motor vehicle operation, 363
movement therapy, 223, 255
moxibustion, 259
MRI studies, 42, 44. See also neuroimaging
MS Contin
　pharmacological properties of, 177t
　withdrawal from, 248
　See also morphine
M3G and M6G. See morphine glucuronides
multidimensional family therapy, 254
Multidimensional Pain Inventory (MPI), 387
multidisciplinary approaches, for fibromyalgia, 228–29
multifocal myoclonus, 180
mu-opioid receptors, 39–40, 74–75, 89, 175–76
　association with craving of, 40, 42
　in endogenous pain relief, 170
　genes for, 54, 186
　intracellular mechanisms of, 186–88
　in opioid addiction, 81–85
　in opioid analgesia, 186–88
　receptor interacting/scaffolding proteins, 93–94
　regulators of, 90
　in reward, 51–52
　See also morphine
muscarinic receptors, 74
muscle conditioning, 223
muscle imbalances, 219
muscle release techniques, 226
muscle strength, 219
musculoskeletal assessment, 217–20
　of balance and stability, 218
　of gait and range of motion, 219
　of illness behavior and Waddell signs, 219–20
　kinetic chains in, 220
　of muscle strength, 219
　of posture, 218
musculoskeletal pain, 191, 317
music therapy, 255
myalgia, HIV-associated, 330
myelopathy, HIV-associated, 330t
myoclonic jerks, 247
myofascial pain syndrome, 225–27, 228t, 234
myofascial trigger points, 225–26, 261
myopathy/myositis, 330t

N-acetylaspartylglutamatea, 73–74
nalbuphine, 194
　pharmacological properties of, 177t, 178–79
　in postoperative settings, 286
naloxone, 51, 176
　abuse of, 370
　in combination with buprenorphine, 179

naloxone (*continued*)
  decreased respiratory rate with, 325
  for inhibition of endogenous pain relief, 170
  in postoperative settings, 286
  as pretreatment for exercise testing, 165
naltrexone, 22, 35–36, 71
  for alcohol abuse, 100, 133, 134
  for opioid tolerance, 110
  in postoperative settings, 286
narcotics
  definition of, 11–12
  historical use of, 161
  See also opioid drugs
Narcotics Anonymous, 273–74
National Consensus Project for Quality Palliative Care, 5t, 321
National Drug Control Policy, 19
National Institute on Alcohol Abuse and Alcoholism, 131
National Sickle Cell Control Act, 339
National Survey on Drug Use and Health, 19, 20–21
nausea and vomiting, 180, 196
nefazodone, for HIV/AIDS-related pain, 333t
negative affectivity pathway, 132
neramexane, 73
Nero, 15
nerve blockade, 233–42, 293–94
  for acute pain, 243
  for cancer pain, 242–43
  CNS electrostimulation for, 239–40
  for complex regional pain syndrome, 241
  disc decompression for, 238–39
  for HIV/AIDS-related pain, 333–34
  intradiscal electrothermal therapy for, 239
  medial branch blocks for, 235
  peripheral blocks for, 234
  pros and cons of, 234t
  radiofrequency lesioning for, 235
  for sacroiliac joint pain, 235–36, 293–94
  spinal drug delivery systems for, 236–38, 240, 242f, 243
  spinal facet joint injections for, 234–35, 293–94
  subarachnoid blockade for, 243
  sympathetic nerve blocks for, 242
  vertebroplasty for, 239
nerve growth factor, 166–71
Network Therapy, 279
neuroimmunomodulatory agents, adjuvant role of, 206
neuroadaptation of addiction, 34–36
neurobehavior of addiction, 59–65
  conditioned stimuli in, 63–64
  habit learning in, 61–63
  incentive sensitization in, 59–61
  therapeutic interventions in, 64–65

VTA-MFB-Acb neural axis, 431
See also behavior of addiction
neurobiology of addiction, 33–36, 49–54, 428–32
  of addictive stimuli, 33, 53, 63–64
  of alcohol dependence, 133
  of craving and anticipation, 40
  CREB transcriptions factor, 83–84
  ΔFosB transcription factor, 84–85
  development of, 33–34, 49–52
  of dopamine, 33–34
  of drug-seeking behavior, 33, 61, 428–30
  effect of chronic pain on, 431–32
  of expression of addiction, 34–36, 52–54
  genetic susceptibility in, 54, 155
  incentive sensitization theory, 59–61
  limbic priming circuit, 34f, 35
  mechanism of analgesia, 428
  motor memory circuit, 34f, 35
  neuroimaging of, 34–35, 39–44
  neurotransmitter systems, 34, 39–40
  of opioid use, 81–85
  of physical dependence, 428
  of relapse, 33, 52–54, 60–61, 429–30
  of rewards and reinforcement, x, 33, 40, 49–52, 428–29
  of risks of addiction, 427–32
  signal transduction, 81
  of tobacco use, 155–56
  of tolerance, 52–54, 81, 89
  in undertreatment of pain, 432
  ventral tegmental area-MFB-Acb neural axis, 431–32
neurobiology of pain and inflammation, 161–72, 428
  intracellular mechanisms of, 186–88
  modulation of, 184–85
  nerve growth factors in, 166–70
  neural pathways of, 183–86
  in perception, 185
  in transduction and transmission, 183–84
neurochemistry of addiction
  of alcohol use, 44
  arrestins, 92
  of cocaine use, 41
  of ecstasy use, 42
  implications for treatment of, 64–65, 71–75
  of marijuana use, 43
  of opioid use, 40
  receptor interacting/scaffolding proteins, 92–94
  regulators of G protein signaling, 81–83, 89–91
  of stimulant use, 41
  See also opioid receptors
neurodynamic therapy, 225
neurogenic inflammation, 171
neuroimaging, 34–35, 39–44
  of alcohol use, 43–44
  of cocaine use, 41–42

of ecstasy use, 42–43
of marijuana use, 43
of opioid drug use, 40
of stimulant use, 41–42
neuroleptic drugs, for HIV/AIDS-related pain, 332
neuropathic pain, 166–70, 317
  astrocytes in, 168
  chemokines in, 168
  complex regional pain syndrome, 241
  HIV-associated, 205, 330
  microglia in, 168
  mirror-image pain, 169
  neural inflammation in, 168
  in reactive gliosis, 167–68
  in sickle-cell disease, 343t, 344
  sympathetically maintained pain (SMP), 169–70
  treatment of, 190, 204, 205
neuroplasticity, 167
  See also learning
neurotensin, 35–36
neurotransmitters
  in development of addiction, 33–34
  imaging of, 34–35, 39–44
  See also SNRIs; SSRIs
nevirapine, drug interactions of, 116
nicotine
  dependence, 155
  receptors, 74
  See also tobacco use
Niebuhr, Reinhold, 277
nightshade, 161
nitrazepam, abuse of, 138–39
NMDA (*N*-methyl-D-aspartate) receptors, 113, 206
  in central sensitization, 170–71
  in cocaine euphoria, 149
  in opioid tolerance, 109–10
NMDA receptor antagonists, 73, 110
  adjuvant role of, 206
  for postoperative pain, 287, 288
nociceptin/orphanin FQ (NOP), 75
nociceptive system, 162–65, 171–72, 183–86
noncardiac chest pain, neurogenic inflammation in, 171
nonmedical use of opioids. *See* addiction; prescription drug abuse
nonsteroidal antiinflammatory drugs (NSAIDs), 110, 192, 292
  for HIV/AIDS-related pain, 331, 336
  pain resistance to, 206, 292
  for postoperative pain, 287
  for sickle-cell disease, 345–46
norepinephrine, 50f, 99
  nicotine stimulation of, 155
  in pain potentiation, 164
  reuptake blockade of, 292
noribogaine, 105
normeperidine, pharmacological properties of, 178t, 179

norpropoxyphene, pharmacological properties of, 178t, 179
nortriptyline
  adjuvant role of, 205
  for chronic pain, 293t
  for HIV/AIDS-related pain, 333t
NOSE. *See* Numeral Opioid Side Effect (NOSE) assessment
Novocaine, in false-positive tests, 356
NRS-11 scale, 192, 389
NSAIDs. *See* nonsteroidal anti-inflammatory drugs
Nubain, pharmacological properties of, 177t. *See also* nalbuphine
nucleoplasty, 239
nucleus acumbens, 71–72
  in relapse, 54, 61
  in rewards, 49–52, 50f
Numeral Opioid Side Effect assessment, 194, 196, 386t, 387
Numorphan, 368–69. *See also* oxymorphone
Nyswander, M., 17

obsessive-compulsive disorder, 99
occupational therapy. *See* physical and occupational therapies
octreotide
  adjuvant role of, 204t, 207
  for opioid detoxification, 250
Office of National Drug Control Policy, 5t
olanzapine
  for cocaine dependency, 149
  for HIV/AIDS-related pain, 333t
Olds, J., 33, 49
oligoanalgesia, 309
oligodendrocytes, 167–68
ondansetron
  for alcohol abuse, 100–101, 134
  for opioid detoxification, 250
Opana
  pharmacological properties of, 177t
opiate reward. *See* reward and reinforcement
opiates, vii, 161
  definition of, 11–12
  drug-retention times, 355t
  historical overview of, 3–7
  urine tests for, 355, 356
  See also opioid drugs
Opinions About Methadone, 118
opioid analgesia, 183–98, 367–75, 422–23
  abuse of, 367–71
  adverse effects of, 116, 117, 179–80, 190, 196–98, 291–92, 325
  assessment of, 194
  at-risk populations for, 370, 371
  clinical background of, 192
  clinical use of. *See* pain management
  combination therapies, 188
  documentation tools for, 385–90

drug interactions with, 195
for end-of-life disorders, 326t
four As of, 370, 385–86
gender differences in, 192
historical overview of, 4–6, 17–18, 367–69
for HIV/AIDS-related pain, 331–32, 336
immediate-release forms, 369, 370–71
intracellular mechanisms of, 186–88
language of pain in, 9–13
long-term opioid therapy, 189, 192–94
Model Guidelines for the Use of Controlled Substances for Pain Management, 18, 378, 382
morphine-like agonists, 176–78
neural pathways of, 183–86
opioid rotation in, 110, 179
opiophobia, vii, 6, 189, 370
in perioperative settings, 285–88
pharmacological properties of, 175–81, 194–96
for postoperative pain, 286–87
preferred drugs for, 369
principle of balance in, 17–18, 23, 189, 379
risks of addiction in, 396–97, 406, 427–32
routes for administration of, 179, 196
screening for substance abuse in, 396–403
for sickle-cell disease, 344–46
tolerance in, 109–14, 125, 180–81, 196, 247
topography of pain in, 371f, 372
trials of, 372–74
See also names of specific opioids
opioid contracts, 359–64
sample contracts, 359, 360f, 362f
specific statement groups in, 361t, 362
trilateral agreements, 362
opioid drugs, 15
categorization of, 194
definition of, 11–12
historical overview of, 15–18, 161–63
medical use of, 17–18
metabolism of, 356f
mixed agonist-antagonist analgesics, 176, 177f
morphine-like agonists, 176–78
pharmacological properties of, 175–81
rotation, 110, 179
trials, 372–74
See also names of specific opioids
opioid-induced hyperalgesia, 7, 109–10, 187, 287–88
opioid receptors, 15, 34, 39–40, 49–50, 81–85, 175–76, 428
in acupuncture analgesia, 261–63
antagonists of, 22, 75, 176, 177

cellular signaling mechanisms of, 89–94, 97–99
delta receptors, 51–52, 81, 175, 186
genetic susceptibility to addiction, 54
G protein coupled receptors, 81–83, 89–91
in inflammation, 164–65
interactions with cannabinoids of, 125–26
intracellular mechanisms of, 186–88
kappa receptors, 51–52, 54, 81, 89, 126, 175, 186
modulation and inhibition systems of, 184–86
mu receptors, 39–40, 42, 51–52, 54, 81–85, 175, 186–88
RanBPM interaction with, 93–94
levels, 39, 50–52
in stress induced analgesia, 176
opioid-responsive pain, 192
Opioid Risk Tool, 397t, 398, 400, 401, 402, 408
opiophobia, vii, 6, 189, 370
opium, vii, 161
historical overview of, 3–7
medical uses of, 4, 5t
poppies, 3–4, 11, 15
oral transmucosal fentanyl citrate, 195, 371
Oramorph SR, pharmacological properties of, 177t. See also morphine
organic mental syndrome, 312f
organomegaly, 330t
orthopedic problems, acupuncture for, 266
Osler, William, 260
osteoarthritis
acupuncture for, 265
physical medicine approaches to, 223–24
Oswestry Disability Questionnaire, 387
Overt Aggression Scale-Modified, 102
15O-water PET, 40, 41, 42, 43
oxazepam, abuse of, 138–39
oxcarbazepine
adjuvant role of, 205
for chronic pain, 204, 293
oxycodone (OxyContin, OxyIR), 3, 5t, 11
abuse of, 19–22, 368, 369, 370
adverse effects of, 197–98
for chronic pain, 191
demographics of abuse of, 19–21, 310
for end-of-life disorders, 326t
for HIV/AIDS-related pain, 331t, 332t
methadone equivalent to, 249t
pharmacological properties of, 177t, 178, 195
in postoperative settings, 287
for sickle-cell disease, 345–46

sustained-release forms of, 6, 21, 22, 368, 369
urine tests for, 355
withdrawal from, 248
oxymorphone
controlled-release formulation of, 368–69
pharmacological properties of, 176, 177t, 178t, 195

pain
classifications of, 192
definitions of, 183
journals, 372f, 373–74
language and terminology of, 9–13, 137, 378–82, 427
See also acute pain management; chronic pain; neurobiology of pain
Pain Assessment and Documentation Tool (PADT), 194, 385–86, 407, 408
pain management
acute. See acute pain management
analgesic adjuvants in, 203–8
behavioral approaches to, 211–14
historical overview of, 4–6, 17–18
interventional pain medicine, 233–42
medical professionalism in, 25–29
neuroplasticity in, 167
pain journals and graphs, 372f, 373–74
pathophysiology of pain, 161–72
physical medicine approaches, 217–29
prevention of addiction in, 423
risk factors and outcomes in, 156, 427–32
smoking in, 156
surgical approaches to, 169
topography of pain, 371f, 372
undertreatment of pain, vii, 6, 334, 360, 431–32
See also opioid analgesia; perioperative pain management
pain management in chemically dependent patients, 21, 419–23
abstinence methods of, 147
acupuncture for, 266–67
adverse effects in, 291–92
analgesic adjuvants for, 292–93
behavioral and psychotherapeutic strategies, 253–55
buprenorphine treatment for, 249–50, 303–6
chemical coping in, 299–301
Chinese herbal formulations for, 267–68
in clinical settings, 291–96
clonidine treatment for, 250
documentation tools for, 385–90
in the emergency department, 309–14

for HIV/AIDS patients, 329–37, 406–7
for incarcerated patients, 324
legal and regulatory aspects of, 377–82
medical detoxification in, 247–51
medical evaluation in, 292
methadone treatment for, 117–18, 249
opioid contracts, 359–64
in palliative care, 321–27
in perioperative settings, 285–88, 305–6
pharmacological approaches to, 291–96
in primary care, 317–20
screening for substance abuse, 396–403
in sickle-cell disease, 25–26, 339–49, 406
support groups/12-step programs for, 271–80, 320
termination of treatment in, 423
tolerance in. See tolerance
urine drug tests, 335, 353–57, 406, 423
WHO views on, 431–32
See also opioid analgesia; treatment of drug dependency
Pain Management in the Emergency Department, 313t
Pain & Policy Studies Group research, 378–82
pain specialists, 317–18
Palladone, 5t, 368. See also hydromorphone
palliative care, 5t, 321–27
anxiety in, 326
definition of, 321
drug dependency in, 322–23
end-of-life tasks, 324
hospice programs for, 324–27
for incarcerated patients, 324
legal guidelines in, 324
management of, 323–27
opioid analgesia in, 192
for sickle-cell disease, 344–45
pamidronate, adjuvant role of, 204t, 207
Papaver somniferum (opium poppy), 3–4, 11, 15
Paracelsus, 5t
paraffin, 221t
parameters of gait, 219t
paraplegia, epidural steroid injections for, 238
paroxetine
adjuvant role of, 205
for HIV/AIDS-related pain, 333t
partial agonist analgesics, 17, 177t, 178t, 179
passive physical therapy modalities, 220–22
cryotherapy, 221t
electrical stimulation (TENS & ICT), 220–22, 227
heat, 221t

patient labels, 12–13
Pavlovian conditioning. *See*
conditioned stimuli
pelvic crossed syndrome, 219
pemoline, for HIV/AIDS-related
pain, 332, 333*t*
pentazocine, 194
for abuse of opioids, 370
pharmacological properties of,
177*t*, 178–79
in postoperative settings, 286
for smokers, 155
Percocet/Percodan
abuse of, 21, 369
prevalence of use of, 310
percutaneous disc decompression,
238–39, 293, 295
perfusion MRI, 40
perioperative pain management,
285–88
assessment of opioid use, 285
buprenorphine for, 305–6
patient-controlled analgesia for,
287
neuraxial analgesia in, 287
non-opioid options for, 287, 288
opioid-induced hyperalgesia in,
287–88
regional analgesia in, 287
peripheralization, 225
peripheral nerve blocks, 234
peripheral nociception, 166
persistent noncancer pain. *See*
chronic pain
personality disorders, 312*f*, 323
PET scans. *See* neuroimaging
Pharmacist's Manual (DEA), 377
pharmacological opioid tolerance,
108
pharmacological synergism, 203–4
phases of gait, 219*t*
phenanthrenes, 194
phencyclidine, drug-retention times,
355*t*
phenobarbitol
abuse of, 138–39
drug interactions of, 116
phenothiazines, for HIV/AIDS-
related pain, 333*t*
phentolamine, for sympathetically
maintained pain (SMP), 169
phenylpiperidines, 194
phenytoin
adjuvant role of, 204*t*
drug interactions of, 116
for HIV/AIDS-related pain, 333*t*
2-(phosphonomethyl)-pentanedioic
acid (2-PMPA), 74
physiatry. *See* rehabilitation
approaches to pain
management
physical and occupational therapies,
217, 220–23
aquatic therapy, 223
exercise, 222–23, 225
for HIV/AIDS-related pain, 333
for low back pain, 224–25
manual techniques, 222

mind-body therapy, 223
mobilization, 222
motor reeducation, 223
muscle conditioning, 223
neurodynamic therapy, 225
for osteoarthritis, 223–24
passive modalities, 220–22
for rheumatoid arthritis, 223–24
stabilization, 225
stretching, 223
See also rehabilitation approaches
to pain management
physical dependence, 181, 428
definitions of, 378, 379*t*, 380, 419
impact of chronic pain on, 431–32
See also addiction
physiological dependence, definition
of, 137
See also addiction
piloerection, 247
pimozide, for HIV/AIDS-related
pain, 332, 333*t*
piroxicam, for sickle-cell disease, 346
placebo effects, 255
pleasure. *See* reward and
reinforcement
2-PMPA [2-(phosphonomethyl)-
pentanedioic acid], 74
point of care testing, 357
polyneuropathies, HIV-associated,
330
polysubstance abuse, 137, 140, 396
POMC derived peptides, 75
pool exercise, 223
poorly opioid responsive pain, 192
poppy seeds, 356
Portenoy, R. K., ix
postherpetic neuralgia, x
post-laminectomy syndrome,
166–67
postoperative pain management,
286–87, 305–6
posttraumatic stress disorder, 99
posture, 218
potentiation, 203–4
prayer, 255
prazepam, abuse of, 138–39
prednisone, adjuvant role of, 204*t*,
206
pregabalin
adjuvant role of, 204*t*, 293
for fibromyalgia, 228
for HIV/AIDS-related pain, 333*t*
for neuropathic pain, 204
pregnancy, 363
Prescription Abuse Checklist, 420
prescription drug abuse, ix, 6, 17,
19–23
availability factor, 21–22
CNS depressants and stimulants
in, 22
demographic data, 19–21
epidemiological data, 17
See also addiction
Prescription Drug Use
Questionnaire (PDUQ),
397*t*, 398, 399*t*, 402, 408
pretreatment, sensitization in, 61

priapism, in sickle-cell disease,
343*t*, 344
primary care clinic management of
pain, 317–20
legal guidelines for, 317–18
long-term management, 319–20
medication contracts in, 362
protocols for, 317
urine drug tests in, 353–57
priming, 52
principle of balance, 17–18, 23,
189, 379
processes of change, 213*t*
prochlorperazine, for opioid
detoxification, 250
prodrugs, 22
professionalism in medical practice,
26–28
proinflammatory interleukins,
adjuvant role of, 206
Project MATCH, 253
proopiomelanocortin, 74–75
propoxyphene, 11, 178*t*, 194
drug-retention times of, 355*t*
efficacy in smokers of, 155
for HIV/AIDS-related pain, 331*t*
propranolol, for cocaine
dependency, 149
prostaglandins, 163–64, 206
protein kinase C, 93–94, 109–10
proteomics technology, 92–94
pruritus, 196
pseudoaddiction, 6, 299*f*, 360,
422, 427
differential diagnosis of, 322–23,
405
in the emergency department,
312–13
in sickle-cell disease, 313
tobacco use in, 154–55
pseudotolerance, 427
psoriasis, neurogenic inflammation
in, 171
psychological dependence, 181
psychostimulants, for HIV/AIDS-
related pain, 332, 333*t*
psychotherapeutic intervention
for alcohol abuse, 134
for chemical coping, 301
for cocaine dependency, 146–48
for craving, 147–48
drug counseling, 254
family therapy, 134, 148, 254,
349
motivation enhancement therapy,
134, 214, 254–55
for opioid withdrawal, 254–55
support groups. *See* support
groups
supportive-expressive psychotherapy, 254
therapeutic contracts, 359–64
See also behavioral approaches to
pain management
Pure Food and Drug Act of 1906, 16

qi, 259, 260–61
qi gong, 255

QT_c intervals, impact of methadone
on, 116, 197

race factors
in prescription drug abuse, 20
in sickle-cell disease, 347–48
radiculopathic pain syndromes
epidural steroid injections for, 238
HIV-associated, 330
radiofrequency lesioning, 235,
293–94
RAFFT, 397*t*, 398
RanBP9/RanBPM, 93–94
range of motion, 219
R-coronaridine, 105
reactive gliosis, 167–68
rebound, definition of, 139
receptor interacting/scaffolding
proteins, 92
Recovery Status Exam, 273, 276, 279
recreational therapists, 220–22
recreational use, definition of, 137
recurrence, definition of, 139
recurrent pain, 309
See also chronic pain
reflex sympathetic dystrophy, 170–71
regional cerebral blood flow. *See*
cerebral blood flow and
metabolism
regional factors. *See* geographic
factors
regulation. *See* legal and regulatory
management
regulators of G protein signaling
(RGS) proteins, 81–83, 85,
89–91
rehabilitation approaches to pain
management, 217–29
for chemical coping, 301
for fibromyalgia, 227–29
for low back pain, 224–25
mind-body therapy, 223
musculoskeletal assessment,
217–20
for myofascial pain syndrome,
225–27, 228*t*
for osteoarthritis, 223–24
physical and occupational
therapy, 220–23
psychological factors, 217, 220
for rheumatoid arthritis, 223–24
Reilly, Richard, 275
reinforcing effects, 412
relapse
biology of, 33, 52–54, 60–61,
429–30
cue-induced, 33, 53
definition of, 52
drug-triggered, 429–30
extinction-reinstatement model, 61
incentive sensitization in, 60–61
neuroadaptation of, 53–54
priming and, 53
psychological prevention
methods, 148
stress-triggered, 53, 430
See also self-administration
paradigm

relaxation techniques, 256–57
reliability, 400
remifentanil, for chronic pain, 190–91
respiratory depression, 179–80
reward and reinforcement
 biology of, x, 33, 40, 49–52, 97, 428–29
 dopamine, 72–73, 97, 429
 incentive sensitization, 60
 learning, 33, 50, 72
 endogenous and exogenous rewards, 97
 impulsology paradigm of, 97–99
 reward cascade in, 155, 263
 in tobacco abuse, 155–56
reward-aversion circuitry, x
RGS (regulators of G protein signaling), 81–83, 85, 89–91
rheumatoid arthritis
 neurogenic inflammation in, 171
 physical medicine approaches to, 223–24
R-ibogamine, 105
rifampin, drug interactions of, 116
riluzole, 74
rimonabant (SR141716A), 74
risk factors for addiction, 396–97, 406
risk management, 5t
ritonavir, drug interactions of, 116
Robiquet, Pierre-Jean, 16
rostral ventromedial medulla, in endogenous pain relief, 170
Roxicodone, pharmacological properties of, 177t. See also oxycodone
Rush, Benjamin, 162

sacroiliac joint pain, 235–36, 293–94
safe harbor laws, 17
saliva testing, 357
Saunders, Cicely, 321
Schedule I drugs, 16–17
Schedule II drugs, 17
sciatic inflammatory neuropathy, 169
Screener and Opioid Assessment for Patients with Pain, 397t, 400, 401t, 402
screening for substance abuse. See assessment
Screening Instrument for Substance Abuse Potential, 397t, 400, 401t, 402
sedation, 180, 196
Self-Administered Alcoholism Screening Test, 397
self-administration paradigm
 of incentive sensitization, 60
 of reward and reinforcement, 51–52
 treatment options, 72
self-medication, 156, 300–301
self-report of drug use, 353, 354, 402
sensation seeking, 300
sensitization, 59–61, 81
 neural pathways of, 183
 in pretreatment, 61

sensory nervous system, neuroplasticity of, 167
serenity prayer, 277
serotonin (5-HT), 34, 42–43, 49–50, 50f
sertraline, for HIV/AIDS-related pain, 333t
Sertürner, Friedrich, 4, 5t, 16
serum testing, 357
Severity of Opiate Dependence Questionnaire (SODQ), 397t, 398
SF-36 outcomes assessment, 387
shen, 260–61
sickle-cell disease, 339–49, 342, 406
 adjuvant therapy for, 346
 anemia in, 344
 cognitive function and learning in, 347
 historical overview of, 339–42
 nonpharmacological management of, 348–49
 opioid analgesia for, 344–46
 pain management in, 25–26, 313
 pain syndromes in, 343–44
 pathophysiology of pain in, 342–43
 polymerization of hemoglobin-S in, 341–42
 psychosocial aspects of, 347–48
 substance abuse in, 346–47
 vasoocclusive crisis in, 343
signal transduction, 81
Single Dose Questionnaire, 411
situational cues. See cue-exposure paradigms
situation-specific outcome expectancies, 154
sleep apnea, 198
smoking. See tobacco use
smoking effect outcome expectancies, 154
SNRIs (serotonin and noradrenaline reuptake inhibitors)
 adjuvant role of, 204t, 205, 292–93
 for fibromyalgia, 228
 for HIV/AIDS-related pain, 332
Social, Analgesia, Function, Emotional (SAFE) scale, 194, 389–90
social stress model of substance use, 156
somatic pain, 163–65
somatization, 300
somatostatin, adjuvant role of, 207
spasticity, intrathecal pumps for, 295
SPECT, 41, 42
spectrum of problematic drug-use behaviors, 299f, 312f
spinal cord injuries
 deafferentation pain, 169
 epidural steroid injections for, 238
spinal cord stimulation (SCS), 240, 242, 293, 295
spinal drug delivery systems, 240, 242f, 293–96
spinal facet joints, 234–35, 293–94

spinal pain
 acupuncture for, 263
 diagnosis of, 233–34
 facet joint syndrome in, 234–35
 interventional approaches for, 233–40, 293–96
 physical medicine approaches to, 217t, 224–25
 sacroiliac joint pain in, 235–36
 See also pain management
spiritual healing, 255
spray and stretch technique, 227
SSRIs (selective serotonin reuptake inhibitors)
 adjuvant role of, 204t, 205
 for benzodiazepine withdrawal, 140
 for fibromyalgia, 228
 for HIV/AIDS-related pain, 333t
stability
 musculoskeletal assessment of, 218
 physical therapy for, 225
Stadol, pharmacological properties of, 177t. See also butorphanol
stages of change, 213t
state policies. See legal and regulatory management
State-Trait Anger Expression Inventory, 102
stavudine, drug interactions of, 116
stellate ganglion blockade, 241, 293–96
steroids
 epidural injections, 236–38, 293
 for sickle-cell disease, 346
 See also nerve blockade
stimulant use, 41–42, 141
 See also benzodiazepines
strengthening, 223
stress, 53, 99
 -induced analgesia, 176
 -induced craving, 147, 149
 -induced pain, 170
 posttraumatic stress disorder, 99
 relapse triggers of, 53, 430
 in responses to pain, 212
 in undertreatment of pain, 432
stretching, 223
structural neuroimaging. See neuroimaging
Structured Clinical Interview, 310–11, 397, 397t, 406–7
subarachnoid blockade, 243
Suboxone, 179, 249–50, 304
 See also buprenorphine
substance abuse, definition, 10, 310
 See also addiction
Substance Abuse and Mental Health Services Administration. See Treatment Episode Data Set
Substance Abuse Subtle Screening Inventory-3, 397t, 398
substance P, 35–36, 164, 166, 171
Subutex, 179
 for opioid detoxification, 249–50, 304

 See also buprenorphine (Buprenex)
sufentanil
 intrathecal administration of, 296t
 in postoperative settings, 286
 reward effects of, 51
support groups, 255, 271–80, 320
 American Chronic Pain Association guidelines, 274–75
 for co-occurrence of chronic pain and addiction, 279–80
 Chronic Pain Association approach, 273, 275–76, 280
 Internet groups, 272
 leadership of, 273, 279
 Network Therapy, 279
 Recovery Status Exam, 273, 276, 279
 role of pain medication in, 279–80
 for sickle-cell disease, 348–49
 for specific disorders, 272–73
 See also 12-step programs
supportive-expressive psychotherapy, 254
surgical resection, for sympathetically maintained pain, 169
sweat testing, 357
Sydenham, Thomas, 15, 162
sympathetically maintained pain (SMP), 169–70
sympathetic nerve blocks, 242, 293–94
synergism, 203–4
synthetic heroin, 368
synthetic opioids, 11

Tabernanthe iboga, 105
tai chi, 223, 255
Talwin
 abuse of, 369
 pharmacological properties of, 177t
 See also pentazocine
tapering, 12, 248–49, 377, 387–89
TCAs. See tricyclic antidepressants
Tc-HMPAO SPECT, 40, 41, 44
temazepam
 abuse of, 138–39
 for end-of-life disorders, 326t
TENS. See transcutaneous electric nerve stimulation
termination of use
 detoxification, 12, 247–51
 discontinuance syndrome, 137
 rebound anxiety, 139
 withdrawal syndrome, 11, 139
 See also detoxification; withdrawal
terminology of pain and addiction, 9–13, 137, 378–82, 427
Texas Intractable Pain Act, 318
thalidomide, adjuvant role of, 206
THC (Δ^9-tetrahydrocannabinol), 123, 206
 See also cannabinoids

therapeutic contracts, 359–64
  samples, 359, 360f, 362f
  specific statement groups in, 361t, 362
  trilateral agreements, 362
therapeutic dependence, 422
therapy for drug dependency. *See* treatment of drug dependency
Thomas Aquinas, Saint, 161
tiagabine, for chronic pain, 204
tic douloureux, 167
tizanidine
  adjuvant role of, 204t, 205
  for chronic pain, 293
tobacco use, 74
  chemical coping in, 156
  co-occurrence of alcohol abuse, 155
  co-occurrence of opioid dependence, 153–56, 273, 396
  cue-specific paradigms in, 154
  neurobiology of, 155–56
  nicotine-induced analgesia, 155–56
  outcome implications of, 154, 156
  in persistent pain contexts, 153–56
  pharmacotherapies for, 99–100
  smoking cessation programs, 99–100
  12-step programs for, 273–74
tolerance in opioid analgesia, 109–14, 125, 180–81, 196, 247
  clinical features of, 109
  clinical management of, 110–11, 335–36
  definitions of, 378, 379t, 380, 419
  disease escalation in, 109, 110
  mechanisms of, 109–10
  methadone for, 110, 113–14
  neurobiology of, 52–54, 81, 89
  opioid-induced hyperalgesia in, 109–10, 187
topiramate
  for alcohol dependency, 101, 134
  for benzodiazepine withdrawal, 140
  for chronic pain, 204, 293
  for cocaine dependency, 149
topography of pain, 371f, 372
Torsade de Pointes, 197
Towns, Charles B., 5t
tramadol hydrochloride
  for chronic pain, 190
  prevalence of use of, 310
transcendental meditation, 256
transcription factor expression, 82f, 83–85, 89
transcutaneous electric nerve stimulation (TENS), 220, 222t, 227, 239–40, 333
transduction of pain, 183–84
Translational Analgesia Score, 194, 387–89

traumatic brain injury, alcohol use in, 132–33
trazodone
  for benzodiazepine withdrawal, 140
  for end-of-life disorders, 326t
  for HIV/AIDS-related pain, 333t
  for sickle-cell disease, 346
Treatment Episode Data Set, 19, 20–21, 137–38
treatment of drug dependency, 419–23
  abstinence methods of, 146–48
  for alcohol abuse, 71, 74, 100–101, 133–34
  alpha-adrenergic receptor agonists in, 110
  aversive therapy for, 71
  for benzodiazepine withdrawal, 140
  for cocaine dependency, 145–50
  detoxification for. *See* detoxification
  goal-directed therapy agreements in, 193
  historical overview of, 4, 17–18, 71
  ibogamines for, 105–7
  maintenance therapy for, 71
  methadone therapy, 110, 113–19, 249
  neurobehavioral approaches to, 64–65
  neurochemical basis of, 64–65, 71–75
  pain management. *See* pain management in chemically dependent patients
  psychological intervention, 134, 146–48
  smoking cessation, 99–100
  withdrawal. *See* withdrawal
treatment of pain. *See* pain management
Treatment Outcomes in Pain Survey, 387
Treaty of Nanking, 16
Trendelenburg sign, 218
tricyclic antidepressants (TCAs)
  adverse effects of, 205
  for chronic pain, 190, 192, 204t, 205, 292–93
  for fibromyalgia, 228
  for HIV/AIDS-related pain, 333t
Tridimensional Personality Questionnaire, 102
trigeminal neuralgia, 204
trigger-point injections, 234
tumor necrosis factor-α, 169, 206
12-step programs, 271, 273–80
  for alcohol abuse, 134
  for chronic pain, 273–80
  for co-occurrence of chronic pain and addiction, 279–80
  leadership of, 279
  meeting formats of, 275–76
  for mental illness, 274
  Network Therapy, 279
  in palliative care, 323

Recovery Status Exam, 273, 276, 279
  role of pain medication in, 279–80
  serenity prayer, 277
  sponsorship in, 276
  for substance abuse, 273–74
  for tobacco use, 273–74
  working the steps, 276–78
The Twelve Steps and Twelve Traditions ("Twelve and Twelve"), 274
12 Steps for Those Afflicted With Chronic Pain (Colameco), 275t
Twelve-Step Sponsorship (Hamilton), 276
Two-Item Conjoint Screening Tool, 396, 397–98
Tylox
  demographics of abuse of, 21
  prevalence of use of, 310
  See also acetaminophen
Type I and II alcoholism, 132

ulcerative colitis, neurogenic inflammation in, 171
ultrasound, 221–22t, 333
undercontrolled behavioral pathway, 132
undertreatment of pain, vii, 6, 334, 360, 432
  See also pseudoaddiction
Uniform Controlled Substances Act, 381
upper crossed syndrome, 219
UPPS Impulsive Behavior Scale, 102
urinary retention, 180
urine drug tests, 335, 353–57, 406, 423
  in abstinence treatment, 147
  documentation of, 385
  drug-retention times, 354–55
  drugs covered by, 354
  immunoassay tests, 355
  reliability of, 355–56
  unexpected negatives in, 356–57
U.S. Food and Drug Administration (FDA), 5t
use, definition of, 9–10
  See also addiction

validity, 400
valproic acid
  for benzodiazepine withdrawal, 140
  for HIV/AIDS-related pain, 333t
varenicline, for smoking cessation, 100
venlafaxine
  adjuvant role of, 205, 292–93
  for fibromyalgia, 228
  for HIV/AIDS-related pain, 333t
ventral palladium, 50f, 72
ventral tegmental area (VTA), 39, 71–72
  CREB activity in, 83–84
  -MFB-Acb neural axis, 431–32
  in opioid dependence, 81–85
  in relapse, 54

  in rewards, 49–52
  See also dopamine; mesolimbic dopamine system
vertebral compression fractures, 295
vertebroplasty, 239, 293, 295
Vicodin
  abuse of, 369
  demographics of abuse of, 20–21
  prevalence of use of, 310
vigabatrin, for alcohol dependency, 134
visceral pain, 165–66, 207–8
vocational rehabilitation, 253
von Economo neurons, x
voxel-based morphometry, 40, 41, 42, 43
VTA. *See* ventral tegmental area

Waddell signs and symptoms, 219–20
weaning, definition of, 12
Webb v. United States, 16
WHO. *See* World Health Organization
withdrawal, 247–51
  buprenorphine for, 249–50, 303–6
  from cocaine, 145
  definitions of, 139, 181
  in HIV/AIDS management, 336
  medical management of, 247–51
  methadone treatment for, 249
  syndromes, 11, 139–40
  tapering, 12, 248–49, 377, 387–89
  See also detoxification
Wood, Alexander, 4, 5t, 16
Woolf, Virginia, 163
working memory, 99
workplace injuries, 225–27
World Health Organization (WHO), 317
  addiction-related terminology of, 378
  analgesic ladder for treatment of cancer pain, 17, 323, 331, 336
  definitions of terms by, 9, 137, 378–80
  statements on opioid analgesia and addiction by, 431–32
Wright, C. Alder, 16

xerostomia, 325

yin and yang, 161, 162, 260–61
yoga, 255
yohimbine, 99
young adults, prescription drug abuse rates in, 20

zidovudine, drug interactions of, 116
zoledronic acid, adjuvant role of, 207
zolendronate, adjuvant role of, 204t
zolpidem
  abuse of, 138–39
  for end-of-life disorders, 326t
zonisamide, for chronic pain, 204, 293
zopiclone, abuse of, 138–39
zygapophysial joints, 234–35